Orthopaedic Knowledge Update®

OKU®

Hip and Knee Reconstruction

6

Orthopaedic Knowledge Update®

OKU® 6

Hip and Knee Reconstruction

EDITED BY

Michael A. Mont, MD, FAAOS
Vice President of Strategic Initiatives
Northwell Health Orthopedics
Lenox Hill Hospital
New York, New York

Michael Tanzer, MD, FRCSC, FAAOS
Jo Miller Chair of Orthopaedic Research
McGill University Hospital Centre
Associate Surgeon-in-Chief
McGill University Hospital Centre
Vice Chair Surgery (Clinical) & Professor
McGill University
Montreal, Quebec, Canada

Wolters Kluwer
Philadelphia • Baltimore • New York • London
Buenos Aires • Hong Kong • Sydney • Tokyo

AAOS
American Academy of Orthopaedic Surgeons

AAOS

AMERICAN ACADEMY OF
ORTHOPAEDIC SURGEONS

Staff
American Academy of Orthopaedic Surgeons

Anna Salt Troise, MBA, *Chief Education Strategist*

Hans Koelsch, PhD, *Director, Publishing*

Lisa Claxton Moore, *Senior Manager, Editorial*

Steven Kellert, *Senior Editor*

Wolters Kluwer Health

Brian Brown, *Director, Medical Practice*

Stacey Sebring, *Senior Development Editor*

Emily Buccieri, *Senior Editorial Coordinator*

Erin Cantino, *Portfolio Marketing Manager*

Catherine Ott, *Production Project Manager*

Stephen Druding, *Design Coordinator*

Margie Orzech, *Senior Manufacturing Coordinator*

TNQ Technologies, *Prepress Vendor*

ISBN 9781975157999

Library of Congress Control Number: Cataloging in Publication data available on request from publisher.

Printed in China

Published 2022 by the American Academy of Orthopaedic Surgeons
9400 West Higgins Road
Rosemont, Illinois 60018

CCS1120

Acknowledgments

Editorial Board, Orthopaedic Knowledge Update®: Hip and Knee Reconstruction 6

Editors

Michael A. Mont, MD, FAAOS
Vice President of Strategic Initiatives
Northwell Health Orthopedics
Lenox Hill Hospital
New York, New York

Michael Tanzer, MD, FRCSC, FAAOS
Jo Miller Chair of Orthopaedic Research
McGill University Hospital Centre
Associate Surgeon-in-Chief
McGill University Hospital Centre
Vice Chair Surgery (Clinical) & Professor
McGill University
Montreal, Quebec, Canada

Contributors

David C. Ayers, MD
The Arthur Pappas Professor and Chair
Department of Orthopedics and Physical Rehabilitation
Medical Director, Orthopedic Center of Excellence
University of Massachusetts Medical School
Orthopedist-in-Chief
UMass Memorial Medical Center
Worcester, Massachusetts

James F. Baker, MD
Resident, Department of Orthopaedic Surgery
University of Louisville
Louisville, Kentucky

Samik Banerjee, MD
Fellow, Department of Orthopaedic Surgery
Thomas Jefferson University
Philadelphia, Pennsylvania

Elexis C. Baral, MS
Research Engineer
Department of Biomechanics
Hospital for Special Surgery
New York, New York

Wael K. Barsoum, MD
Professor, Department of Orthopaedic Surgery
Cleveland Clinic Lerner College of Medicine
Cleveland, Ohio

Keith R. Berend, MD
Vice President, JIS Orthopedics
President, White Fence Surgical Suites
New Albany, Ohio

Daniel J. Berry, MD
L.Z. Gund Professor of Orthopedic Surgery
Mayo Clinic
Rochester, Minnesota

Jordan Bonier, DO, MS
Joint Reconstruction Fellow
Rubin Institute of Advanced Orthopedics
Sinai Hospital of Baltimore
Baltimore, Maryland

Tracy M. Borsinger, MD
Resident, Department of Orthopaedics
Dartmouth-Hitchcock Medical Center
Lebanon, New Hampshire

Mathias Per Gunnar Bostrom, MD
Salvati Professor of Orthopaedic Surgery
Arthroplasty Research Laboratory
Hospital for Special Surgery
New York, New York

Scot A. Brown, MD
Assistant Professor of Orthopaedic Surgery
Rothman Orthopaedic Institute
Thomas Jefferson University
Philadelphia, Pennsylvania

Brian P. Chalmers, MD
Clinical Fellow, Adult Reconstruction and Joint Replacement
Hospital for Special Surgery
New York, New York

Justin S. Chang, MBBS, MRCS, FRCSC
Orthopaedic Surgeon
University College London Hospitals NHS Foundation Trust
University College London
London, England

Henry D. Clarke, MD
Chair, Department of Orthopedic Surgery
Professor of Orthopedics
Mayo Clinic College of Medicine and Science
Mayo Clinic
Phoenix, Arizona

John C. Clohisy, MD
Professor, Department of Orthopaedic Surgery
Washington University School of Medicine
St. Louis, Missouri

Dominick V. Congiusta, MD, MPH
Orthopaedic Surgery Resident
Department of Orthopaedics
Rutgers New Jersey Medical School
Newark, New Jersey

P. Maxwell Courtney, MD
Assistant Professor of Orthopaedic Surgery
Rothman Orthopaedic Institute
Thomas Jefferson University
Philadelphia, Pennsylvania

David A. Crawford, MD
Associate, JIS Orthopedics
New Albany, Ohio

Antonio Cusano, MD
Resident, Department of Surgery
University of Connecticut Health Center
Farmington, Connecticut

Fred D. Cushner, MD
Assistant Clinical Professor
Hospital for Special Surgery
New York, New York

Ronald E. Delanois, MD
Chairman of Orthopedics
Rubin Institute of Advanced Orthopedics
Sinai Hospital of Baltimore
Baltimore, Maryland

Matthew E. Deren, MD
Assistant Professor
Department of Orthopaedics and Physical Rehabilitation
University of Massachusetts Medical School
Worcester, Massachusetts

Christopher A.F. Dodd, FRCS
Consultant Orthopaedic and Knee Surgeon
The Manor Hospital
Oxford, England

Michael J. Dunbar, MD, FRCSC, PhD, FCAHS
Professor, Division of Orthopaedic Surgery
Department of Surgery
Dalhousie University
Halifax, Nova Scotia, Canada

Christian J. Eccles, MD
Resident, Department of Orthopaedic Surgery
University of Louisville
Louisville, Kentucky

Joseph O. Ehiorobo, MD
Research Fellow
Northwell Health Orthopedics
Lenox Hill Hospital
New York, New York

Patricia D. Franklin, MD, MBA, MPH
Professor and Co-Director, Outcomes and Measurement Hub
Department of Medical Social Sciences
Northwestern University Feinberg School of Medicine
Chicago, Illinois

Andrew A. Freiberg, MD
Staff Surgeon
Newton Wellesley Hospital
Mass General Brigham Health
Boston, Massachusetts

Donald S. Garbuz, MDCM, FRCSC
Professor and Head
Division of Lower Limb Reconstruction
Department of Orthopaedics
University of British Columbia
Vancouver, British Columbia, Canada

Elizabeth B. Gausden, MD, MPH
Assistant Professor
Department of Orthopaedic Surgery
Hospital for Special Surgery
New York, New York

Emmanuel Gibon, MD, PhD
Clinical Fellow
Department of Orthopaedic Surgery
New York University
New York, New York

Gregory J. Golladay, MD
Professor, Department of Surgery
Virginia Commonwealth University
Richmond, Virginia

Stuart B. Goodman, MD, PhD
Robert L. and Mary Ellenburg Professor of Surgery
Department of Orthopaedic Surgery and Bioengineering
Stanford University
Stanford, California

Hugh Gorman, BS
Research Assistant
Brigham and Women's Hospital
Department of Orthopaedic Surgery
Boston, Massachusetts

Simon Greenbaum, MD
Fellow, NYU Langone Orthopedic Hospital
Insall Scott Kelly Institute
New York, New York

Steven B. Haas, MD
Chief of the Knee Service
John N. Insall Chair, Knee Surgery
Adult Reconstruction and Joint Replacement
Hospital for Special Surgery
Professor of Clinical Orthopedics
Weill-Cornell Medical Center
New York, New York

Fares S. Haddad, BSc, MD (Res), FRCS
Professor of Orthopaedic Surgery
University College London Hospitals NHS Foundation Trust
University College London
London, England

Mohamad J. Halawi, MD
Associate Professor
Department of Surgery
Baylor College of Medicine
Houston, Texas

Nathanael Heckmann, MD
Assistant Professor
Department of Orthopaedic Surgery
Keck School of Medicine of USC
Los Angeles, California

Matthew S. Hepinstall, MD
Associate Professor
Department of Orthopaedic Surgery
New York University
New York, New York

Daniel Holtzman, MD
Department of Orthopaedic Surgery
The Permanente Medical Group
Kaiser Permanente Medical Center
Redwood City, California

Matthew J.W. Hubble, MBBS, FRCS (Tr&Orth)
Consultant Orthopaedic Surgeon
Princess Elizabeth Orthopaedic Centre
Royal Devon & Exeter Hospital
Exeter, England

Hansel E. Ihn, MD
Resident Physician
Department of Orthopaedic Surgery
University of Southern California
Los Angeles, California

Stephen J. Incavo, MD
Section Chief, Adult Reconstructive Surgery
Houston Methodist Hospital, Houston, Texas
Professor of Clinical Orthopaedic Surgery
Weill Cornell Medical School
New York, New York

Richard Iorio, MD
Chief, Adult Reconstruction and Total Joint Arthroplasty Service
Vice Chairman, Clinical Effectiveness
Richard D. Scott, MD Distinguished Chair in Orthopaedic Surgery
Brigham and Women's Hospital
Department of Orthopaedic Surgery
Boston, Massachusetts

Joshua J. Jacobs, MD
Chairman, Department of Orthopaedic Surgery
Rush University Medical Center
Chicago, Illinois

William A. Jiranek, MD, FACS
Professor and Vice Chair
Department of Orthopaedic Surgery
Duke University School of Medicine
Durham, North Carolina

Babar Kayani, MBBS, BSc, MRCS
Specialist Registrar Trauma and Orthopaedic Surgery
University College London Hospitals NHS Foundation Trust
University College London
London, England

Mick P. Kelly, MD
Resident Physician
Department of Orthopaedic Surgery
Rush University Medical Center
Chicago, Illinois

Yatin Kirane, MD, PhD
Assistant Professor of Orthopedic Surgery
SUNY Upstate Medical University
Attending Orthopedic Surgeon
Syracuse VA Medical Center
Syracuse, New York

Chad A. Krueger, MD
Assistant Professor of Orthopaedic Surgery
Rothman Orthopaedic Institute
Thomas Jefferson University
Philadelphia, Pennsylvania

Emile-Victor Kuyl
Research Technician
Arthroplasty Research Laboratory
Hospital for Special Surgery
New York, New York

Jeffrey K. Lange, MD
Associate Orthopedic Surgeon
Department of Orthopaedic Surgery
Brigham and Women's Hospital
Instructor, Harvard Medical School
Boston, Massachusetts

Jesua I. Law, DO
Fellow, JIS Orthopedics
New Albany, Ohio
Associate, Valley Orthopaedic Bone and Joint
Modesto, California

Jordan Lebovic, MD, MBA
Resident, Department of Surgery
New York University
New York, New York

David G. Lewallen, MD
Professor of Orthopedic Surgery
Mayo Clinic
Rochester, Minnesota

Guoan Li, PhD
Director, Orthopaedic Bioengineering Research Center
Department of Surgery
Newton-Wellesley Hospital
Newton, Massachusetts

Elizabeth G. Lieberman, MD
Orthopaedic Surgeon
Northwest Orthopaedic Specialists
Adventist Health Portland
Portland, Oregon

Jay R. Lieberman, MD
Professor and Chair
Department of Orthopaedic Surgery
University of Southern California
Los Angeles, California

Frank A. Liporace, MD
Chairman and Vice President, Department of Orthopaedic Surgery
Chief, Division of Orthopaedic Trauma and Adult Reconstruction
Department of Orthopaedic Surgery
Jersey City Medical Center - RWJBarnabas Health
Jersey City, New Jersey

Adolph V. Lombardi Jr, MD, FACS
President, JIS Orthopedics
Clinical Assistant Professor
Department of Orthopaedics
The Ohio State University Wexner Medical Center
White Fence Surgical Suites
Mount Carmel New Albany Surgical Hospital
Mount Carmel St. Ann's
Southeast Ohio Surgical Suites
New Albany, Ohio

William J. Long, MD, FRCSC
Senior Director
Clinical Associate Professor
NYU Langone Orthopedic Hospital
Insall Scott Kelly Institute
New York, New York

Jess H. Lonner, MD
Professor, Department of Orthopaedic Surgery
Thomas Jefferson University
Philadelphia, Pennsylvania

Arthur L. Malkani, MD
Chief, Adult Reconstruction, Professor of Orthopaedics
Department of Orthopaedic Surgery
University of Louisville
Louisville, Kentucky

Kevin B. Marchand, BS
Research Fellow
Northwell Health Orthopedics
Lenox Hill Hospital
New York, New York

Kevin K. Mathew, BS
Research Fellow
Northwell Health Orthopedics
Lenox Hill Hospital
New York, New York

Scott McDermott, MD
Joint Reconstruction Fellow
Rubin Institute of Advanced Orthopedics
Sinai Hospital of Baltimore
Baltimore, Maryland

Alexander R. Meldrum, MD, FRCSC
Fellow, Division of Orthopaedic Surgery
Department of Surgery
Dalhousie University
Halifax, Nova Scotia, Canada

William M. Mihalko, MD, PhD
JR Hyde Professor and Joint Graduate Program Chair in Biomedical Engineering
Campbell Clinic Department of Orthopaedic Surgery and Biomedical Engineering
University of Tennessee Health Science Center
Memphis, Tennessee

Nequesha S. Mohamed, MD
Physician Scientist
Department of Orthopedics
Wake Forest Baptist Medical Center
Winston-Salem, North Carolina

Michael A. Mont, MD, FAAOS
Vice President of Strategic Initiatives
Northwell Health Orthopedics
Lenox Hill Hospital
New York, New York

James Nace, DO, MPT
Associate Professor
Rubin Institute of Advanced Orthopedics
Sinai Hospital of Baltimore
Baltimore, Maryland

Jason H. Oh, MD
Assistant Professor
Department of Orthopaedic Surgery
Hofstra University and Lenox Hill Hospital
New York, New York

Andrew B. Old, MD
Attending Surgeon
Premier Orthopedics
West Chester, Pennsylvania

Feroz Osmani, MD
Resident in Pathology
Icahn School of Medicine at Mount Sinai
New York, New York

Douglas E. Padgett, MD
Associate Surgeon in Chief
Associate Professor of Orthopaedic Surgery
Hospital for Special Surgery
Weill Cornell Medical College
New York, New York

Patricia C. Pang, MD
Attending Anesthesiologist
Department of Anesthesiology
Lenox Hill Hospital
New York, New York

Christopher Pedneault, MDCM, FRCSC
Orthopedic Surgeon
Hôpital Honoré-Mercier
Saint-Hyacinthe, Quebec, Canada

Vincent D. Pellegrini Jr, MD
Professor and Vice Chair for Education and Research Affairs
Department of Orthopaedics
Dartmouth-Hitchcock Medical Center
Geisel School of Medicine at Dartmouth
Lebanon, New Hampshire
Adjunct Professor and Emeritus Chair
Department of Orthopaedics and Physical Medicine
Medical University of South Carolina
Adjunct Professor
Department of Bioengineering
Clemson University
Charleston, South Carolina

Christopher E. Pelt, MD
Associate Professor
Department of Orthopaedic Surgery
University of Utah
Salt Lake City, Utah

Christopher L. Peters, MD
Professor
Department of Orthopaedic Surgery
University of Utah
Salt Lake City, Utah

Daniel Pincus, MD, PhD, FRCSC
Assistant Professor
Department of Surgery
University of Toronto
Toronto, Ontario, Canada

Luis Pulido, MD
Assistant Professor
Adult Arthroplasty and Joint Reconstruction
Department of Orthopaedic Surgery
University of Florida
Gainesville, Florida

Amar S. Ranawat, MD
Professor of Clinical Orthopaedic Surgery
Weill Cornell Medical College
Attending Surgeon
Hospital for Special Surgery
New York, New York

Anil S. Ranawat, MD
Associate Professor
Department of Surgery
Weill Cornell Medical College
New York, New York

Ethan A. Remily, DO
Resident Physician
Rubin Institute of Advanced Orthopedics
Sinai Hospital of Baltimore
Baltimore, Maryland

Harry E. Rubash, MD, FAOA
Chief Emeritus Orthopaedic Surgery
Massachusetts General Hospital
Edith M. Ashley Distinguished Professor
Harvard Medical School
Boston, Massachusetts

Hytham S. Salem, MD
Research Fellow
Northwell Health Orthopedics
Lenox Hill Hospital
New York, New York

Jibanananda Satpathy, MD, MRCSEd
Associate Professor
Department of Surgery
Virginia Commonwealth University
Richmond, Virginia

Ran Schwarzkopf, MD, MSc
Associate Professor
Associate Division Chief, Adult Reconstructive Division
Director, Adult Reconstruction Research Center
Department of Orthopedic Surgery
NYU Langone Medical Center
New York, New York

W. Norman Scott, MD, FACS
Founding Director
Department of Orthopaedics and Sports Medicine
Insall Scott Kelly Institute for Orthopaedics and Sports Medicine
Clinical Professor
Department Orthopedic Surgery
NYU Langone Medical Center
NYU Langone Orthopaedic Hospital
New York, New York

Giles R. Scuderi, MD
Professor, Department of Orthopedic Surgery
Zucker School of Medicine at Hofstra/Northwell
New York, New York

Monica Shoji, MD
Resident in Orthopaedic Surgery
Brigham and Women's Hospital
Department of Orthopaedic Surgery
Boston, Massachusetts

Ahmed Siddiqi, MD, MBA
Clinical Fellow
Department of Orthopedics
Cleveland Clinic Foundation
Cleveland, Ohio

Branden R. Sosa
Arthroplasty Research Laboratory
Hospital for Special Surgery
New York, New York

Dylan Tanzer, MD
Department of Surgery
University at Buffalo
Buffalo, New York

Michael Tanzer, MD, FRCSC, FAAOS
Jo Miller Chair of Orthopaedic Research
McGill University Hospital Centre
Associate Surgeon-in-Chief
McGill University Hospital Centre
Vice Chair Surgery (Clinical) & Professor
McGill University
Montreal, Quebec, Canada

John M. Tarazi, MD
Research Fellow
Northwell Health Orthopedics
Lenox Hill Hospital
New York, New York

Savyasachi Thakkar, MD
Assistant Professor of Orthopaedic Surgery
Department of Orthopaedic Surgery
Johns Hopkins Medical Center
Baltimore, Maryland

Robert T. Trousdale, MD
Professor of Orthopaedic Surgery
Department of Orthopaedic Surgery
Mayo Clinic
Rochester, Minnesota

Kartik Mangudi Varadarajan, PhD
Assistant Professor
Department of Orthopaedic Surgery
Massachusetts General Hospital/ Harvard Medical School
Boston, Massachusetts

Kelly G. Vince, MD, FRCSC
Consultant Orthopedic Surgeon
Whangarei Regional Hospital
Northland District Health Board
Whangarei, Northland, New Zealand
Associate Professor Orthopedic Surgery (former)
University of Southern California
Keck School of Medicine
Los Angeles, California

Bradford S. Waddell, MD
Orthopaedic Surgeon
OrthoAtlanta Piedmont and Piedmont West
Atlanta, Georgia

Jennifer S. Wayne, PhD
Professor and Department Head
Department of Biomedical Engineering and Mechanics
Virginia Tech
Blacksburg, Virginia

Geoffrey Westrich, MD
Professor of Clinical Orthopedic Surgery
Hospital for Special Surgery
Weill Medical College of Cornell University
New York, New York

Wayne A. Wilkie, DO, MHSA
Resident Physician
Department of Orthopedics
Philadelphia College of Osteopathic Medicine
Philadelphia, Pennsylvania

Timothy M. Wright, PhD
F. M. Kirby Chair
Department of Biomechanics
Hospital for Special Surgery
New York, New York

Richard S. Yoon, MD
Director, Orthopaedic Research
Division of Orthopaedic Trauma & Adult Reconstruction
Department of Orthopaedic Surgery
Jersey City Medical Center - RWJBarnabas Health
Jersey City, New Jersey

Pierre P. Zaharia, MD, FRCSC
Fellow
Division of Orthopaedic Surgery
Department of Surgery
Dalhousie University
Halifax, Nova Scotia, Canada

Preface

Orthopaedic Knowledge Update®: Hip and Knee Reconstruction 6 complements and updates information that was published in the five previous editions. The first edition was published in 1995, the second in 2000, the third in 2006, the fourth in 2011, and the fifth in 2015. This edition encompasses a comprehensive review of the past 5 years of published literature on hip and knee arthroplasty. This sixth edition serves as an update that can stand on its own.

This edition provides residents, fellows, and practicing orthopaedic surgeons with a clear understanding of the state-of-the-art knowledge relevant to adult hip and knee reconstruction. As with the previous five publications, it can be used as a resource for both general orthopaedic surgeons and hip and knee specialists.

The sixth edition, like the fifth edition, is composed of three distinct sections: basic and applied science relevant to both knee and hip arthroplasty; specific total knee arthroplasty topics; and specific total hip arthroplasty topics. There is updated material related to controversial topics, state-of-the-art technologies, and recent advances in hip and knee arthroplasty. All of the chapters have been written by world-renowned experts in each subject, with a concerted effort to reflect the current state-of-the-art knowledge with objectivity by basing material primarily on evidence-based information from recent reports.

We, the editors, would like to thank all of the authors for their tremendous work to complete their chapters. Their time and commitment to this update is greatly appreciated. We also gratefully acknowledge the invaluable assistance of the publishing team of the American Academy of Orthopaedic Surgeons and Wolters Kluwer Health. This includes Hans Koelsch, PhD, Director; Lisa Claxton Moore, Senior Manager, Editorial; Steven Kellert, Senior Editor at AAOS and Brian Brown, Director, Medical Practice; Stacey Sebring, Senior Development Editor, Medical Practice; and Emily Buccieri, Senior Editorial Coordinator at Wolters Kluwer. Their work and diligence helped to make this book of the highest quality.

Michael A. Mont, MD, FAAOS
Michael Tanzer, MD, FRCSC, FAAOS

Table of Contents

Section 1: Hip and Knee

SECTION EDITORS:

Michael A. Mont, MD, FAAOS and Michael Tanzer, MD, FRCSC, FAAOS

Section 2: Knee

SECTION EDITOR:
Michael A. Mont, MD, FAAOS

Section 3: Hip

SECTION EDITOR:
Michael Tanzer, MD, FRCSC, FAAOS

SECTION 1

Hip and Knee

Section Editors:

Michael A. Mont, MD, FAAOS and
Michael Tanzer, MD, FRCSC, FAAOS

CHAPTER 1

Imaging of the Hip and Knee for Primary and Revision Arthroplasty

LUIS PULIDO, MD • STEPHEN J. INCAVO, MD

ABSTRACT

Imaging of the hip and knee for primary and revision arthroplasty includes conventional radiographs, biplanar low-dose radiation radiograph imaging system, nuclear medicine scans, ultrasonograms, CT scans, and MRI scans. Plain radiographs are the first-line diagnostic test in orthopaedics and the most valuable test in the evaluation of hip and knee arthroplasty patients. A methodical approach to the evaluation of hip and knee radiographs is sufficient to determine a diagnosis and establish a treatment plan. Preoperative planning and templating of calibrated radiographs aids the accuracy and efficiency of joint arthroplasty surgery. Advanced imaging modalities have a complementary role in the evaluation of different clinical scenarios before and after hip and knee arthroplasty.

Keywords: hip arthroplasty; imaging; knee arthroplasty; radiography

INTRODUCTION

The diagnostic imaging modalities available today are important tools for the diagnosis and management of musculoskeletal conditions affecting the hip and knee joints. Orthopaedic surgeons use conventional radiographs as initial imaging study for the diagnosis of patients who have hip and knee pain. A methodical approach in the evaluation of hip and knee radiographs is sufficient to establish a diagnosis and treatment plan. Radiographs allow assessing the severity of degenerative joint disease, which is key in the decision making for hip or knee arthroplasty surgery. The accuracy and efficiency of total hip arthroplasty (THA) and total knee arthroplasty (TKA) is increased using digital templates of calibrated radiographs. Radiographs are fundamental in the evaluation of total hip and knee implants. Other than prosthetic joint infection, the main causes of failure of hip and knee arthroplasties are diagnosed with plain radiographs. Advanced imaging techniques including biplanar low-dose radiation systems, nuclear medicine, ultrasonography, CT, and MRI have complementary roles and are not routinely used. The fundamentals of plain radiographs in primary and revision hip and knee arthroplasty are reviewed. The advances and clinical utility of advanced diagnostic imaging tests are also discussed.

TOTAL HIP ARTHROPLASTY

Conventional radiographs are used to assess the severity of hip osteoarthritis[1] (**Figure 1**). The standard views for the evaluation of hip disorders include a weight-bearing AP pelvis, AP, and cross-table lateral of the hip. Weight-bearing radiographs provide a more reliable evaluation of the joint space and allow for a functional view of the pelvis. The proper technique to obtain a pelvis AP view includes having x-ray beam perpendicular and centered at a midpoint between the symphysis pubis and the anterior superior iliac spine with the lower extremities in 10° to 15° of internal rotation for accurate determination of

Dr. Incavo or an immediate family member has received royalties from Innomed, Kyocera, Osteoremedies, Smith & Nephew, Wright Medical Technology, Inc., and Zimmer and has stock or stock options held in Nimbic Systems. Neither Dr. Pulido nor any immediate family member has received anything of value from or has stock or stock options held in a commercial company or institution related directly or indirectly to the subject of this chapter.

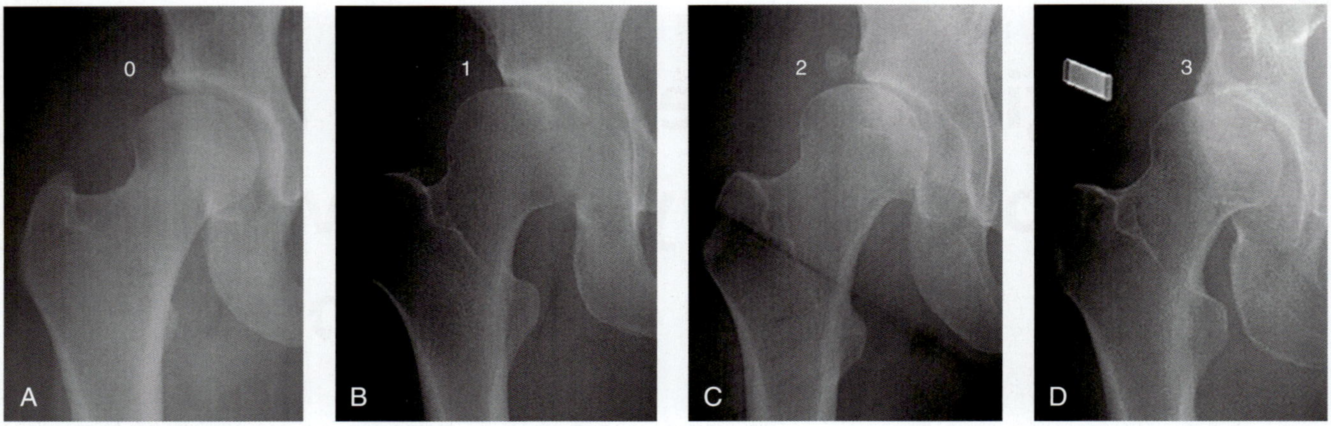

FIGURE 1 Standing AP radiographs of the hip are used in the Tönnis classification to categorize the severity of coxarthrosis. **A**, Preserved hip joints are graded as Tönnis 0. **B**, Tönnis 1, slight joint space narrowing and mild sclerosis of the head and acetabulum. **C**, Tönnis 2, moderate joint space narrowing, moderate femoral head loss of spherecity, and small subchondral cysts. **D**, Tönnis 3, joint space obliteration, large subchondral cysts, severe femoral head deformity, or evidence of necrosis.

neck length and femoral lateral offset. Externally rotated hips increase the neck-shaft angle and decrease the lateral femoral offset affecting the accuracy of the surgical plan in restoring hip biomechanics. The cross-table lateral radiograph is with the patient supine, the contralateral hip flexed, and the affected limb in 15° of internal rotation, with the x-ray beam oriented at 45° to the affected hip. Conventional radiographs help to identify secondary causes of hip arthritis such as osteonecrosis, femoroacetabular impingement, and hip dysplasia. The radiographic evaluation of the young adult with hip pain includes a frog leg lateral, Dunn 45°, and a false profile.[2]

Preoperative Planning and Digital Templating

Digital templating is an important tool in planning primary and revision hip arthroplasty.[3] Digital implant template overlay helps determine the best implant fit, size, and position with the goal of restoring the hip biomechanics. Restoration of the hip center of rotation, the femoral lateral offset, and leg lengths are important goals to achieve in the preoperative planning and execution of THA (**Figure 2**).

Pelvic Obliquity

The pelvic axis orientation is corrected during preoperative templating and surgical execution of THA for accurate acetabular abduction angle placement and for leg length equalization. Restoring the coronal balance of the pelvis following THA is associated with compensation of the spine coronal alignment in the majority of cases. Patients with rigid degenerative scoliosis can develop worsening of the spinal imbalance and back pain after THA.[4] Weight-bearing radiographs obtained using a block on the shortened lower extremity can help determine the target for any planned leg lengthening.

Pelvic Tilt

Pelvic tilt determines the functional anteversion and inclination of the acetabulum. The position of the pelvis in relation to the lumbar spine varies during simple activities such as standing, sitting, or lying down. Functional acetabular position is a difficult and mobile target during THA. There is a role in positioning the acetabular implant based on the functional pelvic tilt seen on weight-bearing radiographs.[5] Patients with rigid lumbopelvic lordosis and kyphosis are associated with greater risk of postoperative dislocation.

Hip Dysplasia

THA for end-stage hip disease secondary to hip dysplasia and developmental dysplasia has unique acetabular and femoral anatomical features.[6,7] The Crowe-Ranawat and the Hartofilakidis classification systems are used to determine the degree of femoroacetabular dysplasia and dislocation (**Figure 3**). The dysplastic acetabulum is shallow, steep, and elongated.[8] The cup should ideally be placed at the true hip center of rotation. Femoral head autograft is used to reconstitute large superolateral acetabular defects. The use of a lateral and high hip center is less favorable because of abnormal hip biomechanics, increased joint reaction forces, and potential higher risk of failure. The dysplastic femur has a high neck-shaft angle with increased femoral anteversion. The use of a femoral stem that allows adjustment of femoral version is preferable.[9] A subtrochanteric shortening osteotomy is a useful technique to manage hip dysplasia with high-grade dislocation and avoid iatrogenic peroneal-sciatic nerve injury from stretching.[10]

Femoral Deformity

Biplanar radiograph with magnification markers of the pelvis and entire femur is recommended in the surgical

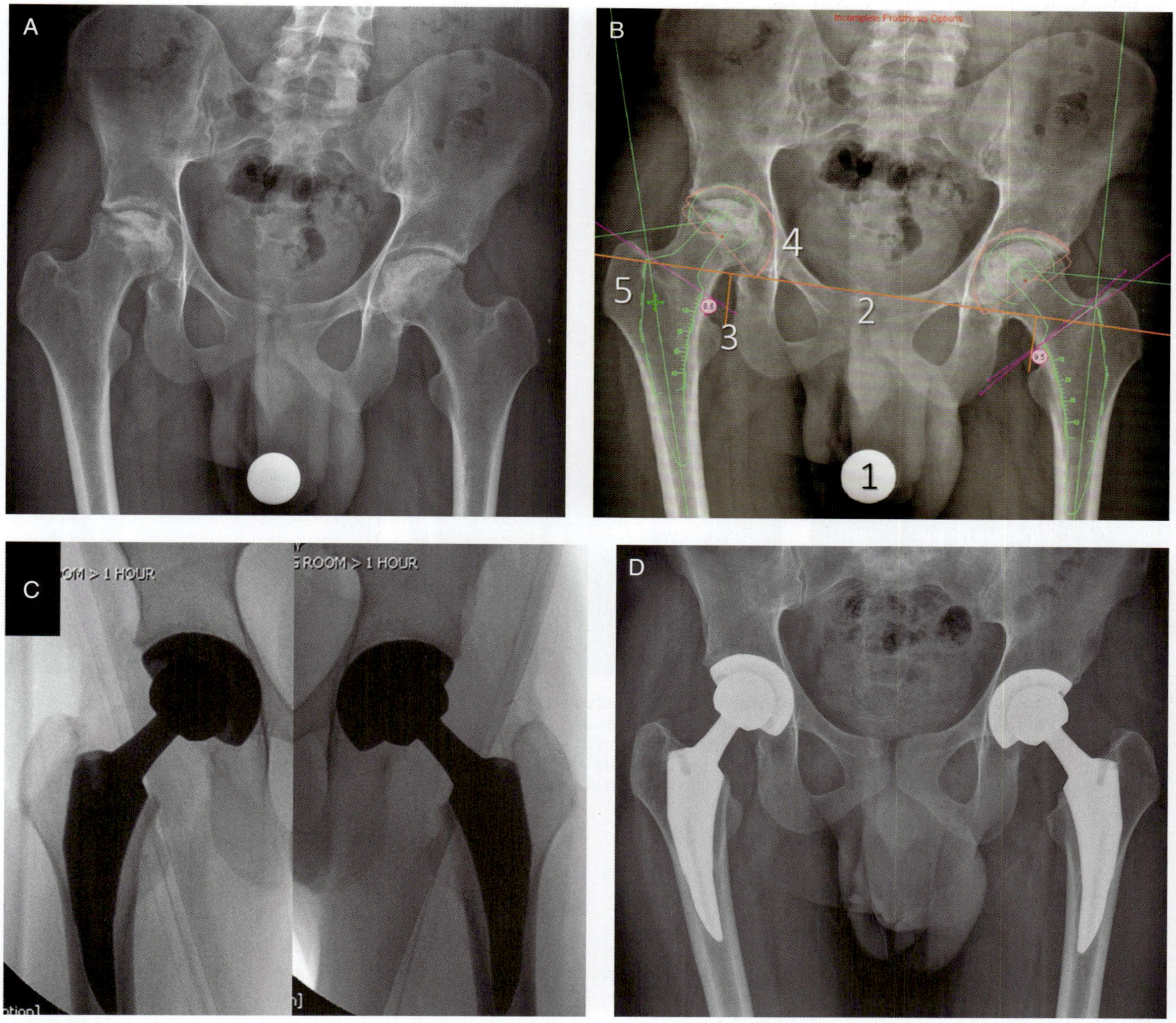

FIGURE 2 **A**, Weight-bearing AP pelvis radiograph in a young patient who had bilateral femoral head osteonecrosis with collapse. **B**, Stepwise approach for templating total hip arthroplasty: (1) Calibrate the digital image with markers. (2) Determine the pelvis axis orientation using a line across the teardrops or ischial tuberosity. (3) Determine the leg lengths using the distance from a line perpendicular to pelvis axis to the top of the lesser trochanters. (4) Place the acetabular implant to restore the hip center of rotation with the cup apex just lateral to the teardrop at 40° to 45° of abduction from the pelvis axis. (5) Template the femoral implant to determine the best fitting stem and the stem size to restore femoral lateral offset and equalize leg lengths. The distance from the lesser trochanter to the neck cut is used intraoperatively to restore leg lengths. **C**, Limited intraoperative fluoroscopy during direct anterior simultaneous bilateral total hip arthroplasty to confirm acetabular position and femoral fit. **D**, Weight-bearing AP pelvis radiograph at 1-year follow-up with well-fixed and positioned bilateral total hip arthroplasty.

planning of THA in patients who have proximal femoral deformity. The use of digital templating allows planning for the management of different deformity sites (ie, greater trochanter, femoral neck, metaphysis, and diaphysis) and types (ie, angular, translational, and torsional). The use of modular stems with distal stability or fixation may become more important in this clinical scenario.

REVISION TOTAL HIP ARTHROPLASTY

Successful revision surgery is based on understanding the cause of failure and determining a treatment plan. The most common causes of failure after hip arthroplasty include dislocation, periprosthetic fractures, deep infection, aseptic loosening, and wear-osteolysis.[11] Plain

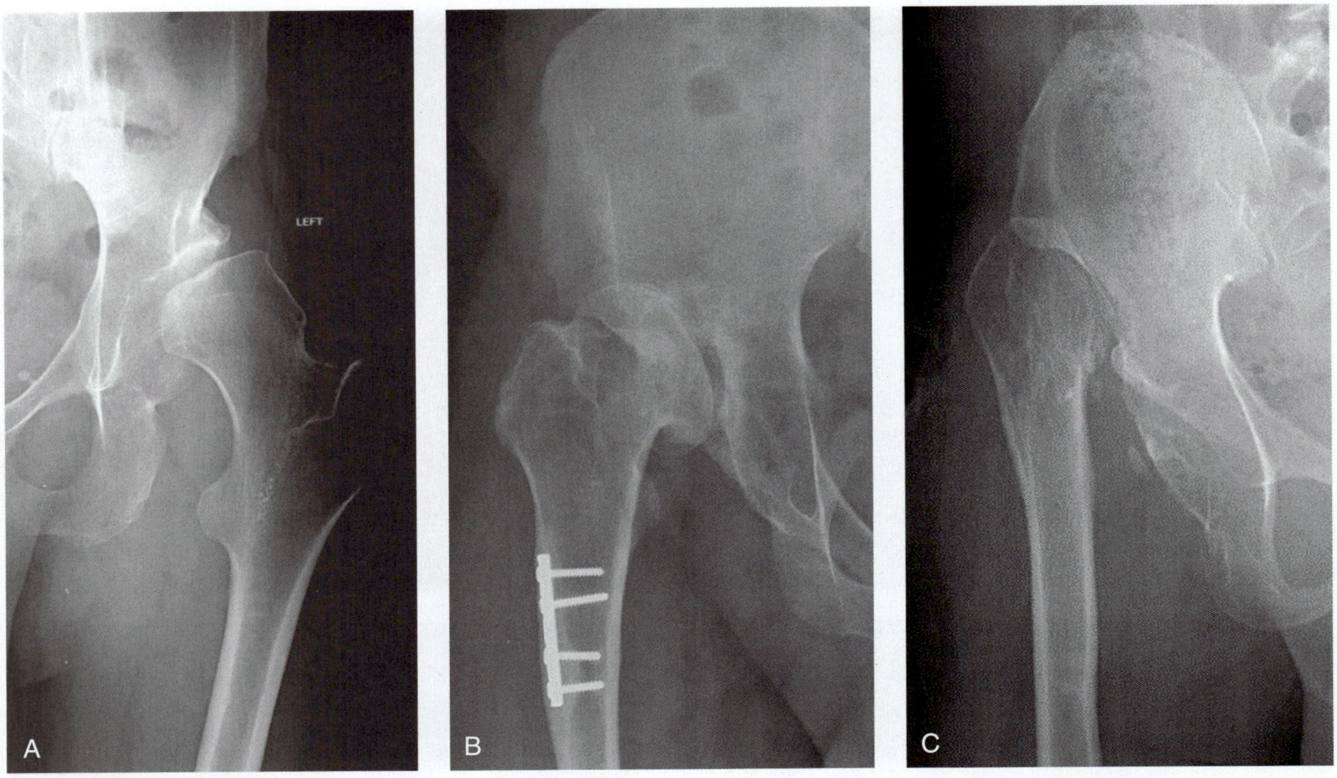

FIGURE 3 Hartofilakidis classification for total hip arthroplasty in congenital dislocation of the hip. **A**, Dysplasia (type A). AP radiographs of the left hip shows a shallow and elongated acetabulum with superior and anterior segmental defects and a contained femoral head in true acetabulum. **B**, Low dislocation (type B). AP radiograph of the right hip shows the femoral head articulating with the false acetabulum and overlapping the true acetabulum. **C**, High dislocation (type C). AP radiographs of the right hip shows a congenital femoroacetabular dislocation where the false acetabulum has no connection with the true acetabulum.

radiographs allow evaluation of the type of prosthesis, implant position, fixation, polywear, osteolysis, periprosthetic bone loss, and fractures. Plain radiographs are used to identify the type of femoral and acetabular implants as well as bearing surfaces. Weight-bearing AP pelvis and cross-table lateral hip radiographs are used to evaluate the acetabular and femoral position and fixation. Serial radiographs are very useful in the evaluation of implant fixation, migration, and remodeling. Full femur radiographs are obtained in certain patients who have long diaphyseal revision stems, long cemented stems, femoral hardware, or deformity. Preoperative templating is also an important aspect of revision hip arthroplasty. Pelvic Judet views are supplemental in the evaluation of pelvic bone loss and column integrity in acetabular revision.

Implant malposition increases the risk of failure because of increased wear, instability, and pain after THA. The etiology of hip instability is multifactorial. Implant factors such as the lack of femoral offset and acetabular malposition due to excessive inclination and version abnormalities can be seen on plain radiographs.

Implant Fixation and Loosening

Serial radiographs are very useful in the evaluation of adequate fixation versus loose implants in primary and revision hip arthroplasty. The ability to identify a loose implant on radiographs is of critical value for the arthroplasty surgeon. Femoral and acetabular loosening is associated with pain, bone loss, and increased risk of fractures. Septic and aseptic loosening are common causes of failure and indication for revision hip surgery. In addition, the treatment plan of postoperative periprosthetic femur fractures after THA depends on the stability of hip implants.

Acetabular fixation is evaluated by determining the areas of lucencies and implant migration. The DeLee and Charnley zones were described for the radiographic analysis of cemented acetabular components[12] (**Figure 4**). The authors of a 1988 study established the positive correlation between the number of radiographic zones of demarcation and the likelihood of intraoperative acetabular loosening in cemented sockets. Seven percent of cups with one zone of demarcation were loose intraoperatively, 71% were loose with two zones of demarcation, and

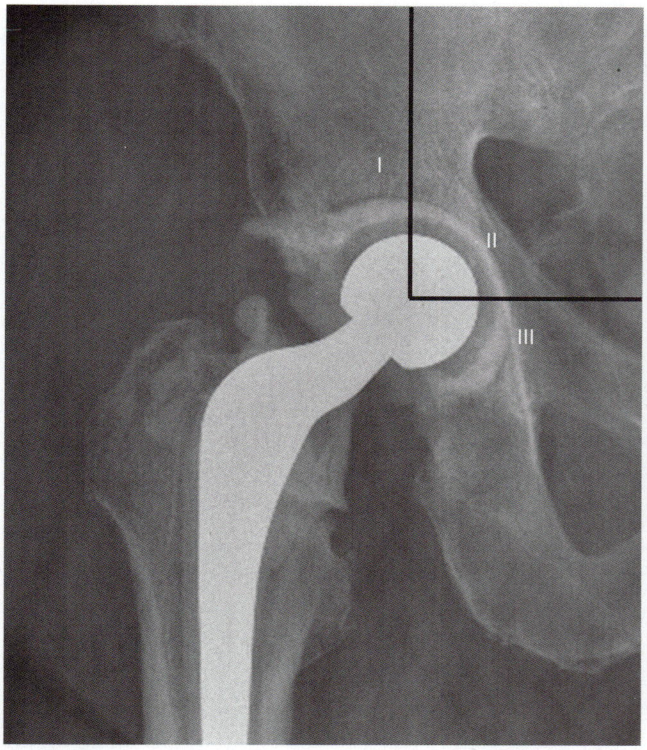

FIGURE 4 Right hip AP radiograph illustrating DeLee and Charnley method to divide the acetabular circumference in zones I, II, and III. Originally described to evaluate acetabular fixation in cemented sockets by determining the depth and location of demarcation at the implant bone-cement interface and the correlation with implant loosening.

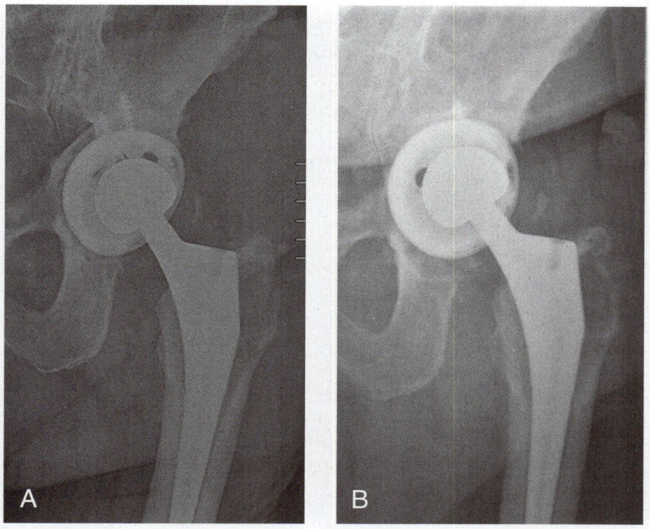

FIGURE 5 Images from an 81-year-old man with a painful left total hip arthroplasty. **A**, AP radiograph of the left hip shows a loose noncemented acetabular implant with radiolucent lines in all three zones. **B**, Serial AP radiograph of the left hip 1-year later shows cup migration. The cup was grossly loose intraoperatively at the time of cup revision.

94% were loose when all three zones had radiographic demarcation. All the sockets that migrated were loose, and the cups with no areas of demarcation were well fixed.[13] The authors of a 2001 study did a similar study in noncemented cups. They evaluated preoperative radiographic findings and their correlation with intraoperative loosening. Loose implants had radiolucent lines that appeared after 2 years, progression of radiolucent lines after 2 years, radiolucent lines in all three zones, radiolucent lines 2 mm or wider in any zone, or cup migration.[14] Broken screws are a common finding in loose sockets secondary to cup migration (**Figure 5**).

Femoral stem fixation and loosening after THA can be determined with plain radiographs. Serial imaging showing evidence of implant migration is probably the most reliable method to evaluate femoral loosening. The authors of a 1979 study[15] studied the modes of failure of cemented stems and described radiographic zones of the femoral implant in the coronal and lateral planes (**Figure 6**). The Gruen zones are commonly used to describe radiographic findings around a femoral stem such as areas of lucencies, demarcation, or osteolytic lesions seen in the coronal plane. The durability of cemented femoral stems is highly dependent on the cementing technique. The authors of a 1992 study classified the quality of cementing technique in THA.[16] They described four grades seen in postoperative radiographs around the femoral implant including grade A, for complete whiteout and dense filling of the intramedullary canal with cement; grade B, if there was a subtle radiolucency in the cement-bone interface; grade C, for incomplete or defective cement mantle involving 50% to 99% of the cement-bone interface; and grade D, when there was failure to fill the canal with cement. The authors of a 1982 study also categorized loosening of cemented stems into definite (migration or fracture of the femoral implant or the cement), probable (100% radiolucency around the cement mantle), and possible (50% to 99% of radiolucency of around the cement-bone interface)[17] (**Figure 7**).

The radiographic criteria used to determine stable fixation in noncemented stems originates from Dr. Engh's evaluation of cylindrical, fully porous-coated cobalt-chromium stems.[18] They classified stable fixation by bone ingrowth when there was no evidence of implant migration, minimal presence of radiopaque reactive lines, and presence of streaming trabeculae in the bone-implant interface. Uniform cortical hypertrophy occurring just distal to the ingrowth surface also indicates the implant is ingrown to the bone and that stress is transferred from the more proximal femur to the femur at the distal portion of the ingrowth surface. Stable fibrous ingrowths were implants with no migration that had a radiopaque reactive line parallel to the stem up to 1 mm and not

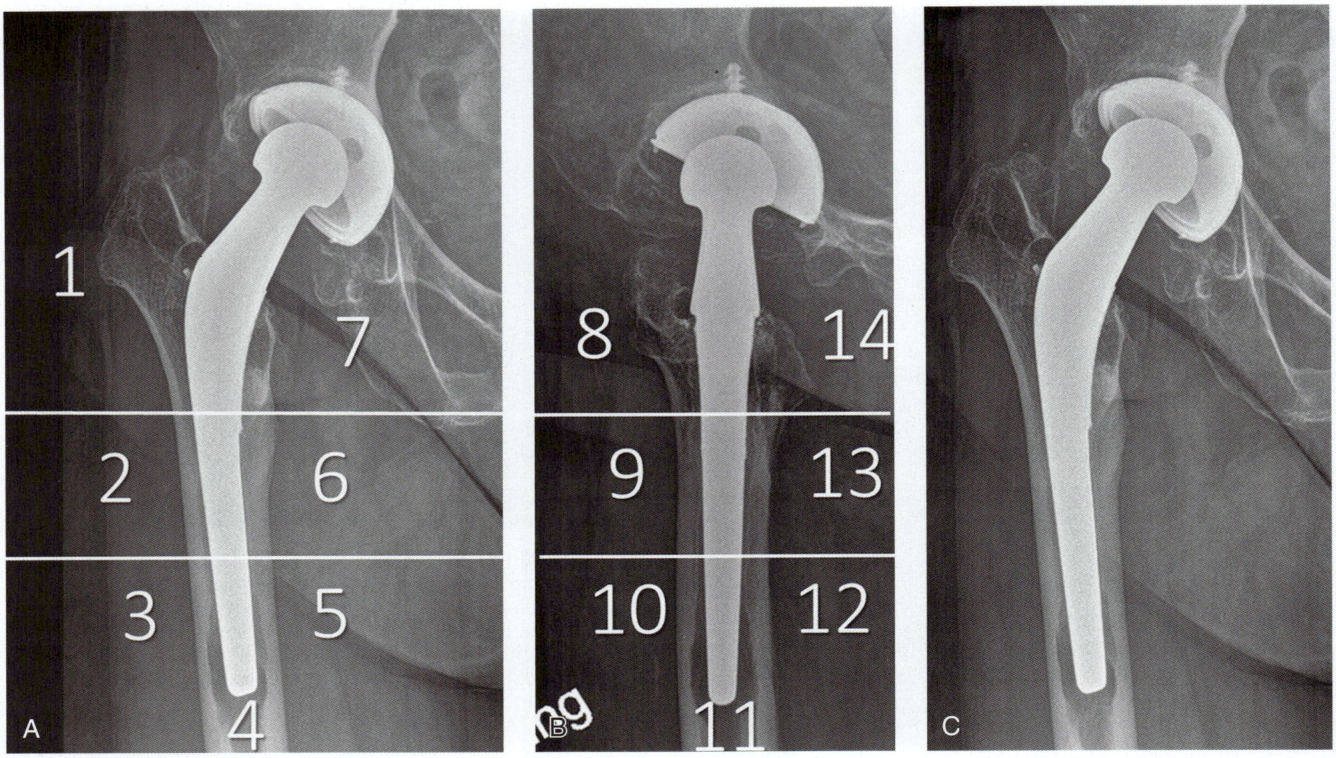

FIGURE 6 The Gruen radiographic zones were described for the analysis of different modes of failure of cemented femoral stems. The Gruen zones are helpful to describe radiographic findings around the femoral implant. **A**, There are seven zones divided in the coronal plane. Zone 1 is located proximal and lateral around the greater trochanter area. Zone 4 is located at the distal end of the prosthesis. Zone 7 is located proximal and medial around the lesser trochanter area. **B**, Gruen's original description included seven additional zones in the lateral plane numbered from 8 to 14. **C**, AP radiograph of the right hip with a right noncemented total hip arthroplasty. The acetabular implant is in a high hip center position, there is polywear, and there is a radiolucent line greater than 2 mm in zone 1, concerning for acetabular loosening. The femoral stem has osteolytic areas in Gruen zones 1, 3, 4, and 5. Magnification of this image shows bead shedding in zones 1 and 7.

cortical hypertrophy. Unstable or loose implants had migration, divergent radiopaque lines or a pedestal, and nonuniform cortical hypertrophy.

Osteolysis and Bone Loss

Plain radiographs tend to underestimate periprosthetic osteolysis and bone loss (**Figure 8**). However, in the setting of mechanical failure, AP pelvis, cross-table lateral, and Judet views can help assess acetabular bone loss, column integrity, and the presence of pelvic discontinuity. The classic radiographic findings of pelvic discontinuity on a true AP pelvis include a fracture line through the anterior and posterior columns, a break in Kohler's line with medial translation of the inferior hemipelvis relative to the superior hemipelvis, and the presence of an asymmetric obturator ring due to rotation of the hemipelvis.[19]

There are multiple systems to classify acetabular bone loss in THA. The Paprosky classification for acetabular defects is widely used and helps guide the reconstruction options.[20] The radiographic and intraoperative findings are categorized to determine the ability of the acetabular rim to provide stability and support for the acetabular implant and reconstruction. The acetabular bone defects are classified as type 1 if the acetabular rim is completely supportive, type 2 if partially supportive, or type 3 if nonsupportive (**Table 1**).

The evaluation of femoral meta-diaphyseal bone loss on radiographs is important in preoperative planning to help define the method used for femoral revision. The quality and length of the isthmus is evaluated as distally fixed tapered conical titanium fluted stems have been universally adopted in femoral revision because of superior clinical results and versatility, which is also the basis for the Paprosky classification for femoral bone loss[21] (**Table 2**).

Extended Trochanteric Osteotomy

Plain radiographs are needed to determine the need, type, and length of femoral osteotomy. Relative indications for extended trochanteric osteotomy in revision hip surgery include femoral varus deformity, trochanteric overhang, removal of long or fully coated stems, long cemented stems, and cement removal.

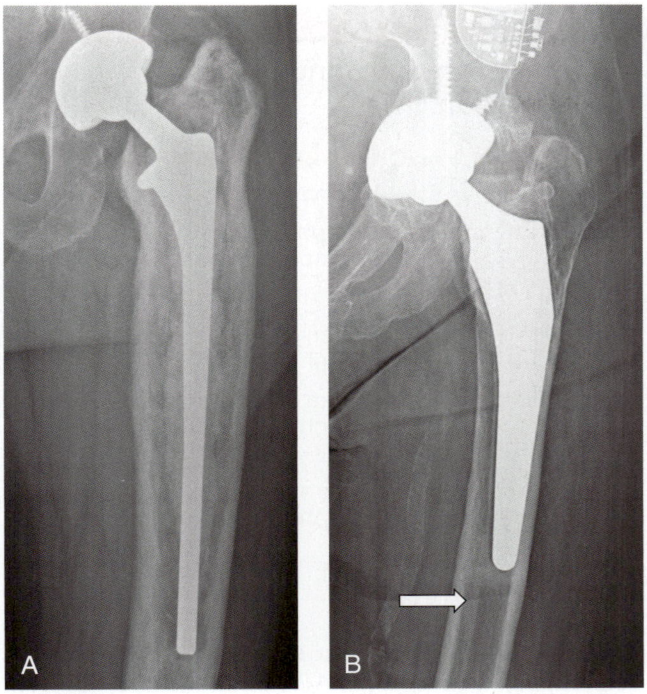

FIGURE 7 **A**, Images from an 85-year-old man with a history of Paget disease and a painful left total hip arthroplasty performed 10 years ago. AP radiograph shows a definite loose cemented femoral prosthesis with implant migration. **B**, Images from an 86-year-old woman with painful left total hip arthroplasty performed 16 years ago. AP radiograph shows a loose noncemented femoral implant with implant migration and divergent pedestal formation (white arrow). There is varus remodeling of the proximal femur and trochanteric overhang.

TOTAL KNEE ARTHROPLASTY

The routine knee radiographs include a standing weight bearing AP in neutral rotation, a lateral view with the knee flexed 30°, and a Merchant axial view. The advantage of a full-length weight-bearing AP view of the lower extremity over shorter images is a more precise measurement of knee anatomic and mechanical axis. These images also provide evidence of possible hip disorders, which must be ruled out in all painful knees, and help identify extra-articular deformities of the femur and/or tibia. The axial alignment of the knee seen in two-dimensional frontal views is influenced by the lower extremity rotation. Excessive internal rotation simulates valgus alignment and excessive external rotation simulates varus alignment.[22] A 45° weight-bearing posteroanterior flexion view (Rosenberg radiograph) is a helpful functional view of the knee that helps to more accurately determine joint space narrowing in the knee.[23]

Conventional radiographs are used to assess the severity of knee osteoarthritis and help in the decision making for TKA. The Kellgren-Lawrence classification system was described to categorize the severity of osteoarthritis seen on AP radiographs.[24] The highest interobserver and intraobserver reliability was seen at the knee joint, for which it has been widely adopted in the evaluation of knee osteoarthritis (**Figure 9**).

In primary TKA, digital templates allow assessment of deformity and help plan the correction using femoral and tibial bone cuts to restore mechanical axis (or axis

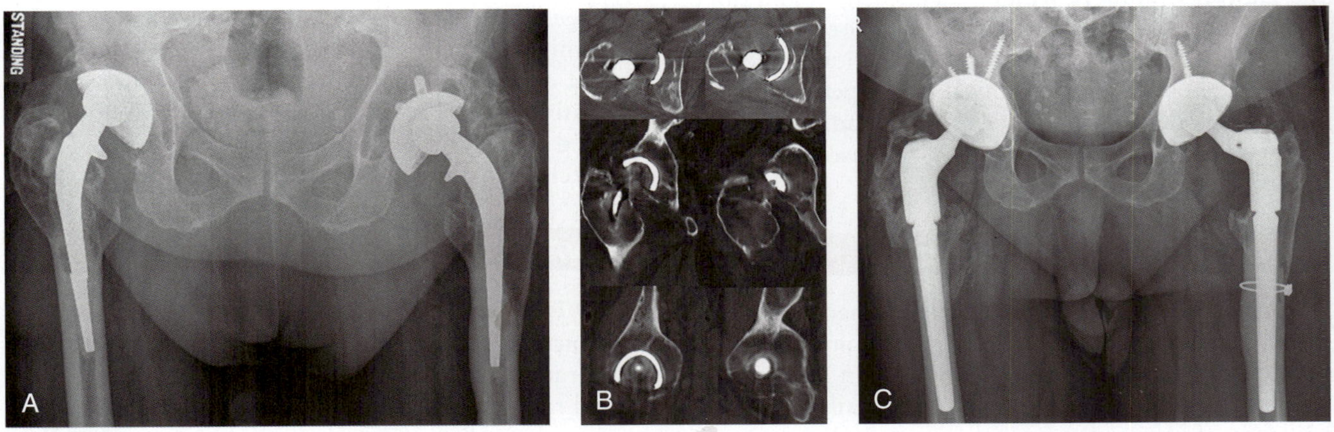

FIGURE 8 **A**, Preoperative radiograph of a 75-year-old man with painful bilateral total hip arthroplasties performed 24 years ago. The right hip has a well-fixed noncemented cup with polywear. There is no gross evidence of periacetabular osteolysis. The right cemented femoral implant is definitely loose with a broken stem. There is an expansile osteolytic lesion affecting the peritrochanteric area. **B**, CT images obtained elsewhere showing extensive osteolysis around the right acetabulum. Plain radiographs underestimated the severity of periacetabular bone loss on the right hip. **C**, Postoperative radiographs after staged bilateral revision hip surgery with tapered fluted modular stems, highly porous acetabular components, and duo-mobility bearing surfaces.

TABLE 1

Paprosky Acetabular Bone Defect Classification

Type	Description
Type 1	No migration, absent ischial lysis and present teardrop
	Intact rim and columns
	Implies near primary situation
Type 2	Destruction of the medial wall or dome
	Cup migration less than 2 cm
	Adequate stability with trial. Greater than 50% contact surface
Type 2A	Superior dome defect
Type 2B	Segmental superolateral defect
Type 2C	Medial defect with cup medial to Kohler line
Type 3	Severe bone loss, ischial lysis, and destruction of the acetabular rim
	Cup migration greater than 2 cm
Type 3A	Up and out. Superior and lateral migration
Type 3B	Up and in. Superior and medial migration. Extensive ischial lysis

TABLE 2

Paprosky Femoral Bone Defect Classification

Type	Description
Type I	Minimal metaphyseal bone loss
Type II	Metaphyseal bone loss and completely intact diaphysis
Type III	Meta-diaphyseal bone loss
Type IIIA	>4 mm of intact cortical diaphyseal bone
Type IIIB	<4 mm of intact cortical diaphyseal bone
Type IV	Extensive meta-diaphyseal bone loss and wide nonsupportive diaphysis

of choice). Digital templating on a lateral view helps with the femoral implant sizing to restore posterior condylar offset and avoid notching. Templating TKAs start with image calibration using markers, followed by femoral sizing on the lateral view and evaluation of the sagittal femoral bowing, patellar height, and tibial slope. For the AP view (long leg or short knee), the distal femoral and proximal tibia resection angles are planned to restore the mechanical axis depending on the surgeon's preferred technique. Long leg radiographs are important to obtain in patients who have extra-articular deformity (**Figure 10**).

REVISION KNEE ARTHROPLASTY

Aseptic loosening, instability, malalignment, and periprosthetic joint infection are the most common causes of failure after knee arthroplasty.[25] Plain radiographs are used to help determine the cause of failure, for surveillance of knee implants and for surgical planning in complex revision TKA.

Implant Position

The knee implant position can be determined using the standard knee series views as noted previously. Neutral, varus, or valgus alignment of the femur and tibia is determined on the coronal AP views. The distance from the medial epicondyle and the adductor tubercle to the medial component is used to determine the femoral joint line in revision TKA. The lateral knee radiographs help determine patellar height, posterior femoral offset, the sagittal position of the femoral implant, and the amount of tibia slope.

IMPLANT FIXATION

Standard knee views, sequential radiographs, and occasionally fluoroscopic views are helpful to determine femoral and tibial loosening after TKA. The size, percentage, and location of radiolucent lines are helpful to determine loosening. Technologies such as radiostereometric analysis are more accurate to measure implant migration after TKA. Radiostereometric analysis has limited clinical use and is mainly used for clinical research.

ADVANCED IMAGING TECHNIQUES

Biplanar Low-Dose Radiation Imaging Systems

Advanced imaging technologies such as biplanar low-dose radiation systems (EOS imaging) provide functional radiographic information in different positions such as standing, squatting, and sitting. The EOS imaging system consists of two pairs of perpendicularly positioned, vertically moving, and linked units of x-ray tubes that produce very thin collimated x-ray beams collected by detectors resulting in a simultaneous and spatially calibrated weight-bearing AP and lateral

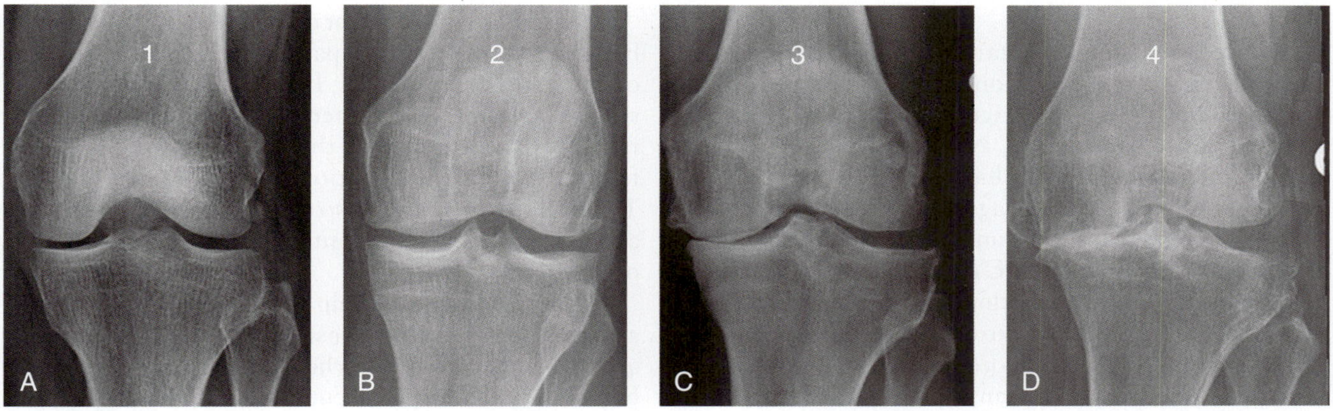

FIGURE 9 The Kellgren-Lawrence classification is a radiographic grading system used to determine the severity of knee osteoarthritis. The radiographic features included joint space narrowing, osteophytes, subchondral sclerosis, periarticular cysts, and deformity. It is a five-grade classification scheme. Grade 0 is no presence of osteoarthritis. **A**, Grade 1, minimal joint space narrowing and possible osteophytes. **B**, Grade 2, mild joint space narrowing with definite osteophytes. **C**, Grade 3, definite joint space narrowing, moderate osteophytes, sclerosis, and possible deformity. **D**, Grade 4, large osteophytes, joint space narrowing, sclerosis, and definite deformity of bone ends.

images. Static functional views in standing, sitting, or squatting positions can be obtained in 10 to 25 seconds with a fraction of the radiation compared with plain radiographs (6 to 9 times less radiation) or CT (600 times less radiation). The EOS system also can create three-dimensional reconstruction models of the spine, pelvis, and lower limbs.[26,27] The role of EOS in THA has not been established. However, EOS has a potential role in the functional position of the acetabulum and determining the hip-spine relationship in THA.[28]

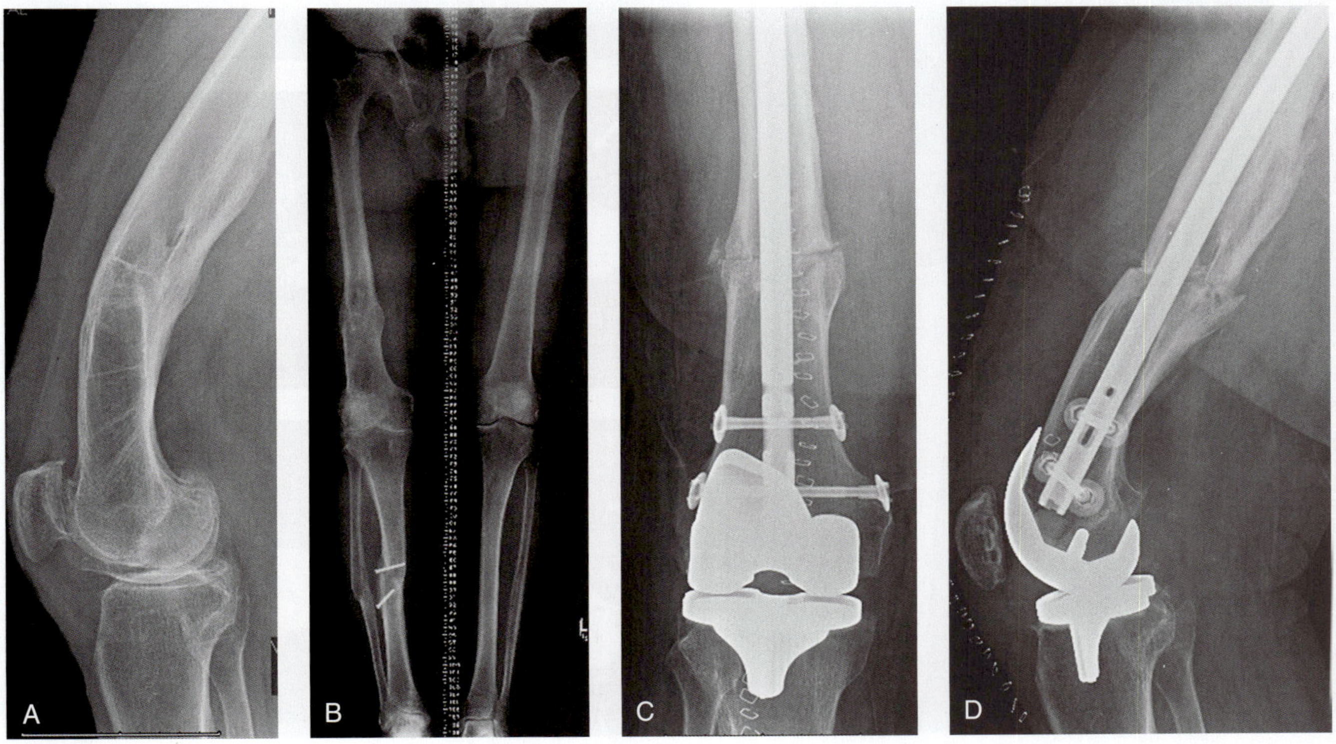

FIGURE 10 Lateral (**A**) and full-length AP weight-bearing (**B**) radiographs demonstrate right knee degenerative joint disease with associated right femoral extra-articular deformity. AP (**C**) and lateral (**D**) radiographs of the right knee demonstrate successful simultaneous total knee arthroplasty and deformity correction with femoral osteotomy and retrograde nail fixation.

Multidetector CT

CT is used as a supplementary diagnostic test to help diagnose prearthritic conditions of the hip, as well as hip and knee implant fixation, fractures, loosening, position, and periprosthetic bone loss. Narrower collimation and low pitch adjustments in multidetector CT reduce metal artifacts and improve the image quality of bone and soft tissues around hip and knee implants. Osteolysis is more accurately determined with CT than plain radiography: CT facilitates better detection, characterization, and quantification of bone loss around acetabular and femoral implants, as well as more accurate determination of implant fixation.[29] CT scans have limited use for the evaluation of periarticular masses and fluid collections following THA. In patients who have failed metal and metal hip arthroplasties, the sensitivity for diagnosis of pseudotumors is only 44%.[30] In this setting, the use of MRI with metal suppression or ultrasonography is recommended.

Rotational malalignment of the femur and/or tibia can be the cause of knee pain, patella maltracking, stiffness, or instability after TKA. Two-dimensional axial CT scan images have weak interobserver and intraobserver reliability in determining the rotation of the tibia and femoral implants in relation with bony landmarks.[31] Three-dimensional reconstruction images are superior and more reliable in obtaining rotational measurements of TKA components.[32]

CT angiography can help with surgical planning and awareness of abnormal vascular anatomy around the acetabulum in patients who have massive acetabular bone loss and intrapelvic cups[33] (**Figure 11**).

Magnetic Resonance Imaging

MRI is used frequently in the evaluation of hip pain in the young adult. The MRI arthrogram has been the preferred imaging test in the evaluation of femoroacetabular

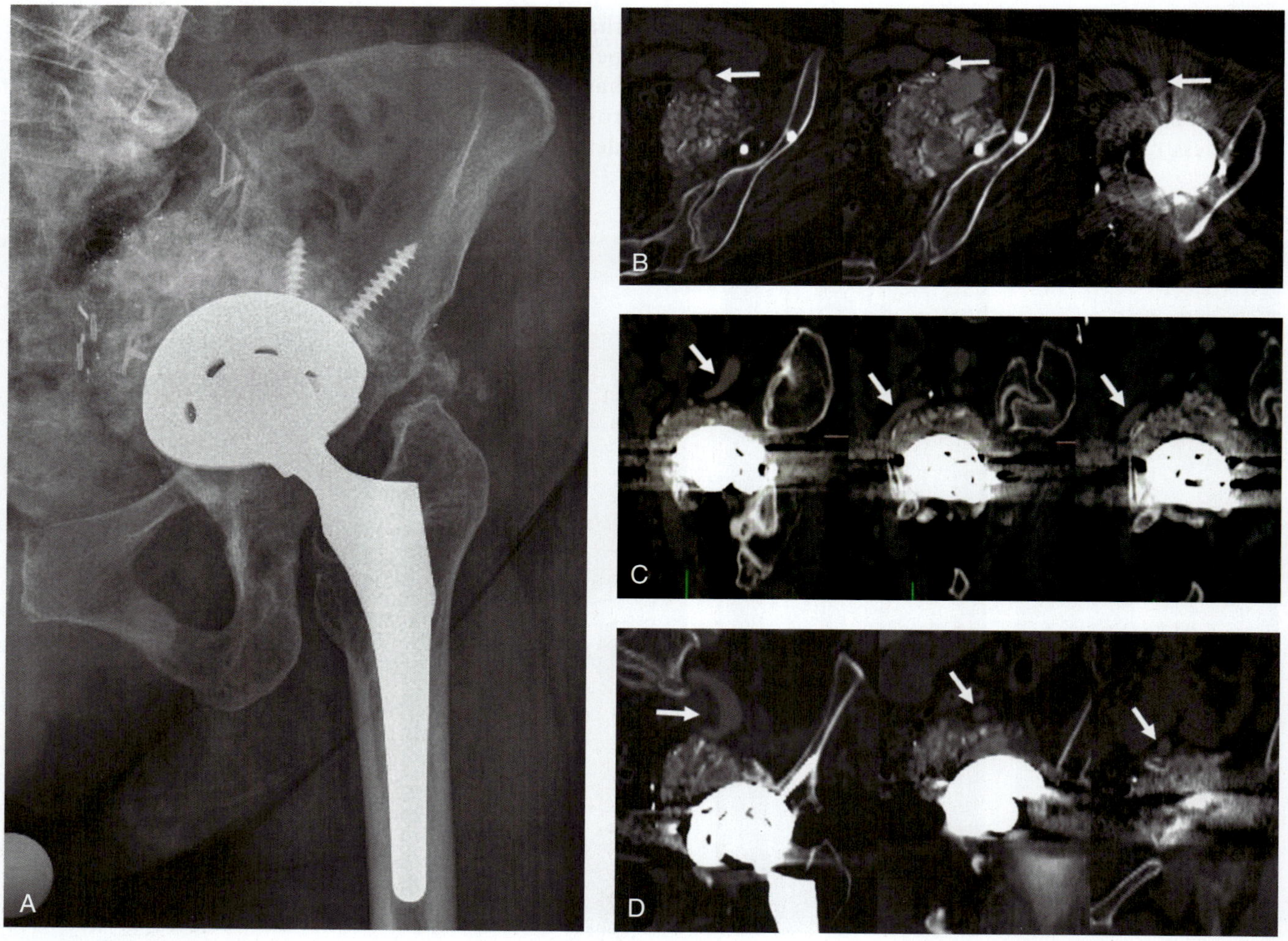

FIGURE 11 **A**, AP radiographs of a 79-year-old woman with a loose cup with medial migration into the pelvis (Paprosky 3B acetabular defect). CT angiography shows the proximity and displacement of the external iliac artery (white arrows) over the intrapelvic particulate acetabular bone grafting in the axial (**B**), sagittal (**C**), and coronal planes (**D**).

impingement and associated labral pathology. However, modern 3T-MRI provides high-quality images of the hip, including osseous and soft-tissue structures. The labrum can be well-visualized without using intra-articular contrast injection. Other advances in MRI include the biochemical imaging techniques such as T2 mapping, T1ρ imaging, and delayed gadolinium-enhanced MRI of cartilage. These techniques were developed to detect cartilage biochemical changes that precede structural damage or degeneration and are used in the evaluation of patients who have hip dysplasia or femoroacetabular impingement.[34]

Metal artifact reduction sequence MRI has the capacity to produce high-resolution images of the periprosthetic tissues in patients who have total hip implants.[35] Metal artifact reduction sequence MRI is recommended when there is suspicion of corrosion-related metal adverse soft-tissue reactions in patients who have metal-on-metal bearings, modular necks, or in patients who have larger metal cobalt-chromium heads[36,37] (**Figure 12**).

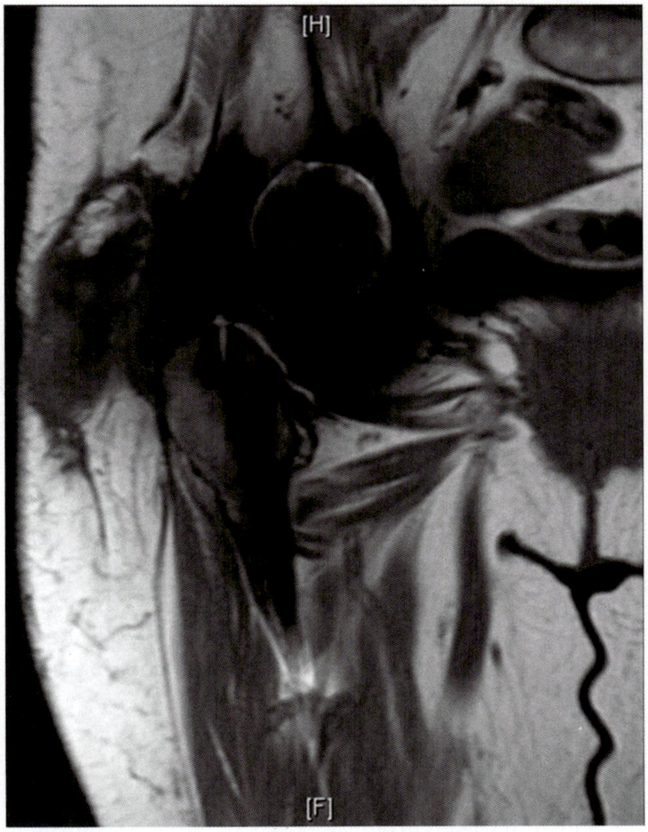

FIGURE 12 Coronal T1-weighted metal artifact reduction sequence magnetic resonance image demonstrates large heterogeneous pseudotumor with disruption of the abductors.

Nuclear Imaging

Nuclear medicine has limited use in total joint arthroplasty because of its low specificity and high cost. Patients who have stress reactions, aseptic loosening, or deep prosthetic joint infections can all have positive bone scans. Bone scintigraphy using labeled leukocytes scans or 18F-fluorodeoxyglucose-positron emission tomography has no role in the diagnosis of prosthetic joint infection.[38] The single photon emission CT–electronic CT technique is a hybrid technique introduced for the evaluation of the painful THA and TKA. This technique can be used in cases for which traditional tests such as radiography, serial radiography, or fluoroscopy views are inconclusive for determining THA and TKA implant loosening. Although this technique is not established in current clinical practice, one study showed promising results with sensitivity of 100%, specificity of 96.0%, positive predictive value of 92.9%, negative predictive value of 100%, and accuracy of 97.4% in the evaluation of aseptic loosening of hip and knee prostheses.[39]

Ultrasonography

Ultrasonography is commonly used to guide intra-articular injections or aspirations of the hip. In clinical practice, ultrasonography-guided intra-articular hip injections are used to differentiate hip pain secondary to hip pathology from other sources of hip pain.[40] Ultrasonography is also used in the evaluation and surveillance of patients who have metal-on-metal total hip arthroplasties, who have modular neck femoral stems, or in whom corrosion-related metal adverse soft-tissue reactions are suspected. This imaging technique is operator dependent, and the sensitivity in detecting pseudotumors varies from 69%[41] to 100%[42] when using MRI findings as reference.

SUMMARY

Plain radiographs are the most valuable diagnostic test in the evaluation of the adult hip and knee. A methodical approach to the evaluation of hip and knee radiographs is sufficient to determine a diagnosis. The most common causes of failure after joint arthroplasty are diagnosed with radiography. Digital templating and preoperative planning is commonly performed in total joint arthroplasty. Serial radiographs are very useful in the evaluation of adequate fixation versus loosening in primary and revision arthroplasty. Advanced imaging techniques, such as CT, MRI, nuclear imaging, and ultrasonography, have a complementary role to radiographs in the evaluation of multiple conditions related to hip and knee arthroplasty issues.

KEY STUDY POINTS

- Plain radiographs are the imaging study of choice in hip and knee primary and revision arthroplasty, not MRI or CT. Weight-bearing radiographs of the hip and knee provide a more reliable determination of osteoarthritis severity. Serial radiographs are useful in the evaluation of fixation and loosening of hip and knee implants.
- Digital templating is an important tool in planning primary and revision THA and TKA.
- Osteolysis is more accurately determined with CT than plain radiography
- Metal artifact reduction sequence MRI is the diagnostic test of choice in patients in whom there is concern for corrosion- related adverse soft-tissue reactions
- Nuclear medicine has limited use in total joint arthroplasty practice.

ANNOTATED REFERENCES

1. Tönnis D: Normal values of the hip joint for the evaluation of X-rays in children and adults. *Clin Orthop Relat Res* 1976;119:39-47.
2. Clohisy JC, Carlisle JC, Beaulé PE, et al: A systematic approach to the plain radiographic evaluation of the young adult hip. *J Bone Joint Surg Am* 2008;90(suppl 4):47-66.
3. Levine B, Fabi D, Deirmengian C: Digital templating in primary total hip and knee arthroplasty. *Orthopedics* 2010;33(11):797.
4. Abe Y, Sato S, Abe S, Masuda T, Yamada K: The impact of the leg-lengthening total hip arthroplasty on the coronal alignment of the spine. *Scoliosis* 2015;10(suppl 2):S4.
5. Maratt JD, Esposito CI, McLawhorn AS, Jerabek SA, Padgett DE, Mayman DJ: Pelvic tilt in patients undergoing total hip arthroplasty: When does it matter? *J Arthroplasty* 2015;30(3):387-391.
6. Crowe JF, Mani VJ, Ranawat CS: Total hip replacement in congenital dislocation and dysplasia of the hip. *J Bone Joint Surg Am* 1979;61(1):15-23.
7. Hartofilakidis G, Stamos K, Ioannidis TT: Low friction arthroplasty for old untreated congenital dislocation of the hip. *J Bone Joint Surg Br* 1988;70(2):182-186.
8. van Bosse H, Wedge JH, Babyn P: How are dysplastic hips different? A three-dimensional CT study. *Clin Orthop Relat Res* 2015;473(5):1712-1723.
9. Tamegai H, Otani T, Fujii H, Kawaguchi Y, Hayama T, Marumo K: A modified S-ROM stem in primary total hip arthroplasty for developmental dysplasia of the hip. *J Arthroplasty* 2013;28(10):1741-1745.
10. Krych AJ, Howard JL, Trousdale RT, Cabanela ME, Berry DJ: Total hip arthroplasty with shortening subtrochanteric osteotomy in Crowe type-IV developmental dysplasia: Surgical technique. *J Bone Joint Surg Am* 2010;92(suppl 1, pt 2):176-187.
11. Melvin JS, Karthikeyan T, Cope R, Fehring TK: Early failures in total hip arthroplasty – A changing paradigm. *J Arthroplasty* 2014;29(6):1285-1288.
12. DeLee JG, Charnley J: Radiological demarcation of cemented sockets in total hip replacement. *Clin Orthop Relat Res* 1976;121:20-32.
13. Hodgkinson JP, Shelley P, Wroblewski BM: The correlation between the roentgenographic appearance and operative findings at the bone-cement junction of the socket in Charnley low friction arthroplasties. *Clin Orthop Relat Res* 1988;228:105-109.
14. Udomkiat P, Wan Z, Dorr LD: Comparison of preoperative radiographs and intraoperative findings of fixation of hemispheric porous-coated sockets. *J Bone Joint Surg Am* 2001;83(12):1865-1870.
15. Gruen TA, McNeice GM, Amstutz HC: "Modes of failure" of cemented stem-type femoral components: A radiographic analysis of loosening. *Clin Orthop Relat Res* 1979;141:17-27.
16. Barrack RL, Mulroy RD Jr, Harris WH: Improved cementing techniques and femoral component loosening in young patients with hip arthroplasty. A 12-year radiographic review. *J Bone Joint Surg Br* 1992;74(3):385-389.
17. Harris WH, McCarthy JC Jr, O'Neill DA: Femoral component loosening using contemporary techniques of femoral cement fixation. *J Bone Joint Surg Am* 1982;64(7):1063-1067.
18. Engh CA, Bobyn JD, Glassman AH: Porous-coated hip replacement. The factors governing bone ingrowth, stress shielding, and clinical results. *J Bone Joint Surg Br* 1987;69(1):45-55.
19. Berry DJ, Lewallen DG, Hanssen AD, Cabanela ME: Pelvic discontinuity in revision total hip arthroplasty. *J Bone Joint Surg Am* 1999;81(12):1692-1702.
20. Paprosky WG, Perona PG, Lawrence JM: Acetabular defect classification and surgical reconstruction in revision arthroplasty. A 6-year follow-up evaluation. *J Arthroplasty* 1994;9(1):33-44.
21. Della Valle CJ, Paprosky WG: The femur in revision total hip arthroplasty evaluation and classification. *Clin Orthop Relat Res* 2004;420:55-62.
22. Radtke K, Becher C, Noll Y, Ostermeier S: Effect of limb rotation on radiographic alignment in total knee arthroplasties. *Arch Orthop Trauma Surg* 2010;130(4):451-457.
23. Rosenberg TD, Paulos LE, Parker RD, Coward DB, Scott SM: The forty-five-degree posteroanterior flexion weight-bearing radiograph of the knee. *J Bone Joint Surg Am* 1988;70(10):1479-1483.
24. Kellgren JH, Lawrence JS: Radiological assessment of osteo-arthrosis. *Ann Rheum Dis* 1957;16(4):494-502.
25. Sharkey PF, Lichstein PM, Shen C, Tokarski AT, Parvizi J: Why are total knee arthroplasties failing today – Has anything changed after 10 years? *J Arthroplasty* 2014;29(9):1774-1778.

26. Illés T, Somoskeöy S: The EOS™ imaging system and its uses in daily orthopaedic practice. *Int Orthop* 2012;36(7):1325-1331.
27. Lazennec JY, Rousseau MA, Brusson A, et al: Total hip prostheses in standing, sitting and squatting positions: An overview of our 8 years practice using the EOS imaging technology. *Open Orthop J* 2015;9:26-44.
28. Lazennec JY, Rousseau MA, Rangel A, et al: Pelvis and total hip arthroplasty acetabular component orientations in sitting and standing positions: Measurements reproductibility with EOS imaging system versus conventional radiographies. *Orthop Traumatol Surg Res* 2011;97(4):373-380.
29. Roth TD, Maertz NA, Parr JA, Buckwalter KA, Choplin RH: CT of the hip prosthesis: Appearance of components, fixation, and complications. *Radiographics* 2012;32(4):1089-1107.
30. Robinson E, Henckel J, Sabah S, Satchithananda K, Skinner J, Hart A: Cross-sectional imaging of metal-on-metal hip arthroplasties. Can we substitute MARS MRI with CT? *Acta Orthop* 2014;85(6):577-584.
31. Konigsberg B, Hess R, Hartman C, Smith L, Garvin KL: Inter- and intraobserver reliability of two-dimensional CT scan for total knee arthroplasty component malrotation. *Clin Orthop Relat Res* 2014;472(1):212-217.
32. Hirschmann MT, Konala P, Amsler F, Iranpour F, Friederich NF, Cobb JP: The position and orientation of total knee replacement components: A comparison of conventional radiographs, transverse 2D-CT slices and 3D-CT reconstruction. *J Bone Joint Surg Br* 2011;93(5):629-633.
33. Kawasaki Y, Egawa H, Hamada D, Takao S, Nakano S, Yasui N: Location of intrapelvic vessels around the acetabulum assessed by three-dimensional computed tomographic angiography: Prevention of vascular-related complications in total hip arthroplasty. *J Orthop Sci* 2012;17(4):397-406.
34. Jazrawi LM, Alaia MJ, Chang G, Fitzgerald EF, Recht MP: Advances in magnetic resonance imaging of articular cartilage. *J Am Acad Orthop Surg* 2011;19(7):420-429.
35. Choi SJ, Koch KM, Hargreaves BA, Stevens KJ, Gold GE: Metal artifact reduction with MAVRIC SL at 3-T MRI in patients with hip arthroplasty. *AJR Am J Roentgenol* 2015;204(1):140-147.
36. Kwon YM, Fehring TK, Lombardi AV, Barnes CL, Cabanela ME, Jacobs JJ: Risk stratification algorithm for management of patients with dual modular taper total hip arthroplasty: Consensus statement of the American Association of Hip and Knee Surgeons, the American Academy of Orthopaedic Surgeons and the Hip Society. *J Arthroplasty* 2014;29(11):2060-2064.
37. Kwon YM, Lombardi AV, Jacobs JJ, Fehring TK, Lewis CG, Cabanela ME: Risk stratification algorithm for management of patients with metal-on-metal hip arthroplasty: Consensus statement of the American Association of Hip and Knee Surgeons, the American Academy of Orthopaedic Surgeons, and the Hip Society. *J Bone Joint Surg Am* 2014;96(1):e4.
38. Workgroup Convened by the Musculoskeletal Infection Society: New definition for periprosthetic joint infection. *J Arthroplasty* 2011;26(8):1136-1138.
39. Abele JT, Swami VG, Russell G, Masson EC, Flemming JP: The accuracy of single photon emission computed tomography/computed tomography arthrography in evaluating aseptic loosening of hip and knee prostheses. *J Arthroplasty* 2015;30(9):1647-1651.
40. Khan W, Khan M, Alradwan H, Williams R, Simunovic N, Ayeni OR: Utility of intra-articular hip injections for femoroacetabular impingement: A systematic review. *Orthop J Sports Med* 2015;3(9):2325967115601030.
41. Siddiqui IA, Sabah SA, Satchithananda K, et al: A comparison of the diagnostic accuracy of MARS MRI and ultrasound of the painful metal-on-metal hip arthroplasty. *Acta Orthop* 2014;85(4):375-382.
42. Garbuz DS, Hargreaves BA, Duncan CP, Masri BA, Wilson DR, Forster BB: The John Charnley Award: Diagnostic accuracy of MRI versus ultrasound for detecting pseudotumors in asymptomatic metal-on-metal THA. *Clin Orthop Relat Res* 2014;472(2):417-423.

CHAPTER 2

Perioperative Assessment and Management

JAY R. LIEBERMAN, MD • HANSEL E. IHN, MD

ABSTRACT

Hip and knee arthroplasty are highly successful procedures that are associated with excellent functional outcomes for most patients. Recently, increased attention has been given to preoperative medical optimization aimed at limiting complications in patients who have specific comorbidities. Venous thromboembolic prophylaxis remains of great interest because of concerns associated with the development of symptomatic pulmonary embolism and death, as well as the potential for excess anticoagulation, which may lead to bleeding. Advancements in neuraxial anesthesia and postoperative multimodal pain regimens have helped minimize postoperative complications, decrease inpatient length of stay, and improve patient satisfaction.

Dr. Lieberman or an immediate family member has received royalties from DePuy, a Johnson & Johnson Company; serves as a paid consultant to or is an employee of DePuy, a Johnson & Johnson Company; has stock or stock options held in Hip Innovation Technology; has received nonincome support (such as equipment or services), commercially derived honoraria, or other non–research-related funding (such as paid travel) from Recro, Inc.; and serves as a board member, owner, officer, or committee member of the American Academy of Orthopaedic Surgeons, the Hip Society, the Musculoskeletal Transplant Foundation, and the Western Orthopaedic Association. Neither Dr. Ihn nor any immediate family member has received anything of value from or has stock or stock options held in a commercial company or institution related directly or indirectly to the subject of this chapter.

Keywords: anesthesia; multimodal pain management; perioperative management; venous thromboembolism prophylaxis

INTRODUCTION

Hip and knee arthroplasty represent two of the largest cost centers in health care. With the shift of the Centers for Medicare & Medicaid Services toward bundled payment programs for total hip arthroplasty (THA) and total knee arthroplasty (TKA), healthcare centers are attempting to minimize perioperative complications, decrease readmission rates, maximize patient outcomes, and reduce costs. The optimization of perioperative medical management, venous thromboembolism (VTE) prophylaxis, anesthesia, and postoperative pain in patients undergoing THA and TKA can have a critical effect on outcomes.

MEDICAL MANAGEMENT AND OPTIMIZATION

Patients undergoing hip and knee arthroplasty are older and often have an increased burden of medical comorbidities[1,2] (**Table 1**). Between 1991 and 2010, the number of comorbidities in this patient population doubled with the prevalence of diabetes increasing from 10% to 24%, and obesity increased from 4% to 10%.[1] Because the increase in comorbidities in this patient population is expected to continue, there is a greater focus on preoperative medical optimization. Risk stratification and preoperative intervention of modifiable risk factors can enhance outcomes and reduce costs.[3]

The identification of preoperative modifiable risk factors for complications depends on a careful review of each patient's medical history, a thorough preoperative

This chapter is adapted from Lieberman JR, Alluri RK: Perioperative assessment and management, in Mont MA, Tanzer M, eds: *Orthopaedic Knowledge Update®: Hip and Knee Reconstruction*, ed 5. Rosemont, IL, American Academy of Orthopaedic Surgeons, 2017, pp 15-26.

TABLE 1

Comorbidity Prevalence in Total Hip and Total Knee Arthroplasty Patients

Comorbidity	Prevalence (%)
Hypertension	60-70
Diabetes mellitus	11-20
Obesity	14-18
Dyslipidemia	35-55
Chronic kidney disease	0.2-4.0
Tobacco use	9-22
Congestive heart failure	0.2-4.0

Data from Yu S, Garvin KL, Healy WL, Pellegrini VD Jr, Iorio R: Preventing hospital readmissions and limiting the complications associated with total joint arthroplasty. *J Am Acad Orthop Surg* 2015;23(11):e60-e71; Gonzalez Della Valle A, Chiu YL, Ma Y, Mazumdar M, Memtsoudis SG: The metabolic syndrome in patients undergoing knee and hip arthroplasty: Trends and in-hospital outcomes in the United States. *J Arthroplasty* 2012;27(10):1743-1749; and Cram P, Lu X, Kates SL, Singh JA, Li Y, Wolf BR: Total knee arthroplasty volume, utilization, and outcomes among Medicare beneficiaries, 1991-2010. *J Am Med Assoc* 2012;308(12):1227-1236.

physical examination, performing basic laboratory studies, and cardiac risk stratification. Several risk prediction models have been developed on the basis of a variety of outcomes, including 30-day complications, readmissions, mortalities, functional outcomes, and discharge dispositions. These models have resulted in the identification of several important risk factors for postoperative complications.

Glycemic Control

Studies have consistently identified diabetes as a risk factor for postoperative complications, and it is included in most risk-stratification algorithms. The preoperative screening of patients who have hyperglycemia by checking hemoglobin A_{1c} (HbA_{1c}) has been an area of increased interest. HbA_{1c} levels greater than 7.5 have been associated with an increased risk of postoperative wound complications and periprosthetic joint infections.[4] However, the target HbA_{1c} level for ideal preoperative optimization remains unclear, and not all patients may be able to achieve a target level.[5] Strict adherence to a certain target level may needlessly delay surgery. Additionally, HbA_{1c} may not be the best surrogate for quantifying the severity of a patient's diabetes, as it is a measure of chronic glycemic control. Other measures of glycemic control have been proposed as superior methods of predicting postoperative complications. When compared with HbA_{1c}, variation in postoperative glucose values was found to be a better predictor of postoperative complications.[6] Fructosamine, a glycated protein, may also be a superior means of monitoring perioperative glucose control.[7]

Obesity

Obesity has been consistently identified as a risk factor for postoperative complications after THA and TKA. Specifically, obesity increases the risk of acute kidney failure, cardiovascular complications, TKA revision, periprosthetic fracture, postoperative infection, and mortality.[8,9] There is no absolute body mass index (BMI) at which a patient's risk of the development of postoperative complications significantly increases; however, many studies stratify patients as having a BMI greater or less than 40 kg/m^2. There is also a question of whether percent body fat is a better predictor of complications than BMI.[10] Additionally, the exact amount or percentage of weight loss needed preoperatively to improve postoperative outcomes remains unclear, and a weight loss greater than 5% may be needed to decrease the risk of postoperative complications.[11] If nonsurgical measures fail, bariatric surgery may be an option though it has had mixed results in the literature when compared with nonsurgical management.[12-14] Current evidence supports delaying arthroplasty for a minimum of 6 months after bariatric surgery.[15]

Nutritional Deficiency

Nutritional deficiency is another commonly cited risk factor for postoperative complications after total joint arthroplasty. A number of studies have shown that hypoalbuminemia, defined as serum values lower than 3.5 g/dL, is associated with increased mortality, periprosthetic joint infection, delayed wound healing, and other complications.[16,17] There is also evidence to support a greater role for nutritional deficiency over obesity in modifying postoperative outcomes in total joint arthroplasty patients.[18] However, the ideal marker for malnutrition is not clear. While albumin is widely used, the ideal cutoff value is also under debate.[19] Addressing perioperative vitamin D levels may be another factor that can be modified, as low levels have been associated with periprosthetic joint infection and increased 90-day complications.[20]

Smoking

Tobacco use is thought to be one of the most important risk factors contributing to postoperative complications, particularly wound complications, which are doubled in active smokers compared with nonsmokers.[21] Preoperative cessation of tobacco use has been associated with a lower likelihood of periprosthetic joint infections.[22] Smoking cessation program started 4 weeks before surgery can decrease postoperative complications.[23] Nicotine screening tests assessing the blood level of cotinine may be a valuable adjunct to smoking cessation. One study demonstrated that checking preoperative serum cotinine levels may encourage patients to quit smoking and allow for the identification of noncompliance with cessation.[24]

Cardiovascular Disease

Cardiovascular complications represent one of the most common systemic adverse events after arthroplasty, and these complications can result in death. Major risk factors for postoperative cardiovascular complications include preoperative cardiovascular disease and older age.[25] Patients who have cardiac stents present a challenging situation for the arthroplasty surgeon, and different stent types mandate different forms of management. The current recommendation is for elective noncardiac surgery to be delayed in patients in whom dual antiplatelet therapy will need to be discontinued within 30 days after bare-metal stent implantation or 6 months after drug-eluting stent implantation.[26]

No evidence-based guidelines exist for antiplatelet therapy cessation and total joint arthroplasty. However, if the surgeon and cardiologist elect to discontinue clopidogrel, it is reasonable to continue aspirin and resume clopidogrel use when the bleeding risk has decreased. Stopping clopidogrel 7 days before surgery may decrease postoperative bleeding-related events and decrease the need for perioperative transfusion from 31.8% to 7.7% without increasing perioperative adverse cardiac events.[27] In general, patients can continue taking aspirin if they are on a dual antiplatelet regimen.

Blood Transfusion

Approximately 25% of all patients undergoing primary arthroplasty procedures may require a perioperative blood transfusion.[28] Perioperative blood transfusions have been previously associated with significant postoperative complications, including sepsis, VTE, readmissions, and mortality.[29] Multiple randomized controlled trials have demonstrated the capability of tranexamic acid (TXA) to decrease intraoperative and postoperative blood loss, thereby minimizing postoperative transfusion rates and decreasing postoperative complications.[30,31] The ideal delivery route is controversial.[30,31] There are data to support administration orally, intravenously, and intra-articularly.[32]

Renal Disease

Patients undergoing THA and TKA are at 10 to 20 times greater risk of experiencing complications when already receiving dialysis.[33] Total hip and knee arthroplasty patients receiving hemodialysis are at increased risk of periprosthetic joint infection compared with those receiving peritoneal dialysis.[34] Evidence also suggests patients with end-stage renal disease receiving dialysis may have improved postoperative outcomes if they elect to undergo renal transplantation before undergoing total joint arthroplasty.[35] In patients undergoing THA or TKA, the comparative risk of transient septicemia during dialysis versus the risk of immunosuppression after kidney transplantation needs to be fully considered.

Methicillin-Resistant *Staphylococcus aureus*

Methicillin-resistant *Staphylococcus aureus* (MRSA) colonization, particularly in the nares, is thought to be a risk factor for postoperative surgical site infections. Some surgeons elect to screen patients for MRSA colonization, and in the setting of a positive test result, decolonization is attempted with various regimens. Both mupirocin ointment and chlorhexidine have demonstrated efficacy in decreasing surgical site infections in some studies,[36] but the overall efficacy of these regimens has not been definitively demonstrated.[37] These patients should receive vancomycin as part of their antibiotic prophylaxis regimen. Postoperatively, the use of extended oral antibiotic prophylaxis in high-risk individuals who tested positive for MRSA may reduce infections.[38]

VTE PROPHYLAXIS

VTE is one the most common perioperative complications after TKA and THA, and orthopaedic surgeons are highly interested in VTE prophylaxis because it can prevent significant postoperative complications, including death.

The American College of Chest Physicians (ACCP) first established VTE prophylaxis guidelines in 1986 and the latest edition to specifically address patients undergoing orthopaedic procedures was published in 2012. Initially, the orthopaedic community had significant concerns regarding these guidelines because of an increased emphasis on efficacy of a prophylaxis regimen and a limited focus on bleeding. However, the most recent guideline for orthopaedic surgery patients recommended a variety of new regimens, including aspirin and portable mechanical compression[39-41] (**Table 2**).

The American Academy of Orthopaedic Surgeons (AAOS) guidelines (2011) do not recommend a specific regimen or duration for VTE prophylaxis after THA and TKA[41] (see **Table 2**). The ACCP recommends one of the following agents: vitamin K antagonists (such as warfarin), low-molecular-weight heparins (LMWHs; such as enoxaparin), aspirin, factor Xa inhibitors (such as apixaban and rivaroxaban), pentasaccharides (such as fondaparinux), direct thrombin inhibitors (such as dabigatran), and mobile portable compression devices (**Table 3**). ACCP guidelines recommend 10 to 14 days of VTE prophylaxis after THA and TKA, with a potential duration for up to 35 days.[39]

Recently, interest has increased regarding the use of aspirin and mobile mechanical compression devices for

VTE prophylaxis as surgeons continue to assess the ideal balance between efficacy and safety. The ideal anticoagulation regimen for each patient needs to be based on risk stratification, attempting to minimize complications caused by inadequate or excessive anticoagulation.

The advantages of aspirin include a high rate of patient compliance, lower bleeding rates, and cost-effectiveness. A potential disadvantage of aspirin is its association with gastrointestinal toxicity.[42] Interest in aspirin as a prophylactic agent was originally driven by the Pulmonary Embolism Prevention trial. This international study demonstrated a significant difference between aspirin and placebo, without an increase in bleeding complications, with respect to the rate of VTE in patients who have a hip fracture treated with arthroplasty.[43] It should be noted that this same study also demonstrated no differences in the symptomatic VTE rates between the aspirin and placebo groups in THA patients.

Aspirin is probably not as powerful an anticoagulant as other available chemoprophylaxis agents, but it appears to be effective and safe in low-risk arthroplasty patients.[44] Similar VTE rates have been noted between use of aspirin and LMWH.[45] Aspirin has been associated with low pulmonary embolism and bleeding rates in a number of studies; however, these were retrospective with the potential for selection bias.[46] In addition, one study comparing aspirin to warfarin found increased rates of VTE complications in the aspirin group after arthroplasty.[47] Another retrospective registry study demonstrated a higher mortality rate in patients receiving aspirin prophylaxis over those receiving LMWH.[48]

Interest has also increased in mobile pneumatic compression devices for VTE prophylaxis following THA and TKA because of shorter hospital lengths of stay. The findings from a 2010 study comparing pharmacologic protocol with the use of a mobile compression device

TABLE 2

Prevention of Venous Thromboembolic Disease After THA and TKA: Select Guidelines

American College of Chest Physicians Recommendations	Grade of Recommendation
In patients undergoing THA or TKA, one of the following agents should be used for a minimum of 10-14 d rather than no venothrombotic prophylaxis:	
LMWH	1B
Fondaparinux	1B
Apixaban	1B
Dabigatran	1B
Rivaroxaban	1B
Low-dose unfractionated heparin	1B
Adjusted-dose vitamin K antagonist	1B
Aspirin	1B
IPCD	1C
In patients undergoing THA or TKA, regardless of the use of an IPCD or length of treatment, LMWH should be used in preference to other alternative agents:	
Fondaparinux	2B
Apixaban	2B
Dabigatran	2B
Rivaroxaban	2B
Low-dose unfractionated heparin	2B
Adjusted-dose vitamin K antagonist	2C
Aspirin	2C
For patients undergoing THA or TKA, thromboprophylaxis should be extended in the outpatient period for up to 35 d following surgery rather than for only 10-14 d.	2B
In patients undergoing THA or TKA, dual prophylaxis with an antithrombotic agent and an IPCD during the hospital stay is recommended.	2C

TABLE 2

Prevention of Venous Thromboembolic Disease After THA and TKA: Select Guidelines (continued)

American Academy of Orthopaedic Surgeons Recommendations	Strength of Recommendation
The workgroup suggests the use of pharmacologic agents, mechanical compressive devices, or both for the prevention of venous thromboembolism in patients undergoing elective THA or TKA who are not at elevated risk beyond that of the surgery itself of experiencing venous thromboembolism or bleeding.	Moderate
The workgroup cannot recommend for or against a specific prophylactic regimen in these patients, as current evidence is unclear about which strategy or strategies is or are optimal or suboptimal.	Consensus
In the absence of reliable evidence regarding the duration of prophylactic strategies, it is the opinion of the panel that patients and physicians should discuss the duration of prophylaxis.	Consensus
In the absence of reliable evidence, it is the opinion of the panel that patients should undergo early mobilization following elective THA or TKA.	Consensus
The use of neuraxial anesthesia for patients undergoing THA or TKA is recommended to help limit blood loss, even though evidence suggests that neuraxial anesthesia does not affect the occurrence of venous thromboembolic disease.	Moderate

IPCD = intermittent pneumatic compression device, LMWH = low-molecular-weight heparin, THA = total hip arthroplasty, TKA = total knee arthroplasty

Data from Falck-Ytter Y, Francis CW, Johanson NA, et al: Prevention of VTE in orthopaedic surgery patients. Antithrombotic therapy and prevention of thrombosis, 9th ed: American College of Chest Physicians evidence-based clinical practice guidelines. *Chest* 2012;141(suppl 2):e278S-e325S; Lieberman JR, Pensak MJ: Prevention of venous thromboembolic disease after total hip and knee arthroplasty. *J Bone Joint Surg Am* 2013;95(19):1801-1811; American Academy of Orthopaedic Surgeons: Clinical Practice Guidelines on *Preventing Venous Thromboembolic Disease in Patients Undergoing Elective Hip and Knee Arthroplasty*. Rosemont, IL, American Academy of Orthopaedic Surgeons, 2011. Available at: http://www.aaos.org/research/guidelines/VTE/VTE_guideline.asp; and Lieberman JR: The new AAOS clinical practice guidelines on venous thromboembolic prophylaxis: How to adapt them to your practice. *J Am Acad Orthop Surg* 2011;19(12):717-721.

suggested similar efficacy between the two modalities.[49] However, in this study, 60% of patients using mobile compression also took aspirin.[49] Similar findings in other studies led to the ACCP recommending (grade IC) mobile pneumatic compression devices as a stand-alone measure for VTE prophylaxis after THA and TKA but only if worn for at least 18 hr/d.[39] Appropriately powered randomized trials are needed to define the true efficacy of mobile compression, and concerns related to the cost of these devices also exist.

TABLE 3

Common Venous Thromboembolism Prophylaxis Dosing Regimens

Pharmacologic Agent	Common Dosing or Therapeutic Level
Warfarin	International normalized ratio, 2.0
Enoxaparin	30 mg subcutaneously two times per day or 40 mg subcutaneously per day
Apixaban	2.5 mg orally two times per day
Rivaroxaban	10 mg orally per day
Fondaparinux	2.5 mg subcutaneously per day
Dabigatran	150 mg orally two times per day
Aspirin	325 mg orally one or two times per day

ANESTHESIA OPTIONS

THA and TKA are commonly performed under neuraxial anesthesia. Neuraxial, or regional, anesthesia has been hypothesized to lower postoperative complications because of decreased sympathetic activation and inflammation, thus decreasing the overall surgical stress response when compared with general anesthesia. However, robust evidence demonstrating the purported benefits of neuraxial anesthesia is lacking, and the optimal anesthetic technique for THA and TKA has not yet been determined.

The potential clinical benefits of neuraxial anesthesia versus general anesthesia have been demonstrated in several studies. The findings of a retrospective registry study demonstrated decreased mortality in THA patients receiving spinal versus general anesthesia; however, a similar study did not demonstrate decreased mortality in TKA patients.[50] Several retrospective database studies have shown neuraxial anesthesia to be associated with decreased surgical time, surgical site infections, postoperative cardiovascular and pulmonary complications, transfusion rates, and overall length of inpatient stay after THA and TKA.[51,52] Prospective studies comparing general versus neuraxial anesthesia in patients undergoing THA and TKA are sparse, but their findings have demonstrated more favorable recovery profiles associated with general anesthesia than with regional anesthesia.[53,54] However, these prospective studies assessed primarily postoperative pain, nausea, and length of stay.[53,54] A recent systematic review and meta-analysis by the International Consensus on Anaesthesia-Related Outcomes after Surgery group provided strong recommendation for use of neuraxial anesthesia in THA.[55] Their recommendation with regard to TKA also favored neuraxial anesthesia, but the evidence to support this was deemed weaker than that in THA.[55]

PAIN MANAGEMENT

The primary goal of postoperative pain management is to reduce pain, thereby improving early postoperative mobilization, patient-perceived outcomes, and length of inpatient hospital stay. These regimens use both pharmacologic and nonpharmacologic interventions that target several different regions of the pain pathway, thus decreasing the total required dose of pain medication. Many of these regimens involve the use of medications with different durations of action and are administered on a scheduled basis.

Oral Medications

Because multimodal pain management regimens have evolved, increased focus has been placed on decreasing postoperative opioid consumption. Many prospective randomized studies assessing the efficacy of multimodal regimens have used opioid consumption as a primary outcome. A major reason for the continued focus on decreasing postarthroplasty opioid intake is that opioid-related adverse effects (sedation, nausea, vomiting, constipation, urinary retention) can have a negative impact on the rehabilitation process, prolong inpatient stays, and increase healthcare resource consumption. The findings of one study demonstrated that more than 50% of postarthroplasty complications were caused by opioid-related adverse drug events.[56] Many of these multimodal pain regimens have decreased opioid consumption during inpatient hospitalization. Orthopaedic surgeons need to limit the use of opioid pain medications to control post-discharge pain.

Oral pain medications may be given before surgery. The use of NSAIDs for preemptive analgesia, particularly selective cyclooxygenase-2 inhibitors, has demonstrated improved postoperative pain scores, decreased opioid consumption, and greater active range of motion without increasing perioperative bleeding.[57] A 2015 randomized controlled trial demonstrated improved short-term pain management with pregabalin use up to 7 days postoperatively; however, pain scores and functional outcome were equivalent at follow-up visits.[58] Acetaminophen facilitates better pain control and a reduced need for rescue analgesia especially in the postoperative period.[59]

Periarticular Injections

Periarticular injections (PAIs) consist of a combination of several medications, including local anesthetics, opioids, NSAIDs, and corticosteroids. These mixtures are injected into the capsule and periarticular tissue during THA and TKA. Comparative studies are difficult to analyze, given the variability of when and where these injections are placed and the different drugs used in these injection cocktails.

There is level I evidence demonstrating that PAIs had equivalent analgesic outcomes as nerve blocks in TKA patients.[60] Furthermore, a recent systematic review demonstrated that PAIs may be superior to adductor canal blocks in terms of postoperative pain scores and postoperative opiate consumption.[61] Either a peripheral nerve block or a PAI can be used for postoperative pain control in these patients, but PAIs may be safer, cheaper, and easier to perform.

The literature assessing the efficacy of PAIs in THA is not as robust as that in the TKA population. In THA, PAIs demonstrated improved postoperative pain control, decreased opioid consumption, and better early functional outcomes when compared with placebo in one study, although another study failed to demonstrate a similar result.[62,63] Effectiveness of PAIs in THA has also been demonstrated as patients were reportedly able to achieve as effective postoperative analgesia as those who received a psoas compartment block.[64] The drugs used in the injection cocktail may influence these results.

Peripheral Nerve Blocks

Both single and continuous peripheral nerve blockades have demonstrated improvement in postoperative pain, length of stay, and patient satisfaction after THA and TKA. A potential disadvantage of these peripheral nerve blocks is the resultant muscular weakness, which potentially increases the risk of postoperative falls. The integration of ultrasonography to facilitate localization of the desired nerve or plexus has enhanced the safety of these blockades.

Common peripheral nerve blocks executed after THA include lumbar plexus blocks, psoas compartment blocks, femoral nerve blocks, and sciatic nerve blocks.

Intraoperative administration of a psoas compartment block by the operating surgeon was found to be as effective at pain control as a preoperatively administered fascia iliaca block by an anesthesiologist.[65] Patients undergoing TKA may receive a femoral nerve, adductor canal, or sciatic nerve block, or a combination thereof. Increased interest in the adductor canal block has developed because of the theory that isolated blockade of sensory nerves with an adductor canal block minimizes the muscular weakness that is associated with femoral nerve blocks. Findings of subsequent studies have demonstrated adductor canal blocks result in better postoperative quadriceps strength and similar levels of pain control as seen with femoral nerve blocks.[66] Single injection adductor canal blocks have also been shown to be noninferior to continuous adductor canal blocks.[67] Some surgeons combine a PAI with an adductor canal block, but the efficacy of this regimen needs to be determined in randomized trials. One retrospective study found no difference in pain control outcomes in patients who received both adductor canal block alone and an adductor canal block with PAIs.[68] The use of a sciatic nerve block after TKA, although controversial, is thought to help decrease posterior knee pain.[69]

SUMMARY

THA and TKA continue to remain some of the most successful surgical procedures, resulting in high patient satisfaction. The burden of comorbidities in patients electing to undergo these procedures is likely to continue rising, and therefore, preoperative optimization is of paramount importance. Recent studies have identified patients at risk for postoperative complications, but further research is needed to determine optimal strategies to modify these factors and improve outcomes. VTE continues to be one of the most common complications after THA and TKA, and recent guidelines do not specify a single agent or regimen for postoperative prophylaxis. Risk stratification is the key in selecting an appropriate VTE prophylaxis regimen, but a definitive risk stratification protocol has not been identified. Furthermore, appropriately powered randomized trials with well-defined parameters for VTE complications are needed to assess the safety of various agents. The choice of general versus neuraxial anesthesia remains important. Neuraxial anesthesia may offer clinically relevant advantages, but adequately powered randomized trials assessing these clinical outcomes are still needed. Multimodal pain regimens after THA and TKA have resulted in decreased postoperative opioid consumption, fewer postoperative complications, shorter inpatient lengths of stay, and higher patient satisfaction.

KEY STUDY POINTS

- As the burden of medical comorbidities in patients undergoing THA and TKA continues to increase, preoperative optimization of modifiable risk factors (ie, diabetes, obesity, smoking, cardiovascular disease, and VTE) is critical for achieving excellent postoperative outcomes.
- Neuraxial versus general anesthesia potentially limits postoperative complications after THA and TKA, but the ideal anesthetic technique needs to be determined.
- VTE prophylaxis after THA and TKA is of paramount importance. The ideal prophylaxis regimen and duration remain undetermined and are dependent on risk stratification of each patient. A validated risk stratification system needs to be developed.
- Multimodal postoperative pain regimens are important in achieving high levels of patient satisfaction and early mobilization and in minimizing opioid-related adverse effects. Preemptive analgesia combined with PAIs are becoming increasingly popular and may be used in addition to or in lieu of peripheral nerve blocks.

ANNOTATED REFERENCES

1. Cram P, Lu X, Kates SL, Singh JA, Li Y, Wolf BR: Total knee arthroplasty volume, utilization, and outcomes among Medicare beneficiaries, 1991-2010. *J Am Med Assoc* 2012;308:1227-1236.

2. Yu S, Garvin KL, Healy WL, Pellegrini VD, Iorio R: Preventing hospital readmissions and limiting the complications associated with total joint arthroplasty. *Instr Course Lect* 2016;65:199-210.

3. Boraiah S, Inneh IA, Rathod P, et al: Management of modifiable risk factors prior to primary hip and knee arthroplasty: A readmission risk assessment tool. *J Bone Joint Surg Am* 2015;97:1921-1928.

4. Cancienne JM, Werner BC, Browne JA: Is there a threshold value of hemoglobin A_{1c} that predicts risk of infection following primary total hip arthroplasty? *J Arthroplasty* 2017;32:S236-S240.

   In this database study, the authors sought to determine a threshold HbA_{1c} above which the risk of periprosthetic joint infection after a THA increased. The PearlDiver database was queried and it was found that patients with an HbA_{1c} greater than 7.5 had a higher risk of periprosthetic joint infection (OR, 2.6; 95% CI, 1.9 to 3.4; $P < 0.0001$). Level of evidence: III.

5. Giori NJ, Ellerbe LS, Bowe T, Gupta S, Harris AHS: Many diabetic total joint arthroplasty candidates are unable to achieve a preoperative hemoglobin A_{1c} goal of 7% or less. *J Bone Joint Surg Am* 2014;96:500-504.

6. Shohat N, Restrepo C, Allierezaie A, Tarabichi M, Goel R, Parvizi J: Increased postoperative glucose variability is associated with adverse outcomes following total joint arthroplasty. *J Bone Joint Surg Am* 2018;100:1110-1117.

The authors of this study sought to find an association between postoperative glucose variability and postoperative complications. In both patients with and without diabetes, they found that postoperative glucose variability was associated with an increased risk of prolonged hospital stay, periprosthetic joint infection, mortality, and surgical site infection. Level of evidence: IV.

7. Shohat N, Tarabichi M, Tan TL, et al: 2019 John Insall Award: Fructosamine is a better glycaemic marker compared with glycated haemoglobin (HbA_{1c}) in predicting adverse outcomes following total knee arthroplasty. A prospective multicentre study. *Bone Joint J* 2019;101-B:3-9.

The authors challenged HbA_{1c} as a standard for predicting postoperative complications related to poor glucose control. They compared fructosamine level with HbA_{1c} levels and found that fructosamine level >293 was a superior predictor of postoperative complications (periprosthetic joint infection, OR, 16.26; readmission, OR, 4.62; revision surgery, OR, 4.37). HbA_{1c} at three thresholds (5.9, 7.0, 7.5) demonstrated no significant association with a postoperative complication. Level of evidence: II.

8. Ward DT, Metz LN, Horst PK, Kim HT, Kuo AC: Complications of morbid obesity in total joint arthroplasty: Risk stratification based on BMI. *J Arthroplasty* 2015;30:42-46.

9. Jeschke E, Citak M, Günster C, et al: Obesity increases the risk of postoperative complications and revision rates following primary total hip arthroplasty: An analysis of 131,576 total hip arthroplasty cases. *J Arthroplasty* 2018;33:2287-2292.e1.

Authors of this study looked at the German insurance database to evaluate the association between increasing BMI and postoperative complications, mortality, and revision rate in the THA population. They found that the higher the BMI category, the higher the likelihood of overall complications, revision within 1 year, and 90-day complications. Level of evidence: III.

10. Ledford CK, Millikan PD, Nickel BT, et al: Percent body fat is more predictive of function after total joint arthroplasty than body mass index. *J Bone Joint Surg Am* 2016;98:849-857.

11. Inacio MCS, Kritz-Silverstein D, Raman R, et al: The impact of pre-operative weight loss on incidence of surgical site infection and readmission rates after total joint arthroplasty. *J Arthroplasty* 2014;29:458-464.

12. Li S, Luo X, Sun H, Wang K, Zhang K, Sun X: Does prior bariatric surgery improve outcomes following total joint arthroplasty in the morbidly obese? A meta-analysis. *J Arthroplasty* 2019;34:577-585.

In this systematic review and meta-analysis, the authors evaluated nine studies comparing bariatric surgery with no bariatric surgery. Overall, patients receiving bariatric surgery had lower odds of suffering a short-term complication compared with patients who had not received bariatric surgery. They noted that patients who received bariatric surgery had more medical comorbidities than those who had not, yet they still had lower odds of short-term complications. Among patients who received bariatric surgery, only those who underwent a TKA had lower odds of short-term periprosthetic infection. This benefit was not seen in THA patients. Long-term complication odds were not significantly different between those who had received bariatric surgery and those who had not. Level of evidence: IV.

13. Severson EP, Singh JA, Browne JA, Trousdale RT, Sarr MG, Lewallen DG: Total knee arthroplasty in morbidly obese patients treated with bariatric surgery. A comparative study. *J Arthroplasty* 2012;27:1696-1700.

14. Nickel BT, Klement MR, Penrose CT, Green CL, Seyler TM, Bolognesi MP: Lingering risk: Bariatric surgery before total knee arthroplasty. *J Arthroplasty* 2016;31:207-211.

15. Schwarzkopf R, Lavery JA, Hooper J, Parikh M, Gold HT: Bariatric surgery and time to total joint arthroplasty: Does it affect readmission and complication rates? *Obes Surg* 2018;28:1395-1401.

The authors of this study evaluated the ideal period to wait after a patient undergoes bariatric surgery before TKA. They queried the SID database and found that 90-day readmission for any cause was lower in those who waited >6 months; however, no difference was seen in 90-day complications. The authors conclude that they are unable to make a recommendation on the optimal time for total joint arthroplasty after bariatric surgery based on this evidence, but waiting 6 months may provide some benefit. Level of evidence: III.

16. Gu A, Malahias MA, Strigelli V, Nocon AA, Sculco TP, Sculco PK: Preoperative malnutrition negatively correlates with postoperative wound complications and infection after total joint arthroplasty: A systematic review and meta-analysis. *J Arthroplasty* 2019;34:1013-1024.

In this systematic review, the authors analyzed the results from 20 studies looking at malnutrition and complications after total joint arthroplasty. All studies cited the use of albumin as a marker, with total lymphocyte count being the second most commonly cited. Level of evidence: III.

17. Blevins K, Aalirezaie A, Shohat N, Parvizi J: Malnutrition and the development of periprosthetic joint infection in patients undergoing primary elective total joint arthroplasty. *J Arthroplasty* 2018;33:2971-2975.

The authors of this study wanted to evaluate the nutritional marker that was associated with a higher likelihood of periprosthetic joint infection after a total joint arthroplasty. They found that hypoalbuminemia had the highest likelihood of being associated with a periprosthetic joint infection (OR, 4.69; 95% CI, 1.100 to 2.718; $P = 0.018$) and was the most specific marker as well (95% CI, 97.8% to 98.4%). Level of evidence: III.

18. Nelson CL, Elkassabany NM, Kamath AF, Liu J: Low albumin levels, more than morbid obesity, are associated with complications after TKA. *Clin Orthop Relat Res* 2015;473:3163-3172.

19. Black CS, Goltz DE, Ryan SP, et al: The role of malnutrition in ninety-day outcomes after total joint arthroplasty. *J Arthroplasty* 2019;34(11):2594-2600.

The authors of this study evaluated the role of hypoalbuminemia (serum value < 3.5 g/dL) in length of stay, 90-day readmission, 90-day emergency department (ED) visits, and rate of discharge to skilled nursing facility. They found that patients with hypoalbuminemia were more likely to have greater lengths of stay, higher rates of 90-day readmission and ED visits, and greater rates of discharge to skilled nursing facility. The authors also demonstrated that an ideal cutoff value for hypoalbuminemia would be 3.94 g/dL based on 90-day outcomes. Level of evidence: III.

20. Traven SA, Chiaramonti AM, Barfield WR, et al: Fewer complications following revision hip and knee arthroplasty in patients with normal vitamin D levels. *J Arthroplasty* 2017;32:S193-S196.

The authors of this study evaluated the association of low preoperative vitamin D levels with rates of complications and readmission in patients undergoing revision hip and knee arthroplasties. Low preoperative vitamin D levels were associated with periprosthetic joint infection and complications within 90 days of surgery. Level of evidence: III.

21. Bedard NA, Dowdle SB, Wilkinson BG, Duchman KR, Gao Y, Callaghan JJ: What is the impact of smoking on revision total knee arthroplasty? *J Arthroplasty* 2018;33:S172-S176.

In this database study, the authors queried the NSQIP database to evaluate the association between tobacco use and revision arthroplasty procedures. They found that current smokers are twice as likely to suffer from any wound complication (OR, 2.1; 95% CI, 1.4 to 3.1) and deep infection (OR, 2.1; 95% CI, 1.2 to 3.6) than nonsmokers. Level of evidence: III.

22. Bedard NA, DeMik DE, Owens JM, Glass NA, DeBerg J, Callaghan JJ: Tobacco use and risk of wound complications and periprosthetic joint infection: A systematic review and meta-analysis of primary total joint arthroplasty procedures. *J Arthroplasty* 2019;34:385-396.e4.

In this systematic review and meta-analysis, the authors evaluated the association between tobacco use and surgical site infection and periprosthetic joint infection after hip and knee arthroplasty procedures. They found that tobacco users were associated with a higher likelihood of surgical site infection and periprosthetic joint infection. Of note, former tobacco users were associated with a lower likelihood of periprosthetic joint infection compared with current tobacco users (OR, 1.52 [1.07 to 2.14]). Level of evidence: III.

23. Lindström D, Azodi OS, Wladis A, et al: Effects of a perioperative smoking cessation intervention on postoperative complications: A randomized trial. *Ann Surg* 2008;248:739-745.

24. Hart A, Rainer WG, Taunton MJ, Mabry TM, Berry DJ, Abdel MP: Cotinine testing improves smoking cessation before total joint arthroplasty. *J Arthroplasty* 2019;34:S148-S151.

The authors of this study retrospectively compared self-reported quit rates between patients who had serum cotinine obtained within 1 month before arthroplasty and those who did not. They found that the proportion of patients who self-reported that they had quit was higher in the cohort who underwent testing. Level of evidence: III.

25. Belmont PJ, Goodman GP, Kusnezov NA, et al: Postoperative myocardial infarction and cardiac arrest following primary total knee and hip arthroplasty: Rates, risk factors, and time of occurrence. *J Bone Joint Surg Am* 2014;96:2025-2031.

26. Levine GN, Bates ER, Bittl JA, et al: 2016 ACC/AHA guideline focused update on duration of dual antiplatelet therapy in patients with coronary artery disease: A report of the American College of Cardiology/American Heart Association Task Force on Clinical Practice Guidelines. *Circulation* 2016;134:e123-e155.

27. Jacob AK, Hurley SP, Loughran SM, Wetsch TM, Trousdale RT: Continuing clopidogrel during elective total hip and knee arthroplasty: Assessment of bleeding risk and adverse outcomes. *J Arthroplasty* 2014;29:325-328.

28. Slover J, Lavery JA, Schwarzkopf R, Iorio R, Bosco J, Gold HT: Incidence and risk factors for blood transfusion in total joint arthroplasty: Analysis of a statewide database. *J Arthroplasty* 2017;32:2684-2687.e1.

This database study investigated the incidence of perioperative blood transfusion and compared transfusion rates among patients undergoing unilateral and bilateral THA or TKA. Almost 25% of the patient population experienced a perioperative blood transfusion. Compared with patients receiving a single TKA, patients receiving a single THA had higher odds of receiving a perioperative transfusion (OR, 1.76). Additionally, the following factors were associated with higher odds of a perioperative transfusion: bilateral total knee (OR, 3.57), bilateral total hip (OR, 6.17), increasing age (odds increased with increasing age group), Medicaid insurance (OR, 1.36), and higher comorbidity index (odds increased with increasing score). Level of evidence: III.

29. Browne JA, Adib F, Brown TE, Novicoff WM: Transfusion rates are increasing following total hip arthroplasty: Risk factors and outcomes. *J Arthroplasty* 2013;28:34-37.

30. Fillingham YA, Ramkumar DB, Jevsevar DS, et al: The efficacy of tranexamic acid in total knee arthroplasty: A network meta-analysis. *J Arthroplasty* 2018;33:3090-3098.e1.

In this systematic review and meta-analysis of 67 studies, the authors evaluated the role of TXA in TKA. They determined that although there was definitive evidence to support the use of TXA in any formulation over a placebo, no definitive evidence was seen to support one formulation over another. The authors did find that preincision dosing of intravenous TXA had a lower risk of transfusion than postincision dosing (risk ratio, 2.05; 95% CI, 1.21 to 3.67). Level of evidence: II.

31. Fillingham YA, Ramkumar DB, Jevsevar DS, et al: The efficacy of tranexamic acid in total hip arthroplasty: A network meta-analysis. *J Arthroplasty* 2018;33:3083-3089.e4.

In this systematic review and meta-analysis of 34 studies, the authors evaluated the role of TXA in THA. Authors determined that although there was definitive evidence to support the use of TXA in any formulation over a placebo, no definitive evidence was seen to support one formulation over another. Level of evidence: II.

32. Zeng WN, Liu JL, Wang FY, Chen C, Zhou Q, Yang L: Low-dose epinephrine plus tranexamic acid reduces early postoperative blood loss and inflammatory response. *J Bone Joint Surg Am* 2018;100:295-304.

In this randomized controlled trial, the authors explored the benefits of adding low-dose intravenous epinephrine to TXA protocol during TKA. All patients received intravenous TXA and topical TXA during the procedure. Depending on the group they were randomized to, these patients also received intravenous low-dose epinephrine, topical epinephrine, or placebo. The authors excluded anyone younger than 65 years as well as those with chronic conditions related to the cardiovascular system (eg, thyrotoxicosis, digoxin therapy). The intravenous epinephrine group demonstrated lower blood transfusion requirements as well as lower postoperative blood loss. Level of evidence: I.

33. Ponnusamy KE, Jain A, Thakkar SC, Sterling RS, Skolasky RL, Khanuja HS: Inpatient mortality and morbidity for dialysis-dependent patients undergoing primary total hip or knee arthroplasty. *J Bone Joint Surg Am* 2015;97:1326-1332.

34. Browne JA, Casp AJ, Cancienne JM, Werner BC: Peritoneal dialysis does not carry the same risk as hemodialysis in patients undergoing hip or knee arthroplasty. *J Bone Joint Surg Am* 2019;101:1271-1277.

In this PearlDiver database study, the authors evaluated the association between mode of dialysis and periprosthetic joint infection after hip or knee arthroplasty. They found that patients who had received a hip or knee arthroplasty and were receiving peritoneal dialysis were 70% and 33%, respectively, less likely to be associated with a periprosthetic joint infection compared with patients receiving hemodialysis. The authors speculated the increased likelihood of infection with hemodialysis was likely related to the increased risk of bacteremia. Level of evidence: III.

35. Cavanaugh PK, Chen AF, Rasouli MR, Post ZD, Orozco FR, Ong AC: Complications and mortality in chronic renal failure patients undergoing total joint arthroplasty: A comparison between dialysis and renal transplant patients. *J Arthroplasty* 2016;31:465-472.

36. Schweizer ML, Chiang HY, Septimus E, et al: Association of a bundled intervention with surgical site infections among patients undergoing cardiac, hip, or knee surgery. *J Am Med Assoc* 2015;313:2162-2171.

37. Tandon T, Tadros BJ, Akehurst H, Avasthi A, Hill R, Rao M: Risk of surgical site infection in elective hip and knee replacements after confirmed eradication of MRSA in chronic carriers. *J Arthroplasty* 2017;32:3711-3717.

The authors compared patients who were documented as being colonized with MRSA and who had undergone eradication protocol with a combo of mupirocin and chlorhexidine. They found that despite documented eradication, those who were colonized with MRSA had a significantly higher rate of infection from a control group. However, no significance was seen when multivariate analysis was performed. Level of evidence: III.

38. Inabathula A, Dilley JE, Ziemba-Davis M, et al: Extended oral antibiotic prophylaxis in high-risk patients substantially reduces primary total hip and knee arthroplasty 90-day infection rate. *J Bone Joint Surg Am* 2018;100:2103-2109.

The authors investigated the use of extended, postoperative oral antibiotics in preventing periprosthetic joint infections in high-risk patients. High-risk individuals received cefadroxil while those who tested positive for MRSA preoperatively received Bactrim DS for 7 days. Those allergic to cephalosporins were given clindamycin for 7 days. The authors found that compared with those who underwent the antibiotic regimen, those who did not receive the regimen were over four times as likely to suffer from a periprosthetic joint infection after a hip or knee arthroplasty. Level of evidence: III.

39. Falck-Ytter Y, Francis CW, Johanson NA, et al: Prevention of VTE in orthopedic surgery patients. Antithrombotic therapy and prevention of thrombosis, 9th ed: American College of Chest Physicians evidence-based clinical practice guidelines. *Chest* 2012;141:e278S-e325S.

40. Lieberman JR, Heckmann N: Venous thromboembolism prophylaxis in total hip arthroplasty and total knee arthroplasty patients: From guidelines to practice. *J Am Acad Orthop Surg* 2017;25:789-798.

This is a review article discussing the most recent AAOS and ACCP guidelines for VTE prophylaxis after total joint arthroplasty. The need for balancing the safety and efficacy of VTE prophylaxis in each individual patient was emphasized. Further appropriately powered head to head trials are still needed to select the optimal prophylaxis regimen. Level of evidence: V.

41. American Academy of Orthopaedic Surgeons: *Clinical Practice Guidelines on Preventing Venous Thromboembolic Disease in Patients Undergoing Elective Hip and Knee Arthroplasty*. Rosemont, IL, American Academy of Orthopaedic Surgeons, 2011. Available at: http://www.orthoguidelines.org/topic?id=1006. Accessed October 2, 2019.

42. Yeomans ND, Lanas AI, Talley NJ, et al: Prevalence and incidence of gastroduodenal ulcers during treatment with vascular protective doses of aspirin. *Aliment Pharmacol Ther* 2005;22:795-801.

43. Rodgers A, MacMahon S, Collins R, Prentice C: Prevention of pulmonary embolism and deep vein thrombosis with low dose aspirin: Pulmonary Embolism Prevention (PEP) trial. *Lancet* 2000;355:1295-1302.

44. Parvizi J, Huang R, Restrepo C, et al: Low-dose aspirin is effective chemoprophylaxis against clinically important venous thromboembolism following total joint arthroplasty: A preliminary analysis. *J Bone Joint Surg Am* 2017;99:91-98.

The authors of this study compared the postoperative VTE-related complications in primary arthroplasty patients who received either higher dose or lower dose aspirin prophylactic regimen. All patients selected for the study were not considered high risk for VTE. The rate of VTE complications in patients receiving a lower dose aspirin protocol was shown to be noninferior to that in the higher dose protocol. Level of evidence: II.

45. Anderson DR, Dunbar M, Murnaghan J, et al: Aspirin or rivaroxaban for VTE prophylaxis after hip or knee arthroplasty. *N Engl J Med* 2018;378:699-707.

The authors of this study compared the 90-day complication rates between low-VTE-risk patients who underwent arthroplasty (both primary and revision) and those who received either a strict rivaroxaban-only prophylactic course or one that involved switching over to low-dose aspirin after the fifth postoperative day. Aspirin therapy was found to be noninferior to rivaroxaban therapy. Level of evidence: I.

46. Hood BR, Cowen ME, Zheng HT, Hughes RE, Singal B, Hallstrom BR: Association of aspirin with prevention of venous thromboembolism in patients after total knee arthroplasty compared with other anticoagulants: A noninferiority analysis. *JAMA Surg* 2019;154(1):65-72.

   In this retrospective database study, the authors compared the outcomes between four different VTE prophylaxis regimens in patients who received total knee arthroplasties. The four regimens were as follows: no anticoagulation therapy, aspirin alone, anticoagulant alone, and combination therapy. Their findings demonstrated that patients who had received aspirin alone had noninferior VTE, death, and bleeding rates relative to anticoagulant and combination therapy. Level of evidence: III.

47. Woller SC, Bertin KC, Stevens SM, et al: A prospective comparison of warfarin to aspirin for thromboprophylaxis in total hip and total knee arthroplasty. *J Arthroplasty* 2012;27:1-9.e2.

48. Jameson SS, Baker PN, Charman SC, et al: The effect of aspirin and low-molecular-weight heparin on venous thromboembolism after knee replacement: A non-randomised comparison using National Joint Registry Data. *J Bone Joint Surg Br* 2012;94:914-918.

49. Colwell CW, Froimson MI, Mont MA, et al: Thrombosis prevention after total hip arthroplasty: A prospective, randomized trial comparing a mobile compression device with low-molecular-weight heparin. *J Bone Joint Surg Am* 2010;92:527-535.

50. Hunt LP, Ben-Shlomo Y, Clark EM, et al: 45-day mortality after 467779 knee replacements for osteoarthritis from the National Joint Registry for England and Wales: An observational study. *Lancet* 2014;384:1429-1436.

51. Helwani MA, Avidan MS, Ben Abdallah A, et al: Effects of regional versus general anesthesia on outcomes after total hip arthroplasty: A retrospective propensity-matched cohort study. *J Bone Joint Surg Am* 2015;97:186-193.

52. Pugely AJ, Martin CT, Gao Y, Mendoza-Lattes S, Callaghan JJ: Differences in short-term complications between spinal and general anesthesia for primary total knee arthroplasty. *J Bone Joint Surg Am* 2013;95:193-199.

53. Harsten A, Kehlet H, Ljung P, Toksvig-Larsen S: Total intravenous general anaesthesia vs. spinal anaesthesia for total hip arthroplasty: A randomised, controlled trial. *Acta Anaesthesiol Scand* 2015;59:298-309.

54. Harsten A, Kehlet H, Toksvig-Larsen S: Recovery after total intravenous general anaesthesia or spinal anaesthesia for total knee arthroplasty: A randomized trial. *Br J Anaesth* 2013;111:391-399.

55. Memtsoudis SG, Cozowicz C, Bekeris J, et al: Anaesthetic care of patients undergoing primary hip and knee arthroplasty: Consensus recommendations from the International Consensus on Anaesthesia-Related Outcomes after Surgery group (ICAROS) based on a systematic review and meta-analysis. *Br J Anaesth* 2019;123:269-287.

   The International Consensus on Anaesthesia-Related Outcomes after Surgery group conducted a systematic review and meta-analysis on the available literature comparing neuraxial anesthesia with general anesthesia. The results supported the use of neuraxial anesthesia with lower odds for almost all complications studied (eg, mortality, acute renal failure, and deep vein thrombosis) except urinary retention. The evidence for this support was rated as stronger for THA than for TKA. Further studies are required to obtain more granular details regarding the varying practices of neuraxial anesthesia across institutions as well as to determine the mechanism behind the perceived advantage over general anesthesia. Level of evidence: V.

56. Halawi MJ, Vovos TJ, Green CL, Wellman SS, Attarian DE, Bolognesi MP: Opioid-based analgesia: Impact on total joint arthroplasty. *J Arthroplasty* 2015;30:2360-2363.

57. Lin J, Zhang L, Yang H: Perioperative administration of selective cyclooxygenase-2 inhibitors for postoperative pain management in patients after total knee arthroplasty. *J Arthroplasty* 2013;28:207-213.

58. Clarke H, Pagé GM, McCartney CJL, et al: Pregabalin reduces postoperative opioid consumption and pain for 1 week after hospital discharge, but does not affect function at 6 weeks or 3 months after total hip arthroplasty. *Br J Anaesth* 2015;115:903-911.

59. Murata-Ooiwa M, Tsukada S, Wakui M: Intravenous acetaminophen in multimodal pain management for patients undergoing total knee arthroplasty: A randomized, double-blind, placebo-controlled trial. *J Arthroplasty* 2017;32:3024-3028.

   The authors of this study looked at the efficacy of intravenous acetaminophen in the postoperative period in TKA patients. They found that early pain scores and quantity of rescue analgesia in the first 17 hours were significantly better in the acetaminophen group. Level of evidence: I.

60. Spangehl MJ, Clarke HD, Hentz JG, Misra L, Blocher JL, Seamans DP: The Chitranjan Ranawat Award: Periarticular injections and femoral & sciatic blocks provide similar pain relief after TKA. A randomized clinical trial. *Clin Orthop Relat Res* 2015;473:45-53.

61. Sardana V, Burzynski JM, Scuderi GR: Adductor canal block or local infiltrate analgesia for pain control after total knee arthroplasty? A systematic review and meta-analysis of randomized controlled trials. *J Arthroplasty* 2019;34:183-189.

   In this systematic review and meta-analysis, the authors reviewed studies that compared the efficacy of PAIs with that of adductor canal block. Six high-quality studies were included for analysis. The patients who received a PAI had significantly lower use of opioids and lower pain scores postoperatively in comparison with those who received an adductor canal block. Level of evidence: I.

62. Liu W, Cong R, Li X, Wu Y, Wu H: Reduced opioid consumption and improved early rehabilitation with local and intraarticular cocktail analgesic injection in total hip arthroplasty: A randomized controlled clinical trial. *Pain Med* 2011;12:387-393.

63. Dobie I, Bennett D, Spence DJ, Murray JM, Beverland DE: Periarticular local anesthesia does not improve pain or mobility after THA. *Clin Orthop Relat Res* 2012;470:1958-1965.

64. Fahs AM, Koueiter DM, Kurdziel MD, Huynh KA, Perry CR, Verner JJ: Psoas compartment block vs periarticular local anesthetic infiltration for pain management after anterior total hip arthroplasty: A prospective, randomized study. *J Arthroplasty* 2018;33:2192-2196.

The authors compared the efficacy of a psoas compartment block with that of a PAI in patients undergoing THA via the direct anterior approach. The PAI consisted of ropivacaine, epinephrine, morphine, and ketorolac. The psoas compartment block consisted of just ropivacaine. The authors found comparable results in terms of postoperative pain control as well as associated complications in both groups. Level of evidence: I.

65. Perry CR, Fahs AM, Kurdziel MD, Koueiter DM, Fayne RJ, Verner JJ: Intraoperative psoas compartment block vs preoperative fascia iliaca block for pain control after direct anterior total hip arthroplasty: A randomized controlled trial. *J Arthroplasty* 2018;33:1770-1774.

The authors compared the efficacy of a preoperatively administered fascia iliaca block and an intraoperatively administered psoas compartment block in patients undergoing total hip arthroplasty via the direct anterior approach. The preoperative administration was carried out by the anesthesiology team. The intraoperative block was carried out by the surgeon. The total sample size was 49 patients. There was no difference in postoperative pain scores, narcotic consumption, or pain scores at 3-week follow-up. Level of evidence: II.

66. Kim DH, Lin Y, Goytizolo EA, et al: Adductor canal block versus femoral nerve block for total knee arthroplasty: A prospective, randomized, controlled trial. *Anesthesiology* 2014;120:540-550.

67. Lee S, Rooban N, Vaghadia H, Sawka AN, Tang R: A randomized non-inferiority trial of adductor canal block for analgesia after total knee arthroplasty: Single injection versus catheter technique. *J Arthroplasty* 2018;33:1045-1051.

Noninferiority trial comparing different adductor canal block modalities including single injection ropivacaine, single injection ropivacaine with an IV dose of dexamethasone, and continuous ropivacaine. The authors found that the single injection formulations with and without dexamethasone provided equivalent levels of analgesia as a continuous adductor canal block. Level of evidence: I.

68. Gwam CU, Mistry JB, Khlopas A, et al: Does addition of multimodal periarticular analgesia to adductor canal block improve lengths of stay, pain, discharge status, and opioid use after total knee arthroplasty? *J Arthroplasty* 2017;32:1470-1473.

The authors compared the management of pain and other outcomes in a TKA patient population who received either adductor canal block alone or PAI. There was no statistically significant difference in any outcome measured including pain scores and opioid consumption. Consequently, adductor canal block on its own was deemed to be likely enough for pain management. Level of evidence: III.

69. Abdallah FW, Brull R: Is sciatic nerve block advantageous when combined with femoral nerve block for postoperative analgesia following total knee arthroplasty? A systematic review. *Reg Anesth Pain Med* 2011;36:493-498.

CHAPTER 3

Blood Management

DOMINICK V. CONGIUSTA, MD, MPH • YATIN KIRANE, MD, PhD • FRED D. CUSHNER, MD

ABSTRACT

Total hip arthroplasty and total knee arthroplasty are associated with marketed perioperative blood loss, resulting in postsurgical anemia that in turn can necessitate blood transfusions. Perioperative blood loss can also result in significant surgical site hemarthrosis, which may lead to wound complications, increased risk of development of infection, and delayed recovery. Allogeneic blood transfusions have been associated with serious complications, such as incorrect blood component transfusion, disease transmission, allergic reactions, fluid overload, transfusion reactions, and immunosuppression. Overall, perioperative anemia and blood transfusions are associated with greater morbidity and mortality, longer hospital stay, and significantly higher hospital costs. Therefore, in this current climate of bundled payments, minimizing surgical blood loss and preventing postoperative anemia are critical to achieving successful clinical outcomes and reducing hospital costs. Numerous interventions have been suggested to minimize perioperative blood loss; however, orthopaedic surgeons lack consensus on the topic, and allogeneic transfusion rates still remain high at some institutions. An evidence-based multimodal individualized approach for blood conservation has been suggested.

Dr. Cushner or an immediate family member has received royalties from Smith & Nephew; is a member of a speakers' bureau or has made paid presentations on behalf of Smith & Nephew; serves as a paid consultant to or is an employee of Acelity and Smith & Nephew; and has stock or stock options held in Canary Medical and Orthalign. Neither of the following authors nor any immediate family member has received anything of value from or has stock or stock options held in a commercial company or institution related directly or indirectly to the subject of this chapter: Dr. Congiusta and Dr. Kirane.

Keywords: blood conservation; total hip arthroplasty; total knee arthroplasty

INTRODUCTION

Total hip arthroplasty (THA) and total knee arthroplasty (TKA) are two of the most commonly performed orthopaedic procedures in the United States and around the world. It has been estimated that more than 500,000 THA and more than 1 million TKA procedures (primary and revision procedures combined) will be performed in the United States alone in 2020.[1] Historically, these procedures have been associated with substantial perioperative blood loss. In addition to the visible blood loss, a substantial amount of hidden blood loss is associated with these procedures as a result of extravasation into the tissues, residual blood accumulation into the joint, and blood loss attributable to hemolysis. The mean total blood loss has been reported to be approximately 1.5 L with both THA and TKA procedures; more hidden blood loss is associated with TKA (49% of total blood loss) than THA (26% of total blood loss).[2]

Revision and bilateral arthroplasty procedures are associated with even greater blood loss. Anemia has been associated with higher rates of postoperative cardiovascular, genitourinary, and other complications, as well as mortality following total joint arthroplasty (TJA).[3] Hemorrhage within the joint and periarticular tissues may result in hematoma formation, leading not only to drainage from the incision site but also delayed wound healing, wound dehiscence, and hence an increased risk of developing infection. Excessive hematoma also contributes to pain, swelling, decreased range of motion, prolonged rehabilitation, and a longer hospital stay. Anemia may further contribute to prolonged recovery by causing fatigue and inability to adequately participate in physical therapy. Furthermore, anemia may cause greater adverse effects in the presence of other coexisting medical conditions among elderly patients, a situation that is quite common in the joint arthroplasty patient population. Approximately 25% of patients undergoing an elective THA or TKA have been reported to have anemia before surgery, whereas the prevalence of postoperative anemia has been reported to be approximately 51%.[4] Perioperative blood loss may result in acute anemia, delayed recovery, and increased mortality risk, all of which may necessitate allogeneic blood transfusion. Blood transfusion rates for postoperative anemia have been reported to be 37% to 53% for primary THA (51% for hip arthritis and 61% following a femur neck fracture), 69% for hip hemiarthroplasty, 43% to 46% for primary TKA, 72% for bilateral TKA, 41% for revision TKA, and 72% for revision THA.[5] With a unit of transfused blood costing an estimated $787.37,[6] the incremental total hospitalization costs have been found to be $2,477, $4,235, and $8,594 higher for patients who underwent primary TKA, bilateral TKA, and revision TKA procedures, respectively, and received blood transfusion compared with those who did not receive transfusion.[7] Furthermore, in addition to higher costs, allogeneic blood transfusion carries a risk—albeit a small risk—of serious complications such as incorrect blood component transfusion, disease transmission, allergic reactions, fluid overload, transfusion reactions, and immunosuppression. In contrast, reduced blood loss translates to better wound healing, quicker rehabilitation, shorter length of hospital stay, higher hemoglobin levels at discharge, fewer medical complications, faster recovery, and improved patient satisfaction. Predictors of marked blood loss necessitating blood transfusion include preoperative anemia, older age, higher body weight, multiple comorbidities, increased surgical time, lateral retinacular release, and use of postoperative anticoagulation.[8,9] Despite known risks, surgical anemia caused by acute blood loss has been considered by many to be a routine and an acceptable complication of major surgical procedures. The need for blood management protocols to reduce the perioperative blood loss, the associated morbidity, and the allogeneic blood transfusion rates and to improve clinical outcomes of joint arthroplasty surgery is increasingly recognized. Minimizing surgical blood loss and preventing postoperative anemia are critical to achieving successful clinical outcomes. Numerous interventions have been suggested to minimize perioperative blood loss; however, orthopaedic surgeons lack consensus on the topic, and allogeneic transfusion rates remain unacceptably high. Several authors have suggested evidence-based multimodal blood management protocols to minimize perioperative blood loss and to achieve improved clinical outcomes, decreased procedural costs, and shorter hospital stays. Furthermore, blood conservation protocols need to be individualized by means of algorithms based on the patient's preoperative hemoglobin level and medical comorbidities, the complexity of the planned procedure, the anticipated blood loss, and the need for transfusion.

BLOOD CONSERVATION STRATEGIES

Preoperative Strategies: Preoperative Screening and Treatment of Anemia

Approximately 24% to 44% of patients have been reported to be anemic before THA or TKA surgery.[4] Preoperative anemia has been associated with higher rates of postoperative complications and mortality following TJA.[3] Therefore, timely detection and management of preoperative anemia, nutritional or metabolic deficiencies, and other modifiable risk factors is extremely important in optimizing patient physiology before surgery. Preoperative assessment should include a complete workup for anemia and nutritional status in addition to routine investigations and consultation with a hematologist or other appropriate specialist if deemed necessary. Authors of a 2016 study recommended hemoglobin screening at the time of indication for arthroplasty by using a noninvasive cutaneous pulse co-oximeter followed by complete blood count. They recommended additional laboratory testing and referral to a hematologist for patients with hemoglobin levels lower than 12.[10] Specifically, the preoperative evaluation should include obtaining patients' personal and family history of bleeding, thromboembolic disease, current medication review, complete blood count with differential, and other appropriate patient-specific laboratory investigations. Optimization of the patient's general health—which may include smoking cessation; weight loss; management of blood pressure and diabetes; prescribing vitamins, iron, and other nutritional supplements; and stopping use of antiplatelet and anticoagulation medications—should be accomplished early.[11] Preoperative hemoglobin levels lower than 11 g/dL, body mass index less than 27 kg/m^2, age older than 75 years, and male sex all are factors that have been associated with an increased requirement for postoperative blood transfusion. Therefore, individualized risk stratification and a multidisciplinary approach have been suggested for early diagnosis and treatment of preoperative anemia. The goal should be to optimize the patient's hemoglobin level above 12 g/dL because lower levels have been correlated with a threefold increase in transfusion requirement.

Nonsteroidal Anti-inflammatory and Anticoagulant Medications

NSAIDs are widely used for perioperative analgesia. Nonselective NSAIDs are known to impair platelet aggregation and prolong bleeding time by acting on cyclooxygenase-1 and -2 enzymes of the prostaglandin formation process. However, cyclooxygenase-2–selective NSAIDs such as celecoxib and etoricoxib are believed to reduce pain and inflammation without affecting platelet aggregation or bleeding time. Cyclooxygenase-2 inhibitors are often an aspect of multimodal pain management after arthroplasty,[12] and they can be safely used in most patients with consideration given to their cardiovascular and other adverse effects. Several other allopathic and alternative herbal medications can prolong bleeding time by affecting various levels of the coagulation cascade and can substantially increase perioperative bleeding. Therefore, all medications with known adverse effects on coagulation should be stopped before surgery. According to the current clinical practice guidelines, anticoagulant and antiplatelet medications such as warfarin, aspirin, clopidogrel, and rivaroxaban should be stopped before the planned surgery to normalize bleeding time.[13] However, benefits of stopping these medications before surgery need to be weighed against the patient's cardiac risk, and the treatment needs to be individualized. To maximize patient safety, the prescribing physician should weigh in regarding if and when to stop these medications rather than use a general rule applied to all patients undergoing arthroplasty procedures.

Vitamins and Iron Supplementation

Patients who have preoperative anemia can be treated with a healthy diet, vitamin B_{12}, folate, oral or intravenous (IV) iron, and erythropoiesis-stimulating agents. Approximately 4 to 6 weeks of nutritional supplementation before the planned surgery is necessary for effective treatment. Lower transfusion and infection rates have been reported following TKA in patients who have hemoglobin levels below 8 mg after receiving daily supplementation of iron (256 mg; 80 mg Fe^{2+}), vitamin C (1,000 mg), and folate (5 mg) for 30 to 45 days.[14] However, higher levels of iron supplementation, especially when administered in the absence of iron deficiency, have been associated with constipation, heartburn, abdominal pain, and other adverse effects.

Erythropoietin

Erythropoietin (EPO), a glycoprotein that is naturally secreted by renal pericapillary cells in response to reduced tissue oxygen tension such as that occurs in an anemic state, acts on bone marrow to increase red blood cell differentiation and maturation. Epoetin α, which is human EPO produced in a laboratory by means of recombinant technology, has the same physiologic effects and is commonly used for patients who have chronic renal disease and those undergoing chemotherapy. Preoperative epoetin injections have been more effective than has preoperative autologous blood donation (PAD) in maximizing preoperative hemoglobin in patients undergoing TKA[15] and reducing the need for allogeneic blood transfusions even in high-risk patients who have anemia.[16] Several preoperative and postoperative dosing regimens have been described[17] (**Table 1**).

Although effective, EPO treatment is expensive: the average price per patient is equivalent to two to three units of PAD or three to four units of allogeneic blood.[18] In a 2015 efficacy/cost-analysis study, EPO treatment was found to have no effect on the length of hospital stay and was not cost effective despite the reduced need for postoperative blood transfusions. Nevertheless, the use of EPO is recommended for patients at higher risk of allogeneic transfusion, such as those who have preoperative anemia (hemoglobin level less than 13 g/dL) and low body weight (less than 50 kg) who are undergoing revision or bilateral surgery for which considerable blood loss is expected.

Autologous Blood

PAD involves procuring one to two units of the patient's own blood before surgery. The donated autologous blood is processed, stored, and transfused back to the patient during or after surgery. PAD can be performed at least 3 weeks before the planned surgery, for anticipated major blood loss in patients who have hemoglobin greater than 11 g/dL and weight greater than 110 pounds.[19] PAD was popular in the United States in the late 1980s, when decreased need for allogeneic blood transfusions with the use of PAD was reported.[20,21] However, in recent years, PAD has become less common for a variety of reasons. First, patients who have preoperative anemia are not candidates for PAD. This severely limits the usefulness of this modality, because patients who have anemia are most likely to require allogeneic transfusion postoperatively. The procedure is inconvenient and expensive; it requires advance planning as well as storage and preparation of the donated blood, and it carries a risk of clerical error. Phlebotomy-induced anemia, bacterial contamination, and infection are additional risks associated with an

TABLE 1

Erythropoietin Dosing Schedules

Dose	Schedule
600 IU/kg	4 doses: preoperative days 21, 14, 7, and 0
300 IU/kg	15 daily doses: preoperative day 10 to postoperative day 4
150 IU/kg	9 daily doses: preoperative day 5 to postoperative day 3

Reproduced from Levine BR, Haughom B, Strong B, Hellman M, Frank RM: Blood management strategies for total knee arthroplasty. *J Am Acad Orthop Surg* 2014;22(6):361-371.

autologous blood donation program. In addition, it may be wasteful and unnecessary for patients who do not have anemia.[22,23] Furthermore, preoperative epoetin α treatment has been more effective than PAD in maximizing preoperative hemoglobin for patients undergoing TKA.[15] There is currently no consensus regarding the efficacy/cost-benefit of PAD, and therefore, its routine use is not recommended.

Hemodilution

Acute normovolemic hemodilution (ANH) involves harvesting a patient's whole blood along with simultaneous infusion of acellular fluids (colloids or crystalloids) at the time of or just before surgery. This is followed by perioperative reinfusion of the procured autologous blood, thereby resulting in a reduced net loss of red blood cells. This procedure has been indicated for patients who have preoperative hemoglobin levels higher than 10 g/dL and for whom procedures in which substantial blood loss is anticipated are planned. Although cumbersome and time consuming, ANH has been found to be equal to PAD in effectiveness for patients undergoing THA and TKA procedures. Furthermore, ANH is less expensive and has a smaller risk of clerical error, bacterial contamination, and blood wastage compared with PAD.[24] The utility of hemodilution currently is limited as a result of considerably reduced blood loss due to multimodal blood conservation protocols and newer drugs such as tranexamic acid (TXA). Hemodilution may still be valuable in patients who refuse allogeneic blood transfusion because of religious beliefs (eg, Jehovah's Witnesses).

Intraoperative Strategies

Tourniquets

Thigh tourniquets have been routinely used for TKA because they allow a bloodless surgical field, improved cement interdigitation, and decreased surgical time. However, the local tissue ischemia and subsequent reactive hyperperfusion with tourniquet use can result in local muscle damage, neurapraxia, thigh pain, delayed wound healing, increased joint swelling and stiffness, and thromboembolic events.[25] There is some controversy regarding the optimal time for release of a tourniquet. Researchers compared clinical outcomes in relation to the timing of tourniquet use in a 2014 nonrandomized prospective cohort study involving 90 patients.[26] The participants were divided into three groups on the basis of the timing of tourniquet use—that is, from incision to wound closure, from incision to after cement hardening, and only during cementing. Use of a tourniquet only during cementing led to lower serum markers for inflammation and muscle damage, such as C-reactive protein, interleukin-6, creatine kinase, and myoglobin. However, there was no difference in the clinical outcomes in terms of Hospital for Special Surgery knee scores, range of motion, estimated blood loss, swelling ratio, visual analog scale pain score, and length of hospital stay. Release of the tourniquet after wound closure has been shown to significantly decrease surgical time without affecting overall perioperative blood loss, or drop in hemoglobin level or transfusion requirement.[27] In a poll at the 2009 Annual Meeting of the American Association of Hip and Knee Surgeons regarding current practice patterns in primary THA and TKA, 37% of the respondents used a tourniquet in all cases irrespective of any prior vascular problems, 58% of the respondents avoided tourniquet use if a patient has known vascular problems, and 5% of the respondents used a tourniquet only during exposure and cementation.[28]

Hypotensive Anesthesia

With the use of hypotensive epidural anesthesia, blood loss is reduced by maintaining a low mean arterial blood pressure (typically 50 to 60 mm Hg) throughout the surgical procedure. This is achieved by decreasing the conduction of the cardioacceleratory fibers of the thoracic sympathetic chain via an epidural dermatome block at T2 level. Hypotensive anesthesia has been shown to effectively reduce intraoperative blood loss by about 38% to 45%; however, it may lead to tissue hypoperfusion, bradycardia, and other serious cardiopulmonary complications, and it should be used with extreme caution in patients who have cardiopulmonary, renal, cerebral, or peripheral vascular diseases.[29,30]

Surgical Technique

The importance of meticulous surgical techniques in limiting the amount of intraoperative blood loss cannot be overstated. Examples of surgical techniques that are particularly helpful for blood conservation include careful dissection, limited incision and soft-tissue release, gentle handling of soft tissues, appropriate use of electrocautery, and administration of periarticular and intra-articular epinephrine mixed with saline and other medications.

Bipolar Sealer Versus Electrocautery

Bipolar sealer uses radiofrequency to achieve coagulation of blood vessels. Because of continuous simultaneous flow of saline, the tip of the bipolar sealer remains cool, causing less damage to the surrounding tissues. There have been mixed reports regarding the efficacy of the bipolar sealer compared with the conventional electrocautery in terms of amount of perioperative blood loss, the need for blood transfusion, and other clinical outcomes. Some authors have reported substantially reduced blood loss, postoperative hemoglobin drop, and transfusion requirement with the use of a bipolar sealer compared with electrocautery in TJA.[31] Bipolar sealers are expensive tools; the incremental costs per case have been estimated to be approximately $676.[32] Researchers in one study observed significantly fewer blood transfusions, lower incidence of hematomas, and significantly shorter lengths of hospital stay after primary THA involving the use of a bipolar sealer. However, no effect on the total hospital costs was found. It was concluded that the higher supply costs associated with the use of a bipolar sealer were likely offset by the reduced hospital inpatient and operating room costs.[32] Another group of investigators reported that the use of a bipolar sealer for simultaneous bilateral TKA was associated with a 35% lower blood transfusion rate compared with the use of conventional electrocautery.[33] However, no significant difference was observed in terms of decrease in hemoglobin level, total blood loss, or length of stay. In other studies by members of the same group of investigators, the use of a saline-coupled bipolar sealing device in revisions of infected THA resulted in shorter surgical times, less blood loss, and smaller perioperative decreases in hemoglobin level.[34] However, the device's use in revision procedures for infected TKA was not clinically or economically justified.[35] The bipolar sealing device shows promise as a blood loss-reduction tool, especially in simultaneous bilateral TKA and revision THA procedures; however, the savings and clinical benefits associated with the reduced transfusion rates need to be evaluated against the per-case expense of the device.

Topical Hemostatic Agents

A variety of topical hemostatic agents such as platelet-rich plasma, fibrin sealant, cellulose, collagen agents, and thrombin have been used to reduce blood loss during TJA. Typically, the selected topical hemostatic agent is sprayed inside the wound before closure. Although there were a few early favorable results regarding efficacy,[36] there is no conclusive evidence in support of routine use of these agents. In a 2014 meta-analysis comprising eight randomized controlled trials (RCTs) involving 641 patients, substantially reduced postoperative drainage and blood transfusion rates were observed, as well as improved postoperative knee range of motion, with the use of a fibrin sealant product.[37] However, there were no substantial differences in terms of total blood loss or other adverse events such as fever, infection, or hematoma. It was concluded that the use of fibrin sealant was effective and safe as a hemostatic therapy during TKA.[37] However, other reports suggest that the fibrin sealant and other topical hemostatic agents do not have any substantial effect on reducing blood loss or transfusion requirement.[38,39] Currently, routine use of these agents remains controversial.

Antifibrinolytic Agent: TXA

Several antifibrinolytic agents have been used to limit blood loss in TJA, including desmopressin, TXA, ε-aminocaproic acid, and aprotin. TXA is by far the most studied and widely accepted drug, and it is being increasingly incorporated into perioperative blood management protocols. Originally discovered in 1962, TXA (trans form of 4-aminomethyl-cyclohexane-carbonic acid) competitively binds to the lysine-binding site on plasminogen, which prevents fibrin from binding to the plasminogen-plasmin tissue activator complex and thus inhibits fibrin clot degradation and bleeding.[40] It is a well-established, safe drug that successfully reduces the amount of blood loss and the likelihood of blood transfusion, with no increased risk of thromboembolic events, regardless of route of administration.[41-44] With a half-life of 80 to 120 minutes, TXA has been reported to rapidly penetrate the synovial fluid and membrane, reaching the same concentration as in plasma within 15 minutes and peak concentration within 1 hour after IV administration.

The IV route continues to be the predominant method of TXA administration, although there may not be a clinically significant difference in rate of transfusions between topical, oral, and IV dosing regimens. The lowest effective dose and route of TXA may therefore be best practice.[45] Low-dose topical TXA (<1.5 g) has not been shown to reduce blood loss compared with placebo in patients undergoing THA but is more successful in patients undergoing TKA. Low-dose IV (<1 g or <20 mg/kg), high-dose IV (>1 g or >20 mg/kg), and high-dose topical (>1.5 g) TXA effectively reduced the amount of blood loss in patients undergoing TJA.[46,47] Other studies demonstrate higher doses of topical TXA (>2 g) may be more effective than lower doses.

The usual dose of IV TXA is 20 mg/kg, and the maximum dose is 2,000 mg. Limited studies report superiority of higher doses of IV or topical TXA administration (3 g versus 1.5 g),[48,49] but other data challenge these conclusions, and a clear benefit has not been demonstrated.[50,51] Similarly, multiple doses of oral or IV TXA have not been shown to reduce hematologic complications in TJA when compared with single-dose administration.[40,52] IV TXA is ideally administered before incision to reduce the risk of blood transfusion in TKA.[47] To date, however, there are no data to suggest administration before incision reduces overall blood loss or has any meaningful effect in patients undergoing THA.

Because the kidneys provide the major route of elimination, the IV dose of TXA needs to be reduced to 50% for patients who have renal impairment for a glomerular filtration rate of 0.5 mL/min, 25% for a glomerular filtration rate 10 to 50 mL/min, and 10% for a glomerular filtration rate of 10 mL/min.[40] The absolute contraindications to TXA include a known allergy to the agent, an ongoing acute venous or arterial thrombosis, and an intrinsic risk or a history of thrombosis or thromboembolism.[42] Caution needs to be exerted when using TXA in the presence of cardiac or peripheral vascular disease, seizures, and acute renal failure, although further studies are needed to fully define all the risks associated with TXA as many trials exclude these patients.[42,53] In patients who have seizures, it has been suggested that higher levels of TXA in cerebrospinal fluid may inhibit glycine and gamma-aminobutyric acid receptors, which have lysine binding sites similar to plasminogen, and thus affect central nervous system inhibition.[54,55]

Studies show that TXA has been associated with decreased perioperative blood loss, higher postoperative hemoglobin levels, lower blood transfusion rates, lower complication rates, and decreased length of hospital stay.[53,56] In patients undergoing TKA, TXA has been shown to decrease total blood loss by 30%, the drainage volume by nearly 50%, and the transfusion requirement by 47%.[57] For patients in whom IV TXA is contraindicated, 2 to 4 g of TXA can be safely injected inside the joint before deflation of the tourniquet. Several studies suggest as low as 1 g intra-articular injection provides lower rates of postoperative blood loss and transfusion rates.[58] Intra-articular administration of TXA has been found to have clinical outcomes comparable with those seen after IV administration, with significantly higher hemoglobin levels during the immediate postoperative period and at discharge.[59] The requirement for blood transfusion was seen to decrease to 5% after intra-articular TXA compared with 22% among those who did not receive TXA.[56] Intra-articular injection of TXA results in 70% of the plasma concentration after IV administration with minimal systemic hypercoagulability effects.[49] Intra-articular use of TXA has been associated with improved knee function in the initial 6 weeks of the immediate postoperative period, as evidenced by significantly improved Knee Society Scores (ability to walk, negotiate stairs up and down, arise from a chair, and the use of support).[56] Furthermore, combined intra-articular administration of TXA and epinephrine significantly reduced total blood loss, hidden blood loss, and transfusion rate compared with TXA alone—without increasing the risks of thromboembolic and hemodynamic complications—in both THA[60] and TKA.[61]

Oral TXA has been used and may be preferred in some instances because of its lower cost compared with IV administration ($75.41 versus $580.83, respectively).[62] In comparison with IV administration, oral doses including 1,950 mg, 2 g, and 20 mg/kg have similar transfusion requirements (4.12% versus 4.06%, respectively).[62] Indeed, recent literature suggests that oral applications are comparable to IV in both hip and knee arthroplasty.[63,64]

There are several recommendations regarding TXA dosing, and further investigations are warranted to determine the optimal dosing and dosing regimen of TXA. Typically, two 20 mg/kg (approximately 2 g) doses of IV TXA are administered; the first dose is given before inflation of the tourniquet, and the other dose is given postoperatively, but recent evidence may call this into question, with 1 dose of 20 mg/kg IV may be the most effective treatment. Recent data also challenge previous notions that additional topical TXA doses higher than 2 g appear to be more efficacious than are lower doses.[46,65] The routes of administration demonstrate similar efficacy in mitigating blood loss and likelihood of transfusions.[44] In per-patient cost analysis studies, TXA ($103.08) was found to be significantly more cost effective than preoperative 3-week iron supplementation ($1,773.48), 1-week EPO regimen ($268.88),[66] and reinfusion drains ($581.89),[67] as well as autologous blood transfusion ($787).[6]

Postoperative Strategies

Wound Drains

Wound drains have been used in orthopaedic surgery for decades to prevent fluid collection and hematoma formation at the surgical site. Traditionally, closed suction drains have been used after TJA to prevent hematoma formation, and thereby to reduce the risk of infection, relieve pain and stiffness, prevent wound dehiscence, improve wound healing, and allow for early mobilization and a shorter length of hospital stay.[68] However, the use of wound drains has become controversial in recent years. Opponents of wound drains consider them a channel for potential retrograde transmission of bacteria. Complications such as accidental suturing of the drain, entrapment, and drain breakage during removal are well known, and these may require reopening the surgical wound in the operating room. Furthermore, closed suction drains are thought to result in increased blood loss because of continuous negative pressure. There have been various recommendations regarding optimal drain management, releasing pressure, clamping, and the timing of drain removal. Typically, patients need to be hospitalized for a day or two for drain management, thus increasing the hospital costs by $538 for THA and $455 for TKA.[69]

Increasing impetus to reduce hospital costs has caused many to reevaluate the postoperative protocol and question the usefulness of wound drains. Several authors now recommend against using wound drains and propose same-day discharge following TJA.[69] With a multimodal blood conservation protocol including medications such as TXA, the risk of hematoma formation and the need for blood transfusion after a TJA are greatly reduced. In a double-blind randomized placebo-controlled trial, investigators reported that TXA treatment without drainage results in substantial reduction in blood loss and the amount of blood transfusions required without increasing the rate of adverse events.[70] In a prospective cohort study, investigators categorized 63 patients undergoing bilateral TKA into bilateral-drain, unilateral-drain, and no-drain groups, and no substantial differences in the short-term or long-term clinical outcomes were observed. It was concluded that wound suction drains are not necessary after TKA.[71] In a meta-analysis of six RCTs, a research team concluded that wound drains did not offer any significant benefits in terms of postoperative recovery.[72] In another meta-analysis of 20 RCTs, investigators observed a reduced need for dressing reinforcement but an increased need for blood transfusion with the use of a closed suction drain after THA, and it was concluded that wound drains following THA likely do more harm than good.[73]

Cold Compressive Dressing

Cold compressive dressing is thought to decrease the amount of internal blood loss, pain, and swelling. Despite the lack of adequate scientific evidence to support these beliefs, cold compressive dressings (such as Cryo/Cuff, DJO Global) are routinely used following TKA.

Blood Salvage and Reinfusion

Blood salvage and reinfusion techniques involve collection of the blood shed during surgery using an intraoperative cell salvage system and postoperatively, using a recollection drain. The collected blood is filtered, washed, and then reinfused into the patient within 6 to 8 hours. There are mixed reports regarding the efficacy of blood salvage and reinfusion. Some authors have reported lower total blood loss and higher postoperative hemoglobin levels with the implementation of reinfusion technique following THA as well as TKA.[74] However, reinfusion systems are expensive and have potential complications, such as contamination, infection, and coagulopathy, due to circulating fibrin-split products and cytokines. In a prospective RCT involving 1,759 patients undergoing THA or TKA procedure, autologous intraoperative and postoperative blood salvage devices were found to be expensive and ineffective.[75] The unit cost of a reinfusion system ($581.89) is substantially higher than those of a standard drain ($7.56) and TXA ($35.91/g).[67] In a recent meta-analysis of 43 RCTs involving 5,631 patients, investigators observed that although cell salvage reduced bleeding and transfusion requirements in THA and TKA in earlier studies, more recently published studies (2010 to 2012) indicate contradictory results. The investigators attributed this finding to the changes in blood transfusion management practices.[76] In another recent meta-analysis, researchers confirmed the efficacy of the reinfusion technique in reducing the need for allogeneic blood transfusion after THA and TKA, but they emphasized that further research is warranted regarding the risks of serious complications and safety of this technique.[77]

Allogeneic Blood Transfusion

Historically, THA and TKA procedures have resulted in substantial perioperative blood loss, often requiring the transfusion of one or more units of blood, which has been a part of the routine postoperative protocol for years. However, allogeneic blood transfusion has significant risks, including incorrect blood component transfusion, disease transmission, allergic reactions, fluid overload, transfusion reaction, and immunosuppression.[78] The risks[17] have been quantified in **Table 2**. Furthermore, allogeneic blood transfusion is associated with significant costs. The costs associated with collecting, testing, processing, storing, and cross-matching one unit of blood have been estimated to be approximately $787.[6] Compared with patients who did not require a blood transfusion, the incremental total hospitalization costs for those who required a transfusion have been estimated to be $2,477 (12%), $4,235 (15%), and $8,594 (35%) higher for a primary TKA, a bilateral TKA, and a revision TKA, respectively.[7] The concept of transfusion triggers has been popular in the past couple of decades. Traditionally, the 10/30 rule dictated that a blood transfusion was required in postsurgical patients if the hemoglobin level fell below 10 g/dL, the hematocrit level fell below 30%, or both. In recent years, more restrictive transfusion triggers have been followed. Evidence-based restrictive transfusion strategy has been recommended by

TABLE 2

Complication Risks Associated With Allogeneic Blood Transfusion

Complication	Incidence
Infectious	
HIV infection	1:1,900,000
Hepatitis B virus infection	1:180,000
Hepatitis C virus infection	1:1,600,000
Bacterial contamination	1:3,000
Cardiopulmonary	
Transfusion-associated circulatory overload	1:5,000
Acute lung injury	1:50,000
Systemic	
Fever or allergic reaction	1:200
Hemolytic transfusion reaction	1:6,000
Fatal hemolytic reaction	1:1,000,000
Anaphylaxis	1:50,000

Reproduced from Levine BR, Haughom B, Strong B, Hellman M, Frank RM: Blood management strategies for total knee arthroplasty. *J Am Acad Orthop Surg* 2014;22(6):361-371.

the American Society of Anesthesiologists Task Force on Perioperative Blood Transfusion and Adjuvant Therapies[79] as well as the AABB (formerly the American Association of Blood Banks).[80] According to these guidelines, the threshold for transfusion for a hemodynamically stable postsurgical patient is a hemoglobin level lower than 7 to 8 g/dL with clinical symptoms of anemia. Thus, the decision to undertake transfusion in a patient is based not only on the laboratory values but also on objective signs and symptoms such as tachycardia, feeling of weakness or dizziness, comorbidities, severity of illness, rate and amount of hemorrhage, and the patient's capacity to cope with the hemorrhage. Blood transfusion rates for postoperative anemia have been reported to be as high as 37% to 53% for primary THA (51% for hip arthritis and 61% after a femoral neck fracture), 69% for hip hemiarthroplasty, 43% to 46% for primary TKA, 72% for bilateral TKA, 41% for revision TKA, and 72% for revision THA.[5] With implementation of an individualized patient blood management protocol, researchers reported a 44% decrease in the transfusion rate and a significant reduction in complications, readmissions, and length of hospital stay.[81] With the implementation of a practical multimodal blood conservation protocol and adherence to evidence-based guidelines, it is possible to significantly reduce blood transfusion rates following TJA.

Complex Cases

Bilateral TJA

An increasing number of patients are undergoing simultaneous bilateral THA (especially via the direct anterior approach) or TKA procedures because of the convenience of a single trip to the operating room, one-time anesthesia, and one-time surgery. However, simultaneous bilateral TJA procedures can result in substantially greater blood loss, and there is an increased risk of requiring a blood transfusion in the perioperative period. Blood transfusion rates for bilateral TKA have been reported to be as high as 72%.[5] A multimodal patient-specific blood conservation protocol becomes critical when planning bilateral THA or TKA procedures. Of all the different modalities, TXA seems to have the greatest effect on blood conservation. In a retrospective study involving 103 patients who underwent simultaneous bilateral TKA, investigators observed significantly higher hemoglobin levels on the first postoperative day and almost a 70% decrease in the incidence of blood transfusion with the administration of TXA.[82]

Revision Knee Arthroplasty

With the growth of the aging population and the increasing number of primary THA and TKA procedures being performed each year, the number of revision arthroplasties is on the rise. Blood transfusion rates for revision arthroplasty procedures have been quite high. Based on nationwide hospital and blood bank data, researchers reported 72% and 41% blood transfusion rates for revision THA and TKA procedures, respectively.[5] A blood conservation protocol incorporating TXA was shown to significantly decrease the blood transfusion rates among patients undergoing revision TKA.[83]

Sickle Cell Anemia

Patients who have sickle cell disease undergoing THA or TKA have an increased risk of perioperative complications, especially when a blood transfusion is required.[84] There is no consensus regarding the optimal blood management for patients who have sickle cell anemia who are undergoing TJA. A multimodal blood conservation protocol is of utmost importance for these patients to avoid a sickle cell crisis. In a 2013 multicenter randomized trial, researchers found that preoperative blood transfusions in patients who have the hemoglobin SS form of sickle cell disease were associated with decreased risks of serious complications, particularly acute chest syndrome.[85] Maintenance of hydration and optimal pain control are essential to prevent sickle cell crisis. In general, these patients should be treated in consultation with a hematologist during the perioperative period.[85]

Religious Objections to Blood Transfusions

Some patients may refuse blood transfusions because of their religious beliefs, such as those who are Jehovah's Witnesses. Therefore, effective blood conservation protocol is critical in these patients to ensure safe and transfusion-free procedures with minimal complications. Researchers reported excellent outcomes of TKA procedures in patients who are Jehovah's Witnesses using a specific blood management strategy.[86] Preoperative evaluation and treatment were conducted by a coordinated team consisting of internists, hematologists, intensivists, and anesthesiologists. Preoperative optimization of patients' red blood cell mass was achieved using iron and folate supplements. Patients with hemoglobin levels between 13 and 15 g/dL were treated with a combination of ANH and EPO therapy. Patients with a hemoglobin level of less than 13 g/dL were initially treated with EPO alone, followed by combination therapy of IV iron and blood salvage if their hemoglobin levels remained lower than 13 g/dL. Surgery was performed using a less invasive approach, with emphasis given to meticulous hemostasis, decreased surgical time, and avoidance of a drain if possible. Postoperative measures included microvenipunctures, iron supplements, and EPO therapy.

SUMMARY

Perioperative management of patients undergoing TJA is evolving. Blood loss following THA or TKA procedures that necessitates postoperative blood transfusion is no longer accepted as routine. Several authors have emphasized the importance of implementing individualized risk stratification and multimodal blood conservation protocols. Such multimodal approaches consist of numerous preoperative, intraoperative, and postoperative measures. Preoperative measures are focused on timely diagnosis and treatment of preoperative anemia, as well as on optimization of the patient's red blood cell mass and general health using iron and vitamin supplementation, EPO injections, or both. Intraoperative strategies focus on minimizing blood loss by means of meticulous surgical technique, hypotensive anesthesia, bipolar sealer, topical hemostatic agents, and antifibrinolytic agents such as TXA. Postoperative measures include reinfusion and allogeneic blood transfusion in select patients. The evidence-based restrictive transfusion trigger strategy is recommended for allogeneic blood transfusion in hemodynamically stable patients to avoid unnecessary risks associated with blood transfusion. The ultimate goal is not only to minimize the need for blood transfusion for patients undergoing TJA procedures but also to limit surgical site hemarthrosis and wound complications.

KEY STUDY POINTS

- TJA procedures are associated with substantial blood loss, which can compromise patient recovery and overall clinical outcomes by causing greater morbidity and mortality, longer hospital stay, and significantly higher hospital costs.
- Multimodal blood conservation strategies comprising preoperative, intraoperative, and postoperative measures can effectively reduce blood loss associated with TJA.
- Preoperative anemia is a major factor in predicting transfusion requirements; therefore, patients should be adequately screened and treated for anemia preoperatively.
- TXA is now the benchmark in blood loss prevention in TJA, and IV or intra-articular TXA should be considered for every patient undergoing TJA.

ANNOTATED REFERENCES

1. Kurtz SM, Ong KL, Lau E, Bozic KJ: Impact of the economic downturn on total joint replacement demand in the United States: Updated projections to 2021. *J Bone Joint Surg Am* 2014;96(8):624-630.
2. Sehat KR, Evans RL, Newman JH: Hidden blood loss following hip and knee arthroplasty. Correct management of blood loss should take hidden loss into account. *J Bone Joint Surg Br* 2004;86(4):561-565.
3. Viola J, Gomez MM, Restrepo C, Maltenfort MG, Parvizi J: Preoperative anemia increases postoperative complications and mortality following total joint arthroplasty. *J Arthroplasty* 2015;30(5):846-848.
4. Spahn DR: Anemia and patient blood management in hip and knee surgery: A systematic review of the literature. *Anesthesiology* 2010;113(2):482-495.
5. Verlicchi F, Desalvo F, Zanotti G, Morotti L, Tomasini I: Red cell transfusion in orthopaedic surgery: A benchmark study performed combining data from different data sources. *Blood Transfus* 2011;9(4):383-387.
6. Tuttle JR, Ritterman SA, Cassidy DB, Anazonwu WA, Froehlich JA, Rubin LE: Cost benefit analysis of topical tranexamic acid in primary total hip and knee arthroplasty. *J Arthroplasty* 2014;29(8):1512-1515.
7. Nichols CI, Vose JG: Comparative risk of transfusion and incremental total hospitalization cost for primary unilateral, bilateral, and revision total knee arthroplasty procedures. *J Arthroplasty* 2016;31(3):583-589.e1.
8. Sizer SC, Cherian JJ, Elmallah RD, Pierce TP, Beaver WB, Mont MA: Predicting blood loss in total knee and hip arthroplasty. *Orthop Clin North Am* 2015;46(4):445-459.
9. Ahmed I, Chan JK, Jenkins P, Brenkel I, Walmsley P: Estimating the transfusion risk following total knee arthroplasty. *Orthopedics* 2012;35(10):e1465-e1471.
10. Holt JB, Miller BJ, Callaghan JJ, Clark CR, Willenborg MD, Noiseux NO: Minimizing blood transfusion in total hip and knee arthroplasty through a multimodal approach. *J Arthroplasty* 2016;31(2):378-382.
11. Bruce W, Campbell D, Daly D, Isbister J: Practical recommendations for patient blood management and the reduction of perioperative transfusion in joint replacement surgery. *ANZ J Surg* 2013;83(4):222-229.
12. Parvizi J, Miller AG, Gandhi K: Multimodal pain management after total joint arthroplasty. *J Bone Joint Surg Am* 2011;93(11):1075-1084.
13. Mont MA, Jacobs JJ, Boggio LN, et al, American Academy of Orthopaedic Surgeons: Preventing venous thromboembolic disease in patients undergoing elective hip and knee arthroplasty. *J Am Acad Orthop Surg* 2011;19(12):768-776.
14. Cuenca J, García-Erce JA, Martínez F, Cardona R, Pérez-Serrano L, Muñoz M: Preoperative haematinics and transfusion protocol reduce the need for transfusion after total knee replacement. *Int J Surg* 2007;5(2):89-94.
15. Cushner FD, Lee GC, Scuderi GR, Arsht SJ, Scott WN: Blood loss management in high-risk patients undergoing total knee arthroplasty: A comparison of two techniques. *J Knee Surg* 2006;19(4):249-253.
16. Weber EW, Slappendel R, Hémon Y, et al: Effects of epoetin alfa on blood transfusions and postoperative recovery in orthopaedic surgery: The European Epoetin Alfa Surgery Trial (EEST). *Eur J Anaesthesiol* 2005;22(4):249-257.
17. Levine BR, Haughom B, Strong B, Hellman M, Frank RM: Blood management strategies for total knee arthroplasty. *J Am Acad Orthop Surg* 2014;22(6):361-371.

18. Bedair H, Yang J, Dwyer MK, McCarthy JC: Preoperative erythropoietin alpha reduces postoperative transfusions in THA and TKA but may not be cost-effective. *Clin Orthop Relat Res* 2015;473(2):590-596.
19. Bezwada HR, Nazarian DG, Henry DH, Booth RE Jr, Mont MA: Blood management in total joint arthroplasty. *Am J Orthop (Belle Mead NJ)* 2006;35(10):458-464.
20. Bou Monsef J, Figgie MP, Mayman D, Boettner F: Targeted preoperative autologous blood donation: A prospective study of two thousand and three hundred and fifty total hip arthroplasties. *Int Orthop* 2014;38(8):1591-1595.
21. Gandini G, Franchini M, Bertuzzo D, et al: Preoperative autologous blood donation by 1073 elderly patients undergoing elective surgery: A safe and effective practice. *Transfusion* 1999;39(2):174-178.
22. Pierson JL, Hannon TJ, Earles DR: A blood-conservation algorithm to reduce blood transfusions after total hip and knee arthroplasty. *J Bone Joint Surg Am* 2004;86(7):1512-1518.
23. Lee GC, Hawes T, Cushner FD, Scott WN: Current trends in blood conservation in total knee arthroplasty. *Clin Orthop Relat Res* 2005;440:170-174.
24. Goodnough LT, Despotis GJ, Merkel K, Monk TG: A randomized trial comparing acute normovolemic hemodilution and preoperative autologous blood donation in total hip arthroplasty. *Transfusion* 2000;40(9):1054-1057.
25. Tai TW, Lin CJ, Jou IM, Chang CW, Lai KA, Yang CY: Tourniquet use in total knee arthroplasty: A meta-analysis. *Knee Surg Sports Traumatol Arthrosc* 2011;19(7):1121-1130.
26. Huang ZY, Pei FX, Ma J, et al: Comparison of three different tourniquet application strategies for minimally invasive total knee arthroplasty: A prospective non-randomized clinical trial. *Arch Orthop Trauma Surg* 2014;134(4):561-570.
27. Hernández-Castaños DM, Ponce VV, Gil F: Release of ischaemia prior to wound closure in total knee arthroplasty: A better method? *Int Orthop* 2008;32(5):635-638.
28. Berry DJ, Bozic KJ: Current practice patterns in primary hip and knee arthroplasty among members of the American Association of Hip and Knee Surgeons. *J Arthroplasty* 2010;25(6 suppl):2-4.
29. Juelsgaard P, Larsen UT, Sørensen JV, Madsen F, Søballe K: Hypotensive epidural anesthesia in total knee replacement without tourniquet: Reduced blood loss and transfusion. *Reg Anesth Pain Med* 2001;26(2):105-110.
30. Eroglu A, Uzunlar H, Erciyes N: Comparison of hypotensive epidural anesthesia and hypotensive total intravenous anesthesia on intraoperative blood loss during total hip replacement. *J Clin Anesth* 2005;17(6):420-425.
31. Suarez JC, Slotkin EM, Szubski CR, Barsoum WK, Patel PD: Prospective, randomized trial to evaluate efficacy of a bipolar sealer in direct anterior approach total hip arthroplasty. *J Arthroplasty* 2015;30(11):1953-1958.
32. Ackerman SJ, Tapia CI, Baik R, Pivec R, Mont MA: Use of a bipolar sealer in total hip arthroplasty: Medical resource use and costs using a hospital administrative database. *Orthopedics* 2014;37(5):e472-e481.
33. Kamath AF, Austin DC, Derman PB, Clement RC, Garino JP, Lee GC: Saline-coupled bipolar sealing in simultaneous bilateral total knee arthroplasty. *Clin Orthop Surg* 2014;6(3):298-304.
34. Clement RC, Kamath AF, Derman PB, Garino JP, Lee GC: Bipolar sealing in revision total hip arthroplasty for infection: Efficacy and cost analysis. *J Arthroplasty* 2012;27(7):1376-1381.
35. Derman PB, Kamath AF, Lee GC: Saline-coupled bipolar sealing in revision total knee arthroplasty for infection. *Am J Orthop (Belle Mead NJ)* 2013;42(9):407-411.
36. Yang TQ, Geng XL, Ding MC, Yang MX, Zhang Q: The efficacy of fibrin sealant in knee surgery: A meta-analysis. *Orthop Traumatol Surg Res* 2015;101(3):331-339.
37. Wang H, Shan L, Zeng H, Sun M, Hua Y, Cai Z: Is fibrin sealant effective and safe in total knee arthroplasty? A meta-analysis of randomized trials. *J Orthop Surg Res* 2014;9:36.
38. Randelli F, D'Anchise R, Ragone V, Serrao L, Cabitza P, Randelli P: Is the newest fibrin sealant an effective strategy to reduce blood loss after total knee arthroplasty? A randomized controlled study. *J Arthroplasty* 2014;29(8):1516-1520.
39. Maheshwari AV, Korshunov Y, Naziri Q, Pivec R, Mont MA, Rasquinha VJ: No additional benefit with use of a fibrin sealant to decrease peri-operative blood loss during primary total knee arthroplasty. *J Arthroplasty* 2014;29(11):2109-2112.
40. Kim C, Park SS, Davey JR: Tranexamic acid for the prevention and management of orthopedic surgical hemorrhage: Current evidence. *J Blood Med* 2015;6:239-244.
41. Boyle JA, Soric MM: Impact of tranexamic acid in total knee and total hip replacement. *J Pharm Pract* 2017;30(1):89-93.

    These authors, both Doctors of Pharmacy, retrospectively evaluated 327 patients who underwent THA or TKA to evaluate the effectiveness of TXA. Over half of their sample population received TXA and was shown to reduce likelihood of hemoglobin change and need for transfusions, but not length of stay. There was no change in risk of venous thromboembolism among these patients. Similar to several 2017 and 2018 studies, this information highlights the utility and safety of TXA in our target population.
42. Goobie SM: Tranexamic acid: Still far to go. *Br J Anaesth* 2017;118(3):293-295.

    The author is affiliated with the Department of Anesthesiology at Boston Children's Hospital. In this editorial, the author acknowledges the limited amount of data on the use of TXA in adult patients undergoing spine surgery and questions its optimal dosing regimen. In the text, however, there is a clear reference to the lack of a link between TXA and thromboembolic events; hence, it adds to the data supporting its safe use.
43. Sabbag OD, Abdel MP, Amundson AW, Larson DR, Pagnano MW: Tranexamic acid was safe in arthroplasty patients with a history of venous thromboembolism: A matched outcome study. *J Arthroplasty* 2017;32(9 suppl):S246-S250.

    The authors retrospectively reviewed 1262 patients with a history of venous thromboembolism who underwent primary joint arthroplasty to identify the safety of use of TXA. They found that, after matching patients to a control group, there was no difference in risk of recurrent venous thromboembolism between those who received TXA compared with those who did not. Although retrospective in nature, this study corroborates with the work of others, including those in 2017 and 2018, and provides data to support its safe use in the total joint population. It is an effective agent that decreases blood loss without increased risk thrombotic events. Level of evidence: III.

44. Fillingham YA, Ramkumar DB, Jevsevar DS, et al: The safety of tranexamic acid in total joint arthroplasty: A direct meta-analysis. *J Arthroplasty* 2018;33(10):3070-3082.e1.

    These authors from multiple institutions based in the United States provide a meta-analysis that compared the effect of oral, topical, and intravenous TXA on arterial and venous thrombotic events. Despite the theoretical risk of increased thrombotic events with use of TXA, these authors provide powerful evidence suggesting that it is safe to use in patients undergoing hip and knee arthroplasty. In the context of this chapter, they corroborate the work of others, including several studies in 2017.

45. Fillingham YA, Darrith B, Calkins TE, et al, Hip Society Research Group: 2019 Mark Coventry Award: A multicentre randomized clinical trial of tranexamic acid in revision total knee arthroplasty. Does the dosing regimen matter? *Bone Joint J* 2019;101-B(7 suppl C):10-16.

    This randomized clinical trial of different dosing regimens for TXA in the use of revision TKA shows that the lowest effective dose of TXA should be used to prevent blood loss without increased risk of adverse events. The authors found no difference in calculated blood loss and transfusion rates between each treatment group, which included groups receiving either a single dose of 1g IV, a double dose of 1g IV, a 1g IV dose along with 1g topical, or three doses of 1950mg oral TXA. Taken along with previous work by these authors, these data suggest that the route of TXA administration may not matter, so long as it is given, particularly in patients undergoing TKA. Level of evidence: I.

46. Fillingham YA, Ramkumar DB, Jevsevar DS, et al: The efficacy of tranexamic acid in total hip arthroplasty: A network meta-analysis. *J Arthroplasty* 2018;33(10):3083-3089.e4.

    In another study by these authors, 34 publications were analyzed to assess differences in administration of TXA and their effect on outcomes in patients undergoing THA. They conclude that each method (topical, intravenous, or oral) resulted in reduced blood loss and transfusion risk compared with those not receiving any TXA, but no method was better between groups. Along with the previous reference, this helps illustrate the notion that the route of TXA administration may not matter, so long as it is given, particularly in patients undergoing TKA.

47. Fillingham YA, Ramkumar DB, Jevsevar DS, et al: The efficacy of tranexamic acid in total knee arthroplasty: A network meta-analysis. *J Arthroplasty* 2018;33(10):3090-3098.e1.

    The authors of this study review 67 publications to assess differences in administration of TXA and their effect on outcomes in patients undergoing TJA. As in the preceding reference, the authors conclude that each method assessed (topical, intravenous, or oral) resulted in reduced blood loss and transfusion risk compared with those not receiving any TXA, but no method was better between groups. This reinforces the utility of TXA in use in arthroplasty procedures but fails to identify a superior mode of administration.

48. Maniar R, Kumar G, Singhi T, Nayak R, Maniar P: Most effective regimen of tranexamic acid in knee arthroplasty: A prospective randomized controlled study in 240 patients. *Clin Orthop Relat Res* 2012;470(9):2605-2612.

49. Wong J, Abrishami A, El Beheiry H, et al: Topical application of tranexamic acid reduces postoperative blood loss in total knee arthroplasty: A randomized, controlled trial. *J Bone Joint Surg Am* 2010;92(15):2503-2513.

50. Sarzaeem MM, Razi M, Kazemian G, Moghaddam ME, Rasi AM, Karimi M: Comparing efficacy of three methods of tranexamic acid administration in reducing hemoglobin drop following total knee arthroplasty. *J Arthroplasty* 2014;29(8):1521-1524.

51. Barrachina B, Lopez-Picado A, Remon M, et al: Tranexamic acid compared with placebo for reducing total blood loss in hip replacement surgery: A randomized clinical trial. *Anesth Analg* 2016;122(4):986-995.

52. Hourlier H, Fennema P: Single tranexamic acid dose to reduce perioperative morbidity in primary total hip replacement: A randomised clinical trial. *Hip Int* 2014;24(1):63-68.

53. Tengborn L, Blombäck M, Berntorp E: Tranexamic acid – An old drug still going strong and making a revival. *Thromb Res* 2015;135(2):231-242.

54. Lecker I, Wang DS, Romaschin AD, Peterson M, Mazer CD, Orser BA: Tranexamic acid concentrations associated with human seizures inhibit glycine receptors. *J Clin Invest* 2012;122(12):4654-4666.

55. Kratzer S, Irl H, Mattusch C, et al: Tranexamic acid impairs γ-aminobutyric acid receptor type A-mediated synaptic transmission in the murine amygdala: A potential mechanism for drug-induced seizures? *Anesthesiology* 2014;120(3):639-649.

56. Serrano Mateo L, Goudarz Mehdikhani K, Cáceres L, Lee YY, Gonzalez Della Valle A: Topical tranexamic acid may improve early functional outcomes of primary total knee arthroplasty. *J Arthroplasty* 2016;31(7):1449-1452.

57. Good L, Peterson E, Lisander B: Tranexamic acid decreases external blood loss but not hidden blood loss in total knee replacement. *Br J Anaesth* 2003;90(5):596-599.

58. Kamatsuki Y, Miyazawa S, Furumatsu T, et al: Intra-articular 1 g tranexamic acid administration during total knee arthroplasty is safe and effective for the reduction of blood loss and blood transfusion. *Eur J Orthop Surg Traumatol* 2019;29(8):1737-1741.

    This retrospective study from Japan analyzed 86 patients who underwent primary TKA, approximately half of whom received TXA. The authors found that patients who received 1g intra-articular TXA had lower rates of transfusion and less blood loss than those who did not receive TXA. Furthermore, no differences regarding deep vein thrombosis and pulmonary embolism were found. The majority of publications and surgeons use IV TXA. Along with previous research by the author of a 2018 study, these data support the idea that administrative route of TXA may not be as important as receiving it by any means overall.

59. Cao G, Chen G, Huang Q, et al: The efficacy and safety of tranexamic acid for reducing blood loss following simultaneous bilateral total knee arthroplasty: A multicenter retrospective study. *BMC Musculoskelet Disord* 2019; 20(1):325.

This article from China is a retrospective study of nearly 600 patients who underwent simultaneous bilateral TKA and received TXA. Similar to that of a 2018 and a 2019 study, there is no significant difference in route of administration of TXA, but giving TXA by any route is better than placebo. There are similar amounts of blood loss, length of stay, hospital expenses, and complications between all routes. In the context of this chapter, it provides another example of how there is no clearly superior method of giving patients TXA in even complicated arthroplasty procedures.

60. Gao F, Sun W, Guo W, Li Z, Wang W, Cheng L: Topical application of tranexamic acid plus diluted epinephrine reduces postoperative hidden blood loss in total hip arthroplasty. *J Arthroplasty* 2015;30(12):2196-2200.

61. Gao F, Sun W, Guo W, Li Z, Wang W, Cheng L: Topical administration of tranexamic acid plus diluted-epinephrine in primary total knee arthroplasty: A randomized double-blinded controlled trial. *J Arthroplasty* 2015;30(8): 1354-1358.

62. Wang N, Xiong X, Xu L, et al: Transfusions and costbenefit of oral versus intravenous tranexamic acid in primary total hip arthroplasty: A meta-analysis of randomized controlled trials. *Medicine (Baltimore)* 2019;98(17):e15279.

These authors from Chongqing, China, performed a meta-analysis investigating the transfusions and cost-benefit of oral and intravenous (IV) TXA in patients undergoing primary THA. Their analysis, which included four studies, concluded that although both oral and IV TXA are effective, oral TXA may be more cost-effective. This information informs the debate on whether mode of administration of TXA matters. In the context of this chapter, it serves to show that oral TXA may be a viable option when used in total joint patients. Level of evidence: I.

63. Wang L, Cao JG, Liu J: Comparison between oral and intravenous application of tranexamic acid for total hip arthroplasty: A meta-analysis. *J Comp Eff Res* 2019;8(6):423-430.

This meta-analysis of four randomized control trials and one retrospective analysis add to the aforementioned studies that concluded that there is no difference in blood loss and hemoglobin reduction between different modes of TXA administration, particularly the oral and IV routes. The authors suggest that oral TXA may be more cost-effective, however, as corroborated by the authors of a 2019 study. In both of these studies, it is noted that the cost of oral TXA is less than IV. With virtually equal efficacy, the argument can be made for oral administration.

64. Zhang LK, Ma JX, Kuang MJ, et al: Comparison of oral versus intravenous application of tranexamic acid in total knee and hip arthroplasty: A systematic review and meta-analysis. *Int J Surg* 2017;45:77-84.

The authors of this study, from China, provide a systematic review and meta-analysis of five studies on the differences between oral and IV TXA in patients undergoing TKA or THA. Similar to several studies, there is no significant difference in efficacy of the route of TXA administration. This study provides a robust population of 3,474 patients that lends credence to the aforementioned claim. The data it provides give more examples of how there is no clearly superior method of giving patients TXA in total joint arthroplasty.

65. Melvin JS, Stryker LS, Sierra RJ: Tranexamic acid in hip and knee arthroplasty. *J Am Acad Orthop Surg* 2015;23(12):732-740.

66. Phan DL, Ani F, Schwarzkopf R: Cost analysis of tranexamic acid in anemic total joint arthroplasty patients. *J Arthroplasty* 2016;31(3):579-582.

67. Springer BD, Odum SM, Fehring TK: What is the benefit of tranexamic acid vs reinfusion drains in total joint arthroplasty? *J Arthroplasty* 2016;31(1):76-80.

68. Koyano G, Jinno T, Koga D, Hoshino C, Muneta T, Okawa A: Is closed suction drainage effective in early recovery of hip joint function? Comparative evaluation in one-stage bilateral total hip arthroplasty. *J Arthroplasty* 2015;30(1):74-78.

69. Bjerke-Kroll BT, Sculco PK, McLawhorn AS, Christ AB, Gladnick BP, Mayman DJ: The increased total cost associated with post-operative drains in total hip and knee arthroplasty. *J Arthroplasty* 2014;29(5):895-899.

70. Wang CG, Sun ZH, Liu J, Cao JG, Li ZJ: Safety and efficacy of intra-articular tranexamic acid injection without drainage on blood loss in total knee arthroplasty: A randomized clinical trial. *Int J Surg* 2015;20:1-7.

71. Watanabe T, Muneta T, Yagishita K, Hara K, Koga H, Sekiya I: Closed suction drainage is not necessary for total knee arthroplasty: A prospective study on simultaneous bilateral surgeries of a mean follow-up of 5.5 years. *J Arthroplasty* 2016;31(3):641-645.

72. Quinn M, Bowe A, Galvin R, Dawson P, O'Byrne J: The use of postoperative suction drainage in total knee arthroplasty: A systematic review. *Int Orthop* 2015;39(4):653-658.

73. Zhou XD, Li J, Xiong Y, Jiang LF, Li WJ, Wu LD: Do we really need closed-suction drainage in total hip arthroplasty? A meta-analysis. *Int Orthop* 2013;37(11):2109-2118.

74. Horstmann W, Kuipers B, Ohanis D, Slappendel R, Kollen B, Verheyen C: Autologous re-transfusion drain compared with no drain in total knee arthroplasty: A randomised controlled trial. *Blood Transfus* 2014;12(suppl 1):s176-s181.

75. So-Osman C, Nelissen RG, Koopman-van Gemert AW, et al: Patient blood management in elective total hip- and knee-replacement surgery (part 2): A randomized controlled trial on blood salvage as transfusion alternative using a restrictive transfusion policy in patients with a preoperative hemoglobin above 13 g/dl. *Anesthesiology* 2014;120(4):852-860.

76. van Bodegom-Vos L, Voorn VM, So-Osman C, et al: Cell salvage in hip and knee arthroplasty: A meta-analysis of randomized controlled trials. *J Bone Joint Surg Am* 2015;97(12):1012-1021.

77. Xie J, Feng X, Ma J, et al: Is postoperative cell salvage necessary in total hip or knee replacement? A meta-analysis of randomized controlled trials. *Int J Surg* 2015;21:135-144.
78. Klein HG: How safe is blood, really? *Biologicals* 2010;38(1):100-104.
79. American Society of Anesthesiologists Task Force on Perioperative Blood Transfusion and Adjuvant Therapies: Practice guidelines for perioperative blood transfusion and adjuvant therapies: An updated report by the American Society of Anesthesiologists Task Force on Perioperative Blood Transfusion and Adjuvant Therapies. *Anesthesiology* 2006;105(1):198-208.
80. Carson JL, Grossman BJ, Kleinman S, et al, Clinical Transfusion Medicine Committee of the AABB: Red blood cell transfusion: A clinical practice guideline from the AABB. *Ann Intern Med* 2012;157(1):49-58.
81. Loftus TJ, Spratling L, Stone BA, Xiao L, Jacofsky DJ: A patient blood management program in prosthetic joint arthroplasty decreases blood use and improves outcomes. *J Arthroplasty* 2016;31(1):11-14.
82. Bagsby DT, Samujh CA, Vissing JL, Empson JA, Pomeroy DL, Malkani AL: Tranexamic acid decreases incidence of blood transfusion in simultaneous bilateral total knee arthroplasty. *J Arthroplasty* 2015;30(12):2106-2109.
83. Samujh C, Falls TD, Wessel R, Smith L, Malkani AL: Decreased blood transfusion following revision total knee arthroplasty using tranexamic acid. *J Arthroplasty* 2014;29(9 suppl):182-185.
84. Perfetti DC, Boylan MR, Naziri Q, Khanuja HS, Urban WP: Does sickle cell disease increase risk of adverse outcomes following total hip and knee arthroplasty? A nationwide database study. *J Arthroplasty* 2015;30(4):547-551.
85. Howard J, Malfroy M, Llewelyn C, et al: The transfusion alternatives preoperatively in sickle cell disease (TAPS) study: A randomised, controlled, multicentre clinical trial. *Lancet* 2013;381(9870):930-938.
86. Issa K, Banerjee S, Rifai A, et al: Blood management strategies in primary and revision total knee arthroplasty for Jehovah's Witness patients. *J Knee Surg* 2013;26(6):401-404.

CHAPTER 4

Thromboprophylaxis

TRACY M. BORSINGER, MD • VINCENT D. PELLEGRINI JR, MD

ABSTRACT

Despite important advances in perioperative care and understanding of the pathophysiology of clot formation, venous thromboembolism (VTE) remains the most common life-threatening postoperative complication after total joint arthroplasty. Nevertheless, current evidence does not permit endorsement of a single optimal regimen for prevention of clinically important deep vein thrombosis and pulmonary embolism. Warfarin remains a popular choice for postoperative VTE prophylaxis because of a low bleeding risk that is likely attributable to its delayed onset of action. Yet, occasionally erratic pharmacokinetics and the need for routine monitoring have largely fueled the search for alternative antithrombotic drugs. Newer anticoagulants, including fractionated heparins, synthetic pentasaccharides, and direct factor Xa and IIa (thrombin) inhibitors, have demonstrated potent actions on reduction of venographic evidence of thrombosis, yet this is accompanied by a substantial increase in major and nonmajor clinically important bleeding without a demonstrable reduction in PE-related deaths. Recommendations regarding aspirin have undergone considerable evolution as it has gained popularity among orthopaedic surgeons, likely because of its low cost and familiarity, ease of administration, and general perception of a low bleeding risk, despite a paucity of contemporary randomized clinical trials interrogating this agent. Although definitive data comparing thromboprophylaxis options are lacking, orthopaedic surgeons remain best positioned to balance the risks of venous thromboembolism with those of perioperative bleeding when prescribing VTE prophylaxis after total joint arthroplasty.

Keywords: anticoagulants; bleeding; deep vein thrombosis; pulmonary embolism; total hip arthroplasty; total knee arthroplasty

Dr. Pellegrini or an immediate family member has received research or institutional support from Synthes and serves as a board member, owner, officer, or committee member of the American Orthopaedic Association, the Association of American Medical Colleges, Board of Directors, Chair, the Council of Faculty and Academic Societies, AAMC, and the Health Volunteers Overseas/Orthopaedics Overseas, Board of Directors. Neither Dr. Borsinger nor any immediate family member has received anything of value from or has stock or stock options held in a commercial company or institution related directly or indirectly to the subject of this chapter.

INTRODUCTION

In an era of continually declining length of stay, and even same-day discharge, after primary total hip arthroplasty (THA) and total knee arthroplasty (TKA), venous thromboembolism (VTE) remains the most common life-threatening postoperative complication (**Figure 1**). A recent 5-year (2011 to 2016) query of the National Surgical Quality Improvement Program database revealed that nearly 0.5% of patients sustained a postoperative pulmonary embolism (PE), more common than a cardiac event, stroke, or death from any cause; after the surgical day, PE was the most commonly occurring of these catastrophic events.[1] Although current available evidence and guidelines promote routine prophylaxis, there is no consensus on a specific chemoprophylactic regimen. As orthopaedic surgeons, it is important to understand the pathophysiology of venous thromboembolic disease (VTED) and prophylaxis options for patients undergoing high-risk procedures such as THA and TKA.

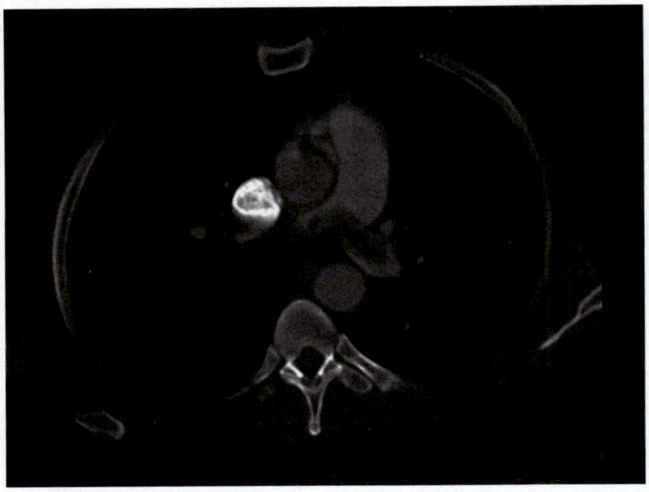

FIGURE 1 Axial view of chest CT with contrast, revealing life-threatening saddle embolus at the bifurcation of the pulmonary artery.

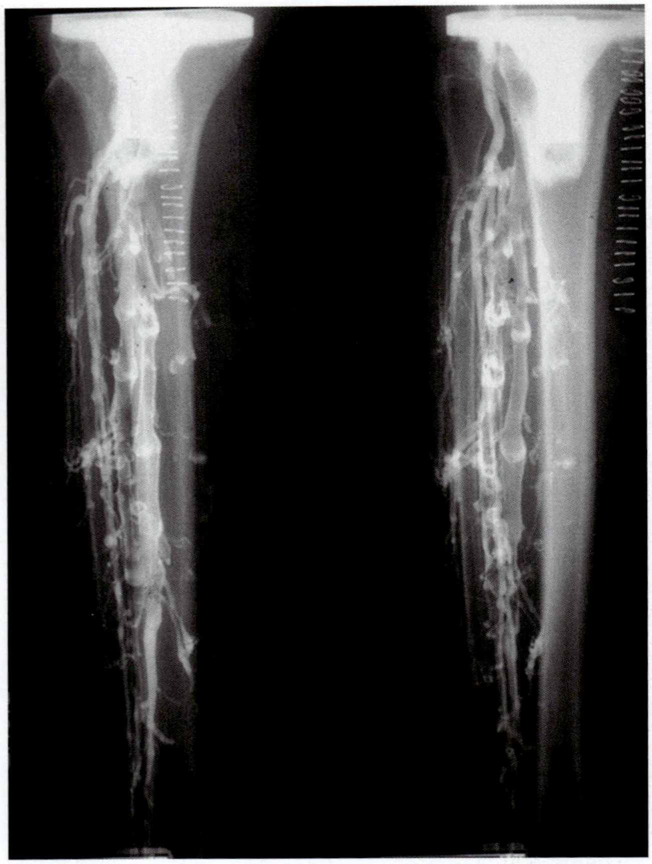

FIGURE 2 Contrast venogram showing extensive calf deep vein thrombosis after total knee arthroplasty.

PATHOPHYSIOLOGY OF DVT/PE IN TKA AND THA

An evolving understanding of the pathophysiology of VTED in patients undergoing TKA and THA can provide the basis for new therapeutic approaches for thrombosis prevention. The underlying mechanism leading to coagulation as described by Virchow triad remains the foundation of current understanding. This identifies the role of stasis, hypercoagulability, and endothelial injury on the clotting cascade, with abnormalities or disturbances in one or all of these elements leading to thrombosis. Orthopaedic procedures are particularly prone to incite VTED because of intimal injury resulting from direct or torsional trauma to the vessel, as well as intravasation of highly thrombogenic marrow fat into the bloodstream following instrumentation of the intramedullary canal.

Thrombogenesis in TKA and THA

The pathophysiology of deep vein thrombosis (DVT) following TKA and THA is thought to be somewhat distinct as evidenced by the different predominant location of thrombus formation. In TKA, nearly all clots occur in the calf distal to the popliteal trifurcation (**Figure 2**), likely initiated by stasis related to intraoperative flexion of the knee resulting in occlusion of the popliteal vein. Proximal DVT in these patients is typically associated with contiguous calf thrombosis (**Figure 3**), suggesting that popliteal and femoral thrombi result from propagation of distal clots in the calf.[2] In contrast to the relatively benign natural history of spontaneous calf thrombus in nonsurgical patients, distal clots in surgical patients have a higher likelihood of proximal propagation, occurring in nearly one-quarter of general surgical patients. Longitudinal surveillance studies found that 17% to 23% of distal thrombi will extend proximally to the thigh veins, where they acquire substantially greater embolic potential. Although mixed data exist, tourniquet use in TKA has also been associated with potential increased risk of DVT, likely related to stasis and intimal injury from hypoxemia.[3]

In contrast to TKA, intimal injury to the femoral vein near the level of the lesser trochanter during THA likely explains the predominantly proximal distribution of DVT after this surgery (**Figure 4**). Both intraoperative femoral medullary canal instrumentation and torsion, or complete obstruction, of the femoral vein are thought to allow for tissue thromboplastin and other procoagulants to aggregate and lead to alterations that promote thrombogenesis.[4] Intraoperatively, elevation of prothrombin F1.2, thrombin-antithrombin complexes, fibrinopeptide A, and D-dimer has been noted to be most pronounced during cemented femoral implant insertion. These increases continue into the postoperative period, specifically over the first hour after surgery. Mean pulmonary artery pressure has been shown to peak and central venous oxygen tension reaches a nadir following

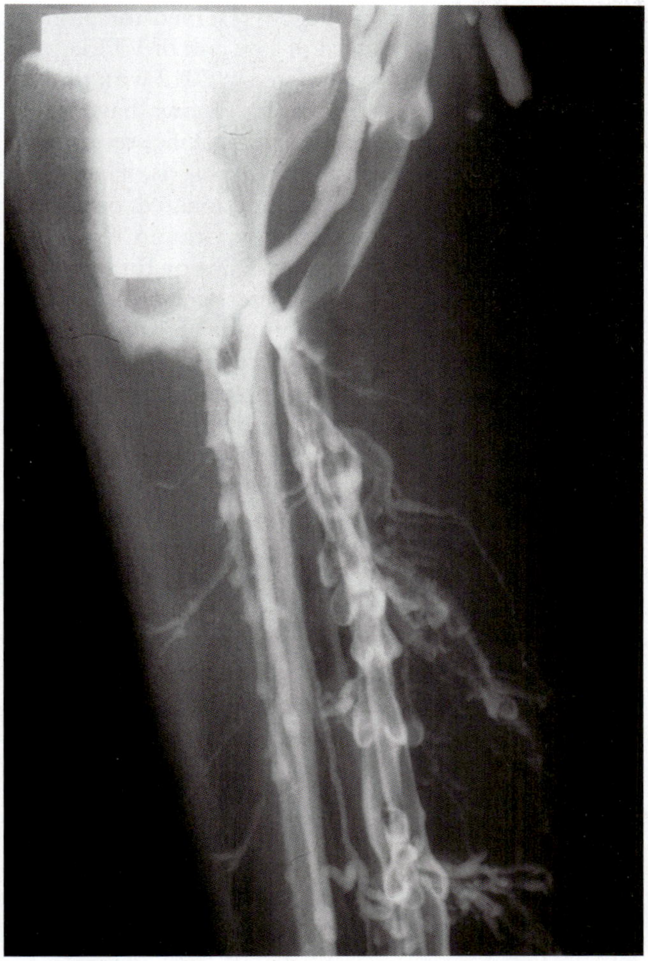

FIGURE 3 Contrast venogram showing calf thrombosis with contiguous extension to the popliteal vein after total knee arthroplasty.

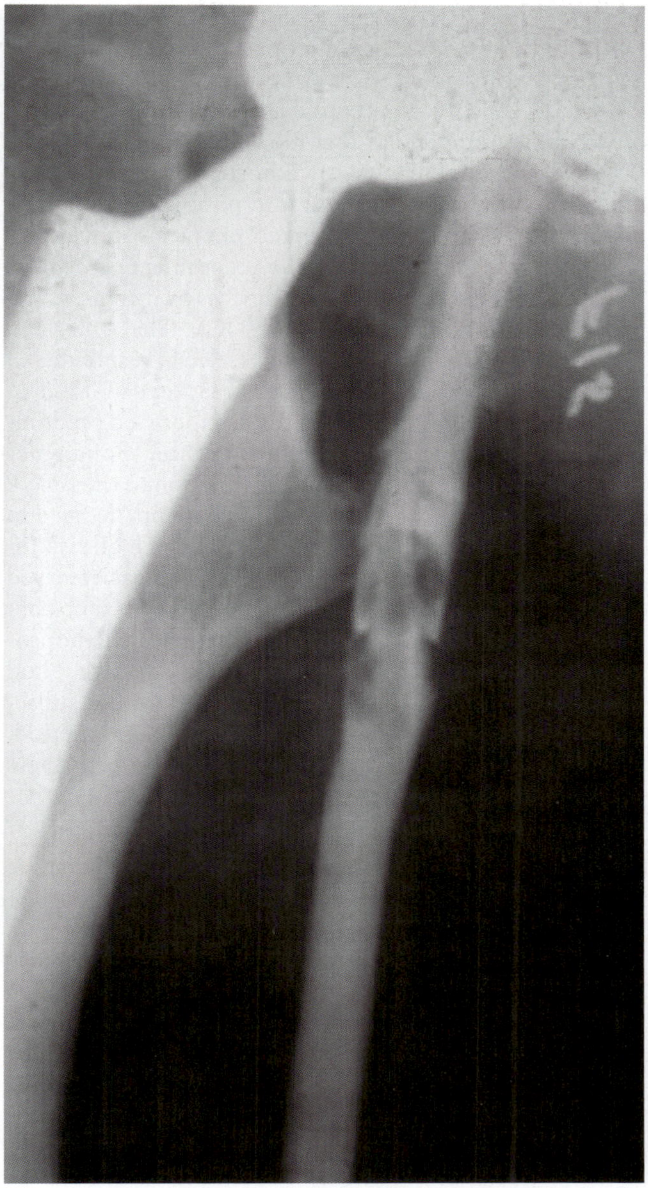

FIGURE 4 Contrast venogram showing discontinuous segmental proximal femoral vein thrombosis at the level of the lesser trochanter after total hip arthroplasty.

reduction of the hip, suggesting transient venous occlusion during the preceding femoral preparation. Kinking of the femoral vein during positioning of the lower limb for canal preparation and component insertion leads to local intimal injury as well as temporary stasis followed by delayed release of embolic medullary contents into the lung, which is thought to be the cause of unique segmental femoral thrombi after THA. Furthermore, because of blood loss and a relative decrease in circulating antithrombin III (ATIII), the intraoperative and postoperative periods represent relatively hypercoagulable states with decreased endogenous fibrinolytic activity.

CURRENT GUIDELINES

Since the last National Institutes of Health–sponsored consensus conference on VTED in 1986, several new potent and highly selective anticoagulant medications have been introduced.[5] Notwithstanding this fact, there has been only modest progress in providing evidence for clinical efficacy of these agents in prevention of fatal PE after THA and TKA. In 1986, prophylaxis was recommended "for high-risk orthopedic patients undergoing elective hip surgery or knee reconstruction…[with] low-dose warfarin, dextran, or adjusted dose-heparin…for at least 7 days." These recommendations quickly became the standard of care in the United States, resulting in an ongoing search for the best agent for routine VTED prophylaxis.

The first notable change in VTED prophylaxis guidelines came in 2008 with the introduction of fractionated heparins, followed by the acceptance of using clinical DVT or PE, rather than asymptomatic venographic DVT, as primary outcomes.[6] The American College of Chest Physicians (ACCP), a perennial authority on VTED prophylaxis, recommended low-molecular-weight heparin (LMWH), fondaparinux, or adjusted-dose vitamin K antagonist (ie, warfarin, goal international normalized ratio [INR] 2 to 3) as preferred chemoprophylaxis.[7] Moreover, the ACCP specifically recommended *against* the use of aspirin or mechanical devices as primary VTE prophylaxis following THA and TKA. The American Academy of Orthopaedic Surgeons (AAOS) responded in the same year with the release of its first set of VTE prophylaxis clinical practice guidelines, supported predominantly by observational studies using clinical outcomes of DVT/PE and death.[8] In contradistinction to the ACCP guidelines, aspirin was endorsed for patients deemed at relatively low, or baseline, risk of VTED and high risk for bleeding complications, whereas warfarin was reserved for patients at unusually high risk for VTED, such that aspirin was thought to provide inadequate chemoprophylaxis. This AAOS recommendation effectively laid the groundwork for the critical interpretation of subsequent observational studies conducted during this period, specifically with respect to the presumed effectiveness of aspirin, which was purposely reserved for patients considered to be at standard or low risk of VTED.[9]

The current guidelines, updated in 2012 with the second AAOS and the ninth ACCP versions, have found commonality in a generic, but nonspecific, recommendation for chemoprophylaxis[10-12] (**Table 1**). The ACCP recommends use of a synthetic, fractionated, or unfractionated heparin; an adjusted-dose vitamin K antagonist (warfarin); a direct oral factor Xa or IIa inhibitor, or aspirin (all grade 1B); and intermittent pneumatic compression devices for a minimum of 10 to 14 days postoperatively. They express a preference for portable compression devices and offer a slight preference for LMWH chemoprophylaxis over other alternatives. The AAOS guidelines likewise offer a moderate-level recommendation for pharmacologic agents and/or mechanical compressive devices for those not at elevated VTE risk, whereas patients who have a history of a VTE are suggested to receive pharmacologic prophylaxis *and* mechanical compressive devices. The AAOS does not endorse any specific chemoprophylaxis agent. Because of the propensity for false-negative studies and the chance of subsequent development of thrombosis, both the AAOS and ACCP recommend strongly against routine postoperative duplex DVT screening.[10]

TABLE 1

Most Recent ACCP (2012)[11] and AAOS (2011)[10,12] Guidelines for VTE Prophylaxis for Patients Undergoing Elective THA or TKA

	Recommendation/Agent	Level of Evidence/Grade of Recommendation	Recommended Duration of Therapy
ACCP	Aspirin	1B	Minimum 10-14 d
	LMWH	1B	Prolong therapy for up to 35 d (grade 2B)
	Low-dose unfractionated heparin	1B	
	Vitamin-K antagonist	1B	
	Apixaban	1B	
	Dabigatran	1B	
	Rivaroxaban	1B	
	Intermittent pneumatic compression	1C	
	Preference for LMWH versus fondaparinux, apixaban, dabigatran, rivaroxaban, low-dose unfractionated heparin	2B	
AAOS	Pharmacologic agents and/or mechanical compressive devices for those not at elevated risk beyond that of the surgery itself for VTE or bleeding	Moderate	No specific recommendation
	Pharmacologic prophylaxis and mechanical compressive devices for those with previous VTE	Consensus	

AAOS = American Academy of Orthopaedic Surgeons, ACCP = American College of Chest Physicians, LMWH = low-molecular-weight heparin, THA = total hip arthroplasty, TKA = total knee arthroplasty, VTE = venous thromboembolism

The Agency for Healthcare Research and Quality also notes a similar indeterminant conclusion for a preferred chemoprophylaxis regimen and calls for future comparative clinical trials to focus on clinically meaningful health outcomes rather than a venographic DVT surrogate. The Joint Commission, Center for Medicare and Medicaid Services, and Surgical Care Improvement Project now all *mandate* routine VTE prophylaxis after THA and TKA according to accepted guidelines.[6] Absent the ideal prophylactic regimen, surgeons are left to balance risk of VTE with the potential for untoward bleeding in each patient and understand the paucity of available data to support stronger recommendations at this time.

PROPHYLAXIS OPTIONS

Mechanical Compression Devices

Although chemoprophylaxis is the predominant focus of VTE prophylaxis, adjunctive use of pneumatic compression devices has been shown to decrease DVT following total joint arthroplasty. These intermittent pneumatic devices are particularly appealing because of their attractive safety profile with minimal adverse impact on postoperative hemostasis. Through local prevention of venous stasis and promotion of endothelium-derived fibrinolysis, calf pneumatic compression devices have demonstrated decreased rates of distal DVT. One prospective randomized trial found that plantar foot compression combined with aspirin reduced proximal DVT after TKA compared with aspirin alone. However, three prior studies comparing pneumatic devices with warfarin after THA revealed a concerning increase in proximal DVT when pneumatic sleeves were used as the sole method of prophylaxis.[13-15] The current body of evidence does not support use of compressive devices alone in most patients, but rather as an adjunct to chemical prophylaxis. Only when the bleeding risk is unacceptably high, do ACCP guidelines support use of pneumatic compression as the sole means of thromboprophylaxis (1A recommendation). They further recommend that chemoprophylaxis be promptly added to, or substituted for, mechanical modalities once the period of elevated bleeding risk has passed.[7]

Newer mobile devices with respiratory synchronization and methods for measuring usage may lead to improved compliance and potentially enhanced efficacy. One observational registry assessing 3,060 nonrandomized and nonconsecutive patients after TKA or THA demonstrated noninferiority relative to reported chemoprophylaxis results. This study was funded by the device manufacturer, did not control for concurrent use of aspirin, and was subject to the vagaries of surgeon selection bias.[16,17] Experience with the patient advisory board of one large ongoing clinical trial suggested use of these devices to not be popular among patients. More research is necessary before mechanical devices can be recommended as sole VTE prophylaxis.

Warfarin

For more than 4 decades, warfarin has been the most commonly used agent for thromboprophylaxis following total joint arthroplasty in the United States, and a 2008 survey revealed a majority of surgeons using warfarin for in-hospital thromboprophylaxis after THA and TKA.[18] Warfarin is an oral vitamin K antagonist that inhibits synthesis of associated procoagulant factors (factors II, VII, IX, and X) and physiologic anticoagulants (proteins C and S) in the liver (**Figure 5**). Its anticoagulant effect lags 48 hours behind initiation of the drug and is readily reversed by administration of fresh frozen plasma or parenteral vitamin K. Proponents of warfarin note its low bleeding risk (1% to 2%) and good efficacy in preventing clinically significant DVT and PE. Alternatively, erratic pharmacokinetics, dietary sensitivity, and the need for routine monitoring have largely fueled the search for alternative anticoagulants for thromboprophylaxis.

Historically, early warfarin studies with a target prothrombin time index of 2.0 or greater reported bleeding rates of 8% to 12%, with occasional life-threatening events. Delayed drug administration and reduction of anticoagulation intensity to a prothrombin time index of 1.3 to 1.5, or an INR of 1.8 to 2.0, reduced the bleeding rate to 1% in subsequent studies.[19,20] Persistent venographic DVT in 9% to 26% after THA and 35% to 55% after TKA, with proximal clot rates of 2% to 5% after THA, and 2% to 14% after TKA, suggest that prevention of DVT has been far more recalcitrant to chemoprophylaxis after TKA than after THA, and warfarin preferentially reduces proximal compared with distal DVT.[21,22]

A recent randomized controlled trial assessing standard (target INR 2.5) and low-intensity (target INR 1.8) warfarin following TKA and THA failed to prove noninferiority of the low-intensity regimen despite a generous noninferiority margin of 3.0%, with lower than expected primary outcome rates that likely resulted in insufficient power to meet noninferiority criteria.[23] Prior studies have shown that continuing low-intensity warfarin (INR 1.5 to 2.0) for 4 to 6 weeks after surgery is an effective method of prophylaxis. One trial of low-intensity warfarin given for 6 weeks postoperatively in THA and TKA *eliminated* the risk of PE (0/844 versus 17/2,449; P = 0.01) and significantly reduced VTE-related readmissions from 1.6% to 0.2% (P = 0.0015).[24-26]

Notwithstanding these favorable results, the prevailing critique of warfarin includes its erratic pharmacokinetics and a need for INR monitoring. Increased bleeding has been reported when combined with nonsteroidal anti-inflammatory medications. One study of 184 THA

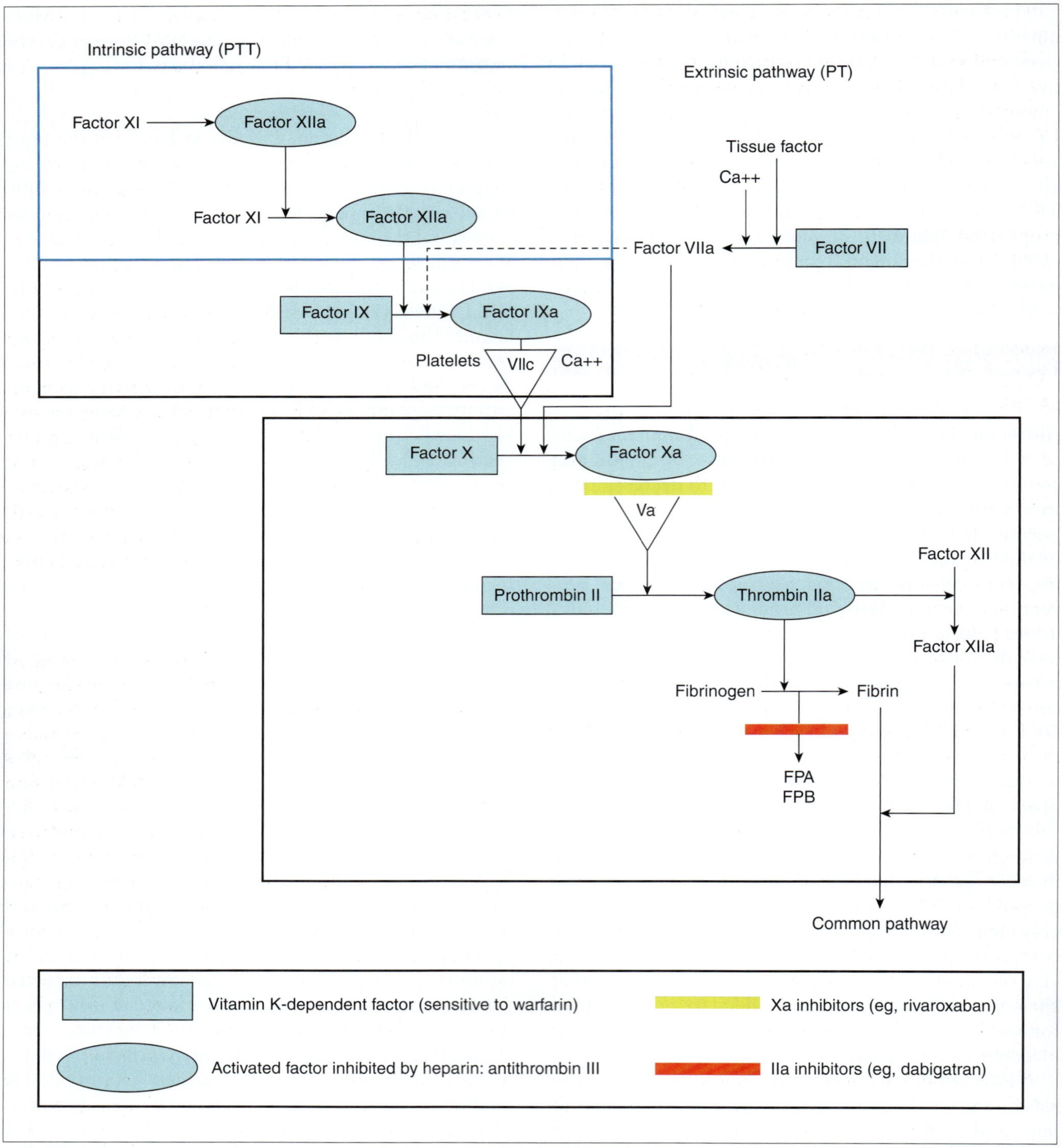

FIGURE 5 Schematic diagram showing the clotting cascade, with critical points of interference by anticoagulant agents. FPA = fibrinopeptide A, FPB = fibrinopeptide B, HMWK = high-molecular-weight kallikrein, KAL = kallikrein. (Adapted with permission from Stead RB: Regulation of hemostasis, in Goldhaber SZ, ed: *Pulmonary Embolism and Deep Venous Thromboembolism*. Philadelphia, PA, WB Saunders, p 32. © Elsevier 1985.)

and TKA patients demonstrated achievement of therapeutic values in only 54.4% with a target INR of 1.7 to 2.7, and even less frequently with a target INR of 2.0 to 3.0.[27] Cost-effectiveness analysis has estimated the adjusted 2013 monthly cost for warfarin, inclusive of monitoring, at $80.78; aspirin had more quality-adjusted life years saved in all age groups assessed.[28]

Heparinoids

Unfractionated heparin (UFH) is naturally occurring in mammalian tissues and consists of glycosaminoglycans with a molecular weight ranging from 3,000 to 40,000 d. LMWH (fractionated heparin) has a molecular weight ranging from 3,000 to 15,000 d (average, 5,000 d). All heparins contain a five-sugar moiety that binds to ATIII and initiates steric transformation of a second ATIII binding site that mates with either factor X or factor II (thrombin). Because of this reliance on ATIII to exert an effect, heparinoids lack any intrinsic fibrinolytic properties. UFH binds reversibly and nonspecifically with factor II and factor X. Unlike UFH, LMWH has a much greater affinity for factor X because of its smaller size and better exposed binding site. Because of the upstream position of factor X in the clotting cascade compared with thrombin, LMWH has a more potent anticoagulant effect than UFH (**Figure 5**). Finally, fondaparinux is a synthetic five-sugar molecule that has specific and singular affinity for the binding site on factor X and, hence, is the most specific in action of all the heparinoids.

Fractionated heparins are given by injection and do not require monitoring; they have less antiplatelet effect and are less bound by plasma proteins than UFH. This translates to a 10-fold reduction in the risk of heparin-induced thrombocytopenia (prevalence of 0.2%) and a nearly threefold increase in bioavailability. Peak plasma concentrations are reached within 90 minutes of administration, with a half-life of 4 to 6 hours and ultimate excretion by the kidneys.

Fractionated heparins have demonstrated efficacy in reducing venographic thrombosis; however, they are associated with a considerably increased risk of perioperative bleeding.[29,30] One comparison of dalteparin with warfarin (INR 2.0 to 3.0) in 406 THA patients demonstrated decreased venographic DVT and comparable symptomatic PE rates with dalteparin, but with more bleeding ($P = 0.03$) and an increased rate of postoperative transfusion ($P = 0.001$).[31] Another study of LMWH after THA and TKA demonstrated a threefold increase in return to the operating room for wound complications and hematoma drainage compared with a prior study with warfarin.[32] Finally, two dalteparin regimens (beginning 2 hours before or 4 hours after surgery) were compared with warfarin (INR 2.0 to 3.0) in 1,472 THA patients, with only the preoperative heparin regimen resulting in a reduced rate of symptomatic DVT compared with warfarin (1.5% versus 4.4%; $P = 0.02$), but preoperative dalteparin produced a twofold greater frequency of major (8.9% versus 4.5%, $P = 0.01$) and surgical site bleeding events (8.3% versus 3.9%, $P = 0.03$).[33]

Fondaparinux produces irreversible inhibition of activated factor X (factor Xa). Several studies have shown a greater than 50% reduction in overall venographic DVT after THA, TKA, and hip fracture repair compared with enoxaparin.[34-36] After elective TKA, DVT was reduced to 12.5% with 2.5 mg of fondaparinux compared with 28% with LMWH (enoxaparin 30 mg twice daily), but was accompanied by a bleeding rate of 3% to 6%, exceeding even the rates associated with LMWH. In one THA study, patients receiving enoxaparin were compared with five different dosing regimens of fondaparinux; the 6.0 and 8.0 mg daily dosing groups were suspended because of unacceptably high bleeding (up to 12%).[35] Although LMWH and fondaparinux convincingly reduce clinical and venographic VTED, routine use of these agents is associated with an increase in frequency of bleeding complications, particularly those related to the surgical wound.

Aspirin

Aspirin recommendations have undergone some of the most dramatic changes in all the guidelines since the initial 1986 National Institutes of Health Consensus Conference concluded that aspirin has not been shown to be beneficial in VTE prophylaxis.[5] This statement cited conflicting data with inconsistent methodology and longstanding conventional wisdom that aspirin was an arterial agent ineffective on the venous side of the circulation. However, in the 1990s, there was a resurgence of enthusiasm for aspirin in orthopaedics, largely because of its better safety profile and lower bleeding risk compared with fractionated heparins introduced during the same period. By 2010, absent any new clinical data for VTED, almost 15% of orthopaedic surgeons used aspirin for inpatient and 35% preferred it for extended prophylaxis after discharge following THA or TKA.[18,37]

Aspirin is an irreversible inhibitor of platelet cyclooxygenase (COX) through acetylation of the serine in COX-1 and COX-2, although its affinity for COX-2 is 170 times lower than that of COX-1. Inhibition of COX-1 decreases synthesis of thromboxane A2 (platelet-activating eicosanoid) and related platelet activation and has demonstrated substantial reduction in arterial thrombotic events as well as survival benefit from stroke and myocardial infarction in high-risk patients.[38,39] Although present in smaller proportions, platelets in venous thrombi have the potential to release proinflammatory mediators and lead to generation of DNA-histone-granule constituent complexes that induce further platelet aggregation.[38] Although the exact mechanism of aspirin on these processes in the venous circulation is not known, the extended use of aspirin following initial treatment of unprovoked DVT or PE with a conventional anticoagulant regimen has been shown to decrease the risk of recurrent VTE by about one-third.[40,41]

Since 2006, observational data from three large single-center studies and a national joint replacement registry have resurrected enthusiasm and provided credence to the belief that aspirin may be an effective agent for prevention of clinically evident PE after total joint arthroplasty, particularly when used in conjunction with regional anesthesia.[42-45] In nearly 2,000 THA patients who have hypotensive epidural anesthesia, and intravenous heparin during femoral preparation combined with in-hospital pneumatic compression followed by 6 weeks of aspirin (325 mg twice daily) or low-intensity warfarin (in 18% of patients deemed to be high risk), overall VTED-related readmission was 3.2% with a PE rate of 0.6% (9/1,599 patients on aspirin, 3/348 patients on warfarin) and no fatal PE.[42] A similar study in more than 3,400 TKA patients who had regional anesthesia continued for 36 hours followed by aspirin (325 mg twice daily for 6 weeks) found overall VTED-related readmission of 0.5% with a clinical PE rate of 0.26% and fatal PE in 0.1%.[43] Only 2% of the patients were considered to be high risk and received warfarin or LMWH instead of aspirin. In a matched cohort propensity analysis of 22,942 patients receiving aspirin or fractionated heparin, there was no difference in 90-day outcomes related to DVT, clinical PE, stroke or gastrointestinal bleeding, or revision surgery.[45] However, there was an all-cause mortality survival benefit with fractionated heparin (0.49% versus 0.65%, relative risk = 0.75, $P = 0.02$).

One notable catalyst for change in the ninth ACCP clinical practice guidelines for thromboprophylaxis after THA and TKA came from reexamination of the Pulmonary Embolism Prevention trial data from 1992 to 1998.[11] The original interpretation in 2000 suggested that aspirin (160 mg daily for 35 days) effected a one-third reduction in overall incidence of PE and DVT compared with placebo (2.3% versus 1.6%, $P = 0.003$) after hip fracture, but no difference was apparent in overall PE-DVT or mortality in arthroplasty patients. This initial interpretation also called out critical methodologic weaknesses including failure to standardize anesthetic type, the supplementary use of fractionated heparin prophylaxis in over one-third of patients, and the commingling of dissimilar fracture and arthroplasty patients. In 2012, reexamination of the study as a pragmatic trial for comparative clinical effectiveness endorsed an overall 19% reduction (1.15% versus 1.4%) in aggregate VTE end points in elective THA and TKA patients.[11]

Although recent studies have advocated for aspirin as an effective VTE prophylaxis agent with increasing enthusiasm, the observational nature of these reports shares a common critical flaw in the selection bias of the surgeon. Because of prevailing AAOS recommendations since 2008 that endorsed risk stratification of patients, only those perceived to be at lowest risk of VTED (eg, without personal history of prior VTE, active cancer diagnosis, or coagulopathy) received aspirin prophylaxis. Therefore, observational databases from this period reflect an inherent selection bias that favors demonstration of lower VTED event rates in patients receiving aspirin prophylaxis.[6] A recent report of 41,537 primary TKA procedures from 29 institutions in the Michigan Arthroplasty Collaborative claimed noninferiority of aspirin VTED prophylaxis, with a margin of 0.3, compared with other classic anticoagulants (LMWH, warfarin, and Xa inhibitors).[46] However, only 30.9% of patients received aspirin prophylaxis alone and 13% received aspirin in combination with an anticoagulant. Overall, less than 44% of patients received aspirin, suggesting a very strong underlying surgeon selection bias. One retrospective review of over 30,000 patients undergoing primary THA or TKA compared aspirin with nonaspirin prophylaxis and demonstrated an almost five times lower risk of cardiac-related death and an overall lower risk of death at 30 days and 1 year in the aspirin group.[47] Only 25.9% of patients received aspirin therapy alone in this series. Another nonconsecutive nonrandomized series of patients undergoing THA or TKA found 81 mg to be noninferior to 325 mg as VTED prophylaxis with a 0.25% noninferiority margin. This work was similarly limited by surgeon bias as patients deemed to be at high risk by the surgeon were excluded from the aspirin protocol.[48] Parenthetically, related literature outside of orthopaedics has shown that higher doses of aspirin (325 to 650 mg daily) are not superior to lower dose aspirin (50 to 100 mg daily) in preventing cerebrovascular events or acute coronary syndrome.[49]

Notwithstanding these favorable observational reports regarding aspirin for VTED prophylaxis after THA and TKA, two *prospective* trials have raised serious concerns about its effectiveness and safety. One randomized trial using AAOS risk stratification to guide aspirin or warfarin prophylaxis was stopped early because of a ninefold increase in PE risk and a sevenfold increase in VTED in the standard risk group receiving aspirin.[50] Another noninferiority trial randomized 1,804 THA and 1,620 TKA patients to receive either aspirin or rivaroxaban after all had received 5 days of rivaroxaban from the time of surgery.[51] Although not adequately powered to detect differences in the groups, the data showed 90-day VTE events to be similar, but the relative risk of major bleeding was 1.6-fold greater in the aspirin than the rivaroxaban

group (0.47% versus 0.29%; $P = 0.42$). Collectively, the data from observational reports are substantially flawed in favor of aspirin because of a selection bias defined by prevailing clinical guidelines, and the available prospective series do not provide sufficiently compelling evidence to endorse broad adoption of aspirin as the sole VTED prophylaxis after THA and TKA at this time. Such clinical equipoise leaves us to seek prospective randomized data to more definitively establish any role for aspirin in orthopaedic VTED prophylaxis.[9]

Direct Oral Anticoagulants

The introduction of direct factor X and II inhibitors represents an appealing opportunity for anticoagulation with oral administration and no need for routine monitoring (**Figure 5**). Of the direct oral anticoagulants, the Xa inhibitor, rivaroxaban, has been the most extensively studied following THA and TKA. Four randomized clinical trials (RECORD 1-4), with similar methodology and a primary efficacy outcome of composite DVT, either symptomatic or detected by mandatory bilateral venography performed at the conclusion of anticoagulant therapy, nonfatal PE, and death from any cause at 30 to 42 days, have compared rivaroxaban with LMWH in patients following THA[52,53] or TKA[54] (**Table 2**). In all four trials, the rivaroxaban dose was 10 mg daily (starting 6 to 8 hours *after* surgery), and in RECORD 1-3 the enoxaparin dose was 40 mg daily (starting 12 hours *before* surgery), whereas in RECORD 4 the enoxaparin dose was 30 mg twice daily (bid) starting 12 hours *after* surgery as practiced in North America. In RECORD-1, a total of 4,541 patients were randomized to 10 mg of oral rivaroxaban daily or 40 mg of enoxaparin subcutaneously daily for 35 days.[53] The primary efficacy outcome occurred in 1.1% of the rivaroxaban group and 3.7% of the enoxaparin group (absolute risk reduction, 2.6%; CI 1.5 to 3.7; $P < 0.001$). Major venous thromboembolism occurred in 0.2% of the rivaroxaban group and 2.0% of the enoxaparin group (absolute risk reduction, 1.7%; CI 1.0 to 2.5; $P < 0.001$), and major bleeding was not significantly different between the groups (0.3% rivaroxaban, 0.1% enoxaparin; $P = 0.18$). RECORD-2 compared THA patients assigned to receive extended oral rivaroxaban 10 mg once daily (for 31 to 39 days) versus enoxaparin 40 mg once daily subcutaneously for 10 to 14 days.[52] The primary outcome occurred in 2.0% in the rivaroxaban group compared with 9.3% in the enoxaparin group (absolute risk reduction 7.3%; CI 5.2 to 9.4; $P < 0.0001$), with no between-group differences in any on-treatment bleeding events. An important limitation of this study was the inability to obtain valid venograms in over a quarter of the patients in each group as well as the lack of power to assess bleeding risk. Similar results were seen in TKA patients receiving oral rivaroxaban compared with LMWH. In RECORD-3 involving 2,531 TKA patients receiving either rivaroxaban or enoxaparin for 12 days, the primary efficacy outcome occurred in 9.6% in the rivaroxaban group compared with 18.9% in the enoxaparin group (absolute risk reduction, 9.2%; CI 5.9 to 12.4; $P < 0.001$) and major bleeding was again similar between groups (0.6% with rivaroxaban versus 0.5% with enoxaparin).[55] Finally, in RECORD-4, the enoxaparin dosing followed the North American protocol of 30 mg bid and both groups received anticoagulation for 12 days. The rivaroxaban group exhibited a reduction in the primary efficacy outcome (6.9% versus 10.1%; absolute risk reduction 3.2%; $P = 0.012$), and rates of major and clinically relevant bleeding were similar between groups (rivaroxaban 3.0% versus enoxaparin 2.3%; $P = 0.179$).[54]

Pooled analysis of the four methodologically similar RECORD trials, including 7,050 THA and 5,679 TKA patients, revealed a 58% reduction in all-cause mortality and symptomatic VTE with rivaroxaban versus enoxaparin (0.6% versus 1.3%; $P < 0.001$), but aggregate bleeding data revealed a worrisome increase in major plus

TABLE 2

Summary of RECORD 1-4 Trial Designs

	Number of Patients	Procedure	Enoxaparin Dosing	Rivaroxaban Dosing
RECORD 1	4,541	THA	40 mg daily starting 12 hr before surgery	10 mg daily starting 6-8 hr after surgery
RECORD 2	2,509	THA	40 mg daily starting 12 hr before surgery	10 mg daily starting 6-8 hr after surgery
RECORD 3	2,531	TKA	40 mg daily starting 12 hr before surgery	10 mg daily starting 6-8 hr after surgery
RECORD 4	3,148	TKA	30 mg bid starting 12 hr after surgery[a]	10 mg daily starting 6-8 hr after surgery

hr = hours, bid = twice daily, THA = total hip arthroplasty, TKA = total knee arthroplasty
[a]Per North American protocol.

clinically relevant nonmajor bleeding events (3.2% versus 2.6%; CI 1.02 to 1.54; $P = 0.039$).[52-56] Importantly, the analysis of bleeding did not account for surgical bleeding and has been under scrutiny for deviating from accepted definitions of bleeding.[57] It is also noteworthy that only RECORD-1 and RECORD-4 trials are applicable to practice guidelines in the North America; considering only these two studies, the aggregate increase in bleeding risk exceeded the reduction in symptomatic VTED with rivaroxaban compared with enoxaparin, and a higher risk of ischemic and cardiovascular events were noted on discontinuation of the treatment regimen with rivaroxaban.[57] Similarly, there have been a number of retrospective studies assessing rivaroxaban in hip and knee arthroplasty, challenged by all of the attendant limitations of such reports that have highlighted an increased bleeding risk with rivaroxaban, including more than double the risk of any reportable postoperative bleeding and more than triple the risk of conventionally defined major bleeding.[58-60]

Apixaban, another direct oral Xa inhibitor, and dabigatran, an oral direct factor II (thrombin) inhibitor, have been less extensively studied in orthopaedic patients but demonstrate comparable efficacy to fractionated heparins with the advantage of an oral preparation.[61-65]

ROLE OF ANESTHESIA

Early studies noted a decreased incidence of VTED in patients managed with epidural or spinal anesthesia compared with general anesthesia.[66] A variety of mechanisms have been proposed, including inhibition of platelet and leukocyte adhesion as well as promotion of endothelial fibrinolysis, although these have not been substantiated in controlled studies. Alternatively, a more important influence of epidural anesthesia is likely its effect on the sympathetic nervous system, resulting in reduced vascular tone and increased lower extremity blood flow intraoperatively and postoperatively, which mitigates the effects of stasis. A 2009 meta-analysis of 21 studies comparing regional and general anesthesia in THA and TKA noted significant reduction in DVT and PE of approximately 50% with regional anesthesia.[67] Importantly, the regional anesthesia group was noted to have significantly lower blood pressure, and subgroup analysis demonstrated elimination of the previously noted difference when this confounder was excluded.[67] It is also important to note the heterogeneity of concomitant chemoprophylaxis agents used in a majority of studies assessing regional anesthesia. A study of warfarin combined with prolonged epidural anesthesia/analgesia for 48 hours reported an overall venographic DVT rate of less than 10%, with proximal thrombi in 2.3% of patients.[68] Similarly, the combination of aspirin and regional anesthesia has been observed to decrease VTE clinical events (specifically, clinical PE) after THA as well as TKA.[42,44,66,68,69] Current evidence suggests an important, although not completely understood, role of regional anesthesia in the multimodal approach to VTED prevention.

SUMMARY

A thorough understanding of the pathophysiology of clot formation as well as the available chemoprophylaxis options is critical to managing orthopaedic arthroplasty patients. Although high-quality data comparing thromboprophylaxis options are lacking, orthopaedic surgeons are best positioned to exercise the clinical judgment necessary to balance the risks of venous thromboembolism with those of perioperative bleeding. Currently, the need for chemoprophylaxis has been established, but no single agent has prevailed in terms of efficacy in preventing clinically important VTED while offering an acceptable safety profile with low bleeding risk. Such clinical equipoise leaves us to seek prospective randomized data to more definitively establish appropriate regimens for orthopaedic VTED prophylaxis.

KEY STUDY POINTS

- The pathophysiology and anatomic distribution of DVT following TKA and THA differ, likely related to intraoperative manipulation resulting in torsion, stasis, and intimal injury, with predominantly distal clots after TKA and proximal femoral vein clots following THA.
- Although initial studies, particularly those guiding early recommendations, used venographic end points to define outcomes for VTED, recent research has focused on more meaningful clinical outcome measures including readmission, symptomatic DVT/PE, or fatal PE.
- Warfarin has remained a mainstay of VTE prophylaxis in the United States likely because of its historically favorable bleeding risk profile, suspected secondary to its delayed onset of action until after the period of greatest perioperative bleeding risk has passed.
- Aspirin has increasingly gained popularity for use as thromboprophylaxis because of its ease of administration and more recent observational studies demonstrating comparable efficacy in reducing VTED rates, although current data are limited by inherent selection bias secondary to prevailing contemporary guidelines.
- Current clinical practice guidelines from AAOS and ACCP acknowledge the need for active intervention and chemoprophylaxis in preventing VTE after THA and TKA, but the scarcity of high-quality outcome data from randomized clinical trials has led to the lack of endorsement of any specific regimen.

ANNOTATED REFERENCES

1. Johnson DJ, Hartwell MJ, Weiner JA, Hardt KD, Manning DW: Which postoperative day after total joint arthroplasty are catastrophic events most likely to occur? *J Arthroplasty* 2019;34(10):2466-2472.

   This retrospective query of a large database registry reports on the incidence as well as timing of four major postoperative outcomes (PE, myocardial infarction or cardiac arrest, cerebrovascular accident, and death) in patients undergoing primary total joint arthroplasty. Level of evidence: III.

2. Stulberg BN, Insall JN, Williams GW, Ghelman B: Deep-vein thrombosis following total knee replacement. An analysis of six hundred and thirty-eight arthroplasties. *J Bone Joint Surg Am* 1984;66(2):194-201.

3. Zan P, Mol MO, Yao JJ, et al: Release of the tourniquet immediately after the implantation of the components reduces the incidence of deep vein thrombosis after primary total knee arthroplasty. *Bone Joint Res* 2017;6(9):535-541.

   The authors prospectively enrolled 200 patients undergoing TKA with tourniquet inflation before incision and deflation after introduction of the components. Outcomes from these patients were compared with retrospectively collected outcomes of patients who underwent TKA with tourniquet inflation before incision, but deflation after application of dressings. Early release of the tourniquet was associated with lower incidence of DVT (4.6% compared with 12% with late release; odds ratio [OR] 0.35, 95% confidence interval [CI] 0.16 to 0.78, $P = 0.008$), although none of the patients received chemoprophylaxis. Level of evidence: II.

4. Sharrock NE, Go G, Harpel PC, Ranawat CS, Sculco TP, Salvati EA: The John Charnley Award. Thrombogenesis during total hip arthroplasty. *Clin Orthop Relat Res* 1995;319:16-27.

5. Prevention of venous thrombosis and pulmonary embolism. *Natl Inst Health Consens Dev Conf Consens Statement* 1986;6(2):1-8.

6. Pellegrini VD: Prophylaxis against venous thromboembolism after total hip and knee arthroplasty: A critical analysis review. *JBJS Rev* 2015;3(9):01874474-201509000-00005.

7. Geerts WH, Bergqvist D, Pineo GF, et al: Prevention of venous thromboembolism: American College of Chest Physicians Evidence-Based Clinical Practice Guidelines (8th edition). *Chest* 2008;133(6 suppl):381S-453S.

8. American Academy of Orthopaedic Surgeons: *American Academy of Orthopaedic Surgeons: Clinical Guideline on Prevention of Symptomatic Pulmonary Embolism in Patients Undergoing Total Hip or Knee Arthroplasty*. Rosemont, IL, American Academy of Orthopaedic Surgeons, 2007.

9. Pellegrini V, Eikelboom J, Franklin P, et al: Selection bias, orthopaedic style: Knowing what we don't know about aspirin. *J Bone Joint Surg Am* 2020;102(7):631-633.

   This article on behalf of the Steering Committee of the PEPPER (Pulmonary Embolism Prevention after Hip and Knee Replacement) trial reviews prior studies regarding aspirin use after hip and knee arthroplasty and highlights the lack of critical data from high-quality studies to support aspirin as a superior VTED prophylactic agent. The authors note that while aspirin has been quickly adopted among the orthopedic community, large comparative effectiveness studies are lacking. They suggest that the PEPPER trial will help to elucidate the role of aspirin in relation to other VTED prophylactic agents. Level of evidence: V.

10. Mont MA, Jacobs JJ: AAOS Clinical Practice Guideline: Preventing venous thromboembolic disease in patients undergoing elective hip and knee arthroplasty. *J Am Acad Orthop Surg* 2011;19(12):777-778.

11. Falck-Ytter Y, Francis CW, Johanson NA, et al: Prevention of VTE in orthopedic surgery patients. Antithrombotic Therapy and Prevention of Thrombosis, 9th ed: American College of Chest Physicians Evidence-Based Clinical Practice Guidelines. *Chest* 2012;141(2 suppl):e278S-e325S.

12. American Academy of Orthopaedic Surgeons: *American Academy of Orthopaedic Surgeons: Clinical Guideline on Preventing Venous Thromboembolic Disease in Patients Undergoing Elective Hip and Knee Arthroplasty*. Rosemont, IL, American Academy of Orthopaedic Surgeons, 2011.

13. Francis CW, Pellegrini VD, Marder VJ, et al: Comparison of warfarin and external pneumatic compression in prevention of venous thrombosis after total hip replacement. *J Am Med Assoc* 1992;267(21):2911-2915.

14. Paiement G, Wessinger SJ, Waltman AC, Harris WH: Low-dose warfarin versus external pneumatic compression for prophylaxis against venous thromboembolism following total hip replacement. *J Arthroplasty* 1987;2(1):23-26.

15. Kaempffe FA, Lifeso RM, Meinking C: Intermittent pneumatic compression versus coumadin. Prevention of deep vein thrombosis in lower-extremity total joint arthroplasty. *Clin Orthop Relat Res* 1991;269:89-97.

16. Colwell CW, Froimson MI, Anseth SD, et al: A mobile compression device for thrombosis prevention in hip and knee arthroplasty. *J Bone Joint Surg Am* 2014;96(3):177-183.

17. Colwell CW, Froimson MI, Mont MA, et al: Thrombosis prevention after total hip arthroplasty: A prospective, randomized trial comparing a mobile compression device with low-molecular-weight heparin. *J Bone Joint Surg Am* 2010;92(3):527-535.

18. Markel DC, York S, Liston MJ, et al: Venous thromboembolism: Management by American Association of Hip and Knee Surgeons. *J Arthroplasty* 2010;25(1):3-9.e1-e2.

19. Coventry MB, Nolan DR, Beckenbaugh RD: 'Delayed' prophylactic anticoagulation: A study of results and complications in 2,012 total hip arthroplasties. *J Bone Joint Surg Am* 1973;55(7):1487-1492.

20. Hirsh J: Optimal intensity and monitoring warfarin. *Am J Cardiol* 1995;75(6):39B-42B.

21. Pellegrini VD, Langhans MJ, Totterman S, Marder VJ, Francis CW: Embolic complications of calf thrombosis following total hip arthroplasty. *J Arthroplasty* 1993;8(5):449-457.

22. Pellegrini VD, Sharrock NE, Paiement GD, Morris R, Warwick DJ: Venous thromboembolic disease after total hip and knee arthroplasty: Current perspectives in a regulated environment. *Instr Course Lect* 2008;57:637-661.

23. Gage BF, Bass AR, Lin H, et al: Effect of low-intensity vs standard-intensity warfarin prophylaxis on venous thromboembolism or death among patients undergoing hip or knee arthroplasty: A randomized clinical trial. *J Am Med Assoc* 2019;322(9):834-842.

This study is a randomized controlled trial comparing warfarin administration in patients who underwent THA and TKA with INR goal of 1.8 compared with 2.5. Perhaps underpowered, the study demonstrated low-intensity INR goal did not meet the noninferiority criterion for composite VTE or death. Level of evidence: I.

24. Pellegrini VD, Donaldson CT, Farber DC, Lehman EB, Evarts CM: The John Charnley Award: Prevention of readmission for venous thromboembolic disease after total hip arthroplasty. *Clin Ortho Relat Res* 2005;441:56-62.

25. Pellegrini VD, Clement D, Lush-Ehmann C, Keller GS, Evarts CM: The John Charnley Award. Natural history of thromboembolic disease after total hip arthroplasty. *Clin Orthop Relat Res* 1996;333:27-40.

26. Pellegrini VD, Donaldson CT, Farber DC, Lehman EB, Evarts CM: The Mark Coventry Award: Prevention of readmission for venous thromboembolism after total knee arthroplasty. *Clin Orthop Relat Res* 2006;452:21-27.

27. Nam D, Sadhu A, Hirsh J, Keeney JA, Nunley RM, Barrack RL: The use of warfarin for DVT prophylaxis following hip and knee arthroplasty: How often are patients within their target INR range? *J Arthroplasty* 2015;30(2):315-319.

28. Mostafavi Tabatabaee R, Rasouli MR, Maltenfort MG, Parvizi J: Cost-effective prophylaxis against venous thromboembolism after total joint arthroplasty: Warfarin versus aspirin. *J Arthroplasty* 2015;30(2):159-164.

29. Planes A, Vochelle N, Darmon JY, Fagola M, Bellaud M, Huet Y: Risk of deep-venous thrombosis after hospital discharge in patients having undergone total hip replacement: Double-blind randomised comparison of enoxaparin versus placebo. *Lancet* 1996;348(9022):224-228.

30. Bergqvist D, Benoni G, Björgell O, et al: Low-molecular-weight heparin (enoxaparin) as prophylaxis against venous thromboembolism after total hip replacement. *N Engl J Med* 1996;335(10):696-700.

31. Francis CW, Pellegrini VD, Totterman S, et al: Prevention of deep-vein thrombosis after total hip arthroplasty. Comparison of warfarin and dalteparin. *J Bone Joint Surg Am* 1997;79(9):1365-1372.

32. Burnett RSJ, Clohisy JC, Wright RW, et al: Failure of the American College of Chest Physicians-1A protocol for Lovenox in clinical outcomes for thromboembolic prophylaxis. *J Arthroplasty* 2007;22(3):317-324.

33. Hull RD: Low-molecular-weight heparin prophylaxis using dalteparin in closeness, proximity to surgery vs warfarin in hip arthroplasty patients: A double-blind, randomized comparison. *Arch Intern Med* 2000;160(14):2199-2207.

34. Bauer KA, Eriksson BI, Lassen MR, Turpie AG, Steering Committee of the Pentasaccharide in Major Knee Surgery Study: Fondaparinux compared with enoxaparin for the prevention of venous thromboembolism after elective major knee surgery. *N Engl J Med* 2001;345(18):1305-1310.

35. Turpie AGG, Gallus AS, Hoek JA, Pentasaccharide Investigators: A synthetic pentasaccharide for the prevention of deep-vein thrombosis after total hip replacement. *N Engl J Med* 2001;344(9):619-625.

36. Eriksson BI, Bauer KA, Lassen MR, Turpie AG, Steering Committee of the Pentasaccharide in Hip-Fracture Surgery Study: Fondaparinux compared with enoxaparin for the prevention of venous thromboembolism after hip-fracture surgery. *N Engl J Med* 2001;345(18):1298-1304.

37. Anderson FA, Huang W, Friedman RJ, Kwong LM, Lieberman JR, Pellegrini VD, Orthopaedic Surgeon's Survey Steering Committee: Prevention of venous thromboembolism after hip or knee arthroplasty: Findings from a 2008 survey of US Orthopedic Surgeons. *J Arthroplasty* 2012;27(5):659-666.e5.

38. Becker RC: Aspirin and the prevention of venous thromboembolism. *N Engl J Med* 2012;366(21):2028-2030.

39. Warkentin TE: Aspirin for dual prevention of venous and arterial thrombosis. *N Engl J Med* 2012;367(21):2039-2041.

40. Simes J, Becattini C, Agnelli G, et al, INSPIRE Study Investigators (International Collaboration of Aspirin Trials for Recurrent Venous Thromboembolism): Aspirin for the prevention of recurrent venous thromboembolism: The INSPIRE collaboration. *Circulation* 2014;130(13):1062-1071.

41. Brighton TA, Eikelboom JW, Mann K, et al, ASPIRE Investigators: Low-dose aspirin for preventing recurrent venous thromboembolism. *N Engl J Med* 2012;367(21):1979-1987.

42. Della Valle AG, Serota A, Go G, et al: Venous thromboembolism is rare with a multimodal prophylaxis protocol after total hip arthroplasty. *Clin Orthop Relat Res* 2006;443:146-153.

43. Lotke PA, Lonner JH: The benefit of aspirin chemoprophylaxis for thromboembolism after total knee arthroplasty. *Clin Orthop Relat Res* 2006;452:175-180.

44. Cusick LA, Beverland DE: The incidence of fatal pulmonary embolism after primary hip and knee replacement in a consecutive series of 4253 patients. *J Bone Joint Surg Br* 2009;91(5):645-648.

45. Jameson SS, Charman SC, Gregg PJ, Reed MR, van der Meulen JH: The effect of aspirin and low-molecular-weight heparin on venous thromboembolism after hip replacement: A non-randomised comparison from information in the National Joint Registry. *J Bone Joint Surg Br* 2011;93(11):1465-1470.

46. Hood BR, Cowen ME, Zheng HT, Hughes RE, Singal B, Hallstrom BR: Association of aspirin with prevention of venous thromboembolism in patients after total knee arthroplasty compared with other anticoagulants: A noninferiority analysis. *JAMA Surg* 2019;154(1):65-72.

This is an observational report of 41,537 primary TKA procedures from 29 institutions in the Michigan Arthroplasty Collaborative. This study claimed noninferiority of aspirin VTED prophylaxis, with a margin of 0.3, compared with other classic anticoagulants (LMWH, warfarin, and Xa inhibitors). However, overall, less than 44% of patients in the collaborative received aspirin, suggesting a very strong underlying surgeon selection bias with only a minority of patients considered of sufficiently low risk. Level of evidence: III.

47. Rondon AJ, Shohat N, Tan TL, Goswami K, Huang RC, Parvizi J: The use of aspirin for prophylaxis against venous thromboembolism decreases mortality following primary total joint arthroplasty. *J Bone Joint Surg Am* 2019;101(6):504-513.

    This retrospective review of over 31,133 patients undergoing primary THA or TKA receiving either aspirin or nonaspirin prophylaxis demonstrated an almost five times lower risk of cardiac-related death in the aspirin group as well as an overall lower risk of death at 30 days and 1 year. However, only 25.9% of patients received aspirin therapy alone in this series, suggesting potential selection bias for patients deemed to be at relatively low VTED risk. Level of evidence: III.

48. Parvizi J, Huang R, Restrepo C, et al: Low-dose aspirin is effective chemoprophylaxis against clinically important venous thromboembolism following total joint arthroplasty: A preliminary analysis. *J Bone Joint Surg Am* 2017;99(2):91-98.

    In this prospective, nonconsecutive nonrandomized study of patients undergoing THA or TKA, 81 mg aspirin dosing was found to be noninferior to 325 mg as VTED prophylaxis with a 0.25% noninferiority margin. Of note, patients deemed to be at high risk by the surgeon were excluded from the aspirin protocol. Level of evidence: II.

49. Hart RG, Harrison MJ: Aspirin wars: The optimal dose of aspirin prevent stroke. *Stroke* 1996;27(4):585-587.

50. Intermountain Joint Replacement Center Writing Committee: A prospective comparison of warfarin to aspirin for thromboprophylaxis in total hip and total knee arthroplasty. *J Arthroplasty* 2012;27(1):1-9.e2.

51. Anderson DR, Dunbar M, Murnaghan J, et al: Aspirin or rivaroxaban for VTE prophylaxis after hip or knee arthroplasty. *N Engl J Med* 2018;378(8):699-707.

    This noninferiority trial of 1,804 THA and 1,620 TKA procedures from 15 centers in Canada randomized patients from January 2013 through April 2016 to receive either aspirin or rivaroxaban for VTED prophylaxis, following all patients receiving 5 days of rivaroxaban from the time of surgery. Analysis of incidence of postoperative DVT and PE found aspirin to be noninferior ($P < 0.001$) but not superior ($P = 0.84$) to rivaroxaban. Although not powered to detect differences, data showed relative risk of a major bleeding event was actually 1.6-fold greater in the aspirin than the rivaroxaban group (0.47% versus 0.29%; $P = 0.42$). Level of evidence: I.

52. Kakkar AK, Brenner B, Dahl OE, et al, RECORD2 Investigators: Extended duration rivaroxaban versus short-term enoxaparin for the prevention of venous thromboembolism after total hip arthroplasty: A double-blind, randomised controlled trial. *Lancet* 2008;372(9632):31-39.

53. Eriksson BI, Borris LC, Friedman RJ, et al, RECORD1 Study Group: Rivaroxaban versus enoxaparin for thromboprophylaxis after hip arthroplasty. *N Engl J Med* 2008;358(26):2765-2775.

54. Turpie AG, Lassen MR, Davidson BL, et al, RECORD4 Investigators: Rivaroxaban versus enoxaparin for thromboprophylaxis after total knee arthroplasty (RECORD4): A randomised trial. *Lancet* 2009;373(9676):1673-1680.

55. Lassen MR, Ageno W, Borris LC, et al, RECORD3 Investigators: Rivaroxaban versus enoxaparin for thromboprophylaxis after total knee arthroplasty. *N Engl J Med* 2008;358(26):2776-2786.

56. Turpie A, Lassen MR, Eriksson B, et al: Rivaroxaban for the prevention of venous thromboembolism after hip or knee arthroplasty: Pooled analysis of four studies. *Thromb Haemost* 2011;105(3):444-453.

57. Van Thiel D, Kalodiki E, Wahi R, Litinas E, Haque W, Rao G: Interpretation of benefit-risk of enoxaparin as comparator in the RECORD Program: Rivaroxaban oral tablets (10 milligrams) for use in prophylaxis in deep vein thrombosis and pulmonary embolism in patients undergoing hip or knee replacement surgery. *Clin Appl Thromb Hemost* 2009;15(4):389-394.

58. Lindquist DE, Stewart DW, Brewster A, et al: Comparison of postoperative bleeding in total hip and knee arthroplasty patients receiving rivaroxaban, enoxaparin, or aspirin for thromboprophylaxis. *Clin Appl Thromb Hemost* 2018;24(8):1315-1321.

    This retrospective cohort analysis assessed 1244 patients receiving either aspirin, enoxaparin, or rivaroxaban for the primary outcome of postoperative bleeding, defined as a composite of clinically overt fatal bleeding, critical organ bleeding, bleeding requiring transfusion of 2 or more units of blood, bleeding that necessitated reoperation, bleeding outside the surgical site that was associated with a Hgb decrease in 2 g/dL, or clinically relevant non major bleeding. In this study, patients receiving aspirin or enoxaparin were noted to have a statistically significantly lower rate of any bleeding compared to those receiving rivaroxaban. The rate of major bleeding between the groups was also similar though the differences did not demonstrate statistical significance. Level of evidence: III.

59. Wood RC, Stewart DW, Slusher L, et al: Retrospective evaluation of postoperative bleeding events in patients receiving rivaroxaban after undergoing total hip and total knee arthroplasty: Comparison with clinical trial data. *Pharmacotherapy* 2015;35(7):663-669.

60. Charters MA, Frisch NB, Wessell NM, Dobson C, Les CM, Silverton CD: Rivaroxaban versus enoxaparin for venous thromboembolism prophylaxis after hip and knee arthroplasty. *J Arthroplasty* 2015;30(7):1277-1280.

61. Eriksson BI, Dahl OE, Rosencher N, et al: Oral dabigatran etexilate vs. subcutaneous enoxaparin for the prevention of venous thromboembolism after total knee replacement: The RE-MODEL randomized trial. *J Thromb Haemost* 2007;5(11):2178-2185.

62. RE-MOBILIZE Writing Committee, Ginsberg JS, Davidson BL, Comp PC, et al: Oral thrombin inhibitor dabigatran etexilate vs North American enoxaparin regimen for prevention of venous thromboembolism after knee arthroplasty surgery. *J Arthroplasty* 2009;24(1):1-9.

63. Eriksson BI, Dahl OE, Huo MH, et al, RE-NOVATE II Study Group: Oral dabigatran versus enoxaparin for thromboprophylaxis after primary total hip arthroplasty (RE-NOVATE II*). A randomised, double-blind, non-inferiority trial. *Thromb Haemost* 2011;105(4):721-729.

64. Eriksson BI, Dahl OE, Rosencher N, et al, RE-NOVATE Study Group: Dabigatran etexilate versus enoxaparin for prevention of venous thromboembolism after total hip replacement: A randomised, double-blind, non-inferiority trial. *Lancet* 2007;370(9591):949-956.

65. Friedman RJ, Dahl OE, Rosencher N, et al, RE-MOBILIZE, RE-MODEL, RE-NOVATE Steering Committees: Dabigatran versus enoxaparin for prevention of venous thromboembolism after hip or knee arthroplasty: A pooled analysis of three trials. *Thromb Res* 2010;126(3):175-182.

66. Sharrock NE, Ranawat CS, Urquhart B, Peterson M: Factors influencing deep vein thrombosis following total hip arthroplasty under epidural anesthesia. *Anesth Analgesia* 1993;76(4):765-771.

67. Hu S, Zhang ZY, Hua YQ, Li J, Cai ZD: A comparison of regional and general anaesthesia for total replacement of the hip or knee: A meta-analysis. *J Bone Joint Surg Br* 2009;91(7):935-942.

68. Dalldorf PG, Perkins FM, Totterman S, Pellegrini VD: Deep venous thrombosis following total hip arthroplasty: Effects of prolonged postoperative epidural anesthesia. *J Arthroplasty* 1994;9(6):611-616.

69. Salvati EA, Pellegrini VD, Sharrock NE, et al: Recent advances in venous thromboembolic prophylaxis during and after total hip replacement. *J Bone Joint Surg Am* 2000;82(2):252-270.

CHAPTER 5

Outpatient Joint Arthroplasty

JESUA I. LAW, DO • DAVID A. CRAWFORD, MD
ADOLPH V. LOMBARDI JR, MD, FACS • KEITH R. BEREND, MD

ABSTRACT

With the advances in perioperative care, rapid recovery protocols, and meticulous surgical technique, outpatient joint arthroplasty is a safe and effective option in many patients. To ensure the best outcome with minimal complications, patients must be properly medically optimized, be appropriately educated, and have adequate support at home. This combination of patient optimization must be combined with comprehensive rapid recovery protocols and multidisciplinary medical and anesthesia teams. Surgeons should use a multimodal pain control protocol, blood conservation, and minimally invasive techniques so that patients may be mobile hours after surgery with minimal complications.

Keywords: multimodal pain control; outpatient; partial knee arthroplasty; rapid recovery protocol; total hip arthroplasty; total knee arthroplasty

Dr. Crawford or an immediate family member serves as a paid consultant to or is an employee of DePuy, a Johnson & Johnson Company and has received research or institutional support from Kinetic Concepts, Inc. and Zimmer. Dr. Lombardi or an immediate family member has received royalties from Innomed and Zimmer Biomet; serves as a paid consultant to or is an employee of Zimmer Biomet; has stock or stock options held in Elute, Inc., Joint Development Corporation, Prescribe Fit, SPR Therapeutics, LLC, and VuMedi; has received research or institutional support from Kinamed, Kinetic Concepts, Inc., SPR Therapeutics, and Zimmer Biomet; and serves as a board member, owner, officer, or committee member of the Central Ohio Orthopaedic Management Company, the Current Concepts in Joint Replacement, the Hip Society, the Knee Society, and the Operation Walk USA. Dr. Berend or an immediate family member has received royalties from Zimmer Biomet; serves as a paid consultant to or is an employee of Zimmer Biomet; has stock or stock options held in Elute, Inc., Joint Development Corporation, Prescribe Fit, SPR Therapeutics, LLC, and VuMedi; has received research or institutional support from SPR Therapeutics and Zimmer Biomet; and serves as a board member, owner, officer, or committee member of the Knee Society. Neither Dr. Law nor any immediate family member has received anything of value from or has stock or stock options held in a commercial company or institution related directly or indirectly to the subject of this chapter.

INTRODUCTION

With an aging population, the American Academy of Orthopaedic Surgeons has estimated an increase of up to 180% in hip and knee arthroplasty in the next 10 years.[1] Improvements in the perioperative care of patients undergoing joint arthroplasty have changed the length of stay from weeks to days and recently to an outpatient setting.[2] This diminished surgical trauma and rapid recovery is gaining popularity worldwide[3] and is attractive to patients and beneficial to controlling the cost of health care. Centers for Medicare and Medicaid has removed total knee and hip arthroplasty from the inpatient-only list and allows partial and total knee arthroplasty to be performed as a same-day surgery at an ambulatory surgery center (ASC). Multiple studies have shown outpatient hip and knee arthroplasty to be safe, effective, and decreasing cost of care.[4] Even though the hospital length of stay has been decreasing over the past decade without an increase in perioperative complications, there is still a persistent concern with perioperative complications going unnoticed or underdocumented.[5] These concerns with outpatient joint arthroplasty include uncontrolled pain after surgery, postoperative medical, or wound complications.[6] However, studies have shown equivalent or even improved outcomes with outpatient joint arthroplasty.[7]

LOCATION OF SURGERY

Outpatient arthroplasty can be performed in the hospital setting or at a free-standing ASC. The benefits of performing outpatient joint arthroplasty at an ASC are numerous. Efficiency is noted to be improved in ASCs when compared with traditional hospital operating rooms in regard to turnover time, ancillary time, procedure time, and exit time.[8] Healthcare costs are noted to be much lower in an ASC,[9] while still maintaining good surgical outcomes and patient safety.[10] Patient satisfaction is higher in the ASC settings[11] partially because the patients enjoy the more personalized experience ASCs offer over a large hospital setting. Patients also benefit from recovering in a familiar environment without continual exposure to nosocomial organisms.[12] In physician-owned ASC, providers are able to make decisions that affect patient care and improve the patient experience without layers of hospital bureaucracy. In this scenario, the healthcare provider has direct control to hire and train staff all with a common goal in mind.

PATIENT SELECTION

Given the fact that hip and knee arthroplasty is an elective procedure, patients have the opportunity for medical optimization before proceeding with surgery. Multiple models have been proposed for selecting patients for outpatient arthroplasty. Some surgeons have developed scoring systems, whereas others have used a more simplified medical optimization model.[10,13,14] With the Outpatient Arthroplasty Risk Assessment, developed by the authors of a 2017 study, the patient is given a score based on hematologic, endocrine, cardiac, and other risk factors.[14] According to this risk assessment score, the surgeon can then determine if the patient is at acceptable risk for an outpatient arthroplasty procedure. In the simplified model, patients with active medical comorbidities that are not optimized have their surgery delayed until such time as their medical condition is appropriately treated. The only hard contraindication in this model to outpatient surgery is a failing organ system such as chronic obstructive pulmonary disease (especially those needing home oxygen), congestive heart failure, chronic kidney disease, or liver cirrhosis.[15] In those patients who have end-organ failure, but are still considered candidates for arthroplasty, the outpatient setting should be avoided and the surgery performed at a hospital where a comprehensive medical team may evaluate and monitor the patient. It should be stressed that the reason a patient would require inpatient monitoring is to monitor the corresponding medical conditions, not for the arthroplasty surgery itself.

All patients who are considering an arthroplasty should have a preoperative evaluation by a medical physician to evaluate for risk and optimize any underlying medical conditions. Studies have reported new diagnoses discovered during the medical prescreening process with 2.5% of these patients not being suitable candidates for elective surgery.[16]

After establishing whether the patient is a candidate for outpatient surgery based on their medical conditions, a discussion must be had with the patient and family regarding home support. It is expected that the patient has family or friends available to ensure they are safe immediately following surgery and have transportation for follow-up visits and physical therapy. Next, the patient should have the appropriate equipment needed to perform their activities of daily living (ADLs) safely. Patients should consider handrails or safety bars in the shower and stairways and have easy access to a walker, cane, or crutches. Gait training and fall prevention should be a focal point for the first few weeks after joint arthroplasty and all loose carpet or cords should be out of common walkways.

Case selection is as important as patient selection when considering outpatient hip and knee arthroplasty, especially at an ASC. The surgeon should consider the complexity of the case and the resources available at the surgical setting. In an ASC, the surgeon should be aware of the limitations of storage space and sterilization capacity to streamline the workflow and instrument trays needed. Although most primary joint arthroplasty cases are easily accomplished at an ASC, complex revisions that require 7 to 10 pans of instrument sets can overwhelm the sterile processing capabilities at an ASC. Even in a hospital-based setting, these complex revisions may not be suitable for outpatient status. Complex cases, such as large hip revisions or radical knee débridements, have a greater propensity for blood loss[17] and need for medical specialties and should be done in a hospital setting. Some revisions can be performed in an outpatient setting such as polyethylene liner changes and single-component hip revisions, but as the complexity of the case increases, the surgeon should consider the need for a hospital-based outpatient surgery center or even inpatient hospitalization.

PATIENT EDUCATION

It is important that patients be properly counseled on the unique aspects of outpatient joint arthroplasty. Many patients will have preconceived notions of what to expect from joint arthroplasty. They may have had these procedures years ago or know a family member who underwent a joint arthroplasty surgery and were admitted to the hospital for multiple days and then discharged to a short-term rehabilitation facility. Inpatient admission and extended care facilities may represent the patient's perceived standard of care, and something different may seem rushed or intimidating to them. Preoperative education will ease these fears and explain the advantages and benefits of recovering from surgery at home.[18] All those who come in contact with the patient, from office staff to hospital/ASC employees, should be of the same mindset so that a unified approach can be delivered and the patient feels comfortable and fully supported by all team members.

Various types of educational formats can be used from simple handout material to organized joint arthroplasty classes. Regardless of the primary source of education, written comprehensive patient education materials should be made available because the patient often does not remember all that were discussed during the visit and/or classes. Furthermore, many new questions may arise after the clinical encounter. Patient education should include a preoperative medical evaluation overview, presurgical and postsurgical physical therapy, exercise, ADL goals for the first few days after surgery, wound care, and hygiene, as well as maintaining adequate hydration leading up to the surgical procedure.[19] The preoperative role of the physical therapists is to outline the stepwise approach to safely performing ADL, to teach patients how to use ambulatory aids, and perform more complex activities such as going up and down stairs. These educational materials should also include presurgical home planning, outline the risks of surgery, and set expectations for pain management and blood clot prevention postsurgery.

Knowledgeable office staff can aid in answering questions that are not covered in the material. Patients should be encouraged to view the facility where surgery is to be performed and meet the staff and postoperative care team (ie, physical therapy). Nursing staff should be available to explain both to the patient and family proper wound/dressing care and what signs to look for if problems arise.

PAIN MANAGEMENT

The primary apprehension patients have about outpatient joint arthroplasty is the ability to manage postoperative pain at home.[20] However, the reality is that uncontrolled pain after outpatient arthroplasty rarely leads to an overnight stay or emergency department visit within 48 hours of surgery.[11,13] To successfully achieve a same-day discharge, a multimodal pain control regimen must be used. These protocols have been shown to be the most effective means of controlling patient pain while limiting postoperative narcotics and their associated adverse effects. Successful high-volume centers have combined minimally invasive surgical techniques with multimodal pain and efficient anesthesia to reduce length of stay and speed recovery.[21] The prime objective is to minimize pain, sedation, and nausea while promoting mobilization and a safe discharge. **Table 1** shows a revised outpatient protocol.

TABLE 1

Outpatient Total Hip and Partial or Total Knee Arthroplasty Protocol

Patient Selection

Orthopaedic evaluation and scheduling for surgery

Preoperative medical history and physical examination, including laboratory testing

Patient Education

Educational materials are provided

Physical therapy evaluation and instruction

Preoperative educational class or video focused on outpatient joint arthroplasty

Pain Management

Night before surgery

- Acetaminophen 1 g orally

Day of surgery

- Acetaminophen 1 g orally
- Celecoxib 400 mg orally (not used if cardiac history or other contraindications)
- Dexamethasone 10 mg IV
- Scopolamine 1.5-mg patch (not used if history of BPH or glaucoma)
- Pregabalin/gabapentin 600 mg orally (300 mg for patients older than 65 yr)

Regional Anesthesia

Hip arthroplasty surgery

- Spinal anesthesia: 50-60 mg of lidocaine

Partial and total knee arthroplasty surgery

- Adductor canal block: 15 mL 0.5% ropivacaine
- IPACK block: 15 mL 0.2% ropivacaine

Intraoperatively

Pericapsular injection: 60 mL 0.5% ropivacaine, 0.5 mL 1:1,000 epinephrine (no posterior capsular injection in knees if IPACK block used)

30 mg ketorolac (not used in patients with renal impairment)

Narcotics are titrated and used sparingly

Postoperatively

Hydromorphone 0.5 mg IV every 10 min as required up to 2 mg

Acetaminophen 1 g orally (4 hr after first dose)

Oxycodone 5 mg orally for pain levels 1-3

Hydrocodone/acetaminophen 5/325 mg 1 pill for pain levels 1-3

(continued)

TABLE 1

Outpatient Total Hip and Partial or Total Knee Arthroplasty Protocol (continued)

Hydrocodone/acetaminophen 5/325 mg 2 pills for pain levels 4-10

Diazepam 2.5 mg IV as required for spasms

Home Medications

Tramadol 50 mg 1-2 pills every 8 hr as required for pain

Oxycodone 5 mg orally 1-2 pills every 4-6 hr as required for severe pain

Hydromorphone 2 mg 1 pill every 4-6 hr as required for breakthrough pain

Celecoxib 200 mg orally daily for 2 wk

Blood Management

Intravenous crystalloid hydration is started preoperatively

Tranexamic acid 1 g IV preoperatively (if no contraindications are present)

Surgery

Light general anesthesia: propofol ± short-acting inhalants

Ketamine 0.5 mg/kg IV before incision

Preoperative IV antibiotics

Minimum of 2 L crystalloid IV hydration

Ondansetron 4 mg IV

Postoperative Care

Minimum 1 L crystalloid IV hydration

Ondansetron 4 mg IV as required for nausea/vomiting

Promethazine 6.25 mg IV as required for nausea/vomiting

Urecholine 20 mg in male patients with BPH or risk of urinary retention

Discharge instructions are provided by the nursing staff

Postoperative antibiotics are administered orally for 3 doses

Aspirin 325 mg orally for 6 wk for DVT prophylaxis (low-molecular-weight heparin is used in obese or high-risk patients)

Battery-powered pneumatic-compression ambulatory calf pumps are worn for 2 wk

Follow-up telephone communication at 24 hr by nursing staff

Office evaluation at 6 wk

BPH = benign prostatic hyperplasia, DVT = deep vein thrombosis, IPACK = infiltration between popliteus artery and capsule of the knee.

The multimodal approach recommended uses a combination of NSAIDs, regional anesthesia, and a nonnarcotic analgesia (acetaminophen), preoperatively. This combination allows for adequate pain control while minimizing the usage and adverse effects of narcotic medication such as hypoventilation, sedation, and nausea, which will delay a safe same-day discharge. Postoperative nausea and vomiting are aggressively treated preemptively by administering dexamethasone (for both anti-inflammatory and antiemetic effects), metoclopramide, and scopolamine patches, while ensuring the patient has maintained adequate hydration before and throughout the procedure. Gabapentin and pregabalin are also useful in decreasing pain by blocking nociceptive receptors, thereby decreasing the need for narcotics.[22]

Regional anesthesia is a vital component to the multimodal protocol. Patients undergoing knee arthroplasty should receive an adductor canal block as well as a block to cover the posterior knee such as an IPACK block (regional anesthesia infiltrated between the posterior capsule and the popliteus artery).[23] With the addition of an IPACK block, the posterior capsule should not be injected with local anesthetic intraoperatively to avoid a peroneal nerve palsy. Femoral nerve blocks are no longer recommended because of the increased fall risk due to quadriceps muscle weakness,[24] and the preference has shifted to using adductor canal.[25] Patients who undergo hip replacement receive spinal anesthesia in combination with sedation or light general anesthesia. It has been previously shown that spinal anesthesia decreases blood loss when compared with general anesthesia.[26] In a 2020 study comparing spinal with general anesthesia, patients who received spinal anesthesia had less short-term complications and fewer nonhome discharges than those who received general anesthesia.[27] Narcotics should be avoided in regional anesthesia blocks because of pruritus, nausea, and sedation, which will also require the patient to stay more than 23 hours for observation. Before closure it is recommended that the patient receive an infiltration of local anesthesia into the periarticular tissue. The combination of peripheral and light general anesthesia has been shown to decrease pain, increase early mobility, decrease the need for narcotics, decrease length of stay, and reduce readmissions.[28]

BLOOD MANAGEMENT

There have been many improvements in the past decade in blood management techniques, which have led to decreased blood transfusion rates. Many ASCs do not have access to blood products, and it is important that patients at risk for bleeding be screened and considered as inpatient surgical candidates rather than for outpatient surgery. The surgeon should be considerate of genetic bleeding disorders as well as home medications that may hypocoagulate the blood. Studies have shown that preoperative blood levels are the greatest indicator for postoperative blood levels after surgery, and that a preoperative hemoglobin level >13 g/dL had a transfusion rate that approached zero.[29] These select patients who have lower overall blood volume at baseline will experience a larger clinical effect to the same drop in blood volume when compared with patients who have a preoperative hemoglobin level above 13 g/dL.

Regional, hypotensive anesthesia, and meticulous surgical dissection are other ways to avoid excessive blood loss and the need for transfusion.[30] The combination of regional blocks along with hypotensive anesthesia with mean arterial pressure around 60 mm Hg has been shown to decrease blood loss and keep transfusion rates low.[31]

The introduction of tranexamic acid (TXA) has nearly eliminated the need for blood transfusion in primary total joint arthroplasty. TXA has been shown to significantly decrease blood loss and transfusions in numerous studies by reducing the rate of clot breakdown while not increasing the rate of clot.[32] TXA can be given orally, topically, or intravenously and all routes have shown to be effective.[33,34] Both intravenous and oral administrations have been shown to be effective at 1 gram before skin incision and then again after surgery; where topical solutions have been described using 2 to 3 grams diluted and infiltrated into the wound at time of closure.

SURGICAL APPROACH

Outpatient surgery and rapid recovery is best achieved when a minimally invasive surgical approach is used. Minimally invasive really is not about a small incision size, but rather mindful handling of the deep soft tissue to minimize trauma and the associated inflammatory response. The anterior approach to the hip, for example, uses a true internervous plane and has been shown in numerous studies to improve early recovery compared with muscle cutting approaches.[35,36]

Prolonged surgical time has various negative consequences including increased infection risk, tourniquet time, amount of general anesthetic, and postoperative pain.[37] Furthermore, for outpatient arthroplasty to be successful, surgeries must be completed at a reasonable hour to allow for postoperative recovery and discharge. To achieve improvements in surgical time, the focus of the surgical team is to optimize efficiency. Efficiency is the ability to produce a desired outcome with minimal expenditure of time, energy, money, and materials. This is different than speed, which is just moving quickly and can lead to mistakes and complications. The operating room should have trained staff well versed in the choreography of a hip or knee arthroplasty to ensure an efficient surgery and best outcome for the patient. The steps should be rehearsed with the staff so that all present are aware of their roles in the procedure, which limits surgical errors and streamlines the recovery process. Processes must run in parallel to create efficiency, and there has to be a teamwork approach.

Postoperative Care and Management

Following surgery, the postoperative care can be divided into two phases: acute and step-down care. The initial postoperative acute phase is where anesthesia and nursing staff treat pain and nausea while stabilizing the patient medically. In this phase, hydration and minimal narcotics are used to ensure the goal of rapid recovery can be accomplished.

Once stabilized, the patient may transition to step-down care where they can sit up, hydrate orally, and be given a light snack. Physical therapists should be available to see the patient at this time and reinforce the proper use of walking aids that were instructed preoperatively as well as assisting the patient in standing and walking to the bathroom. Early ambulation not only aids in building confidence in the newly replaced joint, but can also decrease issues of urinary retention. Physical therapists should work with the patient and family regarding obstacles while at home and how to perform ADL such as stair climbing.

Deep vein thrombosis (DVT) is a concern with any hip or knee arthroplasty and should be assessed based on the patient's risk factors.[38] The goals of anticoagulation are to properly anticoagulate the patient, minimizing the chance of a DVT, while avoiding the risk of postoperative bleeding. Many of the patients can be treated with compression stockings, pneumatic compression devices, and aspirin for chemoprophylaxis.[39] In higher risk patients, stronger chemoprophylaxis may be needed based on a risk stratification approach.[38]

Once the patient has met goals and is ready for discharge, the nursing staff should review the education packets with the patient and family, ensuring that concerns regarding medications prescribed and wound care instructions are clear while all questions are answered appropriately. Within 24 to 48 hours from discharge, a follow-up phone call from an experienced staff member should be made to the patient and family to review medication schedules, ensure proper DVT prophylaxis is in place, and answer any questions. These follow-up calls will ease patient anxiety and likely reduce unnecessary emergency department visits and/or hospital admissions. Patients are encouraged to perform any prescribed physical therapy at an outpatient center as this gets the patient out of the house and allows use of more advanced rehabilitation equipment.

SUMMARY

Many studies have shown successful outcomes with outpatient arthroplasty, low readmission rates, and low complication rates.[40] Developing a successful program starts with establishing a rapid recovery protocol and multimodal approaches to patient care. This transition will give the surgeon and team a safety net to fall back on until outpatient surgery becomes a reality as these rapid recovery protocols become refined.

Outpatient joint arthroplasty is a safe and effective option in many patients. With proper patient selection, education, and multidisciplinary medical assistance, patients are able to have their hip or knee arthroplasty and be ambulatory hours after surgery. It is important that the surgeon considering outpatient joint arthroplasty have a comprehensive rapid recovery protocol and be knowledgeable in multimodal pain control and regional peripheral nerve blocks. At the conclusion of the procedure, the patient should have access to physical therapy, close follow-up in clinic, and risk-appropriate DVT prophylaxis for home.

KEY STUDY POINTS

- Outpatient joint arthroplasty is safe and effective in the properly selected patient.
- Use either simplified model or Outpatient Arthroplasty Risk Assessment scoring to determine if patient is candidate for outpatient surgery.
- Preadmission testing is required to ensure all medical diagnoses are known and medically optimized.
- Proper patient education ensures realistic expectations and keeps the patient from feeling abandoned when at home.

ANNOTATED REFERENCES

1. Sloan M, Premkumar A, Sheth NP: Projected volume of primary total joint arthroplasty in the U.S., 2014 to 2030. *J Bone Joint Surg Am* 2018;100:1455-1460.

   This study gives an updated projection of primary total joint procedures up to 2030. Level of evidence: I.

2. Teeny SM, York SC, Benson C, Perdue ST: Does shortened length of hospital stay affect total knee arthroplasty rehabilitation outcomes? *J Arthroplasty* 2005;20(7 suppl 3):39-45.

3. Tingle C, Berger RA, Bolognesi MP, et al: Same-day outpatient TJR gains popularity, but careful considerations must be made. *Orthop Today* 2015;35(8):1, 10-1.

4. Bertin KC: Minimally invasive outpatient total hip arthroplasty: A financial analysis. *Clin Orthop Relat Res* 2005;435:154-163.

5. Berger RA, Kusuma SK, Sanders SA, Thill ES, Sporer SM: The feasibility and perioperative complications of outpatient knee arthroplasty. *Clin Orthop Relat Res* 2009;467(6):1443-1449.

6. Mabrey JD, Toohey JS, Armstrong DA, Lavery L, Wammack LA: Clinical pathway management of total knee arthroplasty. *Clin Orthop Relat Res* 1997;345:125-133.

7. Kort NP, Bemelmans YFL, Schotanus MGM: Outpatient surgery for unicompartmental knee arthroplasty is effective and safe. *Knee Surg Sports Traumatol Arthrosc* 2017;25: 2659-2667.

   This study illustrates the effectiveness of an outpatient surgical protocol for unicompartmental knee arthroplasties. In properly selected patients with the help of a multidisciplinary team, outpatient joint arthroplasty is safe and effective with acceptable clinical outcomes. Level of evidence: III.

8. Imran JB, Madni TD, Taveras LR, et al: Analysis of operating room efficiency between a hospital-owned ambulatory surgical center and hospital outpatient department. *Am J Surg* 2019;218(5):809-812.

   This study demonstrates the increased efficiency of outpatient joint arthroplasty at an ASC when compared with a hospital-based outpatient surgery center. Level of evidence: III.

9. Reichert JC, von Rottkay E, Roth F, et al: A prospective randomized comparison of the minimally invasive direct anterior and the transgluteal approach for primary total hip arthroplasty. *BMC Musculoskelet Disord* 2018;19(1):241.

   This study demonstrates a higher patient activity in 1 year following a direct anterior total hip arthroplasty when compared with a transgluteal direct lateral approach. Hip functional scores are similar in both groups. Level of evidence: I.

10. Crawford DA, Adams JB, Berend KR, Lombardi AV Jr: Low complication rates in outpatient total knee arthroplasty. *Knee Surg Sports Traumatol Arthrosc* 2020;28(5):1458-1464.

    Outpatient joint arthroplasty is safe and effective in properly selected patients. Certain comorbidities increase the risk of overnight stay. Outpatient total joint arthroplasties had improvements in range of motion and outcome scores while maintaining a low revision rate. Level of evidence: III.

11. Kelly MP, Calkins TE, Culvern C, Kogan M, Della Valle CJ: Inpatient versus outpatient hip and knee arthroplasty: Which has higher patient satisfaction? *J Arthroplasty* 2018;33(11):3402-3406.

    Patient satisfaction scores were high in both inpatient and outpatient total joint arthroplasty groups, but satisfaction scores favored outpatient total joint arthroplasty in an ASC. Level of evidence: III.

12. Giuliano KK, Baker D, Quinn B: The epidemiology of nonventilator hospital-acquired pneumoniain the United States. *Am J Infect Control* 2018;46(3):322-327.

This study illustrates the incidence and influence of nonventilator hospital-acquired pneumonia and its effect on healthcare cost, hospital length of stay, and mortality. Level of evidence: I.

13. Berend KR, Lombardi AV, Berend ME, Adams JB, Morris MJ: Outpatient total hip arthroplasty: A paradigm change. *Bone Joint J* 2018;100-B:31-35.

    This study demonstrates that certain comorbitities were not associated with increased risk of surgical complications but are at an increased risk for overnight stay. Level of evidence: III.

14. Meneghini RM, Ziemba-Davis M, Ishmael MK, Kuzma AL, Caccavallo P: Safe selection of outpatient joint arthroplasty patients with medical risk stratification: The "Outpatient Arthroplasty Risk Assessment score". *J Arthroplasty* 2017;32(8):2325-2331.

    This study provides a numeric scoring system to assist in patient selection for outpatient joint arthroplasty. Level of evidence: III.

15. Courtney PM, Rozell JC, Melnic CM, Lee GC: Who should not undergo short stay hip and knee arthroplasty? Risk factors associated with major medical complications following primary total joint arthroplasty. *J Arthroplasty* 2015;30(9 suppl):1-4.
16. Meding JB, Klay M, Healy A, Ritter MA, Keating EM, Berend ME: The prescreening history and physical in elective total joint arthroplasty. *J Arthroplasty* 2007;22(6 suppl 2): 21-23.
17. Bozic KJ, Katz P, Cisternas M, Ono L, Ries MD, Showstack J: Hospital resource utilization for primary and revision total hip arthroplasty. *J Bone Joint Surg Am* 2005;87(3):570-576.
18. Dowsey MM, Kilgour ML, Santamaria NM, Choong PF: Clinical pathways in hip and knee arthroplasty: A prospective randomized controlled study. *Med J Aust* 1999;170(2):59-62.
19. Hausel J, Nygren J, Thorell A, Lagerkranser M, Ljungqvist O: Randomized clinical trial of the effects of oral preoperative carbohydrates on postoperative nausea and vomiting after laparoscopic cholecystectomy. *Br J Surg* 2005;92:415-421.
20. Adelani MA, Barrack RL: Patient perceptions of the safety of outpatient total knee arthroplasty. *J Arthroplasty* 2019;34(3):462-464.

    This study illustrates the difference between patient safety based on complications and the patient perception of safety based on a select group of patients. Level of evidence: IV.

21. Berend KR, Lombardi AV Jr: Liberal indications for minimally invasive oxford unicondylar arthroplasty provide rapid functional recovery and pain relief. *Surg Technol Int* 2007;16:193-197.
22. Buvanendran A, Kroin JS, Della Valle CJ, Kari M, Moric M, Tuman KJ: Perioperative oral pregabalin reduces chronic pain after total knee arthroplasty: A prospective, randomized, controlled trial. *Anesth Analg* 2010;110(1):199-207.
23. Kandarian B, Indelli P, Sinha S, et al: Implementation of the IPACK (Infiltration between the Popliteal Artery and Capsule of the Knee) block into a multimodal analgesic pathway for total knee replacement. *Korean J Anesthesiol* 2019;72(3):238-244.

    This study demonstrates a novel peripheral block that can be implemented in a multimodal analgesic technique to decrease opioid consumption postoperatively. Level of evidence: III.

24. Sharma S, Iorio R, Specht LM, Davies-Lepie S, Healy WL: Complications of femoral nerve block for total knee arthroplasty. *Clin Orthop Relat Res* 2010;468(1):135-140.
25. Jaeger P, Nielsen ZJ, Henningsen MH, Hilsted KL, Mathiesen O, Dahl JB: Adductor canal block versus femoral nerve block and quadriceps strength: A randomized, double-blind, placebo-controlled, crossover study in healthy volunteers. *Anesthesiology* 2013;118(2):409-415.
26. MacFarlane AJR, Arun Prasad G, Chan VWS, Brull R: Does regional anesthesia improve outcome after total knee arthroplasty? *Clin Orthop Relat Res* 2009;467:2379-2402.
27. Warren J, Sundaram K, Anis H, et al: Spinal anesthesia is associated with decreased complications after total knee and hip arthroplasty. *J Am Acad Orthop Surg* 2020;28(5):e213-e221.

    This study demonstrates that patients with spinal anesthesia have less 30-day complications and are more likely to have a discharge to home when compared with patients with general anesthesia. Level of evidence. III.

28. Beaupre LA, Johnston DB, Dieleman S, Tsui B: Impact of a preemptive multimodal analgesia plus femoral nerve blockade protocol on rehabilitation, hospital length of stay, and postoperative analgesia after primary total knee arthroplasty: A controlled clinical pilot study. *ScientificWorldJournal* 2012;2012:273821.
29. Rosencher N, Kerkkamp HE, Macheras G, et al, OSTHEO Investigation: Orthopedic Surgery Transfusion Hemoglobin European Overview (OSTHEO) study: Blood management in elective knee and hip arthroplasty in Europe. *Transfusion* 2003;43(4):459-469.
30. Sharrock NE, Salvati EA: Hypotensive epidural anesthesia for total hip arthroplasty: A review. *Acta Orthop Scand* 1996;67(1):91-107.
31. Park JH, Rasouli MR, Mortazavi SM, Tokarski AT, Maltenfort MG, Parvizi J: Predictors of perioperative blood loss in total joint arthroplasty. *J Bone Joint Surg Am* 2013;95(19):1777-1783.
32. Duncan CM, Gillette BP, Jacob AK, Sierra RJ, Sanchez-Sotelo J, Smith HM: Venous thromboembolism and mortality associated with tranexamic acid use during total hip and knee arthroplasty. *J Arthroplasty* 2015;30(2):272-276.
33. Alshryda S, Sarda P, Sukeik M, Nargol A, Blenkinsopp J, Mason JM: Tranexamic acid in total knee replacement: A systematic review and meta-analysis. *J Bone Joint Surg Br* 2011;93(12):1577-1585.
34. Irwin A, Khan SK, Jameson SS, Tate RC, Copeland C, Reed MR: Oral versus intravenous tranexamic acid in enhanced-recovery primary total hip and knee replacement: Results of 3000 procedures. *Bone Joint J* 2013;95-B(11): 1556-1561.
35. Alexandrov T, Ahlmann ER, Menendez LR: Early clinical and radiographic results of minimally invasive anterior approach hip arthroplasty. *Adv Orthop* 2014;2014:954208.

36. Matta JM, Shahrdar C, Ferguson T: Single-incision anterior approach for total hip arthroplasty on an orthopedic table. *Clin Orthop Rel Res* 2005;441:115-124.
37. Triantafyllopoulos G, Stundner O, Memtsoudis S, Poultsides L: Patient, surgery, and hospital related risk factors for surgical site infections following total hip arthroplasty. *ScientificWorldJournal* 2015;2015:979560.
38. Jacobs JJ, Mont MA, Bozic KJ, et al: American Academy of Orthopaedic Surgeons clinical practice guideline on: Preventing venous thromboembolic disease in patients undergoing elective hip and knee arthroplasty. *J Bone Joint Surg Am* 2012;94(8):746-747.
39. Falck-Ytter Y, Francis CW, Johanson NA, et al: Prevention of VTE in orthopedic surgery patients: Antithrombotic therapy and prevention of thrombosis, 9th ed., American College of Chest Physicians Evidence-Based Clinical Practice guidelines. *Chest* 2012;141:e278S-e325S.
40. Berger RA, Sanders S, Gerlinger T, Della Valle C, Jacobs JJ, Rosenberg AG: Outpatient total knee arthroplasty with a minimally invasive technique. *J Arthroplasty* 2005;20(7 suppl 3):33-38.

CHAPTER 6

Pain Management

JASON H. OH, MD • PATRICIA C. PANG, MD • MATTHEW S. HEPINSTALL, MD

ABSTRACT

Pain after joint arthroplasty can hinder functional recovery and decrease patient satisfaction. Anesthetic and analgesic regimens can have a significant effect on patient experience and outcomes. Multidisciplinary pain management strategies focusing on opioid-sparing, multimodal analgesia beginning in the preoperative period are growing in favor. The goal is to achieve optimal pain relief while minimizing medication adverse effects and associated complications, thereby expediting recovery. Such perioperative analgesia strategies are multifaceted and should be tailored to meet each patient's needs.

Keywords: multimodal pain management; neuraxial anesthesia; opioids; periarticular injection; regional anesthesia

INTRODUCTION

Although pain relief and improved function are the primary goals of hip and knee arthroplasty, acute postoperative pain remains a major problem for many patients, with a subset at risk for the development of chronic postoperative pain. Furthermore, poorly controlled pain may hinder postoperative rehabilitation and can be associated with increased medical complications, prolonged hospitalization, higher costs, lower rates of discharge home, and lower patient satisfaction. Patients report that fear of postoperative pain is their foremost concern regarding joint arthroplasty and is a primary driver behind decisions to postpone or refuse surgery.[1]

Traditionally relied on as the primary analgesic following joint arthroplasty, opioids are now prescribed with greater caution in light of the escalating opioid crisis in the United States. Multimodal analgesic regimens aim to attenuate acute postoperative pain while minimizing medication adverse effects, decreasing the incidence of chronic postoperative pain, and mitigating the risk of long-term narcotic use and dependence. Thus, orthopaedic surgeons must familiarize themselves with a wide range of analgesic modalities and should be prepared to engage anesthesiologists and behavioral health specialists in the preoperative period to form an interdisciplinary effort to optimize pain management, especially in high-risk patients. It is important to review commonly used treatment modalities, along with practical recommendations for opioid-sparing, multimodal regimens.

PAIN PHYSIOLOGY

Pain may be categorized into nociceptive and neuropathic subtypes. Nociceptive pain is caused by direct tissue trauma in the course of surgical dissection, bone preparation, and implant fixation. Inflammatory pain is a type of nociceptive pain that results from neuronal activation in response to inflammatory cytokines, such as prostaglandins, kinins, histamine, cytokines, leukotrienes, and neuropeptides. Among the most important of these inflammatory mediators are the prostaglandins, which are derived from arachidonic acid via the action

Dr. Hepinstall or an immediate family member is a member of a speakers' bureau or has made paid presentations on behalf of Stryker; serves as a paid consultant to or is an employee of Corin USA, Exactech, Inc., KCI, and Stryker; has received research or institutional support from Cymedica, Flexion Therapeutics, and Stryker; and serves as a board member, owner, officer, or committee member of the American Academy of Orthopaedic Surgeons. Neither of the following authors nor any immediate family member has received anything of value from or has stock or stock options held in a commercial company or institution related directly or indirectly to the subject of this chapter: Dr. Oh and Dr. Pang.

of cyclooxygenase (COX) enzymes. Neuropathic pain is generated by direct injury to the nervous system—central or peripheral.

Noxious stimuli by direct trauma and inflammatory mediators are sensed by Aδ and C nociceptors within the peripheral nerves near the site of tissue damage. The normal physiologic pain response is localized, is time-limited, and follows a predictable stimulus-response relationship. Pathologic pain is associated with peripheral and central sensitization, which lowers the threshold for pain and results in a pain response that is disproportionate to a given stimulus. This is referred to as hyperalgesia. Primary hyperalgesia is defined as hypersensitivity to noxious stimuli at the site of injury (eg, surgical site)—a result of peripheral sensitization of nociceptors. Described as hypersensitivity occurring in surrounding, undamaged tissues, secondary hyperalgesia results from central sensitization—the hyperexcitability of spinal cord neurons due to sustained afferent inputs. In cases of severe central sensitization, pain can be evoked by afferent inputs from Aβ nerve fibers, which normally transmit innocuous mechanosensory inputs. When pain results from normally nonpainful stimuli, this condition is known as allodynia.

This section represents only an abbreviated overview of the pathophysiology of pain. Although acute pain is expected following trauma, the development of chronic pain is complex and risk factors are multifactorial. Pain management strategies for each patient must be considered individually.

MULTIMODAL AND PREEMPTIVE ANALGESIA

Successful pain management encompasses dampening of immediate and delayed local pain responses as well as the prevention of sensitization. Different interventions have variable effects on the responses to both peripheral and central pain, as well as immediate and delayed postoperative pain. As a result, multimodal strategies that use a variety of anesthetic techniques and analgesic agents form the current standard for pain management in joint arthroplasty. Based on the developing understanding of sensitization, medication administration is recommended to begin in the preoperative period before surgical incision. This is termed preemptive analgesia, and large meta-analyses have demonstrated that this strategy is effective for decreasing visual analog scale pain scores, and for patient satisfaction and postoperative opioid utilization in arthroplasty as well as other surgical specialties.[2] Medications appropriate for preoperative administration are presented in **Table 1**.

NONPHARMACOLOGIC ANALGESIA MODALITIES

Cryotherapy

Cryotherapy is one of the simplest means of reducing pain in the postoperative period, involving the application of an ice pack or other cooling device to the surgical site. The temperature of the device should be maintained at or just above 0°C, as direct analgesia results from reversible nerve conduction blockade achieved when the local tissue temperature is between 0° and 10°C. The cryotherapy device should be separated from the skin by a cloth barrier to prevent skin injury. Additional indirect pain relief results from local vasoconstriction that decreases edema and inflammation at the surgical site, thereby reducing cytokine-mediated chemical stimulation of nociceptors. Although there is a paucity of evidence showing significant clinical benefit from cryotherapy with regard to functional outcomes and medication utilization,[3] the low cost, benign adverse effect profile, and ease of use make it a standard intervention in many practice settings—particularly following knee arthroplasty.

Patient Education and Psychotherapy

As previously discussed, the fear of postoperative pain is a primary concern of many patients who have undergone joint arthroplasty. These concerns can be mitigated by preoperative education and discussions regarding

TABLE 1

Oral Agents Suitable for Preoperative Analgesia

Medication	Dose (mg)	Consider Reduced Dose or Alternatives If:
Acetaminophen	500-1,000	Hepatic dysfunction
Celecoxib	200-400	Renal dysfunction; sulfonamide allergy
Meloxicam	15-30	Renal dysfunction
Gabapentin	300-600	Elderly patients; other risk factors for delirium
Pregabalin	75-150	Elderly patients; other risk factors for delirium

expectation management. In addition to consultations in the office, patients can also be referred to formal arthroplasty education classes that have been established at many institutions; these classes may be conducted by a combination of nurses, physical therapists, and physician assistants. These classes have been shown to improve perioperative pain management[4] as well as other clinical parameters, including length of stay and compliance with neuraxial anesthesia.[5]

Studies have shown that psychiatric disorders may have a significant effect on acute and chronic postoperative pain as well as functional recovery. Disorders such as anxiety and depression, as well as pain catastrophizing behavior and somatization disorders, are associated with increased acute postoperative pain—the effects of which may persist longer than 1 year following surgery, if unrecognized.[6] Furthermore, untreated depression has been found to be a risk factor for poor functional recovery following total joint arthroplasty.[7] As such, preoperative screening for psychiatric disorders is integral to identifying for psychiatric disease before surgery. Medical treatment of these conditions with the appropriate antidepressants and anxiolytic agents has been associated with improved functional recovery after arthroplasty.[7] Ideally, proper referrals to psychiatric specialists are made before surgery, such as to initiate care and facilitate expedient postoperative follow-up. Psychiatric co-management is also useful for teaching coping strategies and establishing emotional support systems in the postoperative period.

PHARMACOLOGIC ANALGESIA MODALITIES

Acetaminophen

Acetaminophen is one of the most widely used pharmacologic analgesic agents worldwide, established as an effective analgesic—particularly in conjunction with opioids—with a relatively benign safety profile. Although the precise mechanism of action is still not fully understood, proposed mechanisms include that acetaminophen acts via selective COX-2 and COX-3 inhibition as well as inhibition of endocannabinoid reuptake in the brain.[8] Acetaminophen has antipyretic and analgesic properties but does not have clinically significant anti-inflammatory properties. Because acetaminophen is metabolized in the liver, hepatic disease should be screened before administration. Historically, the maximum daily dose of acetaminophen was 4 g. However, following the publication of studies demonstrating increased incidence of liver injury and acute liver failure from therapeutic levels of acetaminophen intake in the United States,[9] current FDA guidelines now recommend limiting intake of acetaminophen to 3 g/day. Acetaminophen is available in both oral and intravenous formulations. Although intravenous delivery allows for uninterrupted administration during surgery, evidence of superior analgesia over the oral formulation is controversial.[10,11]

Nonsteroidal Anti-inflammatory Drugs

NSAIDs act through inhibition of the COX-1 and COX-2 enzymes. COX-1 mediates production of thromboxane A2, and COX-2 mediates production of prostaglandins, leukotrienes, and prostacyclins; each of these enzymes has various implications on multiple organ systems.

Nonselective NSAIDs (eg, ibuprofen) inhibit both COX-1 and COX-2, whereas selective NSAIDs (eg, celecoxib) preferentially target COX-2. NSAIDs produce their therapeutic analgesic effects by blocking prostaglandin production, thereby directly reducing inflammatory pain at the surgical site. Recent clinical studies have shown comparable analgesic efficacy of NSAIDs compared with opioids for a variety of orthopaedic indications.[12,13] Another beneficial effect of NSAIDs, particularly in hip arthroplasty, is the reduction of postoperative heterotopic ossification.[14] The major adverse effects of nonselective NSAIDs include gastrointestinal mucosal injury and acute renal injury. Patients who have *Helicobacter pylori* infection or concurrent glucocorticoid use, as well as those who have a history of alcohol abuse, are at increased risk for gastrointestinal ulceration and bleeding.

The perioperative use of nonselective NSAIDs is controversial. Increased surgical bleeding is a potential risk because of dysfunction of platelet aggregation, which occurs following inhibition of COX-mediated production of thromboxane A2. Historical evidence suggesting that nonselective NSAIDs were associated with increased perioperative bleeding and hypotension prompted many surgeons to advocate discontinuing NSAIDs either 7 to 10 days or at least five half-lives before surgical procedures. However, the most common source of bleeding in these studies was from the upper gastrointestinal tract, not the surgical site. Many studies across various surgical disciplines have demonstrated no increase in perioperative bleeding with nonselective NSAIDs, such as ketorolac.[15]

Selective COX-2 inhibitors maintain the analgesic effects of nonselective NSAIDs with significantly lower risk of gastrointestinal and bleeding adverse effects. Selective COX-2 inhibitors have also demonstrated equal efficacy as nonselective NSAIDs in decreasing heterotopic ossification.[16] Additionally, studies have shown no increased risk of platelet dysfunction or clinical bleeding, even when used in conjunction with antithrombotic agents such as heparin.[17] However, the risk of renal toxicity with selective COX-2 inhibitors remains unchanged relative to nonselective NSAIDs, so kidney function should be monitored if ongoing therapy with selective COX-2 inhibitors is used, as with nonselective NSAIDs.

Of note, the selective COX-2 inhibitors rofecoxib and valdecoxib were both withdrawn from the US market for being associated with increased risk of cardiovascular thromboembolic events, including myocardial infarction and stroke. Decreased prostacyclin production in the vascular endothelium secondary to COX-2 inhibition likely resulted in increased endothelial injury and thrombosis. This adverse effect appears to be offset, in part, by the accompanying reduction in COX-1-mediated thromboxane A2 production in nonselective and semiselective NSAIDs.[18] Nevertheless, clinical studies demonstrate a dose-dependent risk of cardiovascular events for all NSAIDs—selective and nonselective. Thus, prolonged use of any such medication requires some caution. Currently, celecoxib is the only COX-2 highly selective NSAID approved for human use in the United States. Studies regarding celecoxib's cardiovascular safety profile have shown increased risk of cardiovascular-related death at sustained high dosages,[19] although lower doses (on the order of 200 mg/day) are considered noninferior to nonselective agents such as naproxen.[20]

There is some controversy regarding the effect of NSAIDs—both nonselective and COX-2 selective—on bone healing and implant ingrowth. Although exact mechanisms are not well understood, animal studies have demonstrated that NSAIDs impede the process of fracture healing through endochondral ossification, and also reduce the strength of osseous ingrowth into implant materials.[21,22] Although there is a lack of prospective studies in humans, retrospective analyses from the trauma and spine literature have shown that NSAID use may be associated with impaired healing following intramedullary nailing of diaphyseal femoral fractures and lower success rates in lumbar arthrodesis.[23,24] However, there has been no evidence to date that NSAIDs impair the process of joint implant osseointegration in humans.[25] Given the wide range of benefits provided by NSAIDs with respect to pain control, prevention of heterotopic ossification, and reduction of opioid-related adverse effects, most arthroplasty surgeons continue to use these medications as first-line treatment in most cases (**Table 2**).

TABLE 2

Commonly Used Nonsteroidal Anti-inflammatory Drugs

No COX selectivity	Ibuprofen Ketoprofen Ketorolac Naproxen
Moderate COX-2 selectivity	Diclofenac Etodolac Indomethacin Meloxicam Nabumetone Piroxicam Sulindac
High COX-2 selectivity	Celecoxib

COX = cyclooxygenase

Opioids

Opioid analgesics function as mu-opioid receptor agonists. Mu-opioid receptors are located primarily in central nervous system neurons and mediate changes in neuronal excitability through suppression of presynaptic release of the neurotransmitter gamma-aminobutyric acid, which produces the desired analgesic effect. Conversely, there also exists the phenomenon of opioid-induced hyperalgesia, a condition in which pain nociceptors become paradoxically hypersensitized by exposure to opioids.[26] Opioids have traditionally been used alongside acetaminophen as a first-line surgical analgesic agent, and some protocols still successfully incorporate opioids for both preemptive and postoperative analgesia[27] (**Table 3**). However, concerns regarding opioid sensitization and hyperalgesia have led some surgeons to abandon the practice of preemptive opioid use, instead reserving opioids for postoperative use.[28] Mu-opioid agonists are also associated with a wide range of other adverse effects—the most common of which include nausea, vomiting, constipation, pruritus, somnolence, confusion, and respiratory depression. Furthermore, physical and psychocognitive dependence are major concerns resulting from sustained opioid use and can result from both appropriate and inappropriate use. If long-term opioid use is abruptly discontinued, patients may experience withdrawal symptoms; thus, patient education regarding appropriate use and tapering is integral.

Despite the many drawbacks of opioid use, they are still considered to be the most potent analgesics in many clinical scenarios. With many formulations available of variable administration route and duration of action, opioids are a highly versatile option for pain management (**Table 4**). Opioid metabolism occurs primarily in the liver, with a smaller contribution from the kidneys. Because opioid metabolism varies between patients—especially in those with developed tolerance or impaired hepatic and renal function—most analgesia regimens administer opioids on an as-needed basis rather than a scheduled basis. Barring unique situations in patients who have chronic pain, this practice reduces the likelihood of overdose and severe respiratory depression, which can be fatal. Another option for opioid dosing is patient-controlled analgesia, a modality that allows patients to self-administer intravenous opioids with preset limits

TABLE 3

Oral Medications Suitable for Postoperative Analgesia

Medication	Dose (mg)	Frequency	Consider Reduced Dose or Alternatives If:
Acetaminophen	975	Every 8 hr	Hepatic dysfunction
Celecoxib	200	Every 12 hr	Renal dysfunction; sulfonamide allergy
Meloxicam	15	Every 24 hr	Renal dysfunction
Ketorolac	15-30	Every 6 hr	Renal dysfunction; peptic ulcer disease
Gabapentin	200	Every 8 hr	Elderly patients; other risk factors for delirium
Pregabalin	75	Every 12 hr	Elderly patients; other risk factors for delirium
Oxycodone	5-10	Every 4 hr	—
Tramadol	50-100	Every 8 hr	—

on maximum dosage per unit time. Although patient-controlled analgesia was originally expected to improve pain management by reducing time to intervention, most clinical studies have shown no benefit over nurse-administered opioids.[29]

Tramadol and tapentadol also may be considered for the management of postsurgical pain. These agents bind the mu-opioid receptor with lower affinity than true opioids and thus generate fewer adverse effects such as respiratory depression and drowsiness. A secondary analgesic effect is produced through reuptake blockade of neurotransmitters such as serotonin and norepinephrine, a mechanism similar to some antidepressants. Associated with a favorable adverse effect profile, tramadol can provide adequate analgesia and has been recommended by the American Academy of Orthopaedic Surgeons for treatment of knee osteoarthritis. However, because of the neurotransmitter reuptake blockade, patients should be monitored for serotonin syndrome as well as the development of physical dependence, addiction, and withdrawal symptoms.

TABLE 4

Oral Opioids at Equivalent Dosages

Opioid	Dosage (mg)
Morphine	30
Codeine	200
Oxycodone	20
Oxymorphone	10
Hydrocodone	30
Hydromorphone	7
Methadone	10
Tramadol	300
Tapentadol	75

Compared with opioid-naïve individuals, patients who have preoperative opioid use are at increased risk for the development of postoperative opioid tolerance and dependence. In addition, preoperative opioid usage has been associated with increased surgical complications, increased pain, prolonged hospitalization, and an increased likelihood of being discharged to rehabilitation facilities. All of these negative effects are more pronounced in patients using long-acting opioid formulations compared with those using short-acting formulations.[30] Provided that these high-risk patients are identified, these detrimental effects may be curtailed by initiating a weaning protocol preoperatively, with increasing reliance on nonopioid analgesics. Patients who successfully decrease their opioid requirements by at least 50% preoperatively have been shown to have clinical outcomes similar to opioid-naïve individuals.[31]

Glucocorticoids

Glucocorticoids, such as dexamethasone and methylprednisolone, are commonly used to promote analgesia through reduction of the inflammatory response. A bolus of intravenous corticosteroid is often given when anesthesia is administered, and an additional dose may be given in the periarticular injection (PAI), which will be discussed in further detail later.[32] Glucocorticoids have a favorable safety profile and do not increase the risk of wound complications or infection in the short term.[33] Additionally, glucocorticoids have antiemetic properties, the mechanism of which is not fully understood. However, care should be exercised in patients who have diabetes, because glucocorticoid use can result in acute disruption of glycemic control. Nevertheless, it has been shown that low doses of glucocorticoids may be given to patients who have well-controlled diabetes in the perioperative setting without an increase in adverse events, provided that careful monitoring is in place. One recent retrospective study demonstrated that doses ranging from 6 to 12 mg of intravenous dexamethasone delivered intraoperatively did not cause significant postoperative hyperglycemia in patients who have diabetes with hemoglobin A1c levels below 7%; furthermore, dexamethasone administration did not increase the incidence of periprosthetic joint infection among patients who have diabetes compared who have patients without diabetes.[34]

Gabapentinoids

Gabapentin and pregabalin are calcium channel ligands that act by reducing the gamma-aminobutyric acid–mediated hyperexcitability of activated neurons.[35] Commonly used as adjuncts for treating chronic neuropathic pain, both medications have been evaluated for their potential role in treating acute postsurgical pain. The effectiveness of gabapentinoids in this role is controversial, because some studies have found that these drugs may reduce pain scores and opioid consumption in the immediate postoperative period,[11,36-38] whereas other studies have found no benefit.[39] Perioperative administration of gabapentinoids has not correlated with clinically significant decreases in opioid consumption or chronic pain in the months to years after surgery.[40]

There are significant limitations and drawbacks to gabapentinoid administration that must be considered before use. First, the effective doses appropriate for perioperative gabapentinoid administration are variable, and there is no clear consensus in the literature for initial dosing regimens. The range of typical dosing regimens for gabapentin (150 to 1,300 mg/day) is considerably wider than that of pregabalin (150 to 300 mg/day).[41-43] Second, dose-dependent adverse effects must be accounted for, because gabapentinoids are associated with sedation and dizziness. These effects can lead to impaired exercise tolerance and falls. Gabapentinoids should be used with caution in patients who have other risk factors for delirium and falls, such as advanced age and polypharmacy. Research performed on patients aged 70 years and older who have undergone arthroplasty has demonstrated that this subset of patients may not experience the same benefits as younger patients with regard to pain relief and opioid reduction.[44]

Ketamine

Ketamine is an anesthetic agent commonly used for procedural sedation and for the management of postoperative pain. Ketamine provides analgesia by reducing the production of cytokines such as interleukin 6, thereby contributing to the reduction of primary hyperalgesia.[45] It also reversibly antagonizes *N*-methyl-D-aspartate receptors, thus reducing secondary hyperalgesia as well as central sensitization. In addition, ketamine has a minor local anesthetic effect secondary to blockade of voltage-gated neuronal sodium channels.

Ketamine's utility in joint arthroplasty is a relatively new topic of study, and early clinical results have been mixed. Randomized controlled trials in patients who have undergone total knee arthroplasty suggest that intraoperative ketamine administration in subanesthetic dosages followed by continuous infusion for 24 to 48 hours postoperatively has demonstrated decreased pain scores, lower opioid utilization, and superior mobilization.[46] Perioperative administration of ketamine in patients who had undergone total hip arthroplasty has also correlated with decreased opioid utilization, improved ability to tolerate physical therapy, and reduced rates of chronic pain measured at 6 months postoperatively.[47] Additionally, ketamine appears to reduce the incidence of postoperative nausea and vomiting.[48,49] However, one recent study that examined ketamine's efficacy when used in tandem with spinal anesthesia found minimal improvement in pain relief and no significant reduction in opioid consumption in patients who had undergone knee arthroplasty.[50]

Ketamine has unique adverse effects that can present logistical challenges in its administration. Albeit rare in the subanesthetic doses recommended in the setting of joint arthroplasty, ketamine is associated with dissociative and psychotomimetic adverse effects including somnolence, hallucinations, delirium, and nightmares.[49] Tachycardia, hypertension, hepatotoxicity, and cholangiopathy have also been reported.[51,52] Thus, patients on ketamine infusions must be monitored for these adverse reactions. Depending on facility regulations, admission to an intensive care unit or other monitored setting may be required during and immediately after ketamine infusion. Close cooperation with medical specialists in chronic pain management is recommended if prolonged ketamine usage is planned.

ANESTHESIA CHOICES

Neuraxial Anesthesia and Analgesia

The introduction of neuraxial anesthesia revolutionized joint arthroplasty. Compared with the prior standard of general anesthesia, neuraxial anesthesia decreased pulmonary and renal complications, infections, blood loss, cost, mortality, and hospital length of stay, particularly in patients older than 65 years.[53,54] Additionally, neuraxial anesthesia used in conjunction with sedation decreases associated side effects of opioids and anesthetic gas to which the patient would otherwise be exposed under general anesthesia. If the patient is a candidate, single-shot spinal anesthesia is effective for most primary arthroplasty procedures. Local anesthetic choice is based on expected surgical duration, with the goal of quick resolution postoperatively to facilitate early ambulation. A commonly used agent is bupivacaine, which has a favorable adverse effect profile and a typical duration of action between 3 and 9 hours. If shorter procedural time is expected, then mepivacaine can also be considered. Mepivacaine has a duration of action between 90 and 150 minutes, thereby allowing for earlier ambulation and lower likelihood of urinary retention.[55] Epidural catheter placement can be considered if prolonged surgical time is expected or if the team chooses to maintain the epidural catheter for postoperative analgesia. In such situations, patients may still participate in physical therapy if a dilute local anesthetic infusion produces minimal motor blockade, but extreme caution must be used to avoid falls. However, with the increasing data supporting efficacy of peripheral nerve blockade and PAIs as part of multimodal analgesic regiments, maintenance of epidural catheters postoperatively has become less common.

Regional Anesthesia

Regional techniques represent an important anesthetic modality for patients who have undergone joint arthroplasty. These targeted injections provide focused anesthesia and reduce the need for the systemic administration of opioids and other agents for analgesia in the early postoperative period. Although early regional blocks were associated with problems of motor blockade and subsequently delayed physical therapy and falls, the development of modern ultrasonography-guided techniques has allowed better access to sensory nerves at very low risk with relatively minimal procedural time required. Bupivacaine and ropivacaine are two commonly used agents for regional blocks. Although most studies have demonstrated comparable functional results between the two compounds, there may be a tendency for decreased potency, shorter duration of action, and less profound motor blockade with ropivacaine.[56] Therefore, ropivacaine may not be ideal for single-agent spinal anesthesia, but can have an advantage over bupivacaine in regional blocks. Animal models have also demonstrated decreased risk of cardiotoxicity with ropivacaine compared with bupivacaine.[57]

Although peripheral nerve blockade is not a standard for patients undergoing total hip arthroplasty, the fascia iliaca compartment block is a useful technique for preoperative and postoperative pain relief for hip and proximal femur fractures. Local anesthetic is introduced deep to the fascia of the iliopsoas, with the goal of medial spread to the femoral nerve as well as lateral spread to the lateral femoral cutaneous nerve. Although inconsistent, local anesthetic spread to the obturator nerve can occur as well. Because the fascia iliaca compartment block causes motor blockade to the anterior and medial thigh compartments, careful evaluation must be performed postoperatively before clearing the patient for ambulation therapy.

For knee arthroplasty, the femoral nerve block (FNB) was historically the most commonly used regional technique. In performing an FNB, local anesthetic surrounds the femoral nerve and can spread to the lateral femoral cutaneous nerve and obturator nerves as well; this is referred to as the three-in-one block. Like the fascia iliaca compartment block, FNB is associated with quadriceps weakness and can delay participation in physical therapy. As a result, the adductor canal block (ACB) has gained favor, because it primarily causes sensory nerve blockade. The ACB targets the saphenous nerve within the adductor canal at the level of the midthigh, with the goal of injecting local anesthetic periarterial to the femoral artery. At this level, anatomic studies have demonstrated concomitant spread to the nerve of the vastus medialis, which offers additional analgesic benefit, but can also result in partial motor blockade. Because studies have demonstrated equivalent pain relief between the FNB and ACB, ACBs are preferred given their decreased risk of falls secondary to motor blockade.

Although the FNB and ACB provide efficacious pain relief to the anterior and medial aspects of the knee, residual posterior knee pain is attributed to nerves from the sciatic distribution. Sciatic nerve blockade can be performed at multiple levels along the thigh depending on patient habitus and operator preference. Although studies have demonstrated that the sciatic nerve blockade is effective at decreasing pain scores and reducing opioid utilization, resultant motor blockade will delay ambulation and can increase fall risk. Recent introduction of blockade of the interspace between the popliteal artery and capsule of the posterior knee (ie, IPACK block) has shown favorable results as an opioid-sparing adjunct to curbing posterior knee pain. This block targets the deep genicular nerves that provide sensory innervation to the posterior capsule of the knee. Like the ACB, the IPACK block seeks to avoid motor blockade. Clinical studies have demonstrated that the IPACK block produces clinically significant pain relief and improves patients' ability to participate in physical therapy, particularly when combined with ACB.[58,59]

Periarticular Injection

The PAI is another important adjunct for surgical analgesia in arthroplasty. PAIs are analgesic formulations administered directly by the surgeon into the most sensitive soft tissues of the surgical field, usually following the completion of surgical dissection and bone resection. Typical targets in knee arthroplasty include the tibial and femoral periosteum, the extensor mechanism, the iliotibial band, the infrapatellar fat pad, the meniscal rim, the posterior cruciate ligament, and the posterior capsule. In hip arthroplasty, the PAI is usually delivered to the femoral periosteum, the hip capsule, and other tissues that are divided or retracted during the surgical approach and instrumentation. For example, these would include the tensor fascia lata in the anterior approach, the fascia lata and gluteus medius and minimis in the lateral approach, and the fascia lata and gluteus maximus in the posterior approach.

PAIs were developed to improve pain control within the first days to weeks following surgery, both by providing direct analgesia and by reducing the likelihood of the development of primary and secondary hyperalgesia. Prospective randomized controlled trials have established that the PAI does, in fact, provide significant benefits with regard to pain, function, discharge disposition, and reduction in opioid utilization within the first 24 to 48 hours following surgery,[60] with ongoing benefits through the 10th postoperative day.[61] Although the PAI was originally proposed as an alternative to regional blocks, current literature has shown that combined therapy with neuraxial anesthesia, regional anesthetic techniques, and PAI provides additive rather than redundant benefits.[59,61]

PAIs are frequently composed of multiple drugs, the standard foundation including a long-acting local anesthetic as well as epinephrine for local vasoconstriction. The combination of medications is commonly diluted with normal saline to generate additional volume for improved consistency of injection. NSAIDs, opioids, antibiotics, and corticosteroids can also be added to the injectate, depending on patient situation. Many combinations have been devised and in general all have been found to be superior to placebo;[60,62,63] however, there is no definitive evidence to support the existence of a single best formulation.

Liposomal bupivacaine is a newer medication available for use in the PAI. Liposomal bupivacaine is purported to maintain its analgesic properties for up to 72 hours via delayed release of the active agent from its lipid carrier. Because of its pharmacologic characteristics, liposomal bupivacaine cannot be mixed with nonbupivacaine local anesthetics. Although liposomal bupivacaine should only be mixed with bupivacaine at less than a 1:2 ratio, inclusion with other components of multiagent PAI is permitted. Clinical studies investigating the efficacy of traditional multiagent PAI versus liposomal bupivacaine PAI have had mixed results, with some demonstrating superiority of liposomal bupivacaine and others showing no significant difference.[64,65] Because of lack of standardization with respect to study design, infiltration protocols, patient factors, and outcome measures, there is still no definitive conclusion as to whether the high cost of liposomal bupivacaine is justified by clinically important differences in postoperative pain.

SUMMARY

Optimal perioperative pain management in total joint arthroplasty is best achieved through multimodal analgesic strategies. Modifiable risk factors for postoperative pain such as psychiatric disease should be addressed prior to surgery. Medical management with multiple agents is initiated prior to incision. Neuraxial and regional anesthetic techniques are preferred over general anesthesia whenever possible. PAI administered intraoperatively can reduce oral and parenteral medication requirements postoperatively. Close attention must be paid to analgesic protocols through each perioperative stage in order to minimize adverse effects and optimize outcomes.

KEY STUDY POINTS

- Multimodal pain management methods are preferred to minimize the potential harms of opioid analgesics.
- Patient education and engagement are key goals to assist with pain management.
- Perioperative analgesia should be initiated preemptively to prevent pain sensitization.
- Neuraxial anesthesia is strongly preferred over general anesthesia whenever possible. Close communication and partnership with anesthesia staff are critical.
- There is no consensus regimen for postoperative pain control; treatment must be tailored according to the needs of each case.

ANNOTATED REFERENCES

1. Trousdale RT, McGrory BJ, Berry DJ, Becker MW, Harmsen WS: Patients' concerns prior to undergoing total hip and total knee arthroplasty. *Mayo Clin Proc* 1999;74(10):978-982.

2. Steinberg AC, Schimpf MO, White AB, et al: Preemptive analgesia for postoperative hysterectomy pain control: Systematic review and clinical practice guidelines. *Am J Obstet Gynecol* 2017;217(3):303-313.e6.

   A systematic review of the gynecologic literature investigated the efficacy of preemptive analgesia for patients undergoing total abdominal hysterectomy. Sixty-nine articles were ultimately included in the analysis. Findings: preemptive analgesia with acetaminophen, gabapentin, rofecoxib, ketamine, and opioids reduced postoperative visual analog scale pain scores and opioid requirements.

3. Adie S, Kwan A, Naylor JM, Harris IA, Mittal R: Cryotherapy following total knee replacement. *Cochrane Database Syst Rev* 2012;(9):CD007911.

4. Torisho C, Mohaddes M, Gustafsson K, Rolfson O: Minor influence of patient education and physiotherapy interventions before total hip replacement on patient-reported outcomes: An observational study of 30,756 patients in the Swedish Hip Arthroplasty Register. *Acta Orthop* 2019;90(4):306-311.

This retrospective study used the Swedish Hip Arthroplasty Register to assess the effect of preoperative physical therapy and patient education on pain, satisfaction, and quality of life following total hip arthroplasty. A total of 30,756 patients who underwent surgery from 2012 through 2015 were analyzed. Patient-reported outcome measures were recorded through the end of the first postoperative year. Findings: preoperative physical therapy was associated with lower pain, better quality of life, and higher satisfaction. Preoperative patient education was associated with lower pain and better quality of life.

5. Elkassabany NM, Abraham D, Huang S, et al: Patient education and anesthesia choice for total knee arthroplasty. *Patient Educ Couns* 2017;100(9):1709-1713.

   This retrospective observational study from a single center investigated whether attendance at a preoperative patient education class improved compliance rates with spinal anesthesia for patients undergoing unilateral total knee arthroplasty. A total of 1,010 patients who underwent surgery from April 2013 through December 2014 were included. Thirty-one percent of patients attended the class. Findings: class participants were 70% more likely to receive spinal anesthesia than nonparticipants.

6. Hanusch BC, O'Connor DB, Ions P, Scott A, Gregg PJ: Effects of psychological distress and perceptions of illness on recovery from total knee replacement. *Bone Joint J* 2014;96-B(2):210-216.

7. Kohring JM, Erickson JA, Anderson MB, Gililland JM, Peters CL, Pelt CE: Treated versus untreated depression in total joint arthroplasty impacts outcomes. *J Arthroplasty* 2018;33:S81-S85.

   A retrospective review assessed the effect of depression on outcomes following total joint arthroplasty. A total of 280 cases were reviewed, with patients subdivided into normal, treated depressed, and untreated depressed groups. Primary outcome measure was physical function as assessed on a patient-reported outcome score sheet. Results: patients with untreated depression had significantly less improvement in their physical function following surgery. Treated depressed patients had results more similar to healthy control patients.

8. Hinz B, Cheremina O, Brune K: Acetaminophen (paracetamol) is a selective cyclooxygenase-2 inhibitor in man. *FASEB J* 2008;22(2):383-390.

9. Watkins PB, Kaplowitz N, Slattery JT, et al: Aminotransferase elevations in healthy adults receiving 4 grams of acetaminophen daily: A randomized controlled trial. *J Am Med Assoc* 2006;296:87-93.

10. O'Neal JB, Freiberg AA, Yelle MD, et al: Intravenous vs oral acetaminophen as an adjunct to multimodal analgesia after total knee arthroplasty: A prospective, randomized, double-blind clinical trial. *J Arthroplasty* 2017;32(10):3029-3033.

    A double-blind prospective randomized controlled trial from a single center compared the efficacy of intravenous acetaminophen against oral acetaminophen and placebo for patients undergoing unilateral total knee arthroplasty. A total of 174 patients were randomized into three groups: oral acetaminophen, intravenous acetaminophen, and placebo. All patients also received spinal anesthesia and institutional multimodal pain management. Outcome measures included visual analog scale pain scores, opioid consumption, time to discharge from the recovery room, time to rescue analgesia, and time to breakthrough pain. Findings: there were no statistically significant differences in the outcome measures between all three groups.

11. Sun L, Zhu X, Zou J, Li Y, Han W: Comparison of intravenous and oral acetaminophen for pain control after total knee and hip arthroplasty: A systematic review and meta-analysis. *Medicine (Baltimore)* 2018;97(6):e9751.

    A meta-analysis of randomized controlled trials compared the efficacy of intravenous versus oral acetaminophen for pain relief following total knee and hip arthroplasty in the setting of multimodal analgesia. Two trials were included, with 236 patients. Findings: there were no significant differences found with respect to pain scores or opioid consumption at 12, 24, and 48 hours postoperatively between the two groups.

12. Krebs EE, Gravely A, Nugent S, et al: Effect of opioid vs nonopioid medications on pain-related function in patients with chronic back pain or hip or knee osteoarthritis pain: The SPACE randomized clinical trial. *J Am Med Assoc* 2018;319(9):872-882.

    This is a report of the Strategies for Prescribing Analgesics Comparative Effectiveness (SPACE) study, a prospective randomized trial investigating the effectiveness of opioid versus nonopioid medications for controlling back, hip, or knee pain in patients at Veterans Affairs clinics. A total of 240 patients were randomized into two groups: opioid treatment with morphine, oxycodone, or hydrocodone/acetaminophen, and nonopioid treatment with acetaminophen or an NSAID. Specific drug treatments were subject to adjustment over the course of 12 months. Outcome measures included pain intensity, pain-related function, and adverse events. Findings: pain intensity was lower in the nonopioid group than the opioid group. Adverse events were less likely in the nonopioid group than the opioid group. There was no significant difference between the two groups with regard to pain-related function.

13. Pham H, Pickell M, Yagnatovsky M, et al: The utility of oral nonsteroidal anti-inflammatory drugs compared with standard opioids following arthroscopic meniscectomy: A prospective observational study. *Arthroscopy* 2019;35(3):864-870.e1.

    A prospective, nonrandomized, comparative observational study from a single center investigated the analgesic efficacy of opioids versus NSAIDs with lower doses of opioids. Study population comprised 68 adults (18 to 65 years old) who had undergone arthroscopic meniscectomy. One group received 30 to 40 tablets of oxycodone/acetaminophen 5/325 mg, and the other group received ibuprofen 600 mg as well as 10 tablets of oxycodone/acetaminophen 5/325 mg. Outcome measures recorded at 8 hours, 24 hours, 48 hours, and 1 week postoperative included medication usage, visual analog scale pain scores, adverse events, and satisfaction. Findings: the opioid group consumed significantly more opioids on postoperative day 1 than the NSAID group. There were no significant differences between pain control, satisfaction, and total opioid consumption at 1 week postoperatively between the two groups. Level of evidence: II.

14. Kan SL, Yang B, Ning GZ, et al: Nonsteroidal anti-inflammatory drugs as prophylaxis for heterotopic ossification after total hip arthroplasty. *Medicine (Baltimore)* 2015;94(18):e828.

15. Gobble RM, Hoang HLT, Kachniarz B, Orgill DP: Ketorolac does not increase perioperative bleeding: A meta-analysis of randomized controlled trials. *Plast Reconstr Surg* 2014;133(3):741-755.

16. Zhu XT, Chen L, Lin JH: Selective COX-2 inhibitor versus non-selective COX-2 inhibitor for the prevention of heterotopic ossification after total hip arthroplasty: A meta-analysis. *Medicine (Baltimore)* 2018;97(31):e11649.

A meta-analysis of randomized controlled trials evaluated the efficacy of COX-2-specific NSAIDs for prevention of heterotopic ossification after total hip arthroplasty compared with nonselective NSAIDs. Eight studies with 1,636 patients were included. Findings: no significant differences were found between selective and nonselective NSAIDs with regard to overall incidence of heterotopic ossification, or incidence of heterotopic ossification at every level of severity according to the Brooker classification. There were also no significant differences with respect to excessive bleeding. Selective NSAIDs were less likely to incur gastrointestinal adverse effects.

17. Noveck RJ, Hubbard RC: Parecoxib sodium, an injectable COX-2-specific inhibitor, does not affect unfractionated heparin-regulated blood coagulation parameters. *J Clin Pharmacol* 2004;44(5):474-480.

18. Graham DJ: COX-2 inhibitors, other NSAIDs, and cardiovascular risk: The seduction of common sense. *J Am Med Assoc* 2006;296(13):1653-1656.

19. Solomon SD, McMurray JJV, Pfeffer MA, et al: Cardiovascular risk associated with celecoxib in a clinical trial for colorectal adenoma prevention. *N Engl J Med* 2005;352(11):1071-1080.

20. Nissen SE, Yeomans ND, Solomon DH, et al: Cardiovascular safety of celecoxib, naproxen, or ibuprofen for arthritis. *N Engl J Med* 2016;375(26):2519-2529.

21. Cottrell J, Patrick O'Connor J: Effect of non-steroidal anti-inflammatory drugs on bone healing. *Pharmaceuticals* 2010;3:1668-1693.

22. Jacobsson SA, Djerf K, Ivarsson I, Wahlström O: Effect of diclofenac on fixation of hydroxyapatite-coated implants. An experimental study. *J Bone Joint Surg Br* 1994;76(5):831-833.

23. Giannoudis PV, MacDonald DA, Matthews SJ, Smith RM, Furlong AJ, De Boer P: Nonunion of the femoral diaphysis. The influence of reaming and non-steroidal anti-inflammatory drugs. *J Bone Joint Surg Br* 2000;82(5):655-658.

24. Glassman SD, Rose SM, Dimar JR, Puno RM, Campbell MJ, Johnson JR: The effect of postoperative nonsteroidal anti-inflammatory drug administration on spinal fusion. *Spine (Phila Pa 1976)* 1998;23:834-838.

25. Nizam I, Kohan L, Field C, Kerr D: Do nonsteroidal anti-inflammatory drugs cause endoprosthetic loosening? Mid- to long-term follow-up of 100 total hip arthroplasties after local NSAID infiltration. *Biomed Res Int* 2015;2015:703071.

26. Hayhurst CJ, Durieux ME: Differential opioid tolerance and opioid-induced hyperalgesia: A clinical reality. *Anesthesiology* 2016;124:483-488.

27. Xu Z, Zhang H, Luo J, Zhou A, Zhang J: Preemptive analgesia by using celecoxib combined with tramadol/APAP alleviates post-operative pain of patients undergoing total knee arthroplasty. *Phys Sportsmed* 2017;45:316-322.

This prospective study assessed the effect of preemptive analgesia with celecoxib and low-dose tramadol/acetaminophen on postoperative pain in patients undergoing unilateral total knee arthroplasty. A total of 132 patients were included and separated into a preemptive analgesia group and a standard multimodal analgesia group. The preemptive analgesia group received 3 days of preoperative medication with celecoxib and tramadol/acetaminophen; all intraoperative and postoperative analgesic measures were kept the same between groups. Outcome measures included visual analog scale pain scores for up to 12 months postoperatively, as well as length of stay, cost of care, and complications. Results: experimental group experienced significantly less pain for up to 3 months postoperatively.

28. Cooper HJ, Lakra A, Maniker RB, Hickernell TR, Shah RP, Geller JA: Preemptive analgesia with oxycodone is associated with more pain following total joint arthroplasty. *J Arthroplasty* 2019;34(12):2878-2883.

This retrospective cohort study assessed whether using oxycodone for preemptive analgesia is effective for controlling postoperative pain following total joint arthroplasty. A total of 550 patients who underwent elective primary total joint arthroplasty were identified and divided into one cohort that received oxycodone with a standard multimodal preemptive analgesic regimen and one cohort that received the multimodal analgesic regimen without oxycodone. Outcome measures included visual analog scale pain scores, opioid consumption, length of stay, and ambulation distance. Results: patients in the opioid group experienced more pain on postoperative day 1 and ambulated less than the nonopioid group. They also consumed more opioids in the course of their hospitalizations.

29. Kastanias P, Gowans S, Tumber PS, Snaith K, Robinson S: Patient-controlled oral analgesia for postoperative pain management following total knee replacement. *Pain Res Manag* 2010;15(1):11-16.

30. Sing DC, Barry JJ, Cheah JW, Vail TP, Hansen EN: Long-acting opioid use independently predicts perioperative complication in total joint arthroplasty. *J Arthroplasty* 2016;31(9):170-174.e1.

31. Nguyen L-CL, Sing DC, Bozic KJ: Preoperative reduction of opioid use before total joint arthroplasty. *J Arthroplasty* 2016;31(9 suppl):282-287.

32. Tsukada S, Wakui M, Hoshino A: The impact of including corticosteroid in a periarticular injection for pain control after total knee arthroplasty: A double-blind randomised controlled trial. *Bone Joint J* 2016;98-B(2):194-200.

33. Mathiesen O, Jacobsen LS, Holm HE, et al: Pregabalin and dexamethasone for postoperative pain control: A randomized controlled study in hip arthroplasty. *Br J Anaesth* 2008;101(4):535-541.

34. Godshaw BM, Mehl AE, Shaffer JG, Meyer MS, Thomas LC, Chimento GF: The effects of peri-operative dexamethasone on patients undergoing total hip or knee arthroplasty: Is it safe for diabetics? *J Arthroplasty* 2019;34(4):645-649.

This retrospective review investigated the effect of perioperative dexamethasone on glycemic control and complications of patients who have diabetes undergoing primary total hip and knee arthroplasty. A total of 2,317 patients were included and stratified into diabetic and nondiabetic categories; these were substratified into groups depending on whether they received dexamethasone during surgery. The outcome measures included periprosthetic joint infection (PJI) and serum glucose levels. Findings: dexamethasone was not associated with an increased risk of PJI in the overall study group. There was an overall higher rate of PJI among patients who had diabetes compared to those who did not.; however, there was no significant difference in PJI between these two groups who received dexamethasone. Serum glucose levels rose postoperatively; although diabetes was associated with greater glucose variability, dexamethasone administration did not alter the magnitude of change.

35. Clarke HA, Katz J, McCartney CJL, et al: Perioperative gabapentin reduces 24 h opioid consumption and improves in-hospital rehabilitation but not post-discharge outcomes after total knee arthroplasty with peripheral nerve block. *Br J Anaesth* 2014;113(5):855-864.

36. Zhai L, Song Z, Liu K: The effect of gabapentin on acute postoperative pain in patients undergoing total knee arthroplasty: A meta-analysis. *Medicine (Baltimore)* 2016;95(20):e3673.

37. Han C, Kuang MJ, Ma JX, Ma XL: Is pregabalin effective and safe in total knee arthroplasty? A PRISMA-compliant meta-analysis of randomized-controlled trials. *Medicine (Baltimore)* 2017;96(26):e6947.

This meta-analysis of randomized placebo-controlled trials assessed the safety and efficacy of pregabalin for pain control in total knee arthroplasty. Seven studies were included with 962 patients in the analysis. Outcome measures included visual analog scale pain scores, opioid consumption, knee range of motion, and adverse effects. Results: pregabalin was associated with reduced opioid consumption, increased knee range of motion, and fewer complications such as nausea, pruritus, and constipation.

38. Li F, Ma J, Kuang M, et al: The efficacy of pregabalin for the management of postoperative pain in primary total knee and hip arthroplasty: A meta-analysis. *J Orthop Surg Res* 2017;12(1):49.

This meta-analysis of randomized controlled trials assessed the safety and efficacy of pregabalin for pain control in primary total knee and total hip arthroplasty. Seven studies were included with 823 patients in the analysis. Outcome measures included visual analog scale pain scores, opioid consumption, and adverse effects. Results: pregabalin was associated with lower pain scores at 24 and 48 hours but not at 72 hours compared with placebo.

39. Yik JH, Tham WYW, Tay KH, Shen L, Krishna L: Perioperative pregabalin does not reduce opioid requirements in total knee arthroplasty. *Knee Surg Sports Traumatol Arthrosc* 2019;27:2104-2110.

This prospective randomized double-blind placebo-controlled trial assessed whether pregabalin is effective for reducing pain and opioid consumption following total knee arthroplasty when added to a multimodal analgesia regimen. A total of 87 patients were randomized into two groups: one group received the standard multimodal protocol and the other group received the same interventions with preemptive pregabalin that continued through the second postoperative day. Outcome measures included pain scores and opioid consumption through the first 72 postoperative hours, as well as functional outcome measures through the first 6 months. Results: pregabalin administration was not associated with lower pain scores or reduced opioid consumption at 48 or 72 hours postoperatively. Pregabalin also did not correlate with improved functional outcomes at 3 or 6 months. Level of evidence: II.

40. Kjær Petersen K, Lunn TH, Husted H, et al: The influence of pre- and perioperative administration of gabapentin on pain 3-4 years after total knee arthroplasty. *Scand J Pain* 2018;18:237-245.

This prospective randomized controlled trial assessed the effects of gabapentin on chronic pain and psychologic health at 3 to 4 years following primary total knee arthroplasty. A total of 300 patients were initially enrolled in the study and 215 of these were included in the final follow-up. The patients were divided into three groups: the high-dose group received 1,300 mg of gabapentin daily, the low-dose group received 900 mg of gabapentin daily, and the control group received placebo. Dosing began preemptively and continued through the seventh postoperative day. Outcome measures included pain scores, pain catastrophizing scores, and anxiety and depression scores. Results: gabapentin was not associated with greater improvements in pain, depression, or anxiety at 3 to 4 years following surgery.

41. Lunn TH, Husted H, Laursen MB, Hansen LT, Kehlet H: Analgesic and sedative effects of perioperative gabapentin in total knee arthroplasty: A randomized, double-blind, placebo-controlled dose-finding study. *Pain* 2015;156:2438-2448.

42. Mao Y, Wu L, Ding W: The efficacy of preoperative administration of gabapentin/pregabalin in improving pain after total hip arthroplasty: A meta-analysis. *BMC Musculoskelet Disord* 2016;17:373.

43. Dong J, Li W, Wang Y: The effect of pregabalin on acute postoperative pain in patients undergoing total knee arthroplasty: A meta-analysis. *Int J Surg* 2016;34:148-160.

44. Brooks E, Freter SH, Bowles SK, Amirault D: Multimodal pain management in older elective arthroplasty patients. *Geriatr Orthop Surg Rehabil* 2017;8:151-154.

This prospective observational study assessed the effectiveness of a modern multimodal pain management regimen compared with a traditional regimen for pain control in patients older than 70 years undergoing elective primary arthroplasty. A total of 158 patients were divided into two groups: one group received traditional analgesia with acetaminophen and opioids, whereas the other group received a multimodal regimen with acetaminophen, opioids, gabapentin, and celecoxib. Outcome measures included pain scores, opioid consumption, postoperative delirium, time to independent ambulation, and cost. Results: the multimodal group consumed significantly more morphine equivalents of opioids but did not demonstrate any improvements in pain, delirium, or mobility through the third postoperative day. Costs were higher in the multimodal group.

45. Beilin B, Rusabrov Y, Shapira Y, et al: Low-dose ketamine affects immune responses in humans during the early postoperative period. *Br J Anaesth* 2007;99(4):522-527.

46. Perrin SB, Purcell AN: Intraoperative ketamine may influence persistent pain following knee arthroplasty under combined general and spinal anaesthesia: A pilot study. *Anaesth Intensive Care* 2009;37(2):248-253.

47. Remérand F, Le Tendre C, Baud A, et al: The early and delayed analgesic effects of ketamine after total hip arthroplasty: A prospective, randomized, controlled, double-blind study. *Anesth Analg* 2009;109(6):1963-1971.

48. Li Z, Chen Y: Ketamine reduces pain and opioid consumption after total knee arthroplasty: A meta-analysis of randomized controlled studies. *Int J Surg* 2019;70:70-83.

This meta-analysis of randomized controlled trials investigated the effect of ketamine on pain and opioid utilization following total knee arthroplasty. Six studies with 244 total patients were included in the analysis. Patients who received intraoperative ketamine were compared against those who did not. Outcome measures included visual analog scale pain scores, opioid consumption, length of stay, and complications. Findings: ketamine was associated with lower pain scores in the first 24 hours, lower opioid utilization, and lower incidence of nausea and vomiting.

49. Xu B, Wang Y, Zeng C, et al: Analgesic efficacy and safety of ketamine after total knee or hip arthroplasty: A meta-analysis of randomised placebo-controlled studies. *BMJ Open* 2019;9(9):e028337.

This meta-analysis of prospective randomized controlled trials investigated the efficacy and safety of ketamine in patients undergoing primary total hip and knee arthroplasty. Ten studies with 577 total patients were included. Patients who received intraoperative ketamine were compared with those who did not. Outcome measures included visual analog scale pain scores, opioid consumption, and complications. Findings: ketamine was associated with superior pain relief in the first 8 hours and lower opioid utilization in the first 24 and 48 hours. There was no observed increased risk of gastrointestinal or psychotic adverse effects.

50. Tan TL, Longenecker AS, Rhee JH, et al: Intraoperative ketamine in total knee arthroplasty does not decrease pain and narcotic consumption: A prospective randomized controlled trial. *J Arthroplasty* 2019;34(8):1640-1645.

This prospective randomized controlled trial assessed the effectiveness of ketamine for pain control in total knee arthroplasty when used in tandem with spinal anesthesia. A total of 91 patients undergoing primary total knee arthroplasty with spinal anesthesia were divided into two groups. The experimental group received an intraoperative ketamine infusion at a rate of 6 µg/kg/min for 75 minutes and the control group received a saline placebo. Outcome measures included visual analog scale pain scores and opioid consumption. Results: the ketamine group experienced lower average pain scores on postoperative days 1 and 4, but there were no differences between the two groups in maximum pain or opioid consumption at any time.

51. Hewitt NA, Cox P: Recurrent subanesthetic ketamine infusions for complex regional pain syndrome leading to biliary dilation, jaundice, and cholangitis: A case report. *A A Pract* 2018;10(7):168-170.

This is a case report of a single patient undergoing serial treatment with subcutaneous ketamine infusion for the treatment of type 1 complex regional pain syndrome. During the course of his third 3-day infusion with subanesthetic doses of ketamine, biliary dilatation, jaundice, and cholangitis developed. The symptoms were managed with medical and surgical intervention.

52. Short B, Fong J, Galvez V, Shelker W, Loo CK: Side-effects associated with ketamine use in depression: A systematic review. *Lancet Psychiatry* 2018;5(1):65-78.

This systematic review of the literature assessed the adverse effect profile of ketamine in the treatment of patients with depression. A total of 60 studies were included with 899 patients who received ketamine. The most common adverse effects from ketamine administration included psychiatric and psychomimetic effects such as anxiety, dissociation, and delusions; cardiovascular effects such as hypertension and tachycardia; and neurocognitive effects such as headache, memory loss, and cognitive impairment.

53. Pugely AJ, Martin CT, Gao Y, Mendoza-Lattes S, Callaghan JJ: Differences in short-term complications between spinal and general anesthesia for primary total knee arthroplasty. *J Bone Joint Surg Am* 2013;95(3):193-199.

54. Memtsoudis SG, Cozowicz C, Bekeris J, et al: Anaesthetic care of patients undergoing primary hip and knee arthroplasty: Consensus recommendations from the International Consensus on Anaesthesia-Related Outcomes after Surgery group (ICAROS) based on a systematic review and meta-analysis. *Br J Anaesth* 2019;123(3):269-287.

This systematic review of the anesthesia literature investigated the optimal anesthetic modality for the care of primary total joint arthroplasty patients. A total of 94 studies were included in the review. Outcome measures included mortality and complication rates. Findings: neuraxial anesthesia was statistically superior to general anesthesia with respect to mortality, pulmonary complications, renal complications, thromboembolic complications, infections, and blood transfusion rates. However, neuraxial anesthesia was associated with higher rates of urinary retention.

55. Mahan MC, Jildeh TR, Tenbrunsel TN, Davis JJ: Primary arthroplasty mepivacaine spinal anesthesia facilitates rapid recovery in total knee arthroplasty compared to bupivacaine. *J Arthroplasty* 2018;33:1699-1704.

This retrospective review assessed the efficacy and safety of mepivacaine compared with that of bupivacaine for spinal anesthesia in patients undergoing primary total knee arthroplasty. A total of 156 consecutive patients were divided into two groups: one group received mepivacaine and the other received bupivacaine for single-shot spinal anesthesia. Outcome measures included pain scores, opioid consumption, urinary retention, length of stay, and distance ambulated with physical therapy. Results: mepivacaine was associated with shorter length of stay and lower rates of urinary retention requiring catheterization compared with bupivacaine. Mepivacaine was also associated with higher pain scores and opioid consumption in the postanesthesia care unit, but not through the subsequent hospitalization.

56. Kaur A, Singh RB, Tripathi RK, Choubey S: Comparison between bupivacaine and ropivacaine in patients undergoing forearm surgeries under axillary brachial plexus block: A prospective randomized study. *J Clin Diagn Res* 2015;9:UC01-UC06.

57. Dony P, Dewinde V, Vanderick B, et al: The comparative toxicity of ropivacaine and bupivacaine at equipotent doses in rats. *Anesth Analg* 2000;91:1489-1492.

58. Sankineani SR, Reddy ARC, Kiran Eachempati K, Jangale A, Gurava Reddy AV: Comparison of adductor canal block and IPACK block (interspace between the popliteal artery and the capsule of the posterior knee) with adductor canal block alone after total knee arthroplasty: A prospective control trial on pain and knee function in immediate postoperative period. *Eur J Orthop Surg Traumatol* 2018;28(3):1391-1395.

   This prospective controlled trial investigated the effect of adding an IPACK block to an adductor canal block (ACB) for patients undergoing primary total knee arthroplasty. A total of 120 patients were divided into two study groups: the first 60 received both ACB and IPACK blocks, and the second 60 received ACB alone. Analgesic management was kept otherwise identical. Outcome measures included visual analog scale pain scores through the second postoperative day, range of motion, and ambulation distance. Findings: the combined ACB + IPACK group had significantly lower pain scores, higher range of motion, and greater ambulation distances than the ACB group.

59. Kim DH, Beathe JC, Lin Y, et al: Addition of infiltration between the popliteal artery and the capsule of the posterior knee and adductor canal block to periarticular injection enhances postoperative pain control in total knee arthroplasty. *Anesth Analg* 2018;129(2):1.

   This triple-blind, randomized controlled trial investigated the effect of adding an IPACK block to PAI for patients undergoing primary total knee arthroplasty. A total of 86 patients were divided into two study groups: the first group received the PAI alone, and the second group received both the PAI and an IPACK block. Outcome measures included pain on postoperative day 1, satisfaction ratings, and opioid consumption. Findings: the combined PAI + IPACK group had significantly lower pain scores, higher satisfaction ratings, and lower opioid consumption than the PAI group.

60. Busch CA, Shore BJ, Bhandari R, et al: Efficacy of periarticular multimodal drug injection in total knee arthroplasty. A randomized trial. *J Bone Joint Surg Am* 2006;88(5):959-963.

61. Srampickal GM, Jacob KM, Kandoth JJ, et al: How effective is periarticular drug infiltration in providing pain relief and early functional outcome following total hip arthroplasty? *J Clin Orthop Trauma* 2019;10(3):550-554.

   This prospective randomized trial evaluated the efficacy of PAI versus postoperative epidural analgesia for pain control following primary total hip arthroplasty. A total of 50 patients were divided into two groups: the first group received a PAI consisting of ropivacaine, methylprednisolone, morphine, ketorolac, cefazolin, and saline, and the second group received a lumbar epidural catheter that continuously dispensed bupivacaine and fentanyl for 48 hours postoperatively. Outcome measures included visual analog scale pain scores, satisfaction scores, functional scores, and complications. Findings: the PAI group has significantly lower pain scores through the 10th postoperative day as compared to the epidural group. Functional recovery was also improved in the PAI group. Finally, the PAI group had lower incidence of complications including nausea and vomiting, motor weakness, back pain, and urinary retention. Satisfaction scores were higher in the PAI group.

62. Iwakiri K, Ohta Y, Kobayashi A, Minoda Y, Nakamura H: Local efficacy of periarticular morphine injection in simultaneous bilateral total knee arthroplasty: A prospective, randomized, double-blind trial. *J Arthroplasty* 2017;32:3637-3642.

   This prospective randomized controlled trial assessed the efficacy of periarticular injection of morphine for pain control in simultaneous bilateral total knee arthroplasty. A total of 53 patients undergoing 106 total knee arthroplasties were divided into two groups: the first group received a periarticular injection with morphine and the second group had the same injection with morphine omitted. Outcome measures included visual analog scale pain scores, range of motion, functional outcome scores, and adverse effects. Results: there were no differences between the two groups for any outcome measure at any time point.

63. Ishida K, Shibanuma N, Matsumoto T, Tei K, Kuroda R, Kurosaka M: Periarticular multimodal drug injection improves post-operative pain and functional recovery after total knee arthroplasty. *J Orthop Sci* 2016;21:178-183.

64. Yayac M, Li WT, Ong AC, Courtney PM, Saxena A: The efficacy of liposomal bupivacaine over traditional local anesthetics in periarticular infiltration and regional anesthesia during total knee arthroplasty: A systematic review and meta-analysis. *J Arthroplasty* 2019;34(9):2166-2183.

   This systematic review and meta-analysis of controlled trials investigated the efficacy of liposomal bupivacaine versus older analgesic medications and modalities for controlling pain following primary total knee arthroplasty. A total of 42 studies were included in the systematic review, of which 17 controlled trials were also included in the meta-analysis. Findings: liposomal bupivacaine yielded lower pain scores than peripheral nerve blocks and traditional periarticular injections. However, it was questionable as to whether the benefit was clinically distinguishable.

65. Yu SW, Szulc AL, Walton SL, Davidovitch RI, Bosco JA, Iorio R: Liposomal bupivacaine as an adjunct to postoperative pain control in total hip arthroplasty. *J Arthroplasty* 2016;31(7):1510-1515.

Osteonecrosis of the Hip and Knee

HYTHAM S. SALEM, MD • KEVIN K. MATHEW, BS • KEVIN B. MARCHAND, BS
JOHN M. TARAZI, MD • JOSEPH O. EHIOROBO, MD • MICHAEL A. MONT, MD, FAAOS

ABSTRACT

Osteonecrosis is a debilitating condition that can result in structural collapse. It most commonly affects the femoral head, followed by the knee and shoulder joints. Because osteonecrosis is often progressive in nature, it inevitably requires surgical intervention. The surgeon treating osteonecrosis of the hip and knee joint should understand the etiology, diagnosis, and management of the disease.

Mr. Marchand or an immediate family member is a member of a speakers' bureau or has made paid presentations on behalf of Stryker; serves as a paid consultant to or is an employee of Stryker; and has stock or stock options held in Stryker. Dr. Mont or an immediate family member has received royalties from Microport; serves as a paid consultant to or is an employee of Cymedica, DJ Orthopaedics, Flexion Therapeutics, Johnson & Johnson, Ongoing Care Solutions, Orthosensor, Pacira, Peerwell, Performance Dynamics, Pfizer, Skye Biologics, Stryker, and TissueGene; has stock or stock options held in Peerwell and USMI; has received research or institutional support from DJ Orthopaedics, Johnson & Johnson, National Institutes of Health (NIAMS & NICHD), Ongoing Care Solutions, Orthosensor, Stryker, and TissueGene; and serves as a board member, owner, officer, or committee member of the American Academy of Orthopaedic Surgeons, the American Association of Hip and Knee Surgeons, and the Knee Society. None of the following authors or any immediate family member has received anything of value from or has stock or stock options held in a commercial company or institution related directly or indirectly to the subject of this chapter: Dr. Salem, Mr. Mathew, Dr. Tarazi, and Dr. Ehiorobo.

Keywords: collapse; hip; knee; management; osteonecrosis

INTRODUCTION

Osteonecrosis is a condition with debilitating results that can cause structural collapse of the joints affected. Osteonecrosis most commonly occurs in the femoral head, with an incidence of 20,000 to 30,000 new cases annually in the United States, which is expected to continue to increase.[1,2] Osteonecrosis is seen more commonly in males and typically present in patients 35 to 50 years of age.[3] The knee is the second most common location of osteonecrosis, comprising 10% of all cases, and most frequently the distal femur is affected.[4]

Treatment options can vary depending on the stage of disease at presentation. In the early stage of osteonecrosis, there is little to no structural collapse, and the prognosis is often better compared with advanced stages of the disease. Surgery is often indicated, although occasionally, patients in early stages (precollapse) of the disease can be treated nonsurgically. In osteonecrosis of the hip, almost 80% of cases are bilateral, and the eventual joint destruction and loss of function comprise 10% of all total hip arthroplasties (THAs).[5] Therefore, it is important for orthopaedic surgeons to be comfortable with managing osteonecrosis of both the hip and knee. Understanding the etiology and pathology, evaluation and diagnosis, and treatment (surgical and nonsurgical modalities) all help the surgeon in managing osteonecrosis of the hip and knee.

This chapter is adapted from Patel NK, Mistry JB, Elmallah RK, Chughtai M, Nace J, Mont MA: Osteonecrosis of the hip and knee, in Mont MA, Tanzer M, eds: *Orthopaedic Knowledge Update®: Hip and Knee Reconstruction*, ed 5. Rosemont, IL, American Academy of Orthopaedic Surgeons, 2017, pp 45-61.

OSTEONECROSIS OF THE HIP

Etiology and Pathogenesis

Many risk factors for osteonecrosis have been identified (**Table 1**), although despite much research, the etiology is not well characterized. The process common with all proposed etiologies is circulatory obstruction, the causes of which include coagulation of intraosseous circulation, venous thrombosis, retrograde arterial occlusion, and lipid hypertrophy. In the setting of lipid accumulation within the bone marrow, intraosseous pressure increases causing femoral head ischemia and eventual osteonecrosis. Even when a repair process is initiated, subchondral fracture and collapse are almost always inevitable. Osteonecrosis does not develop in all patients with risk factors, suggesting some genetic predisposition.

Trauma

Hip dislocation and femoral head/neck fractures interrupt the medial circumflex artery, which is the main blood supply to the femoral head. Hip dislocation, which can cause osteonecrosis in 9% to 33% of patients, increases with the degree of initial displacement, and possibly with time to reduction (greater than 12 hours).[6] The rate of osteonecrosis following femoral head fracture (usually with hip dislocation) ranges from 1% to 50%, depending on the location of an associated acetabular fracture and increasing with the Pipkin classification type (commonly used for uncommon femoral head fractures associated with hip dislocations [four types]). The rate of osteonecrosis for femoral neck fracture is as high as 10% in nondisplaced injuries and 30% in displaced injuries, increasing with the Garden classification type (for femoral neck fractures; can help predict risk of osteonecrosis [four types]). The risk of osteonecrosis can be reduced with prompt anatomic reduction and surgical fixation. Less commonly, cervicotrochanteric and intertrochanteric fractures can cause osteonecrosis.[7]

TABLE 1

Risk Factors for the Development of Osteonecrosis

Direct Risk Factors	Indirect Risk Factors
Trauma: fracture or dislocation	Corticosteroids
Sickle cell disease	Alcohol abuse
HIV infection	Tobacco use
Chemotherapy	Systemic lupus erythematosus
Radiation	Organ transplantation
Myeloproliferative disorders	Renal failure
Gaucher disease	Coagulation abnormalities
	Pregnancy
	Genetic factors
	Caisson disease

Data from Mont MA, Cherian JJ, Sierra RJ, Jones LC, Lieberman JR: Nontraumatic osteonecrosis of the femoral head: Where do we stand today? A ten-year update. *J Bone Joint Surg Am* 2015;97(19):1604-1627.

Corticosteroids

High-dose corticosteroid use is a well-known risk factor for osteonecrosis, with rates of 3% to 23% seen in patients following solid organ transplantation.[8,9] The available data are inconsistent in explaining the relationship between osteonecrosis and dosage, route, or treatment; however, several studies have shown the cumulative dose to be an important factor.[8,10] In bone marrow stromal cells, corticosteroids cause cell apoptosis and a decrease in precursor cell proliferation, altering bone homeostasis and causing cellular injury.[11] In addition, corticosteroids can impair blood flow by enhancing femoral head arterial constriction, as seen within 24 hours of methylprednisolone treatment.[12] Moreover, corticosteroids can activate proinflammatory pathways and are linked to various gene alterations (eg, interleukin [IL]-23, IL-1α, transforming growth factor-β, IL-10, and tumor necrosis factor-α).[13] These pathways also include decreased expression of bone-marker genes and increased expression of adipogenic gene *422(aP2)* when bone marrow stromal cells are exposed to dexamethasone. Corticosteroids can also induce extravascular fat deposition, adipocyte hypertrophy, and oxidative stress, suggesting a multifactorial pathophysiology.[13]

Alcohol Abuse

Alcohol abuse is also a well-known risk factor for osteonecrosis of the hip with a clear dose-response relationship.[14,15] Suspected causes of osteonecrosis of the hip and knee include impaired mesenchymal cell differentiation, diminished blood flow, and direct cellular toxicity. Alcohol reduces osteogenic differentiation and increases adipogenic cell differentiation, thus increasing adipogenic volume in the femoral head and hindering circulatory dynamics. Mesenchymal stem cells (MSCs) retrieved from proximal femoral bone marrow from alcoholics with osteonecrosis have demonstrated reduced osteogenic gene expression when cultured with alcohol.[16] Many of the mechanisms are similar to those of corticosteroids, including cell apoptosis and possibly lipopolysaccharide interactions, which activate proinflammatory pathways.

Coagulation Disorders

Coagulation disorders, including inherited thrombophilia and hypofibrinolysis, are risk factors for blood flow interruption.[17] In addition, endothelial progenitor cells required for angiogenesis can become dysfunctional.[11] A study examined 200 patients who have sickle cell disease at 15-year follow-up and reported that the incidence of osteonecrosis was 43% in the SS genotype, 38% in the SC genotype, and 19% in the Sβ^+ thalassemia genotype.[18] Hypofibrinolysis from familial high plasminogen activator inhibition was associated with osteonecrosis, and these patients were more likely to carry a hypofibrinolytic 4G polymorphism of the plasminogen activator inhibitor-1 gene compared with control patients.[17]

Autoimmune Disease

Osteonecrosis has been linked with various conditions such as systemic lupus erythematosus (SLE), Behçet disease, and rheumatoid arthritis. SLE has been shown to be an independent risk factor for osteonecrosis, especially in the presence of Raynaud phenomenon, hyperlipidemia, and raised anticardiolipin/antiphospholipid antibodies. Corticosteroid use in patients who have SLE leads to a significantly higher risk of osteonecrosis compared with nonusers (37% versus 21%).[19]

Evaluation and Diagnosis

Patients who have osteonecrosis may be asymptomatic, but those who present with pain often report deep, throbbing anterior hip and thigh pain with insidious onset.[20] A history of antecedent trauma may not always be present. The pain is typically worse with activity, with weight bearing, and at night. The presence of risk factors should always be explored (**Table 1**). In the early stages of osteonecrosis, physical examination can be normal. Specific joint examination can show an antalgic gait and a positive Trendelenburg sign because of pain. The leg may be held in a position of maximal comfort, with a possible limb-length discrepancy (secondary to collapse) and surgical scars. Range of motion is preserved but is generally painful at the groin.

Imaging

Initially, plain radiographs including AP and frog-lateral views, are required, particularly for staging. The findings on these views are often normal, unless osteonecrosis has progressed enough to show subchondral collapse, acetabular involvement, and secondary osteoarthritis (**Figure 1**). Radiographs can also demonstrate radiolucencies and opacities. MRI has at least 90% sensitivity and specificity and therefore is the benchmark for evaluating osteonecrosis of the femoral head.[21-23] MRI is particularly useful in detecting precollapse lesions that can occur without subchondral fracture[24] (**Figure 2**). Additionally, MRI helps with diagnosis, lesion sizing, and disease staging. Bone marrow edema also can be detected on MRI and has been shown to correlate with the presence of hip pain and disease progression in 61 asymptomatic or minimally symptomatic hips at 60-month follow-up.[25]

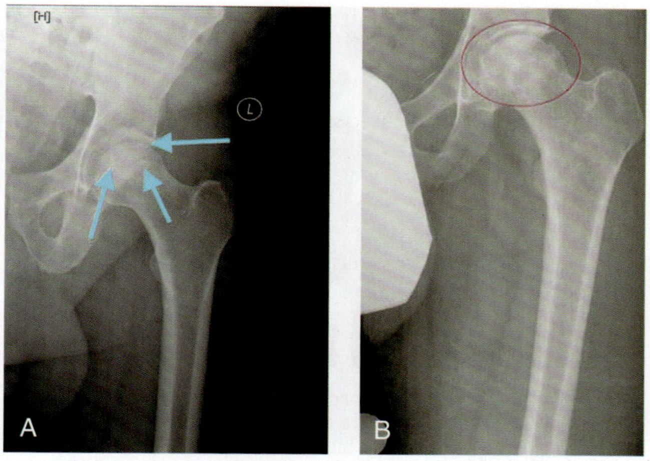

FIGURE 1 Radiographs of a left hip demonstrate femoral head collapse. **A**, AP view shows a subchondral fracture (crescent sign) and precollapse lesion of the femoral head (arrows). **B**, AP view shows a postcollapse lesion of the femoral head (circle). (Reproduced with permission from Mont MA, Cherian JJ, Sierra RJ, Jones LC, Lieberman JR: Nontraumatic osteonecrosis of the femoral head: Where do we stand today? A ten-year update. *J Bone Joint Surg Am* 2015;97[19]:1604-1627.)

If radiographs are normal or unclear, CT also can detect subchondral collapse. Bone scans have a high false-negative rate, and positron emission tomography scan, which is expensive and less commonly available, is sensitive but not specific, making these modalities less useful.[24]

Staging

Disease staging helps to determine prognosis and plan treatment options for osteonecrosis. Various staging systems use radiologic features to stage osteonecrosis. The most frequently used system is Ficat and Arlet, which includes four stages that range from normal radiographic findings (stage 1) to femoral head collapse and acetabular involvement (stage 4). Other commonly used classification systems are the Association Research Circulation Osseous system, the Japanese Orthopaedic Association system, and the University of Pennsylvania system (**Table 2**). The four radiographic factors that are useful in evaluation are stage (before/after collapse), lesion size, amount of femoral head depression, and acetabular involvement.[26] Increased lesion size specifically correlates with poorer prognosis. The Kerboul classification[27] can help delineate prognosis and disease progression by using the combined

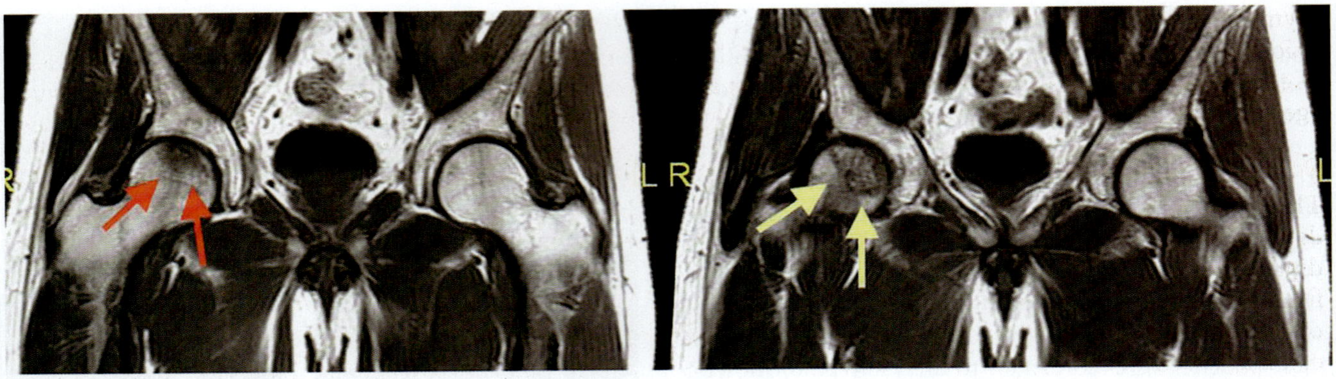

FIGURE 2 T1-weighted coronal magnetic resonance images of the femoral head showing a precollapse lesion of the femoral head (arrows). The separate coronal images demonstrate the extent of the lesion (dark areas). (Reproduced with permission from Mont MA, Cherian JJ, Sierra RJ, Jones LC, Lieberman JR: Nontraumatic osteonecrosis of the femoral head: Where do we stand today? A ten-year update. *J Bone Joint Surg Am* 2015;97[19]:1604-1627.)

necrotic angle, which is defined as the sum of the angles subtended by the necrotic segment in both midcoronal and midsagittal MRIs. Results showed no hip collapse with angles up to 190° in four hips, half-collapsed hips at angles between 190° and 240° in four hips, and fully collapsed hips at angles of 240° or greater in 25 hips.[27] A 2010 study demonstrated 101 asymptomatic hips with medially located small lesions (Kerboul angle less than 200°) had a rate of collapse less than 10%, compared with 25% for the remainder.[28]

Treatment

The course of treatment of osteonecrosis depends on the stage of progression and the presence of symptoms. A study of the contralateral asymptomatic hip in 40 patients showed that 88% of lesions became symptomatic and 73% collapsed in 11 years.[29] Another study showed that 7% of small and 80% of large lesions (Kerboul angle greater than 240°) collapsed in 8 years.[30] Spontaneous resolution can occur in small asymptomatic lesions, and treatment should be considered in moderate to large

TABLE 2

Overview of Commonly Used Plain Radiographic Staging Systems

Association Research Circulation Osseous		Japanese Orthopaedic Association		Ficat and Arlet		University of Pennsylvania	
Stage	**Findings**	**Stage**	**Findings**	**Stage**	**Findings**	**Stage**	**Findings**
0	Normal hip	1	Demarcation line	1	Normal radiograph	0	Normal hip
1	MRI findings only	2	Early femoral head flattening	2	Diffuse sclerotic/cystic lesions	1	MRI findings only
2	Focal osteoporosis, cystic lesions, sclerosis	3	Cystic lesions	3	Crescent sign (subchondral fracture)	2	Diffuse cystic/sclerotic lesions
3	Crescent sign (subchondral fracture)			4	Acetabular involvement, femoral head collapse	3	Subchondral step-off
4	Acetabular involvement					4	Femoral head flattening
						5	Acetabular involvement or joint space narrowing
						6	Advanced joint degeneration

asymptomatic lesions.[28] Small-sized, medially located lesions have the best prognosis, with only 10% ending in collapse.[28] **Figure 3** is a suggested algorithm for management of hip osteonecrosis.

Nonsurgical Management

The use of several drug types such as lipid-lowering drugs, antiplatelet and anticoagulant agents, and diphosphonates has been reported, but there is not sufficient evidence to support their benefit in the setting of osteonecrosis. Lipid-lowering agents such as statins can manipulate lipid deposition and target thrombosis. Antiplatelet and anticoagulant agents have been hypothesized to prevent progression of early osteonecrosis and may improve blood flow, more likely in patients who have inherited coagulation disorders. Diphosphonates are used to increase bone mineral density and improve clinical function. Alternative modalities such as extracorporeal shock wave therapy and hyperbaric oxygen have shown improvement in pain and functional scores. Although these nonsurgical modalities have reported benefits, studies are limited and the evidence to support such claims is insufficient.

Surgical Management

Surgical management includes either joint preservation techniques (core decompression with or without adjunctive procedures and rotational osteotomies) in precollapse lesions or arthroplasty in advanced disease.

Core Decompression

Good outcomes have been demonstrated in hips with symptomatic, precollapse, and small-sized to medium-sized lesions, with failure rates of 14% to 25%.[5] Trephines (8- to 10-mm) are drilled into the area of subchondral necrosis as an attempt to reduce intraosseous pressure and prevent further compression.[31] More selective indications for core decompression (only smaller precollapse lesions) and improved techniques, particularly since 1992,[14] have resulted in better outcomes. Core decompression can be used as the first surgical treatment option for symptomatic small-sized to medium-sized precollapse lesions only. In these cases, core decompression is preferred over nonsurgical management. Adjunctive treatment is sometimes used at the time of core decompression; the various modalities will be discussed in the following sections.

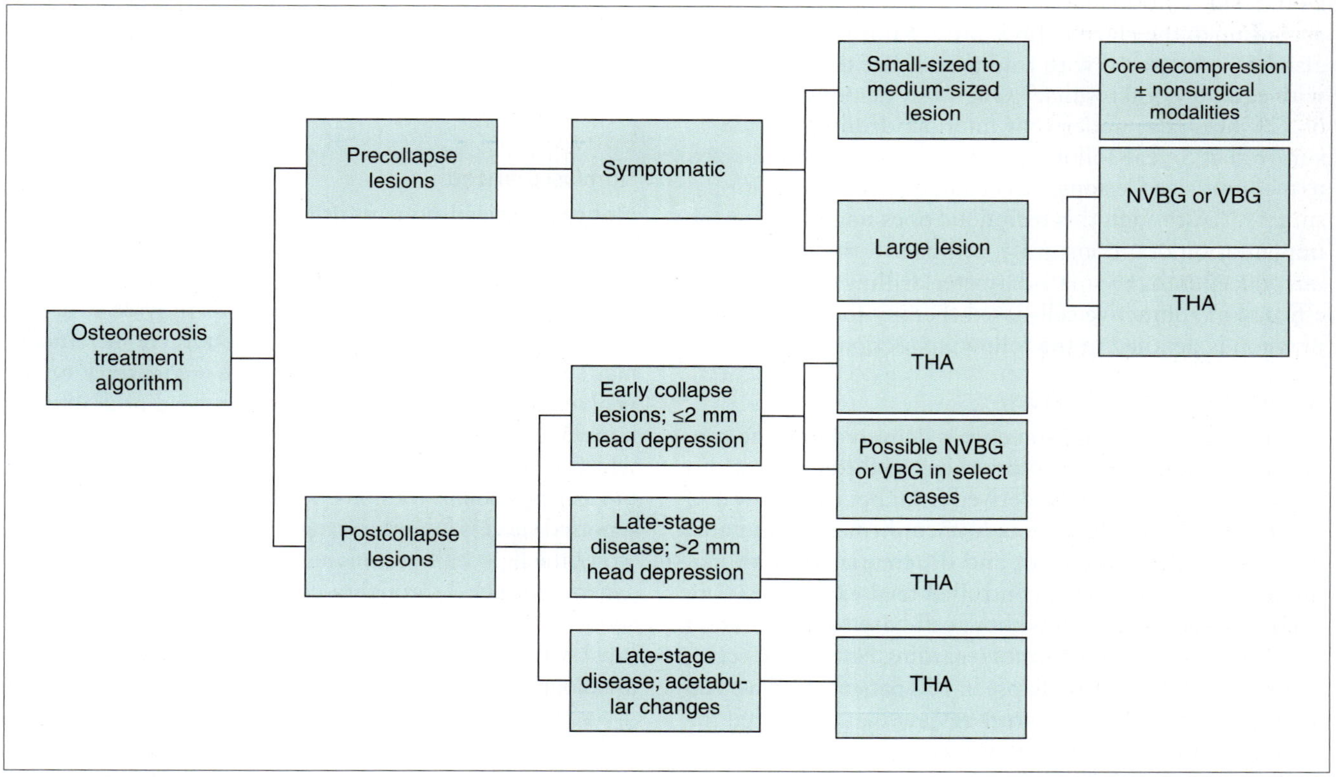

FIGURE 3 Algorithm for the management of hip osteonecrosis. NVBG = nonvascularized bone grafting, THA = total hip arthroplasty, VBG = vascularized bone grafting. (Adapted with permission from Wolters Kluwer Health, Inc.: Mont MA, Cherian JJ, Sierra RJ, Jones LC, Lieberman JR: Nontraumatic osteonecrosis of the femoral head: Where do we stand today? A ten-year update. *J Bone Joint Surg Am* 2015;97[19]:1604-1627.)

Adjunctive Bone Grafting

Implantation of a bone graft into the core decompression tract is sometimes used as an attempt to restore structural integrity and provide a scaffold for new bone growth. In a study of 18 hips that underwent core decompression with fibular bone grafting, mean Harris Hip Score improved from 61.6 to 83.9 after approximately 53 postoperative months.[32] A 2010 study evaluated 76 precollapse hips in patients who underwent treatment with core decompression and implantation of a biomaterial-loaded allograft threaded cage and reported a 91% success rate and significantly improved functional outcomes (63 to 82 points on the Harris Hip Score) compared with core decompression alone.[33] In another study, 28 of 40 hips with stage 2 lesions that underwent fibular grafting did not show radiologic evidence of progression after a mean postoperative period of approximately 53 months.[34]

Multiple Drilling

Decompression with multiple small-diameter drillings may provide the same clinical benefit as a single large-diameter bore. In one report of this technique, multiple 3-mm trephinations were introduced percutaneously at a 45° angle in patients who had precollapse femoral head osteonecrosis. After approximately 2 years postoperatively, 24 of 30 hips (80%) demonstrated good to excellent results according to the Harris Hip Score.[31] Multiple drilling has also been compared with traditional core decompression with equally good results.[35] One study demonstrated that of 120 hips that underwent multiple drilling, 93 (78%) survived at 5-year follow-up; of 59 hips with small-sized to medium-sized lesions, 52 (88%) required no additional surgery.[36] Although this technique does not allow for the implantation of a bone graft, cell-based products can be introduced into the small-diameter drillings. The clinical efficacy of adjunctive cell-based therapy for core decompression is detailed in the following section.

Ancillary Cell-based Therapy

Cell-based products are sometimes delivered into the core decompression track to allow them to differentiate into osteoblasts. MSCs can be derived from bone marrow and adipose tissue which, although unconfirmed in humans, have survived, proliferated, and differentiated in animal models.[37] A randomized controlled trial examining core decompression with and without cell-based augmentation has shown favorable outcomes regarding Harris Hip Score, lesion size, and time to collapse in 100 patients followed up for 60 months.[38] In a literature review that compared the clinical and radiologic improvement of autologous MSC implantation into the core decompression track versus using the core compression alone, it was suggested that the survival of the femoral head improves and the need for hip arthroplasty is minimized when autologous cells are used during the precollapse stages of osteonecrosis of the femoral head.[39] A recent systematic review attempted to assess the efficacy of cell-based therapy for femoral head osteonecrosis.[40] Overall, 24.5% (93/380 hips) that received cell therapy demonstrated radiologic evidence of progression compared with 40% (98/245 hips) in the control group. Among 10 studies that reported THA conversion rate, a lower prevalence was found in the cell therapy group (16%; 62/380 hips) compared with the control group (21%; 52/252 hips). Of the 11 studies that described patient-reported outcomes, 10 showed improved results with ancillary cell treatment compared with control groups.

Femoral Osteotomy

Rotational or angular osteotomies aim to redistribute weight-bearing forces from necrotic areas to healthy cartilage. Success rates range from 82% to 100% at 3- to 15-year follow-up (evidence levels II to IV) for rotational, and 82% to 98% at 6- to 18-year follow-up (evidence levels III and IV) for angular osteotomy.[13,41] One study examined angular osteotomy in 73 hips and reported 92% survivorship at 12 years.[42] Despite good outcomes, the use of femoral osteotomy is less popular because of the inherent technical challenges, limited use in small lesions, associated complications (delayed union and nonunion, loss of position and or/fixation), and complex conversions to THA. One study demonstrated longer surgical time and higher transfusion rates in 14 patients with conversion of osteotomy to THA, compared with routine THA.[41]

Bone Graft

Nonvascularized

Nonvascularized bone grafting (NVBG) is often used in patients in whom core decompression has failed. The necrotic segment is decompressed, and the autograft or allograft material is implanted in the femoral head to provide structural support and allow healing and subchondral bone remodeling.[28] The segment is accessed through a core track or cortical window at the base of the femoral head-neck junction known as the lightbulb, trapdoor, or Phemister technique, which is indicated for medium-sized or larger precollapse or early postcollapse lesions. Several studies of NVBG have reported success rates that range from 67% to 91%. In one study, the light bulb technique (NVBG with bone morphogenetic protein 7 through a cortical window) had a 67% success rate in 39 hips, which improved to 81% (18 of 22 hips) with early-stage lesions.[43] A level II study showed that an allograft procedure had 84% survival (46 of 55 hips) at 3-year follow-up.[33] One study on NVBG used the trapdoor technique in 33 hips and reported at 2-year follow-up that 80% of hips with Ficat and Arlet stage II disease did not need additional surgery.[43] These studies show that NVBG can delay the need for THA in young patients with small-sized to medium-sized precollapse or early postcollapse lesions.

Vascularized

Like NVBG, vascularized bone grafting (VBG) provides structural support to allow subchondral bone healing, remodeling, and restoration of vascular supply (pedicle grafting). This revascularization can be from bone, such as the fibula to the lateral circumflex artery and the iliac crest to deep circumflex iliac vessels. The revascularization could also be from muscle, such as from the quadratus femoris, sartorius, tensor fascia lata, and gluteus medius. VBG is used for early postcollapse lesions, ideally from reversible causes. Survival rates are 80% to 100%; however, outcomes are poorer after collapse occurs.[5] One study followed up 103 patients for a minimum of 5 years following management of osteonecrosis of the hips using a vascularized fibular graft. The study demonstrated that the management of small and medium precollapse lesions had the best results. Of 75 patients who answered a questionnaire, 61 (81%) were satisfied with the results. Among 24 of the 62 hips (39%) with a more advanced lesion, only 5 of 22 hips (23%) had satisfactory results, and 2 of 19 hips (11%) with a precollapse injury were converted to a THA.[44] One study demonstrated an 88% success rate with VBG and the mean Harris Hip Score improved from 50 to 91 points.[38] Another study of 120 hips that underwent multiple drilling reported a 78% survivorship (93 hips) at 5-year follow-up, and 88% of hips (52 of 59) with small-sized to medium-sized lesions required no additional surgery.[36] Age may be a factor with mixed outcomes in patients older than 40 years.[28,33] One study of VBG augmented with MSCs mixed with β-tricalcium-phosphate reported a 94% survival in 30 hips at 99-month follow-up. Despite the lack of randomized controlled trials, VBG results in good outcomes in precollapse disease.

Total Hip Arthroplasty

THA is indicated when there is femoral head collapse with or without secondary osteoarthritis, and nonsurgical management has failed. Advances in techniques and implant technology such as highly cross-linked polyethylene, newer generation ceramic bearings, and more completely porous coated surfaces have improved outcomes and have shown excellent results at short-term to midterm follow-up.[13] A 2013 study reported a 100% survivorship and a mean Harris Hip Score of 93 points (range, 77 to 98 points) for THA patients with osteonecrosis using highly cross-linked polyethylene after a minimum follow-up of 5 years.[45] In addition, a 2017 study reported a 100% survivorship and a mean Harris Hip Score of 90 points (range, 71 to 100 points) for THA patients who have osteonecrosis using highly cross-linked polyethylene after a mean follow-up of 5.6 years.[46] Previously, THA performed for osteonecrosis has had poor outcomes, with rates of aseptic loosening between 8% and 37% and a revision rate of 17% at 9 years.[47] These patients tended to be younger and placed high demands on their THAs, risking polyethylene wear, osteolysis, and ceramic fracture. Newer studies with follow-up of more than 10 years[48,49] demonstrate low wear rates on radiostereometric analyses, suggesting that osteonecrosis is no longer a substantially negative factor for THA.[48,49]

Previously, concerns existed that osteonecrosis could hinder ingrowth in cementless implants. However, a 2013 study reported significantly lower rates of aseptic loosening in cementless implants compared with cemented implants.[48] In addition, a 2013 study of cementless implants in 64 hips showed survival rates of 100% for aseptic loosening and 94% for all causes at a mean follow-up of 15.8 years.[49] The etiology of the osteonecrosis may influence the rate of aseptic loosening. In a meta-analysis of 3,277 hips, higher failure rates were reported in patients who had osteonecrosis secondary to sickle cell disease, Gaucher disease, and renal transplantation. Lower rates of osteonecrosis were seen in patients who had idiopathic disease, SLE, and heart transplantation.[47] The overall quality of the bone stock remains an important factor that may influence outcomes.

OSTEONECROSIS OF THE KNEE

The specific cause of osteonecrosis of the knee is still largely unknown. There are three types of knee osteonecrosis: primary (or spontaneous osteonecrosis of the knee [SONK]), secondary (also called atraumatic, idiopathic, or ischemic osteonecrosis), and postarthroscopic. SONK has an incidence of 9.4% in women older than 65 years.[50] Secondary osteonecrosis affects younger patients (younger than 45 years) and women more often than men (a ratio of 4:1), similarly to hip osteonecrosis.[51] Few cases of postarthroscopic osteonecrosis are reported each year, usually occurring in patients in their fifth decade, and it commonly occurs at the medial femoral condyle (**Table 3**). One study of 50 patients reported that in 2 patients (4%), postarthroscopic osteonecrosis developed.[52]

In the acute phase, most patients present with an effusion and reduced range of motion. Plain weight-bearing radiographs should be obtained initially with all types of osteonecrosis, although the images typically appear normal in the early stages of disease.[51] Alternatively, radiographs may show increased bone density from new bone formation next to the necrotic bone, accentuated by surrounding osteopenia. Diagnosis of each type of osteonecrosis is confirmed using MRI, which has positive findings in the early stages of disease for bone edema, focal epiphyseal depressions, and low-signal subchondral and deep linear signal intensities on T2-weighted images.[53]

Management of osteonecrosis of the knee depends on the type, symptoms, and stage of disease. Classification systems (**Table 4**) can help guide staging: the Koshino classification[54] was later modified so that stage 1 is

TABLE 3

Clinical Presentation and Etiology in Osteonecrosis of the Knee

Type	Age	Bilaterality	Other Joint Involvement	Associated Risk Factors	Lesion Description
Spontaneous osteonecrosis of the knee	Older than 50 yr	<5%	No	Microtrauma, chronic mechanical stress, idiopathic	Bony fibrosis, healing fracture, osteoarthritis, osteopenia, necrosis only at distal portion of fractured segment
Secondary osteonecrosis	Younger than 45 yr	>80%	>90% (commonly shoulder, hip, ankle)	Indirect causes: corticosteroid use, inflammatory bowel disease, smoking, systemic lupus erythematosus, coagulation abnormalities (hypofibrinolysis, thrombophilia) Direct causes: chemotherapy, radiation, trauma, Caisson disease, Gaucher disease	Necrotic bone
Postarthroscopic osteonecrosis	Any	No	No	Anterior cruciate ligament reconstruction, meniscectomy, laser-assisted or radiofrequency-assisted surgery, or cartilage débridement	Healing fracture and bony fibrosis; bone necrosis after direct thermal or acoustic injury

TABLE 4

Staging Systems for Osteonecrosis of the Knee

Classification and Stage	Description
Koshino	**For primary/spontaneous osteonecrosis of the knee**
I	Knee symptoms, radiographs normal
II	Radiographic flattening and subchondral lucencies on weight-bearing area, surrounded by osteosclerosis
III	Radiographic extension of subchondral lucencies around affected area and subchondral collapse
IV	Radiographic degenerative change with osteosclerosis and osteophyte formation
Modified Ficat and Arlet	**For secondary and postarthroscopic**
I	Normal joint space, no subchondral collapse, osteoporosis mottled areas
II	Normal joint space, no subchondral collapse, wedge sclerosis in trabeculae
III	Normal or slightly narrowed joint space, subchondral collapse, trabecular sequestration (crescent sign)
IV	Narrowed joint space, subchondral collapse, extensive destruction

Data from Woehnl AN, Naziri Q, Costa C, et al: Osteonecrosis of the knee. *Orthop Knowl Online J* 2012;10(5) and Koshino T, Okamoto R, Takamura K, Tsuchiya K: Arthroscopy in spontaneous osteonecrosis of the knee. *Orthop Clin North Am* 1979;10(3):609-618.

normal, stage 2 is a mild flattening of weight-bearing surface, stage 3 is a subchondral lucency, stage 4 is a collapse of the subchondral bone, and stage 5 is characterized by secondary degenerative change.[55]

The size of the osteonecrotic lesion is prognostic, and various methods are available for measurement. The first method multiplies the width of the lesion measured on AP and lateral radiographs. Small lesions (less than 3.5 cm^2) usually regress, medium lesions (range, 3.5 to 5.0 cm^2) may or may not progress, and large lesions (larger than 5 cm^2) usually progress to condylar collapse.[55,56] The second method calculates the lesion size as a percentage of the affected femoral condyle on the AP radiograph. One study showed that 6 of 23 patients (26%) who had a mean involvement of 32% of the medial femoral condyle required surgery, whereas all 79 patients who had more than 50% involvement progressed to collapse without surgery and ultimately required arthroplasty.[57] In secondary osteonecrosis, large epiphyseal lesions were found to have a substantially worse prognosis than metaphyseal or diaphyseal lesions.[51] Postarthroscopic osteonecrosis does not correlate as well with lesion size. Algorithms can be used to plan the management of primary (**Figure 4**), secondary (**Figure 5**), and postarthroscopic (**Figure 6**) osteonecrosis of the knee.

Spontaneous Osteonecrosis of the Knee

Etiology and Pathogenesis

SONK typically presents as a unilateral, focal, subchondral lesion affecting a single joint and condyle. The medial femoral condyle is most commonly involved (more than 90% of cases). It is theorized that minor trauma in the setting of osteopenic bone, which affects 75% of patients who have SONK, causes subchondral insufficiency fractures. Fluid accumulates in these potential spaces, causing edema, focal ischemia, and eventual necrosis.[50,51] A 2009 study of 22 patient specimens reported no evidence of osteonecrosis was found; however, 64% (14 of 22) showed evidence of osteopenia and 68% showed evidence of osteoarthritis (15 of 22).[50] Overall, SONK is thought to be underdiagnosed, and many patients who present with osteoarthritis may actually have occult SONK.

Evaluation and Diagnosis

SONK causes acute, severe medial knee pain, which is worse on weight bearing and typically occurs at night. Usually, no history of trauma is reported, although a few patients report preceding trauma. With SONK, tenderness is found on the medial femoral condyle (or affected area).

Imaging

On plain radiographs, radiolucencies with a surrounding sclerotic halo and flattening of the femoral condyle may be seen, mainly affecting the epiphysis. Late disease stages show a crescent sign from collapse of the necrotic bone segment from the subchondral bone, followed by full collapse, femoral condyle flattening, and osteoarthritis (**Figure 7**). An early MRI for SONK may have normal findings; therefore, it should be performed 4 to 6 weeks following symptom onset. Usually, one necrotic

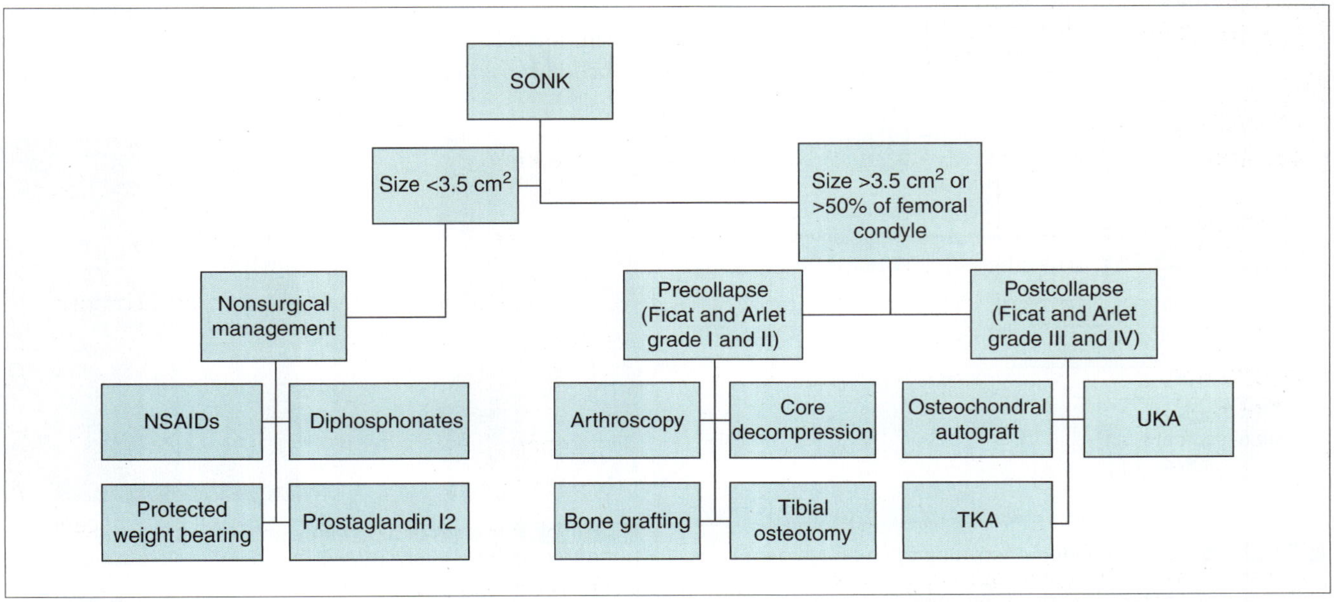

FIGURE 4 Algorithm for the management of spontaneous osteonecrosis of the knee. SONK = spontaneous osteonecrosis of the knee, TKA = total knee arthroplasty, UKA = unicompartmental knee arthroplasty. (Adapted with permission from Karim AR, Cherian JJ, Jauregui JJ, Pierce T, Mont MA: Osteonecrosis of the knee: Review. *Ann Transl Med* 2015;3[1]:6.)

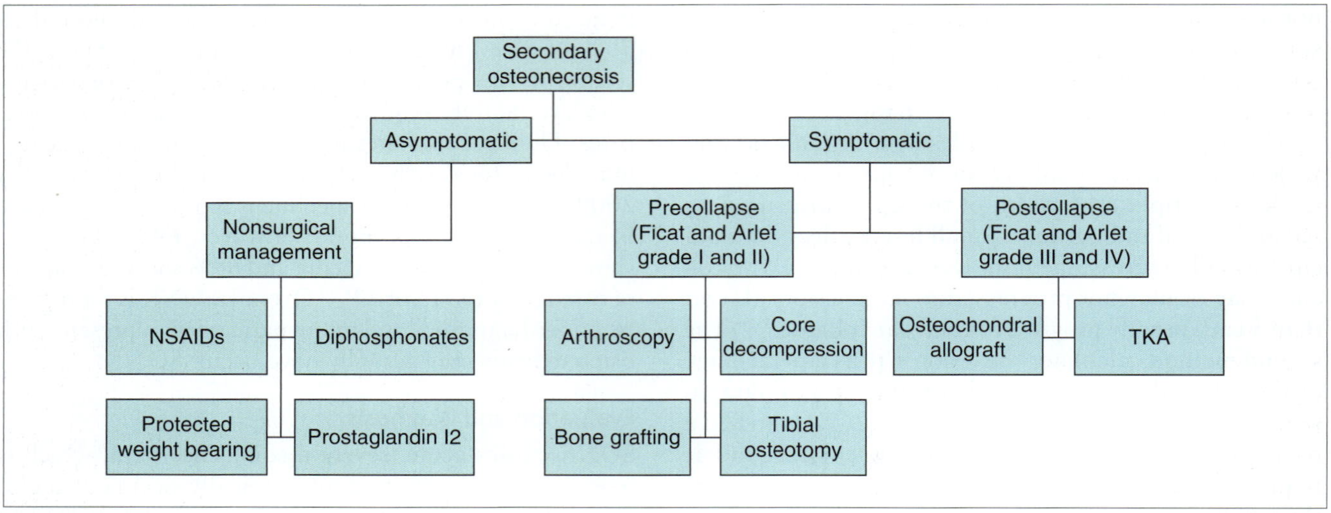

FIGURE 5 Illustration demonstrating the management of secondary osteonecrosis of the knee. TKA = total knee arthroplasty. (Adapted with permission from Karim AR, Cherian JJ, Jauregui JJ, Pierce T, Mont MA: Osteonecrosis of the knee: Review. *Ann Transl Med* 2015;3[1]:6.)

lesion with a low signal intensity is seen on T1-weighted and T2-weighted images, surrounded by marrow edema, affecting the whole condyle. Other findings can include articular cartilage abnormalities, loose bodies, and sclerosis.

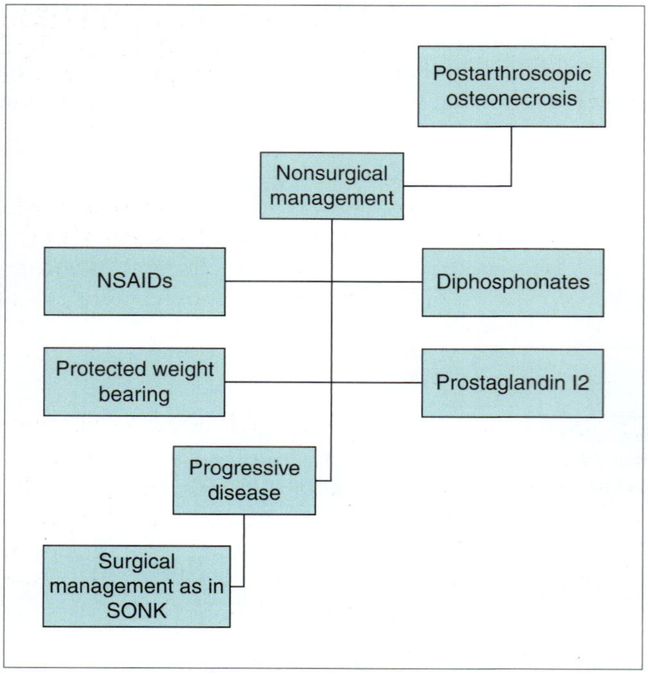

FIGURE 6 Illustration demonstrating the management of postarthroscopic osteonecrosis of the knee. SONK = spontaneous osteonecrosis of the knee. (Reproduced with permission from Karim AR, Cherian JJ, Jauregui JJ, Pierce T, Mont MA: Osteonecrosis of the knee: Review. *Ann Transl Med* 2015;3[1]:6.)

Nonsurgical Treatment

Protected weight bearing for 4 to 6 weeks, physical therapy, analgesics, and NSAIDs are indicated for small lesions (less than 3.5 cm^2). Some patients in the early stages of SONK who are treated nonsurgically usually experience resolution of symptoms and MRI findings within 3 to 8 months.[4] One study showed none of the 10 patients who had less than 20% involvement required surgery at 9-year follow-up.[58] Another study of 79 cases of stage 1 SONK of the medial femoral condyle showed 89% resolution after nonsurgical treatment; only one patient required TKA.[57] Diphosphonates can prevent or delay the need for surgery by inhibiting bone resorption and were shown to prevent subchondral collapse in femoral head osteonecrosis.[59] After

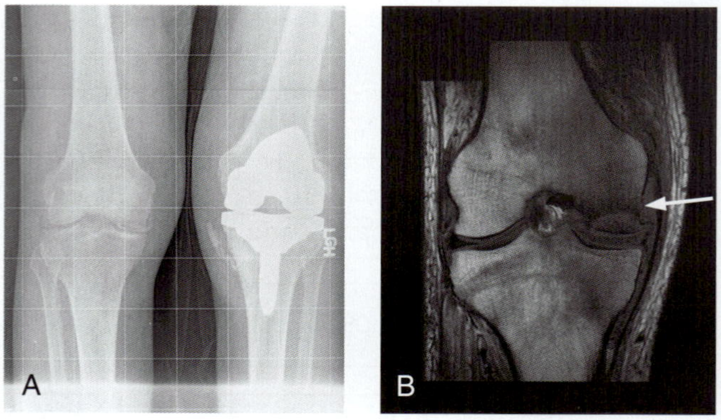

FIGURE 7 Images of a patient with secondary osteonecrosis undergoing hemodialysis. **A**, Bilateral AP radiographs demonstrate collapse of the medial femoral condyle in the right knee and total knee arthroplasty in the left. **B**, T1-weighted coronal magnetic resonance image of the right knee shows osteonecrosis and collapse of the medial femoral condyle from secondary osteonecrosis (arrow).

a minimum of 6 months of treatment with alendronate, subchondral collapse developed in 3 of 17 patients (18%) who had SONK (all 3 stopped treatment prematurely).[58] However, a randomized controlled trial compared diphosphonates with NSAIDs for early SONK and reported no benefit regarding pain scores and radiologic outcomes.[60] A promising nonsurgical treatment is pulsed electromagnetic field therapy, which has been shown to reduce pain and the size of the necrotic lesion in SONK at 6 months.[61]

Surgical Treatment

Surgery is indicated when no clinical or radiographic improvement is seen after 3 months of nonsurgical treatment or in patients with large osteonecrotic lesions (larger than 3.5 cm^2 or greater than 50% of the condyle). However, the risk of progression to collapse is high.[51,57] Initially, joint preservation techniques can be used, ideally in the precollapse state, including arthroscopy (microfracture, chondroplasty, or meniscectomy), core decompression, osteochondral allograft techniques, and high tibial osteotomy.

Using the Cincinnati Knee Rating System, microfracture resulted in clinical improvement in 25 of 26 patients (96%) with SONK at 27-month follow-up.[62] In another study, core decompression improved immediate postoperative knee pain in all 16 patients (15 who had stages 1 and 2, 1 who had stage 3), and those who had early-stage disease had normalization of bone marrow signal intensity on latest follow-up MRI.[63] Core decompression is effective in delaying the need for TKA, and the addition of calcium hydroxyapatite bone graft to the core track has also demonstrated good outcomes.[64] Osteochondral allograft techniques allow restoration of the articular cartilage following subchondral collapse. The principles of osteochondral allografting are to remove the collapsed tissue and replace it with structurally sound osteochondral tissue. Outcomes have been excellent, despite small numbers, including a study in which eight of nine patients had SONK had a successful outcome with postoperative mean Knee Society Score (KSS) of 85 points at 40-month follow-up.[64] For younger, more active patients, high tibial osteotomy shifts the weight-bearing axis to offload the affected condyle, reduces pain, and potentially allows healing. One study of 78 knees (in 64 patients) that underwent high tibial osteotomy with bone substitute reported significantly improved mean scores (KSS knee, 50 points preoperatively to 88 points postoperatively; KSS functional, 57 points preoperatively to 89 points postoperatively) at 6.5-year follow-up.[65] Importantly, the results were equally good in those older than 70 years. Core decompression can also be successfully implemented with this technique.[4] In advanced disease with collapse, and/or when joint preservation techniques fail, arthroplasty should be considered.

Unicompartmental knee arthroplasty (UKA) is an option for involvement of only one condyle, but historically has had poor outcomes. In 2006 study, outcomes have been good with improved techniques and implants.[65] A retrospective study of 52 patients who underwent UKA for SONK demonstrated improved KSS from 85 points preoperatively to 173 points at 10-year follow-up.[66] Survival was 93% and 91% at 10 and 15 years, respectively. Another study compared the medial Oxford UKA (Biomet) in 29 knees (27 patients) with SONK in 28 knees (26 patients) with osteoarthritis and reported similar Oxford UKA knee scores at 5 years postoperatively (38 and 40 points, respectively). No failures were reported in either group at 5-year follow-up.[67] When more than one compartment is affected, TKA is recommended. A systematic review of 148 patients reported those who underwent TKA for SONK had the best outcomes compared with TKA for secondary osteonecrosis and UKA for SONK; those who underwent TKA for SONK had better postoperative knee scores and lower revision rates,[65] making them comparable to patients who had osteoarthritis.

Secondary Osteonecrosis

Etiology and Pathogenesis

With secondary osteonecrosis, multiple diffuse lesions are usually seen in both the femoral and tibial condyles (bilateral in 80% of cases), possibly extending into the diaphysis and metaphysis. Multiple joints can be involved including the femoral head and proximal humerus. As with the hip, numerous risk factors, both direct and indirect, are involved.

Evaluation and Diagnosis

Secondary osteonecrosis presents with gradual onset of pain, usually over the femoral condyles, but also the proximal tibia and other sites. Secondary osteonecrosis presents with more diffuse tenderness from possible multifocal lesions.

Imaging

Secondary osteonecrosis has multiple larger lesions with serpentine appearance of radiodense bony infarcts on radiographs. A similar appearance can be noted on MRI and bone scintigraphy: multiple areas of central fatty marrow signal intensity surrounded by a serpentine border of reactive bone with low signal intensity on T1-weighted and high signal intensity on T2-weighted images.

Nonsurgical Treatment

Nonsurgical treatment is only recommended in asymptomatic cases of secondary osteonecrosis because symptomatic patients tend to be younger, with larger lesions and poor prognosis. In one study, 8 of 10 asymptomatic patients had no disease progression on radiographs and did not require surgery at 8-year follow-up.[56] The same study also had 41 symptomatic patients, 8 (19%) of whom had satisfactory outcomes (KSS greater than 80 and no surgery) with this approach, and 29 patients (70%) required TKA. Diphosphonates may also play a role in secondary osteonecrosis. One study[67] of 28 symptomatic patients treated with pamidronate followed by alendronate reported improvements in pain scores at 6 weeks and greater improvements at 6 months. In addition, 15 patients (53%) had complete resolution of pain and 18 patients (64%) had complete reversal of bone marrow edema on MRI at 6-month follow-up. Prostaglandin I2 has been shown to improve pain, function, and bone marrow edema in early disease, but not in advanced disease.[67]

Surgical Management

Secondary osteonecrosis of the knee can be managed using joint-preservation techniques in precollapse disease stages. In addition, bone impaction grafting can be performed to help delay the need for arthroplasty. Arthroscopy treats any coexisting chondral and/or meniscal pathologies and is also useful to assess the chondral surface. Core decompression can be performed with a small (3 mm) drill into the affected condyle via the metaphysis, under fluoroscopic guidance, followed by partial weight bearing for 4 to 6 weeks. This technique relieves pain with low morbidity and delays further surgery. One study reported a 92% success rate after core decompression, defined as a KSS higher than 80 points in 56 of 61 knees (38 patients): of these, success was noted in all small lesions as well as in 86% of large lesions (32 of 37 knees) at 3-year follow-up.[54] In addition, only 2 knees (3%) required TKA at 3-year follow-up.[68] Impaction bone grafting is used in solitary early lesions, because it involves removal of the osteonecrotic area via a metaphyseal window, and impaction of autograft or allograft to prevent collapse and restore condylar sphericity.[51]

Although there are few studies assessing impaction bone grafting, early results demonstrate that it may delay the need for TKA in early collapse disease. A study of three patients demonstrated improvements in mean KSS from 63 points preoperatively to 89 points and functional KSS from 19 points preoperatively to 81 points at 2-year follow-up, with no complications and near-normal function and activity levels.[69] Another prospective study of nine patients reported no progression of collapse: three patients had signs of early osteoarthritis and overall scores (KSS objective, 63 points preoperatively to 89 points postoperatively; functional, 19 points preoperatively to 81 points postoperatively) improved at 51-month follow-up, and none required TKA.[70] Osteochondral allograft transplantation restores the articular cartilage and subchondral bone, including that affected by large lesions. Current data are limited; however, one study with 28 patients demonstrated an 89% success rate in postcollapse disease at 2-year follow-up, with an increase in functional KSS preoperatively from 60 to 86 points at final follow-up.[71] Importantly, caution is recommended in corticosteroid-related osteonecrosis because graft subsidence may occur in patients who have inadequate graft revascularization.

Finally, arthroplasty should be considered with joint collapse and when joint preservation techniques have failed. Unlike SONK, more diffuse disease occurs in secondary osteonecrosis, warranting TKA. One study reported a survival rate of 97% in 30 patients, with an increase in mean KSS from 54 points preoperatively to 95 points at 108-month follow-up.[72]

Postarthroscopic Osteonecrosis

Etiology and Pathogenesis

Postarthroscopic osteonecrosis of the knee is usually seen following meniscectomy, chondroplasty, and less commonly, anterior cruciate ligament reconstruction. In one study of medial meniscal root tears, elevated hoop stresses caused increased tibiofemoral contact pressures and subchondral insufficiency fractures in 80% of cases.[73] Synovial fluid ingress causes edema, subchondral vascular insufficiency, and necrosis. In addition, overly aggressive early rehabilitation before adequate postoperative remodeling has occurred can also cause insufficiency fractures.

Evaluation and Diagnosis

Postarthroscopic osteonecrosis also results in acute onset of pain in the area of pathology and surgery, usually 6 to 8 weeks postoperatively, which becomes persistent.[73] Each patient will have stiffness and swelling, with potentially worsening pain from progressive collapse. Postarthroscopic osteonecrosis presents with tenderness in the area of the lesion and/or surgical compartment.[4]

Imaging

Two criteria must be fulfilled for diagnosis of postarthroscopic osteonecrosis: absence of osteonecrosis on preoperative MRI 4 to 6 weeks after symptom onset and a recent history of arthroscopy and development of suspicious bone marrow edema pattern in the surgical compartment on postoperative MRI.[51,73] In one study, edema was shown to occur in 32 of 93 patients (34%) undergoing arthroscopic meniscectomy within 8 months, and osteonecrosis developed in none.[74] Bone scans show uptake in the affected condyle in all three phases after 72 hours, but are not recommended because of poor sensitivity and specificity. Scintigraphy detects only 56% of multifocal lesions seen on MRI and confirmed histopathologically.[4]

Nonsurgical Treatment

Nonsurgical treatment should be used only in patients with early-stage, precollapse lesions and includes protected weight bearing, NSAIDs, and analgesics. One study showed that 44 of 47 patients (97.6%) continued to have the same MRI appearance after 6 weeks of protected weight bearing.[73] Diphosphonates such as intravenous pamidronate followed by oral alendronate for 4 to 6 months resulted in a decreased pain score at 6 weeks and at 6 months (80% reduction) in 22 patients who had osteonecrosis following meniscectomy.[75]

Surgical Management

Surgical intervention is indicated when there is collapse and/or degeneration of the articular surface. With early symptomatic disease, joint preservation techniques are indicated. However, the outcomes of the limited studies on these techniques are less than optimal. In a study of six patients, repeat arthroscopy and core decompression were performed in one patient at 9 months and failed; UKA was necessary 1 year postoperatively.[75] With advanced disease and osteoarthritis, knee arthroplasty is indicated, depending on the number of compartments affected.

SUMMARY

Osteonecrosis is a challenging condition because it affects young patients who have high activity levels and has an unclear etiology. Despite multiple pathophysiologic theories, the final common pathway is ischemia and cell death. The hip is a load-bearing joint and osteonecrosis may result in collapse and secondary osteoarthritis. Small-sized to medium-sized precollapse lesions can be managed nonsurgically or with core decompression; larger lesions can be managed with bone grafting. Early postcollapse hips may be amenable to joint preservation; however, those with late collapse and secondary osteoarthritis require arthroplasty. Secondary osteonecrosis is related to medical conditions and risk factors such as vascular occlusion and bone marrow crowding, whereas primary and postarthroscopic osteonecroses of the knee are thought to be associated with subchondral insufficiency fractures. Osteonecrosis of the hip and knee is diagnosed by using radiographs and MRIs, with management guided by the presence of symptoms, lesion size, and collapse. Outcomes in these patients have improved over the past several decades, which are reflected in advancements in both surgical and nonsurgical modalities. Further research with longer follow-up should focus on early detection and intervention to minimize joint destruction.

KEY STUDY POINTS

- Osteonecrosis of the hip and knee can have various etiologies; however, interruption of the blood supply ultimately is the main culprit.
- A high index of suspicion is the key to an early diagnosis in patients who are at risk of developing osteonecrosis.
- Effective imaging modalities for osteonecrosis of the hip or knee include plain radiographs, MRI, and CT. Bone scintigraphy and positron emission tomography do not yet have definitive roles in diagnosis.
- In general, nonsurgical treatment is not appropriate and joint-preserving procedures should be considered as an attempt to preserve the native joint. Small-sized, medially located lesions of the femoral head may have a better prognosis and could potentially heal without surgery.
- Joint arthroplasty is indicated in the setting of collapse and/or degeneration of the articular surface. The outcomes of arthroplasty for patients who have osteonecrosis are excellent, with results similar to patients in whom osteoarthritis is the underlying diagnosis.

ANNOTATED REFERENCES

1. Jacobs B: Epidemiology of traumatic and nontraumatic osteonecrosis. *Clin Orthop Relat Res* 1978;130:51-67.
2. Mont MA, Hungerford DS: Non-traumatic avascular necrosis of the femoral head. *J Bone Joint Surg Am* 1995;77(3):459-474.
3. Cooper C, Steinbuch M, Stevenson R, Miday R, Watts NB: The epidemiology of osteonecrosis: Findings from the GPRD and THIN databases in the UK. *Osteoporos Int* 2010;21(4):569-577.
4. Karim AR, Cherian JJ, Jauregui JJ, Pierce T, Mont MA: Osteonecrosis of the knee: Review. *Ann Transl Med* 2015;3(1):6.
5. Mont MA, Jones LC, Hungerford DS: Nontraumatic osteonecrosis of the femoral head: Ten years later. *J Bone Joint Surg Am* 2006;88(5):1117-1132.
6. Kellam P, Ostrum RF: Systematic review and meta-analysis of avascular necrosis and posttraumatic arthritis after traumatic hip dislocation. *J Orthop Trauma* 2016;30(1):10-16.
7. Baixauli EJ, Baixauli F Jr, Baixauli F, Lozano JA: Avascular necrosis of the femoral head after intertrochanteric fractures. *J Orthop Trauma* 1999;13(2):134-137.
8. Aaron RK, Voisinet A, Racine J, Ali Y, Feller ER: Corticosteroid-associated avascular necrosis: Dose relationships and early diagnosis. *Ann N Y Acad Sci* 2011;1240:38-46.
9. Zhao FC, Guo KJ, Li ZR: Osteonecrosis of the femoral head in SARS patients: Seven years later. *Eur J Orthop Surg Traumatol* 2013;23(6):671-677.

10. Chan KL, Mok CC: Glucocorticoid-induced avascular bone necrosis: Diagnosis and management. *Open Orthop J* 2012;6:449-457.

11. Chen C, Yang S, Feng Y, et al: Impairment of two types of circulating endothelial progenitor cells in patients with glucocorticoid-induced avascular osteonecrosis of the femoral head. *Joint Bone Spine* 2013;80(1):70-76.

12. Drescher W, Bunger MH, Weigert K, Bunger C, Hansen ES: Methylprednisolone enhances contraction of porcine femoral head epiphyseal arteries. *Clin Orthop Relat Res* 2004;423:112-117.

13. Mont MA, Cherian JJ, Sierra RJ, Jones LC, Lieberman JR: Nontraumatic osteonecrosis of the femoral head: Where do we stand today? A ten-year update. *J Bone Joint Surg Am* 2015;97(19):1604-1627.

14. Marker DR, Seyler TM, Ulrich SD, Srivastava S, Mont MA: Do modern techniques improve core decompression outcomes for hip osteonecrosis? *Clin Orthop Relat Res* 2008;466(5):1093-1103.

15. Yoon BH, Kim TY, Shin IS, Lee HY, Lee YJ, Koo KH: Alcohol intake and the risk of osteonecrosis of the femoral head in Japanese populations: A dose-response meta-analysis of case-control studies. *Clin Rheumatol* 2017;36(11): 2517-2524.

    This meta-analysis determined the association of alcohol consumption with the development of femoral head osteonecrosis. It was found that the risk of osteonecrosis increased 35.3% for every 100 g/wk increase in alcohol intake. Level of evidence: III.

16. Cui Q, Wang Y, Saleh KJ, Wang GJ, Balian G: Alcohol-induced adipogenesis in a cloned bone-marrow stem cell. *J Bone Joint Surg Am* 2006;88(suppl 3):148-154.

17. Glueck CJ, Freiberg RA, Wang P: Heritable thrombophilia-hypofibrinolysis and osteonecrosis of the femoral head. *Clin Orthop Relat Res* 2008;466(5):1034-1040.

18. Flouzat-Lachaniete CH, Roussignol X, Poignard A, Mukasa MM, Manicom O, Hernigou P: Multifocal joint osteonecrosis in sickle cell disease. *Open Orthop J* 2009;3:32-35.

19. Shigemura T, Nakamura J, Kishida S, et al: Incidence of osteonecrosis associated with corticosteroid therapy among different underlying diseases: Prospective MRI study. *Rheumatology (Oxford)* 2011;50(11):2023-2028.

20. Nakamura J, Konno K, Orita S, et al: Distribution of hip pain in patients with idiopathic osteonecrosis of the femoral head. *Mod Rheumatol* 2017;27(3):503-507.

    This prospective evaluation of 119 hips in 90 patients found that the most common presenting symptoms of femoral head osteonecrosis in descending order are groin pain, knee pain, anterior thigh pain, and buttock pain. Level of evidence: IV.

21. Zhang YZ, Cao XY, Li XC, et al: Accuracy of MRI diagnosis of early osteonecrosis of the femoral head: A meta-analysis and systematic review. *J Orthop Surg Res* 2018;13(1):167.

    This meta-analysis of 43 studies determined the overall sensitivity (93%) and specificity (91%) of MRI for the early detection of femoral head osteonecrosis. Level of evidence: III.

22. Pierce TP, Jauregui JJ, Cherian JJ, Elmallah RK, Mont MA: Imaging evaluation of patients with osteonecrosis of the femoral head. *Curr Rev Musculoskelet Med* 2015;8(3):221-227.

23. Hauzeur JP, Pasteels JL, Schoutens A, et al: The diagnostic value of magnetic resonance imaging in non-traumatic osteonecrosis of the femoral head. *J Bone Joint Surg Am* 1989;71(5):641-649.

24. Lee GC, Khoury V, Steinberg D, Kim W, Dalinka M, Steinberg M: How do radiologists evaluate osteonecrosis? *Skeletal Radiol* 2014;43(5):607-614.

25. Ito H, Matsuno T, Minami A: Relationship between bone marrow edema and development of symptoms in patients with osteonecrosis of the femoral head. *AJR Am J Roentgenol* 2006;186(6):1761-1770.

26. Lee GC, Steinberg ME: Are we evaluating osteonecrosis adequately? *Int Orthop* 2012;36(12):2433-2439.

27. Ha YC, Jung WH, Kim JR, Seong NH, Kim SY, Koo KH: Prediction of collapse in femoral head osteonecrosis: A modified Kerboul method with use of magnetic resonance images. *J Bone Joint Surg Am* 2006;88(suppl 3):35-40.

28. Mont MA, Zywiel MG, Marker DR, McGrath MS, Delanois RE: The natural history of untreated asymptomatic osteonecrosis of the femoral head: A systematic literature review. *J Bone Joint Surg Am* 2010;92(12):2165-2170.

29. Hernigou P, Poignard A, Nogier A, Manicom O: Fate of very small asymptomatic stage-I osteonecrotic lesions of the hip. *J Bone Joint Surg Am* 2004;86(12):2589-2593.

30. Nakamura J, Harada Y, Oinuma K, Iida S, Kishida S, Takahashi K: Spontaneous repair of asymptomatic osteonecrosis associated with corticosteroid therapy in systemic lupus erythematosus: 10-year minimum follow-up with MRI. *Lupus* 2010;19(11):1307-1314.

31. Mont MA, Ragland PS, Etienne G: Core decompression of the femoral head for osteonecrosis using percutaneous multiple small-diameter drilling. *Clin Orthop Relat Res* 2004;429:131-138.

32. Zeng Y, Qi X, Feng W, et al: One-sided hip-preserving and concurrent contralateral total hip arthroplasty for the treatment of bilateral osteonecrosis of the femoral head in different stages: Short-medium term outcomes. *BMC Musculoskelet Disord* 2015;16:133.

33. Yang S, Wu X, Xu W, Ye S, Liu X, Liu X: Structural augmentation with biomaterial-loaded allograft threaded cage for the treatment of femoral head osteonecrosis. *J Arthroplasty* 2010;25(8):1223-1230.

34. Lakshminarayana S, Dhammi IK, Jain AK, Bhayana H, Kumar S, Anshuman R: Outcomes of core decompression with or without nonvascularized fibular grafting in avascular necrosis of femoral head: Short term followup study. *Indian J Orthop* 2019;53(3):420-425.

    Patients who had stage 1 osteonecrosis (n = 36) received core decompression while those who had stage 2 disease (n = 40) also received a nonvascularized fibular bone graft. After a mean follow-up period of 53.5 months, radiologic progression and collapse was noted in 25% ($n = 9$) of patients who underwent core decompression alone and 30% ($n = 12$) of those who underwent ancillary bone grafting. Level of evidence: III.

35. Al Omran A: Multiple drilling compared with standard core decompression for avascular necrosis of the femoral head in sickle cell disease patients. *Arch Orthop Trauma Surg* 2013;133(5):609-613.

36. Song WS, Yoo JJ, Kim YM, Kim HJ: Results of multiple drilling compared with those of conventional methods of core decompression. *Clin Orthop Relat Res* 2007;454:139-146.

37. Wang B, Zhao D, Liu B, Wang W: Treatment of osteonecrosis of the femoral head by using the greater trochanteric bone flap with double vascular pedicles. *Microsurgery* 2013;33(8):593-599.

38. Zhao D, Cui D, Wang B, et al: Treatment of early stage osteonecrosis of the femoral head with autologous implantation of bone marrow-derived and cultured mesenchymal stem cells. *Bone* 2012;50(1):325-330.

39. Papakostidis C, Tosounidis TH, Jones E, Giannoudis PV: The role of "cell therapy" in osteonecrosis of the femoral head. A systematic review of the literature and meta-analysis of 7 studies. *Acta Orthop* 2016;87(1):72-78.

40. Piuzzi NS, Chahla J, Jiandong H, et al: Analysis of cell therapies used in clinical trials for the treatment of osteonecrosis of the femoral head: A systematic review of the literature. *J Arthroplasty* 2017;32(8):2612-2618.

    This systematic review attempted to assess the clinical benefit of cell-based therapy for femoral head osteonecrosis. Ten of the 11 included studies described patient-reported outcomes, all 10 of which showed improved results with cell-therapy compared to controls. However, the authors noted a high level of heterogeneity among studies in the type of cell-based treatments that were used. Level of evidence: III.

41. Issa K, Johnson AJ, Naziri Q, Khanuja HS, Delanois RE, Mont MA: Hip osteonecrosis: Does prior hip surgery alter outcomes compared to an initial primary total hip arthroplasty? *J Arthroplasty* 2014;29(1):162-166.

42. Zhao G, Yamamoto T, Ikemura S, et al: Radiological outcome analysis of transtrochanteric curved varus osteotomy for osteonecrosis of the femoral head at a mean follow-up of 12.4 years. *J Bone Joint Surg Br* 2010;92(6):781-786.

43. Seyler TM, Marker DR, Ulrich SD, Fatscher T, Mont MA: Nonvascularized bone grafting defers joint arthroplasty in hip osteonecrosis. *Clin Orthop Relat Res* 2008;466(5):1125-1132.

44. Urbaniak JR, Coogan PG, Gunneson EB, Nunley JA: Treatment of osteonecrosis of the femoral head with free vascularized fibular grafting. A long-term follow-up study of one hundred and three hips. *J Bone Joint Surg Am* 1995;77(5):681-694.

45. Min BW, Lee KJ, Song KS, Bae KC, Cho CH: Highly cross-linked polyethylene in total hip arthroplasty for osteonecrosis of the femoral head: A minimum 5-year follow-up study. *J Arthroplasty* 2013;28(3):526-530.

46. Capone A, Bienati F, Torchia S, Podda D, Marongiu G: Short stem total hip arthroplasty for osteonecrosis of the femoral head in patients 60 years or younger: A 3- to 10-year follow-up study. *BMC Musculoskelet Disord* 2017;18(1):301.

    Among 30 patients younger than 60 years who had osteonecrosis, excellent clinical results and radiologic evidence of fixation was demonstrated in all patients at mean 5.6-year follow-up. Level of evidence: IV.

47. Johannson HR, Zywiel MG, Marker DR, Jones LC, McGrath MS, Mont MA: Osteonecrosis is not a predictor of poor outcomes in primary total hip arthroplasty: A systematic literature review. *Int Orthop* 2011;35(4):465-473.

48. Bedard NA, Callaghan JJ, Liu SS, Greiner JJ, Klaassen AL, Johnston RC: Cementless THA for the treatment of osteonecrosis at 10-year follow-up: Have we improved compared to cemented THA? *J Arthroplasty* 2013;28(7):1192-1199.

49. Kim SM, Lim SJ, Moon YW, Kim YT, Ko KR, Park YS: Cementless modular total hip arthroplasty in patients younger than fifty with femoral head osteonecrosis: Minimum fifteen-year follow-up. *J Arthroplasty* 2013;28(3):504-509.

50. Mears SC, McCarthy EF, Jones LC, Hungerford DS, Mont MA: Characterization and pathological characteristics of spontaneous osteonecrosis of the knee. *Iowa Orthop J* 2009;29:38-42.

51. Mont MA, Marker DR, Zywiel MG, Carrino JA: Osteonecrosis of the knee and related conditions. *J Am Acad Orthop Surg* 2011;19(8):482-494.

52. Cetik O, Cift H, Comert B, Cirpar M: Risk of osteonecrosis of the femoral condyle after arthroscopic chondroplasty using radiofrequency: A prospective clinical series. *Knee Surg Sports Traumatol Arthrosc* 2009;17(1):24-29.

53. Fotiadou A, Karantanas A: Acute nontraumatic adult knee pain: The role of MR imaging. *Radiol Med* 2009;114(3):437-447.

54. Koshino T, Okamoto R, Takamura K, Tsuchiya K: Arthroscopy in spontaneous osteonecrosis of the knee. *Orthop Clin North Am* 1979;10(3):609-618.

55. Aglietti P, Insall JN, Buzzi R, Deschamps G: Idiopathic osteonecrosis of the knee. Aetiology, prognosis and treatment. *J Bone Joint Surg Br* 1983;65(5):588-597.

56. Mont MA, Baumgarten KM, Rifai A, Bluemke DA, Jones LC, Hungerford DS: Atraumatic osteonecrosis of the knee. *J Bone Joint Surg Am* 2000;82(9):1279-1290.

57. Lotke PA, Abend JA, Ecker ML: The treatment of osteonecrosis of the medial femoral condyle. *Clin Orthop Relat Res* 1982;171:109-116.

58. Jureus J, Lindstrand A, Geijer M, Robertsson O, Tagil M: The natural course of spontaneous osteonecrosis of the knee (SPONK): A 1- to 27-year follow-up of 40 patients. *Acta Orthop* 2013;84(4):410-414.

59. Lee YK, Ha YC, Cho YJ, et al: Does zoledronate prevent femoral head collapse from osteonecrosis? A prospective, randomized, open-label, multicenter study. *J Bone Joint Surg Am* 2015;97(14):1142-1148.

60. Meier C, Kraenzlin C, Friederich NF, et al: Effect of ibandronate on spontaneous osteonecrosis of the knee: A randomized, double-blind, placebo-controlled trial. *Osteoporos Int* 2014;25(1):359-366.

61. Marcheggiani Muccioli GM, Grassi A, Setti S, et al: Conservative treatment of spontaneous osteonecrosis of the knee in the early stage: Pulsed electromagnetic fields therapy. *Eur J Radiol* 2013;82(3):530-537.

62. Akgun I, Kesmezacar H, Ogut T, Kebudi A, Kanberoglu K: Arthroscopic microfracture treatment for osteonecrosis of the knee. *Arthroscopy* 2005;21(7):834-843.

63. Forst J, Forst R, Heller KD, Adam G: Spontaneous osteonecrosis of the femoral condyle: Causal treatment by early core decompression. *Arch Orthop Trauma Surg* 1998;117(1-2):18-22.

64. Duany NG, Zywiel MG, McGrath MS, et al: Joint-preserving surgical treatment of spontaneous osteonecrosis of the knee. *Arch Orthop Trauma Surg* 2010;130(1):11-16.

65. Myers TG, Cui Q, Kuskowski M, Mihalko WM, Saleh KJ: Outcomes of total and unicompartmental knee arthroplasty for secondary and spontaneous osteonecrosis of the knee. *J Bone Joint Surg Am* 2006;88(suppl 3):76-82.

66. Langdown AJ, Pandit H, Price AJ, et al: Oxford medial unicompartmental arthroplasty for focal spontaneous osteonecrosis of the knee. *Acta Orthop* 2005;76(5):688-692.

67. Marulanda G, Seyler TM, Sheikh NH, Mont MA: Percutaneous drilling for the treatment of secondary osteonecrosis of the knee. *J Bone Joint Surg Br* 2006;88(6):740-746.

68. Lee K, Goodman SB: Cell therapy for secondary osteonecrosis of the femoral condyles using the Cellect DBM System: A preliminary report. *J Arthroplasty* 2009;24(1):43-48.

69. Rijnen WH, Luttjeboer JS, Schreurs BW, Gardeniers JW: Bone impaction grafting for corticosteroid-associated osteonecrosis of the knee. *J Bone Joint Surg Am* 2006;88(suppl 3):62-68.

70. Gortz S, De Young AJ, Bugbee WD: Fresh osteochondral allografting for steroid-associated osteonecrosis of the femoral condyles. *Clin Orthop Relat Res* 2010;468(5):1269-1278.

71. Mont MA, Rifai A, Baumgarten KM, Sheldon M, Hungerford DS: Total knee arthroplasty for osteonecrosis. *J Bone Joint Surg Am* 2002;84(4):599-603.

72. Pape D, Seil R, Anagnostakos K, Kohn D: Postarthroscopic osteonecrosis of the knee. *Arthroscopy* 2007;23(4):428-438.

73. Kobayashi Y, Kimura M, Higuchi H, Terauchi M, Shirakura K, Takagishi K: Juxta-articular bone marrow signal changes on magnetic resonance imaging following arthroscopic meniscectomy. *Arthroscopy* 2002;18(3):238-245.

74. Kraenzlin ME, Graf C, Meier C, Kraenzlin C, Friedrich NF: Possible beneficial effect of bisphosphonates in osteonecrosis of the knee. *Knee Surg Sports Traumatol Arthrosc* 2010;18(12):1638-1644.

75. Garino JP, Lotke PA, Sapega AA, Reilly PJ, Esterhai JL Jr: Osteonecrosis of the knee following laser-assisted arthroscopic surgery: A report of six cases. *Arthroscopy* 1995;11(4):467-474.

CHAPTER 8

Economics and Cost Implications of Total Hip and Total Knee Arthroplasty

MONICA SHOJI, MD • HUGH GORMAN, BS • FEROZ OSMANI, MD
SAVYASACHI THAKKAR, MD • JEFFREY K. LANGE, MD • RICHARD IORIO, MD

ABSTRACT

Total joint arthroplasty (TJA) is a successful, cost-effective procedure that requires an increasing amount of healthcare resources. Decreased hospital and physician reimbursement and increased costs have put a financial strain on stakeholders involved in the delivery of TJA. Cost analysis of TJA procedures across the United States shows a wide variation in the cost of the surgery. The development of innovative technologies such as patient-specific instrumentation and robot-assisted arthroplasty systems adds further complexity to the evaluation of cost effectiveness, as these technologies have the potential to improve outcomes and ultimately decrease longitudinal costs despite increased initial fixed costs. Medicare and Medicaid have implemented alternative payment models such as the Bundled Payments for Care Improvement initiative and the Comprehensive Care for Joint Arthroplasty, with the purpose of improving the quality of TJA care while reducing cost. Various quality and cost effectiveness improvement measures have been implemented by surgeons and hospitals, including comanagement models, patient risk optimization, multimodal pain management, implant cost reduction programs, and care management initiatives. The goal of these programs is to deliver TJA in a more cost-effective manner without sacrificing quality. In the future, TJA in a value-based purchasing environment will require more attention to cost-effective care delivery. Other important cost implications include hospital stay, implant pricing, pain management strategies, revision burden, perioperative complications, and bundled payment programs. Stakeholders should take notice of the numerous aspects of TJA episodes of care, their cost implications, and the potential for transmitting value to patients. TJA has a potential episode duration of 30 to 40 years, which makes the current emphasis on episode length of 30 to 90 days seem short-sighted.

Keywords: alternative payment models; bundled payments; cost effectiveness; total joint arthroplasty

Dr. Thakkar or an immediate family member serves as a paid consultant to or is an employee of KCI and OrthAlign and serves as a board member, owner, officer, or committee member of the American Association of Hip and Knee Surgeons. Dr. Lange or an immediate family member serves as a board member, owner, officer, or committee member of the American Association of Hip and Knee Surgeons. Dr. Iorio or an immediate family member serves as a paid consultant to or is an employee of Johnson & Johnson, MedTel, Medtronic, Muve Health, Pacira, Recro Pharma, and Zimmer; has stock or stock options held in Covina, Force Therapeutics, MedTel, Muve Health, and Wellbe; and serves as a board member, owner, officer, or committee member of the American Association of Hip and Knee Surgeons, the Hip Society, and the Knee Society. None of the following authors or any immediate family member has received anything of value from or has stock or stock options held in a commercial company or institution related directly or indirectly to the subject of this chapter: Dr. Shoji, Mr. Gorman, and Dr. Osmani.

INTRODUCTION

Total joint arthroplasty (TJA) is one of the most commonly performed and successful procedures in the United

States. The number of primary TJA procedures performed annually is expected to increase to approximately 2 million by the year 2030 with a projected 71% increase in total hip arthroplasty (THA) and 85% growth in primary total knee arthroplasty (TKA).[1] Many patients undergoing these procedures are insured through the Centers for Medicare and Medicaid Services (CMS), which is challenged by financial constraints. This issue is further exacerbated by the Patient Protection and Affordable Care Act of 2010, which has increased insurance coverage of 11 million formerly uninsured patients, with additional modifications to insurance requirements based on the American Healthcare Act in 2017. Despite these changes in insurance coverage, Medicare payments to hospitals and physicians have not increased to match inflation.[2] These recent payment adjustments and the increasing adoption of novel technologies surrounding the TJA episode of care have affected the value equation for TJA procedures. Other important cost implications include hospital stay, implant pricing, pain management strategies, revision burden, perioperative complications, and bundled payment programs. Stakeholders should take notice of the numerous aspects of TJA episodes of care, their cost implications, and the potential for transmitting value to patients. TJA has a potential episode duration of 30 to 40 years, which makes the current emphasis on episode length of 30 to 90 days seem short-sighted.

REDUCING COSTS ASSOCIATED WITH TJA

The Medicare hospital payment for primary TJA has increased at 50% of the rate of inflation over the past 2 decades, whereas hospital and implant costs have continued to increase at higher rates.[2] TJA costs account for a higher percentage of Medicare spending than any other inpatient procedure. Medicare funding for TJA is a continual target for cost containment.[2] TJA is the largest diagnosis-related group (DRG) expenditure for CMS.[2] Additional projected cuts in Medicare reimbursement for TJA and the downstream effects on other healthcare insurance products have potentially negative effects on access to an orthopaedic surgeon specializing in adult reconstruction for TJA.[2] In 1992, the national Medicare physician reimbursement rate for TKA was $2,102. In 2010, the reimbursement had declined by 30% to $1,470.45.[3] An inflation-adjusted comparison performed using the dollar value in 1992 reported that the reimbursement for TKA in 2010 is equivalent to $666.58, a 68% reduction in Medicare reimbursement of TKA.[3] For the 2014 fiscal year, the average Medicare Physician Fee Schedule cut in payments for orthopaedic procedures was 1%. For 2018, the unadjusted payment rate for TKA was $1,408.30.[3] The American Academy of Orthopaedic Surgeons and the American Association of Hip and Knee Surgeons have worked to minimize these cuts. However, in January 2018, CMS removed the Current Procedural Terminology code describing TKA procedures from Medicare's Inpatient-Only List to allow Medicare payments to hospitals for TKA procedures regardless of inpatient or outpatient status.[4] Although the implementation of outpatient TJA could lead to significant cost savings in appropriate circumstances, a myriad of factors must be addressed including appropriate patient selection, preoperative patient education, social support, clinical experience of the surgical, anesthesia, recovery teams, and evidence-based protocols for safe outcomes. Although models exist for safe same-day discharge in specific practice settings and for specific patient populations,[5] safe same-day discharge is not yet a generalizable goal. Moreover, despite providers' best efforts to designate admission status according to CMS rules, confusion still surrounds the designation of CMS beneficiaries as observation status versus inpatient, because CMS has not yet clarified which patients qualify for these designations. Clarification of this point will be imperative for safe, effective, and transparent care delivery. Surgeons and hospital systems will need to navigate these changes to minimize costs while delivering the appropriate level of care for individual patients.

Cost Analysis

According to a BlueCross BlueShield report published in January 2019, the average price in 2017 for an inpatient TKA is $30,249 compared with $19,002 in an outpatient setting, whereas the average price for an inpatient THA is $30,685 compared with $22,078 in an outpatient setting.[6] Of note, only 11% of knee procedures and 8% of hip procedures were performed on an outpatient basis in BlueCross BlueShield patients, and the report did not distinguish TKA from unicompartmental knee arthroplasty (UKA). Additionally, the report demonstrated wide price variation depending on geographic location. Between Des Moines, IA, and New York, NY, the prices of knee and hip arthroplasty procedures can vary by more than threefold.[6]

Previous studies have reported that more than 75% of hospital expenditures for TJA derive from three main sources: the hospital room cost, the operating room cost, and the implant cost.[7-9] Efforts to control these costs can result in substantial improvement in the overall hospital economic performance for TJA.[2,9]

Inpatient Costs

Hospital revenues for TJA increased at a lower rate than did inflation; hospital expenses increased at a rate greater than that of inflation.[9] The hospital economics of primary TKA and THA were reported on for an 18-year period between 1990 and 2008 at a single teaching hospital.[8,9]

The hospital room, operating room, and supplies (medical and surgical) were the three most cost-intensive service centers, comprising more than 70% of hospital expenditures related to primary TJA.[8,9] The hospital cost allocation to the hospital room service center decreased 42% in TKA and 5% in THA in inflation-adjusted dollars, primarily because of a reduction in hospital length of stay. The cost allocation to the operating room service center decreased 38.0% for TKA in inflation-adjusted dollars because of reduced surgical time; however, the cost allocation increased slightly by 2.4% in THA during the same interval. The supplies service center decreased 53.0% in TKA and 2.4% in THA in inflation-adjusted dollars because of a reduction in knee and hip implant costs.[8,9] Overall, the hospital converted a $2,172 loss per case for primary TKA into a $2,986 profit per case and a $3,848 loss per case for primary THA into a $2,359 profit per case.[8,9]

Additional changes in utilization and unit costs were also made to improve economic results with good effect.[10] Clinical pathways focused on reducing hospital length of stay were implemented:[9] operating room routines were standardized to reduce length of surgery; routine pathologic evaluation of surgical specimens was eliminated;[10] wound drains were eliminated; urinary catheter utilization was standardized; routine postoperative TKA radiographs were eliminated;[9] routine postoperative noninvasive testing for thromboembolic disease was eliminated;[11] and autologous transfusions, reinfusion drains, and cell savers were reduced. In addition, methods were implemented to reduce unit costs of services and supplies associated with TKA such as standardizing operating room packs, reducing inventory, stocking implants on consignment, and reducing cost of implants by developing a single-price/case-price implant purchasing program.[9]

Similar cost control strategies were used for THA cases.[8] However, THA-related hospital economics also merit a discussion of alternative joint-bearing surfaces. Several studies suggest that reduced wear rates are related to alternative bearing surfaces, but little long-term clinical benefit exists from such surfaces.[12] The cost effectiveness of alternative bearing surfaces depends highly on patient age at the time of surgery, implant cost, and associated reduction in the probability of revision relative to conventional bearing surfaces.[12] The cost burden of alternative bearing surfaces was calculated, and the hospital would have lost $1,147 per patient for ceramic-on-ceramic implants and $534 per patient for metal-on-metal implants.[8]

Implant Costs

The total cost of THA in the United States has been reported as twice the cost of the same procedure in Canada, and higher direct costs were explained by the great disparity in implant costs.[3] Previous emphasis to contain in-hospital costs relied on reducing length of stay, but such reductions do not necessarily translate to substantial decreases in hospital costs, because the volume of services rendered is not substantially reduced by shorter hospitalization.[8] Modern cost containment efforts should include controlling the costs of hospital supplies, especially implants, because a large national variation has been reported in the cost of THA prostheses, with identical implants from a single manufacturer varying by as much as 700%.[13] A 2013 cost effectiveness study for innovative TKA implants showed that newer implants must reduce TKA failure by 50% to 55% to be considered cost effective and that patient comorbidities and their remaining lifespan are important variables to keep in mind while developing new implants.[14] Several factors are associated with implant costs. Patient-specific factors including age and comorbidities are minor factors, but hospital characteristics and physician preference are major considerations.[2,9] Establishing a price ceiling on implants is recommended as one method to control and forecast costs. Another effect of standardizing prices was that cost variability among physicians decreased by 50% to 90% in all categories.[2] In addition, 96% of requests for higher cost implants were approved because of patient-specific anatomic variations, and surgeons collaborated on the process of price standardization. Vendors were amenable to negotiation because of the threat of price competition.[2] Therefore, newer technology should be adopted on the basis of evidence of cost effectiveness or the solution of a documented clinical problem not addressed by current technology.

Computer and Robot-assisted Technologies

Newer innovations including computer and robot-assisted technologies have been developed with the intent of improving clinical and functional outcomes by reducing human error and improving surgical precision for component alignment and soft-tissue balancing. For TKA, current evidence demonstrates no proven benefit of computer navigation over conventional techniques with respect to clinical function or implant survivorship at 10 years.[15] In a randomized controlled trial between conventional and computer-assisted (CAS) TKA, the patient-reported outcome scores at 2-year follow-up showed statistically significant improvement for CAS TKA in two subsets of the Knee injury and Osteoarthritis Outcome Score: symptoms and sport and recreational function.[16] However, a causal relationship between these improvements in clinical outcome scores and improved alignment in CAS TKA could not be established in this study.[16] For THA, navigation systems have been shown to improve positioning of acetabular components, which theoretically may prevent impingement, decrease dislocation rates, and minimize overall wear rates.[17,18] However, the long-term clinical outcomes and economic implications are yet to be clearly defined.

Robotic technologies for UKA have been shown to improve accuracy of implant positioning in UKA with robot-assisted surgeries compared with conventional surgical techniques.[19] The expectation is that an improvement in accuracy of component positioning will decrease revision rates from technical errors;[20] however, this has not yet been demonstrated. These technologies are now being applied to TJA, and evidence of efficacy remains to be demonstrated.

Despite the data supporting improvement in component positioning with robot-assisted technologies, the question of its cost effectiveness remains. The cost of implementation and capital expenditure can be a major impediment to the early adoption of robot-assisted technology, as the upfront costs of the technology hardware and software in combination with service contract costs can be expensive. Listed capital investment prices are unique to the particular robotic system and can further vary depending on negotiated pricing. These prices generally range from $400,000 to $1,200,000.[21] Required annual maintenance contracts and software licensing have been reported to cost an additional $40,000 to $150,000 annually.[21] The per-case disposable fees of a robot-assisted procedure are estimated to range from $600 to $1,300.[21] Additionally, some systems require nonreimbursed advanced imaging such as CT scans, which can further challenge the return on investment, particularly in a bundled care arrangement. As with any new technology, as adoption increases, costs of implementation will decrease. Unfortunately, the vendors have adopted closed platform models for robotics (limiting each robot to one manufacturer), which limits the ability of hospitals to control implant costs.

Although robot-assisted technology may have marked upfront economic burden, some analyses have identified economic advantages of its utilization. A recent study evaluating 246 robotic versus 492 manual matched UKAs found patients who underwent robot-assisted UKA had fewer revisions (0.81% versus 5.28% $P = 0.002$), shorter mean lengths of stay (2.00 versus 2.33 days; $P > 0.05$), and lower mean costs for the index stay plus revisions ($26,001 versus $27,915).[22] In a Markov analysis of one robotic system, a 2016 study found that if one assumes a system cost of $1.362 million, value can be generated using robot-assisted technologies because of slightly better outcomes despite being more expensive than traditional methods.[23] This value may also be volume-dependent; the robotic system was found to be cost effective at high-volume centers that perform greater than 94 UKA procedures per year,[23] which may limit utility and implementation in centers with relatively low procedural volumes. Additionally, a Markov analysis of the Mako system estimated that each robot-assisted UKA case cost $19,219, compared with $16,476 for traditional UKA, and was associated with an incremental benefit of $47,180 per quality-adjusted life-year based on the assumption of a decreased probability of revision with the robot-assisted UKA.[23] The cost and value of robotic technology also varies depending on not only capital costs and annual service charges but also avoidance of unnecessary preoperative scans.[17,20] Assuming a cost of $500,000 for an image-free system, return on investment was calculated to be achievable within 25 cases annually, roughly one-quarter of the cases necessary with the image-based system,[20] and implementing robotic technology in a hospital setting with a high-volume arthroplasty surgeons demonstrated that the capital needed for the robot could potentially be recuperated in 2 years with increased revenues. However, that model assumed reimbursement for CT planning, which is often no longer provided in most markets, particularly with bundled care arrangements. Robotic surgery is a promising technology that requires further investigation to determine cost effectiveness based on balancing its significant upfront and service costs with potential improvements in patient outcomes, potential for improved revision rates, and avoidance of unnecessary preoperative imaging.

Implant Price Negotiation

Because CMS does not get involved in setting markets for implants or drugs, the hospital must negotiate the best price possible to limit the cost of TJA.[24] An economic analysis demonstrated that although implant cost was affected by hospital factors including volume, number of vendors present, and hospital bed size, a substantial amount for cost variation among hospitals could not be accounted for.[24] Additionally, substantial cost variation was reported as a result of physician preference.[24] Typically, hospitals pay a portion of the list price of an implant, a portion that can vary by case and by hospital. This makes defining the prices paid for implants difficult. List price is generally the starting point in implant negotiations and is not the price paid by most hospitals. Most hospital purchasing contracts have confidentiality clauses that make transparency on average implant costs difficult to determine.

The price of TKA implants has been defined as a percentage of hospital reimbursement.[25] The increasing price of TJA implants offset the gains made in cost control with utilization review. In the 1990s at Lahey Clinic and the Hospital for Joint Diseases, an education program was instituted for surgeons, and a hospital prosthesis procurement program that began a competitive bid system to decrease the price of TJA implants was instituted.[24]

The *Journal of Bone and Joint Surgery* endorsed these cost-containment methods, but only if quality of care remained as the focus of any implant selection decision-making process. This philosophy has been extended to the current value-based purchasing movement.

In 2000, the Lahey Clinic developed a Single Price/Case Price Purchasing Program[26] to eliminate potential conflicts between hospital administrators and surgeons regarding the price and selection of TJA implants. The vendor provided a single price for knee implants for every case regardless of the implant used based on 3 years of historical implant selection data. The cost of knee implants decreased 23% without switching vendors. Similar findings were reported for THA implants, suggesting that price ceilings of implants may successfully reduce costs.

In 2012, the New York University Langone Medical Center (NYULMC) Hospital for Joint Diseases implemented a price ceiling implant cost control program.[24] The average implant cost per case was effectively reduced by 22% to 33%. In addition, cost variability among physicians decreased by 50% to 90% in all categories. The program resulted in over $2 million saved within its first year.

Although the price capitation program was initially successful, vendors rejected further reductions in the price ceilings without a volume guarantee.[27] By 2017, NYULMC transitioned to a volume-guarantee model that partnered with a single preferred vendor in exchange for reductions in implant pricing. Through this model, NYULMC was able to further reduce implant costs by 23% per case for the preferred-vendor cases and 17% overall for all TJA cases regardless of the vendor used. This example shows both the potential benefits and challenges associated with a price capitation model, as implant pricing costs decreased but required significant negotiation with vendors who may be reluctant to participate in this program.

Physician alignment with the hospital as well as other physicians is crucial for effective ceiling price implementation. If alignment is not achieved, vendors will continue to sell higher priced implants, and the implant companies may not limit available implant models and will provide whatever physicians request.[24] Physicians must be educated on cost consciousness and the value of patient care. Implants with higher price and newer technology must either demonstrate a solution to a clinical problem not treated by using standard implants or improved patient benefit.

Defining new technology and preventing rising costs resulting from innovation are important factors to consider. If the contract is defined by specific components and the components change in any way during the contract, the institution is vulnerable to the implant vendor as to how that new component or part is priced.[24] Defining truly new technology and how it is to be implemented are important components of any cost containment program. If truly new technology with improved outcome performance is introduced during the contract, then a price for that technology can be agreed on. New technology introduced during an existing contract should not be accepted at higher prices without clinical performance justification.[24]

Another method of implant cost control is to ensure proper demand matching. Demand matching provides the appropriate implant based on the functional demand of the patient. It is difficult to demonstrate in the literature that more expensive implants have better survivorship than less expensive implants.[26] Implant selection guidelines tend to direct more expensive, newer technology implants for younger, heavier, higher activity patients. Defining these selection guidelines is highly controversial. The Lahey Clinic developed a cost reduction and implant selection program based on demand matching.[25] Patients were assigned to demand groups based on five measures: age, weight, bone stock, general health, and the expected postoperative patient activity as determined by the surgeon. The implants were assigned to demand function categories based on an implant's expected capacity to manage the patient's predicted demand. This program was used in primary TKA. The use of all-polyethylene tibial components in lower demand categories afforded the greatest cost savings. A follow-up study assessed the use of a clinical pathway and the TKA implant standardization program as a regulator of resource utilization and hospital costs for TKA.[9] The hospital cost, adjusted for medical inflation, was reduced 19%, whereas short-term patient outcome remained unaffected. A similar program was successful in decreasing THA hospital costs.

Pain Management. Postoperative pain can affect hospital stay, patient satisfaction, postsurgical rehabilitation, and a range of other clinical and administrative outcomes.[28] The emergence of procedure-specific multimodal pain management has been one of the most important advances in hip and knee arthroplasty. The goal of multimodal pain management is to allow accelerated postoperative recovery while reducing the use of parenteral narcotics with the adverse effects of nausea, pruritus, constipation, delirium, and urinary retention.

Multimodal preemptive analgesics are important adjuncts in pain management for patients undergoing TJA. The average length of hospital stay for patients in the preemptive analgesia group was 2.74 days versus 3.28 days for patient-controlled analgesia (PCA) in patients undergoing TJA.[29] Patients in the PCA group used substantially more intravenous morphine (17.7 mg versus 7.2 mg) and experienced a threefold increase in nausea. In addition, those in the PCA group were twice as likely to miss therapy and almost two times more likely to be discharged to an extended care facility. The use of preemptive oxycodone and a selective cyclooxygenase-2 inhibitor decreased postoperative narcotic requirements and increased participation in rehabilitation. In addition, patients who received preemptive analgesics had decreased hospital length of stay and reduced likelihood of discharge to a skilled nursing facility.[29]

To facilitate rapid recovery after TJA, a single-dose spinal anesthetic is preferred to avoid the complications of other neuraxial anesthetics such as hypotension, urinary retention, poor muscle control, and delayed mobilization.[30] Postoperatively, peripheral nerve blockade has become widely available for inclusion in multimodal regimens, but it is costly and has some important limitations, including an increased incidence of falls, inefficient use of the operating room, muscular weakness, and associated delays in physical therapy and rapid rehabilitation.[28] Recently, periarticular injection of anesthetic and analgesic medications has gained importance and appears to offer comparable benefits to nerve blocks in joint arthroplasty without the limitations associated with peripheral motor blockade. The benefits of local periarticular injection are that it is simple to administer, surgeon directed, and allows an infiltration of anesthetic directly into the pain source.[30] Ropivacaine-based periarticular injections were compared with peripheral nerve blocks (continuous femoral and single-injection sciatic), and both methods were found to be equally effective in controlling postoperative pain, but the patients who underwent periarticular injection had a shorter length of stay and decreased peripheral nerve dysesthesia.[31] Another study that compared postoperative epidural analgesia with periarticular injection after TKA with spinal anesthesia found that patients who underwent periarticular injection had better postoperative pain relief, earlier recovery of knee flexion, and a lower incidence of postoperative nausea.[32] Optimizing these parameters is important when trying to enable rapid recovery after TJA. The use of liposomal bupivacaine as a longer acting local anesthetic after TJA remains controversial and depends greatly on technique.[33] Some studies have indicated that liposomal bupivacaine decreases narcotic use and results in earlier achievement of physiotherapeutic milestones.[34,35] The use of episode of care costs to evaluate the cost effectiveness of components of care pathways is a useful tool for comparing new additions to protocols for TJA episode management. In a retrospective review of the cost effectiveness of different pain management protocols following TKA, the replacement of femoral nerve block injections and PCA with intraoperative periarticular liposomal bupivacaine injections resulted in a higher percentage of patients discharged home compared with rehab, a significantly shorter length of stay, and consequently significantly reduced hospital costs while maintaining equivalent pain scores and increasing patient satisfaction.[35] The authors reported a mean saving of 2.63% for the hospitalization of patients with liposomal bupivacaine injections compared with patients who received a femoral nerve block intraoperatively and a PCA for the first 24 hours postoperatively, and a mean saving of 4.81% compared with patients who received liposomal bupivacaine and a PCA.[35] Further studies are necessary to substantiate the cost effectiveness of liposomal bupivacaine and determine its optimal incorporation into a multimodal postoperative pain regimen.

Revision Surgery. The cost of revision arthroplasty has been found to be more difficult to regulate than the cost of primary TJA. Revision arthroplasty procedures are not suitable for a demand-matching system because of substantial differences in case severity and implant requirements. Implant price has been identified as a major contributing factor to the direct cost of revision arthroplasty. In a recently published retrospective analysis, implant costs comprised approximately 28% of the total hospital cost of a revision TKA.[36] If all three components of the knee arthroplasty were revised, the average cost of implants was $13,640, comprising 33% of the total hospital cost. Alternative implant pricing models such as direct to hospital implant and fixed price implant models may significantly reduce cost;[36] however, these have not yet been established. Whether alternative revision implant systems will deliver value to patients is still undetermined.

Recent studies have shown that the revision burden for TKA has remained relatively constant between 2014 and 2016,[37] whereas the overall revision THA burden has recently decreased in the setting of highly cross-linked polyethylene and cessation of metal on metal implants. Between 2014 and 2016, the American Joint Replacement Registry reported a decrease in the revision THA burden from 13.9% to 8.6%.[37] The 2017 Annual Report of the Australian Orthopaedic Association National Joint Replacement Registry delineated that the cumulative all-cause revision rate for THA with a metal femoral head articulating with a highly cross-linked polyethylene liner was 6.3% of 721 hip arthroplasties.[38] This contrasts to the revision rate of 10.5% of 3,096 THAs with conventional polyethylene liners.[38] In a recently published article, the cost savings implications for utilization of highly cross-linked polyethylene in the United States was estimated to be as much as one billion dollars per annual cohort of THA over their 15-year duration.[39] Additionally, the decreased number of revisions secondary to adverse reactions to metal debris for metal-on-metal hip arthroplasties in recent years has contributed to the decline in the revision burden for THAs.[40] At a single high-volume center in Finland, the trend of revisions in metal-on-metal hips showed a peak in 2012 and gradually decreased afterward.

Although the revision burden has remained constant for TKAs and decreased for THAs,[37] the total number of revision TJAs has increased in recent years, which is most likely a result of the increasing prevalence of primary TJA, expansion of indications to younger patients, more high-demand patients, and an increasing presence of patient factors such as obesity and diabetes.[41] The economic burden of revision THA in the United States was estimated to be $4 billion annually in 2017[42] and may continue to rise as the number of TJAs performed annually and the number of patients able to outlive their implants continue to increase. In this context, it is essential to implement strategies that will minimize revision burden and therefore maximize the cost effectiveness of TJA. For example, the newest iterations of dual-mobility components have been approved for use in the United States since 2009.[43] Dual-mobility implants have reduced dislocation risk compared with smaller diameter femoral heads and appear to be cost effective in both primary and revision THA.[44-47] Additionally, the authors of a 2018 study demonstrated that patients undergoing revision THA with a dual-mobility implant had a reduced rate of subsequent revision compared with patients undergoing revision THA with large conventional femoral head constructs (8.7% versus 19%, respectively).[48] The decreased rate of reinterventions resulted in payer savings of $1,500 to $2,500 per case when using dual-mobility implant compared with large femoral head constructs.[48] Thus, the introduction of new implants such as dual-mobility constructs to reduce revision rates may ultimately contribute to cost savings if used in the appropriate clinical setting.

BUNDLED PAYMENTS AND ALTERNATIVE PAYMENT MODELS

Traditionally, TJA services have been reimbursed with the fee-for-service model, which incentivizes the delivery of healthcare services in volume without much regard for quality and outcomes related to those services.[49] However, financial challenges have shifted the focus to creating more value for the money allocated to TJA services and these new measures strive to reward the delivery of high-quality care with improved outcomes. In 2011, the CMS created a Bundled Payments for Care Improvement (BPCI) initiative that focused on high-quality coordinated care that is outcome based.[50,51]

The BPCI Initiative

Through the BPCI initiative, hospitals are paid one standard predetermined sum for an all-inclusive episode of care, or bundle, that can begin a certain time before an episode and continues for an established length of time after surgery. For TJA, the episode includes preoperative services 72 hours before surgery, inpatient services including surgery, and postoperative care for a period of 30, 60, or 90 days from surgery.[52] In this risk-sharing model, the healthcare provider is responsible for all care episodes within the at-risk postoperative period, including readmissions, without any additional reimbursement. Under this program, if the total costs of all services rendered in that episode are less than the bundled payment, the provider is entitled to the remainder. However, if the costs exceed the bundled payment target price, the provider will sustain a financial loss. The bundled care model incentivizes high-quality care with the goal of reducing readmissions and improving cost effectiveness.[3] This alternative payment model will also shift a higher burden of costs to the provider in cases where patients have complications, require extended post–acute care, are readmitted, or require repeat procedures within the 90-day postoperative period after the index procedure.[51]

In addition to risk sharing, CMS also specifically authorizes gain sharing with stakeholders, with the idea that healthcare providers should be rewarded for restructuring their services to become more coordinated and cost effective.[51] Gain sharing can vary depending on the negotiations between hospitals, surgeons, other episode initiators, or stakeholders. The American Association of Hip and Knee Surgeons Bundled Payment Task Force advises that for gain-sharing arrangements, a specific baseline should be used to measure cost savings and quality measurements.[51] Also, hospitals and surgeons must look beyond just implant-related costs to focus on streamlining the entire episode of care to maximize the benefits of the BPCI model.[51]

Results of BPCI in TJA

Early findings were published on BPCI model 2 for a 90-day TJA episode of care at an urban, academic, orthopaedic specialty hospital.[50] In the first year of the program, the average length of hospital stay for 721 patients decreased from 4.27 to 3.53 days. Discharge to inpatient facilities for rehabilitation also decreased from 65% to 43%. The total 90-day readmission rate was 11%. Readmissions from a facility were higher (13.7%) when compared with readmissions from home (9.0%). Medicare costs were reduced by up to 10% using the BPCI model.[50] Infrastructure costs and the costs of implementing the program were not included in these calculations.[50] The implementation of clinical care pathways and intensive care management services for TJA patients to improve efficiency and quality of care were important factors in generating cost reductions in BPCI.[51]

After year 1 of the BPCI program, an unacceptably high 90-day readmission of 11% was reported.[53] Ninety percent of patients requiring readmission had at least one modifiable risk factor, which could have been optimized before surgery, and 50% of patients had two or more.[53] Therefore, a risk factor stratification and modification program known as the Perioperative Orthopaedic Surgical Home (POSH), designed to delay surgery in high-risk patients with potentially modifiable risk factors, was instituted as a voluntary program for the surgeons involved in BPCI.[54] Preliminary results demonstrated that readmission rates were lowered from 15% in 2009 and 17% in 2011 to 11% at 90 days in 2013, but still remained unacceptably high. The average length of stay decreased from 4.27 to 3.58 days and discharge to inpatient post–acute care facilities decreased from 71% to 44%.[50]

In addition to the POSH preoperative risk factor optimization program, other programs were implemented after year 1 of the initiative including enhanced care coordination and home services, a change in venous thromboembolic disease prophylaxis to a risk-stratified protocol, infection-prevention measures, and a continued emphasis on discharge to home rather than to an inpatient facility. The effect of these changes on cost and quality of patient care has been dramatic. After year 3 of these programs, the average hospital length of stay decreased from 3.58 to 2.96 days.[55] The rate of discharge to an inpatient facility decreased from 44% to 28%. The average 90-day cost per episode decreased by 20%, as the 90-day all-cause readmission rate decreased from 13% to 8%. These results suggest that continued improvements to increase value by improving patient outcomes and simultaneously reducing cost burden are possible.

In 2018, the BPCI initiative concluded and CMS initiated a new bundle payment model known as BPCI Advanced (BPCI-A),[4] building off the successes of the previous payment model iteration. The primary objectives of reducing cost to CMS while improving patient quality of care remain; however, several differences have been incorporated in BPCI-A. Now, a 90-day standard post–acute care period exists for every participant. Payment is linked to the quality of care provided as measured by seven quality measures in the first 2 years. There are both positive and negative financial incentives for healthcare organizations: if quality criteria are met, then the organization can be reimbursed up to an additional 10%, whereas the organization can be penalized 10% if quality criteria are not fulfilled. The first cohort of participants started on October 1, 2018 and will run through December 31, 2023. The effectiveness of this new model is yet to be determined, but will likely guide future payment models. Because of decreased target pricing for the voluntary BPCI-A program, participation has been very low. The elimination of outpatient designated TJA patients from BPCI-A also decreased the opportunity to be successful in the program.

Reducing Readmissions

Alternative payment models are based on a risk-sharing system in which the healthcare provider and institution are compensated based on outcome for the entire episode of care. The episode can include inpatient services such as surgery and postoperative care for a period of up to 90 days following surgery. The at-risk postoperative period under BPCI includes readmissions, which are usually unplanned after TJA procedures. The initiator of the episode is responsible for all related costs within the agreed-on postoperative period, including readmissions, without any additional reimbursement.[51,52]

Reducing readmissions involves managing preoperative comorbidities that are associated with postoperative complications, which can be surgical and medical in nature. Providers must be able to select appropriate patients for TJA and identify high-risk patients and potentially modify risk factors that can be associated with worse outcomes. This selection process has obvious ethical implications, because some patients may need to delay surgery until their health status is optimized and some patients may be incapable or unwilling to modify their risk factors.

Short-term Readmissions

Healthcare providers must understand the nuances of the risk-sharing model focused on an episode of care. The cost burden of 30-day readmissions after primary and revision THA and TKA procedures was studied at a high-volume orthopaedic subspecialty hospital.[2] Using a hospital database for primary and revision TJA procedures performed from 2009 to 2012, direct costs were obtained for each unplanned admission along with the total Part A Medicare payments. The 30-day readmission rate was 2.4 per 100 cases for primary TJA, 9.5 per 100 cases for revision THA, and 11.9 per 100 cases for revision TKA. The mean cost for readmission after primary THA and TKA was $17,103 and $13,008, respectively. The mean cost of readmission was $27,272 per case following revision THA and $29,893 per case following revision TKA. The readmission cost burdens per admission were 4.3% for THA, 2.8% for TKA, 8.3% for revision THA, and 11.9% for revision TKA.

The three primary causes for readmission following TJA are wound complications, surgical site infections, and medical problems.[56-58] Readmission risk is related to a patient's severity of illness (SOI) and preoperative comorbidities. The readmission burden was stratified by SOI using the All Patients-Refined–Diagnosis-Related Group (APR-DRG) severity classification system.[53] The APR-DRG-SOI system has four categories of severity: minor, moderate, major, and extreme.[59] Among 2,026 patients, the readmission rate was as low as 2.6% for patients with moderate SOI and as high as 26.1% for patients with extreme SOI. The average readmission costs were directly proportional to the SOI scale, with $12,781 for minor SOI, $17,575 for moderate SOI, $19,120 for major SOI, and $21,216 for extreme SOI. The readmission burden was also directly proportional to SOI with lower categories of SOI bearing a burden of approximately 4% to 5% and the extreme SOI group, with a readmission burden of 18.5%.

In addition to risk factor modification, it is also essential to understand the preventable causes for readmissions. One study stated that, "for readmission rates to be a useful measure in assessing quality of care, they must capture only those readmissions that could have been prevented."[57] The major causes for readmission are infections, wound issues, workup of deep vein thrombosis and/or pulmonary emboli, and other medical complications.[57,58,60] Current strategies to tackle infection prevention include timely, weight-based administration of preoperative antibiotics, prescreening and treatment of methicillin-resistant *Staphylococcus aureus* carriers, hepatitis C screening and treatment, ensuring adequate perioperative glucose control, creating hand hygiene programs, and maintaining normothermia and patient oxygenation.[57,58] Another potential strategy aimed at reducing readmissions may involve outpatient deep vein thrombosis screening and treatment.

In an effort to identify and optimize medical comorbidities before TJA and prevent readmission, NYULMC developed a surgeon-led screening and optimization pathway known as Perioperative Orthopaedic Surgical Home (POSH).[61] POSH targets eight modifiable comorbidities as previously defined by the validated Readmission Risk Assessment Tool: infection risk factors, smoking, obesity/malnutrition, cardiovascular disease, history of a venous thrombosis, neurocognitive/psychological or substance abuse-related problems, physical deconditioning, and diabetes.[61] Patients identified as high risk (Readmission Risk Assessment Tool score ≥ 3) for poor postoperative outcomes and hospital readmission were approached at the discretion of their orthopaedic surgeon and encouraged to participate in shared decision-making discussions to maximize optimization opportunities. Patients with Readmission Risk Assessment Tool scores between 3 and 5 who participated in the POSH initiative demonstrated significantly lower 30- and 90-day readmission rates compared with the non-POSH cohort. On average, non-POSH Medicare 90-day episode of care costs were 14.9% greater than the POSH TJA recipients. This is the first study to provide evidence demonstrating that prophylactic medical optimization of preexisting comorbidities before elective TJA reduces 30- and 90-day readmissions and cost associated with TJA. Further studies to develop a more formalized screening and referral process are necessary to determine the future implications and potential greater impact of patient optimization through integrated care pathways.

Long-term Readmissions

A study that compared the 30- and 90-day readmission data at a tertiary care urban hospital reported that surgical reasons accounted for slightly more than one-half of overall readmissions.[60] However, the study also reported that medical reasons for readmissions including problems such as cardiac complications, pulmonary complications, and venous thromboses became more important factors in the 90-day postoperative period. The authors found that age (younger than 50 years and older than 80 years), Medicare or self-payer status, coronary artery disease, diabetes mellitus, weight (body mass index less than 18.5 kg/m^2 and greater than 30 kg/m^2), and increased length of hospital stay (more than 5 days) were associated with substantial readmissions in the 90-day period.[60] Similar findings have been reported in other studies.[58] One study reported a direct correlation between increasing SOI and increasing costs of TJA-related readmissions.[62] Patients who are transferred from rehabilitation facilities or outside hospitals tend to have higher categories of SOI and are more likely to be associated with higher readmission costs than patients who do not originate from such facilities.[62]

One study evaluated readmissions, revisions, infections, and hospital resource use in the first year after TJA.[63] The study also examined hospitalization rates before elective TJA and reported that 12.9% of patients undergoing elective THA and 10.2% of patients undergoing elective TKA were hospitalized in the year before their index surgery. Hospitalizations increased to 14.8% of patients undergoing elective THA and 15.5% of patients undergoing elective TKA in the year following surgery, indicating 15% and 52% increases, respectively. Patients undergoing emergency THA (usually hip fractures treated using a prosthesis) were the most resource intensive: 26.7% had hospital admissions before THA and 27.8% were readmitted in the year after surgery. For all patients, the most common reason for readmission was an implant-related complication followed by complications associated with the procedure. However, for patients undergoing emergency THA, the second most common reason for readmission was cardiac complications. Revision surgery within 1 year was 1.3% for patients undergoing elective surgery and 2.0% for patients undergoing emergency surgery. Most commonly, THA cases were revised for mechanical complications and TKA cases were revised for infections. In addition, a 2015 study showed that TKA revision has an 8.5% higher rate and THA revision has a 3.4% higher rate of repeat procedures such as irrigation and débridement or modular components exchange in the 90-day postoperative period. CMS does not proportionately compensate surgeons for the increased time and effort associated with performing revision TJA.[64] The current reimbursement model makes it financially challenging for surgeons to provide revision TJA services to patients.[8,9,64] Alternative payment models have not yet been applied to revision TJA.

SUMMARY

The economics and cost implications of TJA are becoming increasingly challenging to understand, implement, and control. Creating value for patients undergoing arthroplasty requires efficient, integrated, and evidence-based clinical pathways that can deliver services to patients in a cost-effective manner. Intensive patient education, care management, optimization of health status, and alignment of stakeholder incentives will provide more value to patients undergoing TJA. Alternative payment models may help facilitate these care delivery improvements. Value-based purchasing will be integral to the cost-effective delivery of care in the future.

KEY STUDY POINTS

- TJA is a successful, cost-effective procedure that requires an increasing amount of healthcare resources; however, decreasing reimbursement and increased costs of these procedures have resulted in financial strain on the healthcare system.
- Cost analysis of TJA procedures across the United States shows a wide variation in the cost of surgery.
- New technologies, such as surgical robotics, have the potential to improve cost effectiveness of TJA if improved clinical outcomes and reduced long-term complications are demonstrated. Additionally, adjustments to implant design have the potential to reduce long-term cost and improve outcomes (eg, modern dual-mobility implants). Long-term outcomes are necessary to measure these potential benefits.
- Medicare and Medicaid have implemented alternative payment models such as the Bundled Payment for Care Improvement initiative and the Comprehensive Care for Joint Replacement, with the purpose of improving the quality of TJA care while reducing cost.
- Various quality and cost effectiveness improvement measures include patient risk optimization, multimodal pain management, blood management protocols, implant cost negotiation, and care management initiatives. As healthcare models shift toward value-based purchasing, evaluation of cost-effective delivery of TJA is essential.

ANNOTATED REFERENCES

1. Sloan M, Premkumar A, Sheth NP: Projected volume of primary total joint arthroplasty in the U.S., 2014 to 2030. *J Bone Joint Surg Am* 2018;100(17):1455-1460.

   This study used retrospective TJA data (annual procedure incidence rate, population age and sex) from 2000 to 2014 to project future volume of TJA procedures. Using a linear regression of growth rates from 2000 to 2014, THA is projected to increase 71% (635,000 procedures), and TKA is projected to grow 85% (1.26 million procedures) by 2030. Level of evidence: III.

2. Bosco JA, Karkenny AJ, Hutzler LH, Slover JD, Iorio R: Cost burden of 30-day readmissions following Medicare total hip and knee arthroplasty. *J Arthroplasty* 2014;29(5):903-905.

3. Nordt JG: *As Medicare Costs Rise, Reimbursements Drop.* Available at: http://www.aaos.org/news/aaosnow/dec12/cover1.asp. Accessed October 6, 2015.

4. Center for Medicare & Medicaid Services: *BPCI Advanced.* Available at: https://innovation.cms.gov/initiatives/bpci-advanced. Accessed October 20, 2019.

   Across all model 2 episodes, the percentage of BPCI patients discharged to a post–acute care facility declined from 66% to 47%, and the proportion discharged home remained steady. Although not significant, the largest relative declines in payments occurred during the anchor hospital stay (consistent with the reduced length of stay) and for physician evaluation and treatment visits. Level of evidence: III.

5. Kort NP, Bemelmans YFL, van der Kuy PHM, Jansen J, Schotanus MGM: Patient selection criteria for outpatient joint arthroplasty. *Knee Surg Sports Traumatol Arthrosc* 2017;25(9):2668-2675.

   Fourteen studies were reviewed to determine a general consensus for patient selection criteria for outpatient joint arthroplasty. Level of evidence: III.

6. Blue Cross Blue Shield Association: *Planned Knee and Hip Replacement Surgeries are on the Rise in the U.S.* Blue Cross Blue Shield. Available at: https://www.bcbs.com/the-health-of-america/reports/planned-knee-and-hip-replacement-surgeries-are-the-rise-the-us. Accessed October 20, 2019.

   This is a summary of the number of planned hip and knee arthroplasties in the United States Level of evidence: III.

7. Antoniou J, Martineau P, Filion K, et al: In-hospital cost of total hip arthroplasty in Canada and the United States. *J Bone Joint Surg Am* 2004;86A(11):2435-2439.

8. Rana AJ, Iorio R, Healy WL: Hospital economics of primary THA decreasing reimbursement and increasing cost, 1990 to 2008. *Clin Orthop Relat Res* 2011;469(2):355-361.

9. Healy WL, Iorio R, Ko J, Appleby D, Lemos DW: Impact of cost reduction programs on short-term patient outcome and hospital cost of total knee arthroplasty. *J Bone Joint Surg Am* 2002;84(3):348-353.

10. Kocher MS, Erens G, Thornhill TS, Ready JE: Cost and effectiveness of routine pathological examination of operative specimens obtained during primary total hip and knee replacement in patients with osteoarthritis. *J Bone Joint Surg Am* 2000;82(11):1531-1535.

11. Schwarcz TH, Matthews MR, Hartford JM, et al: Surveillance venous duplex is not clinically useful after total joint arthroplasty when effective deep venous thrombosis prophylaxis is used. *Ann Vasc Surg* 2004;18(2):193-198.

12. Bozic K, Morshed S, Silverstein M, Rubash H, Kahn J: Use of cost-effectiveness analysis to evaluate new technologies in orthopaedics: The case of alternative bearing surfaces in total hip arthroplasty. *J Bone Joint Surg Am* 2006;88(4):706-714.

13. Metz CM, Freiberg AA: An international comparative study of total hip arthroplasty cost and practice patterns. *J Arthroplasty* 1998;13(3):296-298.

14. Suter LG, Paltiel AD, Rome BN, et al: Placing a price on medical device innovation: The example of total knee arthroplasty. *PLoS One* 2013;8(5):e62709.

15. Kim YH, Park JW, Kim JS: The clinical outcome of computer-navigated compared with conventional knee arthroplasty in the same patients: A prospective, randomized, double-blind, long-term study. *J Bone Joint Surg Am* 2017;99(12): 989-996.

    The clinical outcomes of 162 patients (153 women and 9 men) who underwent bilateral TKA with computer-navigated arthroplasty in one knee and traditional arthroplasty in the other were observed. Average length of follow-up was 12.3 years, with follow-up appointments occurring at 3 months, 1 year, and every 2 or 3 years thereafter. There was no significant difference in component position or loosening at the 12.3-year follow-up point. Level of evidence: II.

16. Petursson G, Fenstad AM, Gøthesen Ø, et al: Computer-assisted compared with conventional total knee replacement: A multicenter parallel-group randomized controlled trial. *J Bone Joint Surg Am* 2018;100(15):1265-1274.

    A randomized controlled trial comparing 2-year clinical results of CAS versus conventional TKA showed significantly more improvement in the CAS group than in the conventional group in two subscales of the Knee Injury and Osteoarthritis Outcome Score and better pain relief. Level of evidence: I.

17. Kelley TC, Swank ML: Role of navigation in total hip arthroplasty. *J Bone Joint Surg Am* 2009;91(suppl 1):153-158.

18. Najarian BC, Kilgore JE, Markel DC: Evaluation of component positioning in primary total hip arthroplasty using an imageless navigation device compared with traditional methods. *J Arthroplasty* 2009;24(1):15-21.

19. Bell SW, Anthony I, Jones B, MacLean A, Rowe P, Blyth M: Improved accuracy of component positioning with robotic-assisted unicompartmental knee arthroplasty: Data from a prospective, randomized controlled study. *J Bone Joint Surg Am* 2016;98(8):627-635.

20. Lonner JH, Moretti VM: The evolution of image-free robotic assistance in unicompartmental knee arthroplasty. *Am J Orthop (Belle Mead NJ)* 2016;45(4):249-254.

21. Bellemans J, Vandenneucker H, Vanlauwe J: Robot-assisted total knee arthroplasty. *Clin Orthop Relat Res* 2007;464:111-116.

22. Cool CL, Needham KA, Khlopas A, Mont MA: Revision analysis of robotic arm–assisted and manual unicompartmental knee arthroplasty. *J Arthroplasty* 2019;34(5):926-931.

    In a retrospective longitudinal review, the authors demonstrated that robotic arm–assisted UKAs resulted in fewer revision procedures, shorter length of stay, and lower mean costs during the index procedure and at 24 months postoperatively. Level of evidence: III.

23. Moschetti WE, Konopka JF, Rubash HE, Genuario JW: Can robot-assisted unicompartmental knee arthroplasty be cost-effective? A Markov decision analysis. *J Arthroplasty* 2016;31(4):759-765.

24. Bosco JA, Alvarado CM, Slover JD, Iorio R, Hutzler LH: Decreasing total joint implant costs and physician specific cost variation through negotiation. *J Arthroplasty* 2014;29(4):678-680.

25. Iorio R, Healy WL, Kirven FM, Patch DA, Pfeifer BA: Knee implant standardization: An implant selection and cost reduction program. *Am J Knee Surg* 1998;11(2):73-79.

26. Healy WL, Iorio R, Lemos MJ, et al: Single Price/Case Price Purchasing in orthopaedic surgery: Experience at the Lahey Clinic. *J Bone Joint Surg Am* 2000;82(5):607-612.

27. Boylan MR, Chadda A, Slover JD, Zuckerman JD, Iorio R, Bosco JA: Preferred single-vendor program for total joint arthroplasty implants: Surgeon adoption, outcomes, and cost savings. *J Bone Joint Surg Am* 2019;101(15):1381-1387.

    The utilization of a preferred single-vendor model for hip and knee arthroplasty implants led to a decrease in mean cost per case by 23% in the first year. No significant changes were observed with regard to quality metrics. Level of evidence: III.

28. Springer BD: Transition from nerve blocks to periarticular injections and emerging techniques in total joint arthroplasty. *Am J Orthop (Belle Mead NJ)* 2014;43(suppl 10):S6-S9.

29. Duellman TJ, Gaffigan C, Milbrandt JC, Allan DG: Multimodal, pre-emptive analgesia decreases the length of hospital stay following total joint arthroplasty. *Orthopedics* 2009;32(3):167.

30. Sculco PK, Pagnano MW: Perioperative solutions for rapid recovery joint arthroplasty: Get ahead and stay ahead. *J Arthroplasty* 2015;30(4):518-520.

31. Spangehl MJ, Clarke HD, Hentz JG, Misra L, Blocher JL, Seamans DP: The Chitranjan Ranawat Award: Periarticular injections and femoral & sciatic blocks provide similar pain relief after TKA. A randomized clinical trial. *Clin Orthop Relat Res* 2015;473(1):45-53.

32. Tsukada S, Wakui M, Hoshino A: Postoperative epidural analgesia compared with intraoperative periarticular injection for pain control following total knee arthroplasty under spinal anesthesia: A randomized controlled trial. *J Bone Joint Surg Am* 2014;96(17):1433-1438.

33. Joshi GP, Cushner FD, Barrington JW, et al: Techniques for periarticular infiltration with liposomal bupivacaine for the management of pain after hip and knee arthroplasty: A consensus recommendation. *J Surg Orthop Adv* 2015;24(1):27-35.

34. Yu SW, Szulc AL, Walton SL, Davidovitch RI, Bosco JA, Iorio R: Liposomal bupivacaine as an adjunct to postoperative pain control in total hip arthroplasty. *J Arthroplasty* 2016;31(7):1510-1515.

35. Kim K, Elbuluk A, Yu S, Iorio R: Cost-effective peri-operative pain management: Assuring a happy patient after total knee arthroplasty. *Bone Joint J* 2018;100-B(1 suppl A):55-61.

    In an effort to determine the optimal regimen for pain management following TKA, the addition of periarticular injections of liposomal bupivacaine to a multimodal pain regimen and elimination of PCA and femoral nerve blocks led to shorter length of stay and a significantly higher percentage of patients who were discharged to their home. Additionally, liposomal bupivacaine was proven to be cost effective. Level of evidence: II.

36. Elbuluk AM, Old AB, Bosco JA, Schwarzkopf R, Iorio R: Strategies for reducing implant costs in the revision total knee arthroplasty episode of care. *Arthroplast Today* 2017;3(4):286-288.

    This review analyzed implant cost in revision TKA and investigated cost saving with two alternative pricing models. Retrospective analysis showed that 28% of total hospital cost was spent on total knee revision implants. Results suggest that direct to hospital and fixed pricing models on implants could potentially save up to $8,000 per case. Level of evidence: III.

37. Heckmann N, Ihn H, Stefl M, et al: Early results from the American Joint Replacement Registry: A comparison with other National Registries. *J Arthroplasty* 2019;34(7 suppl):S125-S134.e1.

    TJA data from Australia, New Zealand, American Joint Replacement Registry, the United Kingdom, Norway, and Sweden between 2014 and 2016 were compared with results from the United States. Variables including polyethylene type, type of surgery, mobile bearings, and revision burden were compared. Level of evidence: III.

38. Australian Orthopaedic Association National Joint Replacement Registry: *Annual Reports 2018*. Availabel at: https://aoanjrr.sahmri.com/annual-reports-2018. Accessed October 23, 2019.

    This study includes the annual reports of TJA (hip knee and shoulder) from the Australian Orthopaedic Association National Joint Replacement Registry. Statistics include revision rate, failure rate, and number of surgeries. Level of evidence: III.

39. Harris WH, Muratoglu OK: The role of crosslinked polyethylene in reducing aggregated costs of total hip arthroplasty in the United States. *J Arthroplasty* 2019;34(6):1089-1092.

    This study evaluates the use of cross-linked polyethylene as a method of cost saving for THA. Results suggest that use reduces cost. Level of evidence: III.

40. Lainiala OS, Reito AP, Nieminen JJ, Eskelinen AP: Declining revision burden of metal-on-metal hip arthroplasties. *J Arthroplasty* 2019;34(9):2058-2064.e1.

    This study is a retrospective analysis of patients with metal-on-metal hip arthroplasties for implant survivorship. Results suggest that the rate of adverse reactions to metal debris has been decreasing since 2013. Level of evidence III.

41. Kurtz SM, Lau E, Ong K, Zhao K, Kelly M, Bozic KJ: Future young patient demand for primary and revision joint replacement: National projections from 2010 to 2030. *Clin Orthop Relat Res* 2009;467(10):2606-2612.

42. Kurtz SM, Lau EC, Ong KL, Adler EM, Kolisek FR, Manley MT: Which clinical and patient factors influence the national economic burden of hospital readmissions after total joint arthroplasty? *Clin Orthop Relat Res* 2017;475(12):2926-2937.

    Patient factors that influence economic burden were analyzed in this retrospective study. Results suggest that readmissions within 90 days of TJA represent a massive economic burden, and half of the related cases are due to procedural complications. Level of evidence: III.

43. De Martino I, Triantafyllopoulos GK, Sculco PK, Sculco TP: Dual mobility cups in total hip arthroplasty. *World J Orthop* 2014;5(3):180-187.

44. Garbuz DS, Masri BA, Duncan CP, et al: The Frank Stinchfield Award. Dislocation in revision THA: Do large heads (36 and 40 mm) result in reduced dislocation rates in a randomized clinical trial? *Clin Orthop Relat Res* 2012;470(2):351-356.

45. Plummer DR, Christy JM, Sporer SM, Paprosky WG, Della Valle CJ: Dual-mobility articulations for patients at high risk for dislocation. *J Arthroplasty* 2016;31(9 suppl):131-135.

46. Barlow BT, McLawhorn AS, Westrich GH: The cost-effectiveness of dual mobility implants for primary total hip arthroplasty: A computer-based cost-utility model. *J Bone Joint Surg Am* 2017;99(9):768-777.

    Using a Markov model, this study investigated the cost effectiveness of dual-mobility implants compared with conventional implants in the context of primary THA. In the base case, dual-mobility implants showed absolute dominance over conventional THA implants. The study cited increased quality-adjusted life years and lower accrued cost, both indicating cost savings. Level of evidence: III.

47. Epinette J-A, Lafuma A, Robert J, Doz M: Cost-effectiveness model comparing dual-mobility to fixed-bearing designs for total hip replacement in France. *Orthop Traumatol Surg Res* 2016;102(2):143-148.

48. Abdel MP: Dual-mobility constructs in revision total hip arthroplasties. *J Arthroplasty* 2018;33(5):1328-1330.

    The use of dual-mobility implants is shown to reduce the rate of dislocation in THA cases. This type of implant is implied to be useful in revision THA cases to reduce readmission for dislocation. Level of evidence: III.

49. Luft HS: Economic incentives to promote innovation in healthcare delivery. *Clin Orthop Relat Res* 2009;467(10):2497-2505.

50. Iorio R, Clair AJ, Inneh IA, Slover JD, Bosco JA, Zuckerman JD: Early results of Medicare's bundled payment initiative for a 90-day total joint arthroplasty episode of care. *J Arthroplasty* 2016;31(2):343-350.

51. Froimson MI, Rana A, White RE, et al: Bundled payments for care improvement initiative: The next evolution of payment formulations. AAHKS Bundled Payment Task Force. *J Arthroplasty* 2013;28(8 suppl):157-165.

52. Kiridly DN, Karkenny AJ, Hutzler LH, Slover JD, Iorio R, Bosco JA: The effect of severity of disease on cost burden of 30-day readmissions following total joint arthroplasty (TJA). *J Arthroplasty* 2014;29(8):1545-1547.
53. Yu S, Garvin KL, Healy WL, Pellegrini VD, Iorio R: Preventing hospital readmissions and limiting the complications associated with total joint arthroplasty. *J Am Acad Orthop Surg* 2015;23(11):e60-e71.
54. Boraiah S, Joo L, Inneh IA, et al: Management of modifiable risk factors prior to primary hip and knee arthroplasty: A readmission risk assessment tool. *J Bone Joint Surg Am* 2015;97(23):1921-1928.
55. Dundon JM, Bosco J, Slover J, Yu S, Sayeed Y, Iorio R: Improvement in total joint replacement quality metrics: Year one versus year three of the bundled payments for care improvement initiative. *J Bone Joint Surg Am* 2016;98(23):1949-1953.
56. McCormack R, Michels R, Ramos N, Hutzler L, Slover JD, Bosco JA: Thirty-day readmission rates as a measure of quality: Causes of readmission after orthopedic surgeries and accuracy of administrative data. *J Healthc Manag* 2013;58(1):64-76, discussion 76-77.
57. Shah AN, Vail TP, Taylor D, Pietrobon R: Comorbid illness affects hospital costs related to hip arthroplasty: Quantification of health status and implications for fair reimbursement and surgeon comparisons. *J Arthroplasty* 2004;19(6):700-705.
58. Husted H, Otte KS, Kristensen BB, Orsnes T, Kehlet H: Readmissions after fast-track hip and knee arthroplasty. *Arch Orthop Trauma Surg* 2010;130(9):1185-1191.
59. Mehta S, Hadley S, Hutzler L, Slover J, Phillips M, Bosco JA: Impact of preoperative MRSA screening and decolonization on hospital-acquired MRSA burden. *Clin Orthop Relat Res* 2013;471(7):2367-2371.
60. Saucedo JM, Marecek GS, Wanke TR, Lee J, Stulberg SD, Puri L: Understanding readmission after primary total hip and knee arthroplasty: Who's at risk? *J Arthroplasty* 2014;29(2):256-260.
61. Kim KY, Anoushiravani AA, Chen KK, et al: Perioperative Orthopedic Surgical Home: Optimizing total joint arthroplasty candidates and preventing readmission. *J Arthroplasty* 2019;34(7 suppl):S91-S96.

    The benefits of delaying elective TJA surgeries for patients with modifiable comorbidities to optimize health and outcomes are discussed in this article. The utility of preoperative comorbidity screening using the perioperative orthopaedic surgical home initiative showed that use of the POSH initiative may enhance the value of care TJA patients receive while reducing cost associated with the procedure. Level of evidence: III.
62. Plate JF, Brown ML, Wohler AD, Seyler TM, Lang JE: Patient factors and cost associated with 90-day readmission following total hip arthroplasty. *J Arthroplasty* 2016;31(1):49-52.
63. Bohm ER, Dunbar MJ, Frood JJ, Johnson TM, Morris KA: Rehospitalizations, early revisions, infections, and hospital resource use in the first year after hip and knee arthroplasties. *J Arthroplasty* 2012;27(2):232-237.e1.
64. Tokarski AT, Deirmengian CA, Lichstein PM, Austin MS, Deirmengian GK: Medicare fails to compensate additional surgical time and effort associated with revision arthroplasty. *J Arthroplasty* 2015;30(4):535-538.

National Joint Registries

DANIEL J. BERRY, MD • DAVID G. LEWALLEN, MD • FARES S. HADDAD, BSc, MD (RES), FRCS

ABSTRACT

National joint registries can provide descriptive information about patients undergoing joint arthroplasty, including survivorship rates and outcomes data about joint arthroplasty based on patient, hospital, and implant factors. Registries also can provide information about the most common reasons for implant failure and associated complications. These data can provide a real-time feedback loop to all stakeholders—patients, surgeons, hospitals, payers, and implant manufacturers—that can lead to quality improvement. It is helpful to be aware of the current status and what has been learned from the American Joint Replacement Registry and the United Kingdom National Joint Registry. Registries have limitations, however; the most important limitation is that although they provide information about associations between outcomes and patient and implant factors, they cannot prove such associations as being causal.

Keywords: American Joint Replacement Registry (AJRR); arthroplasty; joint registries; National Joint Registry (NJR) for England; Northern Ireland; the Isle of Man; Wales

Dr. Berry or an immediate family member has received royalties from DePuy, A Johnson & Johnson Company; serves as a paid consultant to or is an employee of Bodycad and DePuy, A Johnson & Johnson Company; has stock or stock options held in Bodycad; has received research or institutional support from DePuy, A Johnson & Johnson Company; and serves as a board member, owner, officer, or committee member of the Current Concepts in Joint Replacement (Hip Society and Knee Society), the International Hip Society, the Mayo Clinic Board of Governors, and the Orthopaedic Research and Education Foundation. Dr. Lewallen or an immediate family member has received royalties from Zimmer Biomet; serves as a paid consultant to or is an employee of Zimmer Biomet; has stock or stock options held in Acuitive Technologies and Ketai Medical Devices; has received research or institutional support from Corin USA; and serves as a board member, owner, officer, or committee member of American Joint Replacement Registry and Orthopaedic Research and Education Foundation. Dr. Haddad or an immediate family member has received royalties from Corin, MatOrtho, Smith & Nephew, and Stryker; serves as a paid consultant to or is an employee of Smith & Nephew and Stryker; has received research or institutional support from Smith & Nephew and Stryker; and serves as a board member, owner, officer, or committee member of BOSTAA.

INTRODUCTION

Registries for hip and knee arthroplasty have been used for 4 decades and have a profound and increasing effect on the clinical practice of total hip arthroplasty (THA) and total knee arthroplasty (TKA). Registries come in many categories, including national registries, regional or state registries, institutional registries, and industry-based registries. Each type of registry has its own advantages, disadvantages, limitations, and applications.

Registries are designed to enroll patients who have undergone joint arthroplasty and systematically collect structured data related to the patient, the procedure, and the outcomes of the procedure. Registries can provide many useful functions to both the orthopaedic community and patients. Registries can provide descriptive data about patients being treated with joint arthroplasty and the characteristics of the joint arthroplasties being used. Registries can provide valuable information on contemporary practice trends in selected orthopaedic communities.[1] This information provides real-time observations about the practice of joint arthroplasty.

Registries can provide high-level data about the overall revision rate for hip and knee replacement and how demographic factors[2] and generic implant characteristics affect rates of implant revision. Registries can provide information on the most common reasons for implant failure and the rates of the most common complications, thereby guiding thoughtful innovation aimed at solving real problems. For example, a recent study from the American Joint Replacement Registry (AJRR) demonstrated a strong correlation between type of implant fixation and risk of revision for periprosthetic fracture after THA.[3] The huge population size in large registries provides powerful information about associations between surgical techniques or implant categories and procedure outcome that would not be identified reliably in smaller data sets.[4,5] Registries show how specific implants are performing (thereby guiding implant selection) and also serve as a trigger to identify implants that are not performing well.[6] Registries can examine associations between specific patient characteristics and comorbidities and the risks of adverse outcomes, which can result in risk stratification. Increasingly, registries may collect global or joint-specific patient-reported outcome measures or clinical joint scores that provide a more nuanced understanding of the results of joint arthroplasty compared with revision as the main end point. In all these roles, registries provide a feedback loop to stakeholders (patients, surgeons, hospitals, and implant manufacturers), which allows stakeholders to compare relevant outcomes with benchmarks and subsequently make choices or changes that improve the results of joint arthroplasty.[7]

REGISTRY END POINTS

The most common registry end point has been revision surgery. Revision is a hard end point that is not subject to interpretation. However, the way in which revisions are categorized from one registry to another varies considerably, which has consequences for what can be learned.[8,9] One registry may combine revisions for osteolysis with revisions for aseptic loosening, whereas another may consider the two as separate categories. More specific categorization may not only be valuable for interpreting results but also increase the risk of miscategorization at the time of data entry. Many registries cannot identify which of several implant parts in a joint arthroplasty have failed and required revision. Therefore, separating failures such as aseptic loosening for a specific implant (eg, acetabular versus femoral components of a THA) may not be possible.

Because many registries consider only revision as the end point, some important complications may not be identified. If only infections that result in revision are captured, then all infections treated without implant revision are overlooked. If only hip dislocations resulting in revision are captured, all other dislocations are not identified.[10]

Some registries collect clinical outcome scores, including patient-reported data, which can provide valuable information about the results of surgery that is more nuanced than just revision as an end point.[11,12] However, for such outcome measures to be useful for comparison purposes, considerable patient information is needed to allow risk stratification. Registries are increasingly trying to gain more detail about patient characteristics, including comorbidities before surgery (so-called level 2 data) to allow the development of better risk stratification models.

LIMITATIONS OF REGISTRIES

Registries can provide big-picture information about what is being done and the results being produced. They also can provide associations between outcomes and patient and implant characteristics. However, it is important to understand that such associations do not necessarily arise from causality, and confounding variables often are present.[13] Registries are subject to selection bias; that is, some procedures or implants may be used disproportionately in certain types of patients or by certain surgeons, with better or worse results, which results in bias in outcomes. Registries primarily reporting revision as an end point will not pick up failures that do not lead—or have not yet led—to revision. This can affect results, particularly if revision surgery is delayed in a systematic fashion, such as in countries with long waiting lists for such surgical procedures. Registries also are limited by the data collected for each registry. For example, a lack of specificity about what part of an implant has failed and the reasons for that failure may limit the conclusions that can be drawn.

National registries have the advantage of extremely large numbers, but for practical reasons, they cannot collect data at the level of detail of some institutional registries. For this reason, institutional registries that collect detailed surgical patient data often can address different questions compared with those of national registries. Likewise, many questions cannot be answered by a registry; therefore, well-designed randomized controlled trials, case-control studies, and detailed case series complement the work of registries.[14] Data from registries may provide information that results in hypothesis generation that can be proven or refuted by subsequent prospective or more in-depth studies.

TRENDS IN REGISTRIES

Registries allow surgeons and hospitals to compare their individual results with large national cohorts. For this comparison to be meaningful, the cohorts must be risk stratified. Risk stratification for different end points is complex and is still being optimized. To perform good risk stratification, registries are increasingly collecting more data about medical comorbidities, patient characteristics, and orthopaedic factors that can influence hip and knee replacement outcomes.

Patient-reported outcome measures and joint-specific outcome measures are being collected more commonly because surgeons, payers, regulatory agencies, and patients seek more nuanced measures of the results of joint arthroplasty versus only revision. Although these measures have great value, they are time consuming and expensive to collect; simplifying how these measures are collected, reducing the number of questions to minimal necessary data sets, and identifying the circumstances under which outcome measures are most valuable to collect is an ongoing effort.

Large, national registries with established infrastructure to collect and analyze arthroplasty data increasingly will serve as a platform for nested randomized trials to explore questions of causality that cannot be answered with routine registry data.[15,16] Registries have the great benefit of collecting structured data, which helps ensure certain data elements are collected and are thus available for analysis. Increasingly natural language processing, which is becoming more available and powerful, will be used to search nonstructured electronic medical records to provide useful information that can be linked to registry data. Likewise the increasing availability and power of artificial intelligence will be harnessed to analyze registry data and associated data in the electronic record, further increasing the clinical relevance and utility of those large databases.

Each registry has its own advantages and disadvantages. Merging or linking data between different registries can provide synergies. Linking databases also allows exploration of associations beyond the scope of a joint registry such as the association of joint replacement procedures with important medical conditions.[3,17] Currently, the International Society of Arthroplasty Registries is working to standardize terminology and define minimal collected data sets. These efforts may allow collaboration of registries to evaluate serious problems that arise infrequently, identify concerns with respect to specific implants or procedures earlier, and confirm or deny observations reported from just one registry.

NATIONAL JOINT REGISTRIES

The American Joint Replacement Registry

Background

The AJRR is a not-for-profit 501(c)(3) tax-exempt organization established in 2009 to collect data on THAs and TKAs performed in the United States to improve the quality of care. It was established as the result of a multiple stakeholder collaborative effort by the American Academy of Orthopaedic Surgeons; the American Association of Hip and Knee Surgeons; the Hip Society; the Knee Society; hospitals within the American Hospital Association; individual participating institutions, health insurance plans, and medical device manufacturers; and both volunteer and direct financial contributions from individual orthopaedic surgeons. All stakeholders and the public are represented on the AJRR board of directors. In 2019 the AJRR formally joined with the AAOS to become the cornerstone of the AAOS family of orthopaedic subspecialty registries.

The goal of the AJRR is to capture data on more than 90% of all hip and knee arthroplasties performed in the United States, while also developing the comprehensive data needed to enhance orthopaedic quality of care, thereby improving patient outcomes and safety, reducing costs, and advancing orthopaedic science and bioengineering.

The American Academy of Orthopaedic Surgeons provided initial support for the AJRR. After formalizing the multiple-stakeholder model, the AJRR evolved to include varying levels of support from virtually all the participating stakeholder groups. It is currently under the direction of the AAOS and is mainly supported by subscriptions or software licensing fees, which are currently paid by a subset of hospitals and, more recently, some physician practice groups (and soon to include individual surgeons) desiring on-demand access and display of their own data benchmarked to the national sample.

Current Status

As of July 2020, the AJRR had gathered level 1 data on more than 2 million procedures performed by more than 11,000 surgeons as reported by 670 participating hospitals located in all 50 states. Level 1 data represent the minimum information required on all cases for participation in the AJRR and include details on the patient, the procedure, the hospital, the surgeon, and the implant itself to allow long-term tracking of implant survivorship. Level 2 data on comorbidities and complications and level 3 data on patient-reported outcomes also are being collected by the AJRR on an expanding subset of patients from hospitals that have elected to collect and report these data.

In the AJRR annual report published in November 2019, information on the cumulative experience from 2012 through the end of 2018 was summarized. This report presented data on hip and knee arthroplasty procedures of all types, totaling more than 1.5 million cases through the end of 2014. These procedures were performed at institutions that represented the full range of hospital types, sizes, and locations. Patients undergoing arthroplasty in this large US sample were predominantly female (59.0%), with a mean age of 65.6 years for hip arthroplasty and 67 years for knee arthroplasty. Thus, almost one-half of all procedures in the United States were performed in individuals younger than 65 years and were not well represented in studies solely of Medicare data sets. In this sample of the national experience, osteoarthritis was the predominant diagnosis prompting arthroplasty. Rheumatoid arthritis was indicated in fewer than 1% of these procedures, likely related to advances in the medical management of inflammatory arthropathies during the past decade.

In the initial few years of any registry operation, data available are mainly descriptive, pending longer term follow-up and survivorship data on implant performance (which can be further studied by hospital, surgeon, surgical technique, and patient factors). Another example of important descriptive information on the national experience is the most recent annual report that demonstrated that femoral neck fracture accounts for 8.2% of hip arthroplasties currently performed in the United States. Short-term shifts in practice patterns also can be documented. For surface replacement arthroplasty, which was once widely performed, the percentage decreased to less than 1% of hip procedures between 2012 and 2014 and was limited to a handful of hospitals and surgeons. Implant-specific information and patterns of use of specific implant technology can be documented as such technology evolves in the initial years of a registry such as the AJRR, which is shown by the example of ceramic head use in THA (**Figure 1**). The relative percentage of ceramic versus cobalt-chromium heads used in hip arthroplasty in the United States from 2012 to 2014 can be tracked by year (**Figure 1**).

Ceramic head usage also can be shown to be biased toward younger patients, comprising most arthroplasties in those younger than 60 years and diminishing usage with each decade of patient age thereafter (**Figure 2**); however, the percentage of older patients receiving a ceramic femoral head has grown each year since 2012.

Data on knee arthroplasties have shown that these procedures are performed almost exclusively for osteoarthritis, with tricompartmental replacement and posterior-stabilized components used in most primary knee arthroplasties. Cruciate-retaining implants were used in less than one-third of the procedures.

Revision burden also can be tracked by a national registry effort such as AJRR, and it is defined as the percentage of total joint arthroplasty cases performed per year that were revisions of prior implants. Revision burden is one measure of the success and long-term durability of these procedures. In the AJRR annual report, the cumulative revision burden was 7.3% of all hip arthroplasties reported to AJRR; for knee arthroplasties, the revision burden was similar at 6.5% to 7.5% per year from 2012 to 2018 of all knee arthroplasties per year.

The AJRR is actively expanding data collection from hospitals with comprehensive level 2 (comorbidity and complications) and optional level 3 (patient-reported outcome measures) data available for local data analysis needs to support the extramural payment and quality reporting needs of institutions and providers. A surge in interest and participation in the AJRR has followed the introduction of incentives by payers and certifying bodies for registry participation as a quality improvement

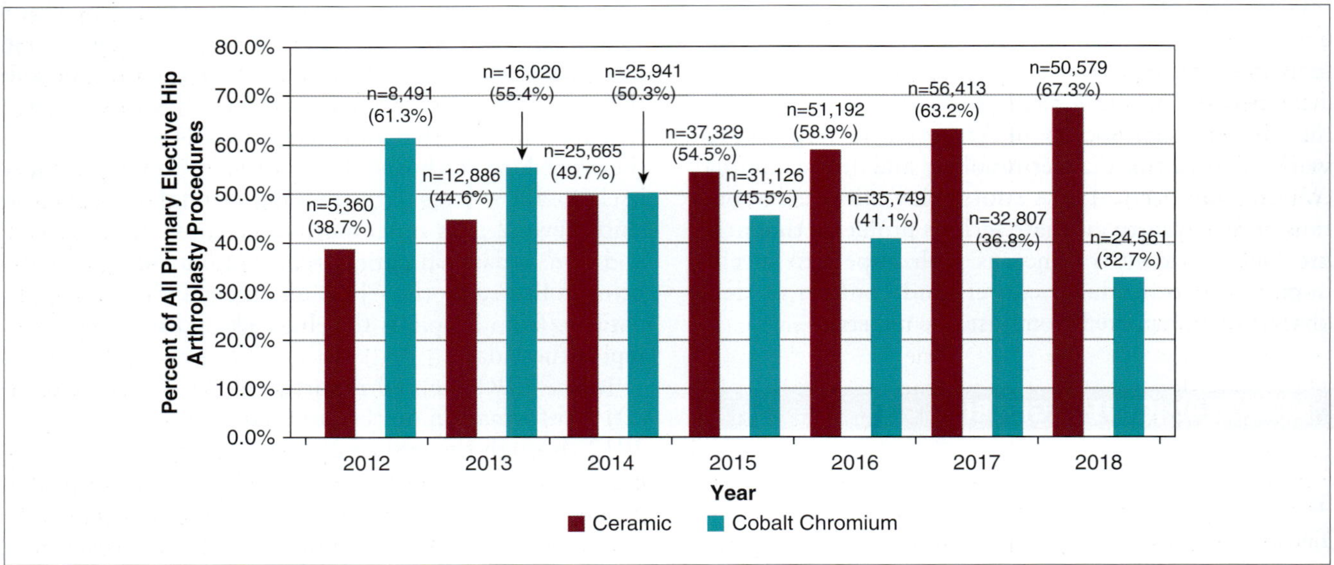

FIGURE 1 Bar graph of ceramic versus cobalt-chromium femoral head usage between 2012 and 2018. (Adapted with permission from the American Joint Replacement Registry Annual Report *2019*. Rosemont, IL, American Joint Replacement Registry, 2019: p 30.)

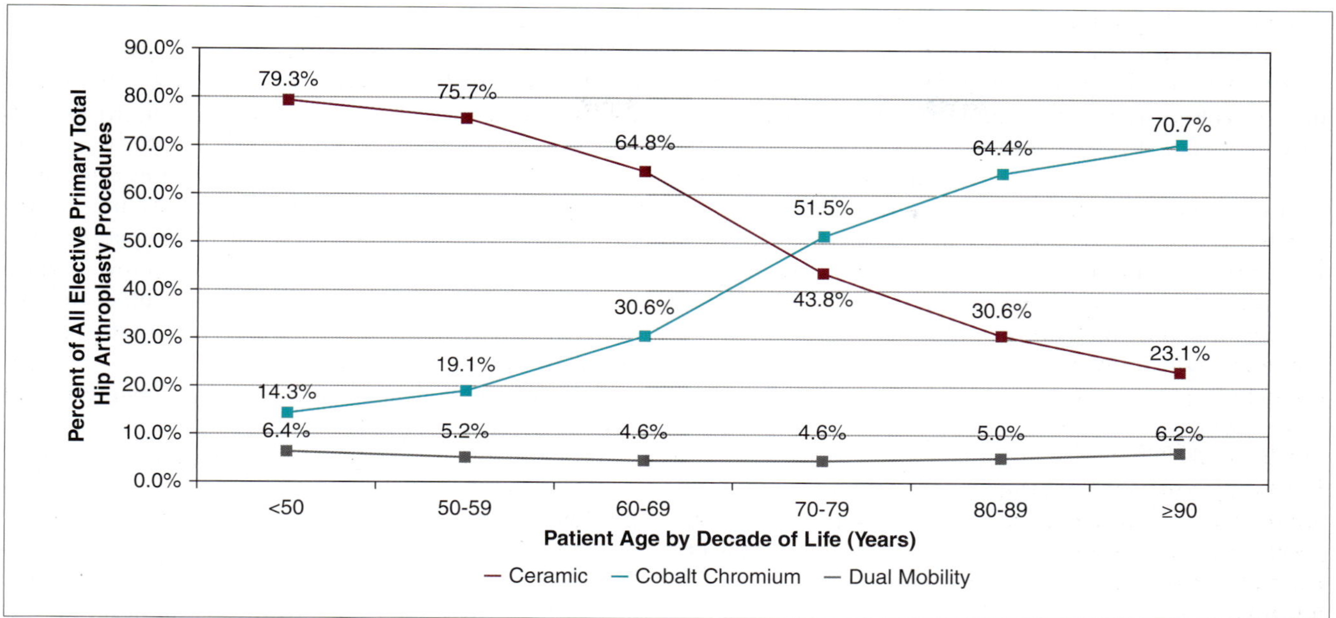

FIGURE 2 Line graph of Ceramic versus Cobalt Chromium head usage by decade of life (N = 384,959). (Adapted with permission from the American Joint Replacement Registry Annual Report 2019. Rosemont, IL, American Joint Replacement Registry, 2019: p 30.)

indicator. The AJRR currently provides a robust foundation for the collection of hospital-specific and provider-specific information that can be benchmarked against national data. Such data will become increasingly valuable in the next several years with the addition of risk-adjusted implant survivorship and complication data, helping to further drive improvements in care for patients undergoing arthroplasty.[18]

The United Kingdom and International Experience

Background

Hip, knee, ankle, elbow, and shoulder joint arthroplasties have become common and highly successful procedures that bring many patients improved mobility and pain relief. The National Joint Registry (NJR) for England, Wales, Northern Ireland, and the Isle of Man has been in existence for more than a decade and was developed based on the success of the Scandinavian registries. During the same period, the Australian registry developed a useful output of information from the Southern Hemisphere, and the hope is that multiple registries will be developed worldwide, for not only hip and knee arthroplasty but also other orthopaedic subspecialties, and harmonized in such a way that they can be assessed together and information gleaned across cohorts and populations.[19,20]

Registry data are now clearly a valuable part of the orthopaedic surgeon's armamentarium. In orthopaedic medicine, physicians have significantly relied on expert opinion and the outcome of case series to guide management. More recently, physicians have increasingly recognized the importance of prospective randomized studies, but these are expensive and not always practical, focusing on specific refined questions. Registry data and studies add great value because they provide information regarding the entire population.[21]

Registry analysis helps identify trends and potential problems. The great advantages of any registry are that registries are cross-sectional across an entire population and provide objective primary data on what happens to patients or implants and procedures. The registries also provide a real-time view, because the data come from more than just major centers or design surgeons. In effect, the data are a real-time check of the generalizability of a procedure or an implant. It also has been shown that feedback improves performance.[22-26]

If a registry has good compliance and produces clean validated data, the optimal treatment modalities (approaches, implants, or procedures) can be identified. Great learning and research potential is possible for the entire community, at potentially large savings for health-care providers, which is predicated on clear, impartial, statistically sound, and unbiased interpretation. Such potential has been effectively shown in the Scandinavian model.[27-31]

Registries have great potential for identifying early failure of a new implant or technique. Registries also can be used to identify a poor performer within a subgroup; for example, a certain type of knee replacement or hip resurfacing. Registries also can identify outlying implants or surgeon performance, which should generate questions related to why outliers are occurring and what, if anything, should be done.[32-34]

The NJR has an Outlier Committee that examines both outlier surgeon and implant performance. This system effectively alerts surgeons and units to potential problems with performance. The data can be checked locally, and changes in practice can be made. This system has improved performance and outcomes for both surgeons and patients. The process also is confidential initially; although it is perhaps important that such evaluations and their outcomes are within the public domain, the process itself does not need to be revealed publicly.[35]

The Remit of NJR

The NJR collects information on joint arthroplasty surgery and monitors the performance of joint arthroplasty implants. It was established in 2002 by the UK Department of Health. The registry helps monitor the performance of implants and the effectiveness of different types of surgery. It currently collects data on all hip, knee, ankle, elbow, and shoulder joint arthroplasties across the National Health Service and the independent healthcare sector and has more than 1 million procedures registered.[36]

The six goals of the NJR are as follows: (1) monitor in real time the outcomes achieved by brand of prosthesis, hospital, and surgeon and highlight where these fall below an expected performance to allow prompt investigation and support follow-up action; (2) inform patients, clinicians, providers, and commissioners of healthcare, regulators, and implant suppliers of the outcomes achieved in joint arthroplasty surgery; (3) showcase variations in outcomes achieved across surgical practices to inform best practice; (4) enhance patient awareness of joint arthroplasty outcomes to better inform patient choice and patients' quality of experience by engaging with patients and patient organizations; (5) support evidence-based purchasing of joint arthroplasty implants for healthcare providers to support quality and cost-effectiveness; and (6) support suppliers in the routine after-market surveillance of implants and provide information to clinicians, patients, hospital management, and the regulatory authorities.

Orthopaedic Registries and Data Interpretation

The NJR is a powerful resource that can contribute to research into the full range of biologic, mechanical, clinical, economic, and social factors influencing the outcome of joint arthroplasty. The data also can help establish the effect of joint arthroplasty on the well-being of patients and the general population. However, problems and challenges exist with some registries. Many have limited data capture and data quality, which makes data interpretation and use difficult.

Registries are now a critical part of surgeon decision making, but it is important to interpret registries given that they are not always necessarily relevant to individual practice and do not prove causation. They merely provide a means for analysis and to generate hypotheses.

Registries also need to be studied longitudinally. Certain aspects, such as cementation of the femoral stem that makes one type of implant, the cemented femoral stem, might look much better than aspects for a noncemented stem in the first decade, but follow-up during the second decade may show that noncemented arthroplasty comes to the fore later.[37,38]

Any data set within a registry needs to be interpreted in light of confounders. For example, using registry data to promote one approach or anesthetic technique over another needs to somehow control for the type of patients in each group and some form of selection bias.[39,40]

An important issue is that the end point in registries is revision, not clinical outcome or function. Because of a large bias toward revision as the key end point for any arthroplasty, it is difficult to say whether a procedure or an implant that has functioned well for 10 years should be discarded in favor of one that functions poorly but survives 10 or 15 years or longer because it is difficult to revise. Moreover, if the data are analyzed poorly, a single poor performer in a subgroup can negatively affect the remainder of the subgroup and skew the data.

Registries are strongly affected by revision bias. Data can be either misinterpreted or overinterpreted, thus opening registries to inappropriate use by colleagues, industry, and politicians.[40,41]

Revisions and other complications also vary with case complexity and orthopaedic and medical comorbidity. Limitations in the accuracy of any inferred conclusions include difficulties in adjusting for case-mix complexity, inaccuracy of propensity scores, a lack of data validation, missing data, incomplete capture of preexisting covariates, limitations of Cox regression analysis, and inferring causation from observational data.[42,43]

One key issue is that registries are not sufficiently developed for patient-level analysis. They provide population data that are ideal for hypothesis generation. The findings from such data need to be tested in appropriately constructed studies. When circumstances determine that this is not possible, the data need to be interpreted for what they are and acted on appropriately. In the United Kingdom, NJR data are not owned by the profession, which creates a disadvantage. Data can be published without knowledge, agreement, or validation by the profession.

Risks and Challenges

Although physicians are aware of the many potential benefits of registries, they continue to grapple with the difficulties that registry data can present. Recent information demonstrating that some retrieved metal-on-metal revision procedures were not incorporated into the NJR implants survival curve is concerning,[8,44-48] and two articles highlighted missing data from the national registry.[45,46] Such instances should be interpreted in light of ongoing initiatives to validate NJR data locally, setting up a more robust and centralized process to understand and evaluate the data in a more transparent way. Nevertheless, these studies raise questions about the potential use of NJR (and other registry) data and particularly about the publication of surgeon-level data.

The headline outcome results of the NJR are similar to those of all other national registries. With 1.7 million entries, even 1,000 missing cases will have little effect. At the individual surgeon level, however, where the denominator may be only a few hundred procedures, the effect may be greater. Using parametric statistical techniques and standard deviations about a norm, to rank and compare surgeon performance, is problematic. There will always be a bottom 1%, 2%, 5%, and 10%. If these are removed, then the process starts again with a new bottom of 1%, 2%, 5%, and 10%. Such parameters may not be what the exercise is aiming to achieve. It would be a detriment if surgeons started avoiding the most complex cases.

The data have not yet been validated, and in the first 10 years of the registry, data capture was inconsistent.[45,46] The data to separate and control for orthopaedic and medical case mix complexity are inadequate and limited to age, body mass index, American Society of Anesthesiologists grade, and the use of bone graft. The data set is incomplete: the national average is 92% complete; although some units have 100% compliance, several are much closer to 50%, which should raise concerns regarding any inferences made at individual surgeon-level reporting. It is fully appreciated that the NJR is getting better each year, but another 10 years may be necessary before the data set is sufficiently validated and appropriately evaluated to consider the publication of surgeon-level data.

The Future

The NJR recently celebrated its 10th anniversary and has registered more than 1.7 million procedures. Combined with other national registries, the NJR has had a huge effect on the practice of joint arthroplasty worldwide. Registries realize the epidemiologic goals of enhancing general awareness; supporting evidence-based practice; providing after-market implant surveillance; and monitoring outcomes achieved by brands of prosthesis, hospitals, and surgeons. Therefore, registries cater to the patients, clinicians, providers, and commissioners of healthcare, regulators, and implant suppliers. The ability to link registry data to patient-reported outcome measures as well as other population-based data sources enhances their usefulness for monitoring outcomes and trends.

Registries, and the NJR in particular, have inherent disadvantages that limit the interpretation of the data made available by them. Compliance issues associated with any data collection and the reporting process limit the quality of the registry data. No robust system is in place to tackle confounding data and capture underreported data or unreported outcomes. Registries were set up to capture survival, but the ancillary data that have been collected are not validated. Caution must be exercised when using registries as high-level evidence. Registry-based study results cannot infer causative explanations. Any trend identified should be used to test hypotheses, not as a study conclusion. Focused studies also will be necessary to introduce new technology, because registries only are surrogates to this process.

The best registry data are complete, validated, and peer-reviewed and have good source data verification. Such data have systems in place to determine the appropriate research questions and methods to be used; high-level database integration techniques and outputs are required to create important messages and result in practice change.

Registries have an ongoing role. They will get improved as good practice is integrated across different medical societies. It is important that registries are used appropriately to avoid politically biased interpretations or poor health economic analyses. Ultimately, registries should help surgeons make their decisions by providing needed and desired data.

SUMMARY

National registries are becoming more common and are maturing. The data provided by these registries are having more beneficial effects on orthopaedic practices. The advantages and limitations of joint registries are important to understand when evaluating data.

KEY STUDY POINTS

- National joint registries can provide descriptive information about patients undergoing joint arthroplasty, survivorship rates, and outcomes data about joint arthroplasty based on patient, hospital, and implant factors.
- Registries also can provide information about the most common reasons for implant failure and complications.

- Data provide a real-time feedback loop to all stakeholders (patients, surgeons, hospitals, payers, and implant manufacturers), which can result in quality improvement.
- Registries have limitations, the most important of which is that they provide information about associations between outcomes and patient and implant factors, but they cannot prove that such associations are causal.

ANNOTATED REFERENCES

1. Heckmann N, Ihn H, Stefl M, et al: Early results from the American Joint Replacement Registry: A comparison with other national registries. *J Arthroplasty* 2019;34(7S):S125-S134.

   Important differences in practice patterns with respect to implant fixation and bearing surface choices were found in different national joint registries. Level of evidence: III.

2. Lenguerrand E, Whitehouse MR, Beswick AD, et al, National Joint Registry for England, Wales, Northern Ireland and the Isle of Man: Risk factors associated with revision for prosthetic joint infection following knee replacement: An observational cohort study from England and Wales. *Lancet Infect Dis* 2019;19(6):589-600.

   The association between numerous demographic and operative variables, some of which are modifiable, is explored in over 600,000 THAs in the NJR.

3. Springer BD, Etkin CD, Shores PB, Gioe TJ, Lewallen DG, Bozic KJ: Perioperative periprosthetic femur fractures are strongly correlated with fixation method: An analysis from the American Joint Replacement Registry. *J Arthroplasty* 2019;34(7S):S352-S354.

   In over 10,000 linked revisions in the AJRR, the risk of early revision for periprosthetic fracture was 2.6% higher than for noncemented compared with cemented stems.

4. Nugent M, Wyatt MC, Frampton CM, Hooper GJ: Despite improved survivorship of uncemented fixation in total knee arthroplasty for osteoarthritis, cemented fixation remains the gold standard: An analysis of a National Joint Registry. *J Arthroplasty* 2019;34(8):1626-1633.

   The New Zealand Joint Registry demonstrated an association between superior survivorship of cemented compared with noncemented TKA in both younger and older patient groups.

5. Jameson SS, Asaad A, Diament M, et al: Antibiotic-loaded bone cement is associated with a lower risk of revision following primary cemented total knee arthroplasty: An analysis of 731,214 cases using Nation Joint Registry data. *Bone Joint J* 2019;101B(11):1331-1347.

   In over 700,000 TKAs, the use of antibiotic-loaded cement was associated with a lower risk of infection compared with plain cement.

6. de Steiger RN, Miller LN, Davidson DC, Ryan P, Graves SE: Joint registry approach for identification of outlier prostheses. *Acta Orthop* 2013;84(4):348-352.

7. Delaunay C: Registries in orthopaedics. *Orthop Traumatol Surg Res* 2015;101(1 suppl):S69-S75.

8. Liebs TR, Splietker F, Hassenpflug J: Is a revision a revision? An analysis of national arthroplasty registries' definitions of revision. *Clin Orthop Relat Res* 2015;473(11):3421-3430.

9. Niinimäki TT: The reasons for knee arthroplasty revisions are incomparable in the different arthroplasty registries. *Knee* 2015;22(2):142-144.

10. Devane PA, Wraighte PJ, Ong DC, Horne JG: Do joint registries report true rates of hip dislocation? *Clin Orthop Relat Res* 2012;470(11):3003-3006.

11. Patel J, Lee JH, Li Z, SooHoo NF, Bozic K, Huddleston JI III: Predictors of low patient-reported outcomes response rates in the California Joint Replacement Registry. *J Arthroplasty* 2015;30(12):2071-2075.

12. Wilson I, Bohm E, Lubbeke A, et al: Orthopaedic registries with patient-reported outcome measures. *EFORT Open Rev* 2019;4(6):357-367.

    Patient-reported outcomes provide a different perspective than revision rates on the success of a procedure, but collection can be expensive and burdensome.

13. Whitehouse SL, Bolland BJ, Howell JR, Crawford RW, Timperley AJ: Mortality following hip arthroplasty—Inappropriate use of National Joint Registry (NJR) data. *J Arthroplasty* 2014;29(9):1827-1834.

14. Inacio MC, Paxton EW, Dillon MT: Understanding orthopaedic registry studies: A comparison with clinical studies. *J Bone Joint Surg Am* 2016;98(1):e3.

15. Sidhu VS, Graves SE, Buchbinder R, et al: CRISTAL: Protocol for a cluster randomized, crossover, non-inferiority trial of aspirin compared to low molecular weight heparin for venous thromboembolism prophylaxis in hip or knee arthroplasty, a registry nested study. *BMJ Open* 2019;9(11):e031657.

    A nested trial of venous thromboembolism risk comparing aspirin with low-molecular-weight heparin is being performed in the Australian Orthopaedic Association National Joint Replacement Registry.

16. Vertullo CJ, Graves SE, Cuthbert AR, Lewis PL: The effect of surgeon preference for selective patellar resurfacing on revision risk in total knee replacement: An instrumental variable analysis of 136,116 procedures from the Australian Orthopaedic Association National Joint Replacement Registry. *J Bone Joint Surg* 2019;101A(14):1261-1270.

    In over 130,000 TKAs, the authors found selective patellar resurfacing had a higher patellar revision rate than routine resurfacing. Level of evidence: III.

17. Sabah SA, Moon JC, Jenkins-Jones S, et al: The risk of cardiac failure following metal-on-metal hip arthroplasty. *Bone Joint J* 2018;100B(1):20-17.

Following metal-on-metal THA, the risk of cardiac failure was not increased in patients with metal-on-metal THA.

18. American Joint Replacement Registry: Annual Report 2014: Second AJRR Annual Report on Hip and Knee Arthroplasty Data. Available at: http://www.ajrr.net/images/annual_reports/AJRR_2014_Annual_Report_final_11-11-15.pdf. Accessed July 10, 2016.
19. Malchau H, Porter ML: Editorial comment: 2014 Meeting of the International Society of Arthroplasty Registers. *Clin Orthop Relat Res* 2015;473(11):3368-3369.
20. Graves SE: The value of arthroplasty registry data. *Acta Orthop* 2010;81(1):8-9.
21. Bedair H, Lawless B, Malchau H: Are implant designer series believable? Comparison of survivorship between designer series and national registries. *J Arthroplasty* 2013;28(5):728-731.
22. Hunt LP, Ben-Shlomo Y, Clark EM, et al, National Joint Registry for England and Wales: 45-day mortality after 467,779 knee replacements for osteoarthritis from the National Joint Registry for England and Wales: An observational study. *Lancet* 2014;384(9952):1429-1436.
23. Hunt LP, Ben-Shlomo Y, Clark EM, et al, on behalf of the National Joint Registry for England, Wales and Northern Ireland: 90-day mortality after 409,096 total hip replacements for osteoarthritis, from the National Joint Registry for England and Wales: A retrospective analysis. *Lancet* 2013;382(9898):1097-1104.
24. Jameson SS, Charman SC, Gregg PJ, Reed MR, van der Meulen JH: The effect of aspirin and low-molecular-weight heparin on venous thromboembolism after hip replacement: A non-randomised comparison from information in the National Joint Registry. *J Bone Joint Surg Br* 2011;93(11): 1465-1470.
25. Malchau H, Garellick G, Eisler T, Kärrholm J, Herberts P: Presidential guest address: The Swedish Hip Registry. Increasing the sensitivity by patient outcome data. *Clin Orthop Relat Res* 2005;441:19-29.
26. Smith AJ, Dieppe P, Porter M, Blom AW, on behalf of the National Joint Registry of England and Wales: Risk of cancer in first seven years after metal-on-metal hip replacement compared with other bearings and general population: Linkage study between the National Joint Registry of England and Wales and hospital episode statistics. *Br Med J* 2012;344:e2383.
27. Gøthesen O, Espehaug B, Havelin L, et al: Survival rates and causes of revision in cemented primary total knee replacement: A report from the Norwegian Arthroplasty Register 1994-2009. *Bone Joint J* 2013;95-B(5):636-642.
28. Jameson SS, Lees D, James P, et al: Lower rates of dislocation with increased femoral head size after primary total hip replacement: A five-year analysis of NHS patients in England. *J Bone Joint Surg Br* 2011;93(7):876-880.
29. Mäkelä KT, Matilainen M, Pulkkinen P, et al: Countrywise results of total hip replacement: An analysis of 438,733 hips based on the Nordic Arthroplasty Register Association database. *Acta Orthop* 2014;85(2):107-116.
30. Malchau H, Graves SE, Porter M, Harris WH, Troelsen A: The next critical role of orthopedic registries. *Acta Orthop* 2015;86(1):3-4.
31. Pedersen AB, Baron JA, Overgaard S, Johnsen SP: Short- and long-term mortality following primary total hip replacement for osteoarthritis: A Danish Nationwide Epidemiological Study. *J Bone Joint Surg Br* 2011;93(2):172-177.
32. Jameson SS, Baker PN, Mason J, et al: The design of the acetabular component and size of the femoral head influence the risk of revision following 34 721 single-brand cemented hip replacements: A retrospective cohort study of medium-term data from a National Joint Registry. *J Bone Joint Surg Br* 2012;94(12):1611-1617.
33. Jameson SS, Baker PN, Mason J, Porter ML, Deehan DJ, Reed MR: Independent predictors of revision following metal-on-metal hip resurfacing: A retrospective cohort study using National Joint Registry data. *J Bone Joint Surg Br* 2012;94(6):746-754.
34. Smith AJ, Dieppe P, Vernon K, Porter M, Blom AW, on behalf of the National Joint Registry of England and Wales: Failure rates of stemmed metal-on-metal hip replacements: Analysis of data from the National Joint Registry of England and Wales. *Lancet* 2012;379(9822):1199-1204.
35. Rowden NJ, Harrison JA, Graves SE, Miller LN, de Steiger RN, Davidson DC: Loss to follow-up after arthroplasty: A new use for registry data. *J Bone Joint Surg Br* 2012;94(4):493-496.
36. National Joint Registry: NJR Annual Report. Available at: http://www.njrcentre.org.uk/njrcentre/Reports,PublicationsandMinutes/Anualreports/tabid/86/Default.aspx. Accessed August 15, 2016.
37. Mäkelä KT, Matilainen M, Pulkkinen P, et al: Failure rate of cemented and uncemented total hip replacements: Register study of combined Nordic database of four nations. *Br Med J* 2014;348:f7592.
38. Troelsen A, Malchau E, Sillesen N, Malchau H: A review of current fixation use and registry outcomes in total hip arthroplasty: The uncemented paradox. *Clin Orthop Relat Res* 2013;471(7):2052-2059.
39. de Steiger RN, Liu YL, Graves SE: Computer navigation for total knee arthroplasty reduces revision rate for patients less than sixty-five years of age. *J Bone Joint Surg Am* 2015;97(8):635-642.
40. Anand R, Graves SE, de Steiger RN, et al: What is the benefit of introducing new hip and knee prostheses? *J Bone Joint Surg Am* 2011;93(suppl 3):51-54.
41. Griffiths EJ, Stevenson D, Porteous MJ: Cost savings of using a cemented total hip replacement: An analysis of the National Joint Registry data. *J Bone Joint Surg Br* 2012;94(8):1032-1035.
42. Konan S, Haddad FS: Joint registries: A Ptolemaic model of data interpretation? *Bone Joint J* 2013;95-B(12):1585-1586.
43. Perry DC, Parsons N, Costa ML: 'Big data' reporting guidelines: How to answer big questions, yet avoid big problems. *Bone Joint J* 2014;96-B(12):1575-1577.

44. Huotari K, Peltola M, Jämsen E: The incidence of late prosthetic joint infections: A registry-based study of 112,708 primary hip and knee replacements. *Acta Orthop* 2015;86(3):321-325.

45. Sabah SA, Henckel J, Cook E, et al: Validation of primary metal-on-metal hip arthroplasties on the National Joint Registry for England, Wales and Northern Ireland using data from the London Implant Retrieval Centre: A study using the NJR dataset. *Bone Joint J* 2015;97-B(1):10-18.

46. Sabah SA, Henckel J, Koutsouris S, et al: Are all metal-on-metal hip revision operations contributing to the National Joint Registry implant survival curves? A study comparing the London Implant Retrieval Centre and National Joint Registry datasets. *Bone Joint J* 2016;98-B(1):33-39.

47. Witso E: The rate of prosthetic joint infection is underestimated in the arthroplasty registers. *Acta Orthop* 2015;86(3):277-278.

48. Gundtoft PH, Pedersen AB, Schønheyder HC, Overgaard S: Validation of the diagnosis "prosthetic joint infection" in the Danish Hip Arthroplasty Register. *Bone Joint J* 2016;98-B(3):320-325.

CHAPTER 10

Retrieval Analysis—Hip and Knee

TIMOTHY M. WRIGHT, PhD • ELEXIS C. BARAL, MS • DOUGLAS E. PADGETT, MD

ABSTRACT

Retrieval analysis, in which subjective observations and quantitative measurements are made on implant components recovered at revision surgery, provides an important performance measure. All retrieval analyses are, by definition, retrospective and may not always represent well-functioning components. Despite these limitations, examinations of retrieved implants have led to clinically relevant conclusions that are useful to arthroplasty surgeons. Two notable examples are the mechanically assisted crevice corrosion that may occur at the junction between modular components, most commonly at the head-neck connection in total hip arthroplasty and the wear behavior of highly cross-linked polyethylene components in hip and knee arthroplasties. Retrieval analyses of modular connections have shown fretting, and corrosion may be a potentially significant problem and may be influenced by variables such as mating materials and taper design. Conversely, analyses of the highly cross-linked polyethylene components confirm the excellent properties of this material, and concurrently the outstanding longer term clinical results show the durability of this bearing.

Keywords: component fracture; component wear; corrosion; retrieval analysis

Dr. Wright or an immediate family member has received royalties from Exactech, Inc., Lima, and Mathys Ltd; has stock or stock options held in Orthobond; has received research or institutional support from Lima Corporate; and serves as a board member, owner, officer, or committee member of the American Joint Replacement Registry, the Knee Society, and Orthopaedic Research and Education Foundation. Dr. Padgett or an immediate family member has received royalties from DJ the Orthopaedics; is a member of a speakers' bureau or has made paid presentations on behalf of DJ Orthopaedics; serves as a paid consultant to or is an employee of DJ Orthopaedics; has stock or stock options held in Evolve Orthopaedics, Orthophor, Parvizi Surgical Innovations, and Tangen; and serves as a board member, owner, officer, or committee member of the Hospital for Special Surgery and the Hip Society. Neither Ms. Baral nor any immediate family member has received anything of value from or has stock or stock options held in a commercial company or institution related directly or indirectly to the subject of this chapter.

INTRODUCTION

The analysis of total hip and knee components retrieved at revision surgery is often considered as failure analysis—something catastrophic and unexpected has occurred, and the source of the failure can be determined from examining the broken parts, similar to reconstructing structural failures such as a fallen roadway bridge or a building collapse. Indeed, early examples of orthopaedic implant failure analyses were fundamental to discovering material defects, such as oversized grains and porosity in cast metallic femoral stems for hip arthroplasty. However, the more important role for retrieval analysis has been as a performance measure in assessing how implant components fared while they were implanted in the body. The success of such an assessment depends on a meaningful number of retrieved implants together with pertinent implant, demographic, clinical, surgical, and radiographic data.

FUNDAMENTALS OF RETRIEVAL ANALYSIS

An adequate source of implants from revision surgery or at autopsy is fundamental to pursuing research questions or hypotheses concerning implant performance. To ensure the veracity of the analysis requires several additional steps (**Figure 1**). Retrieved components should be handled and stored with care from the operating room to the pathology department and the retrieval laboratory to prevent additional damage that might be misconstrued as having occurred in vivo. Once in the laboratory, retrieved components can undergo gentle cleaning with a soft brush and mild detergent to remove extraneous blood and tissue. Ultrahigh-molecular-weight polyethylene (UHMWPE) components should be stored at temperatures below 0°C, particularly if research questions concerning oxidation are anticipated. The oxidative process is essentially stopped at those temperatures,[1] ensuring that any measured oxidation had occurred before the implant removal in the operating room. Retrieval analysis can occasionally become part of litigation, so a chain of custody (for example, signatures from everyone handling the device between the operating room and the retrieval laboratory) is important to safeguard the interests of all involved parties.

Retrieval analysis has inherent limitations in that studies of retrieved components are retrospective for which certain variables such as reason for revision and length of implantation cannot be controlled. Furthermore, retrieved components are associated with the failure of a joint arthroplasty that required revision surgery and thus may not reflect well-functioning devices. Although postmortem analysis of implants provides valuable information on what are presumed to be well-functioning devices, they unfortunately are not readily available.

To improve the overall utility of retrieved implants, linking these devices with the unique factors from the case is crucial to unraveling the mechanisms of failure. These factors include the reason for removing the components along with prerevision radiographs and advanced imaging studies, which can help determine whether the failure of the joint arthroplasty was directly related to the implant components. Additional data pertinent to any thorough retrieval analyses are the original diagnosis, patient age, sex, and body mass index; the length of time that the components had been implanted; and descriptive information about the implant components (eg, design type, material from which the component was fabricated, and any identifying markings such as a manufacturer's name or logo and a part or lot number). Depending on the research question or hypothesis of the retrieval study, access to biologic tissues removed at surgery and subsequent pathologic studies of these tissues can be quite helpful. Indeed, the ASTM Standard Practice[2] for retrieval analysis of medical devices emphasizes the collection of accompanying tissues and fluids.

Once the retrieved components have been procured and cleaned, a wide range of examination tools can be applied to determine the performance or reason for failure of the component. These include macroscopic and light and scanning microscopy examination of the component's surfaces, profilometry to measure changes in surface roughness, laser and white light three-dimensional scanning to determine dimensional changes, advanced imaging techniques such as microcomputed tomography, chemical analyses such as Fourier transform infrared spectroscopy, and swell ratio measurements of cross-link density of UHMWPE components.

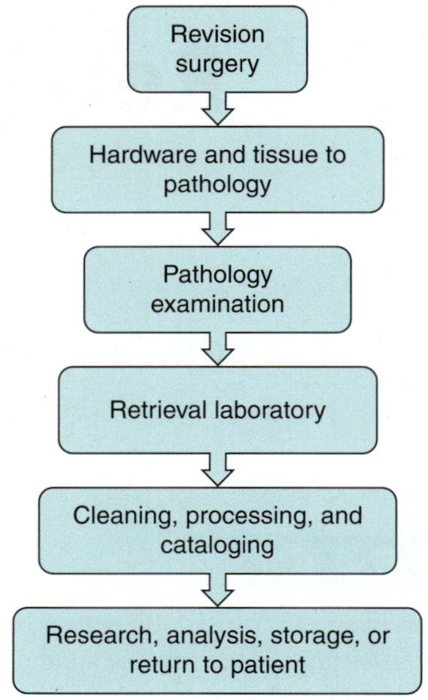

FIGURE 1 Illustration of a typical workflow for retrieval analysis.

The limitation of some of these examination tools is that they allow measurements and observations on small regions of a retrieved component, making thorough examination of an entire component or a region of the component such as the entire articulating surface too time consuming. Nonetheless, important observations on implant performance, such as the effects of material or design differences among manufacturers or implant types, often require a considerable number of retrieved implants. For this reason, subjective systems for grading the presence and severity of surface damage and wear[3] of UHMWPE bearing surfaces and fretting and corrosion of metal-metal and metal-ceramic modular connections[4] have proved effective for comparisons across large numbers of retrieved components, thus providing the statistical power to determine differences in performance while accounting for confounding variables.

The important role of retrieval analysis in hip and knee arthroplasty can be best appreciated by describing two timely examples in which such analyses are providing important insights into implant performance, insights

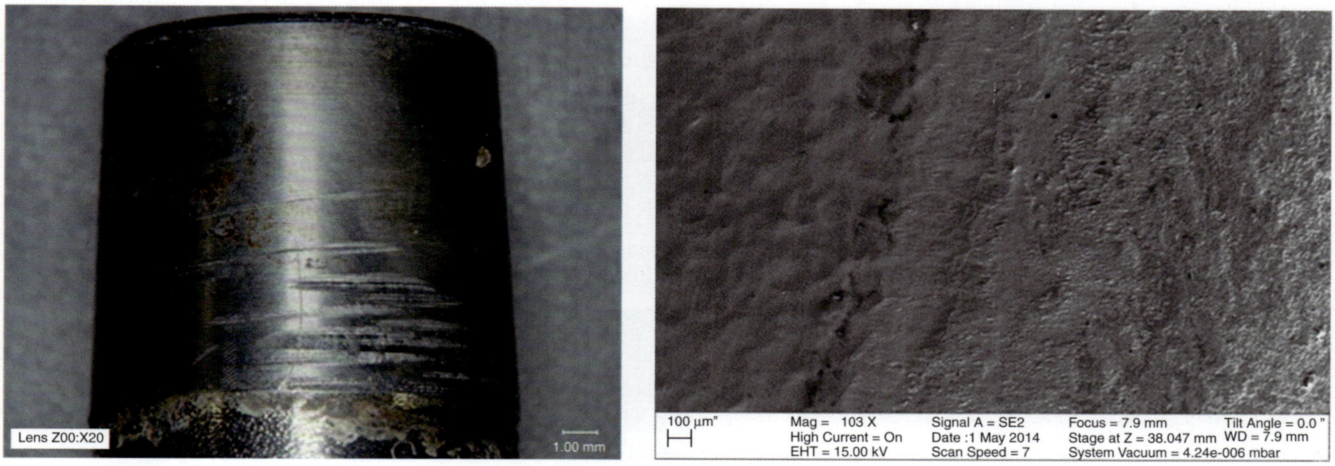

FIGURE 2 Light microscope photograph showing a stem trunnion damaged by fretting and corrosion (left) and a typical scanning electron microscope photograph showing fretting and corrosion damage (right) alongside an undamaged portion of the remaining trunnion.

that can directly affect the clinical practice of an arthroplasty surgeon. The first is the concern for adverse local tissue reactions surrounding modular connections in hip and knee constructs. The theoretical concern for mechanically assisted crevice corrosion (MACC) at the junctions between mechanically mated parts (**Figure 2**) has been known for more than 20 years,[5] but the recent clinical connection made between corrosion and adverse local tissue reaction has drawn attention to this problem.[6] The second is the ongoing monitoring of the performance of highly cross-linked UHMWPE components for hip and knee arthroplasty. The adoption of cross-linked materials has led to dramatic decreases in wear and the associated osteolysis caused by local biologic reaction to particulate polyethylene debris. However, questions remain as to long-term stability of these new polyethylenes, especially concern for continued oxidative degradation.

MACC AT MODULAR CONNECTIONS

Much of what is known about the problem of MACC at modular connections in total hip joints has been learned from observations and measurements made on retrieved implant components. Subjective grading of modular surfaces has been used to assess damage from fretting wear and corrosion (such as surface pitting and discoloration). Scanning techniques have been used to determine the amounts of material removed by the wear and corrosion processes from both the male taper (trunnion) and the female bore of the femoral head. Scanning electron microscopy studies have been used for high magnification examinations of the damaged regions and to chemically identify corrosion products.

Studies of large numbers of retrieved hip implants suggest many factors that may affect the severity of MACC.[4,7] The effects of some factors are intuitive. For example, the severity of fretting damage increases with the length of time that the implant was in situ, consistent with increased wear with increased number of loading cycles. Conversely, corrosion severity does not change as markedly with implantation time, demonstrating that the chemical reactions of the corrosion process proceed from early in the damage process and continue unabated with time.

The design of the taper is another factor that affects the corrosion severity at head-stem modular connections. Several features of taper design, including taper material, taper thickness, and taper engagement length, may affect fretting and corrosion. Taper stiffness, or specifically flexural rigidity, is a function of the modulus of elasticity of the taper material and the amount of material at the location of the deforming force. In the case of a cylindrical taper, the distribution of the material resisting deformation (the area moment of inertia) is proportional to the fourth power of the taper diameter. Therefore, small differences in diameter greatly influence the flexural rigidity of the taper. Tapers with larger diameters have higher flexural rigidities (**Figure 3**), so will deform less under cyclic loads. The result is less micromotion at the modular interface, less fretting, and thus less corrosion.[4,7]

The material combination used to form the modular connection also affects the possibility for MACC with dissimilar materials creating more corrosion than similar material.[4,5,7] Although MACC has been observed with similar materials (cobalt-chromium [CoCr] heads on CoCr stems), there appears to be a greater prevalence between titanium and CoCr alloys. Literature supports that MACC may be mitigated but not eliminated by use of nonmetallic articulating head materials such as ceramics. A 2018 study of autopsy retrievals extending

Flexural rigidity $\propto$ Modulus and d^4

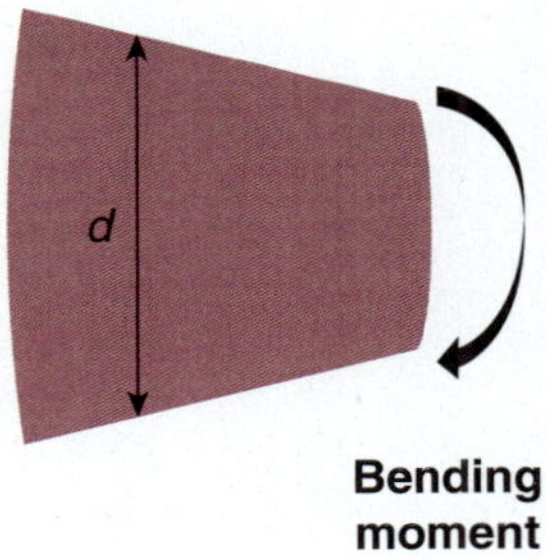

V40 Tapers	Co-Cr (E = 241 GPa)	TMZF (E = 80 GPa)
Rigidity (N m^2)	296 ± 24	96 ± 4
Diameter (mm)	12.6 ± 0.3	12.5 ± 0.1

PCA Tapers	Co-Cr (E = 241 GPa)
Rigidity (N m^2)	386 ± 12
Diameter (mm)	13.4 ± 0.1

FIGURE 3 Illustration showing that the flexural rigidity of a circular cross section similar to the taper on the end of a femoral stem depends on the elastic modulus (*E*) of the material from which it was fabricated and the fourth power of the diameter (*d*). Two tapers of the same geometry (top row) made from materials that differ substantially in modulus will differ substantially in flexural rigidity. Similarly, two tapers made from the same material, but that differ even by a small amount in diameter (left column), will likewise differ substantially in rigidity. (Data from Triantafyllopoulos GK, Elpers ME, Burket JC, Esposito CI, Padgett DE, Wright TM: Otto Aufranc Award: Large heads do not increase damage at the head-neck taper of metal-on-polyethylene total hip arthroplasties. *Clin Orthop Relat Res* 2016;474[2]:330-338.)

beyond 20 years of service with ceramic heads connected to large tapers on cobalt alloy stems showed essentially no corrosion,[8] suggesting that indeed material combination and taper design can be protective against MACC.

The effect of femoral head size on the development of MACC is somewhat controversial. In theory, a larger femoral head size should be related to increased fretting given that the lever arm of the applied load through the head should increase with head size. A larger lever arm would cause greater bending moments at the modular connection with more micromotion and fretting at the interface. Nonetheless, retrieval studies have presented conflicting results on the effect of head size. Some studies have shown no effect, whether by subjective grading[7] or by the measured amount of material removed by the corrosion process,[9] whereas others have supported the hypothesis that larger head sizes are more prone to corrosion.[10] Such conflicting conclusions show the difficulty in researching the effect of one variable in the retrospective, uncontrolled nature of retrieval analyses, where many other patient and implant factors (eg, patient body mass index, taper design, head materials, and bearing combinations) are simultaneously varying along with head size.

UHMWPE IN HIP AND KNEE RECONSTRUCTION

Perhaps the single greatest contribution to hip and knee reconstruction over the past 2 decades has been the introduction of highly cross-linked UHMWPE as a bearing material. Highly cross-linked polyethylenes are manufactured by exposing the polymer to ionizing radiation. The effect of the radiation is to initially cause the polymer chains to break down (scission) but subsequently, in the absence of oxygen, these smaller chains reunite, resulting in both longer chains of the polymer as well as chemical bonding between chains. This cross-linked polymer has been shown to be markedly resistant to the abrasive and adhesive wear modes that can damage bearing surfaces. Long-term results continue to show a marked clinical advantage of even the earliest forms of highly cross-linked polyethylene in randomized controlled trials compared with conventional UHMWPE.[11,12] The outstanding results stem from the improved wear resistance and the accompanying reduction in osteolysis. But what do retrieved highly cross-linked hip and knee components reveal about performance and how performance might differ between hip and knee arthroplasties?

A primary concern for highly cross-linked polyethylenes is their continued susceptibility to oxidative degradation that plagued earlier conventional polyethylene components that had been radiation sterilized and packaged in air. Polyethylenes exposed to high doses of radiation may nonetheless undergo chain scission, creating free radicals. Two thermal postirradiation processes are used to rid the material of free radicals: annealing and remelting. Annealing (heating the cross-linked material to temperatures below the melting temperature) does not quench the material of all the remaining free radicals, but has the advantage of maintaining more of the crystallinity that imparts important mechanical properties to the material. Remelting (heating the material beyond the melting temperature) quenches all the free radicals, but also decreases crystallinity, so it adversely affects important mechanical properties.

Unfortunately, no two commercial highly cross-linked polyethylenes are the same; manufacturers' processes differ between annealing and remelting, in the temperatures that are used for annealing or remelting, and in rate of cooling after thermal processing. Thus, general conclusions such as between annealed and remelted components depend nonetheless on findings from specific types of highly cross-linked UHMWPE from specific manufacturers.

Acetabular components of the same annealed highly cross-linked UHMWPE retrieved from consecutive total hip revision surgeries showed strikingly different amounts of oxidation at the bearing surface (**Figure 4**) compared with at the rim of the components, with greater oxidation at the rim of components that had been implanted for longer times.[13] These results suggest that the bearing surface is protected from oxidation because of its nearly constant contact with the femoral head, allowing little ingress of oxidative species. Although the clinical significance of the in vivo oxidation is unclear, such continued oxidation at the component rim could bode poorly for the mechanical integrity of locking mechanisms that rely on polyethylene strength and ductility, as these properties are adversely affected by oxidation.[14] Surprisingly, in a similar series of remelted highly cross-linked UHMWPE retrieved acetabular components, some showed measurable oxidation after an average of more than 2 years of being implanted.[15]

Similar results have been reported for tibial components retrieved from total knee revision surgeries. For annealed highly cross-linked tibial components, oxidation levels suggested a time-dependent degradative process.[16] A similar finding was found in an analysis of tibial inserts made from remelted highly cross-linked UHMWPE.[17] Oxidation was worse in inserts that had longer in vivo durations, and the increased oxidation was accompanied by a significant decrease in cross-link density. These results suggest that in vivo oxidation is causing material degradation. In yet another study, oxidation and cross-link density were measured in both annealed and remelted tibial inserts and in both loaded regions (as denoted by burnishing of the bearing surface) and unloaded (as denoted by a pristine, unburnished surface).[18] Oxidation increases and cross-link density decreases were greatest in the loaded regions and were more severe in annealed compared with remelted inserts (**Figure 5**). These findings suggest that a mechanical breakdown of cross-links is occurring, because greater changes were found in loaded regions, although lipid absorption into the polyethylene could cause oxidation even in the absence of free radicals.

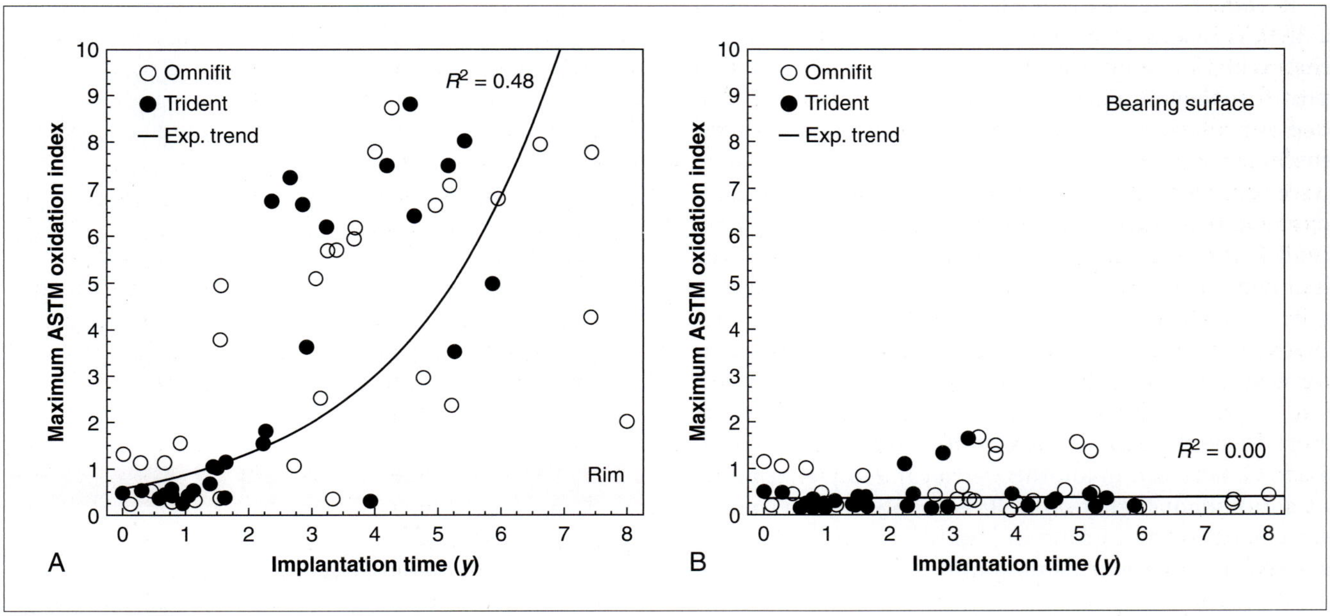

FIGURE 4 Graphs showing the progression of maximum in vivo oxidation (as determined by infrared spectroscopy) with implantation time at the rim (**A**) and at the articulating surface (**B**) for retrieved annealed ultrahigh-molecular-weight polyethylene liners of two different designs (Omnifit and Trident) from the same manufacturer. (Reproduced with permission from *J Arthroplasty* 25[4]. Kurtz SM, Austin MS, Azzam K, et al: Mechanical properties, oxidation, and clinical performance of retrieved highly cross-linked Crossfire liners after intermediate-term implantation 614-623. Copyright © 2010, with permission from Elsevier.)

Section 1: Hip and Knee

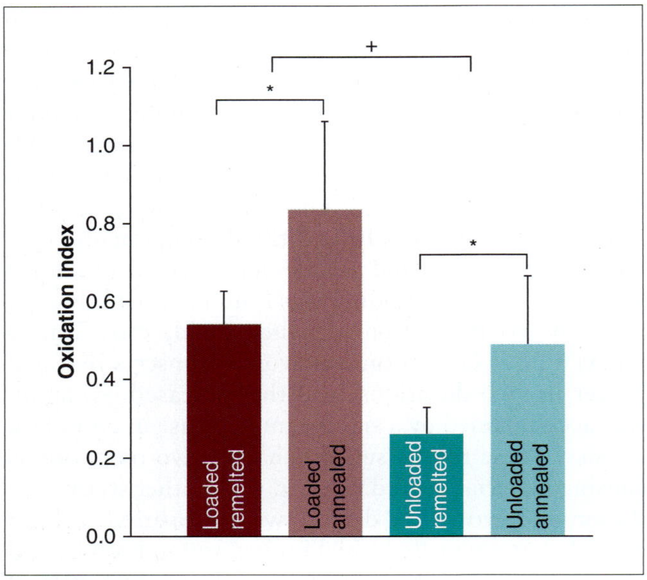

FIGURE 5 A bar chart showing differences in peak oxidation index between remelted and annealed retrieved polyethylene tibial components in areas that were loaded or unloaded in vivo. Significant differences between remelted and annealed polyethylenes are shown with an asterisk. A significant difference in peak oxidation was found between loaded and unloaded groups (shown with +). (Reproduced with permission from Liu T, Esposito CI, Burket JC, Wright TM: Crosslink density is reduced and oxidation is increased in retrieved highly crosslinked polyethylene TKA tibial inserts. *Clin Orthop Relat Res* 2017;475[1]:128-136.)

Retrieval studies to date have been short term, typically less than 5 years of implantation, but the concern that oxidation of highly cross-linked polyethylene might prove problematic with long-term use has led to the introduction of antioxidants (such as vitamin E) to stabilize the material against further oxidation. Recent studies have provided mixed results as to the effect of antioxidants on oxidation. For example, in a 2019 study, more than 100 tibial inserts made from vitamin E-stabilized highly cross-linked polyethylene were compared with a similar number of remelted highly cross-linked inserts that served as a control cohort.[19] The vitamin E inserts showed less oxidation and less surface damage. A second study found similar results with retrieved inserts from three different antioxidant polyethylene materials.[20] Conversely, in another retrieval analysis, a group of antioxidant highly cross-linked polyethylene inserts were matched to a group of highly cross-linked inserts according to patient demographics.[21] The addition of antioxidant was not reflected in the damage on the insert's articulating surface or in the cross-link density or oxidation in either the loaded or unloaded regions of the surface. These conflicting results suggest that the beneficial effects of antioxidants have not yet been realized. Longer term retrieval analysis will be required to demonstrate the effectiveness of antioxidants in providing continued resistance to oxidative degradation.

SUMMARY

Much has been learned about the performance of hip and knee arthroplasties by examining the individual components retrieved at revision surgery. Careful observations of surface features have been combined with an array of objective measures of surface roughness, wear damage, and chemical alterations. Together, they provide clinicians with important conclusions about how material and implant design factors affect problems such as MACC and polyethylene degradation.

KEY STUDY POINTS

- Retrieval analysis of hip and knee components can provide important measures of mechanical performance and of degradation that can occur through chemical processes such as MACC. Accounting for confounding influences of patient and surgical variables can strengthen the conclusions that can be drawn from retrieval studies.
- MACC at modular connections is a multifactorial problem that can lead to implant failure through the creation of adverse local tissue reactions to corrosion and wear debris. Important factors shown by retrieval analyses to have a negative effect on MACC include connections between dissimilar materials and the use of a smaller stem trunnion.
- Oxidative degradation of UHMWPE has been markedly reduced since the now-abandoned practice of radiation sterilization and packaging in air. The adoption of highly cross-linked polyethylenes through additional radiation followed by subsequent thermal treatments to quench free radicals has improved the wear resistance of these materials. But retrieval studies have shown that degradation and loss of cross-link density still occur, suggesting continued vigilance is needed as longer term retrievals become available for examination.

ANNOTATED REFERENCES

1. Kurtz SM, Pruitt LA, Crane DJ, Edidin AA: Evolution of morphology in UHMWPE following accelerated aging: The effect of heating rates. *J Biomed Mater Res* 1999;46(1):112-120.
2. American Society for Testing and Materials International F561-19: *Standard Practice for Retrieval and Analysis of Medical Devices, and Associated Tissues and Fluids.* West Conshohocken, PA, American Society for Testing and Materials International, 2019.

This report highlights basic practices for the retrieval, handling, and analysis of explanted devices and associated tissues and fluids, to limit damage to them and therefore help ensure investigational results. Methodology and explanation are provided.

3. Hood RW, Wright TM, Burstein AH: Retrieval analysis of total knee prostheses: A method and its application to 48 total condylar prostheses. *J Biomed Mater Res* 1983;17(5):829-842.
4. Goldberg JR, Gilbert JL, Jacobs JJ, Bauer TW, Paprosky W, Leurgans S: A multicenter retrieval study of the taper interfaces of modular hip prostheses. *Clin Orthop Relat Res* 2002;401:149-161.
5. Gilbert JL, Buckley CA, Jacobs JJ: In vivo corrosion of modular hip prosthesis components in mixed and similar metal combinations. The effect of crevice, stress, motion, and alloy coupling. *J Biomed Mater Res* 1993;27(12):1533-1544.
6. Ricciardi BF, Nocon AA, Jerabek SA, et al: Histopathological characterization of corrosion product associated adverse local tissue reaction in hip implants: A study of 285 cases. *BMC Clin Pathol* 2016;16:3.
7. Triantafyllopoulos GK, Elpers ME, Burket JC, Esposito CI, Padgett DE, Wright TM: Otto Aufranc Award: Large heads do not increase damage at the head-neck taper of metal-on-polyethylene total hip arthroplasties. *Clin Orthop Relat Res* 2016;474(2):330-338.
8. Lange J, Wach A, Koch CN, et al: Do well-functioning THAs retrieved at autopsy exhibit evidence of fretting and corrosion? *Clin Orthop Relat Res* 2018;476(10):2017-2024.

   This study found little evidence of fretting and corrosion in a cohort of well-functioning CoCr-CoCr and alumina-CoCr head-neck couples retrieved from well-functioning total hip arthroplasties at autopsy, suggesting that patients who have these CoCr alloy stems and trunnion geometries would be at low risk for trunnion corrosion. Level of evidence: IV.
9. Valente G, Lanting B, MacDonald S, Teeter MG, Van Citters D, Howard J: Femoral head material loss at the head-neck junction in total hip arthroplasty: The effect of head size, stem material and stem offset. *Hip Int* 2019;29(6):647-651.

   No difference was found in femoral head maximum linear corrosion depth (as measured with a coordinate measuring machine) at the head-neck junction between 28- and 32-mm matched paired femoral heads, similar or mixed alloy coupled femoral head stem constructs, and regular or high-offset stems. Level of evidence: IV.
10. Siljander MP, Baker EA, Baker KC, Salisbury MR, Thor CC, Verner JJ: Fretting and corrosion damage in retrieved metal-on-polyethylene modular total hip arthroplasty systems: What is the importance of femoral head size? *J Arthroplasty* 2018;33(3):931-938.

    Larger femoral head sizes were correlated with less severe head corrosion and head fretting in this retrieval study of 92 retrieved metal-on-polyethylene hip components. Level of evidence: IV.
11. Hopper RH Jr, Ho H, Sritulanondha S, Williams AC, Engh CA Jr: Otto Aufranc Award: Crosslinking reduces THA wear, osteolysis, and revision rates at 15-year followup compared with noncrosslinked polyethylene. *Clin Orthop Relat Res* 2018;476(2):279-290.

    This long-term, randomized controlled study demonstrated reductions in revision, wear, and osteolysis associated with the use of remelted highly cross-linked polyethylene, affirming durability of these components even though they did not incorporate antioxidants. Level of evidence: I.
12. Teeter MG, Yuan X, Somerville LE, MacDonald SJ, McCalden RW, Naudie DD: Thirteen-year wear rate comparison of highly crosslinked and conventional polyethylene in total hip arthroplasty: Long-term follow-up of a prospective randomized controlled trial. *Can J Surg* 2017;60(3):212-216.

    A randomized controlled trial of first-generation highly cross-linked versus conventional polyethylene in total hip arthroplasties at a minimum of 13 years' follow-up showed that the cross-linked material demonstrated greater wear resistance than conventional polyethylene as measured with radiostereometric analysis. Level of evidence: II.
13. Kurtz SM, Austin MS, Azzam K, et al: Mechanical properties, oxidation, and clinical performance of retrieved highly cross-linked Crossfire liners after intermediate-term implantation. *J Arthroplasty* 2010;25(4):614-623.
14. Rimnac C, Pruitt L: How do material properties influence wear and fracture mechanisms? *J Am Acad Orthop Surg* 2008;16(suppl 1):S94-S100.
15. Currier BH, Van Citters DW, Currier JH, Collier JP: In vivo oxidation in remelted highly cross-linked retrievals. *J Bone Joint Surg Am* 2010;92(14):2409-2418.
16. Kop AM, Pabbruwe MB, Keogh C, Swarts E: Oxidation of second generation sequentially irradiated and annealed highly cross-linked X3™ polyethylene tibial bearings. *J Arthroplasty* 2015;30(10):1842-1846.
17. Reinitz SD, Currier BH, Levine RA, Collier JP, Van Citters DW: Oxidation and other property changes of a remelted highly crosslinked UHMWPE in retrieved tibial bearings. *J Biomed Mater Res B Appl Biomater* 2017;105(1):39-45.

    Oxidation increased with in vivo duration, and cross-link density significantly decreased in a series of retrieved tibial inserts, suggesting that in vivo oxidation is causing material degradation. Level of evidence: IV.
18. Liu T, Esposito CI, Burket JC, Wright TM: Crosslink density is reduced and oxidation is increased in retrieved highly crosslinked polyethylene TKA tibial inserts. *Clin Orthop Relat Res* 2017;475(1):128-136.

    Increased oxidation and decreased cross-link density levels were measured in the worn as opposed to the unworn regions of the articular surfaces of retrieved tibial inserts. Level of evidence: IV.
19. Spece H, Schachtner JT, MacDonald DW, et al: Reasons for revision, oxidation, and damage mechanisms of retrieved vitamin E-stabilized highly crosslinked polyethylene in total knee arthroplasty. *J Arthroplasty* 2019;34(12):3088-3093.

    Comparisons of retrieved highly cross-linked tibial inserts with and without vitamin E revealed that oxidation tended to be less for the vitamin E group at the articular and backside surfaces, although the median differences were minimal and may not be clinically significant. Level of evidence: IV.

20. Currier BH, Currier JH, Holdcroft LA, Van Citters DW: Effectiveness of anti-oxidant polyethylene: What early retrievals can tell us. *J Biomed Mater Res B Appl Biomater* 2018;106(1):353-359.

Retrieved components made from three different antioxidant polyethylenes were compared with remelted highly cross-linked and conventional polyethylene components, with the antioxidant materials demonstrating more effective resistance to oxidation. Level of evidence: IV.

21. Ponzio DY, Weitzler L, deMeireles A, Esposito CI, Wright TM, Padgett DE: Antioxidant-stabilized highly crosslinked polyethylene in total knee arthroplasty: A retrieval analysis. *Bone Joint J* 2018;100-B(10):1330-1335.

Retrieval analysis of tibial inserts fabricated from antioxidant highly cross-linked polyethylene did not reflect a clinically relevant difference in surface damage, cross-link density, or oxidation compared with plain highly cross-linked polyethylene tibial inserts at short-term evaluation. Level of evidence: IV.

CHAPTER 11

The Biologic Response to Bearing Materials

EMMANUEL GIBON, *MD, PhD* • STUART B. GOODMAN, *MD, PhD*

ABSTRACT

Total joint arthroplasty (TJA) is a common and highly successful orthopaedic procedure, for which surgeons have a large choice of different bearing materials. The materials used for TJA must be both biocompatible to minimize adverse local tissue reactions and robust enough to support weight bearing during common daily activities. Modern bearing materials for TJA are made from metals and their alloys, polymers, and ceramics. The biologic response to the different bearing materials used for TJA, as well as the wear byproducts generated, is reviewed.

Keywords: biocompatibility; foreign-body response; hypersensitivity; inflammation; orthopaedic bearing materials

INTRODUCTION

The use of implanted devices in orthopaedic surgery has increased dramatically; when considering this field alone, the underlying industry is expected to grow to $55 billion by 2025.[1] Bearing materials are permanent biomaterials and generally intended to be used for joint arthroplasty. The biologic response to bearing materials used for total joint arthroplasty is reviewed.

Since the first interposition arthroplasties made with tissues such as muscle, fat, or pig bladder, current bearing materials for total joint arthroplasty have become much more complex. Briefly, the goals of these implants are to be efficacious, not lead to any local or systemic adverse effects and be cost effective. Several bearing materials are currently available for consideration for the design of an artificial joint. These materials include metals and their alloys, polymers, and ceramics. The most frequent metal used for bearing surfaces in joint arthroplasty is cobalt-chromium (CoCr) alloy. Polymers include polyethylene: mainly ultra-high–molecular-weight polyethylene (UHMWPE), highly cross-linked polyethylene (HXLPE), and vitamin E-doped HXLPE (VE-HXLPE). The other main material group is ceramics, either alumina or alumina combined with zirconia.

THE USE OF POLYETHYLENE AS PART OF THE BEARING COUPLE

Ceramic-on-polyethylene (COP) and metal-on-polyethylene (MOP) are the most widely used bearing couples for total hip arthroplasty (THA) in the United States, with the former now surpassing the latter.[2] Second-generation HXLPE includes the doping of an antioxidant such as vitamin E within the polyethylene and repeated treatment with heating and annealing of the polymer. The size of the polyethylene particles generated by COP or MOP joint surfaces is generally submicron. These particles are often needlelike and may be up to a 1 mm or longer, but most of the particulate debris is in the range of 0.3 to 5 µm in length. Polyethylene particles will interact with local cells, mainly macrophages,[3] and trigger a foreign-body inflammatory response, leading to a granuloma, if the particles are not cleared and remain locally in sufficient numbers. The cascade of proinflammatory responses is initiated after activation of the macrophages by the particles,

Dr. Goodman or an immediate family member serves as a paid consultant to or is an employee of DePuy, a Johnson & Johnson Company, Integra, Pluristem, and Wishbone Medical; serves as an unpaid consultant to Accelalox and Biomimedica; has stock or stock options held in Accelalox, Arquos, and Biomimedica; and serves as a board member, owner, officer, or committee member of ARCO. Neither Dr. Gibon nor any immediate family member has received anything of value from or has stock or stock options held in a commercial company or institution related directly or indirectly to the subject of this chapter.

either through phagocytosis or through cell contact with the polyethylene particles. Cell contact activation occurs through different membrane receptors known as Toll-like receptors (TLRs). TLR2 and TLR4 have been found to be critical for polyethylene-induced osteolysis.[4] After polyethylene particle–induced activation, TLRs act primarily through an adapter protein called myeloid differentiation primary response gene 88 (MyD88) to induce the transcription factor nuclear factor-κB (NFκB) and others. This transcription factor has been shown to have great relevance to periprosthetic osteolysis associated with wear particles. Activation of the NFκB leads to the release of a plethora of proinflammatory factors including chemokines (macrophage inflammatory protein-1α, monocyte chemoattractant protein [MCP-1]), cytokines (such as tumor necrosis factor alpha [TNF-α], interleukins [ILs] 1β, 6, 8, and others), prostaglandins (especially prostaglandin E_2), nitric oxide, and peroxide metabolic intermediates. High levels of polyethylene-induced inflammatory factors will have consequences on the local and systemic tissues. Release of MCP-1 and macrophage inflammatory protein-1α induces the systemic recruitment of macrophages and mesenchymal stem cells.[5,6] Locally activated macrophages undergo polarization toward the M1 (proinflammatory) phenotype.[7] M1 macrophages produce primarily proinflammatory mediators including TNF-α, IL-1, and IL-6 and express inducible nitric oxide synthase.[8] TNF-α released by locally activated macrophages will stimulate osteoblasts to release granulocyte macrophage colony-stimulating factor, IL-6, and prostaglandin E_2. Granulocyte macrophage colony-stimulating factor will enhance the release of reactive oxygen species such as nitric oxide, which, in turn, activates osteoclastic bone resorption. Locally, osteoclast-like cell growth and differentiation is enhanced by transforming growth factor-α and osteoclastic bone resorption. Osteoclast mobility is also increased by local release of IL-8 from activated macrophages, mesenchymal stem cells, and osteoblasts. Retrieval studies have documented that particles derived from XLPE bearings are significantly smaller than those from UHMWPE. When challenged with XLPE particles, macrophages have been shown to release significantly more TNF-α than with UHMWPE particles. However, it must be kept in mind that for the same bearing surface, many more UHMWPE particles are generated, than with XLPE.

Retrieval studies have helped in understanding the effects of polyethylene particles on the surrounding tissues. Foreign-body giant cells, also called multinucleated giant cells or polykaryons, have been identified within the bone-implant interface. Locally, the presence of multinucleated giant cells increases both osteoclastic bone resorption and osteoclast-like cell growth and differentiation because of their ability to release transforming growth factor-α and other factors. Interestingly, the authors of a 2010 study[9] compared retrieved tissues from loosened aseptic and septic MOP hip implants and synovial membrane samples from osteoarthritic patients. In samples obtained from aseptic loosening, the authors found an intense foreign-body reaction with large infiltrates of CD68+ and CD163+ monocyte/macrophages, foreign-body giant cells, sometimes organized into foreign-body granulomas. Macrophages mostly expressed TLR4 and 9. Macrophages outnumbered other cell types and only scattered T cells, B cells, and neutrophils were seen. In another retrieval study in 2010, the authors[10] investigated the inflammatory processes at the protein level in periprosthetic tissues from loosened MOP THAs. When compared with patients with primary THAs, patients with loosened THAs had higher receptor activator of nuclear factor-κB ligand (RANKL) expression on osteoblastic stromal cells and higher levels of RANKL, IL-6, IL-8, IL-10, interferon-γ-inducible protein-10, MCP-1, and monokine induced by interferon-γ in the synovial fluid from the hip joint.

Taken together, polyethylene particles may be responsible for initiating periprosthetic inflammation. With the intense macrophage particle-induced secretion of chemokines and cytokines, the local inflammation may progress to periprosthetic osteolysis, jeopardizing mechanical support of the implant, limiting its longevity. **Figure 1** summarizes the main biologic effects associated with MOP bearing surfaces.

New Polyethylenes: HXLPE and Vitamin E-doped Polyethylene

The authors of a 2014 study[11] compared two clinically relevant sized particles from VE-HXLPE and virgin HXLPE (average 1.12 and 1.22 μm, respectively). Particles were surgically implanted into mouse calvaria, and osteolysis and biologic activity were later analyzed. Micro-CT showed significantly less osteolysis for VE-HXLPE compared with standard HXLPE. Histologic analysis showed a greater amount of inflammatory tissue for standard HXLPE ($P < 0.0001$). However, the number of osteoclasts in each group was not significantly different. The authors of a 2016 study[12] investigated the biologic reaction of conventional UHMWPE, standard HXLPE, and VE-HXLPE using the mouse calvarial model. Bone mineral density significantly decreased in the HXLPE group compared with the two other groups. HXLPE particles induced the highest number of infiltrated osteoclasts. The authors concluded that VE-HXLPE did not appear to affect the inflammatory and osteolytic responses in this model. The biocompatibility of VE-HXLPE particles was shown to be comparable to that of conventional UHMWPE.[13] The authors showed similar levels of marker of bone resorption (DKK-1 protein) and bone formation (osteoprotegerin). Interestingly, the authors of a 2017 study[14] demonstrated that when murine RAW 264.7 MΦ were challenged with

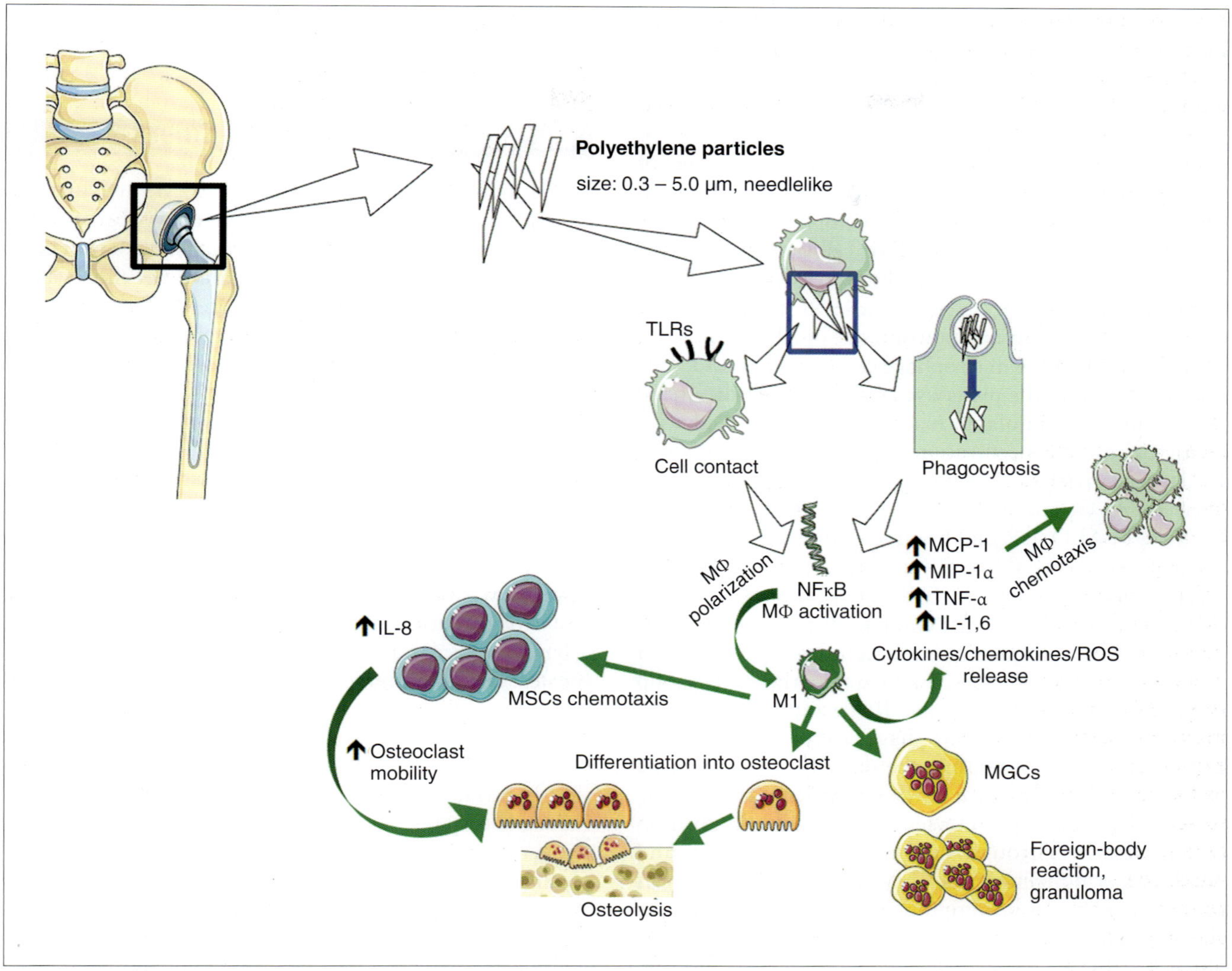

FIGURE 1 Illustration showing the biologic reaction to metal-on-polyethylene bearing surfaces. IL = interleukin, MCP-1 = monocyte chemoattractant protein 1, MGCs = multinucleated giant cells, MIP-1 = macrophage inflammatory protein 1, MSCs = mesenchymal stem cells, MΦ = macrophages, ROS = reactive oxygen species, TLRs = Toll-like receptors, TNF-α = tumor necrosis factor alpha

VE-HXLPE particles, they secreted less TNF-α and responded more effectively against *Staphylococcus aureus* compared with exposure to conventional UHMWPE particles. The authors of a 2018 study[15] investigated the biologic reaction of osteoblasts exposed to VE-XLPE versus conventional UHMWPE particles. Enzyme-linked immunosorbent assay analysis showed that VE-XLPE particles significantly decreased the bone resorption markers RANKL and sclerostin and increased osteoprotegerin, an inhibitor of bone resorption. Another group speculated that the antiosteolytic mechanism associated with VE-doped polyethylene may be due to IL-27.[16] Although the research concerning the newer polyethylenes is not entirely conclusive, the improved wear characteristics and biologic activity of these novel materials suggest an improvement compared with conventional polyethylene.

THE USE OF CERAMICS AS PART OF THE BEARING COUPLE

As a bulk material, ceramics has been shown to be nonimmunogenic and induces a very minor fibrotic response. However, when the ceramic particles are in high quantity, the induced biologic response is similar to that seen with PE particles.

Regarding the size of the particles, the authors of a 2002 study[17] showed that the ceramic particles follow a bimodal distribution. Particles are either nanometric, ranging from 5 to 90 nm, or micrometric ranging from 0.05 to 3.2 μm. Thus, the size of the ceramic wear particles differs dramatically from that of the PE particles generated at the bearing surface. Current ceramics used for joint arthroplasty are made of two compounds: alumina

(Al2O3) and zirconia (ZrO2). Alumina is the primary or continuous phase (70% to 95%) and zirconia is the secondary phase (30% to 5%).[18] Using clinically relevant alumina particles, the authors of a 2003 study[19] showed that these particles exhibit cytotoxicity to human histiocytes. The authors of a 2004 study[20] analyzed the effect of two different sizes of ceramic particles (23 versus 179 nm) on the viability of osteoblasts. The nanophase particles (23 nm) showed no significant effects on cell viability, whereas larger sized particles dramatically decreased the viability of the osteoblasts. The authors of a 1998 study[21] focused on the effects of concentration and size of Al_2O_3 and ZrO_2 particles on the J774 macrophage cell line. For Al_2O_3 particles up to 2 μm, the phagocytosis index (an indicator of the number of stimulated macrophages) increased with particle size and concentration and then reached a plateau for larger particles. No significant difference was found between Al_2O_3 and ZrO_2. Regarding cytotoxicity, large particles of Al_2O_3 (>2 μm) became significantly cytotoxic for concentrations above 500 particles per macrophage. There was no difference in TNF-α release between Al_2O_3 and ZrO_2. However, when compared with polyethylene particles, Al_2O_3 particles induced significantly less TNF-α release from macrophages. Surprisingly, the same group did not measure any detectable IL-1α and IL-1β production after exposure of macrophages to ceramic as well as polyethylene particles. Using the same J774 macrophage cell line, the authors of a 1999 study[22] investigated the effects of particle size, concentration, and composition on cell death. Through fluorescence microscopy and DNA laddering techniques, they showed that the effect of ceramic particles on apoptotic nuclear morphology was size dependent and concentration-dependent and reached a plateau above 150 particles per macrophage at 1.3 μm.

TLRs also play a role in the biologic response to ceramic particles. Nanoparticles of ZrO_2 have a selective capacity for inducing/increasing expression of TLR3, TLR7, and TLR10 on macrophages. Moreover, there was a limited stimulatory effect on IL-1β, no effect on TNF-α production, and a proinflammatory effect of ZrO_2 nanoparticles, with decreased production of IL-1ra (a marker of M2 anti-inflammatory macrophages) by M1 polarized macrophages. The authors of a 2008 study[23] challenged human macrophages with commercial alumina particles (mean size 0.23 μm ± 0.1) and found a limited increase in IL-1β and MCP-1 production. In another study, RANK, TNF-α, and osteoprotegerin mRNA were only slightly upregulated when human monocytic cells were challenged with alumina particles. The authors of a 2010 study[24] have shown that alumina particles are only weakly genotoxic to primary human fibroblasts.

In summary, ceramic particles might be harmful, especially when they are in the nanometer size range and in large numbers. However, this is rarely the case. **Figure 2** summarizes the main biologic effects of ceramic bearing surfaces.

METAL-ON-METAL BEARING COUPLES

Well-functioning metal-on-metal (MOM) articulations generate very low volumes of wear debris because the smaller clearance of the articulation generates a thin fluid-film lubrication and self-polishing ability of this bearing couple. With an estimated wear rate of 2 μm per year for MOM articulations, approximately 10^{12} particles are released within the peri-implant area. The size of the metal particles generated by MOM implant surfaces is substantially smaller than polyethylene particles and is reported to be 40 to 50 nm. Alloys used for MOM implants for joint arthroplasty are CoCr alloys, either cast or wrought, with either a low or high carbon content. The effect of metallic particles on the surrounding bone and soft tissues has been studied extensively. The authors of a 2001 study[25] have shown that metalloprotein complexes made from CoCr degradation byproducts are capable of inducing a lymphocytic proliferative response. This reaction was greatest with high-molecular-weight protein (180 to 250 kd); a possible trigger for the response is cross-linking of the metal-protein complex with lymphocyte receptors (BV17 or CDR1 T-cell receptor). Studies demonstrated that byproducts from CoCr alloy materials induced an inflammatory response via activation of the intracellular danger signaling mechanism called the NLRP3 inflammasome.[26,27] Moreover, as demonstrated in a 2007 study,[28] the size of the particles matters. When comparing nanoparticles and microparticles in an in vitro study with human fibroblasts, the authors showed that nanoparticles released significantly more free radicals and induced more DNA damage than micron-sized particles. Furthermore, challenge with CoCr particles did not increase the release of IL-6, IL-10, TNF-α, or FGF-23, possibly because of cell death. This was confirmed by the authors of a 2008 study[23] who challenged human macrophages with CoCr particles (mean size ± SD: 0.48 μm ± 0.3). They showed that CoCr particles were mildly stimulatory for cytokine release: challenged macrophages released two fold to fivefold greater levels of IL-1α, IL-6, IL-10, and GM-CSF compared with unchallenged cells. The authors of a 2014 study[29] challenged MLO-Y4 osteocytes (a murine cell line) with Co^{2+} and Ni^{2+} ions at various clinically relevant concentrations. Their results showed that Co^{2+} and Ni^{2+} ions had a significant cytotoxic effect on MLO-Y4 cells above 0.05 and 0.10 mM, respectively.

Human implant retrieval studies of more modern MOM implants were first reported by the authors of a 2005 study[30] who harvested and analyzed tissues from 19 second-generation MOM hip revision surgeries. The

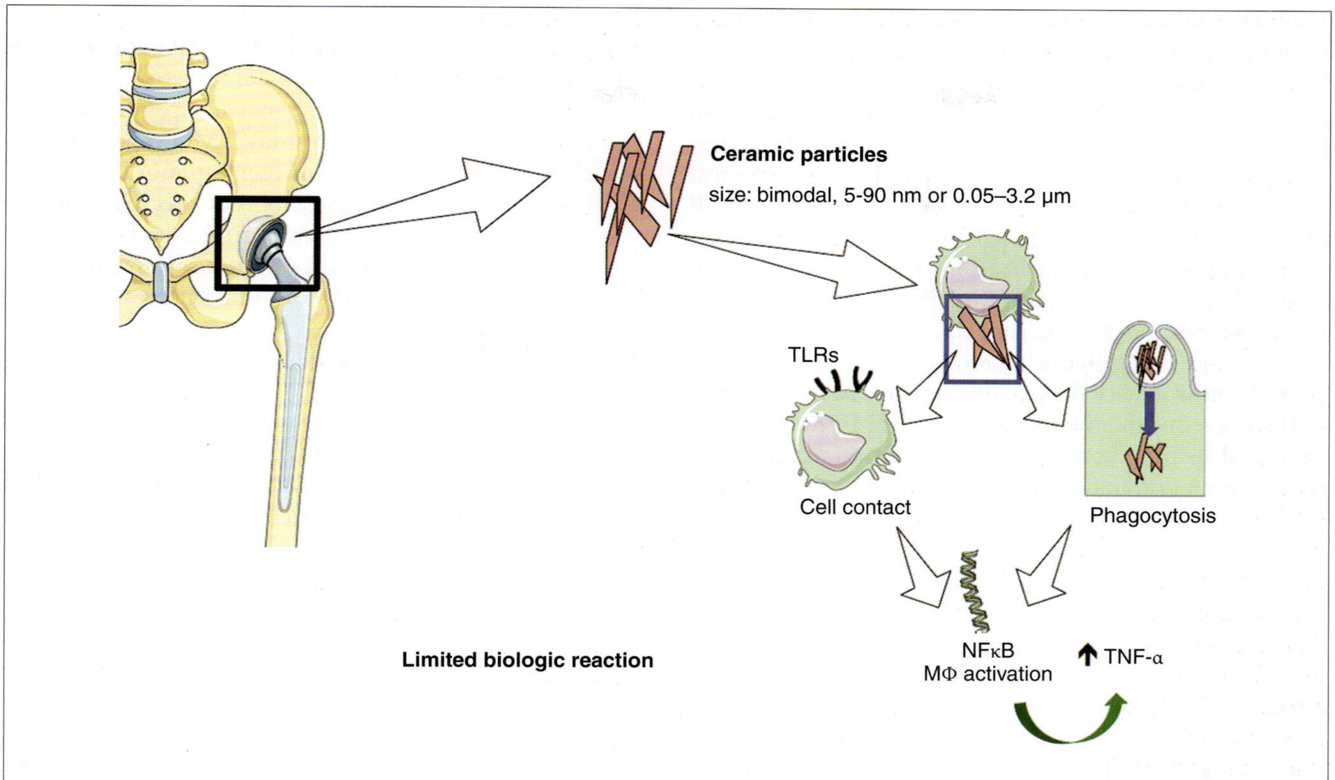

FIGURE 2 Illustration showing the biologic reaction to ceramic-on-ceramic bearing surfaces. MΦ = macrophages, NFκB = nuclear factor-κB, TLRs = Toll-like receptors, TNF-α = tumor necrosis factor alpha

indications for revision were increasing pain and the occurrence of osteolysis. At surgery, the hip implants were well fixed in nine patients. In a classic description of the findings, they reported the following: "the characteristic histologic features were diffuse and perivascular infiltrates of T and B lymphocytes and plasma cells, high endothelial venules, massive fibrin exudation, accumulation of macrophages with drop-like inclusions, and infiltrates of eosinophilic granulocytes and necrosis." The authors of a 2005 study[31] analyzed tissues from 25 MOM hips, including 14 THA and 11 surface-replacement designs, and compared these results with those of tissues retrieved from MOP implants. The MOM retrievals showed pronounced ulceration superficial to the areas demonstrating perilymphocytic vascular infiltration; lymphocytic infiltration was more pronounced in specimens from MOM cases with prosthesis loosening compared with autopsy specimens or those undergoing arthrotomy for primary THA (controls). The authors of another 2005 study[32] studied retrieved tissues from MOM hip arthroplasties demonstrating osteolysis. They found perivascular accumulation of CD3+ T cells, CD68 macrophages, and high levels of IL-1β and TNF-α. They also performed skin-patch tests to assess hypersensitivity to metal, which were positive (higher rate of hypersensitivity) for patients with early osteolysis. The authors of a 2007 study[33] analyzed neo-capsule tissue samples from 46 hips with modern second-generation MOM articulations. The authors found a distinct lymphocytic infiltration in all cases consisting of CD20+ B-lymphocytes and CD3+ T-lymphocytes. These different retrieval studies are suggestive of a type IV delayed hypersensitivity immune reaction. Metal ion studies reported elevation of serum Co and Cr in patients with MOM THA. Although high levels of ions are associated with specific types of cancer in animal models, to date there is no conclusive association of cancer in humans with MOM prostheses.

Pseudotumors associated with MOM implants are small or more extensive, solid or fluid-filled periprosthetic masses that can be painful and lead to substantial destruction of the surrounding tissues. In conjunction with resurfacing or THA implants with MOM bearings, the pseudotumors are composed of granulomatous masses of inflammatory cells (macrophages, T lymphocytes, plasma cells), fibrous tissue, and widespread tissue necrosis. Failed MOM implants with pseudotumors have been associated with alterations in circulating adaptive immune cells.[34] Several risk factors have been identified for pseudotumor formation including young age, female sex especially with small-sized implants, bilateral implants, hip dysplasia, suboptimal implant position, edge loading, and impingement of the implants. Interestingly, the authors of a 2018 study[35] showed that CoCrMo particles induced 120% more inflammatory bone loss in female mice compared with male, which suggests gender differences for particle-induced osteolysis.

Pseudotumors have also been reported with MOP implants. The authors of a 2015 study[36] reported a case of crevice corrosion of the head-neck junction in a MOP leading to a pseudotumor around the joint. Similar cases having trunnionosis been reported.[37-39] The author of a 2012 study[40] described a case of pseudotumor around a MOP arthroplasty due to an extensive eccentric wear of the polyethylene liner that led a MOM articulation.

MOM bearing couples simulate a nonspecific innate macrophage-dominated immune reaction and, in some patients, a type IV delayed hypersensitivity immune reaction as well (see following sections). MOM failures have been associated with delayed hypersensitivity immune reactions including aseptic lymphocytic vasculitis-associated lesion, and dermal and functional lymphocyte hypersensitivity, as shown by the author of a 2015 study.[34] MOM bearing couples carry the worrisome risk of pseudotumor that is now well established and often compromises later function. For this reason, MOM bearing couples are generally limited to resurfacing procedures in males. **Figure 3** summarizes the main biologic effects of MOM bearing surfaces.

BEARING MATERIALS AND HYPERSENSITIVITY

The immune system is a highly complex network of cells and molecules whose goal is to maintain homeostasis and mitigate/eradicate noxious stimuli that jeopardize the organism. The immune response to orthopaedic wear

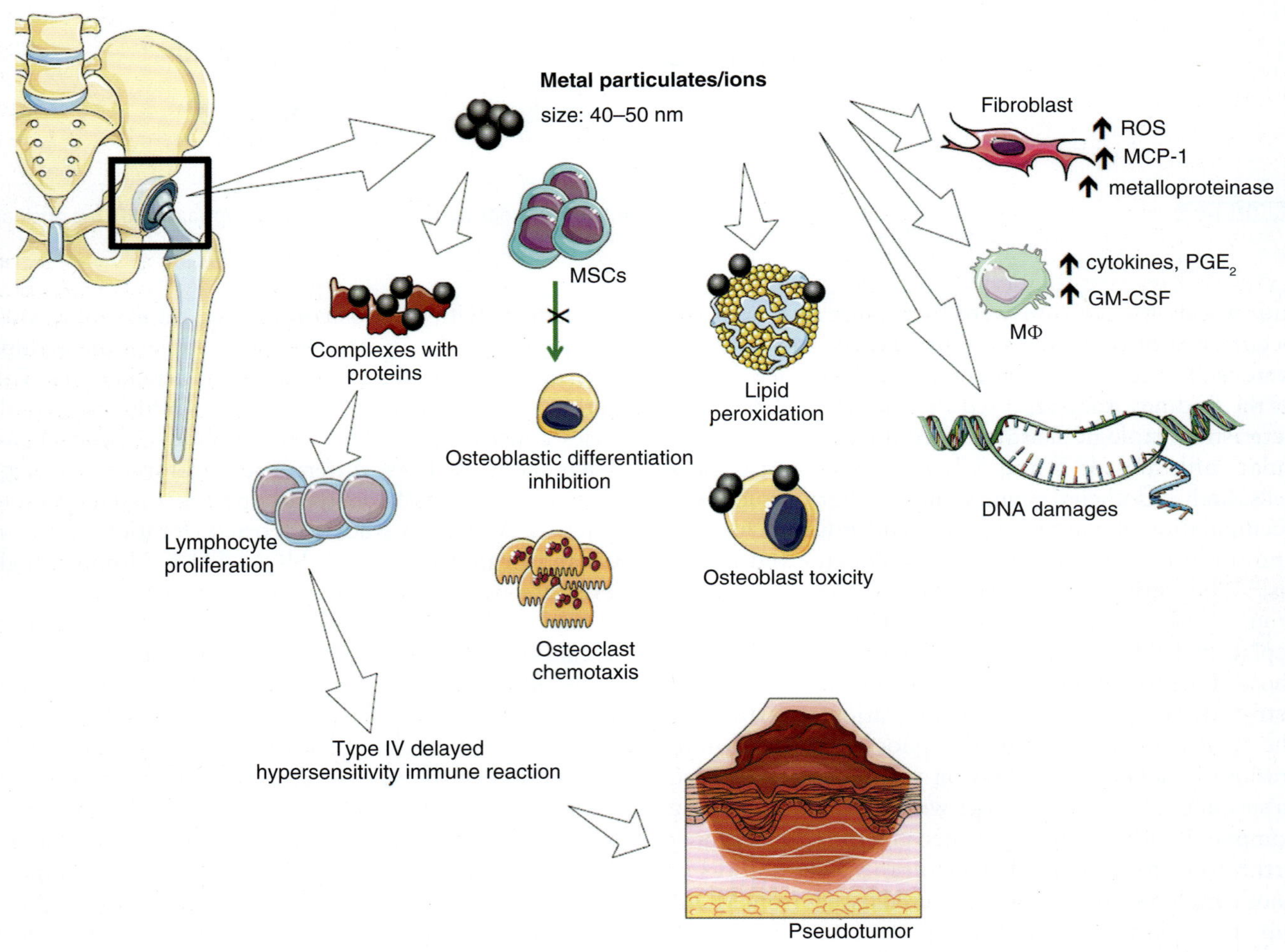

FIGURE 3 Illustration showing the biologic reaction to metal-on-metal bearing surfaces. GM-CSF = granulocyte macrophage colony-stimulating factor, MCP-1 = monocyte chemoattractant protein 1, MSCs = mesenchymal stem cells, PGE_2 = prostaglandin E_2, ROS = reactive oxygen species

debris from bearing materials may stimulate the innate or the adaptive immune systems, or both simultaneously. Whereas the innate immune system reacts in a nonspecific manner to a potentially injurious stimulus, the adaptive immune system is antigen-specific.

The innate immune response to orthopaedic wear debris was first described by the authors of a 1977 study.[41] The key cells in the innate immune system are macrophages, neutrophils, and dendritic cells.[42] The adaptive immune system is composed of four different types of reaction. Regarding bearing materials, the cell-mediated type IV immunologic reaction is most important. This hypersensitivity reaction has been estimated by the authors of a 2001 study[43] to be less than 1% of patients undergoing a joint arthroplasty. In addition to antigen-presenting cells, T-lymphocytes are the key cells for the type IV immunologic response. T-lymphocytes may be activated through antigen-presenting cells (CD68+ macrophages, dendritic cells or others). Indeed, metal-protein complexes are formed through a binding between metal ions (the hapten) and specific serum proteins (eg, albumin, chromodulin, nickel/cobalt transporters). Thereafter, these new metal-protein complexes may act as antigens. Moreover, T cells may be activated by metal ions alone, without any metal-protein complexes, by tyrosine kinase activation induced by cross-linking of thiols of cell surface proteins. Locally, metal particles are phagocytized by CD68 macrophages, which will act as antigen-presenting cells to T lymphocytes, leading to a cell-mediated type IV immunologic reaction. High levels of IL-2 receptor expression (a sign of T lymphocyte activation) are found when tissues (retrieved tissues or blood cells) were challenged with metal particles. Following activation, T lymphocyte responses are increased by costimulation with CD28/CD86 between antigen-presenting cells and activated T cells. Keys points are summarized in **Table 1**.

DRUG-ELUTING IMPLANTS: FUTURE AVENUES TO MITIGATE THE BIOLOGIC RESPONSE TO BYPRODUCTS OF BEARING MATERIALS

Implants with an active coating represent a way to alleviate or suppress particle-associated inflammation and osteolysis or infection.[47] This idea has made its way to the benches of multiple laboratories worldwide. The authors of a 2017 study[48] implanted IL-4-coated polypropylene mesh subcutaneously to successfully increase the M2 to M1 ratio to decrease local inflammation. The authors of a 2018 study[49] coated titanium implants with IL-4 first. Then genipin cross-linked gelatin hydrogel was coated onto the surface to delay the release of IL-4; the implants were cultured with macrophages (MΦ) that were activated to the M1 proinflammatory phenotype by exposure to interferon-gamma. The subsequent delayed release of IL-4 increased the expression of M2 markers, such as IL-10, arginase-1, and platelet-derived growth factor-BB. The authors of a 2014 study[50] showed that a mutant MCP-1, also called 7ND, dramatically reduced the chemotactic effect of human MΦ when exposed to a conditioned media obtained after challenging murine MΦ with polymethyl methacrylate particles. 7ND acts by blocking the chemokine receptor CCR2, which is the receptor for MCP-1. The authors of a 2013 study[51] coated 7ND protein onto titanium rods; using a layer-by-layer technique, 7ND protein was effectively released and remained bioactive by decreasing MΦ trafficking toward MCP-1 in vitro. The concept was then validated in in-vivo studies;[52-54] biologically active rods coated with 7ND mitigated UHMWPE particle–induced osteolysis and decreased systemic MΦ recruitment. The authors of a 2016 study[53] also showed that the continuous delivery of IL-4 led to increased trabecular bone volume in the presence of UHMWPE particles. These studies point to

TABLE 1

Key Points in the Interaction Between Bearing Materials and the Immune System

Immune Reaction	Innate (Nonspecific)	Adaptive (Antigen Specific) Type IV (Cell Mediated)
Specific immunes	PAMPs, PRRs, TLRs, DAMPs, NLRs, RLRs	IL-2R, CD69 activation antigen
Cells	Macrophages, neutrophils, dendritic cells	Lymphocytes
Wear particles involved	Polymers, ceramics, metals	In some cases, metals
Ultimate adverse reaction	Foreign-body granuloma	Necrosis, fibrosis, possible pseudotumor
References	44-46	—

DAMPs = damage-associated molecular paterns, IL-2R = interleukin 2 receptor, NLRs = nucleotide-binding oligomerization domain (NOD)-like receptors, PAMPs = pathogen-associated molecular patterns, PRRs = pattern recognition receptors, RLRs = retinoid acid inducible gene (RIG)-I-like receptors, TLRs = Toll-like receptors novel methods to increase osseointegration and mitigate unwanted chronic inflammation using biologic coatings of implants.

SUMMARY

The biologic response to orthopaedic bearings is driven by the immune system. Byproducts from MOP bearings, which are currently most commonly used, induce a nonspecific innate immune response driven by macrophages. Debris from MOP may be associated with a foreign-body granuloma and periprosthetic osteolysis, depending on the amount and type of particles generated and patient characteristics. Ceramic bearings usually generate little wear debris, but if high amounts of ceramic particles are generated, the subsequent biologic response is similar to that of MOP bearings. MOM bearings release metallic ions and nano-sized particles, triggering in some patients a delayed type IV immune response with the risk of inducing local pain, allergic reactions, and in some cases, tissue destruction and pseudotumor. Because of the aforementioned reasons, the use of MOM bearings is now very limited. Bioactive (coated) implants and other methods of drug delivery, which could modulate the local periprosthetic environment, represent novel technologies to potentially improve the longevity of joint arthroplasties. Research studies are currently ongoing to test these promising technologies.

KEY STUDY POINTS

- Polyethylene particles activate macrophages through phagocytosis or direct cell contact.
- When compared with polyethylene particles, alumina particles induced significantly less TNF-α release from macrophages.
- Metalloprotein complexes made from CoCr degradation byproducts are capable of inducing a chronic inflammatory and lymphocytic proliferative response.
- Regarding hypersensitivity to bearing materials, the cell-mediated type IV immunologic reaction is most important.

ANNOTATED REFERENCES

1. *Orthopedic Devices Market Growth Analysis 2019-2025 Share Report.* Available at: https://www.gminsights.com/industry-analysis/orthopedic-devices-market. Accessed January 21, 2020.

   This website provides up-to-date information and projections regarding the projected growth of the orthopaedic devices market.

2. Heckmann ND, Sivasundaram L, Stefl MD, Kang HP, Basler ET, Lieberman JR: Total hip arthroplasty bearing surface trends in the United States from 2007 to 2014: The rise of ceramic on polyethylene. *J Arthroplasty* 2018;33(6):1757-1763.e1.

   This study used the nationwide inpatient sample database to investigate the epidemiology of THA bearing surface trends in the period 2007 to 2014. The authors showed that ceramic-on-polyethylene is now the most widely used bearings. Level of evidence: III.

3. Nich C, Goodman SB: Role of macrophages in the biological reaction to wear debris from joint replacements. *J Long Term Eff Med Implants* 2014;24(4):259-265.
4. Valladares RD, Nich C, Zwingenberger S, et al: Toll-like receptors-2 and 4 are overexpressed in an experimental model of particle-induced osteolysis. *J Biomed Mater Res A* 2014;102(9):3004-3011.
5. Gibon E, Ma T, Ren P-G, et al: Selective inhibition of the MCP-1-CCR2 ligand-receptor axis decreases systemic trafficking of macrophages in the presence of UHMWPE particles. *J Orthop Res* 2012;30(4):547-553.
6. Gibon E, Yao Z, Rao AJ, et al: Effect of a CCR1 receptor antagonist on systemic trafficking of MSCs and polyethylene particle-associated bone loss. *Biomaterials* 2012;33(14):3632-3638.
7. Mantovani A, Biswas SK, Galdiero MR, Sica A, Locati M: Macrophage plasticity and polarization in tissue repair and remodelling. *J Pathol* 2013;229(2):176-185.
8. Murray PJ, Allen JE, Biswas SK, et al: Macrophage activation and polarization: Nomenclature and experimental guidelines. *Immunity* 2014;41(1):14-20.
9. Pajarinen J, Cenni E, Savarino L, et al: Profile of toll-like receptor-positive cells in septic and aseptic loosening of total hip arthroplasty implants. *J Biomed Mater Res A* 2010;94(1):84-92.
10. Wang C-T, Lin Y-T, Chiang B-L, Lee S-S, Hou S-M. Overexpression of receptor activator of nuclear factor-kappaB ligand (RANKL), inflammatory cytokines, and chemokines in periprosthetic osteolysis of loosened total hip arthroplasty. *Biomaterials* 2010;31(1):77-82.
11. Bichara DA, Malchau E, Sillesen NH, Cakmak S, Nielsen GP, Muratoglu OK: Vitamin E-diffused highly cross-linked UHMWPE particles induce less osteolysis compared to highly cross-linked virgin UHMWPE particles in vivo. *J Arthroplasty* 2014;29(9 suppl):232-237.
12. Huang C-H, Lu Y-C, Chang T-K, et al: In vivo biological response to highly cross-linked and vitamin e-doped polyethylene – A particle-induced osteolysis animal study. *J Biomed Mater Res B Appl Biomater* 2016;104(3):561-567.
13. Neuerburg C, Loer T, Mittlmeier L, et al: Impact of vitamin E-blended UHMWPE wear particles on the osseous microenvironment in polyethylene particle-induced osteolysis. *Int J Mol Med* 2016;38(6):1652-1660.
14. Chen W, Bichara DA, Suhardi J, Sheng P, Muratoglu OK: Effects of vitamin E-diffused highly cross-linked UHMWPE particles on inflammation, apoptosis and immune response against *S. aureus*. *Biomaterials* 2017;143:46-56.

In this work, the authors assessed the biologic activity (apoptosis, inflammation, bactericidal activities) of vitamin E polyethylene (VE-PE) and virgin polyethylene on murine macrophages and murine calvaria. The results showed that VE-PE caused less inflammation, apoptosis, and osteolysis. Level of evidence: animal study.

15. Galliera E, Ragone V, Marazzi MG, Selmin F, Banci L, Corsi Romanelli MM: Vitamin E-stabilized UHMWPE: Biological response on human osteoblasts to wear debris. *Clin Chim Acta* 2018;486:18-25.

In this article, the researchers challenged human osteoblastic SaOS2 cells with vitamin E polyethylene (VE-PE) and conventional polyethylene. The authors showed that VE-PE reduced the production of RANKL and increased the production of osteoprotegerin, thereby protecting against osteolysis. Level of evidence: lab study.

16. Terkawi MA, Kadoya K, Takahashi D, et al: Identification of IL-27 as potent regulator of inflammatory osteolysis associated with vitamin E-blended ultra-high molecular weight polyethylene debris of orthopedic implants. *Acta Biomater* 2019;89:242-251.

In this in vivo work, the authors assessed possible antiosteolytic mechanisms associated with vitamin E polyethylene (VE-PE) as opposed to conventional polyethylene. The results showed that VE-PE upregulated the IL-27 gene in human macrophages. Administration of IL-27 onto murine calvaria mitigated the development of osteolytic lesions. IL-27 is a potent regulator of inflammatory osteolysis. Level of evidence: lab/animal study.

17. Hatton A, Nevelos JE, Nevelos AA, Banks RE, Fisher J, Ingham E: Alumina-alumina artificial hip joints. Part I: A histological analysis and characterisation of wear debris by laser capture microdissection of tissues retrieved at revision. *Biomaterials* 2002;23(16):3429-3440.

18. Kurtz SM, Kocagoz S, Arnholt C, Huet R, Ueno M, Walter WL: Advances in zirconia toughened alumina biomaterials for total joint replacement. *J Mech Behav Biomed Mater* 2014;31:107-116.

19. Germain MA, Hatton A, Williams S, et al: Comparison of the cytotoxicity of clinically relevant cobalt-chromium and alumina ceramic wear particles in vitro. *Biomaterials* 2003;24(3):469-479.

20. Gutwein LG, Webster TJ: Increased viable osteoblast density in the presence of nanophase compared to conventional alumina and titania particles. *Biomaterials* 2004;25(18):4175-4183.

21. Catelas I, Huk OL, Petit A, Zukor DJ, Marchand R, Yahia L: Flow cytometric analysis of macrophage response to ceramic and polyethylene particles: Effects of size, concentration, and composition. *J Biomed Mater Res* 1998;41(4):600-607.

22. Catelas I, Petit A, Zukor DJ, Marchand R, Yahia L, Huk OL: Induction of macrophage apoptosis by ceramic and polyethylene particles in vitro. *Biomaterials* 1999;20(7): 625-630.

23. Kaufman AM, Alabre CI, Rubash HE, Shanbhag AS: Human macrophage response to UHMWPE, TiAlV, CoCr, and alumina particles: Analysis of multiple cytokines using protein arrays. *J Biomed Mater Res A* 2008;84(2):464-474.

24. Tsaousi A, Jones E, Case CP: The in vitro genotoxicity of orthopaedic ceramic (Al_2O_3) and metal (CoCr alloy) particles. *Mutat Res* 2010;697(1-2):1-9.

25. Hallab NJ, Mikecz K, Vermes C, Skipor A, Jacobs JJ: Orthopaedic implant related metal toxicity in terms of human lymphocyte reactivity to metal-protein complexes produced from cobalt-base and titanium-base implant alloy degradation. *Mol Cell Biochem* 2001;222(1-2): 127-136.

26. Samelko L, Landgraeber S, McAllister K, Jacobs J, Hallab NJ: Cobalt alloy implant debris induces inflammation and bone loss primarily through danger signaling, not TLR4 activation: Implications for DAMP-ening implant related inflammation. *PLoS One* 2016;11(7):e0160141.

27. Samelko L, Caicedo MS, Jacobs J, Hallab NJ: Transition from metal-DTH resistance to susceptibility is facilitated by NLRP3 inflammasome signaling induced Th17 reactivity: Implications for orthopedic implants. *PLoS One* 2019;14(1): e0210336.

This in vitro and in vivo study investigated the etiology of metal hypersensitivity responses in joint arthroplasties. The authors showed that metal debris activated the NLRP3 inflammasome that triggered the production of IL-17A/F by CD4+ T cells and eventually led to hypersensitivity reactions. Level of evidence: lab/animal study.

28. Papageorgiou I, Brown C, Schins R, et al: The effect of nano- and micron-sized particles of cobalt-chromium alloy on human fibroblasts in vitro. *Biomaterials* 2007;28(19): 2946-2958.

29. Kanaji A, Orhue V, Caicedo MS, et al: Cytotoxic effects of cobalt and nickel ions on osteocytes in vitro. *J Orthop Surg Res* 2014;9:91.

30. Willert H-G, Buchhorn GH, Fayyazi A, et al: Metal-on-metal bearings and hypersensitivity in patients with artificial hip joints. A clinical and histomorphological study. *J Bone Joint Surg Am Vol* 2005;87(1):28-36.

31. Davies AP, Willert HG, Campbell PA, Learmonth ID, Case CP: An unusual lymphocytic perivascular infiltration in tissues around contemporary metal-on-metal joint replacements. *J Bone Joint Surg Am Vol* 2005;87(1):18-27.

32. Park Y-S, Moon Y-W, Lim S-J, Yang J-M, Ahn G, Choi Y-L. Early osteolysis following second-generation metal-on-metal hip replacement. *J Bone Joint Surg Am Vol* 2005;87(7):1515-1521.

33. Witzleb W-C, Hanisch U, Kolar N, Krummenauer F, Guenther K-P: Neo-capsule tissue reactions in metal-on-metal hip arthroplasty. *Acta Orthop* 2007;78(2):211-220.

34. Hallab NJ: CORR Insights®: Do patients with a failed metal-on-metal hip implant with a pseudotumor present differences in their peripheral blood lymphocyte subpopulations? *Clin Orthop Relat Res* 2015;473(12):3915-3917.

35. Landgraeber S, Samelko L, McAllister K, Putz S, Jacobs JJ, Hallab NJ: CoCrMo alloy vs. UHMWPE particulate implant debris induces sex dependent aseptic osteolysis responses in vivo using a murine model. *Open Orthop J* 2018;12: 115-124.

Using C57BL/6J male and female mice, the authors investigated the sex dependence of osteolysis for CoCrMo alloy and polyethylene particles. Female mice had significantly more osteolysis with CoCrMo particles than male mice. No differences were found for polyethylene particles. Level of evidence: animal study.

36. Watanabe H, Takahashi K, Takenouchi K, et al: Pseudotumor and deep venous thrombosis due to crevice corrosion of the head-neck junction in metal-on-polyethylene total hip arthroplasty. *J Orthop Sci* 2015;20(6):1142-1147.

37. Stahnke JT, Sharpe KP: Pseudotumor formation in a metal-on-polyethylene total hip arthroplasty due to trunnionosis at the head-neck taper. *Surg Technol Int* 2015;27:245-250.

38. Scully WF, Teeny SM: Pseudotumor associated with metal-on-polyethylene total hip arthroplasty. *Orthopedics* 2013;36(5):e666-e670.

39. Mao X, Tay GH, Godbolt DB, Crawford RW: Pseudotumor in a well-fixed metal-on-polyethylene uncemented hip arthroplasty. *J Arthroplasty* 2012;27(3):493.e13-493.e17.

40. Murgatroyd SE: Pseudotumor presenting as a pelvic mass: A complication of eccentric wear of a metal on polyethylene hip arthroplasty. *J Arthroplasty* 2012;27(5):820.e1-820.e4.

41. Willert HG, Semlitsch M: Reactions of the articular capsule to wear products of artificial joint prostheses. *J Biomed Mater Res* 1977;11(2):157-164.

42. Goodman SB, Konttinen YT, Takagi M: Joint replacement surgery and the innate immune system. *J Long Term Eff Med Implants* 2014;24(4):253-257.

43. Hallab N, Merritt K, Jacobs JJ: Metal sensitivity in patients with orthopaedic implants. *J Bone Joint Surg Am Vol* 2001;83-A(3):428-436.

44. Kawai T, Akira S: Toll-like receptors and their crosstalk with other innate receptors in infection and immunity. *Immunity* 2011;34(5):637-650.

45. Kumar H, Kawai T, Akira S: Pathogen recognition by the innate immune system. *Int Rev Immunol* 2011;30(1):16-34.

46. Takagi M: Toll-like receptor – A potent driving force behind rheumatoid arthritis. *J Clin Exp Hematop* 2011;51(2):77-92.

47. Suhardi VJ, Bichara DA, Kwok S, et al: A fully functional drug-eluting joint implant. *Nat Biomed Eng* 2017;1(6):0080.

The goal of this study was to assess the functionality of an antibiotic-eluting polyethylene implant. Using infected rabbit knees, the authors showed complete bacterial eradication with this implant. Level of evidence: animal study.

48. Hachim D, LoPresti ST, Yates CC, Brown BN: Shifts in macrophage phenotype at the biomaterial interface via IL-4 eluting coatings are associated with improved implant integration. *Biomaterials* 2017;112:95-107.

In this in vivo and in vitro study, the authors investigated the effect of an IL-4-eluting implant on macrophage polarization. The results showed that the implant successfully promoted polarization to an anti-inflammatory M2 phenotype. Level of evidence: lab/animal study.

49. Yang CL, Sun YH, Yu WH, Yin XZ, Weng J, Feng B: Modulation of macrophage phenotype through controlled release of interleukin-4 from gelatine coatings on titanium surfaces. *Eur Cells Mater* 2018;36:15-29.

In this work, macrophages were challenged with an IL-4-coated titanium implant. A cross-linked hydrogel was added on top of the titanium implant to control the release of IL-4. After several days in culture, the authors showed a prompt switch of macrophages from an M1 proinflammatory to an M2 anti-inflammatory phenotype. Level of evidence: lab study.

50. Yao Z, Keeney M, Lin T-H, et al: Mutant monocyte chemoattractant protein 1 protein attenuates migration of and inflammatory cytokine release by macrophages exposed to orthopedic implant wear particles. *J Biomed Mater Res A* 2014;102(9):3291-3297.

51. Keeney M, Waters H, Barcay K, et al: Mutant MCP-1 protein delivery from layer-by-layer coatings on orthopedic implants to modulate inflammatory response. *Biomaterials* 2013;34(38):10287-10295.

52. Nabeshima A, Pajarinen J, Lin T-H, et al: Mutant CCL2 protein coating mitigates wear particle-induced bone loss in a murine continuous polyethylene infusion model. *Biomaterials* 2017;117:1-9.

In this in vivo study, the authors investigated the effect of a mutant CCL2 protein (7ND) on polyethylene-associated osteolysis. After implantation of a 7ND-coated rod into the distal femur of mice and tail vein injection of reporter RAW 264.7 macrophages, the results showed a decrease in systemic macrophage homing to the implant site and the number of osteoclasts and reduced wear particle–induced osteolysis. Level of evidence: animal study.

53. Sato T, Pajarinen J, Behn A, et al: The effect of local IL-4 delivery or CCL2 blockade on implant fixation and bone structural properties in a mouse model of wear particle induced osteolysis. *J Biomed Mater Res A* 2016;104(9):2255-2262.

54. Jiang X, Sato T, Yao Z, et al: Local delivery of mutant CCL2 protein-reduced orthopaedic implant wear particle-induced osteolysis and inflammation in vivo. *J Orthop Res* 2016;34(1):58-64.

CHAPTER 12

Medical and Biologic Treatments for Knee and Hip Osteoarthritis

KEVIN K. MATHEW, BS • KEVIN B. MARCHAND, BS
JOHN M. TARAZI, MD • HYTHAM S. SALEM, MD
JOSEPH O. EHIOROBO, MD • MICHAEL A. MONT, MD, FAAOS

ABSTRACT

Osteoarthritis of the knee and hip is a chronic and progressive disease that has a substantial effect on the healthcare system and the quality of life of affected patients. Less invasive treatments exist that aim to decrease pain and improve functionality for the patient. These treatments can be separated into medical and biologic therapies. Medical management can be further stratified into oral pharmacologic treatments such as acetaminophen, NSAIDs, and opioid/opiates. Oral supplements such as chondroitin sulfate and glucosamine are also commonly used. Medical treatment also includes intra-articular injections of either corticosteroids or hyaluronic acid. Alternatively, biologic therapies are more novel options that have garnered recent interest in orthopaedics. The biologic treatments include platelet-rich plasma and mesenchymal stem cell treatments that are derived from either bone marrow, amnion, or adipose tissue. It is important to be aware of the evidence and general consensus regarding the role of these aforementioned therapies in the management of knee and hip osteoarthritis. Currently, platelet-rich plasma, mesenchymal stem cell treatments, and other biologic agents are not recommended by the American Academy of Orthopaedic Surgeons, American Association of Hip and Knee Surgeons, Knee Society, and Hip Society for the management of knee and hip osteoarthritis.

Keywords: biologic management; hip osteoarthritis; knee osteoarthritis; medical management; mesenchymal stem cell treatment

Dr. Mont or an immediate family member has received royalties from Stryker; serves as a paid consultant to or is an employee of Cymedica, Flexion Therapeutics, Johnson & Johnson, Pfizer, Stryker, and Tissue Gene; has stock or stock options held in Peerwell and USMI; has received research or institutional support from Johnson & Johnson, National Institutes of Health (NIAMS & NICHD), and Stryker; and serves as a board member, owner, officer, or committee member of the American Academy of Orthopaedic Surgeons, the American Association of Hip and Knee Surgeons, and the Knee Society. None of the following authors or any immediate family member has received anything of value from or has stock or stock options held in a commercial company or institution related directly or indirectly to the subject of this chapter: Mr. Mathew, Mr. Marchand, Dr. Tarazi, Dr. Salem, and Dr. Ehiorobo.

INTRODUCTION

Osteoarthritis is the most prevalent joint disorder in the United States with an economic burden of over $300 billion annually.[1] As a chronic and continuously progressive disease, osteoarthritis undoubtedly has an immense effect on the healthcare system and the quality of life of affected patients. Consequently, there is urgency to implement measures for the management of osteoarthritis other than the last recourse of joint arthroplasty. Typically, the first stage of care begins with weight management to reduce stress across the knee and hip. Physical therapy and exercise programs are also recommended to promote muscle strengthening to improve functionality. Other nonmedical therapies such as knee braces and heel wedge insoles are also commonly used by the patient. If the safest and least invasive methods are found to be unsuccessful, more invasive interventions are considered. The most common and widely accessible therapies are usually medical and supplemental treatments for osteoarthritis (**Table 1**). However, in recent years, there has been increased interest in the use of biologic agents for the management of osteoarthritis. Specifically, there is available evidence and general consensus recommendations for both medical, supplemental, and biologic interventions for knee and hip osteoarthritis. These include (1) acetaminophen; (2) NSAIDs; (3) opioids and opiates; (4) chondroitin sulfate and glucosamine; (5) corticosteroid injections; (6) hyaluronic acid injections; (7) platelet-rich plasma (PRP) injections; and (8) mesenchymal stem cell (MSC) treatments.

MEDICAL AND SUPPLEMENTAL TREATMENTS

As a chronic and progressively debilitating disease, most medical management for knee and hip osteoarthritis is aimed at providing symptomatic relief rather than a cure. The American Academy of Family Physicians and the American College of Rheumatology have similar recommendations in the progression of medical management of osteoarthritis.[2,3] The first-line pharmacologic recommendation is to begin with acetaminophen therapy followed by NSAIDs if the patient has no contraindications for NSAID therapy. However, recently there are disagreements whether acetaminophen should still be considered in osteoarthritis management. Supplements such as chondroitin sulfate and glucosamine may be considered and continued only if the patient is experiencing relief. The use of intra-articular corticosteroid and hyaluronic acid injections are also considered after typical oral medications have failed. Last, opioids may be considered for severe pain management on a case-by-case basis if prior pharmacologic treatment has failed and if the patient's comorbidities preclude him or her from joint arthroplasty.[2,3]

Acetaminophen and NSAIDs

Acetaminophen (paracetamol) and NSAIDs are the most common pharmacologic treatments for osteoarthritis of the hip and knee, with acetaminophen long being considered as the first-line treatment.[4] The precise mechanism by which acetaminophen provides pain relief is still not clear. It is likely a combination of pathways involving inhibition of prostaglandin synthesis and activation of descending serotonin pathways to modulate pain.[5] NSAIDs, however, work by inhibiting cyclooxygenase enzymes that prevent transformation into various prostacyclins and prostaglandins, which promote inflammation and pain in the joint.[6]

Despite acetaminophen being considered as a first-line treatment, whether acetaminophen should remain a mainstay in arthritis management is a topic of debate. In 2006, a Cochrane review of acetaminophen for arthritis supported that it is an effective measure of pain reduction with no statistically significant increase in toxicity risk when compared with a placebo.[7] However, it was not as effective in pain reduction and improvements in functionality

TABLE 1

Medical and Supplemental Treatments for Osteoarthritis of Hip and Knee

Treatment	Mechanism of Action	Current AAOS Recommendation for Knee	Current AAOS Recommendation for Hip
Acetaminophen	Believed to be through the inhibition of prostaglandin synthesis and activation of descending serotonin pathways to modulate pain	Inconclusive	Inconclusive
NSAIDs	Inhibits cyclooxygenase enzymes that prevent transformation into various prostacyclins and prostaglandins, which promote inflammation and pain in the joint	Recommended	Recommended
Opioids and opiates	Modulate opioid receptors within the central nervous system to reduce pain	Inconclusive	Inconclusive
Chondroitin sulfate and glucosamine	Supplements that are believed to improve bioavailability of substrates necessary in proteoglycan synthesis	Do not recommend	Do not recommend
Intra-articular corticosteroids	Prevents activation of the inflammatory pathway by inhibiting the arachidonic acid cascade and its subsequent prostaglandins	Inconclusive	Inconclusive
Intra-articular hyaluronic acid	A therapeutic effect that is provided by providing lubrication to the articular surface of the joint	Do not recommend	Do not recommend

when compared with NSAIDs. The other key difference between the two medications was the increased risk of gastrointestinal adverse events with NSAIDs.[7] As a result, acetaminophen was originally recommended and still continues to receive support as a primary treatment option for osteoarthritis of the knee and hip by the American Academy of Family Physicians and the American College of Rheumatology.[2,3]

However, a 2019 Cochrane review of 10 randomized controlled trials (RCTs) involving acetaminophen for knee and hip osteoarthritis concluded that there is moderate to strong evidence that the difference between placebo and acetaminophen is too small to be of any clinical significance in patients with arthritis.[8] Another recent and large systematic review also supported that acetaminophen had a clinically insignificant effect on pain and functionality in patients with knee and hip osteoarthritis. Alternatively, NSAIDs such as diclofenac, celecoxib, ibuprofen, and naproxen were effective for pain management and physical disability.[9] As a result, the Osteoarthritis Research Society International and the American Academy of Orthopaedic Surgeons (AAOS) no longer recommend the use of acetaminophen for hip and knee osteoarthritis because of its limited efficacy, and instead support the use of NSAIDs.[10-12]

With the well-established knowledge of gastrointestinal and cardiovascular harm involved with NSAIDs, regular long-term therapy is not recommended. Therefore, the best recommendation is to use NSAIDs intermittently and on an as-needed basis.[9] For patients with associated comorbidities and risk for upper gastrointestinal bleeds, concomitant use of proton pump inhibitors and NSAIDs may reduce the risk.[13] However, the co-prescription of NSAIDs and proton pump inhibitors may have negative effects on small bowel mucosa; therefore, the use of a selective cyclooxygenase-2 inhibitor NSAID may be recommended for those with increased risk for both upper and lower gastrointestinal bleeds.[14]

Opioids and Opiates

Opioids and opiates enact their analgesic effect by modulating opioid receptors within the central nervous system and therefore have no effect on the role of osteoarthritis in producing pain. Considering the growing opioid epidemic in the United States, the regular use of such medications for knee and hip osteoarthritis has largely fallen out of favor. The AAOS and the American Association of Hip and Knee Surgeons have made position statements recommending that the use of opioids for the management of knee and hip osteoarthritis should be limited.[11,12,15] Opioids may be considered on a case-by-case basis if the patient has contraindications to other management options or if other options have failed. If prescribed, it is necessary to use opioids with caution and with close monitoring.

Chondroitin Sulfate and Glucosamine

Chondroitin sulfate and glucosamine are natural compounds that serve as the necessary substrates in the production of proteoglycans, which is essential in the formation of cartilage. As a result, these two compounds have been extracted from animal products to create some of the most widely used dietary supplements on the market. Easily absorbed from the gastrointestinal system and with an excellent safety profile, these products are believed to increase the bioavailability of the substrates in the synovial fluid of the joint and improve proteoglycan synthesis.[16] Although the hypothesis behind the use of chondroitin sulfate and glucosamine is theoretically sound, the evidence behind the efficacy of these products is inconclusive.

In a meta-analysis of 15 studies that evaluated either chondroitin sulfate or glucosamine for the management of osteoarthritis, it was found that there may be a moderate to large improvement in pain and/or mobility. However, many of the available studies that were analyzed in this meta-analysis were poorly designed or had financial support from the manufacturer. Therefore, the true efficacy of these products may be more modest. In contrast, the results from an independent, double-blind RCT of more than 1,500 patients that compared chondroitin sulfate and/or glucosamine with placebo and celecoxib in patients with knee osteoarthritis were inconclusive. It was found that chondroitin sulfate or glucosamine alone did not reduce knee pain by a clinically significant amount compared with a placebo. In this study, a clinically significant difference was determined by a 20% decrease in the Western Ontario and McMaster Universities Osteoarthritis Index (WOMAC) scores. However, when chondroitin and glucosamine are used together, there may be some clinically significant improvement in WOMAC scores in a specific subset of patients with moderate to severe knee pain.[17]

With a limited number of high-quality studies that describe any clinically significant improvement with the use of these supplements, it is difficult to recommend these products for the management of hip and knee osteoarthritis.[11,12] Considering that a particular supplement is a safe product, the patient can decide whether or not to try the product and/or continue with the supplements if they provide relief. If the patient is not experiencing any improvement in pain or mobility, then it is advisable to completely discontinue the use of the product.

Intra-articular Corticosteroids

Intra-articular corticosteroid injections have become commonplace in the management of pain from knee and hip osteoarthritis. Along with the immunosuppressive effects, corticosteroids reduce inflammation by decreasing the production of prostaglandins and other inflammatory mediators. Corticosteroids bind to receptors that translocate into the nucleus and increase transcription of products, which inhibit the activity of phospholipase A2. By inhibiting phospholipase A2, the arachidonic acid cascade that forms prostaglandins is not initiated.[18]

There are a number of US FDA–approved intra-articular corticosteroid injections available for use. Some of the most commonly used corticosteroids are methylprednisolone acetate, triamcinolone hexacetonide, and triamcinolone acetonide. However, there is limited evidence that supports one type of intra-articular steroid as being more efficacious than the others.[19] Intra-articular steroids have been shown to be effective at reducing pain and improving mobility in the short term for hip and knee osteoarthritis, with the greatest effects typically experienced for 1 or 2 weeks after injection.[20,21] After 1 to 2 weeks, it is inconclusive that the use of intra-articular corticosteroids results in outcomes that are significantly better than placebo. There is also limited to no evidence that suggests that corticosteroids are effective after 6 months.[22]

With corticosteroid injections being a common form of management for knee and hip osteoarthritis, there have been concerns regarding the risk of chondrotoxicity—especially after repeated injections. There are a number of in vitro and ex vivo studies that show adverse effects when articular chondrocytes are exposed to corticosteroids and local anesthetic.[23,24] However, in human studies, there is still no consensus. One RCT noted no radiographic decrease in mean knee joint width after corticosteroid injections every 3 months for 2 years compared with a saline control.[25] However, in a more recent similarly designed RCT, significantly greater cartilage loss was noted by MRI in the corticosteroid group compared with the saline group.[26]

After a number of studies of efficacy and safety, the AAOS recommends the use of intra-articular corticosteroids for hip osteoarthritis while providing an inconclusive recommendation for knee osteoarthritis.[11,12] It is evident that patients have experienced relief in the short term from corticosteroids. If the clinician chooses to use corticosteroid injections as part of his or her normal clinical practice, it should be given on an as-needed basis for considerable symptoms instead of as a regularly scheduled intervention.

Intra-articular Hyaluronic Acid

Patients who have knee osteoarthritis and in whom the aforementioned treatment modalities fail may derive benefit from intra-articular hyaluronic acid injection. Hyaluronic acid is a naturally occurring compound found in the synovial fluid of joints. It is thought to provide its therapeutic effect by lubricating the articular surfaces, dissipating frictional energy, and absorbing shock.[27] Viscosupplementation with hyaluronic acid produces a variable effect among patients, with some experiencing pain relief and others reporting no clinical improvement.[28] The AAOS does not recommend the use of hyaluronic acid for patients with symptomatic knee osteoarthritis because according to the available literature, it does not meet the minimum clinically important improvement measures.[29] Although less commonly used, viscosupplementation has also been used for hip osteoarthritis. However, its clinical efficacy for this indication has not been clearly established. According to the AAOS guidelines, there is no strong evidence supporting the use of intra-articular hyaluronic acid because it does not outperform placebo in improving function, mobility, or pain measures in patients who have symptomatic osteoarthritis of the hip.

BIOLOGIC TREATMENTS

Biologic therapy typically involves compounds or therapies that are extracted from living systems that are often a heterogeneous combination of large molecules. These treatments can range from products extracted from different mammalian cell lines to products from a person's own body. This is unlike medical treatments, which are chemically synthesized and are typically a concentration of a specific molecule. The use of biologic therapies has started to garner attention in the orthopaedic space. Particularly, research has been directed toward finding treatments that are capable of mitigating the progression of or even reversing osteoarthritis in hopes of avoiding the need for joint arthroplasty. A couple of these biologic treatments that have shown promise and continue to be researched are PRP and MSC treatments derived from bone marrow, amnion, or adipose tissue.[30]

Platelet-Rich Plasma

PRP is a concentrated source of autologous platelets containing growth factors and cytokines that may inhibit the inflammatory cascades and possibly heal various tissues. Currently, PRP preparation systems are approved by the FDA for use in mixing with bone graft material to complement bone graft properties.[31] Because of the potential anti-inflammatory characteristics and cellular anabolic advantages of PRP, it has also been used as an intra-articular therapy for osteoarthritis in the hip and knee. However, this is considered by the FDA as an off-label use of PRP. PRP is made through centrifugation of whole blood products into constituent elements, which are then divided based on numerous separation systems to formulate the desired concentration. For osteoarthritis, the most commonly used PRP final product is one that is leukocyte poor and platelet rich, PRP as it has shown to have improved functional outcomes.[32]

In recent years, there has been an increase in the number of studies investigating the efficacy of PRP for osteoarthritis in the knee and hip. PRP is most often compared with a placebo, corticosteroid, hyaluronic acid, or a combination of hyaluronic acid and PRP. The number, timing, and quantity of injections can differ based on manufacturer protocols. Because of this variation, it is sometimes difficult to interpret and extrapolate the data to a specific patient.

For the knee, efficacy studies have used pain, function, and quality-of-life measures to analyze PRP effectiveness. PRP has been associated with significant improvements from baseline scores in visual analog scale (VAS), WOMAC, and the Timed-Up and Go test scores when patients with Kellgren-Lawrence (K-L) grade II and III received at least two PRP injections in 2-week intervals.[33,34] Similarly, when compared with corticosteroid injections, a single injection of PRP was found to significantly improve VAS, daily activities, and quality of life over the course of 6 months in patients with K-L grade II or III osteoarthritis.[35] In 2019, a meta-analysis of 15 RCTs comparing PRP and hyaluronic acid in patients who have K-L grade II or III was conducted. The authors found no significant differences in pain relief and function between the two groups within the first 3 months after injection. However, when these metrics were evaluated over 1 year, patients in the PRP group had significantly better scores, indicating there may be some long-term benefit.[36] Conversely, the literature has shown no significant difference when comparing PRP with corticosteroids or hyaluronic acid in patients with more advanced (K-L grades III/IV) osteoarthritis.[37]

Overall, PRP intra-articular hip injections have also received mixed outcomes when evaluating function and pain scores. In K-L grade I and II osteoarthritis, significantly improved VAS scores were seen over 6 months following a PRP injection. Patients who had K-L grade III and IV osteoarthritis did not have a reduction in pain at any time interval. All patients did have significant improvements in the Hip Disability and Osteoarthritis Outcome Scale over 6 months. However, K-L grade I and II patients showed the greatest improvements, suggesting that early intervention with PRP could have a greater effect.[38] In 2016, two studies reported VAS and WOMAC scores of patients who either underwent PRP or hyaluronic acid hip injections. In both studies, the patients receiving PRP had the most improved VAS scores, whereas one study had reported significantly improved WOMAC scores.[39,40]

Many studies have reported improved early pain relief and functional scores in both the knee and hip, but there has been no evidence that suggests that PRP regenerates damaged cartilage. As mentioned earlier, the variety of outcomes, metrics, and study protocols used in collecting PRP data prevents generalizability between different studies. Therefore, it is currently not recommended as part of standard care, but future consistent studies may provide more insight on PRP's role in knee and hip osteoarthritis management.

Stem Cell Treatments

Bone Marrow Aspirate Concentrate and Bone Marrow–Derived MSCs

Bone marrow aspirate concentrate (BMAC) is an FDA-approved form of MSCs, progenitor cells, and growth factors.[41] BMAC is commonly prepared by extracting bone marrow percutaneously from the iliac crest via a bone marrow aspiration needle and syringe preloaded with heparin to prevent coagulation of the marrow. Typically, 60 to 100 mL of bone marrow is aspirated during the procedure. The aspirated bone marrow is filtered and then centrifuged to separate the platelet-poor plasma, buffy coat layer, and red blood cells to acquire the BMAC product. Either BMAC or the bone marrow–derived mesenchymal stem cells (BMSCs) in BMAC are expanded in culture and then injected into the knee.[42]

The precise mechanism by which BMAC enacts its effect on articular cartilage is still being defined. The hypothesis behind its use in osteoarthritis is multifactorial. The BMSCs in BMAC are believed to differentiate into varying cell lines such as chondrocytes that can help renew the damaged articular cartilage.[42] BMAC also contains a high concentration of growth factors that include but are not limited to vascular endothelial growth factor, platelet-derived growth factor, and transforming growth factor beta that are believed to promote chondrocyte repair. BMSC may also downregulate inflammatory cytokines such as interleukin-1 and tumor necrosis factor alpha, which may promote cartilage healing and reduce pain.[43]

However, the widespread use of BMAC or BMSC for knee and hip osteoarthritis is a topic of debate. It is still considered an investigational treatment and therefore not currently covered by insurance. The most recent literature does show that the bone marrow–derived products may have promise in reducing cartilage damage. Two RCTs using culturally expanded BMSC have shown statistically significant improvements in pain and functionality compared with a hyaluronic acid control. These studies reported either no radiographic changes in joint space with the use of BMSC or a decrease in poor cartilage index identified by T2-weighted MRI.[44,45] A systematic review of three articles shows that the use of BMAC in knee osteoarthritis has also shown improvements in pain and functionality.[46] However, in another RCT, no statistical difference was noted between BMAC and placebo in improving pain. But it should be noted that both the placebo and BMAC resulted in significant improvements in pain in this study.[47] The available research on the use of BMACs for hip osteoarthritis is more limited. In a short-term case series of four patients with mild to severe hip osteoarthritis, patients received a total of four BMAC injections each. All four patients reported less pain and improved functional ability after BMAC intervention with an average of at least 60% total improvement, but better designed studies will be needed to confirm.

Although most of the available studies on the use of BMAC on knee and hip osteoarthritis have been positive, they have a number of limitations. The use of small sample sizes and short-term follow-up resulted in evidence that cannot support with great confidence that bone marrow–derived stem cell products are effective and lasting measures for knee osteoarthritis management. The variations in how the bone marrow products are derived, the concentrations that are used, the frequency of injections, and the outcomes that were measured make the generalizability of the evidence difficult. What is clear is that there may be potential in the use of BMAC or BMSC and therefore further investigation with stronger designed studies is warranted. Future research should be performed with larger sample sizes, longer follow-up, and standardized methods involved in treatment and its administration.

Adipose-Derived Stem Cells

Adipose-derived stem cells (ADSCs) have recently gained popularity in orthopaedics as a source of MSCs in hopes of cartilage regeneration. This source of stem cells is usually obtained from fat found in the abdomen or the fat pad of the knee. These stem cells, known as lipoaspirates, are collected through minimally invasive techniques such as liposuction or lipoaspiration.[48] The lipoaspirate is incubated with collagenase to form the final product of stromal vascular fraction, which contains blood vessel–rich extracellular matrix and adipocytes. Currently, stromal vascular fraction is the only ADSC allowed for clinical use in humans.[49] The extracellular matrix has the ability to regenerate cartilage in vitro by adhering to cartilage lesions and releasing various growth factors and cytokines. By having positive effects on neighboring progenitor cells and serving as a scaffold, it is believed that the extracellular matrix can potentially enhance the survival and development of the injected ADSCs.[50]

Compared with BMSC, some studies suggest that ADSC has an increased number of MSCs per unit volume of tissue.[51] However, it is still unclear whether the regenerative potential of ADSC is dependent on the quantity of MSCs.[52] The current literature on ADSC is limited. There is only one level I study reporting on the safety and efficacy of in vitro expanded MSC derived from human donor adipose tissue for intra-articular injections without arthroscopy or microfracture procedures.[53,54] In this study of 20 patients, there were improvements in VAS pain, WOMAC, and mobility scores. There was also less lateral tibial cartilage loss after 12 months. Although there is equivocal radiographic outcomes at 12 months, there were improved clinical outcomes.[53]

Given the paucity of high-power studies on intra-articular injections with ADSC, additional level I studies with larger sample sizes and longer follow-up times are required to further understand the effect and outcomes of these particular stem cells on degenerating hip and knee joints. Although many published animal models have been used toward understanding the regenerative mechanism and effect of ADSC with regard to osteoarthritis, most of these models do not reflect osteoarthritis of the human hip or knee joint. Although there is promise, it is currently difficult to infer the effect of ADSC in clinical practice.

Amnion-Derived Stem Cells

MSC derived from the placenta presents a noninvasive alternative to ADSC or BMAC. Placental cells, including amniotic fluid, amnion, chorion, and the umbilical cord and its blood are rich sources of MSC and growth factors that can be harvested immediately after a delivery.[55] Placental or amnion-derived MSCs have been shown to proliferate at a higher rate and have greater differentiation potential than MSC sourced from different types of adult tissues.[56] It has also been shown that older adult stem cells have a negative correlation with MSC function and therefore, amnion-derived MSCs have shown greater healing and regenerative potential.[57] In addition, amnion-derived MSCs have demonstrated a greater affinity to differentiate into bone and cartilage when compared with ADSC.[58]

The preparation of amnion-derived MSC may include concentration, cryopreservation, freeze-drying, packaging, and thawing, which results in tissues that contain no live stem cells. As a result, the FDA does not necessarily consider it as a biologic product, and the use is not regulated by the FDA. Research into the efficacy of amnion-derived MSC intra-articular injections for osteoarthritis of the knee and hip remains ongoing. Similar to other biologics, there is little standardization in type of placental tissue used, concentration, timing, and number of injections. The one available study used a single intra-articular knee injection of cryopreserved amniotic suspension. This study reported improved Knee Injury and Osteoarthritis Outcome Survey and International Knee Documentation Committee scores from baseline over the course of 1 year in patients with K-L grade III and IV knee osteoarthritis.[59] There is promise with the use of amnion-derived MSC in orthopaedics, but more extensive research is needed to determine if it can become part of common practice in the management of knee and hip osteoarthritis.

SUMMARY

There are a number of nonsurgical treatment options for the management of knee and hip osteoarthritis. Early treatment typically includes weight loss and a combination of aerobic and strength training. There have been recent changes in preferences for the pharmacologic management of hip and knee osteoarthritis. The AAOS currently recommends the use of NSAIDs on an as-needed basis over the use of acetaminophen for pain management. The use of opiates is discouraged. Oral chondroitin sulfate and glucosamine supplements have limited data supporting their efficacy and therefore are not recommended. Intra-articular corticosteroid injections have demonstrated short-term improvements in pain and functionality, but the long-term effect is more varied. If used, intra-articular corticosteroid injections should be administered on an as-needed basis for severe symptoms rather than regularly scheduled injections. In contrast, intra-articular hyaluronic injections showed variable responses in patients and therefore are not recommended. Biologic therapies such as intra-articular PRP and stem cell treatments have gained increased interest in recent years. Initial studies show that there is promise, but the evidence is still too limited to implement these therapies as part of standard care. As of June 2019, the American Association of Hip and Knee Surgeons, the Hip Society, and the Knee Society released a joint position statement expressing that stem cell or PRP injections for the management of advanced hip or knee osteoarthritis cannot be currently recommended.[60]

KEY STUDY POINTS

- NSAIDs are the recommended first-line medical management for knee and hip osteoarthritis over acetaminophen.
- Intra-articular corticosteroid injections have benefits in the short term but do not provide long-term relief. They should be used on an as-needed basis for severe symptoms instead of regularly scheduled treatments.
- Chondroitin sulfate and glucosamine supplements are safe products but have shown limited efficacy in knee and hip osteoarthritis, and therefore not recommended.
- Biologic treatments such as PRP and stem cell treatments have shown promise, but are not currently recommended as part of standard care. Further study is required to decide its role in management of knee and hip osteoarthritis.

ANNOTATED REFERENCES

1. Vina ER, Kwoh CK: Epidemiology of osteoarthritis: Literature update. *Curr Opin Rheumatol* 2018;30(2):160-167.

   A literature review of recent studies investigated osteoarthritis epidemiology such as prevalence, disease impact, and risk factors. Osteoarthritis is a leading cause of disability, and there may be different phenotypes that show there may be different mechanisms in the development of the disease. Level of evidence: V.

2. Sinusas K: Osteoarthritis: Diagnosis and treatment. *Am Fam Physician* 2012;85(1):49-56.
3. Hochberg MC, Altman RD, April KT, et al: American College of Rheumatology 2012 recommendations for the use of nonpharmacologic and pharmacologic therapies in osteoarthritis of the hand, hip, and knee. *Arthritis Care Res* 2012;64(4):465-474.
4. Jordan KM, Arden NK, Doherty M, et al: EULAR Recommendations 2003: An evidence based approach to the management of knee osteoarthritis. Report of a Task Force of the Standing Committee for International Clinical Studies Including Therapeutic Trials (ESCISIT). *Ann Rheum Dis* 2003;62(12):1145-1155.
5. Sharma CV, Mehta V: Paracetamol: Mechanisms and updates. *Contin Educ Anaesth Crit Care Pain* 2014;14(4):153-158.
6. Vane JR: Inhibition of prostaglandin synthesis as a mechanism of action for aspirin-like drugs. *Nat New Biol* 1971;231(25):232-235.
7. Towheed T, Maxwell L, Judd M, Catton M, Hochberg MC, Wells GA: Acetaminophen for osteoarthritis. *Cochrane Database Syst Rev* 2006;(1):CD004257.
8. Leopoldino A, Machado G, Ferreira P, et al: Paracetamol versus placebo for knee and hip osteoarthritis. *Cochrane Database Syst Rev* 2019;(2):CD013273. CD013273. Available at: www.cochranelibrary.com.

   A Cochrane review of the literature assessed benefits and harms of paracetamol (acetaminophen) for the treatment of knee and hip osteoarthritis and showed that paracetamol may not be the best first-line medication for knee and hip osteoarthritis. Level of evidence: I.

9. da Costa BR, Reichenbach S, Keller N, et al: Effectiveness of non-steroidal anti-inflammatory drugs for the treatment of pain in knee and hip osteoarthritis: A network meta-analysis. *Lancet* 2017;390(10090):e21-e33.

   A meta-analysis of 76 studies showed paracetamol is not effective for osteoarthritis, and NSAIDs should be considered as a treatment option. Level of evidence: I.

10. Bannuru RR, Osani MC, Vaysbrot EE, et al: OARSI guidelines for the non-surgical management of knee, hip, and polyarticular osteoarthritis. *Osteoarthr Cartil* 2019;27(11): 1578-1589.

    A presentation of the Osteoarthritis Research Society International patient-focused treatment guidelines for knee, hip, and polyarticular osteoarthritis was developed from higher level studies. Level of evidence: IV.

11. *Treatment of Osteoarthritis of the Knee: Evidence-based Guideline, ed 2*. American Academy of Orthopaedic Surgeons, 2013. Available at: https://aaos.org/globalassets/quality-and-practice-resources/osteoarthritis-of-the-knee/osteoarthritis-of-the-knee-2nd-editiion-clinical-practice-guideline.pdf.

12. *Management of Osteoarthritis of the Hip: Evidence-based Clinical Practice Guideline*. American Academy of Orthopaedic Surgeons, 2017. Available at: https://aaos.org/quality/quality-programs/lower-extremity-programs/osteoarthritis-of-the-hip/.

    The guidelines and recommendations by the American Academy of Orthopaedic Surgeons on management of hip osteoarthritis are presented. There is an inconclusive recommendation for the use of acetaminophen for hip osteoarthritis.

13. Spiegel BMR, Farid M, Dulai GS, Gralnek IM, Kanwal F: Comparing rates of dyspepsia with Coxibs vs NSAID+PPI: A meta-analysis. *Am J Med* 2006;119(5):448.e27-448.e36.

14. Gwee KA, Goh V, Lima G, Setia S: Coprescribing proton-pump inhibitors with nonsteroidal anti-inflammatory drugs: Risks versus benefits. *J Pain Res* 2018;11:361-374.

    A review of literature shows that concomitant use of proton pump inhibitors may help potentiate the effect of NSAIDs in certain cases. Level of evidence: V.

15. *Opioid Use for the Treatment of Osteoarthritis of the Hip and Knee*. American Association of Hip and Knee Surgeons, 2019. Available at: http://www.aahks.org/wp-content/uploads/2019/01/AAHKS-Opioids-Treatment-Position-Statement-01.19.pdf.

    This position statement from the American Association of Hip and Knee Surgeons does not recommend the use of opioids in the normal management of osteoarthritis.

16. Vasiliadis HS, Tsikopoulos K: Glucosamine and chondroitin for the treatment of osteoarthritis. *World J Orthop* 2017;8(1):1-11.

    This study is a review of literature on the efficacy and safety of glucosamine and chondroitin sulfate supplements in the management of osteoarthritis of the knee and hip. This review finds that these products are safe but have limited evidence showing efficacy. Level of evidence: V.

17. Clegg D, Reda D, Harris C, et al: Glucosamine, chondroitin sulfate, and the two in combination for painful knee osteoarthritis. *N Engl J Med* 2006;354(8):795-808.

18. Ramamoorthy S, Cidlowski JA: Corticosteroids: Mechanisms of action in health and disease. *Rheum Dis Clin North Am* 2016;42(1):15-31.

19. Lomonte ABV, de Morais MGV, de Carvalho LO, de Freitas Zerbini CA: Efficacy of triamcinolone hexacetonide versus methylprednisolone acetate intraarticular injections in knee osteoarthritis: A randomized, double-blinded, 24-week study. *J Rheumatol* 2015;42(9):1677-1684.

20. Arroll B, Goodyear-Smith F: Corticosteroid injections for osteoarthritis of the knee: Meta-analysis. *Br Med J* 2004;328(7444):869-870.

21. Lai WC, Arshi A, Wang D, et al: Efficacy of intraarticular corticosteroid hip injections for osteoarthritis and subsequent surgery. *Skeletal Radiol* 2018;47(12):1635-1640.

    A retrospective study of 82 intra-articular corticocosteroid hip injections of the osteoarthritic hip shows that they are not effective for long-term management. Level of evidence: V.

22. Jüni P, Hari R, Aws R, et al: Intra-articular corticosteroid for knee osteoarthritis: Summary of findings for the main comparison. *Cochrane Database Syst Rev* 2015;(10):2-3. CD005328.pub3. Available at: www.cochranelibrary.com.

23. Jayaram P, Kennedy DJ, Yeh P, Dragoo J: Chondrotoxic effects of local anesthetics on human knee articular cartilage: A systematic review. *PM R* 2019;11(4):379-400.

    A systematic review of 16 studies shows local anesthetics have dose-dependent and time-dependent adverse effects on chondrocytes in human articular cartilage. Level of evidence: I.

24. Sherman SL, Khazai RS, James CH, Stoker AM, Flood DL, Cook JL: In vivo toxicity of local anesthetics and corticosteroids on chondrocyte and synoviocyte viability and metabolism. *Cartilage* 2015;6(4):233-240.

25. Raynauld JP, Buckland-Wright C, Ward R, et al: Safety and efficacy of long-term intraarticular steroid injections in osteoarthritis of the knee: A randomized, double-blind, placebo-controlled trial. *Arthritis Rheum* 2003;48(2):370-377.

26. McAlindon TE, LaValley MP, Harvey WF, et al: Effect of intra-articular triamcinolone vs saline on knee cartilage volume and pain in patients with knee osteoarthritis: A randomized clinical trial. *J Am Med Assoc* 2017;317(19):1967-1975.

    An RCT of intra-articular corticosteroid and saline shows that corticosteroid was associated with significantly greater cartilage volume loss compared with saline. Level of evidence: I.

27. Balazs EA: Viscosupplementation for treatment of osteoarthritis: From initial discovery to current status and results. *Surg Technol Int* 2004;12:278-289.

28. Bellamy N, Campbell J, Welch V, Gee TL, Bourne R, Wells GA: Viscosupplementation for the treatment of osteoarthritis of the knee. *Cochrane Database Syst Rev* 2006;(2):CD005321.

29. Jevsevar DS, Brown GA, Jones DL, et al: The American Academy of Orthopaedic Surgeons evidence-based guideline on treatment of osteoarthritis of the knee, 2nd edition. *J Bone Joint Surg Am* 2013;95(20):1885-1886.

30. Holton J, Imam M, Ward J, Snow M: The basic science of bone marrow aspirate concentrate in chondral injuries. *Orthop Rev (Pavia)* 2016;8(3):80-84.

31. Beitzel K, Allen D, Apostolakos J, et al: US definitions, current use, and FDA stance on use of platelet-rich plasma in sports medicine. *J Knee Surg* 2014;28(1):29-34.

32. Piuzzi N, Chughtai M, Khlopas A, et al: Platelet-rich plasma for the treatment of knee osteoarthritis: A review. *J Knee Surg* 2017;30(7):627-633.

    This review of 15 RCTs assessed knee osteoarthritis, and three RCTs in hip osteoarthritis compared PRP injections with various other injection therapies and found PRP to be safe with potential to provide symptomatic relief from osteoarthritis. Level of evidence: V.

33. Kavadar G, Demircioglu DT, Celik MY, Emre TY: Effectiveness of platelet-rich plasma in the treatment of moderate knee osteoarthritis: A randomized prospective study. *J Phys Ther Sci* 2015;27(12):3863-3867.

34. Smith PA: Intra-articular autologous conditioned plasma injections provide safe and efficacious treatment for knee osteoarthritis: An FDA-sanctioned, randomized, double-blind, placebo-controlled clinical trial. *Am J Sports Med* 2016;44(4):884-891.

35. Forogh B, Mianehsaz E, Shoaee S, Ahadi T, Raissi GR, Sajadi S: Effect of single injection of platelet-rich plasma in comparison with corticosteroid on knee osteoarthritis: A double-blind randomized clinical trial. *J Sports Med Phys Fitness* 2016;56(7-8):901-908.

36. Han Y, Huang H, Pan J, et al: Meta-analysis comparing platelet-rich plasma vs hyaluronic acid injection in patients with knee osteoarthritis. *Pain Med* 2019;20(7): 1418-1429.

    This meta-analysis found PRP to be more effective in treating pain and improving function than hyaluronic acid in patients with knee osteoarthritis. Level of evidence: I.

37. Filardo G, Di Matteo B, Di Martino A, et al: Platelet-rich plasma intra-articular knee injections show no superiority versus viscosupplementation: A randomized controlled trial. *Am J Sports Med* 2015;43(7):1575-1582.

38. Singh JR, Haffey P, Valimahomed A, Gellhorn AC: The effectiveness of autologous platelet-rich plasma for osteoarthritis of the hip: A retrospective analysis. *Pain Med* 2019;20(8):1611-1618.

    This retrospective analysis reviewed 36 patients who received PRP for hip osteoarthritis and found significant improvement from baseline at 6 months in patients with mild/moderate hip osteoarthritis. Level of evidence: III.

39. Di Sante L, Villani C, Santilli V, et al: Intra-articular hyaluronic acid vs platelet-rich plasma in the treatment of hip osteoarthritis. *Med Ultrason* 2016;18(4):463-468.

40. Dallari D, Stagni C, Rani N, et al: Ultrasound-guided injection of platelet-rich plasma and hyaluronic acid, separately and in combination, for hip osteoarthritis: A randomized controlled study. *Am J Sports Med* 2016;44(3): 664-671.

41. Youn GM, Woodall BM, Elena N, et al: Arthroscopic bone marrow aspirate concentrate harvesting from the intercondylar notch of the knee. *Arthrosc Tech* 2018;7(11):e1173-e1176.

    This technical note and video describe the technique for arthroscopically aspirating bone marrow from the intercondylar femoral notch as an alternative to harvesting from the iliac crest for BMAC. Level of evidence: V.

42. Themistocleous GS, Chloros GD, Kyrantzoulis IM, et al: Effectiveness of a single intra-articular bone marrow aspirate concentrate (BMAC) injection in patients with grade 3 and 4 knee osteoarthritis. *Heliyon* 2018;4(10):e00871.

    A retrospective study of 233 patients reports that single intra-articular BMAC injection is an effective and safe procedure for knee osteoarthritis. Level of evidence: III.

43. Carr JB II, Rodeo SA: The role of biologic agents in the management of common shoulder pathologies: Current state and future directions. *J Shoulder Elbow Surg* 2019;28(11):2041-2052.

    This study reviews preclinical and clinical evidence for the most commonly used biologic agents including PRP for the management of shoulder pathologies. Level of evidence: V.

44. Lamo-Espinosa JM, Mora G, Blanco JF, et al: Intra-articular injection of two different doses of autologous bone marrow mesenchymal stem cells versus hyaluronic acid in the treatment of knee osteoarthritis: Long-term follow up of a multicenter randomized controlled clinical trial (phase I/II). *J Transl Med* 2018;16(1):213.

    This is an RCT involving 30 patients with knee osteoarthritis who were randomly assigned to a control group, hyaluronic acid, and to a combined treatment of hyaluronic acid with different concentrations of bone marrow derived MSCs. Bone marrow derived MSCs were found to be safe and feasible in long-term clinical and functional improvement of knee OA. Level of evidence: I.

45. Vega A, Martín-Ferrero MA, Del Canto F, et al: Treatment of knee osteoarthritis with allogeneic bone marrow mesenchymal stem cells: A randomized controlled trial. *Transplantation* 2015;99(8):1681-1690.

46. Chahla J, Dean CS, Moatshe G, Pascual-Garrido C, Serra Cruz R, LaPrade RF: Concentrated bone marrow aspirate for the treatment of chondral injuries and osteoarthritis of the knee: A systematic review of outcomes. *Orthop J Sports Med* 2016;4(1):1-8.

47. Shapiro SA, Kazmerchak SE, Heckman MG, Zubair AC, O'Connor MI: A prospective, single-blind, placebo-controlled trial of bone marrow aspirate concentrate for knee osteoarthritis. *Am J Sports Med* 2017;45(1):82-90.

    This RCT of 25 patients with bilateral symptomatic knee osteoarthritis has shown that both saline and BMAC were associated with a similar relief of pain. Level of evidence: II.

48. Huebner K, Frank RM, Getgood A: Ortho-biologics for osteoarthritis. *Clin Sports Med* 2019;38(1):123-141.

    The authors reviewed five key orthobiologics for the treatment of osteoarthritis: viscosupplementation, platelet-rich plasma, autologous conditioned serum, BMAC, and ADSC therapy. Level of evidence: V.

49. Pak J, Lee JH, Kartolo WA, Lee SH: Cartilage regeneration in human with adipose tissue-derived stem cells: Current status in clinical implications. *Biomed Res Int* 2016;2016:4702674.

50. Zuk PA, Zhu M, Ashjian P, et al: Human adipose tissue is a source of multipotent stem cells. *Mol Biol Cell* 2002;13(12):4279-4295.

51. Zhu Y, Liu T, Song K, Fan X, Ma X, Cui Z: Adipose-derived stem cell: A better stem cell than BMSC. *Cell Biochem Funct* 2008;26(6):664-675.

52. Jayaram P, Ikpeama U, Rothenberg JB, Malanga GA: Bone marrow–derived and adipose-derived mesenchymal stem cell therapy in primary knee osteoarthritis: A narrative review. *PM R* 2019;11(2):177-191.

    The authors studied MSC-derived therapy for the management of primary knee osteoarthritis while comparing adipose-derived and bone marrow–derived MSC therapy. Level of evidence: IV.

53. Kuah D, Sivell S, Longworth T, et al: Safety, tolerability and efficacy of intra-articular Progenza in knee osteoarthritis: A randomized double-blind placebo-controlled single ascending dose study. *J Transl Med* 2018;16(1):49.

    The authors investigated a potential disease-modifying treatment by using in vitro expanded MSCs derived from human donor adipose tissue. Level of evidence: I.

54. Koh YG, Kwon OR, Kim YS, Choi YJ, Tak DH: Adipose-derived mesenchymal stem cells with microfracture versus microfracture alone: 2-year follow-up of a prospective randomized trial. *Arthroscopy* 2016;32(1):97-109.

55. Ha CW, Park YB, Chung JY, Park YG: Cartilage repair using composites of human umbilical cord blood-derived mesenchymal stem cells and hyaluronic acid hydrogel in a minipig model. *Stem Cell Transl Med* 2015;4(9):1044-1051.

56. Sung HJ, Hong SC, Yoo JH, et al: Stemness evaluation of mesenchymal stem cells from placentas according to developmental stage: Comparison to those from adult bone marrow. *J Korean Med Sci* 2010;25(10):1418-1426.

57. Yao B, Huang S, Gao D, Xie J, Liu N, Fu X: Age-associated changes in regenerative capabilities of mesenchymal stem cell: Impact on chronic wounds repair. *Int Wound J* 2016;13(6):1252-1259.

58. Topoluk N, Hawkins R, Tokish J, Mercuri J: Amniotic mesenchymal stromal cells exhibit preferential osteogenic and chondrogenic differentiation and enhanced matrix production compared with adipose mesenchymal stromal cells. *Am J Sports Med* 2017;45(11):2637-2646.

    This laboratory study found amnion-derived MSCs to show greater differentiation potential toward bone and cartilage compared with adipose-derived MSCs. Level of evidence: II.

59. Vines JB, Aliprantis AO, Gomoll AH, Farr J: Cryopreserved amniotic suspension for the treatment of knee osteoarthritis. *J Knee Surg* 2016;29(6):443-450.

60. Browne JA, Nho SJ, Goodman SB, Della Valle CJ: American Association of Hip and Knee Surgeons, Hip Society, and Knee Society position statement on biologics for advanced hip and knee arthritis. *J Arthroplasty* 2019;34(6):1051-1052.

    This statement by the American Association of Hip and Knee Surgeons, Hip Society, and Knee Society states that although biologic therapies may have promising applications in orthopaedics, currently they cannot be recommended for advanced hip or knee osteoarthritis. Level of evidence: V.

CHAPTER 13

Nonarthroplasty Management of the Knee

ETHAN A. REMILY, DO • NEQUESHA S. MOHAMED, MD
WAYNE A. WILKIE, DO, MHSA • JORDAN BONIER, DO, MS
SCOTT McDERMOTT, MD • JAMES NACE, DO, MPT • RONALD E. DELANOIS, MD

ABSTRACT

Nonarthroplasty management of symptomatic knee osteoarthritis attempts to improve quality of life in patients by decreasing pain and increasing mobility, with the goal of delaying or even completely avoiding the procedure of total knee arthroplasty. Many interventions can be used, which include lifestyle changes, mechanical devices, pharmacologic therapy, and nonarthroplasty surgical procedures. Lifestyle changes include weight loss and exercise, which emphasize strengthening the periarticular musculature. Pharmacologic therapy includes oral formulations addressing pain and inflammation, in addition to intra-articular injections consisting of corticosteroids, viscosupplementation, platelet-rich plasma, or mesenchymal stem cells. For individuals who have unicompartmental osteoarthritis resulting from angular limb deformities, distal femoral and tibial osteotomies may be performed.

Dr. Nace or an immediate family member serves as a paid consultant to or is an employee of Microport; has received research or institutional support from Microport, Stryker, and United Orthopedics; and serves as a board member, owner, officer, or committee member of the Arthritis Foundation. Dr. Delanois or an immediate family member has received research or institutional support from Flexion therapeutics, Orthofix, Inc., Stryker, Tissue Gene, and United Orthopedics and serves as a board member, owner, officer, or committee member of the Baltimore City Medical Society. None of the following authors or any immediate family member has received anything of value from or has stock or stock options held in a commercial company or institution related directly or indirectly to the subject of this chapter: Dr. Remily, Dr. Mohamed, Dr. Wilkie, Dr. Bonier, and Dr. McDermott.

Keywords: corticosteroids; knee osteoarthritis; nonarthroplasty management; nonsurgical management; NSAIDs; viscosupplementation

INTRODUCTION

Osteoarthritis, the most common cause of disability in the United States, is also the most common indication for total knee arthroplasty (TKA), accounting for 94% to 97% of all annual TKAs performed.[1,2] As the average age and weight in the United States continues to increase, the number of patients who have knee osteoarthritis is expected to increase substantially.[3] Consequently, the annual utilization of TKA is expected to exponentially grow to 3.5 million by 2030.[1,4] Despite the success of this surgical procedure, the suitability of TKA in some candidates has been called into question, as an analysis using validated appropriateness criteria concluded that nearly one-third of patients were unnecessarily undergoing this procedure.[5] As the US healthcare system shifts to models emphasizing cost-saving measures, nonarthroplasty management of knee osteoarthritis is of paramount importance to reduce cost, improve quality of life, and delay the use of TKA.

NONARTHROPLASTY MANAGEMENT OF UNICOMPARTMENTAL OSTEOARTHRITIS

Lifestyle Changes

Patients who have increased weight and decreased strength are subjected to higher levels of stress within the knee, which can compromise the integrity of the articular cartilage and subsequently decrease function. Weight status has an effect beyond objective measures, as those who experienced a 5% to 10% loss in weight reported a decrease in pain, decrease in disability, and increase in quality of life.[6] When considering certain resistance programs (eg, high-intensity or low-intensity training regimens), a meta-analysis revealed no difference in Western Ontario and McMaster Universities Osteoarthritis Index (WOMAC) pain and function scores.[7] Moreover, a single-blind, 18-month randomized controlled trial (RCT) compared weight loss, fat composition, and WOMAC scores in three cohorts (intensive diet, exercise, and intensive diet plus exercise) consisting of overweight and obese individuals who have knee osteoarthritis.[8] The diet plus exercise group demonstrated the most significant differences in degree of weight loss, reductions in fat mass, and improved WOMAC pain and function scores. This group also had greater levels of mobility, although this was not significantly different from the other groups.

Although the benefits of strength training have been repeatedly validated, the mechanism in which strength training relieves pain remains unclear. Numerous physiologic factors, such as muscular strength, proprioception, and joint stability, have been proposed as reasons why patients experience pain relief. A systematic review of 94 studies investigated the aforementioned physiologic factors, in addition to several others, in patients presenting with knee osteoarthritis.[9] The participants had their respective factor measured before and after the exercise regimen, which varied from walking programs to strength training. Although several factors were investigated, only increasing quadriceps strength, decreasing extension impairments, and increasing proprioception consistently demonstrated significant reductions in pain. Another recent meta-analysis examined 45 studies investigating knee extensor strengthening in comparison with no intervention.[10] A significant difference in strength was observed between the groups, although no differences were observed with regard to pain relief as measured by the WOMAC pain scale. Despite the lack of significance, meta-regression allowed the authors to estimate that a 30% increase in knee extensor strength would likely provide a beneficial effect on knee pain. In another meta-analysis of RCTs, the effect of physical exercise on quality of life was measured in patients who have knee osteoarthritis.[11] After the completion of exercise regimens, WOMAC and Short Form 36 scores significantly increased, indicating the intervention may be effective in improving overall health status and quality of life. Exercise clearly has an important role in the management of symptomatic knee osteoarthritis, as it is cost-effective and provides both objective and subjective benefits to the patient.

Mechanical Therapies

Treatment modalities involving mechanical therapies include compressive knee sleeves and corrective knee braces. Accommodative bracing treatment is often the first measure taken by patients to treat their knee pain, because braces are easily accessible and available over the counter. One such device, the rigid realignment brace, has been used with the goal of redistributing the force load of the knee from the affected compartment to the unaffected compartment. In a Cochrane review investigating corrective braces as the management of medial compartment knee osteoarthritis, evidence surrounding the device was considered inconclusive concerning symptom relief, stiffness, function, and quality of life.[12] Furthermore, the American Academy of Orthopaedic Surgeons is unable to recommend valgus-directing braces, because the current literature provides inconclusive evidence against these therapies.[13] Thus, these modalities appear to have limited utility because they fail to provide any significant relief of pain in patients who have osteoarthritis and are associated with increased costs.

Oral and Topical Medications

Oral medications represent an integral facet of nonarthroplasty management in knee osteoarthritis. When an adjunct treatment to lifestyle changes and mechanical therapies is needed to sufficiently remedy pain, oral analgesics are routinely used (**Table 1**). The selection of pharmaceutical agents varies greatly, ranging from over-the-counter dietary supplementation to opioid prescriptions, with many of them providing adequate pain relief. However, the type of drug selected must be patient specific, because many of these formulations have unique adverse effect profiles, limiting their use in certain populations.

Oral NSAIDs

Oral medications are the most common nonsurgical treatment used in patients who have symptomatic knee osteoarthritis, with NSAIDs and acetaminophen being two of the drugs most often used for treatment. A meta-analysis analyzing 15 RCTs compared the two drugs, concluding that the routine administration of NSAIDs appears to provide better benefits with regard to reduction in pain and improvement in functional status.[14] However, the use of these oral medications is not without risks. Osteoarthritis primarily occurs in elderly patients, and clinicians must be aware of the possible adverse effects and associated drug interactions. Likewise, older individuals are often on multiple medications such as anticoagulants, and therefore at higher risk for adverse effects.

Long-term, high-dose NSAID use confers an increased risk of gastrointestinal (peptic ulcers, bleeding) and cardiovascular (heart attack, stroke) adverse effects, and high doses of acetaminophen can cause liver damage. Both drugs have been demonstrated to have a negative effect on kidney function, although the effect of acetaminophen is far less than that of NSAIDs. Regardless, caution should be taken when prescribing acetaminophen to those with renal disease. Having a thorough knowledge of these medications' adverse effect profiles is important. A multicenter observational study determined

TABLE 1

Pharmacologic Therapies

- NSAIDs
  - Ketorolac
  - Meloxicam
  - Diclofenac
  - Celecoxib
  - Naproxen
  - Ibuprofen
- Acetaminophen
- Opioids
  - Tramadol
- Injections
  - Viscosupplementation
    - Hyaluronic acid
  - Corticosteroids
    - Betamethasone acetate
    - Betamethasone sodium phosphate
    - Dexamethasone
    - Triamcinolone acetate
    - Triamcinolone hexacetonide
  - Biologic therapies
    - Platelet-rich plasma
    - Mesenchymal stem cells

that 86.6% of patients who would benefit from NSAID use were at increased risk for gastrointestinal adverse effects, and 44.2% were at high risk for cardiovascular adverse effects.[15] Despite the risk, more than 80% of patients received nonselective NSAIDs. The underestimation of NSAID's adverse effects has large implications, as approximately 103,000 NSAID-related hospitalizations and more than 16,000 NSAID-related deaths occur annually in the United States, amounting to a cost in excess of $2 billion.[16]

In an Agency for Healthcare Research and Quality review of oral analgesics for osteoarthritis,[17] nonselective NSAIDs, such as ibuprofen and naproxen, demonstrated an increased risk for both cardiovascular and gastrointestinal complications, but more so with regard to gastrointestinal complications. Because of these heightened risks, several studies have analyzed NSAID use with various gastroprotective agents, such as misoprostol, H2 antagonists, or proton pump inhibitors, and found a significant reduction in the number of gastrointestinal events when compared with placebos. Thus, clinicians may consider using these agents in patients with increased risk. In contrast, selective cyclooxygenase-2 (COX-2) inhibitors, such as celecoxib, have decreased gastrointestinal risk profiles, but heighten the risk for cardiovascular complications. The concomitant use of aspirin in high-risk individuals has been investigated but has not been found to be beneficial and may actually be harmful. In the multicenter Prospective Randomized Evaluation of Celecoxib Integrated Safety versus Ibuprofen or Naproxen trial, approximately 24,000 patients who have osteoarthritis or rheumatoid arthritis who were at increased cardiovascular risk were randomized into treatment arms of celecoxib, ibuprofen, or naproxen, with or without aspirin.[18] When these NSAIDs were not taken with aspirin, celecoxib displayed a better overall safety profile than the other two drugs as a result of fewer adverse cardiovascular events. However, with the addition of aspirin, the COX-2 inhibitor lost the safety advantage because an increased number of patients experienced adverse events. A viable alternative to the traditional NSAIDs is meloxicam, which is a partially selective COX-2 NSAID. This drug has exhibited a lower risk of gastrointestinal adverse effects when compared with nonselective and selective NSAIDs, while also demonstrating a lower risk of cardiovascular and renal events when compared with other COX-2 inhibitors.[17] Irrespective of NSAID choice, the lowest effective dose should be used to mitigate the risk for adverse effects.

Topical NSAIDs

Other formulations of NSAIDs have been proposed as alternatives, such as topical diclofenac sodium gel. This medication is enticing because the formulation provides local pain relief with decreased levels of systemic exposure, thereby reducing the risk of adverse effects. A randomized crossover study comparing oral and topical formulations of diclofenac demonstrated the topical formulation to have a 17-fold decrease in systemic levels when compared with the oral formulation.[19] Moreover, the observed systemic levels in topical administrations failed to affect the aggregatory effect of platelets. A double-blind RCT compared topical 1% diclofenac sodium gel with a placebo in individuals who have mild to moderate knee osteoarthritis for 12 weeks.[20] Although improved WOMAC pain and function scores were observed with the diclofenac gel, participants experienced higher overall adverse event rates (60.2% versus 53.8%). Despite a higher rate of adverse events overall, topical diclofenac has been validated in those with elevated risk profiles. A study performing a post hoc analysis on five randomized, double-blind, parallel-group trials revealed no increase in risk for individuals who have mild to moderate knee osteoarthritis who have certain comorbidities, such as hypertension, type 2 diabetes, and cardiovascular disease.[21] Furthermore, topical diclofenac sodium gel can be used for prolonged periods in these high-risk individuals, as a multicenter prospective study noted no differences in adverse event rates throughout the 12 months of treatment.[22] The number of studies on topical diclofenac illustrate its viability as an alternative to oral NSAIDs in those who have mild to moderate knee osteoarthritis.

Opioids

Opioid medications are effective in controlling osteoarthritic pain, but their addictive potential and risk for adverse effects outweigh their benefit, as the number of deaths resulting from opioid overdoses continues to increase. Approximately 30% of patients taking opioids experience gastrointestinal adverse effects such as nausea and vomiting, while urinary retention and respiratory depression have also been observed, albeit less commonly.[23] The lack of superiority opioids have over NSAIDs also deters its usage. In the Strategies for Prescribing Analgesics Comparative Effectiveness RCT, opioid-based analgesic regimens were compared with nonopioid-based regimens in patients who have chronic back pain, hip pain, or knee pain.[24] Opioids not only failed to provide superior relief in terms of pain-related function or pain intensity over 12 months, but also caused significantly more medication-related adverse effects when compared with NSAIDs. Although opioids alleviate pain, long-term administration has been demonstrated to decrease pain tolerance in patients, necessitating the need for higher dosages and potentiating the risk of adverse events. The possibility for negative effects, in addition to the lack of superiority over NSAIDs, makes opioids a last-line medication for the management of knee osteoarthritis.

An atypical opioid, tramadol, has been commonly prescribed to treat symptomatic knee osteoarthritis, as it has been demonstrated to relieve pain despite its lesser potency compared with other opioids. However, recent research suggests tramadol may not be as useful as once perceived. In a Cochrane meta-analysis of 22 studies, tramadol was found to have no clinically significant benefit on pain reduction when compared to a placebo, while also demonstrating a greater risk for adverse events.[25] Conversely, a meta-analysis of 44 studies analyzed the efficacies of various pharmacologic interventions for knee osteoarthritis, finding tramadol to reduce pain as effectively as NSAIDs.[26] The literature has also explored mortality rates with tramadol. In a sequential propensity-matched cohort study of 88,902 patients, 1-year mortality rates were compared between tramadol, naproxen, diclofenac, celecoxib, and codeine.[27] Mortality rates were found to be higher with tramadol when compared with each NSAID, but not against codeine. Although this was a high-power study, it did not control for several potential confounding variables, and the conclusions should be taken with a degree of suspicion. Interestingly, preoperative exposure of tramadol appears to influence the postoperative recovery of patients who have undergone TKA. One study compared postoperative outcomes in patients who were preoperatively opioid naïve or tramadol users, finding those who used tramadol preoperatively had higher pain levels and lower function scores at 12 weeks postoperatively.[28] Tramadol may be a capable medication for the management of knee osteoarthritis, although its lack of advantages over other nonopioid oral medications and potential for increased risk of mortality make the use of this medication questionable. Therefore, this medication should be reserved for patients who have knee osteoarthritis not benefitting from or unable to tolerate NSAIDs.

Injection Therapies

Knee injections have been a mainstay in the nonsurgical management of knee osteoarthritis. Because injections are more invasive than other methods of treatment, this therapy has been regarded as the next level in the hierarchy of care after attempts have been made to reduce pain with lifestyle modifications, physical therapy, and oral medications (**Table 2**). Intra-articular injections have been demonstrated to be rapidly cleared from the joint by way of lymphatic drainage, with the rate of clearance dependent on the molecular weight of the drug.[29] Hyaluronic acid, a large glycosaminoglycan, has been demonstrated to take approximately 26 hours to clear the joint, with injectable NSAIDs and corticosteroids ranging from 1 to 4 hours.[30,31] Despite the rapid eradication of drugs, the pain-relieving effect has been demonstrated to last considerably longer.[32]

Corticosteroid Injections

The exact mechanism of action of corticosteroids is complex but believed to primarily act on nuclear steroid receptors, interrupting the transcription of several inflammatory genes and thus attenuating the inflammatory response on a multitude of levels. The inflammatory mediators produced from compromised bone, cartilage, and synovium cause pain and facilitate the progression of structural changes observed throughout the arthritic process. The effect of corticosteroids on these inflammatory mediators is believed to be the reason behind its ability to relieve pain. The benefits of pain relief do not come without risk, as corticosteroids have demonstrated gross cartilage damage and chondrotoxic effects with doses greater than 3 mg.[33] Furthermore, the effect of corticosteroids in patients who have diabetes should not be overlooked, because studies have demonstrated these patients to experience increased insulin resistance and blood glucose levels for a short period following the injection.[34]

The US FDA has approved five injectable formulations of corticosteroids for the management of knee osteoarthritis, which include betamethasone acetate, betamethasone sodium phosphate, dexamethasone, triamcinolone acetate, and triamcinolone hexacetonide.[35] Several studies

TABLE 2

Stepwise Algorithmic Approach to Nonarthroplasty Management of Knee Osteoarthritis

Step 1. Nonpharmacologic Therapy

- Lifestyle modifications
  - Centering around weight loss and exercise
- Physical therapy

Step 2. Pharmacologic Therapy

- NSAIDs
  - Medication selection should be dependent on the patient-specific risk profile
- Acetaminophen
- Tramadol
  - For refractory pain

Step 3. Injection Therapies

- Viscosupplementation
- Corticosteroids
- Biologic therapies
  - Platelet-rich plasma, stem cells

Step 4. Nonarthroplasty Surgical Intervention

- Distal femoral osteotomy
  - For valgus deformities
- High tibial osteotomy
  - For varus deformities

have demonstrated the effect of intra-articular corticosteroids on pain relief in the affected knee. A systematic review investigated the aforementioned corticosteroids in an attempt to determine if any certain formulation holds superiority over the other.[36] Triamcinolone hexacetonide may be more efficacious than methylprednisolone, as triamcinolone demonstrated a faster onset of action and similar duration of pain relief. Moreover, no significant difference was observed when triamcinolone acetate and betamethasone sodium phosphate were compared with methylprednisolone.

One obstacle is the duration in which these patients experience pain relief. Most patients experience relatively short-term relief for 2 to 4 weeks, although this effect has been demonstrated to last longer.[32,35] In an effort to prolong the therapeutic effect, triamcinolone acetate has been synthesized as an extended-released formulation. The drug is suspended in a poly(lactic-*co*-glycolic acid) microsphere–based solution, which is different from the traditional crystalline formulation. In a phase 2 trial comparing the two drugs, triamcinolone acetate-extended release was noted to have prolonged intra-articular residence time, reduced peak plasma levels, and decreased systemic exposure compared with the standard crystalline formulation.[37] In a phase 3, double-blind, 24-week single-dose study, average daily pain and WOMAC scores were compared in patients receiving triamcinolone acetate-extended release, crystalline triamcinolone acetate, or saline injections.[38] The extended-release formulation consistently outperformed saline injections and crystalline triamcinolone acetate with regard to average daily pain intensity and WOMAC pain score reductions for 24 weeks. Concerning glucose tolerance, a double-blind randomized phase 2 study analyzed the effect of triamcinolone acetate-extended release on blood glucose levels compared with crystalline triamcinolone acetate in patients who have type 2 diabetes.[39] The extended-release formulation was found to have a smaller effect on blood glucose levels, with fewer individuals experiencing glycemic spikes over 180 mg/dL. Newer extended-release formulations of corticosteroids appear to be improving by reducing adverse effects and prolonging therapeutic effects and may be a useful therapy to delay the need for TKA.

Viscosupplementation

Hyaluronic acid is a naturally occurring glycosaminoglycan that functions as a lubricant and shock absorber during movement, while also reducing stress and friction between cartilaginous surfaces. In the setting of osteoarthritis, synovial inflammation and defects within the cartilage allow for extravasation of hyaluronic acid, leading to decreased concentrations and lost viscoelastic properties within the joint. Hyaluronic acid injections are meant to replace these lost functions and increase the intra-articular fluid viscosity within the knee. Currently, this polysaccharide is the only FDA-approved glycosaminoglycan to be injected into the knee joint with three formulations: sodium hyaluronate, hylan G-F 20, and high-molecular-weight hyaluronan.[35] Injection schedules vary based on the formulation, but typically consist of one to five weekly injections. These injections are generally well tolerated; however, pseudoseptic reactions have been observed in 2% to 4% of procedures.[35]

Despite FDA approval and various formulations, the benefit of viscosupplementation remains inconclusive. In a meta-analysis of five RCTs comparing intra-articular hyaluronic acid injections with continuous oral NSAIDs, no statistical difference was observed between the two therapies at 4 and 12 weeks with regard to function and stiffness.[40] Despite the lack of difference between the two modalities, hyaluronic acid injections may be an alternative for those unwilling or unable to tolerate oral NSAIDs for knee osteoarthritis. A meta-analysis of seven RCTs compared the effect of pain relief between hyaluronic acid and corticosteroids at various timepoints for 26 weeks.[41]

Corticosteroids were superior at 2 weeks, the two therapies were equal at 4 weeks, and then hyaluronic acid was found to be superior thereafter. These findings suggest that corticosteroids may have better utility for short-term relief, whereas viscosupplementation may provide long-term relief. These conclusions should be heeded with caution, as moderate levels of heterogeneity were observed and most of the analyzed RCTs were sponsored by manufacturers of hyaluronic acid. As a result of the discrepant nature of the current literature, the American Academy of Orthopaedic Surgeons strongly recommends against this therapy in the management of knee osteoarthritis.[13]

Platelet-Rich Plasma

Platelet-rich plasma (PRP) is a relatively new therapy that has been gaining traction as a treatment option for knee osteoarthritis. This biologic therapy is derived from autologous blood containing four to five times the concentration of growth factors (eg, vascular endothelial growth factor, transforming growth factor beta, epidermal growth factor, fibroblast growth factor, and platelet-derived growth factor) than normal blood.[42] The high concentration of factors is thought to promote local angiogenesis, attenuate inflammation, and recruit local stem cells and fibroblasts to the joint.[42] The FDA initially approved PRP for the purpose of enhancing the handling properties in bone graft materials and not for intra-articular injection, although the procedure can be legally performed off-label in the clinical setting for knee osteoarthritis. As a result, many insurance companies refuse to pay for the procedure, resulting in high out-of-pocket expenses for patients.

Despite a variety of studies investigating this therapy for osteoarthritis, a lack of standardization exists with respect to PRP processing, nomenclature, and classification, thus making comparisons between studies challenging. Nevertheless, meta-analyses have been performed on the modality. A 2017 systematic review and meta-analysis analyzed 14 RCTs comparing PRP with varying controls (saline, hyaluronic acid, ozone, corticosteroids) and measured their effects on pain relief and function.[43] PRP was superior to every control at 3, 6, and 12 months with regard to pain and function and did not significantly increase the risk of adverse events. Despite these promising results, a considerable risk of performance and attrition bias, in addition to a large amount of heterogeneity, was observed. A 2019 systematic review of 11 PRP studies determined that PRP had a modest effect in reducing pain and increasing function in early osteoarthritis.[44] However, the study was critical of the other currently available RCTs performed on PRP, as small sample sizes, short-term follow-up, and the lack of protocol standardization make the conclusions regarding PRP dubious. As a result, various orthopaedic societies, including the American Academy of Orthopaedic Surgeons, American Association of Hip and Knee Surgeons, Knee Society, and Hip Society, do not currently recommend PRP in the management of knee osteoarthritis. PRP may be a viable treatment to decrease pain and increase function in early osteoarthritis, although the financial burden to the patient must be considered because these injections typically are not covered by health insurance plans.

Stem Cell Therapy

Mesenchymal stem cell (MSC) injections have gained popularity in recent years, as these injections have been theorized to attenuate the inflammatory cascade while promoting cartilaginous healing through the release of growth factors and differentiation of stem cells into chondrocytes. Stem cell injections can be derived from either bone marrow stem cells or adipose stem cells, because both stem cell lines demonstrate similar phenotypes and morphologies, although adipose stem cells have recently been shown to provide higher levels of stem cells and increased proliferation capacity.[45] Regardless of cell source, stem cell injections have been demonstrated to improve clinical and functional outcomes, as a 2020 systematic review of 18 studies revealed improvements in mean visual analog scale scores, WOMAC scores, and Knee injury and Osteoarthritis Outcome Score at 6 and 12 months postinjection.[46] MSC injections may be more efficacious than the hyaluronic acid injections. One RCT compared 4-year clinical and functional outcomes in 30 individuals randomized into treatment arms of hyaluronic acid only, hyaluronic acid plus low-dose MSCs (10×10^6 cells), or hyaluronic acid plus high-dose MSCs (100×10^6 cells).[47] The addition of MSCs to hyaluronic acid significantly improved both clinical and functional outcomes, although low-dose MSCs appeared to demonstrate higher benefits. The literature on stem cell therapy for knee osteoarthritis is encouraging but sparse, and the lack of FDA approval and high costs substantially limit the number of patients able to benefit from this treatment.

SURGICAL MANAGEMENT OF UNICOMPARTMENTAL OSTEOARTHRITIS

The distribution of forces within the knee is highly dependent on the lower limb mechanical alignment, and deviations influence cartilaginous wear patterns. Therefore, varus or valgus deformities can predispose an individual to unicompartmental osteoarthritis, because the distribution of forces becomes centered on the compartment in which the lower leg is deviated toward. Because cross-sectional studies have demonstrated varus deformities as the more common malalignment, isolated medial compartment osteoarthritis is more commonly observed.[48] Osteotomies were once often used to restore the normal joint alignment, which decompressed forces within the affected compartment. However, as TKA implants and outcomes continue to improve, the use of osteotomy has been progressively declining. Furthermore, the inconsistency of pain relief associated with osteotomy has also deterred its use in recent years. The procedure is typically reserved for individuals younger than 60 years who are nonobese, have adequate range of motion (flexion greater than 120°), and are more active. In addition to those who do not meet the aforementioned criteria, patients with tricompartmental disease or inflammatory arthritis preclude consideration for this procedure.

Distal Femoral Osteotomy

For valgus deformities, a distal femoral osteotomy (DFO) can be performed with lateral opening wedges or medial closing wedges. For a valgus deformity less than 10°, an opening-wedge DFO can be performed, whereas greater deformities should be managed with a closing-wedge DFO. A systematic review of 16 studies examined both variations of DFO by analyzing union rates, outcomes, and revision surgery rates in patients with varying follow-up periods (3.75 to 15 years).[49] Nonunion rates and patient-reported outcomes demonstrated similar results between the two procedures. Additionally, more patients with lateral opening-wedge procedures required hardware removal and more patients with medial closing wedges required conversion to arthroplasty. However, it should be noted that the studies reporting on medial closing wedges had longer follow-up, and many of those patients did not require such a procedure until more than 10 years after their index osteotomy. These conclusions are reassuring, although this systematic review comprised case series only, and a large amount of heterogeneity and confounding factors may have skewed the results. Both types of DFO appear to provide sizeable benefits to patients and sufficiently delay arthroplasty, although neither procedure demonstrates superiority over the other. Therefore, the type of osteotomy performed is solely based on physician preference.

High Tibial Osteotomy

High tibial osteotomies (HTOs) can be performed through medial opening-wedge or lateral closing-wedge osteotomies and are typically reserved for individuals with varus deformities less than 15°. A meta-analysis of nine RCTs compared clinical outcomes, radiographic outcomes, complications, and survivorship between closing-wedge and opening-wedge HTO.[50] Clinically, both types of HTO demonstrated similar improvements in pain and function scores at both short-term and long-term follow-up. Radiographically, there was no difference between hip-knee-ankle angles at short-term and midterm analysis. Although an increased mean posterior tibial slope was observed in opening-wedge HTO, closing wedge HTO demonstrated a reduced slope. The clinical relevance of these variations is uncertain, because no differences in complications and survival rates were noted. Nonetheless, the results of this meta-analysis portray similar outcomes between the two HTO approaches. These findings should be interpreted cautiously, because most analyzed studies had small sample sizes and presented a high level of heterogeneity. Indeed, similar to DFO, the type of HTO performed is likely dependent on physician preference.

SUMMARY

A number of nonarthroplasty options exist for the management of knee osteoarthritis. Lifestyle changes such as weight loss and strength training should be used as the first line of treatment. Mechanical therapies such as knee sleeves, knee braces, and heel wedges have been used, but their use has not been demonstrated to be beneficial and may create unnecessary costs to the patient. Several nonopioid analgesic medications such as acetaminophen and NSAIDs exist for the management of knee osteoarthritis. However, a keen awareness of the adverse effects and patient risk factors should dictate selection of these oral medications. Opioid medications should be avoided when possible. Intra-articular injections, such as viscosupplementation, corticosteroids, local anesthetics, PRP, and MSCs, represent the next level in management of knee osteoarthritis and have been demonstrated to provide pain relief. Newer formulations of corticosteroids have prolonged the duration of pain relief, while research on viscosupplementation remains inconclusive. Furthermore, PRP and MSCs have demonstrated benefits in pain relief and function; however, the high out-of-pocket costs make these therapies less appealing. For unicompartmental osteoarthritis, DFOs and HTOs may be performed for valgus and varus deformities, respectively. The type of osteotomy (opening versus closing) is dependent on physician preference, because each type does not appear to be clinically superior over the other.

KEY STUDY POINTS

- Weight loss combined with strength training is the first line of management for knee osteoarthritis.
- A patient-specific approach should be taken when considering oral analgesic medications, because many have potentially serious adverse effects.
- The literature on viscosupplementation is inconclusive and viscosupplementation may not provide clinically significant relief when compared with other treatments.
- Despite the promising results of PRP, the lack of standardization and FDA approval limits the therapy's applicability for knee osteoarthritis.

ANNOTATED REFERENCES

1. Centers for Disease Control and Prevention (CDC): Prevalence and most common causes of disability among adults – United States, 2005. *MMWR Morb Mortal Wkly Rep* 2009;58:421-426.
2. Carr AJ, Robertsson O, Graves S, et al: Knee replacement. *Lancet* 2012;379:1331-1340.
3. Pereira D, Severo M, Ramos E, et al: Potential role of age, sex, body mass index and pain to identify patients with knee osteoarthritis. *Int J Rheum Dis* 2017;20:190-198.

   This cross-sectional study assessed the role age, sex, and body mass index has on knee osteoarthritis and pain and found all to be correlated with higher pain scores.
4. Kurtz S, Ong K, Lau E, Mowat F, Halpern M: Projections of primary and revision hip and knee arthroplasty in the United States from 2005 to 2030. *J Bone Joint Surg Am* 2007;89:780-785.
5. Riddle DL, Jiranek WA, Hayes CW: Use of a validated algorithm to judge the appropriateness of total knee arthroplasty in the United States: A multicenter longitudinal cohort study. *Arthritis Rheumatol* 2014;66:2134-2143.
6. Chu IJH, Lim AYT, Ng CLW: Effects of meaningful weight loss beyond symptomatic relief in adults with knee osteoarthritis and obesity: A systematic review and meta-analysis. *Obes Rev* 2018;19:1597-1607.

   This systematic review and meta-analysis investigated the effect of weight loss on knee pain, function, and quality of life in 7 articles consisting of 1,105 patients. A 5% to 10% reduction in weight loss was determined to significantly improve pain; however, its effect on function was inconclusive. Level of evidence: I.
7. Regnaux JP, Lefevre-Colau MM, Trinquart L, et al: High-intensity versus low-intensity physical activity or exercise in people with hip or knee osteoarthritis. *Cochrane Database Syst Rev* 2015;(10):CD010203.
8. Messier SP, Mihalko SL, Legault C, et al: Effects of intensive diet and exercise on knee joint loads, inflammation, and clinical outcomes among overweight and obese adults with knee osteoarthritis: The IDEA randomized clinical trial. *J Am Med Assoc* 2013;310:1263-1273.
9. Runhaar J, Luijsterburg P, Dekker J, Bierma-Zeinstra SMA: Identifying potential working mechanisms behind the positive effects of exercise therapy on pain and function in osteoarthritis; a systematic review. *Osteoarthr Cartil* 2015;23:1071-1082.
10. Bartholdy C, Juhl C, Christensen R, Lund H, Zhang W, Henriksen M: The role of muscle strengthening in exercise therapy for knee osteoarthritis: A systematic review and meta-regression analysis of randomized trials. *Semin Arthritis Rheum* 2017;47:9-21.

    This systematic review and meta-analysis of 45 RCTs evaluated exercise regimens following the American College of Sports Medicine definition of muscle strength training, finding significant increases in knee extensor strength but no difference in pain or disability. Level of evidence: I.
11. Tanaka R, Ozawa J, Kito N, Moriyama H: Does exercise therapy improve the health-related quality of life of people with knee osteoarthritis? A systematic review and meta-analysis of randomized controlled trials. *J Phys Ther Sci* 2015;27:3309-3314.
12. Duivenvoorden T, Brouwer RW, van Raaij TM, Verhagen AP, Verhaar JAN, Bierma-Zeinstra SMA: Braces and orthoses for treating osteoarthritis of the knee. *Cochrane Database Syst Rev* 2015;(3):CD004020.
13. Jevsevar DS: Treatment of osteoarthritis of the knee: Evidence-based guideline, 2nd edition. *J Am Acad Orthop Surg* 2013;21:571-576.
14. Towheed T, Maxwell L, Judd M, Catton M, Hochberg MC, Wells GA: Acetaminophen for osteoarthritis. *Cochrane Database Syst Rev* 2006;(1):CD004257.
15. Lanas A, Tornero J, Zamorano JL: Assessment of gastrointestinal and cardiovascular risk in patients with osteoarthritis who require NSAIDs: The LOGICA study. *Ann Rheum Dis* 2010;69:1453-1458.
16. Singh G: Gastrointestinal complications of prescription and over-the-counter nonsteroidal anti-inflammatory drugs: A view from the ARAMIS database. Arthritis, Rheumatism, and Aging Medical Information System. *Am J Ther* 2000;7:115-121.
17. Chou R, McDonagh M, Nakamoto E, Griffin J: *Analgesics for Osteoarthritis: An Update of the 2006 Comparative Effectiveness Review.* Rockville, MD, Agency for Healthcare Research and Quality, 2011.
18. Reed GW, Abdallah MS, Shao M, et al: Effect of aspirin coadministration on the safety of celecoxib, naproxen, or ibuprofen. *J Am Coll Cardiol* 2018;71:1741-1751.

    The Prospective Randomized Evaluation of Celecoxib Integrated Safety versus Ibuprofen or Naproxen trial looked at various NSAID analgesics with or without the coadministration of aspirin. Results demonstrated celecoxib to have a better overall safety profile than other NSAIDs, although the effect was attenuated when taking aspirin. Level of evidence: I.
19. Kienzler JL, Gold M, Nollevaux F: Systemic bioavailability of topical diclofenac sodium gel 1% versus oral diclofenac sodium in healthy volunteers. *J Clin Pharmacol* 2010;50:50-61.
20. Barthel HR, Haselwood D, Longley S, Gold MS, Altman RD: Randomized controlled trial of diclofenac sodium gel in knee osteoarthritis. *Semin Arthritis Rheum* 2009;39:203-212.
21. Baraf HSB, Gold MS, Petruschke RA, Wieman MS: Tolerability of topical diclofenac sodium 1% gel for osteoarthritis in seniors and patients with comorbidities. *Am J Geriatr Pharmacother* 2012;10:47-60.
22. Peniston JH, Gold MS, Wieman MS, Alwine LK: Long-term tolerability of topical diclofenac sodium 1% gel for osteoarthritis in seniors and patients with comorbidities. *Clin Interv Aging* 2012;7:517-523.
23. Wheeler M, Oderda GM, Ashburn MA, Lipman AG: Adverse events associated with postoperative opioid analgesia: A systematic review. *J Pain* 2002;3:159-180.

24. Krebs EE, Gravely A, Nugent S, et al: Effect of opioid vs nonopioid medications on pain-related function in patients with chronic back pain or hip or knee osteoarthritis pain: The SPACE randomized clinical trial. *J Am Med Assoc* 2018;319:872-882.

    The Strategies for Prescribing Analgesics Comparative Effectiveness trial was a 12-month RCT comparing opioid-based pain regimens with nonopioid-based regimens in patients with moderate to severe chronic back pain or hip or knee osteoarthritis pain. Nonopioid-based therapies were found to be as effective as opioid therapies with regard to pain relief, while demonstrating fewer adverse medication-related symptoms. Level of evidence: I.

25. Toupin April K, Bisaillon J, Welch V, et al: Tramadol for osteoarthritis. *Cochrane Database Syst Rev* 2019;(5):CD005522.

    This 2019 Cochrane database review of 22 RCTs (n = 3,871) evaluated the effect tramadol has on pain. Conclusions suggest the drug has no clinically meaningful impact on pain relief and that a substantially higher amount of patients stop taking this drug as a result of medication-related adverse events. Level of evidence: I.

26. Jung SY, Jang EJ, Nam SW, et al: Comparative effectiveness of oral pharmacologic interventions for knee osteoarthritis: A network meta-analysis. *Mod Rheumatol* 2018;28:1021-1028.

    This systematic review and meta-analysis of 44 studies investigated the therapeutic effect of various oral pharmacologic therapies for knee osteoarthritis. Results demonstrated WOMAC pain scores are most improved with etoricoxib, celecoxib, and aceclofenac. Level of evidence: I.

27. Zeng C, Dubreuil M, Larochelle MR, et al: Association of tramadol with all-cause mortality among patients with osteoarthritis. *J Am Med Assoc* 2019;321:969-982.

    This sequential propensity-matched cohort study of 88,902 patients evaluated all-cause mortality in tramadol, naproxen, diclofenac, celecoxib, etoricoxib, and codeine at 1 year. Tramadol was associated with a significantly higher rate of mortality than NSAIDs, but the rate was not significantly different from codeine. Level of evidence: II.

28. Driesman A, Kaplan D, Feng JE, et al: Tramadol in knee osteoarthritis: Does preoperative use affect patient-reported outcomes after total knee arthroplasty? *J Arthroplasty* 2019;34(8):1662-1666.

    This retrospective study explored the effect of preoperative tramadol use on postoperative outcomes, concluding the drug may result in significantly less improvement in functional outcomes in the short-term postoperative period. Level of evidence: III.

29. Sterner B, Harms M, Wöll S, Weigandt M, Windbergs M, Lehr CM: The effect of polymer size and charge of molecules on permeation through synovial membrane and accumulation in hyaline articular cartilage. *Eur J Pharm Biopharm* 2016;101:126-136.

30. Gerwin N, Hops C, Lucke A: Intraarticular drug delivery in osteoarthritis. *Adv Drug Deliv Rev* 2006;58:226-242.

31. Larsen C, Østergaard J, Larsen SW, et al: Intra-articular depot formulation principles: Role in the management of postoperative pain and arthritic disorders. *J Pharm Sci* 2008;97:4622-4654.

32. Arden NK, Reading IC, Jordan KM, et al: A randomised controlled trial of tidal irrigation vs corticosteroid injection in knee osteoarthritis: The KIVIS Study. *Osteoarthr Cartil* 2008;16:733-739.

33. Wernecke C, Braun HJ, Dragoo JL: The effect of intra-articular corticosteroids on articular cartilage: A systematic review. *Orthop J Sports Med* 2015;3:2325967115581163.

34. Twu J, Patel N, Wolf JM, Conti Mica M: Impact of variation of corticosteroid dose, injection site, and multiple injections on blood glucose measurement in diabetic patients. *J Hand Surg Am* 2018;43:738-744.

    Seventy patients were enrolled in a prospective study evaluating the effect of corticosteroid injections on blood glucose. Only those receiving injections within the knee joint demonstrated significantly higher increases in fasting blood glucose, whereas preoperative hemoglobin A1c was positively correlated with increase in postinjection glucose levels. Level of evidence: II.

35. Ayhan E, Kesmezacar H, Akgun I: Intraarticular injections (corticosteroid, hyaluronic acid, platelet rich plasma) for the knee osteoarthritis. *World J Orthop* 2014;5:351-361.

36. Garg N, Perry L, Deodhar A: Intra-articular and soft tissue injections, a systematic review of relative efficacy of various corticosteroids. *Clin Rheumatol* 2014;33:1695-1706.

37. Kraus VB, Conaghan PG, Aazami HA, et al: Synovial and systemic pharmacokinetics (PK) of triamcinolone acetonide (TA) following intra-articular (IA) injection of an extended-release microsphere-based formulation (FX006) or standard crystalline suspension in patients with knee osteoarthritis (OA). *Osteoarthr Cartil* 2018;26:34-42.

    Eighty-one patients were enrolled in this phase 2 open-label study analyzing pharmacokinetics of the microsphere-based formulation of triamcinolone acetonide in comparison with triamcinolone acetonide crystalline formulation. The extended-release version demonstrated prolonged joint residency and reduced systemic exposure than the traditional crystalline formulation. Level of evidence: II.

38. Langworthy MJ, Conaghan PG, Ruane JJ, et al: Efficacy of triamcinolone acetonide extended-release in participants with unilateral knee osteoarthritis: A post hoc analysis. *Adv Ther* 2019;36:1398-1411.

    This phase 3 study compared the extended-release formulation of triamcinolone acetonide with crystalline-based triamcinolone acetonide and a saline-placebo in patients with knee osteoarthritis. Results demonstrated the extended-release formulation consistently provided superior levels of pain relief for 5 to 6 months. Level of evidence: I.

39. Russell SJ, Sala R, Conaghan PG, et al: Triamcinolone acetonide extended-release in patients with osteoarthritis and type 2 diabetes: A randomized, phase 2 study. *Rheumatology (Oxford)* 2018;57:2235-2241.

    This double-blind, randomized, phase 2 study investigated the effect of microsphere-based triamcinolone acetonide on glucose levels in comparison with that of the crystalline formulation of triamcinolone acetonide, finding the microsphere formulation demonstrating a smaller mean glucose change postinjection. Level of evidence: I.

40. Bannuru RR, Vaysbrot EE, Sullivan MC, McAlindon TE: Relative efficacy of hyaluronic acid in comparison with NSAIDs for knee osteoarthritis: A systematic review and meta-analysis. *Semin Arthritis Rheum* 2014;43:593-599.

41. Bannuru RR, Natov NS, Obadan IE, Price LL, Schmid CH, McAlindon TE: Therapeutic trajectory of hyaluronic acid versus corticosteroids in the treatment of knee osteoarthritis: A systematic review and meta-analysis. *Arthritis Care Res* 2009;61:1704-1711.

42. Hall MP, Band PA, Meislin RJ, Jazrawi LM, Cardone DA: Platelet-rich plasma: Current concepts and application in sports medicine. *J Am Acad Orthop Surg* 2009;17:602-608.

43. Shen L, Yuan T, Chen S, Xie X, Zhang C: The temporal effect of platelet-rich plasma on pain and physical function in the treatment of knee osteoarthritis: Systematic review and meta-analysis of randomized controlled trials. *J Orthop Surg Res* 2017;12:16.

This systematic review and meta-analysis of 14 RCTs (n = 1,423) evaluated various controls in comparison with PRP, finding the treatment to possibly be superior to all controls at 3, 6, and 12 months posttherapy. Level of evidence: I.

44. Delanois RE, Etcheson JI, Sodhi N, et al: Biologic therapies for the treatment of knee osteoarthritis. *J Arthroplasty* 2019;34:801-813.

This systematic review of biologic therapies (PRP and MSC injections) determined the modalities to improve pain and function. However, much of the published literature available for analysis is limited and higher powered studies are needed. Level of evidence: I.

45. Jayaram P, Ikpeama U, Rothenberg JB, Malanga GA: Bone marrow–derived and adipose-derived mesenchymal stem cell therapy in primary knee osteoarthritis: A narrative review. *PM R* 2019;11(2):177-191.

This level IV narrative review of 34 studies investigated MSCs of various origins, demonstrating the therapy to have an excellent safety profile and significant improvements in pain and function. Level of evidence: IV.

46. Migliorini F, Rath B, Colarossi G, et al: Improved outcomes after mesenchymal stem cells injections for knee osteoarthritis: Results at 12-months follow-up. A systematic review of the literature. *Arch Orthop Trauma Surg* 2020;140(7):853-868.

Eighteen studies were incorporated for this systematic review analyzing MSC injections of various origins. Pain scores, function scores, and quality of life all demonstrated improvements at 6- and 12-month intervals regardless of cell source. Level of evidence: I.

47. Lamo-Espinosa JM, Mora G, Blanco JF, et al: Intra-articular injection of two different doses of autologous bone marrow mesenchymal stem cells versus hyaluronic acid in the treatment of knee osteoarthritis: Long-term follow up of a multicenter randomized controlled clinical trial (phase I/II). *J Transl Med* 2018;16(1):213.

This RCT compared 4-year clinical and functional outcomes in 30 individuals randomized into treatment arms of hyaluronic acid only, hyaluronic acid plus low-dose MSCs (10×10^6 cells), or hyaluronic acid plus high-dose MSCs (100×10^6 cells). The addition of MSCs to hyaluronic acid significantly improved both clinical and functional outcomes. Level of evidence: I.

48. Wise BL, Niu J, Yang M, et al: Patterns of compartment involvement in tibiofemoral osteoarthritis in men and women and in whites and African Americans. *Arthritis Care Res* 2012;64:847-852.

49. Wylie JD, Jones DL, Hartley MK, et al: Distal femoral osteotomy for the valgus knee: Medial closing wedge versus lateral opening wedge. A systematic review. *Arthroscopy* 2016;32:2141-2147.

50. Wang Z, Zeng Y, She W, Luo X, Cai L: Is opening-wedge high tibial osteotomy superior to closing-wedge high tibial osteotomy in treatment of unicompartmental osteoarthritis? A meta-analysis of randomized controlled trials. *Int J Surg* 2018;60:153-163.

This meta-analysis of nine RCTs compared closing-wedge with opening-wedge HTO in patients with isolated unicompartmental osteoarthritis. Clinical outcomes, complication rates, and survival rates demonstrated no difference between the two approaches. Level of evidence: I.

CHAPTER 14

Nonarthroplasty Management of the Hip Including Joint-Preserving Surgery

ELIZABETH G. LIEBERMAN, MD • JOHN C. CLOHISY, MD

ABSTRACT

The field of hip preservation has grown substantially in recent years because of increased understanding of abnormal hip morphologies as well as technical innovations in diagnosis and treatment. Diagnostic tools, including physical examination, radiography, CT, and MRI, can safely identify hip pathology before the development of advanced osteoarthritis. Nonarthroplasty surgical techniques, such as hip arthroscopy, surgical dislocation, and periacetabular osteotomy, have been shown to reduce pain, restore joint kinematics, and improve outcomes in young or very active patients. There is increasing evidence supporting the durability of these procedures, which can delay or even avoid the need for hip arthroplasty. It is important to also be aware of nonsurgical treatments, such as stem cell therapies, platelet-rich plasma, long-acting intra-articular corticosteroid injections, and nerve blockade therapies, which are rapidly advancing and becoming increasingly available to patients.

Keywords: dysplasia; impingement; labral tear; periacetabular osteotomy

Dr. Clohisy or an immediate family member has received royalties from Microport; serves as a paid consultant to or is an employee of Microport Orthopedics, Inc. and Zimmer; and has received research or institutional support from Department of Defense Grant and Zimmer. Neither Dr. Lieberman nor any immediate family member has received anything of value from or has stock or stock options held in a commercial company or institution related directly or indirectly to the subject of this chapter.

INTRODUCTION

The morphology and pathologic variants of the hip have been examined extensively in recent years, leading to improved understanding of abnormal patterns associated with hip pain, dysfunction, and accelerated degeneration. These abnormalities can be broadly grouped into categories, including impingement, instability, residual childhood deformity, and soft-tissue conditions. Nonarthroplasty surgical options for many of these problems are advancing with evidence supporting good outcomes. The number of surgeons performing hip arthroscopy, surgical hip dislocation, and periacetabular osteotomy (PAO) has grown, increasing the accessibility of these procedures to patients. Given this, understanding the indications for nonarthroplasty hip-preserving surgery as well as the expected outcomes of these procedures is essential.

FEMOROACETABULAR IMPINGEMENT

Etiology

Femoroacetabular impingement (FAI) syndrome is a dynamic disorder of the hip, with symptoms that result from repetitive abnormal contact of the proximal femur and the acetabulum.[1] There are two broad categories of morphologies causing impingement that have been described: cam type and pincer type. The cam type is described as an aspherical femoral head or decreased concavity of the femoral head-neck junction, which can impinge at the acetabular rim causing damage to the acetabular cartilage and/or labrum as the hip moves into flexion. The pincer type is caused by acetabular overcoverage, often due to either acetabular retroversion or acetabular protrusio. These processes are dynamic and can exist independently or combined. FAI is theorized to be a precursor to osteoarthritis, which develops secondary to bony deformity and abnormal motion leading to cartilage damage. The etiology of FAI remains under investigation. Genetic factors may play a role in development or susceptibility to develop FAI, but genetic transmission has not yet been proven. Prevalence studies have identified higher rates of FAI in athletes, suggesting an acquired component to FAI pathology.[2] A patient may also report a history of Legg-Calve-Perthes disease or slipped capital femoral epiphysis, which are possible causes of FAI. In a systematic review, the authors found 37% prevalence of radiographic cam deformity and 67% prevalence of radiographic pincer deformity in asymptomatic individuals.[2] Given the large proportion of the normal population who have radiographic abnormalities consistent with FAI, correlation with clinical history and physical examination is paramount in diagnosis and treatment.

Presentation and Examination

Patients with FAI are often young and active and present with insidious onset of pain usually in the groin. Pain may also be reported in the lateral hip, anterior thigh, buttock, knee, lower back, or lateral and posterior thigh.[3] Pain may be referred or multifactorial in origin and is typically aggravated by activity or prolonged sitting. Physical examination is paramount to diagnosis because there is high variability in the association of symptom severity and degree of morphologic abnormality. In addition to pain, patients may also describe clicking, catching, locking, stiffness, or giving way.[1] Examination should include observation of gait, hip range of motion and strength, and palpation for tenderness. Patients with FAI may have antalgic or pain-avoiding gait as well as loss of motion, especially flexion and internal rotation. Clinical examination maneuvers have been described, which are aimed at provoking intra-articular hip pathology. These include FABER (flexion, abduction, external rotation), FADIR (flexion adduction internal rotation), and Stinchfield test (resisted hip flexion). The FADIR and FABER tests have been found to be sensitive for FAI, but not specific. Evidence supporting the diagnostic accuracy of clinical tests is limited because of lack of study heterogeneity and uniformity.[1,3]

Imaging

Image evaluation in suspected FAI begins with radiographs including an AP pelvis and orthogonal view of the femoral neck (cross-table lateral, Dunn, or frog lateral). The AP radiograph should be examined for all potentially painful conditions, including fracture, acetabular dysplasia, and osteoarthritis. An ideal radiograph will be centered on the pubic symphysis, have symmetric obturator foramina indicating no rotation, and will have neutral pelvic tilt.[4] The shape of the acetabulum can be interpreted from the AP radiograph, which is particularly helpful in identifying pincer deformity. Common signs of pincer, or acetabular, overcoverage include a crossover sign, ischial spine sign, negative Tönnis angle (<0°), and lateral center-edge angle (LCEA) greater than 40°.[4] Coxa profunda has been previously described as an indicator of pincer-type deformity; however, newer research identified it as a common finding in asymptomatic individuals, especially females. Additionally, there is low correlation between coxa profunda and other radiographic signs of impingement; thus, it should not be considered a sign of impingement when found in isolation.[5]

Lateral views of the proximal femur are useful for assessment of joint space, anterior acetabular coverage, and the head-neck junction. The false profile view is useful for assessment of joint space, anterior acetabular coverage, and the subspine region. Cross-table and frog lateral images provide good views of the anterior head-neck junction. The 45° Dunn view is particularly helpful in assessing the anterolateral head-neck junction where cam deformity is often identified. With this view, an alpha angle can be calculated to quantify the cam deformity; alpha angle greater than 55° is often viewed as a threshold value consistent with cam morphology.

Plain radiography cannot fully characterize the three-dimensional morphology of the hip. Therefore, if FAI is suspected based on history, examination, and radiography, a cross-sectional examination, such as CT and/or MRI can be obtained. MRI is the examination of choice to identify abnormalities of the labrum, cartilage, joint space, subchondral bone, and soft tissue surrounding the hip joint. The alpha angle was first described as a measurement from an axial-oblique plane of the femoral neck; however, it has been shown that radial views provide a more complete field of vision to quantify the cam deformity.[6] In orthopaedic literature, the threshold value for the alpha angle is typically 50° to 55°. However, one study found high variability (up to 10°) based on the position or cut the angle is measured from. This study also found abnormal alpha angles in many asymptomatic volunteers; thus, these measurements should be interpreted in the context of other clinical factors with caution to avoid overdiagnosis.[6]

CT, including three-dimensional reformatting, can provide better understanding of focal morphologic abnormalities in cam and pincer FAI. CT data can also be used to print to scale three-dimensional models, which can influence surgical planning for FAI. Another application for MRI and CT includes examination of femoral version, which has been recognized as a potential contributing factor to FAI. In both MRI and CT, femoral version can be reliably measured by obtaining limited images of the distal femoral condyles.[7] There are concerns about radiation exposure from CT scans, especially in adolescent patients. However, recent advances in technology and imaging protocols have led to low-dose CT imaging protocols, which have been shown to reduce radiation exposure up to 90% compared with traditional hip CT scan protocols.[8]

CHONDRAL INJURY

Intra-articular cartilage lesions are common in patients with FAI and can also occur with hip conditions, including dysplasia, osteonecrosis, trauma, or dislocation, and sequelae of childhood conditions, such as slipped capital femoral epiphysis (SCFE) or Legg-Calve-Perthes disease. The pattern and location of articular wear is dependent on hip morphology. More frequent and severe articular damage has been shown in patients with cam or mixed impingement compared with pincer.[9] Chondral lesions are most frequently located in the anterosuperior acetabulum and are frequently associated with a labral tear.[10] The etiology of cartilage injury in patients with cam-type FAI is thought to be due to shearing forces across the articular surfaces from an aspherical femoral head that impinges on the acetabular rim as it forces itself into the acetabulum. The authors of a recent study[11] refer to this as an outside-in mechanism of chondral damage because there is disruption first at the anterosuperior chondrolabral junction, which results in a debonding of cartilage from the chondrolabral junction and progressive delamination from subchondral bone (**Figures 1** and **2**). This differs from inside-out cartilage wear patterns in the dysplastic hip, which result from superior migration of the femoral head resulting in more central articular shearing that advances outward with progressive disease (**Figures 3** and **4**). Pincer-type FAI usually presents with relatively maintained articular cartilage, and the increased force is applied around the acetabular rim, resulting in labral hypoplasia, osseous metaplasia, and damage mainly confined to the rim.[11]

The current benchmark imaging modalities for evaluation of hip chondral damage include plain radiography and magnetic resonance arthrography (MRA). Pooled data from multiple studies comparing conventional MRI and MRA show that although specificity is generally high (94% and 86%, respectively), sensitivity of both modalities remains low (59% and 62%, respectively).[12] Advances in imaging technology have shown promising results in improving diagnostic accuracy. 3T conventional MRI has been found to have 94% sensitivity and 100% (femoral) and 67% (acetabular) specificity in diagnosing chondral and labral injury.[13] Advanced MRI techniques, including delayed gadolinium-enhanced MRI of cartilage and T1 rho mapping, have been shown to be sensitive in detecting early osteoarthritis through identifying molecular changes in cartilage, which may be present before the morphologic changes that are detected in traditional radiography.[12] Another potential tool for identifying cartilage pathology is the use of biomarkers, such as cartilage oligomeric matrix protein, C-reactive protein, or fibronectin-aggrecan complex. Increased levels of these inflammatory markers and cartilage breakdown products have been shown to correlate with symptomatic cartilage breakdown and may be useful in identifying pathology and predicting outcomes for patients with FAI.[12]

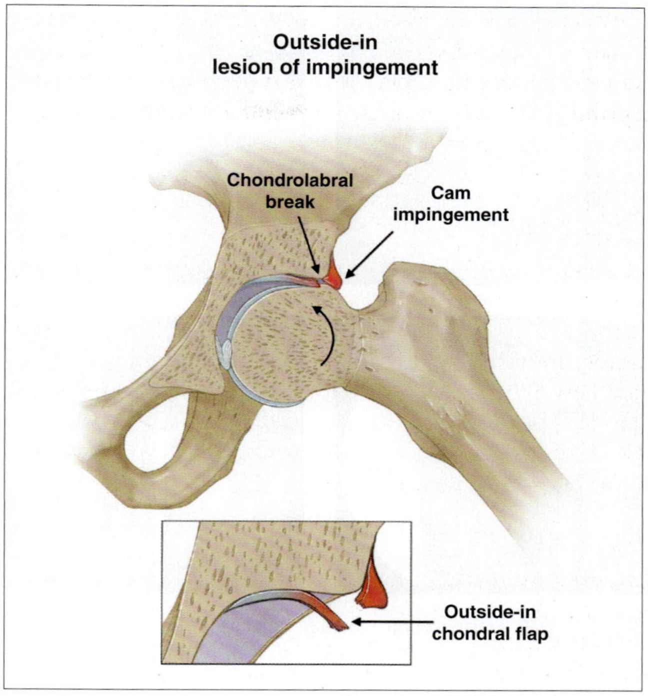

FIGURE 1 Schematic drawing of a left hip and pelvis demonstrating cam impingement and the pathomechanics underlying the development of an outside-in acetabular chondral flap (inset). The outside-in designation is made for centrally anchored flaps exhibiting a break in the chondrolabral junction. (Reprinted with permission from Kraeutler MJ, Goodrich JA, Fioravanti MJ, Garabekyan T, Mei-Dan O: The "outside-in" lesion of hip impingement and the "inside-out" lesion of hip dysplasia: two distinct patterns of acetabular chondral injury. *J Sports Med* 2019;47(12): 2978-2984. Copyright © 2019, © SAGE Publications.)

There are multiple classification systems described for intraoperative grading of chondral injury; the most commonly referenced are detailed in **Table 1**.[14] These classification systems can help guide surgical treatment and have shown correlation between chondral lesion severity and long-term success after joint-preserving treatments.

LABRAL TEAR

In recent years, interest and understanding of the acetabular labrum has increased significantly; however, the function and consequences of labral injury are still not fully understood. The labrum is a fibrocartilaginous

Section 1: Hip and Knee

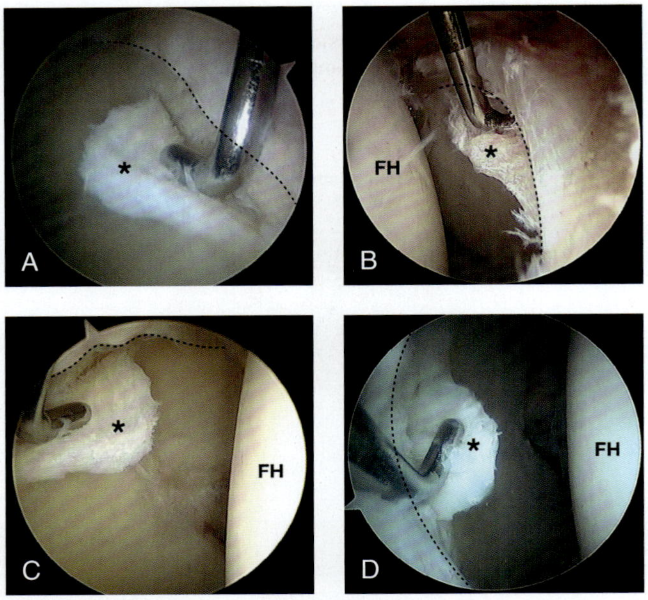

FIGURE 2 Arthroscopic views of two right hips (**A** and **B**) and two left hips (**C** and **D**) with cam impingement demonstrating different cases of the outside-in chondral flap with a break in the chondrolabral junction. The asterisk indicates the outside-in flap, and the dashed line indicates the chondrolabral junction. FH = femoral head. (Reprinted with permission from Kraeutler MJ, Goodrich JA, Fioravanti MJ, Garabekyan T, Mei-Dan O: The "outside-in" lesion of hip impingement and the "inside-out" lesion of hip dysplasia: two distinct patterns of acetabular chondral injury. *J Sports Med* 2019;47(12):2978-2984. Copyright © 2019, © SAGE Publications.)

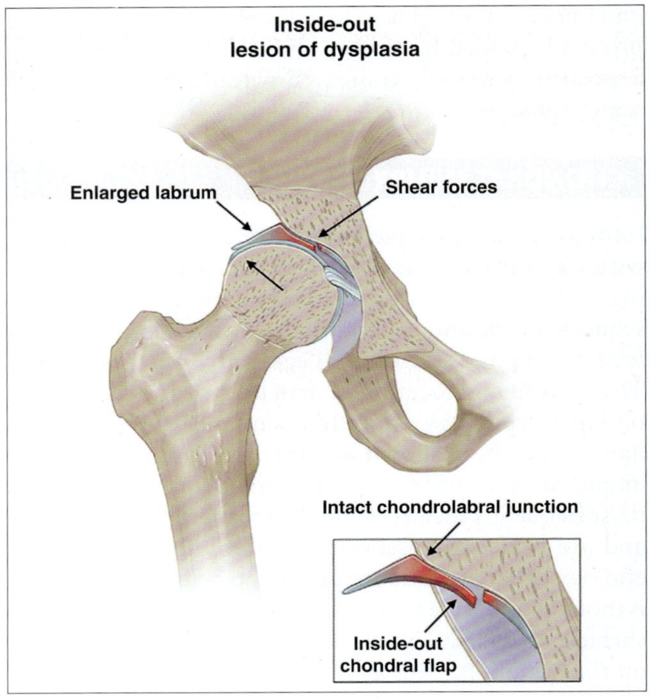

FIGURE 3 Schematic drawing of a dysplastic right hip and pelvis demonstrating the pathomechanics underlying the development of an inside-out acetabular chondral flap (inset). The inside-out flap is characterized by an intact chondrolabral junction with a detached sleeve of chondrolabral tissue from the central acetabulum. (Reprinted with permission from Kraeutler MJ, Goodrich JA, Fioravanti MJ, Garabekyan T, Mei-Dan O: The "outside-in" lesion of hip impingement and the "inside-out" lesion of hip dysplasia: two distinct patterns of acetabular chondral injury. *J Sports Med* 2019;47(12): 2978-2984. Copyright © 2019, © SAGE Publications.)

structure, which joins the transverse acetabular ligament, forming a continuous ring around the rim of the acetabulum (**Figure 5**). Unlike in the shoulder, there is no capsulolabral complex in the hip; the capsule attaches to the rim of the acetabulum, separate from the labrum. In the hip, the labrum functions as a seal, maintaining a layer of cartilage protective pressurized synovial fluid. It also maintains hip stability through a suction effect created between the acetabulum and femoral head and increases the contact area of the hip joint, reducing contact pressure. A histologic study found the labrum to contain nerve fibers with nociceptive and proprioceptive function, suggesting the labrum may be a source of hip pain when injured.[15]

Labral tears are most commonly associated with cam-type and pincer-type FAI and are also found in hips with dysplasia, hips subject to repetitive extremes of motion, such as in ballet dancers, and following trauma or dislocation. Patients typically report insidious onset of activity-related groin, anterior thigh, or lateral hip pain. In a study reviewing presenting symptoms, the authors found approximately one-half of patients reported mechanical symptoms, including snapping, popping, or locking, and 89% of patients reported limping.[16] Imaging evaluation of the acetabular labrum includes plain radiography and MRI for evaluation of cartilage injury. There are normal anatomic variants of the labrum, including a sublabral sulcus, which may be mistaken for a tear. Labral tears appear as intrasubstance signal and may be full thickness if the contrast extends to the articular surface or degenerative if it does not. Paralabral cysts and cartilage delamination can occur in conjunction with labral tears and may be visualized with MRI techniques.

MANAGEMENT

The management of FAI should be directed based on the etiology of impingement (cam or pincer) and associated pathology, such as chondral injury or labral tear. Before surgical treatments, nonsurgical measures, including activity modification, physical therapy, nonsteroidal anti-inflammatory medications, and intra-articular injections, should be considered. In a recently published randomized, multicenter clinical trial, the authors found

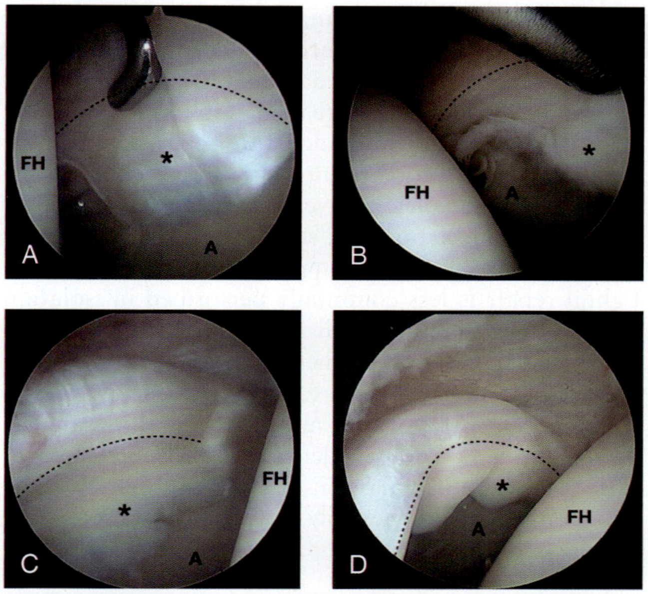

FIGURE 4 Arthroscopic views of (**A** and **B**) two left and (**C** and **D**) two right dysplastic hips demonstrating different cases of the inside-out chondral flap with intact chondrolabral junction. The asterisk indicates the inside-out flap, and the dashed line indicates the chondrolabral junction. A = acetabulum, FH = femoral head. (Reprinted with permission from Kraeutler MJ, Goodrich JA, Fioravanti MJ, Garabekyan T, Mei-Dan O: The "outside-in" lesion of hip impingement and the "inside-out" lesion of hip dysplasia: two distinct patterns of acetabular chondral injury. *J Sports Med* 2019;47(12):2978-2984. Copyright © 2019, © SAGE Publications.)

significant improvement in outcomes in patients who underwent hip arthroscopy compared with best conservative care.[17] The improvement in patient-reported outcomes exceeded the minimum clinically important difference at 12 months after randomization, leading the study authors to conclude that hip arthroscopy is clinically more effective than conservative care, including personalized hip therapy.

Surgical management of FAI may be performed arthroscopically, open, or combined. With advancing technology, evolving indications, and increased surgeon training, there has been an exponential increase in hip arthroscopy surgery in the United States and worldwide. According to a US database study, incidence of hip arthroscopies increased from 3.6 per 100,000 in 2005 to 16.7 per 100,000 in 2013 (465% increase).[18] In patients with FAI, hip arthroscopy has become standard surgical technique for most cases and can be used to address osseous lesions, labral tears, and chondral pathology. The most common reason for revision hip preservation surgery after hip arthroscopy is residual FAI deformity.[19] Intraoperative fluoroscopy techniques can help identify bony deformity and evaluate correction. When resecting cam deformity, the goal is to remove impinging bone while preserving perfusing retinacular vessels. Acetabuloplasty to address pincer deformity can reduce contact between the acetabular rim and femoral neck; however, resection of more than 4 to 6 mm has been shown to alter hip biomechanics and can lead to chondrolabral degeneration.[20]

TABLE 1

Classification Systems for Intraoperative Grading of Macroscopic Chondral Injury

Classification	Grade	Description
Outerbridge	0	Macroscopically normal cartilage
	1	Cartilage softening and swelling
	2	Fragmentation and fissuring involving area <1.5 cm in diameter
	3	Fragmentation and fissuring involving area >1.5 cm in diameter
	4	Loss of cartilage and exposed subchondral bone
Beck	0	Macroscopically normal cartilage
	1	Malacia: Roughening of surface, fibrillation
	2	Pitting malacia: Roughening, partially thinning and full-thickness defects or deep fissuring to bone
	3	Debonding: Loss of fixation to subchondral bone, macroscopically sound cartilage (carpet phenomenon)
	4	Cleavage: Loss of fixation to subchondral bone, frayed edges, thinning of cartilage
	5	Defect: Full-thickness defect
ALAD	0	Macroscopically normal cartilage
	1	Cartilage softening
	2	Early peel back of cartilage
	3	Large flap of cartilage or delamination
	4	Complete loss of cartilage and exposed subchondral bone

ALAD = acetabular labrum articular disruption

Data from El Bitar YF, Linder D, Jackson TJ, Domb BG: Joint-preserving surgical options for management of chondral injuries of the hip. *J Am Acad Orthop Surg* 2014;22(1):46-56.

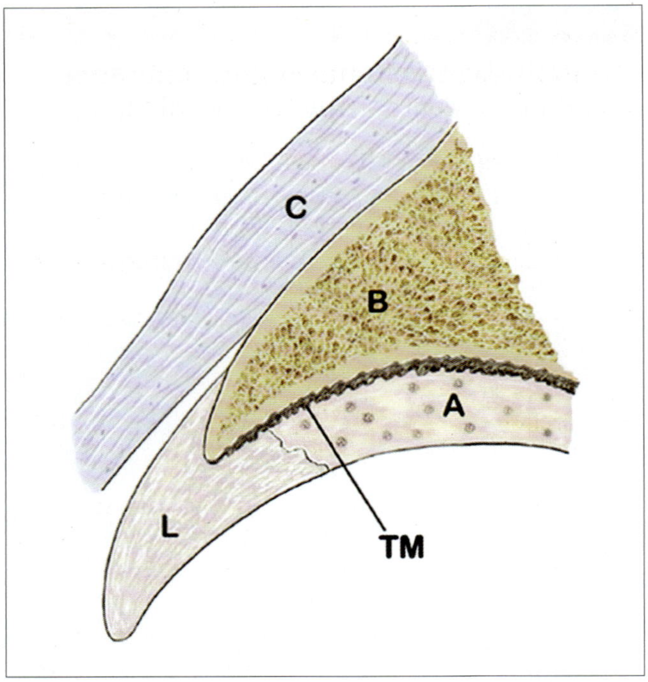

FIGURE 5 Illustration shows the relationship of the acetabular labrum and capsule including the bone of the acetabulum (B), labrum (L), articular cartilage (A), tidemark (TM), and capsule (C). (Reprinted with permission from Byrd JWT: Labral management: An overview, in Byrd JWT, ed: *Operative Hip Arthroscopy*, ed 3. New York, NY, Springer, 2012, pp 171-184. © JW Thomas Byrd, MD)

As described in a 2001 study, the surgical hip dislocation can provide circumferential access to the proximal femur and acetabulum.[21] This technique has been shown to be safe and should be used in complex deformity, which cannot be fully managed or assessed via arthroscopy. Combined open and arthroscopic approaches have been described for management of FAI, including a mini-anterior approach, which allows for better visualization of the anterior head-neck junction without having to dislocate the joint.[22]

Treatment options for cartilage lesions can include débridement or chondroplasty, microplasty, or cartilage transplant. The degree of cartilage degeneration is associated with long-term success; focal lesions may be more amenable to joint-preserving treatments. New techniques are emerging, which incorporate orthobiologics, such as autologous chondrocytes, platelet-rich plasma, and mesenchymal stem cells with cartilage transplant. A summary of treatment options and indications[23] is given in **Table 2**. There remains significant controversy regarding management of high-grade acetabular defects. Additional factors, such as etiology of the cartilage lesion, patient comorbidities, examination findings, and coexisting hip pathology, must be taken into consideration when discussing nonarthroplasty treatment for chondral lesions.

Surgical options for managing labral tears include débridement, repair, or reconstruction. The goal of débridement is to remove damaged tissue, while preserving healthy tissue to create a stable transition and decrease risk of further tearing. Historically, débridement has demonstrated good results. However, techniques for labral repair/refixation have advanced, and as repair has become more popular, some studies have variably shown improved results compared with débridement.[24] Labral repair is less commonly performed in isolation and is often combined with acetabuloplasty for pincer deformity. In cases when there is deficient labral tissue for repair or previous failure, labral reconstruction is a viable option. Use of both autograft and allograft has been described without evidence that one source is superior[25] (**Figure 6**). Labral reconstruction has been shown to have noninferior and possibly better outcomes compared with resection and refixation.[25]

OUTCOMES

A recent meta-analysis of 81 studies found improvement in patient-reported outcomes following hip arthroscopy surgery for FAI in 90% of patients studied.[26] Despite these high rates of successful treatment, clinical failures do occur, so it is important to identify risk factors for failure. In patients undergoing joint-preserving procedures for FAI, increasing age and severity of arthritis are associated with worse outcomes and higher rate of progression to arthroplasty.[23] Other potential factors associated with decreased improvement or failure of surgical management of FAI include elevated body mass index, female sex, failure to respond to intra-articular hip injections, and prior ipsilateral surgery. Radiographic measures have been studied to evaluate outcomes following hip arthroscopy for FAI. Reported predictors of negative outcomes include Tönnis grade ≥1, decreased joint space (≤2 mm), LCEA >40°, coxa profunda, acetabular index <3°, excessive femoral retroversion, chondral defects, and increased head-neck offset in the superior femoral neck. Patients with FAI and significant risk factors for failure can be considered for alternate open hip preservation procedures or total hip arthroplasty (THA) if secondary arthritis is advanced.

HIP INSTABILITY (DYSPLASIA)

Etiology

Developmental dysplasia of the hip (DDH) has been identified as one of the leading causes of secondary osteoarthritis.[3] DDH is thought to be a developmental condition with known risk factors including female sex, primiparity, breech position, and family history. Screening for DDH in newborns is routine; however, a significant proportion of cases are not diagnosed until adulthood.

TABLE 2

Summary of Treatment Procedures, Indications, Contraindications, and Notes for Chondral Lesions in the Hip

Procedure	Indications	Contraindications	Comments
Chondroplasty (débridement)	Low-grade, partial-thickness lesions		Radiofrequency ablation should not be performed
Microfracture	Lesions <2-4 cm²	Partial-thickness chondral defects or underlying bony pathology	Take into account the patient's age, activity level, and adherence to postoperative rehabilitation plan
ACI	Lesions too large for microfracture alone		Potential for serious complications if hip dislocation necessary
AMIC	Grades 3 and 4 acetabular chondral defects, 2-4 cm², patients 18-55 yr of age		
MCC in a PRP matrix	Used in conjunction with microfracture		
Intra-articular injections of expanded MSCs	Diffuse chondral damage, mild osteoarthritis, patients seeking a nonarthroplasty treatment		
OAT	Lesions too large for microfracture, subchondral damage, microfracture or abrasion chondroplasty have failed	Patients older than 50 yr, signs of osteoarthritis	Potential for serious complications if hip dislocation necessary
Mosaicplasty	Multiple smaller lesions on the femoral head		Hip dislocation complications possible
OCA transplant	Young patients with osteonecrosis and segmental collapse of the femoral head		Systemic steroids risk for failure in the procedure, hip dislocation complications possible
Fibrin adhesive	Delaminated, viable cartilage (wave or carpet sign)		Suture repair and scaffold implantation lasts longer than fibrin glue alone

ACI = autologous chondrocyte implantation, AMIC = autologous matrix-induced chondrogenesis, MCC in PRP = mononuclear concentrate in a platelet-rich plasma matrix, MSCs = matrix expanded mesenchymal stem cells, OAT = osteochondral autograft transfer, OCA = osteochondral allograft transplant

Reprinted with permission from Dallich AA, Rath E, Atzmon R, Radpavar JR, Fontana A, Sharfman Z, Amar E: Chondral lesions in the hip: A review of relevant anatomy, imaging, and treatment modalities. *J Hip Preserv Surg* 2019;6(1):3-15, by permission of Oxford University Press.

The morphology of DDH is variable and can involve both the acetabulum and femur. The dysplastic acetabulum is typically characterized as having insufficient femoral head coverage and superolateral inclination of the superior acetabular articular surface. This deformity results in structural instability with increased forces and mechanical overloading of the acetabular rim leading to progressive hip destruction. In addition to the dysmorphic acetabulum, there may be abnormalities in the proximal femur in DDH hips. The femoral head is often small and aspheric, whereas the femur may have increased anteversion and a valgus neck-shaft angle. The acetabular labrum may be hypertrophied because of increased load bearing in the unstable hip. Early recognition and surgical correction of morphologic abnormalities can decrease pain, improve function, and decrease risk of osteoarthritis and need for arthroplasty.

Presentation and Examination

Symptomatic dysplasia commonly presents with insidious onset of activity-related groin or lateral hip pain. In one study, patients undergoing surgical treatment for dysplasia were predominately female (72%) and with average age of 24 years at the time of presentation.[27] Typical

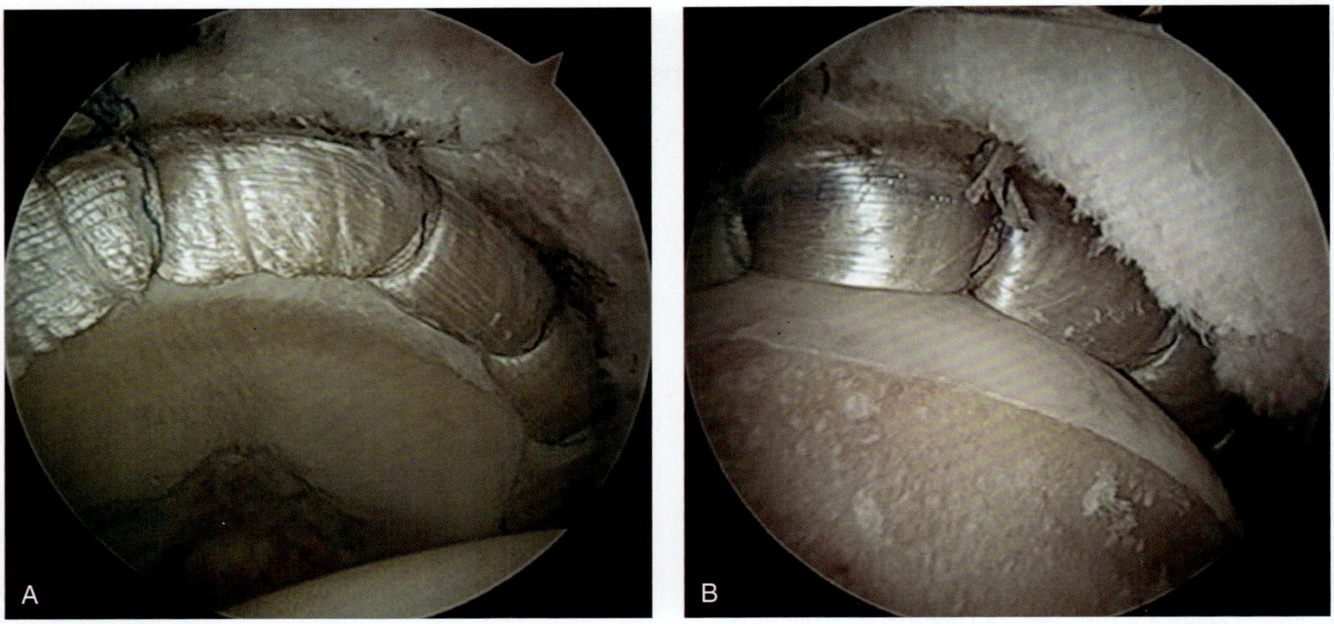

FIGURE 6 Arthroscopic view from the anterolateral portal of the right hip reveals an 8-cm fascia lata allograft fixed with seven anchors. **A**, View with the joint in traction. **B**, View with traction released and the joint reduced demonstrates restoration of the labral seal coapted against the articular surface. (Reprinted from *Arthroscopy* 32[1]. White BJ, Stapleford AB, Hawkes TK, Finger MJ, Herzog MM: Allograft use in arthroscopic labral reconstruction of the hip with front-to-back fixation technique: Minimum 2-year follow up, 26-32. Copyright © 2016 Arthroscopy Association of North America.)

complaints include activity-related groin or lateral hip pain. Examination findings may be variable; however, most patients who have DDH have a positive impingement sign (97%) and often will have a limp (48% to 77%) and positive Trendelenburg sign (38%).[27] Range of motion may be normal, increased, or decreased. Increased range of motion can be secondary to subluxation, whereas limited range of motion in dysplastic patients can indicate combined impingement or underlying arthrosis.

Imaging

Similar to FAI, image evaluation in suspected DDH begins with radiography, including an AP pelvis, false profile view, and orthogonal view of the femoral neck (cross-table lateral, Dunn, or frog lateral).[4] Acetabular depth and inclination can be measured with the LCEA, acetabular index (Tönnis angle), and anterior center-edge angle. There is agreement in current literature that LCEA values <20°, acetabular index <10°, and anterior center-edge angle values <20° are consistent with a diagnosis of structural instability in most cases. Radiographs can also be evaluated for joint congruity and superior subluxation of the femoral head. Shenton line is an arc drawn from the medial aspect of the femoral neck through the superior margin of the obturator foramen and is a reliable and accurate radiographic marker to detect femoral head subluxation.[4]

CT with three-dimensional reconstruction is increasingly being used to characterize morphologic patterns of dysplasia. One study defined three patterns of acetabular deficiency using two-dimensional CT scans: anteriosuperior deficiency (30%), global deficiency (36%), and posterosuperior deficiency (34%).[28] Femoral and acetabular version can also be measured from CT scan, which is critical when planning surgical reorientation. MRI or MRA can provide additional information about chondrolabral pathology as in FAI. Cross-sectional imaging should be obtained in patients with complex deformity to assist with preoperative planning.

Treatment

When left untreated, the structural instability and acetabular rim overload in DDH can lead to progressive hip degeneration. Therefore, surgical interventions, including corrective hip osteotomies as well as open and arthroscopic techniques for chondrolabral pathology, have been proposed for symptomatic hip dysplasia.

PELVIC OSTEOTOMY

In patients with closed triradiate cartilage, the Bernese PAO is the most commonly used surgical procedure for correction of acetabular dysplasia. Indications for PAO include active, physiologically young, and relatively healthy patients with radiographically proven, symptomatic dysplasia. Preexisting arthritis (Tönnis grade 2 or greater), limited range of motion, or comorbidities are considered contraindications for PAO.

The technique for PAO, as described in a 1988 study, included four orthogonal periacetabular cuts.[29] This procedure is performed through one incision, maintains posterior column integrity, preserves the acetabular blood supply, enables powerful multiplanar acetabular reorientation, and provides reliable healing. Surgery is typically performed in a supine position on a radiolucent table using a modified Smith-Petersen approach. Acetabular reduction is performed under intraoperative fluoroscopy. The PAO allows for restoration of femoral head coverage, acetabular inclination, congruency (joint space), acetabular version, and medial translation of the femoral head. The multiplanar correction is technically challenging, and surgeons must pay careful attention to avoid retroversion, which is already present in approximately one in six patients with dysplasia.[30] Secondary impingement may be present following acetabular correction. In this case, femoral head-neck osteochondroplasty may be required. In recent years, modifications to the original technique have been described, including muscle-sparing approaches, multimodal pain management, and concomitant surgeries to address intra-articular pathology, chondrolabral injury, and femoral deformity.[31]

FEMORAL OSTEOTOMY

Patients with hip dysplasia may have coexisting femoral deformity. Most often caused by excessive femoral anteversion, instability due to femoral deformity should be managed with derotational proximal femoral osteotomy. This can be performed independently or in conjunction with periacetabular osteotomy. Additionally, if there is significant coxa valga, a varus correction osteotomy may be performed. Outcomes of combined PAO and proximal femoral osteotomy are similar to those of PAO alone.[32]

Hip arthroscopy alone for management of DDH is associated with poor outcomes. However, there may be a role of hip arthroscopy combined with PAO. Patients with dysplasia who undergo PAO have high reported prevalence of intra-articular pathology, which may lead to continued symptoms if not addressed during correction of the bony deformity.[33] Arthroscopy allows for a less invasive approach to address intra-articular pathology compared with open arthrotomy. When comparing PAO and hip arthroscopy with PAO alone, authors have found similar improvements in outcomes scores and no increase in complication rates with minimum 5-year follow-up.[33]

OUTCOMES

There are reports of favorable midterm and long-term outcomes when PAO is performed by experienced surgeons for management of symptomatic hip dysplasia. Results in 135 hips (109 patients) were available for retrospective review at an average of 9 years postoperatively, with clinical failure defined as conversion to THA or a pain score of 10 or more. Survivorship, using conversion to THA as the end point, was 96% at 5 years and 84% at 10 years.[34] Using the same survivorship criteria, a separate study reported 92% survival rate at 15 years in patients undergoing PAO at a single institution.[35] In a study examining 20-year outcomes of 68 hips after PAO, survival was reported at 75% in hips with a preoperative Tönnis grade of 0 or 1; however, when the same 68 hips were followed up for another 10 years, survival decreased to 29%. In 71% of hips, arthritis had developed, significant pain was reported, or THA had been performed.[36] Risk factors for poor outcomes are similar among these studies and include older patients, lower preoperative function scores, positive impingement test, and poor joint congruency.[34,36] Another retrospective review of 39 hips with preoperative University of California at Los Angeles activity scores of 7 or greater evaluated patients for return to high-level athletic activity following PAO. Most patients reported satisfaction following surgery (97%), and 71% reported return to presurgical or higher activity level after surgery.[37] The Academic Network of Conservational Hip Outcomes Research reported their combined experience with PAO performed by experienced surgeons and found the procedure to be safe with approximately 6% complication rate. The most common complications were asymptomatic heterotopic ossification and lateral femoral cutaneous nerve dysesthesia. Other reported complications include peroneal nerve palsy, infection, thromboembolic complication, nonunion, and hardware complication.[36] The Academic Network of Conservational Hip Outcomes Research group recently published a report of minimum 2-year follow-up from the first 391 patients enrolled in this multicenter study cohort and found clinically important improvements in pain, function, and quality of life with high (93%) patient satisfaction following surgery.[38] Indications and negative prognostic factors for PAO are detailed in **Table 3**.

RESIDUAL CHILDHOOD DEFORMITIES

SCFE and Legg-Calve-Perthes disease (Perthes) are childhood hip conditions, which can result in residual deformity and accelerated arthritis. In SCFE, there is typically a prominent anterior femoral metaphysis. Clinical observations and mechanical modeling have shown anterior impaction leading to cartilage damage and labral tears.

TABLE 3

Indications and Negative Prognostic Factors for Bernese Periacetabular Osteotomy

Indications	Negative Prognostic Factors
Lateral central-edge angle <20°, acetabular index >10°, anterior center-edge angle <18°	Obesity (body mass index >30 kg/m²)
Adequate range of motion (flexion >95°, abduction >30°)	Secondary arthritis (Tönnis grade ≥2)
Active and healthy	Medical comorbidities
Physiologically young (<35 yr)	Previous reconstructive surgery
Severe or secondary dysplasia	Suboptimal joint congruity
Acetabular retroversion	Poor preoperative hip function

This form of impingement leads to a levering of the femoral head posteriorly, and there is high prevalence of posterior wear and labral tearing in SCFE compared with idiopathic FAI.[39] Patients presenting with the sequelae of SCFE are often young and may have significant cartilage damage at the time of presentation. Surgical treatment options include arthroscopic surgery for mild to moderate deformities, realignment osteotomies for major deformities with preserved cartilage, or arthroplasty for patients with advanced cartilage wear.

Perthes deformity can result in femoral head abnormalities, including coxa magna, coxa vara, and coxa plana, as well as secondary acetabular dysplasia or retroversion. These deformities may result in impingement, instability, or both. Additionally, osteochondral lesions may result directly from vascular insult. Long-term observational studies have shown high rates of development of osteoarthritis in patients with childhood Perthes deformity. Surgical options for post-Perthes deformity include trochanteric advancement with relative femoral neck lengthening, femoral head reduction, osteochondroplasty of the femoral head-neck junction, or acetabular osteotomy, depending on the deformity. Joint-preserving procedures have higher rates of failure in patients with sequelae of Perthes deformity compared with surgical correction for other hip pathology. However, in one study, authors studied surgical dislocation combined with PAO for symptomatic Perthes deformity and found 87.5% patients had significant improvement in reported outcomes following surgery.[40] Patients who have sequelae of SCFE or Perthes deformity often have complex morphologic deformity; therefore, it is essential to consider symptoms, hip range of motion, radiographic measurements, cartilage assessment, and goals of treatment. With careful preoperative planning, surgical hip dislocation, femoral, and acetabular osteotomies can result in durable pain relief and improved function in these patients.[27]

SOFT-TISSUE CONDITIONS

General

In patients who present with a painful hip without obvious bony abnormality, soft-tissue conditions must be included in the differential diagnosis. Advances in ultrasonography, MRI, and hip arthroscopy have led to improved understanding of the functional anatomy of the hip. Soft-tissue pathology may be isolated or present in conjunction with dysplasia or FAI. Most of it can be managed with nonsurgical treatments, including rest, NSAIDs, physical therapy, and steroid injections, with surgery reserved for refractory cases.

Ligamentum Teres Rupture

Historically, the ligamentum teres has been thought of as a vestigial structure; however, investigations have identified it as a potential secondary hip stabilizer and possible pain generator.[41] The ligamentum teres is a pyramidal-shaped structure, which originates from the acetabular fossa and inserts on the fovea capitis of the femoral head. Its role as a stabilizer of the hip is controversial. In a cadaver study, the authors found ultimate failure at 204 N and after approximately 15 mm of elongation. This suggests injury is unlikely during routine joint distraction for hip arthroscopy.[42] It has been proposed that microinstability and altered contact forces from ligamentum teres disruption can result in progressive cartilage wear.[43] Risk factors for ligamentum teres tear include older age and abnormal acetabular bony morphology: dysplasia or FAI. Patients may present with variable symptoms; however, most often the patients complain of hip or groin pain and instability. Evaluation of the ligamentum teres may be with MRI or with direct visualization at the time of hip arthroscopy. Injury can be classified according to the classification described in a 1997 study, which includes three groups: complete tear, partial tear, or degenerate tear.[44] Treatment for ligamentum teres rupture includes débridement versus reconstruction. Ligamentum teres débridement has been shown to result in improved outcomes in patients who have tendinopathy or partial tearing. In patients who have complete tears, reconstruction using synthetic grafts, autografts, or allografts may be considered. Data to support ligamentum teres reconstruction are limited and warrant further investigation.[45]

TROCHANTERIC BURSITIS

Trochanteric bursitis is a common cause of lateral hip pain. Other symptoms include pain with direct palpation, pain laying on the affected side, and sometimes snapping of the iliotibial band. Diagnosis of trochanteric bursitis is typically clinical, with imaging to rule out other causes of hip pain. MRI or ultrasonography are not necessary for diagnosis, but may show increased signal or fluid within the trochanteric bursa. Nonsurgical modalities result in resolution of symptoms for most patients and may include rest, activity modification, anti-inflammatory medication, physical therapy including abductor strengthening, and steroid injections. Alternative therapies, including slow-wave therapy and platelet-rich plasma, have also been described. In patients who have persistent symptoms, surgical options include open or arthroscopic bursectomy, iliotibial band release, or gluteal muscle repair. In a series of 25 patients with recalcitrant trochanteric bursitis who underwent arthroscopic bursectomy and iliotibial band release, improvements were noted in physical function (54 versus 33.6) and pain (51.5 versus 28.7) on Medical Outcomes Study 36-Item Short Form subscale scores and on the Harris Hip Score (77 versus 51) at a minimum follow-up of 13 months.[46]

ILIOPSOAS TENDON DISORDERS

The iliopsoas muscle is a hip flexor muscle, which acts as a secondary stabilizer of the hip. The iliopsoas tendon is a conjoint tendon of the psoas major and iliacus muscles; however, there is significant anatomic variability in the size, location, and number of tendinous components. The variable anatomy of the iliopsoas tendon can result in multiple pathologic conditions, including iliopsoas bursitis, tendinitis, impingement, or snapping. Patients who have iliopsoas conditions typically present with anterior groin pain. They may report painful snapping sensations, which are reproduced moving the leg into extension from a position of flexion, abduction, and external rotation.[47] Clinical examination is paramount in the diagnosis of iliopsoas disorders. Other workup should include radiography to rule out bony abnormality. Ultrasonography can be useful in obtaining dynamic evaluation when snapping is suspected. MRI can be used to evaluate acute traumatic injury, bursal inflammation, or tendinopathy. The first line in managing iliopsoas conditions is usually nonsurgical and includes rest, activity modification, anti-inflammatory medications, and physical therapy. Steroid injections may be used as treatment or to aid in diagnosis. Surgical options for patients in whom nonsurgical management fails include open versus arthroscopic iliopsoas tendon release or lengthening. Multiple surgical techniques have been described, including fractional lengthening versus complete release, which may be performed at the level of the labrum, via a transcapsular approach through the central compartment, or at the level of tendon insertion on the lesser trochanter.[48] Surgical treatment has been shown to improve pain and is associated with positive outcomes; however, there are high rates of recurrence and significant concern for postoperative hip flexor weakness and/or hip instability.[49] Therefore, surgery is rarely indicated and should be strictly reserved for patients who have trialed prolonged nonsurgical treatment, have normal bony anatomy, and have consistent signs and symptoms.

SUMMARY

FAI and hip dysplasia are relatively common conditions, which can cause pain in young adults. These structural abnormalities may lead to labral tears and cartilage injury, which can predispose individuals to premature arthritis. Other causes of hip pain, including soft-tissue conditions and sequelae of childhood deformity, must be also be considered in the painful hip. Examination of gait, range of motion, and pain location can help localize pathology. Imaging techniques, including plain radiography, MRI/MRA, and CT, also aid in diagnosis. There are arthroscopic and open surgical procedures to manage FAI, dysplasia, and other hip conditions in young adults, which are joint sparing and have been shown to have good midterm to long-term outcomes.

KEY STUDY POINTS

- FAI commonly includes pathology on the femoral and acetabular side of the hip joint.
- Management of FAI can be arthroscopic or open depending on the morphologic abnormality.
- Acetabular dysplasia is a developmental condition and may be found in combination with abnormal femoral version and/or head/neck offset deformities.
- Surgical management of symptomatic acetabular dysplasia includes acetabular reorientation osteotomy, which has shown good outcomes and excellent survivorship in most patients.

ANNOTATED REFERENCES

1. Griffin DR, Dickenson EJ, O'Donnell J, et al: The Warwick Agreement on femoroacetabular impingement syndrome (FAI syndrome): An international consensus statement. *Br J Sports Med* 2016;50(19):1169-1176.
2. Frank JM, Harris JD, Erickson BJ, et al: Prevalence of femoroacetabular impingement imaging findings in asymptomatic volunteers: A systematic review 2015;31(6):1199-1204.

3. Clohisy JC, Knaus ER, Hunt DM, Lesher JM, Harris-Hayes M, Prather H: Clinical presentation of patients with symptomatic anterior hip impingement. *Clin Orthop Relat Res* 2009;467(3):638-644.
4. Clohisy JC, Carlisle JC, Beaule PE, et al: A systematic approach to the plain radiographic evaluation of the young adult hip. *J Bone Joint Surg Am* 2008;90(suppl 4):47-66.
5. Nepple JJ, Lehmann CL, Ross JR, Schoenecker PL, Clohisy JC: Coxa profunda is not a useful radiographic parameter for diagnosing pincer-type femoroacetabular impingement. *J Bone Joint Surg Am* 2013;95(5):417-423.
6. Sutter R, Dietrich TJ, Zingg PO, Pfirrmann CW: How useful is the alpha angle for discriminating between symptomatic patients with cam-type femoroacetabular impingement and asymptomatic volunteers? *Radiology* 2012;264(2):514-521.
7. Sutter R, Dietrich TJ, Zingg PO, et al: Femoral antetorsion: Comparing asymptomatic volunteers and patients with femoroacetabular impingement. *Radiology* 2012;263:475-483.
8. Su AW, Hillen TJ, Eutsler EP, et al: Low-dose computed tomography reduces radiation exposure by 90% compared with traditional computed tomography among patients undergoing hip-preservation surgery. *Arthroscopy* 2019;35(5):1385-1392.

   This article describes the author's protocol for low-dose CT and compares radiation exposure with traditional hip CT. They found a 90% reduction in total effective dose radiation using the low-dose protocol compared with traditional CT. Level of evidence: II.
9. Pascual-Garrido C, Li DJ, Grammatopoulos G, Yanik EL, Clohisy JC, ANCHOR Group: The pattern of articular cartilage wear is hip-morphology dependent and patient demographic-dependent. *Clin Orthop Relat Res* 2019;477(5):1021-1033.

   This is a multicenter study of patients undergoing hip arthroscopy for symptomatic FAI. The authors found associations between FAI pathology and acetabular wear patterns. Cartilage injury was more frequent and more severe in cam-type and mixed-type impingement. Level of evidence: III.
10. Suarez-Ahedo C, Gui C, Rabe SM, Chandrasekaran S, Lodhia P, Domb BG: Acetabular condral lesions in hip arthroscopy: Relationships between grade, topography, and demographics. *Am J Sports Med* 2017;45(11):2501-2506.

    The authors review the associations between chondral lesions, acetabular labral articular disruption, and labral tears. Labral tears are identified in 98% of patients who have acetabular labral articular damage at the time of hip arthroscopy. Level of evidence: III.
11. Kraeutler MJ, Goodrich JA, Fioravanti MJ, Garabekyan T, Mei-Dan O: The "outside-in" lesion of hip impingement and the "inside-out" lesion of hip dysplasia: two distinct patterns of acetabular chondral injury. *J Sports Med* 2019;47(12):2978-2984.

    This study aims to associate mechanism of cartilage injury with wear pattern. The authors define two patterns of cartilage wear: outside-in, which results from cam-type impingement, and inside-out, which results from instability or dysplasia. Level of evidence: III.
12. Naraghi A, White LM: MRI of labral and chondral lesions of the hip. *AJR Am J Roentgenol* 2015;205(3):479-490.
13. White LM, Naraghi A, Murnaghan L, Whelan DB, Linda D: Femoroacetabular impingement: Accuracy of non-arthrographic 3T MR imaging in evaluation of intra-articular pathology of the hip. *Skeletal Radiol* 2014;43(12):1794-1795.
14. El Bitar YF, Lindner D, Jackson TJ, Domb BG: Joint-preserving surgical options for management of chondral injuries of the hip. *J Am Acad Orthop Surg* 2014;22(1):46-56.
15. Haversath M, Hanke J, Landgraeber S, et al: The distribution of nociceptive innervation in the painful hip: A histological investigation. *Bone Joint J* 2013;95-B:770-776.
16. Burnett RS, Della Rocca GJ, Prather H, Curry M, Maloney WJ, Clohisy JC: Clinical presentation of patients with tears of the acetabular labrum. *J Bone Joint Surg Am* 2006;88(7):1448-1457.
17. Griffin DR, Dickenson EJ, Wall PDH, et al, FASHIoN Study Group: Hip arthroscopy versus best conservative care for the treatment of femoroacetabular impingement syndrome (UK FASHIoN): a multicenter randomized controlled trial. *Lancet* 2018;391(10136):2225-2235.

    This is a multicenter study comparing outcomes 1 year after randomization to hip arthroscopy versus best conservative care. Significant improvement in outcomes in the hip scope group, which exceeded minimum clinically important difference, was observed. Level of evidence: I.
18. Maradit Kremers H, Schilz SR, Van Houten, et al: Trends in utilization and outcomes of hip arthroscopy in the United States between 2005 and 2013. *J Arthroplasty* 2017;32(3):750-755.

    The authors report the incidence of hip arthroscopy based on database information. They include demographics and results of arthroscopy. Level of evidence: III.
19. Ross JR, Larson CM, Adeoye O, Kelly BT, Bedi A: Residual deformity is the most common reason for revision hip arthroscopy: A three-dimensional CT study. *Clin Orthop Relat Res* 2015;473(4):1388-1395.
20. Bhatia S, Lee S, Shewman E, et al: Effects of acetabular rim trimming on hip joint contact pressures: How much is too much? *Am J Sports* 2015;43(9):2138-2145.
21. Ganz R, Gill TJ, Gautier E, Ganz K, Krugel N, Berlemann U: Surgical dislocation of the adult hip a technique with full access to the femoral head and acetabulum without the risk of avascular necrosis. *J Bone Joint Surg Br* 2001;83(8):1119-1124.
22. Nassif NA, Clohisy JC: *Combined techniques in FAI: Hip arthroscopy followed by mini-anterior approach*, in *Femoroacetabular Impingement*. Berlin, Germany, Springer, 2012, pp 159-166.
23. Griffin DW, Kinnard MJ, Formby PM, McCabe MP, Anderson TD: Outcomes of hip arthroscopy in the older adult: A systematic review of the literature. *Am J Sports Med* 2017;45(8):1928-1936.

    The authors found hip arthroscopy to be safe and result in improved outcomes in patients older than 40 years based on review of current literature. Studies reviewed did find high rates of conversion to THA. Level of evidence: II.

24. Krych AJ, Thompson M, Knutson Z, Scoon J, Coleman SH: Arthroscopic labral repair versus selective labral debridement in female patients with femoroacetabular impingement: A prospective randomized study. *Arthroscopy* 2013;29(1):46-53.

25. Rahl MD, LaPorte C, Steinl GK, O'Connor M, Lynch TS, Menge TJ: Outcomes after arthroscopic hip labral reconstruction: A systematic review and meta-analysis. *Am J Sports Med* 2020;48(7):1748-1755.

    No difference between graft type in labral reconstruction was shown in this large review. Level of evidence: II.

26. Levy DM, Kuhns BD, Chahal J, Philippon MJ, Kelly BT, Nho SJ: Hip arthroscopy outcomes with respect to patient acceptable symptomatic state and minimal clinically important difference. *Arthroscopy* 2016;32(9):1877-1886.

27. Nunley RM, Prather H, Hunt D, Schoenecker PL, Clohisy JC: Clinical presentation of symptomatic acetabular dysplasia in skeletally mature patients. *J Bone Joint Surg Am* 2011;93(suppl 2):17-21.

28. Nepple JJ, Wells J, Ross JR, Bedi A, Schoenecker PL, Clohisy JC: Three patterns of acetabular deficiency are common in young adult patients with acetabular dysplasia. *Clin Orthop Relat Res* 2017;475(4):1037-1104.

    Authors analyzed data from 153 hips that ultimately underwent PAO to measure and describe patterns of deficiency and version. This was correlated with range of motion. Three patterns were described to help guide surgical management. Level of evidence: III.

29. Ganz R, Klaue K, Vinh TS, Mast JW: A new periacetabular osteotomy for the treatment of hip dysplasias: Technique and preliminary results. *Clin Orthop Relat Res* 1988;1988(232):26-36.

30. Li PL, Ganz R: Morphologic features of congenital acetabular dysplasia: One in six is retroverted. *Clin Orthop Relat Res* 2003;416:245-253.

31. Pascual-Garrido C, Harris MD, Clohisy JC: Innovations in joint preservation procedures for the dysplastic hip "the periacetabular osteotomy". *J Arthroplasty* 2017;32(9 suppl):S32-S37.

    The authors review indications for PAO and provide an update on modifications to the originally described technique. Innovations include adjunctive hip arthroscopy, femoral procedures, pain management protocols, and rapid recovery programs.

32. Clohisy JC, St John LC, Nunley RM, Schutz AL, Schoenecker PL: Combined periacetabular and femoral osteotomies for severe hip deformities. *Clin Orthop Relat Res* 2009:467;2221-2227

33. Maldonado DR, LaReau JM, Perets I, et al: Outcomes of hip arthroscopy with concomitant periacetabular osteotomy, minimum 5-year follow-up. *Arthroscopy* 2019;35(3):826-834.

    In a case series, authors compared outcomes and complication rates between PAO alone and PAO with hip arthroscopy. There were no differences in outcomes or complication rates at minimum 5-year follow-up. Level of evidence: IV.

34. Matheney T, Kim YJ, Zurakowski D, Matero C, Millis M: Intermediate to long-term results following Bernese periacetabular osteotomy and predictors of clinical outcome. *J Bone Joint Surg Am* 2009;91:2113-2123.

35. Wells J, Schoeneker P, Duncan S, Goss CW, Thomason K, Clohisy J: Intermediate-temr hip survivorship and patient-reported outcomes of periacetabular osteotomy: The Washington University experience. *J Bone Joint Surg Am* 2018;100(3):218-225

    About 92% PAO survivorship was reported at average 15-year follow-up in patient cohort from a single institution. Level of evidence: IV.

36. Lerch TD, Steppacher SD, Liechti EF, Tannast M, Siebenrock KA: One-third of hips after periacetabular osteotomy survive 30 years with good clinical results, no progression of arthritis, or conversion to THA. *Clin Orthop Relat Res* 2017;475(4):1154-1168.

    The first 75 hips performed at the institution where PAO was first described were reevaluated at average 19 years. Forty-one hips were preserved at 20 years, 26 were converted to THA, and 1 was fused. Risk factors for failure were older age, preexisting arthritis, and positive anterior impingement test. This is a follow-up study examining a cohort of 75 hips with follow-up extended to 30 years. About 71% of hips developed arthritis or pain or had undergone THA. Thus, survival after PAO was reported at 29% at 30-year follow-up. Level of evidence: III.

37. Bogunovic L, Hunt D, Prather H, Schoenecker PL, Clohisy JC: Activity tolerance after periacetabular osteotomy. *Am J Sports Med* 2014;42(8):1791-1795.

38. Clohisy JC, Ackerman J, Baca G, et al: Patient-reported outcomes of periacetabular osteotomy from the prospective ANCHOR cohort study. *J Bone Joint Surg Am* 2017;99(1):33-41.

    This is a prospective, multicenter study of the Academic Network of Conservational Hip Outcomes Research cohort reporting 2-year minimum patient-reported outcomes. The study found improved patient-reported outcome measure scores. Female gender and overweight body mass index were associated with greatest improvements. Level of evidence: IV.

39. Sink EL, Zaltz I, Heare T, Dayton M: Acetabular cartilage and labral damage observed during surgical hip dislocation for stable slipped capital femoral epiphysis. *J Pediatr Orthop* 2010;30(1):26-30.

40. Clohisy JC, Nepple JJ, Ross JR, Pashos G, Schoenecker PL: Does surgical hip dislocation and PAO improve pain in patients with perthers-like deformityes and acetabular dysplasia. *Clin Orthop Relat Res* 2015;473(4):1370-1377.

41. Bardakos NV, Villar RN: The ligamentum teres of the adult hip. *J Bone Joint Surg Br* 2009;91(1):8-15.

42. Philippon MJ, Rasmussen MT, Turnbull TL, et al: Structural properties of the native ligamentum teres. *Orthop J Sports Med* 2014;2(12):2325967114561962.

43. Kaya M, Suziki T, Minowa T, Yamashita T: Ligamentum teres injury is associated with the articular damage pattern in patients with femoroacetabular impingement. *Arthroscopy* 2014;30(12):1582-1587.

44. Gray AJ, Villar RN: The ligamentum teres of the hip: An arthroscopic classification of its pathology. *Arthroscopy* 1997;13(5):575-578.

45. de SA D, Phillips M, Philippon MJ, Letkemann S, Simunovic N, Ayeni OR: Ligamentum teres injuries of the hip: A systematic review examining surgical indications, treatment options, and outcomes. *Arthroscopy* 2014;30(12):1634-1641.

46. Baker CL Jr, Massie RV, Hurt WG, Savory CG: Arthroscopic bursectomy for recalcitrant trochanteric bursitis. *Arthroscopy* 2007;23(8):827-832.

47. Domb BG, Shindle MK, McArthur B, Voos JE, Magennis EM, Kelly BT: Iliopsoas impingement: A newly identified cause of labral pathology in the hip. *HSS J* 2011;7(2):145-150.

48. Ilizaliturri VM Jr, Buganza-Tepole M, Olivos-Meza A, Acuna M, Acosta-Rodriguez E: Central compartment release versus lesser trochanter release of the iliopsoas tendon for the treatment of internal snapping hip: A comparative study. *Arthroscopy* 2014;30(7):790-795.

49. Hain KS, Blankenbaker DG, De Smet AA, Keene JS, Del Rio AM: MR appearance and clinical significance of changes in the hip muscles and iliopsoas tendon after arthroscopic iliopsoas tenotomy in symptomatic patients. *HSS J* 2013;9(3):236-241.

CHAPTER 15

Infection

CHAD A. KRUEGER, MD • SCOT A. BROWN, MD • P. MAXWELL COURTNEY, MD

ABSTRACT

Periprosthetic joint infections continue to occur at 0.5% to 1.5% of all primary total hip and knee arthroplasties with rates approaching 10% for revision surgeries. Despite many recent advances within this field, periprosthetic joint infections continue to challenge surgeons from a preventive, diagnostic, and treatment standpoint. It is important to know about an update on the incidence of, risk factors associated with, diagnostic modalities of, and treatment options for periprosthetic joint infections.

Keywords: diagnosing arthroplasty infection; infected total hip arthroplasty; infected total knee arthroplasty; periprosthetic infection

INTRODUCTION

Periprosthetic joint infection (PJI) remains a challenging complication to manage following total hip arthroplasty (THA) and total knee arthroplasty (TKA). Although the incidence remains low at approximately 1% following primary procedures, PJI presents both a substantial clinical and financial burden to the health system and the patients. Diagnosis has classically relied on imperfect criteria such as culture and synovial fluid analysis; however, new research into infection biomarkers and next-generation sequencing has shown promise. Although standard management of PJI has been a two-stage exchange arthroplasty, recent literature has evaluated the role for single-stage exchange arthroplasty and débridement and implant retention (DAIR). Because of the difficulty and limited success in definitive treatment of PJI, perioperative optimization protocols should be developed to focus on prevention. Modifiable risk factors such as smoking, obesity, malnutrition, and glycemic control should be corrected before undergoing elective THA or TKA to minimize the risk of this devastating complication.

INCIDENCE

The incidence of PJI ranges from 0.74% to 1.38% for primary TKA and from 0.69% to 1.09% for primary THA.[1] Despite the low incidence, PJIs account for up to 50% of revisions within 2 years after primary TKA and THA,[2] making PJI the most common reason for early failure and the second most common reason for revision overall.[3] Infections following a revision THA or TKA are even more prevalent, with rates approaching 3% to 10%.[4] These infections are incredibly morbid for many patients and can carry a 5-year mortality rate of over 25%.[5] With months of missed time from work and multiple hospitalizations often required for treatment, PJI also presents a substantial financial burden to the patient and the health system.[6] The increase in popularity of alternative payment models such as bundled payments have further emphasized the need to prevent PJI following THA and TKA. With the overall number and economic burden of these

Dr. Krueger or an immediate family member serves as a board member, owner, officer, or committee member of the American Association of Hip and Knee Surgeons. Dr. Courtney or an immediate family member serves as a paid consultant to or is an employee of DePuy, A Johnson & Johnson Company, Hip Innovation Technology, and Zimmer; has stock or stock options held in Parvizi Surgical Innovation; and serves as a board member, owner, officer, or committee member of the American Association of Hip and Knee Surgeons. Neither Dr. Brown nor any immediate family member has received anything of value from or has stock or stock options held in a commercial company or institution related directly or indirectly to the subject of this chapter.

infections increasing,[1,7] it is of paramount importance that surgeons understand how to best prevent, diagnose, and manage these infections.

RISK FACTORS

Several studies have identified both modifiable and nonmodifiable risk factors for PJI (**Table 1**). Previous data have shown an increased risk of PJI in patients with rheumatologic disease, coagulopathies, immune dysfunction, and preoperative anemia.[8] Although many of these conditions cannot be improved before undergoing THA or TKA, patients should be counseled on the elevated risks of infection. Modifiable risk factors present an opportunity for counseling and intervention to optimize at-risk patients before undergoing elective arthroplasty. Although there are strong data linking obesity to an increased incidence of PJI, controversy surrounds the use of body mass index (BMI) cutoffs and access to arthroplasty care for obese patients. Obese patients may also be more likely to be malnourished than patients with BMI below 40 kg/m^2. Patients with preoperative serum albumin levels <35 g/L are at markedly increased risk for PJI as well. Preoperative screening of at-risk patients for malnutrition with serum albumin, prealbumin, and transferrin levels may provide a target for intervention to help modify nutritional intake before surgery.

Tobacco use has long been associated with adverse outcomes after TJA, and a recent meta-analysis found that tobacco users had a significantly increased risk of wound complication (odds ratio 1.78) and PJI (odds ratio 2.02) compared with non–tobacco users and former tobacco users.[9] Preoperative weight loss is commonly believed to lead to decreased risks of PJI. However, some studies have found that THA patients who lost weight preoperatively had an odds ratio of 3.77 for a deep surgical site infection postoperatively.[10] This finding may speak to the importance of maintaining optimal nutrition in the perioperative period for purposes of wound healing and infection prevention and suggest that such nutrition is more important than weight loss itself. With the increasing incidence of diabetes mellitus in the United States, glycemic control is important to manage before THA or TKA. The largest multicenter trial looking at the optimum HbA1c level found that the cutoff should be 7.7, above which there is an increased risk of PJI.[11] To better evaluate the blood glucose levels of patients who recently underwent a TJA, blood glucose measurements should be obtained at 5 and 9 PM on the night of the surgery.[12] Because HbA1c measures blood glucose level over a 3-month period, fructosamine may be a better indicator of perioperative glycemic control and may also be used as a screening test.[13]

TABLE 1

Risk Factors Associated With Increased Risk of Periprosthetic Joint Infection

Modifiable	Nonmodifiable
Diabetes	Age
Malnutrition	Male gender
Obesity	Socioeconomic status
Smoking	History of infection
Oral hygiene	Bacterial colonization
Anemia	Allergy to cephalosporin
Inflammatory arthropathies	Renal disease
Operating room traffic	Cirrhosis
Antibiotic prophylaxis	Active cancer
Skin wounds	Revision arthroplasty
Anticoagulants	

Patients who have already sustained a PJI after a primary TKA were significantly more likely to sustain a PJI in their contralateral TKA (6.1%) compared with a matched cohort who had a previous primary TKA without an associated PJI (2.6%). This study also found that patients on chronic suppressive antibiotics at the time of their contralateral TKA were at a significantly increased risk of infection (21.4% versus 1.4%) despite not having a worse host grade than the control group.[14] These findings are in line with previous data that have shown an increased risk of PJI for primary cases performed in the same operating room after an infected case.[15] Another factor found to increase the risk of PJI after THA is when a conversion THA takes place. One study found that the incidence of PJI after these procedures was 8.6% during a single-stage conversion compared with a 3.8% incidence during which the hardware removal and THA were performed in separate procedures.[16] These findings differed from previous studies looking at the topic of increased risk of THA infection following hardware removal but raise the point as to whether these procedures should be performed as a single-staged or multistaged procedure. However, there does appear to be a well-established increase in risk for TKA after previous knee surgery.[17,18]

Other factors such the previous injection of corticosteroid into a knee within 3 months of a TKA,[19] increased surgical case time,[20] and persistent wound drainage have also been found to contribute to an increased risk of PJI (**Table 2**).

TABLE 2

Various Perioperative Routines and Procedures That Are Associated With Infection Risk Categorized by the Level of Evidence Supporting their Use

Perioperative Strategies		
Strong Evidence	**Moderate Evidence**	**Limited Evidence**
Preoperative antibiotics	Chlorhexadine wipes	Ultraviolet light
Dilute betadine	Laminar flow	Forced air flow warmers
Surgical site cleaning	Hair removal	Topical irrigation with antibiotics
Neuraxial anesthesia	Iodine-impregnated skin drapes	Changing knife blade after skin incision
Operating room traffic	Electrocautery tip and suction tip changing	Topical incisional sealants
Operating room temperature	Suture-type for skin closure	
Surgical case length	Negative pressure wound dressings	
Splash basin contamination	Surgical dressing selection	

PREVENTION

Patient optimization plays an important role in decreasing PJIs. Previous work has found that optimizing HbA1c levels, Hb levels, BMI, and albumin preoperatively leads to a decreased risk of developing PJI.[21] Glucose control is also important in the postoperative phase as levels above 137 mg/dL were associated with an increased risk of infection. Interestingly, patients in that study who did not have diabetes were found to be significantly more likely to develop a postoperative infection related to elevated blood glucose levels compared with those who had diabetes.[22] Although there is little evidence suggesting a direct link between periodontal disease and orthopaedic infection, routine screening of patients who are at high risk of dental infections may be beneficial. Although preoperative antiseptic showering has been associated with decreased *Staphylococcus aureus* and methicillin-resistant *S aureus* (MRSA) infections, it has not been found to decrease the total incidence of surgical site infection in all studies.[23] Still, there appears to be enough data to support the decolonization of patients before undergoing a TKA or THA and that chlorhexidine wipes may be superior to soaps and baths with a potential cost savings per 1,000 patients of over $2.1 million.[24]

Outside of patient-specific optimization, there have been many studies looking at perioperative factors that may influence the incidence of PJI. Studies have not shown that laminar flow or surgical helmet systems significantly decrease the risk of PJI after TKA.[17] However, studies have shown that there is a substantial amount of operating room traffic during TJAs with an average of 60 operating room door openings during primary joints and 135 for revisions. These changes in airflow secondary to operating room door opening may increase the risk of infection for TJA patients.[25]

Intraoperative strategies can also be used to decrease the risk of PJI. Reapplication of sterile skin preparation solution after draping but before the application of iodophor-impregnated incisive draping results in significantly lower rate of surgical site infection.[26] Several studies have found that the intraoperative splash basin is a common source of contamination during TJA[27] and that adding dilute betadine or chlorhexidine to the splash basin mixture can decrease the contamination rate of this piece of equipment.[27] Although there was one large retrospective study questioning its utility,[28,29] a recent randomized controlled trial found that betadine lavage of a surgical wound before closure for primary THA and TKA significantly decreased the risk of PJI.[30] There are mixed data regarding the effects that skin closure may have on the risks of infection, but previous studies have found that using a Hydrofiber dressing significantly decreased the risk of wound infection compared with a standard dressing.[31] One recently completed prospective randomized clinical trial found that using a closed, incisional negative pressure wound dressing postoperatively on patients significantly decreased wound complications. These findings are in line with other studies that have negative pressure wound therapy to significantly decrease wound complications in primary THA and TKA as well.[32]

Strong evidence supports the use of first-generation cephalosporins such as cefazolin administered within 60 minutes of incision to reduce the incidence of PJI. Cephalosporins alone may be inadequate at some institutions with high rates of MRSA or gram-negative bacteria as up to 30% of PJIs in some studies have been related to gram-negative bacteria.[24] The American Academy of Orthopaedic Surgeons has recommended the addition of vancomycin for prophylactic antibiotics at institutions where MRSA infection rates are above 10%.[24] However, caution should be used with the universal administration of vancomycin because of acute kidney injury and antibiotic resistance. One recently published study found that PJIs are significantly more likely when a noncefazolin antibiotic is used for TKA and THA prophylaxis. That study also found that more than 96% of patients with a reported allergy to penicillin or cephalosporin did not actually have a true allergy. Therefore, the authors recommended that allergy testing for patients with a reported allergy should be completed before abandoning the use of cephalosporins for preoperative antibiosis.[33]

One recent retrospective study looked at giving patients who were at higher risk of developing PJI (BMI >35 kg/m^2, diabetes, smoking, chronic kidney disease, autoimmune disease, and/or nasal colonization with MRSA/methicillin-sensitive *S aureus*) an extended dose of oral antibiotics postoperatively. The authors found that high-risk patients who did not receive this extended oral antibiotic course were 4.9 and 4.0 times more likely to develop a PJI after TKA and THA, respectively.[21] Although the Centers for Disease Control and Prevention guidelines published in 2017 recommend against postoperative antibiotics, the limitations of the data used to formulate these conclusions should be noted.[34] Other studies have found that there may be no additional benefit to patients receiving a single dose of postoperative antibiotics compared with those receiving multiple doses, as the PJI rate was not significantly different between both groups (0.6% and 0.88%).[35]

DEFINITION

The Musculoskeletal Infection Society criteria use both major (sinus tract formation, pathogen isolation from two separate cultures) and minor criteria (four of the following: elevated serum C-reactive protein [CRP], serum erythrocyte sedimentation rate [ESR], synovial white blood cell [WBC], synovial polymorphonuclear leukocyte [PMN], synovial CRP, + alpha-defensin, positive intraoperative histology, or purulence) in their predictive model. One recent study focused solely on the diagnostic capabilities of the minor criteria and found that the area under the curve for their receiver operator curve was 0.98. This would suggest excellent diagnostic capabilities for these minor criteria.[36] The minor criterion found to be most predictive of a PJI was a positive culture, whereas an elevated ESR was found to be least predictive.[36]

In an effort to validate these major and minor criteria, a recent study suggested that the following values should be used for the diagnosis of a PJI.[37] First, if a patient has two positive cultures or the presence of a sinus tract, there is an infection present. If neither of those criteria are met, an elevated CRP (>1 mg/dL), D-Dimer (>860 ng/mL) were given 2 points. Elevated ESR (>30 mm/hr) was given 1 point. Elevated synovial fluid WBC count (>3,000 cells/µL) 3 points, alpha-defensin (>1) 3 points, leukocyte esterase (2+) 3 points, PMN% (>80%) 2 points, and synovial CRP (>6.9 mg/L) 1 point. An aggregate score of 6+ was considered an infection with a sensitivity of 97.7% and a specificity of 99.5%.[37] This scoring system has been further validated by more recent literature.[38]

DIAGNOSIS

It is important to remember that basic clinical findings such as fever, pain, effusion, and surrounding wound erythema are positive predictors of infection. Fever and erythema have a likelihood ratio of infection of 10.78 and 8.08 when a patient presents for evaluation following a TKA.[39] A recent systematic review found that synovial leukocyte esterase reagent strips (2+) and alpha-defensin tests were the best tests for diagnosing PJI along with synovial CRP and the percentage of PMNs. However, the authors also found that many of the tests evaluated were studied under conditions that put them at high risk for bias and that improved transparency should be available when evaluating these tests in the literature.[40] Suggested cutoffs for synovial fluid analysis of the hip are 3,966 WBCs and PMN% of 80+.[41] For the knee, these values are 1,630 WBCs with PMN% of 61%.[42] However, it appears that the current thresholds for WBC, PMN%, and CRP miss about half of all PJIs,[43] and newer tests such as alpha-defensin may have substantial value when it comes to PJI diagnosis.[44] It is also important to note that patients with a metal-on-metal prosthesis may also have artificially elevated levels. Other factors that can artificially lower synovial WBC counts include local anesthetics, volume of synovial fluid, bloody aspirations, bacterial type, and length of transport of the sample to the laboratory.[42] Previous administration of antibiotics before obtaining serum and synovial infectious markers can change the results. However, the leukocyte esterase strip test was found to maintain its performance in the face of this setting.[45]

When obtaining cultures to evaluate the presence of a PJI, previous work has determined that at least five cultures should be taken from the operative field and that all cultures should be held for at least 8 days.[46] Some studies suggest that over 50% of PJIs may be culture negative and that some of these culture-negative infections end up growing bacteria at later dates, with over 60% of those being *Staphylococcus*.[47,48] Next-generation sequencing is more sensitive than culture for identifying infectious organisms, but also less specific and quite expensive.[49] Until its role is better defined within the domain of PJI, it is recommended that it is only used when there is a high pretest probability of an infection to better identify the organism.[49]

MANAGEMENT OF PJI

The first step in any type of management of a PJI is performing a thorough débridement of any compromised tissue. This is usually accomplished through an extensile exposure that allows a full view of the infected joint. Injecting methylene blue into the affected joint before arthrotomy may allow the surgeon a more accurate view of the progress with débridement.[50] A variety of topical agents (betadine, acetic acid, dilute chlorohexidine, hydrogen peroxide, etc) have been used to remove the bacteria and biofilms associated with PJI with all of these solutions having their own specific strengths and weaknesses.[51] There is no consensus within the literature as to which agents should be used for which cases to decrease infection risk. However, dilute betadine is the most studied of these agents and seems to have enough supporting literature to be used confidently in this regard if the surgeon desires.[30]

DÉBRIDEMENT AND IMPLANT RETENTION

There has been much written recently about performing DAIR for PJIs. This is likely due to the obvious benefits of such a procedure if it is successful. The authors of one study found the 2-year infection-free survival rate to be 85%, 88%, and 60% for patients who underwent a DAIR within 28, 42, and 90 days after their index procedure.[52] Another recent study looked at a two-stage débridement with retention of implants for both THA and TKA patients who had a minimum of 1-year follow-up. Following the described protocol, success rates of 82.9% in THA and 89.6% of TKA were observed.[4] The authors found that joints that remained infection free were treated an average of 4 days sooner after the onset of symptoms than those that were subsequently infected after the procedure.[4] These studies contrast the findings of another study, which found that the 4-year failure rate was 57% and that the 5-year mortality rate was almost 20%.[53] There are also some studies suggesting improved results with DAIR procedures when multiple débridement and irrigations are performed.[4]

The expected outcome of a DAIR needs to be tempered if the patient has a positive blood culture as one study found that only 36% of patients who had a positive blood culture remained infection free 1 year status post DAIR.[54] Similarly, DAIR is associated with a high rate of failure for patients who had acute hematogenous PJI, because the rate was over 50% in one study—a failure rate that was almost two times higher than that found for acute postsurgical infections.[55] Patients with diabetes, MRSA, *Pseudomonas*, and polymicrobial infections are also more likely to experience failure after treatment with DAIR.[55,56] Furthermore, a DAIR was successful in only 35% of patients who had a CRIME80 (chronic obstructive pulmonary disease [2], CRP > 150 mg/L [1], rheumatoid arthritis [3], prosthesis for fracture [3], male gender [1], exchange of mobile components [−1], age older than 80 years [2]) score of 3 or more.[57] These are important factors to consider, because there are data suggesting that a prior failed DAIR increases the risk of a failed two-stage exchange arthroplasty by up to 100%.[4,56]

When looking at the use of DAIR in patients who underwent a unicompartmental knee arthroplasty, the authors found that DAIR was associated with a lower infection-free 5-year survivorship than those who were treated with a two-stage exchange and conversion to a TKA. However, there were only 15 patients in the entire cohort, so the study conclusion remains uncertain.[58]

ONE-STAGE EXCHANGE ARTHROPLASTY (FIGURE 1)

There has also been renewed interest in the use of a single-stage exchange arthroplasty for the definitive treatment of PJIs. A systematic review found that the risk of reinfection after a two-stage exchange arthroplasty was between zero and 41% and the risk of reinfection after a one-stage exchange arthroplasty was between zero and 11%.[59] One study found that one-stage exchange arthroplasty provides greater health utility and cost-effectiveness than two-stage revisions for revision TKA for PJI.[60] If it is found to be as effective as two-stage revisions at eradicating the infection, this provides further support that one-stage revision decreases the overall costs to the healthcare system for PJI treatment. When looking at reasons for why a one-stage exchange TKA failed, the surgeons at the ENDO-Klinik found that a history of a failed exchange arthroplasty and infection with enterococci or streptococci bacteria were significant risk factors.[59] Previous studies have also found that elevated BMI above 100 kg/m^2 increases the risk of failure for both one-stage and two-stage exchange arthroplasties.[59]

TWO-STAGE EXCHANGE ARTHROPLASTY (FIGURE 2)

A staged exchange arthroplasty procedure, in which components are removed and the wound is débrided during one surgery, the patient is placed on parental

Section 1: Hip and Knee

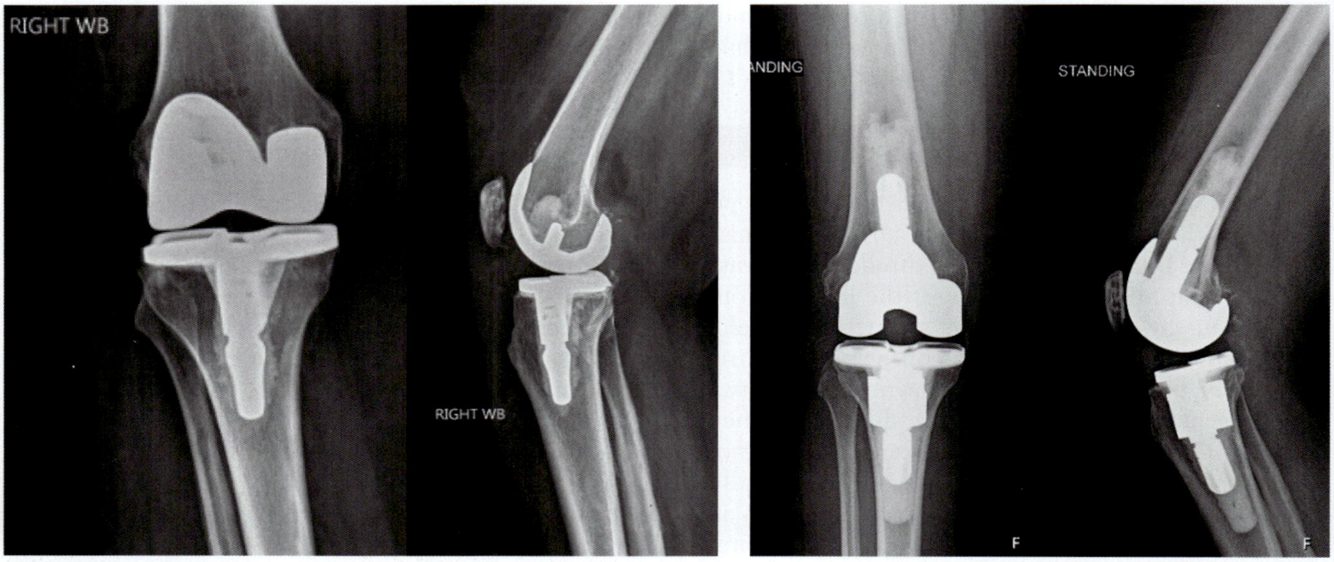

FIGURE 1 Preoperative and postoperative radiographs of a patient who underwent a single-stage exchange for an infected total knee arthroplasty.

antibiotics, and another surgical débridement with reimplantation of components is performed after 6 to 12 weeks, has traditionally been the treatment for PJIs. These two-stage exchange arthroplasties have been reported to have a success rate of 91% at 2 years and 84% at 5 years.[61] BMI above 30 kg/m^2, surgical time >4 hours, gout, and the presence of *Enterococcus* species during the initial procedure all are associated with significant increases in failure rate.[61] Prior studies have also shown that a polymicrobial infection leads to increased failure rates after single-stage and two-stage exchange arthroplasties.[59]

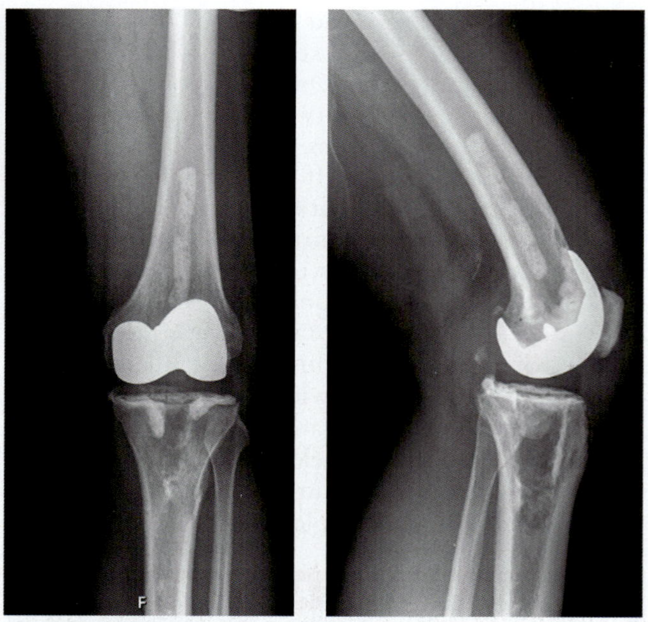

FIGURE 2 Example of radiographs of a functional spacer for a two-stage exchange arthroplasty. For this case, a prosthetic femur and all-polyethylene tibial component were implanted with high-dose antibiotics. A cement dowel was also placed up the femoral canal.

These procedures are resource intensive, are difficult for patients to tolerate, and have been reported to cost as much as four primary TKAs.[60] There also appears to be a difference in infection-free survival for PJIs depending on the type of bacteria found to be infecting the wound. One recent study found that the 2-year infection-free rate for PJIs associated with TKAs differed between methicillin-sensitive *S aureus* (93%), methicillin-sensitive *Staphylococcus epidermidis* (95%), MRSA (80%), and methicillin-resistant *S epidermidis* (54%).[62]

Such factors along with the growing body of literature suggesting relatively equivalent outcomes with a single-stage functional spacer are some of the reasons that the single-stage exchange arthroplasty is gaining interest.[48] In addition, 17% of patients who are planning to undergo a two-stage exchange arthroplasty end up needing an additional spacer exchange before the final implant can be placed. These patients have much higher failure rates and reinfection rates than those not undergoing the additional spacer exchange.[63] Furthermore, almost 20% of patients never undergo the intended replantation part of the two-stage exchange arthroplasty, which may lower the true success rate of a two-stage exchange.[64]

When trying to determine when a patient undergoing a two-stage exchange arthroplasty may be ready for their definitive treatment, surgeons often try a variety of tests and clinical examinations to determine if the infection has been appropriately eradicated. A patient's ESR and CRP do not appear to be useful markers for this purpose.[65] The alpha-defensin test has also fared poorly at predicting the success or failure of reimplantation when used before the definitive procedure.[66] To this day, there is still no benchmark for determining when the definitive treatment should take place.

When performing a two-stage exchange arthroplasty for the hip, it is important to remember that spacer complications are quite common, with an overall complication rate of 26% in some series, and can lead to significant morbidity for many patients.[67]

FUNGAL INFECTIONS

Fungal infections represent about 1% of all PJI.[68] A recent meta-analysis of fungal PJIs found that patients only have elevated serum ESR, CRP, and WBC count about 50% of the time, making their diagnosis more difficult. In addition, leukocyte esterase analysis of the synovial fluid is not positive, and alpha-defensin has not been extensively studied with fungal PJI.[68] Fungal infections typically form more dense biofilms than bacterial infections making DAIR a less attractive (and a less successful) option.[68] The literature on two-stage revision of PJIs with fungal infections suggests that the failure rate is between 20% and 40%.[68] When considering a cement spacer for a fungal infection, it should be noted that amphotericin B forms covalent cross-links in polymethyl methacrylate, which can limit its elution. In that light, surgeons can use fluconazole or voriconazole within the cement for better elution outcomes.[68]

FAILED MANAGEMENT OF PJI (FIGURES 3 AND 4)

There are patients who, despite receiving optimal care and exhausting all treatment options, continue to have an infected TKA or THA. In those situations, patients can be placed on lifelong suppressive antibiotics, undergo a resection arthroplasty, elect for an amputation, or consider an arthrodesis.[69] None of these options are particularly attractive, but many are effective. For instance, one study that evaluated recalcitrant infections of TKA found that a resection arthroplasty successfully resolved the infection in 84% of patients.[70] Although these patients typically need bracing treatment and assistive devices for ambulation, a resection arthroplasty may be a more attractive option to some patients than an amputation.[70] Similarly, there are many of the same complications present for patients whether they undergo a knee arthrodesis or an amputation for a chronically infected TKA.[70] This is also true for patients with persistently infected THAs—although a hip resection arthroplasty may successfully eradicate the infection, functional expectations after such a procedure should be limited.[71] In light of these findings, it is important to have a lengthy discussion with patients regarding their treatment options to try to maximize their acceptance of this incredibly difficult situation.

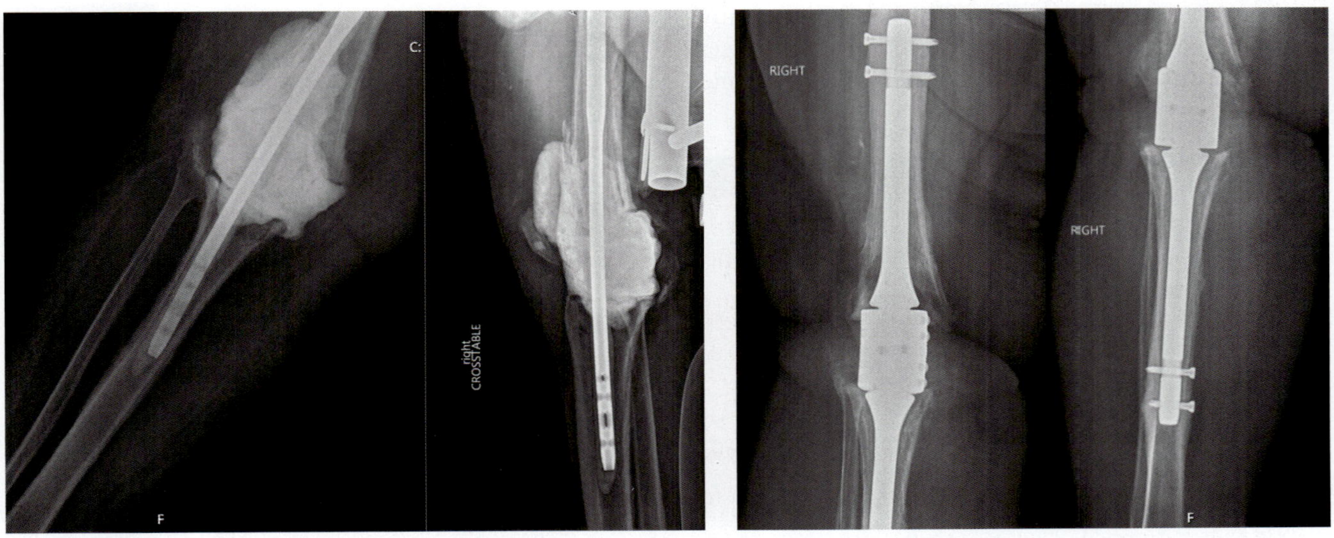

FIGURE 3 Preoperative and postoperative radiographs of a patient who underwent two previous failed exchange arthroplasties for chronic infection and eventually underwent a successful knee arthrodesis.

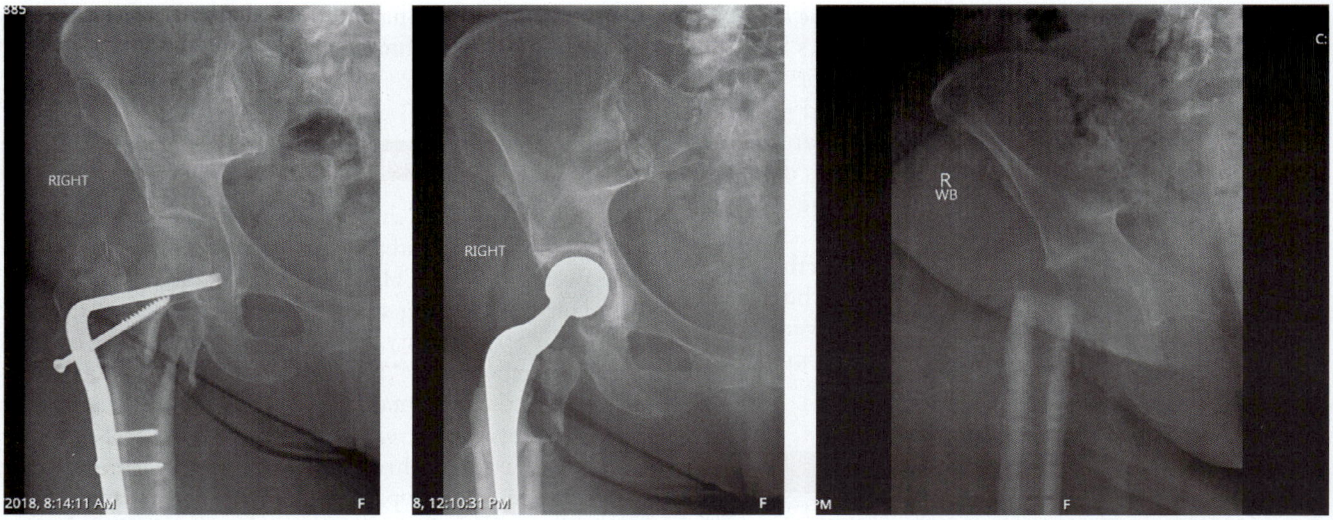

FIGURE 4 Radiographs of a patient who had multiple failed surgeries on her right hip and eventually developed a chronic infection. She was treated with an exchange spacer and eventually underwent a hip resection arthroplasty.

SUMMARY

With the continued demand for, and expanding indications of, both TKA and THA, the number of PJIs is likely to dramatically increase. These are exceedingly challenging cases that require extensive resources and incur a significant morbidity and mortality on the patient. There continues to be a large amount of research devoted to this topic, but the basic principles of patient selection, patient optimization, and sterile technique will likely always form the foundation of any infection prevention strategy. Although the consensus as to what constitutes a PJI continues to be refined, there remains a large chasm between diagnosis and definitive treatment. There is likely not a one-size-fits-all treatment of PJI, and it is imperative that determining the best treatment strategies for each of the patients be continued to optimize their outcome.

KEY STUDY POINTS

- The incidence of PJIs has remained largely unchanged despite advances in preventive strategies, patient optimization, and surgical technique.
- Surgeons should use a variety of clinically studied tests as part of their algorithm for determining if a total hip or knee arthroplasty is infected.
- There are emerging data challenging the long-held belief that a two-stage exchange arthroplasty should be considered the benchmark for the management of PJI. The treatment option for each infection should be tailored specifically to each patient, infectious pathogen, and soft-tissue envelope.
- The management of recalcitrant PJIs should be proceeded by very honest conversations with the patient regarding various options. Patient expectations should be clearly managed as patient outcomes for these procedures are guarded.

ANNOTATED REFERENCES

1. Kurtz SM, Lau EC, Son MS, Chang ET, Zimmerli W, Parvizi J: Are we winning or losing the battle with periprosthetic joint infection: Trends in periprosthetic joint infection and mortality risk for the medicare population. *J Arthroplasty* 2018;33(10):3238-3245.

   In this retrospective review, the authors evaluated the rate of PJIs from 2005 to 2015. They found that the rate of PJIs has not declined in recent years. However, mortality after PJI has decreased. Level of evidence: IV.

2. Koh CK, Zeng I, Ravi S, Zhu M, Vince KG, Young SW: Periprosthetic joint infection is the main cause of failure for modern knee arthroplasty: An analysis of 11,134 knees. *Clin Orthop Relat Res* 2017;475(9):2194-2201.

   This study evaluated over 11,000 primary total knee arthroplasties and found that the infection rate was 2%. PJI was the most common reason for revision surgery in their study. Level of evidence: III.

3. Parvizi J, Shohat N, Gehrke T: Prevention of periprosthetic joint infection. *Bone Joint J* 2017;99-B(suppl 4):3-10.

   This article summarizes the strategies for prevention of PJI. Level of evidence: IV.

4. Chung AS, Niesen MC, Graber TJ, et al: Two-stage debridement with prosthesis retention for acute periprosthetic joint infections. *J Arthroplasty* 2019;34(6):1207-1213.

This retrospective study evaluated the success of infection prevention at 1 year after a two-staged débridement with implant retention. The authors found that 83% of THA and 90% of TKA patients remained infection free at 1 year after their protocol. Level of evidence: IV.

5. Patel VP, Walsh M, Sehgal B, Preston C, DeWal H, Di Cesare P: Factors associated with prolonged wound drainage after primary total hip and knee arthroplasty. *J Bone Joint Surg Am* 2007;89(1):33-38.
6. Kamath AF, Ong KL, Lau E, et al: Quantifying the burden of revision total joint arthroplasty for periprosthetic infection. *J Arthroplasty* 2015;30(9):1492-1497.
7. Kurtz SM, Lau E, Watson H, Schmier JK, Parvizi J: Economic burden of periprosthetic joint infection in the United States. *J Arthroplasty* 2012;27(suppl 8):61-65.e1.
8. Bozic KJ, Lau E, Kurtz S, et al: Patient-related risk factors for periprosthetic joint infection and postoperative mortality following total hip arthroplasty in Medicare patients. *J Bone Joint Surg Am* 2012;94(9):794-800.
9. Bedard NA, DeMik DE, Owens JM, Glass NA, DeBerg J, Cllaghan JJ: Tobacco use and risk of wound complications and periprosthetic joint infection: A systematic review and meta-analysis of primary total joint arthroplasty procedures. *J Arthroplasty* 2019;34(2):385-396.e4.

   This systematic review found that tobacco users had significantly higher rates of wound complications and PJI compared with non-tobacco users and that current tobacco users have significantly higher risk of infection compared with former tobacco users. Level of evidence: III.
10. Inacio MCS, Kritz-Silverstein D, Raman R, et al: The risk of surgical site infection and re-admission in obese patients undergoing total joint replacement who lose weight before surgery and keep it off post-operatively. *Bone Joint J* 2014;96-B(5):629-635.
11. Tarabichi M, Shohat N, Kheir MM, et al: Determining the threshold for HbA1c as a predictor for adverse outcomes after total joint arthroplasty: A multicenter, retrospective study. *J Arthroplasty* 2017;32(suppl 9):S263-S267.e1.

    This is a retrospective study of more than 1,500 TJAs from multiple centers. Using the analyses, it was determined that patients with an HbA1c above 7.7 had a roughly six times increase in PJI. Level of evidence: III.
12. Varady NH, Schwab PE, Jones T, Collins JE, Fitz W, Chen AF: Optimal timing of glucose measurements after total joint arthroplasty. *J Arthroplasty* 2019;34(7 suppl):S152-S158.

    This study of more than 300 patients demonstrated that most TJA patients, both those with diabetes and those without diabetes, are hyperglycemic during the postoperative period. Level of evidence: IV.
13. Shohat N, Tarabichi M, Tischler EH, Jabbour S, Parvizi J: Serum fructosamine: A simple and inexpensive test for assessing preoperative glycemic control. *J Bone Joint Surg Am* 2017;99(22):1900-1907.

    This study of more than 800 patients showed that a patient's fructosamine levels correlated better with the risk of deep infection, readmission, and revision surgery than the HbA1c level. Level of evidence: III.
14. Chalmers BP, Weston JT, Osmon DR, Hanssen AD, Berry DJ, Abdel MP: Prior hip or knee prosthetic joint infection in another joint increases risk three-fold of prosthetic joint infection after primary total knee arthroplasty: A matched control study. *Bone Joint J* 2019;101-B(7 suppl C):91-97.

    This study of more than 100 TKA patients showed that patients who had previously had a PJI of TKA were three times more likely to develop a subsequent PJI than patients who had previously had a TKA and not a PJI. Level of evidence: III.
15. Chen AF, Kheir MM, Greenbaum JM, Restrepo C, Maltenfort MG, Parvizi J: Surgical case order has an effect on the risk of subsequent periprosthetic joint infection. *J Arthroplasty* 2017;32(7):2234-2238.

    In this study of more than 31,000 TJAs, the authors demonstrated that cases following an infected case in the same operative room on the same operative day had a higher risk of PJI than cases performed when not following an infected case. The authors suggest that terminal cleaning appears to be effective at reducing bioburden in TJA cases. Level of evidence: III.
16. Scholten R, Füssenich W, Somford MP, van Susante JLC: High incidence of early periprosthetic joint infection following total hip arthroplasty with concomitant or previous hardware removal. *Arch Orthop Trauma Surg* 2019;139(8):1051-1056.

    The authors of this study found that when a THA conversion took place in one stage, the incidence of PJI was 6.9%. This was a much higher percentage than when the THA conversion took place in two stages (3.8%). Level of evidence: IV.
17. Tayton ER, Frampton C, Hooper GJ, Young SW: The impact of patient and surgical factors on the rate of infection after primary total knee arthroplasty: An analysis of 64,566 joints from the New Zealand Joint Registry. *Bone Joint J* 2016;98-B(3):334-340.
18. Watters TS, Zhen Y, Martin JR, Levy DL, Jennings JM, Dennis DA: Total knee arthroplasty after anterior cruciate ligament reconstruction: Not just a routine primary arthroplasty. *J Bone Joint Surg Am* 2017;99(3):185-189.

    In this matched cohort study of 122 patients undergoing TKA who had previously had an ACL reconstruction, the authors found that previously having an ACL reconstruction increased a patient's risk of revision surgery. Level of evidence: III.
19. Richardson SS, Schairer WW, Sculco TP, Sculco PK: Comparison of infection risk with corticosteroid or hyaluronic acid injection prior to total knee arthroplasty. *J Bone Joint Surg Am* 2019;101(2):112-118.

    These authors looked at almost 19,000 patients who received an injection of hyaluronic acid or corticosteroid before TKA. They found that patients who received the injection within 3 months of TKA had an increased risk of infection. Level of evidence: III.
20. Wang Q, Goswami K, Shohat N, Aalirezaie A, Manrique J, Parvizi J: Longer operative time results in a higher rate of subsequent periprosthetic joint infection in patients undergoing primary joint arthroplasty. *J Arthroplasty* 2019;34(5):947-953.

The authors retrospectively reviewed more than 17,000 patients and found that each 20-minute increase in surgical time increased the infection risk of a primary TKA by almost 25%. Level of evidence: IV.

21. Inabathula A, Dilley JE, Ziemba-Davis M, et al: Extended oral antibiotic prophylaxis in high-risk patients substantially reduces primary total hip and knee arthroplasty 90-day infection rate. *J Bone Joint Surg Am* 2018;100(24):2103-2109.

    A retrospective study of more than 2,100 patients showed 7 days of extended antibiotic prophylaxis in high-risk patients undergoing primary TJA decreased infection risk almost five times compared with the same patients undergoing primary TJA without extended antibiotics. Level of evidence: III.

22. Kheir MM, Tan TL, Kheir M, Maltenfort MG, Chen AF: Postoperative blood glucose levels predict infection after total joint arthroplasty. *J Bone Joint Surg Am* 2018;100(16):1423-1431.

    This retrospective review of more than 13,000 patients showed that there was an increase in PJI for patients who had a blood glucose level above 137 mg/dL postoperatively. Level of evidence: III.

23. Farber NJ, Chen AF, Bartsch SM, Feigel JL, Klatt BA: No infection reduction using chlorhexidine wipes in total joint arthroplasty. *Clin Orthop Relat Res* 2013;471(10):3120-3125.

24. Elbuluk AM, Novikov D, Gotlin M, Schwarzkopf R, Iorio R, Vigdorchik J: Control strategies for infection prevention in total joint arthroplasty. *Orthop Clin North Am* 2019;50(1):1-11.

    This review discusses current strategies to decrease the risk of PJI. Level of evidence: IV.

25. Panahi P, Stroh M, Casper DS, Parvizi J, Austin MS: Operating room traffic is a major concern during total joint arthroplasty. *Clin Orthop Relat Res* 2012;470(10):2690-2694.

26. Morrison TN, Chen AF, Taneja M, Küçükdurmaz F, Rothman RH, Parvizi J: Single vs repeat surgical skin preparations for reducing surgical site infection after total joint arthroplasty: A prospective, randomized, double-blinded study. *J Arthroplasty* 2016;31(6):1289-1294.

27. Nazal MR, Galloway JL, Dhaliwal KK, Nishiyama SK, Shields JS: Dilute povidone-iodine solution prevents intraoperative contamination of sterile water basins during total joint arthroplasty. *J Arthroplasty* 2020;35(1):241-246.

    In this randomized controlled trial, the authors found that a splash basin treated with dilute povidone-iodine solution eliminated splash basin contamination in TJA. Level of evidence: I.

28. Hernandez NM, Hart A, Taunton MJ, et al: Use of povidone-iodine irrigation prior to wound closure in primary total hip and knee arthroplasty: An analysis of 11,738 cases. *J Bone Joint Surg Am* 2019;101(13):1144-1150.

    A retrospective review of more than 11,000 patients found that using povidone iodine irrigation during primary THA and TKA did not reduce risk of PJI at 3 and 12 months postoperatively. Level of evidence: III.

29. Hart A, Hernandez NM, Abdel MP, Mabry TM, Hanssen AD, Perry KI: Povidone-iodine wound lavage to prevent infection after revision total hip and knee arthroplasty: An analysis of 2,884 cases. *J Bone Joint Surg Am* 2019;101(13):1151-1159.

    This retrospective review of more than 2,800 revision THA and TKA cases demonstrated no decrease in PJI risk when povidone-iodine was used during the surgical case for irrigation. Level of evidence: III.

30. Calkins TE, Culvem C, Nam D, et al: Dilute betadine lavage reduces the risk of acute postoperative periprosthetic joint infection in aseptic revision total knee and hip arthroplasty: A randomized controlled trial. *J Arthroplasty* 2020;35(2):538-543.e1.

    This is a prospective study including close to 500 patients that found that performing a dilute betadine lavage before surgical wound closure in aseptic revision TKA and THA significantly decreased the risk of infection. Level of evidence: I.

31. Grosso MJ, Berg A, LaRussa S, Murtaugh T, Trofa DP, Geller JA: Silver-impregnated occlusive dressing reduces rates of acute periprosthetic joint infection after total joint arthroplasty. *J Arthroplasty* 2017;32(3):929-932.

    This is a retrospective study showing a reduction in infection rates with a silver-impregnated dressing. Level of evidence: III.

32. Newman JM, Siqueira MBP, Klika AK, Molloy RM, Barsoum WK, Higuera CA: Use of closed incisional negative pressure wound therapy after revision total hip and knee arthroplasty in patients at high risk for infection: A prospective, randomized clinical trial. *J Arthroplasty* 2019;34(3):554-559.e1.

    This is a prospective randomized trial that demonstrated closed incisional negative pressure wound therapy decreased wound complications after revision TKA or THA. Level of evidence: II.

33. Wyles CC, Hevesi M, Osmon DR, et al: 2019 John Charnley Award: Increased risk of prosthetic joint infection following primary total knee and hip arthroplasty with the use of alternative antibiotics to cefazolin. The value of allergy testing for antibiotic prophylaxis. *Bone Joint J* 2019;101-B(6 suppl B):9-15.

    This is a retrospective review of almost 30,000 TJAs that demonstrated a significantly increased risk of PJI when patients received a preoperative antibiotic besides cefazolin. The authors also found that 97% of patients who reported being allergic to cefazolin were not actually allergic to cefazolin on testing. Level of evidence: III.

34. Siddiqi A, Forte SA, Docter S, Bryant D, Sheth NP, Chen AF: Perioperative antibiotic prophylaxis in total joint arthroplasty: A systematic review and meta-analysis. *J Bone Joint Surg Am* 2019;101(9):828-842.

    This is a meta-analysis that did not find benefit to extended postoperative antibiotic prophylaxis after TJA. Level of evidence: III.

35. Tan TL, Shohat N, Rondon AJ, et al: Perioperative antibiotic prophylaxis in total joint arthroplasty: A single dose is as effective as multiple doses. *J Bone Joint Surg Am* 2019;101(5):429-437.

This retrospective study of more than than 20,000 patients did not find any difference in PJI rates between patients who received a single dose of postoperative antibiotics and multiple doses. Level of evidence: III.

36. Bingham JS, Salib CG, McQuivey K, Temkit MH, Spangehl MJ: An evidence-based clinical prediction algorithm for the Musculoskeletal Infection Society minor criteria. *J Arthroplasty* 2018;33(9):2993-2996.

This study aimed to develop a predictive algorithm that could predict a PJI by using only the five minor criteria associated with the Musculoskeletal Infection Society definition of PJI. Their algorithm showed an area under the curve of 98% when all five minor criteria were met. Level of evidence: III.

37. Parvizi J, Tan TL, Goswami K, et al: The 2018 definition of periprosthetic hip and knee infection: An evidence-based and validated criteria. *J Arthroplasty* 2018;33(5):1309-1314.e2.

This study provides an evidence-based algorithm that can be used to predict PJI. Level of evidence: IV.

38. Shohat N, Tan TL, Della Valle CJ, et al: Development and validation of an evidence-based algorithm for diagnosing periprosthetic joint infection. *J Arthroplasty* 2019;34(11):2730-2736.e1.

This study evaluates the validity of a previously developed algorithm for the diagnosis of periprosthetic joint infections. evidence-based algorithm that can be used to predict PJI. Level of evidence: III.

39. Shohat N, Goswami K, Tan TL, et al: Fever and erythema are specific findings in detecting infection following total knee arthroplasty. *J Bone Jt Infect* 2019;4(2):92-98.

This retrospective review found that fever and wound erythema were the most important sign and symptom for PJI. Level of evidence: IV.

40. Carli AV, Abdelbary H, Ahmadzai N, et al: Diagnostic accuracy of serum, synovial, and tissue testing for chronic periprosthetic joint infection after hip and knee replacements: A systematic review. *J Bone Joint Surg Am* 2019;101(7):635-649.

This systemic review looked at the accuracy of various diagnostic tests meant to diagnose PJI. The authors found that many studies are at high risk of bias but that synovial fluid–based tests perform the best for diagnosing chronic PJI. Level of evidence: III.

41. Higuera CA, Zmistowski B, Malcom T, et al: Synovial fluid cell count for diagnosis of chronic periprosthetic hip infection. *J Bone Joint Surg Am* 2017;99(9):753-759.

This study evaluated 374 aseptic revision THAs and 79 septic THAs. The authors found that optimal threshold for diagnosing PJI based on synovial WBC and %PMNs was 3,966 cells/µg and 80% PMNs. Level of evidence: III.

42. Ottink KD, Strahm C, Muller-Kobold A, Sendi P, Wouthuyzen-Bakker M: Factors to consider when assessing the diagnostic accuracy of synovial leukocyte count in periprosthetic joint infection. *J Bone Jt Infect* 2019;4(4):167-173.

This article provides an overview of different variables that can affect the accuracy of WBC counts and %PMNs on synovial fluid aspirates. Level of evidence: IV.

43. Xu C, Tan TL, Kuo FC, Goswami K, Wang Q, Parvizi J: Reevaluating current cutoffs for acute periprosthetic joint infection: Current thresholds are insensitive. *J Arthroplasty* 2019;34(11):2744-2748.

The authors retrospectively evaluated 218 patients with acute PJIs that occurred within 6 weeks of the index surgery. They found the sensitivity of CRP, synovial WBC and %PMNs to be 55%, 60% and 51%, respectively. They also found that coagulase-negative *Staphylococcus* as an independent risk factor for false-negative CRP readings. Therefore, they recommend reconsidering these thresholds for acute PJI. Level of evidence: IV.

44. Miyamae Y, George J, Klika AK, Barsoum WK, Higuera CA: Diagnostic accuracy of the alpha-defensin test for periprosthetic joint infection in patients with inflammatory diseases. *J Arthroplasty* 2019;34(8):1767-1771.

The authors of this retrospective review of more than 1,300 patients found that the alpha defensin test had a high accuracy for diagnosing PJI in patients with inflammatory disease. Level of evidence: IV.

45. Shahi A, Alvand A, Ghanem E, Restrepo C, Parvizi J: The leukocyte esterase test for periprosthetic joint infection is not affected by prior antibiotic administration. *J Bone Joint Surg Am* 2019;101(8):739-744.

The authors of this study evaluated 121 patients with PJI according to Musculoskeletal Infection Society. They found the patients who received antibiotics before diagnostic testing had lower values of all tests except for leukocyte esterase. Level of evidence: III.

46. Kheir MM, Tan TL, Ackerman CT, Modi R, Foltz C, Parvizi J: Culturing periprosthetic joint infection: Number of samples, growth duration, and organisms. *J Arthroplasty* 2018;33(11):3531-3536.e1.

The authors of this study evaluated the cultures of more than 700 patients and determined that at least five cultures should be taken from suspected cases of PJI and that cultures should be held for at least 8 days. Level of evidence: IV.

47. Hersh BL, Shah NB, Rothenberger SD, Zlotnicki JP, Klatt BA, Urish KL: Do culture negative periprosthetic joint infections remain culture negative? *J Arthroplasty* 2019;34(11):2757-2762.

The authors of this multicenter cohort study found that more than 50% of culture-negative infections treated with irrigation and débridement that failed eventually grew bacteria after the failed treatment. Level of evidence: IV.

48. Siddiqi A, Nace J, George NE, et al: Primary total knee arthroplasty implants as functional prosthetic spacers for definitive management of periprosthetic joint infection: A multicenter study. *J Arthroplasty* 2019;34(12):3040-3047.

The authors of this multicenter study found that functional prosthetic spacers had improved cost-effectiveness and a similar success rate (79%) compared with two-stage exchange (71%). Level of evidence: III.

49. Torchia MT, Austin DC, Kunkel ST, Dwyer KW, Moschetti W: Next-generation sequencing vs culture-based methods for diagnosing periprosthetic joint infection after total knee arthroplasty: A cost-effectiveness analysis. *J Arthroplasty* 2019;34(7):1333-1341.

The authors of this study found that the effectiveness of next-generation sequencing to diagnose PJI depends largely on the pretest probability of the patient having an infection. Level of evidence: III.

50. Shaw JD, Miller S, Plourde A, Shaw DL, Wustrack R, Hansen EN: Methylene blue-guided debridement as an intraoperative adjunct for the surgical treatment of periprosthetic joint infection. *J Arthroplasty* 2017;32(12):3718-3723.

In this study, the authors analyzed tissue samples from patients who had a PJI. They found that injecting methylene blue into the infected joint before the débridement allowed surgeons to better identify infected tissue than in those without. Level of evidence: IV.

51. Tsang STJ, Gwynne PJ, Gallagher MP, Simpson AHRW: The biofilm eradication activity of acetic acid in the management of periprosthetic joint infection. *Bone Joint Res* 2018;7(8):517-523.

The authors of this preclinical study found that using a 5% concentration of acetic acid was able to eliminate 96% of methicillin-sensitive *Staphylococcus aureus* following a 20-minute treatment time. The authors caution that using concentrations above 5% may be harmful to native tissues. Level of evidence: IV.

52. Ottesen CS, Troelsen A, Sandholdt H, Jacobsen S, Husted H, Gromov K: Acceptable success rate in patients with periprosthetic knee joint infection treated with debridement, antibiotics, and implant retention. *J Arthroplasty* 2019;34(2):365-368.

This study of 67 patients found that 84% of patients who underwent a débridement irrigation and retention of implants remained infection free at 2 years postoperatively. Level of evidence: IV.

53. Urish KL, Bullock AG, Kreger AM, Shah NB, Jeong K, Rothenberger SD: A multicenter study of irrigation and debridement in total knee arthroplasty periprosthetic joint infection: Treatment failure is high. *J Arthroplasty* 2018;33(4):1154-1159.

In this multicenter study of patients undergoing débridement irrigation and component retention, the authors report that the 4-year failure rate was 57% and the 5-year mortality was 19.9%. Level of evidence: III.

54. Kuo FC, Goswami K, Klement MR, Shohat N, Parvizi J: Positive blood cultures decrease the treatment success in acute hematogenous periprosthetic joint infection treated with debridement, antibiotics, and implant retention. *J Arthroplasty* 2019;34(12):3030-3034.e1.

In this retrospective study of 49 patients who had an acute hematogenous PJI, the authors found that those with a positive blood culture had a higher failure rate after débridement irrigation and retention (36%). Level of evidence: III.

55. Shohat N, Goswami K, Tan TL, Fillingham Y, Parvizi J: Increased failure after irrigation and debridement for acute hematogenous periprosthetic joint infection. *J Bone Joint Surg Am* 2019;101(8):696-703.

This retrospective study found that failure rate for patients who undergo débridement irrigation and retention of components after acute hematogenous infection was two times higher than that of patients who underwent the procedure for an acute postoperative infection. Level of evidence: IV.

56. Rajgopal A, Panda I, Rao A, Dahiya V, Gupta H: Does prior failed debridement compromise the outcome of subsequent two-stage revision done for periprosthetic joint infection following total knee arthroplasty? *J Arthroplasty* 2018;33(8):2588-2594.

The authors of this study found that a prior failed débridement irrigation and implant retention procedure was associated with an almost doubling of the failure rate of a subsequent two-stage exchange revision compared with patients who underwent a two-stage exchange directly without first undergoing a DAIR. Level of evidence: III.

57. Wouthuyzen-Bakker M, Sebillotte M, Lomas J, et al, on behalf of the ESCMID Study Group for Implant-Associated Infections (ESGIAI): Timing of implant-removal in late acute periprosthetic joint infection: A multicenter observational study. *J Infect* 2019;79(3):199-205.

The authors found that DAIR is a good option for acute PJI but that patients with a CRIME80 score above 3 should be considered for a two-stage exchange. Level of evidence: III.

58. Hernandez NM, Petis SM, Hanssen AD, Sierra RJ, Abdel MP, Pagnano MW: Infection after unicompartmental knee arthroplasty: A high risk of subsequent complications. *Clin Orthop Relat Res* 2019;477(1):70-77.

The authors of this study evaluated 15 patients who sustained a PJI for unicompartmental knee arthroplasty. Patients who underwent a DAIR for the procedure had more subsequent revisions and complications compared with patients who underwent a two-stage exchange for a TKA. Level of evidence: IV.

59. Citak M, Friedenstab J, Abdelaziz H, et al: Risk factors for failure after 1-stage exchange total knee arthroplasty in the management of periprosthetic joint infection. *J Bone Joint Surg Am* 2019;101(12):1061-1069.

This study looked at 91 patients in whom a one-stage revision arthroplasty had failed. They found several risk factors that were associated with failure to include *Enterococcus* or *Streptococcus* infections. Level of evidence: III.

60. Srivastava K, Bozic KJ, Silverton C, Nelson AJ, Makhni EC, Davis JJ: Reconsidering strategies for managing chronic periprosthetic joint infection in total knee arthroplasty: Using decision analytics to find the optimal strategy between one-stage and two-stage total knee revision. *J Bone Joint Surg Am* 2019;101(1):14-24.

The authors of this study looked at quality-adjusted life years and costs associated with both one-stage and two-stage revision surgery for infection. They found that a one-stage revision was associated with the highest quality of life at a lower cost. Level of evidence: IV.

61. Ma CY, Lu YD, Bell KL, et al: Predictors of treatment failure after 2-stage reimplantation for infected total knee arthroplasty: A 2- to 10-year follow-up. *J Arthroplasty* 2018;33(7):2234-2239.

The authors of this study found that BMI above 30 kg/m^2, surgical time over 4 hours, gout, and the presence of *Enterococcus* species were associated with increased failure of two-stage revision arthroplasty for PJI. Level of evidence: IV.

62. Hischebeth GT, Randau TM, Ploeger MM, et al: *Staphylococcus aureus* versus *Staphylococcus epidermidis* in periprosthetic joint infection-Outcome analysis of methicillin-resistant versus methicillin-susceptible strains. *Diagn Microbiol Infect Dis* 2019;93(2):125-130.

This study found that patients who sustained a PJI associated with methicillin-resistant coagulase-negative *Staphylococcus* were significantly less likely to be definitively free of infection at 2 years compared with other MRSA, methicillin-sensitive *S epidermidis*, and MRSA. Level of evidence: III.

63. Tan TL, Goswami K, Kheir MM, Xu C, Wang Q, Parvizi J: Surgical treatment of chronic periprosthetic joint infection: Fate of spacer exchanges. *J Arthroplasty* 2019;34(9):2085-2090.e1.

These authors evaluated 90 patients who underwent an unplanned spacer exchange as part of their two-stage exchange arthroplasty. They found that these patients were associated with worse outcomes compared with those who underwent a regular two-stage exchange arthroplasty. Level of evidence: IV.

64. Wang Q, Goswami K, Kuo FC, Xu C, Tan TL, Parvizi J: Two-stage exchange arthroplasty for periprosthetic joint infection: The rate and reason for the attrition after the first stage. *J Arthroplasty* 2019;34(11):2749-2756.

An analysis of more than 600 patients found that almost 20% of patients never receive their intended replantation as part of a two-stage treatment protocol for PJI. These patients need to be considered when evaluating the efficacy of this procedure. Level of evidence: IV.

65. Stambough JB, Curtin BM, Odum SM, Cross MB, Martin JR, Fehring TK: Does change in ESR and CRP guide the timing of two-stage arthroplasty reimplantation? *Clin Orthop Relat Res* 2019;477(2):364-371.

The authors of this study conclude that ESR and CRP are not reliable markers for when a patient should undergo the second stage of their planned two-stage reimplantation for PJI. Level of evidence: III.

66. Samuel LT, Sultan AA, Kheir M, et al: Positive alpha-defensin at reimplantation of a two-stage revision arthroplasty is not associated with infection at 1 year. *Clin Orthop Relat Res* 2019;477(7):1615-1621.

This study found that a positive alpha defensin result at the time of reimplantation did not correlate with persistent infection at 1 year after a two-stage revision for PJI. Level of evidence: IV.

67. Jones CW, Selemon N, Nocon A, Bostrom M, Westrich G, Sculco PK: The influence of spacer design on the rate of complications in two-stage revision hip arthroplasty. *J Arthroplasty* 2019;34(6):1201-1206.

In this study looking at two-stage exchanges for THA PJI, 185 patients were reviewed. The authors found that 26% of patients had a complication secondary to their spacer. Level of evidence: IV.

68. Nace J, Siddiqi A, Talmo CT, Chen AF: Diagnosis and management of fungal periprosthetic joint infections. *J Am Acad Orthop Surg* 2019;27(18):e804-e818.

This review focuses on fungal PJIs. Level of evidence: IV.

69. Wouthuyzen-Bakker M, Nijman JM, Kampinga GA, van Assen S, Jutte PC: Efficacy of antibiotic suppressive therapy in patients with a prosthetic joint infection. *J Bone Jt Infect* 2017;2(2):77-83.

In this study, the authors found that antibiotic suppressive therapy was successful in 67% of patients. The authors recommend it as a good option for patients who are not good candidates for implant removal or revision. Level of evidence: IV.

70. Goldman AH, Clark NJ, Taunton MJ, Lewallen DG, Berry DJ, Abdel MP: Definitive resection arthroplasty of the knee: A surprisingly viable treatment to manage intractable infection in selected patients. *J Arthroplasty* 2020;35(3):855-858.

The authors of this study found that resection arthroplasty successfully eradicated the infection in 84% of patients with previously recalcitrant PJI. Level of evidence: IV.

71. Vincenten CM, Den Oudsten BL, Bos PK, Bolder SBT, Gosens T: Quality of life and health status after Girdlestone resection arthroplasty in patients with an infected total hip prosthesis. *J Bone Jt Infect* 2019;4(1):10-15.

This evaluation of 63 patients with a Girdlestone found that their health status and quality-of-life scores were significantly lower than those of patients who had sustained a myocardial infarction or underwent a lower limb amputation. Level of evidence: IV.

CHAPTER 16

Periprosthetic Fractures—Hip and Knee

RICHARD S. YOON, MD • FRANK A. LIPORACE, MD

ABSTRACT

With younger, more active patients undergoing total hip arthroplasty (THA) and total knee arthroplasty (TKA), as they get older, an increasing incidence of periprosthetic fractures is also expected. Periprosthetic fractures around THAs and TKAs can have devastating consequences, and goals of surgical intervention should revolve around constructs that allow for immediate weight bearing and mobilization. Surgical management is predicated on fracture location, implant stability, and the amount and quality of bone available. Preparation should include options for fixation, revision, or some combination of both. The evaluation, management, and technical aspects of fixation and revision of periprosthetic fractures about THA and TKA are reviewed.

Keywords: periprosthetic fracture; revision total hip arthroplasty; revision total knee arthroplasty; total hip arthroplasty; total knee arthroplasty

Dr. Yoon or an immediate family member is a member of a speakers' bureau or has made paid presentations on behalf of Surgical Care Affiliates (SCA); serves as a paid consultant to or is an employee of Arthrex, Inc., DePuy, A Johnson & Johnson Company, LifeNet Health, Orthobullets, OrthoXel, Synthes, Use-Lab, and Wright Medical Technology, Inc.; serves as an unpaid consultant to BuiltLean; has stock or stock options held in Taithera Inc.; and has received research or institutional support from Biomet, Coventus, Synthes, and Wright Medical Technology, Inc. Dr. Liporace or an immediate family member has received royalties from Biomet and Wright Medical Technology, Inc.; is a member of a speakers' bureau or has made paid presentations on behalf of Biomet and Synthes; serves as a paid consultant to or is an employee of Biomet and Synthes; and serves as an unpaid consultant to AO.

INTRODUCTION

By 2060, the patient population older than 44 years is estimated to be approximately 140 million.[1] With a recent emphasis on health, wellness, and improvements in modern medicine, patients are living longer and staying more active. Combined with improvements in metallurgy and wear properties, a concomitant rise in the number of total hip arthroplasties (THAs) and total knee arthroplasties (TKAs) is expected. Furthermore, with younger patients undergoing THA and/or TKA and living longer, leading more active lives, an increase in the incidence of periprosthetic hip and knee fractures is inevitable.[1]

Recent studies have shown that morbidity and mortality of periprosthetic THA and TKA fractures are comparable to the hip fracture demographic.[2,3] Similarly, expeditious medical optimization minimizing time to the operating room is of paramount importance. If possible, identification and review of any previous associated surgeries including complications should be performed before surgery. Knowing the prior surgical approach and specific implant knowledge can aid in offering a smooth surgical course. Last, intimate knowledge of the patient's mental status, code status, functional activity level, and goals of care are important potential discussion points to consider in a rising elderly population.

Surgical management of periprosthetic fractures about the hip and knee can be approached by implementing a systematic assessment and approach. There are several key points that can be determined to facilitate a viable and successful surgical plan (**Table 1**).

FRACTURE LOCATION AND IMPLANT STABILITY

Typically, fracture location around the implant can help dictate the definitive plan. Generally speaking, fractures very proximal or distal in relation to a stable implant can usually be fixed. However, the surgeon should never assume a well-fixed implant. CT can identify fracture

TABLE 1

Key Factors in Surgical Planning for Periprosthetic THA/TKA Fractures

1. Fracture location
2. Implant stability
3. Presence of cement mantle
4. Presence of potential infection
5. Bone quality and expected amount of bone loss
6. Be prepared to fix or revise or both

THA = total hip arthroplasty, TKA = total knee arthroplasty

lines extending into the implant, which may infer a loose implant; however, assessment of overall implant stability should be routinely performed intraoperatively, regardless of fracture location. The surgeon should always err on the side of caution and be prepared for a loose implant with a plan for revision. Planning in this strategic manner can lead to more decisive decision making and lower overall surgical time, blood loss, and time under anesthesia.

Presence of Cement Mantle

Addressing a cement mantle can adversely affect surgical time, increasing risk of associated complications. Tools to remove cement, particularly around the fracture, should be available. Especially when planning for a possible revision, appropriate cement removal instruments and tools should be available to improve case efficiency.[4] Furthermore, to avoid prolonged surgical time, appropriate cement-in-cement technique can be used with good results.[4,5]

Presence of Potential Infection

Even in the fracture setting, a prudent surgeon should always consider concomitant infection and should have a low threshold for an associated workup. Preexisting prodromal pain, intermittent drainage, and/or the presence of a draining sinus or associated wound dehiscence should warn of an infection. Preparing to execute several strategies, such as antibiotic-coated locking plates and using antibiotic hip or knee spacers, can allow for definitive treatment while allowing for reliable fracture fixation, allowing for even immediate, partial weight bearing.[6-8]

Bone Quality, Expected Amount of Bone Loss, and Being Prepared to Fix, Revise, or Both

Critical assessment of bone quality and the expected amount of bone loss, arguably the most important factor in preoperative planning, should complete the preoperative list of implants and fixation devices needed for each case. Even if surgical fixation seems attainable, having available potential revision implants that may not necessarily be readily available can help one be prepared for any clinical scenario in which fixation fails. Bone quality and stock assessment yielding to decisive decision making leads to a more efficient surgical case, which can minimize postoperative complications. It is important to remember that immediate weight bearing and early mobilization are the most important goals; therefore, the final construct should reflect and allow for these goals.

PERIPROSTHETIC FRACTURES ASSOCIATED WITH HIP ARTHROPLASTY

Periprosthetic fractures can occur around THA, hemiarthroplasty, and hip resurfacing. The focus of this discussion will be regarding fractures about THA, addressing both the acetabular and femoral sides. For periprosthetic fractures about hemiarthroplasty, they can be treated based on the recommendations for treating the femoral side for a THA. Typically, for fractures occurring around hip resurfacing, they will require revision to THA.

Periprosthetic Hip Fractures on the Acetabular Side

Fixation of periprosthetic acetabular fractures depends on implant stability, which is determined by fracture displacement, column involvement, and available bone stock. Summarizing recommendations based on these characteristics, the Paprosky classification provides an algorithm for addressing periprosthetic fractures about the acetabulum[9] (**Table 2**). For both intraoperative and postoperative fractures about the cup, assessment of fracture displacement and available bone stock can dictate management—stable, minimally displaced fractures can usually be treated without additional fixation; however, unstable components with displaced fractures with or without bone stock require either revision components and/or supplemental plate fixation.[9]

For unstable intraoperative acetabular fractures, upsizing to a larger revision cup may be enough to provide a stable construct; however, if there is any question about cup stability, even with screw fixation, an additional posterior column buttress should be provided. This can be achieved via further proximal and distal dissection and contouring and placing a reconstruction plate along the posterior column for additional buttress.

For periprosthetic fractures that occur with an obviously loose cup, a thorough preoperative assessment with CT should be performed to assess any amount of associated bone loss as well as the fracture lines to help in surgical planning. Although an anterior approach (eg, ilioinguinal or modified Stoppa) to the inner table is rarely required for surgical treatment of these fractures, depending on the fracture pattern, access to the quadrilateral plate may be necessary to achieve adequate

TABLE 2

Paprosky Classification of Periprosthetic Acetabular Fractures

Type and Subtype	Location and Characteristics
Intraoperative (During Insertion)	
A	Recognized, stable, nondisplaced fracture
B	Recognized, unstable, displaced fracture
C	Unrecognized
Intraoperative (During Removal)	
A	Less than 50% bone stock
B	Greater than 50% bone stock
Traumatic	
A	Stable component
B	Unstable component
Spontaneous	
A	Less than 50% bone stock
B	Greater than 50% bone stock
Pelvic Discontinuity	
A	Less than 50% bone stock
B	Greater than 50% bone stock
C	Associated with pelvic radiation

fixation, especially if gross acute discontinuity is noted between the anterior and posterior columns. However, depending on the amount of bone loss, there should be a low threshold not only to revise the cup to a jumbo cup, but also to use a cage construct to help restore columnar stability.

Periprosthetic Hip Fractures on the Femoral Side

Management of periprosthetic fractures that occur around the femoral implant can often be reasonably guided by its classification (**Table 3**). The Vancouver classification, similar to the others, separates the fracture patterns by location. For fractures about the stem, the classification is further stratified by implant stability and available bone stock, classification principles that also help dictate treatment. Additionally, preoperative assessment of the acetabular implant should also be performed, and there should be a low threshold to revise the cup in the same setting to obtain longevity of the hip.

Vancouver type A fracture subtypes depend on location, either about the greater (AG) or lesser trochanters (AL, **Table 3**). Intraoperative fractures that occur about

TABLE 3

Vancouver Classification

Type and Subtype	Location and Characteristics
Type A	—
AG	Greater trochanter
AL	Lesser trochanter
Type B	—
B1	Around stem/tip, well fixed
B2	Around stem/tip, loose stem
B3	Around stem/tip, loose stem, poor bone stock
Type C	Distal to stem

the trochanters can typically be addressed with cerclage wiring. However, it is imperative to assess the integrity of the calcar. If the calcar is fractured or unstable, it may result in subsidence and subsequent instability and lead to dislocation or potential implant instability. Thus, there should be a low threshold to change the femoral stem to a calcar-replacing, diaphyseal fitting, or modular diaphyseal fitting stem to avoid such complications. When occurring postoperatively, many fractures about the trochanters are often minimally displaced and can be managed nonsurgically with motion restrictions. However, with substantial displacement, nonunion can occur, and surgical fixation with a trochanteric grip plate (with or without cerclage wires) is recommended. Again, it is imperative to assess implant stability intraoperatively, and if there is any question that the stem is loose, revision is recommended.

Of note, if there is a greater trochanteric fracture with concomitant lesser trochanteric involvement, then the surgeon should be highly suspicious of the potential for implant loosening, because the fracture line may be continuous and hidden by the implant on plain radiographs. CT scan may help in evaluation but the femoral implant may obstruct the ability to make a full evaluation; ordering a three-dimensional reconstruction can often unmask unnoticeable fracture propagation (**Figure 1**).

Vancouver type B fractures are generally surgical fractures. Definitive classification of stem stability is usually made intraoperatively; thus, the surgeon should be prepared for fixation and implant revision. Type B fractures, by definition, occur about the distal tip of the stem, and each subclassification depends on the stability of the implant and the surrounding bone stock. Type B1 fractures are about well-fixed implants with good bone stock and are most often amenable to surgical

Section 1: Hip and Knee

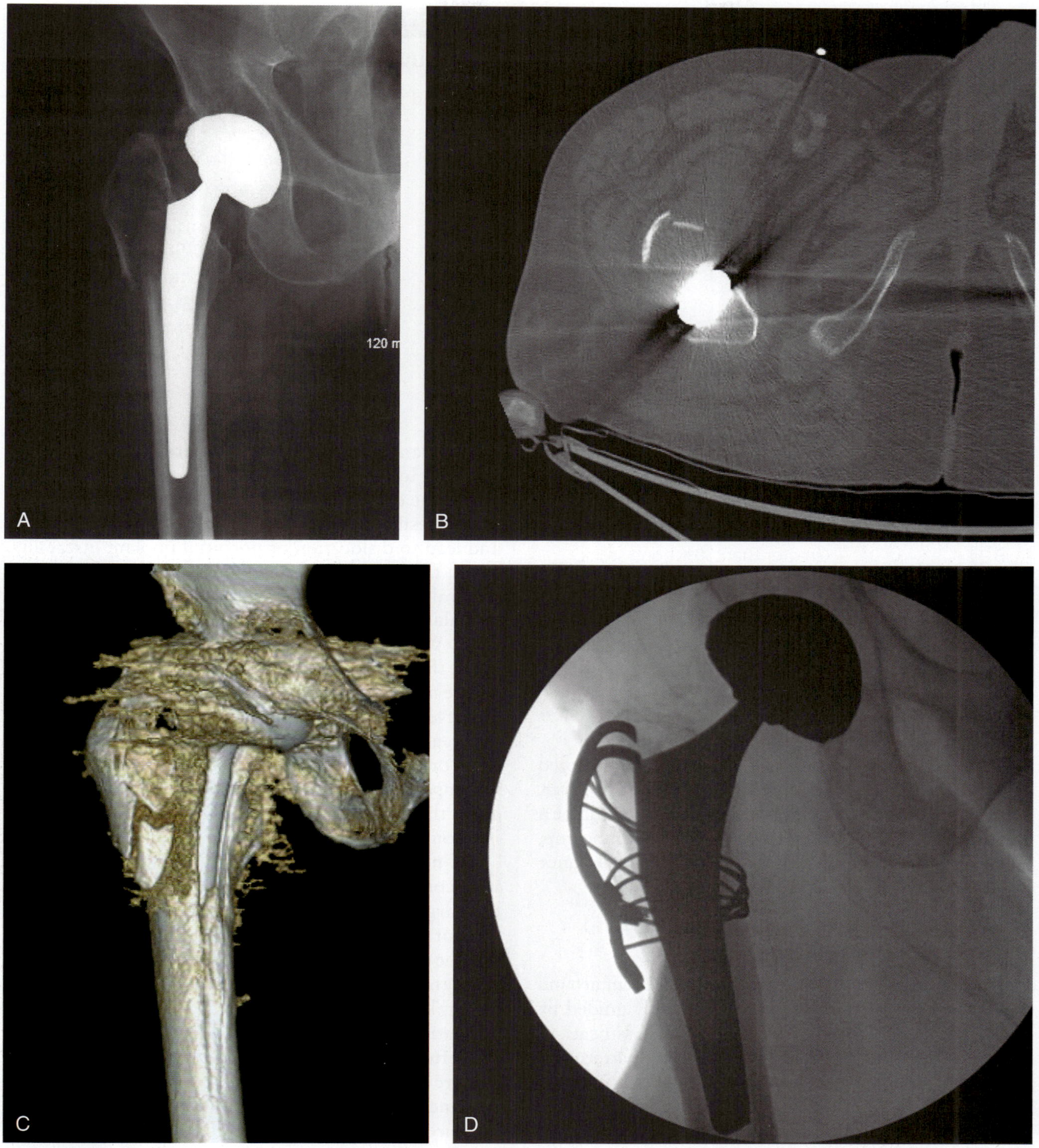

FIGURE 1 A 67-year-old man with a well-functioning right total hip arthroplasty for 7 years sustains a fall. **A**, Radiograph exhibits a presumed, isolated greater trochanter fracture. CT on both axial (**B**) and three-dimensional reconstruction (**C**) shows a more extensive proximal periprosthetic femur fracture requiring surgical intervention. Intraoperative assessment indicated a stable implant, requiring only fixation of the proximal fracture component. **D,** Fluoroscopic AP view of the hip exhibiting proximal fragment fixation with a claw plate and cables.

fracture fixation after intraoperative assessment of the stem. An extensile lateral approach to the femur without devascularizing the muscle is a powerful approach that allows full visualization of the fracture. Fixation strategies typically recommend that the surgeon apply an appropriate amount of plate/implant overlap, which has been a topic of debate. With increased distance of fixation past the overlap between the plate and the stem, the potential development of a stress riser at the tip of the stem becomes negligible.[10] However, the ideal plate length to use is still an unknown entity and controversial because of the lack of high-level evidence.[11-14] Proximally, biomechanical studies fail to find significant differences between plates that reach the greater trochanter and those that stop short. Some have recommended maximizing distance from overlap based on the availability of intact bone, thus maximizing the working length of the fixation.[11-13,15-17] Distally, there is emerging literature that spanning the entire femur from the femoral condyles with or without an additional intramedullary nail (nail-plate combination technique) may further decrease nonunion rates and allow for prophylactic fixation to avoid future injury[18-20] (**Figure 2**).

The ideal fixation strategy also remains controversial. Although biomechanically superior to conventional plating, locked plating has not consistently decreased nonunion rates in all case series.[11,13] Although locked plating did not yield significantly higher complication or nonunion rates, a significantly higher rate of failure and infection with concomitant allograft use was reported.[13]

Recent studies have attempted to compare the results between open reduction and internal fixation and revision to determine whether one modality was superior to the other.[2,21] The authors of one study compared the two treatment methods and reported a twofold higher rate of complications in the open reduction and internal fixation cohort.[22] Another study similarly compared the two cohorts and reported a significantly

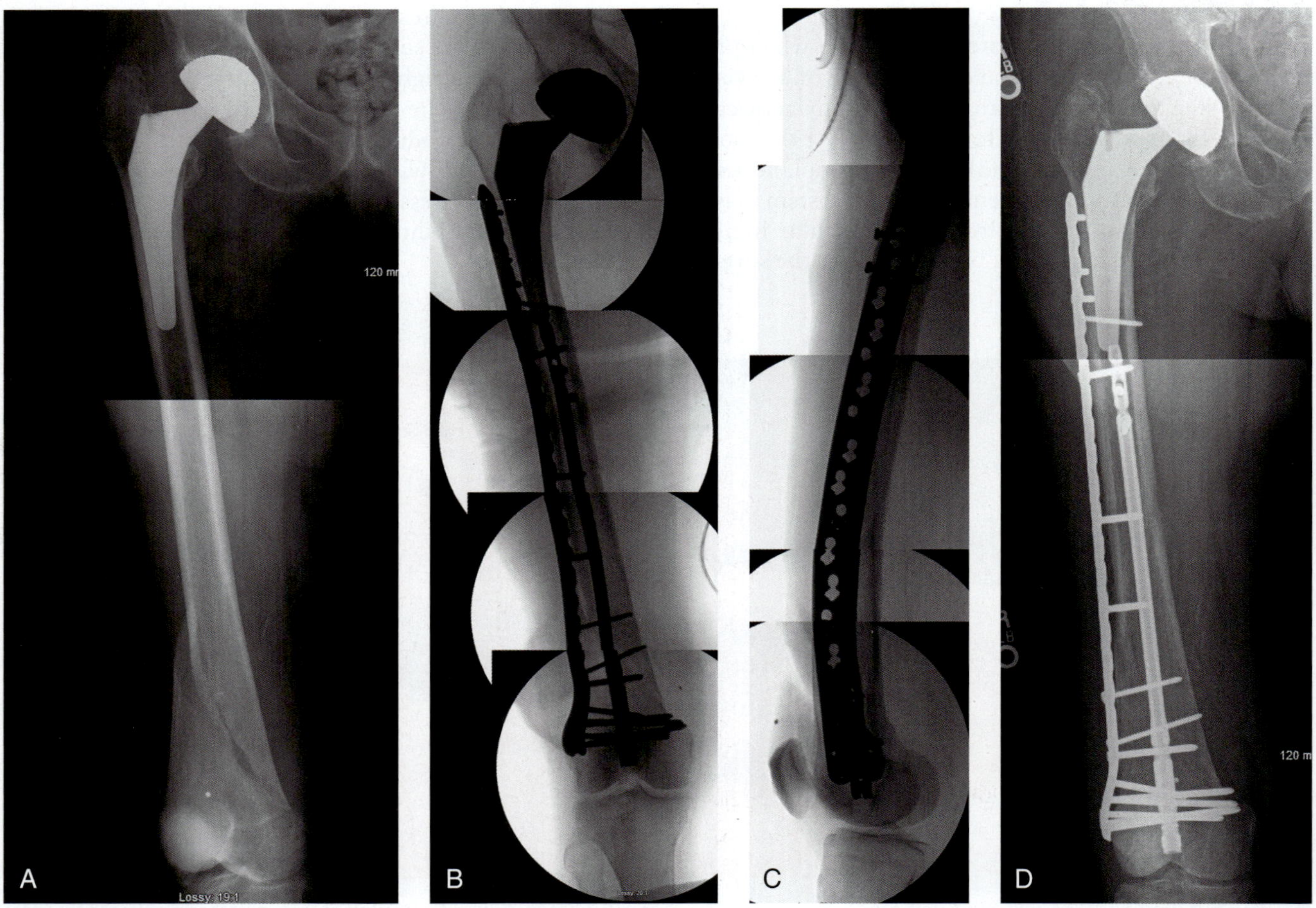

FIGURE 2 Radiographs of the femur of an 87-year-old man after twisting from standing height. He reports a well-functioning right total hip arthroplasty for the past 7 years. **A**, Radiograph showing a distal Vancouver C femur fracture. **B** and **C**, Radiographs showing an independent nail-plate combination technique was ideal to allow community ambulation and to offer enough stability to allow for immediate bearing leading to uneventful healing, at 3-month follow-up. **D**, AP femur radiograph exhibiting the nail-plate combination technique for Vancouver C type periprosthetic fracture.

Section 1: Hip and Knee

higher mortality rate in the open reduction and internal fixation group when compared with revision.[2] In these studies, authors have suggested that revision with or without supplementary fixation may prove beneficial to the geriatric patient by allowing for earlier mobilization and at least immediate partial weight bearing.[2,21] However, both of these studies perform severely underpowered subgroup comparisons with inherent selection biases that likely represent statistical error. Larger prospective comparative studies are required to offer a definitive comparison.

Treatment of type B2 fractures is often more extensive in complexity and exposure. Here, implant removal can be facilitated by using the fracture analogous to an extended trochanteric osteotomy.[14] With an open-book fracture site, removing the implant may be facilitated. Revisions, in this setting, often use diaphyseal fitting stems, many of which are modular.[23-25] The standard proximal posterolateral approach can be extended distally into an extensile lateral femoral approach acting as the workhorse to accomplish the goals of surgical management (**Figure 3**).

To protect against fracture propagation when prepping the intact femur for the distal aspect of a revision femoral stem, the surgeon can place a prophylactic cable distal to the fracture site before reaming. At this point, reaming and potting the distal end of the implant before reducing the fracture fragments around the stem may be beneficial. Potting the diaphysis of a modular implant not only confirms a good fit, but also allows the surgeon to temporarily build the trial proximal body while using the greater trochanter as a reference for overall sizing before trialing stability.

Type B3 fractures are characterized by poor proximal bone stock and a loose stem. Depending on the amount of proximal bone stock available, options for revision include full-coated stems, fluted tapered stems, prosthesis-strut allograft composite constructs, and proximal femoral replacements (PFRs).[23-26] Although frequently used in the past, prosthesis-strut allografts are becoming less common because of prolonged time to incorporation, infection risk, and modern improvements in fixation as well as revision implants. Implant removal strategies are similar to those described previously. Encouraging short-term and midterm survivorship and function with modular, fluted tapered stems have been reported, even in the setting of poor proximal bone stock.[25-27]

In type B3 fractures, however, definitive assessment of available bone typically does not occur until after the incision is made. Thus, having a PFR on stand-by is recommended. Especially in the elderly, low-demand patients, a low threshold to proceed with PFR is advocated, to minimize surgical time and blood loss and allow for immediate weight bearing (**Figure 4**). Similar to any revision setting, the surgeon should not only assess the integrity of the abductors, but also assess cup position and stability. Following assessment, there should be a low threshold to address the acetabular side via revision or use of a dual mobility or a constrained liner to minimize dislocation risk.

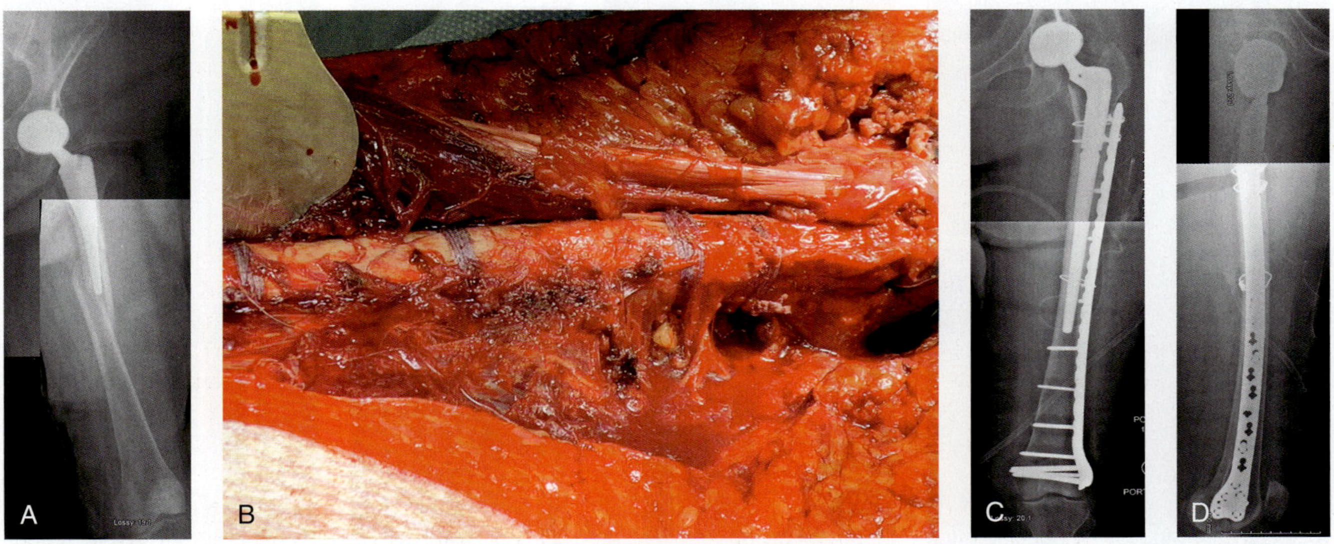

FIGURE 3 Radiographs and clinical photograph from an 84-year-old woman 4 weeks after left total hip arthroplasty for femoral neck fracture. She was independent and discharged home, but fell down the stairs on the way to outpatient therapy. Only 4 weeks later, by definition, the stem was loose. **A**, Radiograph shows subsidence, which indicates the stem was loose. **B**, Clinical photograph exhibits an extensile lateral approach using a combination of nonabsorbable cerclage suture to maintain reduction during revision to a diaphyseal fitting prosthesis and distal femoral locked plating. **C** and **D**, AP postoperative radiographs.

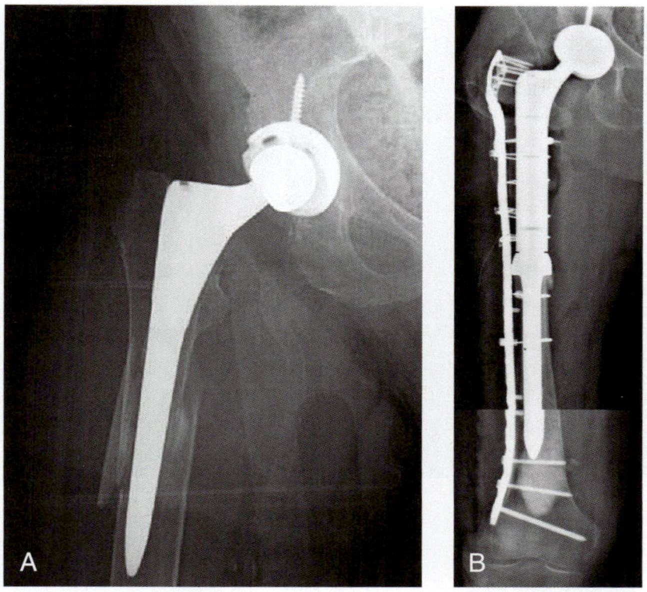

FIGURE 4 Radiographs of the hip and femur of a 91-year-old woman who fell at home. **A**, Radiograph shows Vancouver B3 periprosthetic total hip arthroplasty fracture with excessive stress-shielding in extremely poor bone stock. Achieving goals of efficient surgical time, immediate weight bearing, and early mobilization, postoperative radiograph (**B**) shows a revision to proximal femoral replacement with a spanning, distal femoral locking plate, providing additional fixation for the greater trochanter.

Type C fractures, which occur distal to the stem, are often treated as distal femur fractures, with many surgeons using distal femoral plates. Similar to the controversy that lies with type B1 fracture types, adequate overlap with the femoral stem and the plate (with a combination of cables and screws) is also recommended to provide the best biomechanical construct. However, there is no general consensus on the ideal length and construct.[16]

PERIPROSTHETIC FRACTURES ASSOCIATED WITH KNEE ARTHROPLASTY

For periprosthetic TKA fractures, treatment is guided by location (above or below the implant), bone quality, and implant stability.[22,28] Similarly, surgical goals are to achieve a fixation and/or revision construct that allows for immediate weight bearing and early mobility in this elderly population.

Periprosthetic Knee Fractures on the Femoral Side

Management of fractures occurring on the femoral side of a TKA depends on the stability of the implant[28] (**Table 4**). Lewis and Rorabeck classified periprosthetic TKA fractures into three types: Type I is nondisplaced with a stable implant. Type II is a displaced fracture with a stable implant. Type III fractures are displaced (IIIA) or nondisplaced (IIIB) fractures with unstable or loose implants.

TABLE 4

Lewis and Rorabeck Classification of Periprosthetic Supracondylar Fractures (TKA)

Type	Characteristics
Type I	Nondisplaced, stable prosthesis
Type II	Displaced, stable prosthesis
Type III	
IIIA	Displaced, loose prosthesis
IIIB	Nondisplaced, loose prosthesis

TKA = total knee arthroplasty

Type I fractures can occasionally be treated nonsurgically, especially in those patients with severe comorbidities. However, even in the most minimally displaced fracture, fixation may provide a more stable construct to promote earlier mobilization and avoid progressive deformity. Type I and II fractures are treated similarly, with options including either the use of a lateral plate or a retrograde nail. There is a paucity of definitive level I or II evidence to support one over the other. Both are well accepted depending on surgeon preference.[29,30] Several key pearls dictate implant choice. First and foremost, the presence of an implant in the proximal femur, whether it is a femoral stem or a short intramedullary nail, should dictate the use of a construct that spans the entire femur. In other words, if a lateral plate is used, it should extend proximally enough to overlap with the femoral implant.[16] If a retrograde intramedullary nail is used and stopped short of the femoral implant, a plate may be placed to overlap both implants and avoid creation of a stress riser. Recently evidence denoting the biomechanical benefits of linking these implants together has been published.[20,31]

For grossly loose implants with concomitant fractures, revision is recommended. With good bone stock and an easily removable femoral implant, fixing the fracture and placing another primary component is certainly possible but rare. Typically, the femur is revised with a stemmed component with or without augments for areas of defects and to match flexion/extension gaps. Although some implant companies allow mating of revision to primary components, typically revising the femur also means revising the tibial component to have a mated system (**Figure 5**). For fractures extending far distally into the flange, with questionably stable implants with or without poor bone stock, a distal femoral replacement can offer a faster, lower morbidity procedure that also allows immediate weight bearing and mobilization in the elderly.[32]

Section 1: Hip and Knee

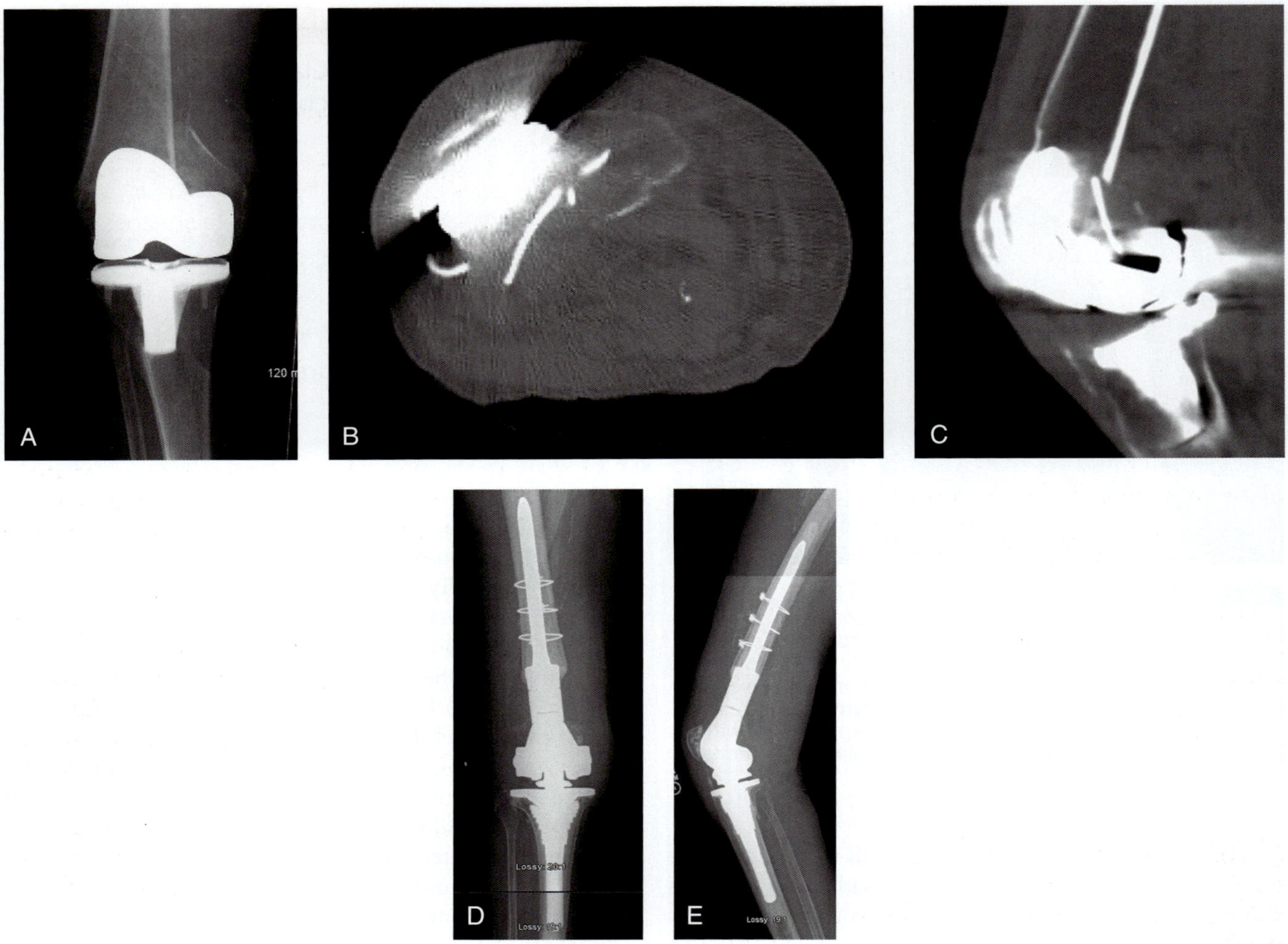

FIGURE 5 Imaging studies from an 88-year-old woman with a well-functioning right total knee arthroplasty for 9 years who fell down two steps. **A**, Radiograph shows a periprosthetic supracondylar fracture with distal extension. **B**, CT axial and **C**, sagittal reconstructions detailing comminution, impaction, and likely loose femoral implant. With proximal extension of the fracture, cable fixation along with revision to distal femoral replacement allowed for immediate weight bearing and early mobilization. **D** and **E**, AP and lateral knee radiographs at 6-month follow-up during which the patient was ambulating with a walker for long distances and a four-prong cane at home with no pain.

Periprosthetic Knee Fractures About the Patellar Component

Periprosthetic fractures that occur around the patellar component are rare, but can occur. Surgical versus nonsurgical intervention is dependent on integrity of the extensor mechanism. Even for injuries with an extensor lag, attention to patellar thickness must be taken into account before offering surgical intervention. Commonly, immobilization in full extension (via cast or brace) with gradual return of range of motion with guided physical therapy can offer a nonsurgical solution in this unique clinical scenario. When indicating surgical intervention, osteonecrosis, nonunion, and need for revision surgery are true risks, and early failure can cause functional deficits. Therefore, either augmentation of patellar fracture repair or performing a partial or full patellectomy with Marlex mesh extensor mechanism reconstruction may offer the best clinical outcome with low risk of attenuation.[32,33]

Periprosthetic Knee Fractures on the Tibial Side

Very little has been written about periprosthetic fractures that occur on the tibial side of a TKA; however, the principles remain the same as for other periprosthetic fractures. Nondisplaced fractures around stable implants can often be managed nonsurgically in either a cast or brace with protected weight bearing. Many have a low threshold for fixation in these cases, to allow immediate mobilization and prevent joint contracture. Minimally invasive fixation techniques can deliver this stability with low morbidity. A stable implant with a displaced fracture typically can be fixed with plate and screw constructs. It is imperative to assess the anatomic axis and restore the appropriate parameters about the joint line. Also, when plating around the tibial component, variable angle locked screws can be helpful in obtaining good purchase while avoiding the stem. Nonanatomic reduction may lead to increased wear and failure of the TKA. A loose implant warrants revision with long-stemmed components with or without augments. Again, although some companies allow for mixed mating of their primary and revision components, typically revising one side requires revising the other to create a mated system.

Midshaft and distal tibial fractures occur rarely in association with TKA and typically occur independent of the implant. However, proper assessment of the implant, the mechanical and anatomical axis, should occur, and there should be a low threshold to fix the fracture (**Figure 6**). Plate and screw constructs can provide excellent fixation with minimal soft-tissue disruption, especially in the setting of poor bone quality, when the surgeon may opt to span the entire length of the bone to avoid stress risers and future fracture.

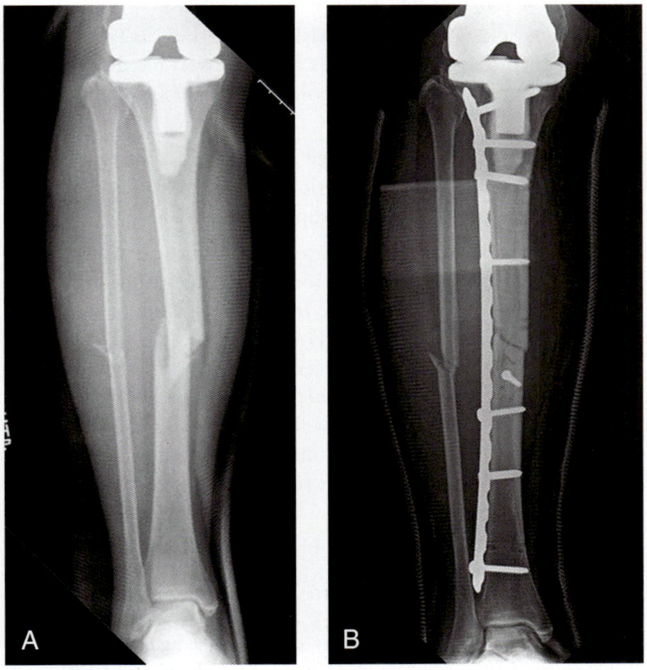

FIGURE 6 Radiographs from a 63-year-old woman who tripped and fell down subway stairs. **A**, AP radiograph showing tibial shaft fracture distal to the tibial component. **B**, AP postoperative radiograph shows a contoured plate placed via minimally invasive, percutaneous technique to restore length, alignment, and rotation.

SUMMARY

The incidence of periprosthetic hip and knee fractures is rising. It requires a systematic approach: identify the location of the fracture relative to the prosthesis; assess the inherent implant stability; and consider the surrounding bone quality and available bone stock. The surgeon should consider and be prepared for revision arthroplasty. Especially in the elderly population, constructs that allow for immediate weight bearing and early mobilization are preferred. For proximal and distal femur fractures with significant bone loss, the surgeon should have a low threshold to revise to a PFR and distal femoral replacement. When dealing with patella fractures, the surgeon should be prepared to augment with a Marlex mesh construct to avoid repeat extensor mechanism failure. When performing internal fixation, extensile approaches should be used and the surgeon should have little hesitation to span the entire long bone to increase stability, and avoid creating stress risers.

KEY STUDY POINTS

- Treatment is determined by fracture location, implant stability, available bone stock, and bone quality.
- The surgeon should always be prepared to revise, and in certain situations, use end segment replacing prostheses.
- Patients should be treated in a manner similar to those with geriatric hip fractures—optimization and mobilization are key principles to maximize outcomes.

ANNOTATED REFERENCES

1. Della Rocca GJ, Leung KS, Pape HC: Periprosthetic fractures: Epidemiology and future projections. *J Orthop Trauma* 2011;25(suppl 2):S66-S70.
2. Bhattacharyya T, Chang D, Meigs JB, Estok DM II, Malchau H: Mortality after periprosthetic fracture of the femur. *J Bone Joint Surg Am* 2007;89:2658-2662.
3. Boylan MR, Riesgo AM, Paulino CB, Slover JD, Zuckerman JD, Egol KA: Mortality following periprosthetic proximal femoral fractures versus native hip fractures. *J Bone Joint Surg Am* 2018;100:578-585.

   In this epidemiologic analysis comparing the mortality outcomes between patients with periprosthetic proximal femur fractures and patients with native hip fractures, there was no difference in mortality rate at 1 month (3.2% versus 4.6%). This statistic indicates the need for early mobilization and weight bearing, even in the periprosthetic fracture population. Level of evidence: III.
4. Liddle A, Webb M, Clement N, et al: Ultrasonic cement removal in cement-in-cement revision total hip arthroplasty: What is the effect on the final cement-in-cement bond? *Bone Joint Res* 2019;8:246-252.

In this cadaver study of 24 specimens, the authors tested the porosity and strength of cement preparation in cement-in-cement technique. Comparing strength and porosity in cement removed with a burr, ultrasonic means, or no removal, the authors noted that there was increased porosity and weaker bonds in cement removed via ultrasonic technique. Translating this to the clinical arena, the authors warned against a potentially weaker cement mantle when using ultrasonic removal before cement-in-cement technique. Level of evidence: n/a.

5. Woodbridge AB, Hubble MJ, Whitehouse SL, Wilson MJ, Howell JR, Timperley AJ: The Exeter short revision stem for cement-in-cement femoral revision: A five to twelve year review. *J Arthroplasty* 2019;34:S297-S301.

   In this retrospective survivorship analysis, the authors followed up 166 cases in which a cement-in-cement technique was performed with the Exeter hip stem. The Exeter hip stem was used because of its short stem, which can be used in the revision setting. The authors reported Kaplan-Meier survivorship at 10 years to be 100% for aseptic loosening, 96.8% for stem failure, and overall 88.9% survivorship for all causes. Level of evidence: IV.

6. Liporace FA, Yoon RS, Frank MA, et al: Use of an "antibiotic plate" for infected periprosthetic fracture in total hip arthroplasty. *J Orthop Trauma* 2012;26:e18-e23.

7. Maceroli MA, Yoon RS, Liporace FA: Use of antibiotic plates and spacers for fracture in the setting of periprosthetic infection. *J Orthop Trauma* 2019;33(suppl 6):S21-S24.

   In this case-based, technical article, the authors describe successful treatment of a patient with a periprosthetic femur fracture in the setting of an active infection. Following débridement and removal of an infected allograft, the authors successfully treated the patient with a stage-one mold hip spacer with an antibiotic plate, with subsequent two-stage revision to a proximal femoral replacement. Level of evidence: V.

8. Patel JN, Pizzo RA, Yoon RS, Liporace FA: Addressing antibiotic hip spacer instability via hybrid screw-cement fixation of a constrained liner and cement-rebar interface techniques: A technical narrative. *J Am Acad Orthop Surg* 2020;28:166-170.

   In this retrospective case series, the authors described a modified technique in using a constrained liner and a stage one molded hip spacer for infection. This technique uses countersunk 3.5 mm screws through the constrained liner to provide additional fixation and also describes the creation of a cement-rebar wall that can be helpful in scenarios with posterior wall bone loss with or without periprosthetic infection. Level of evidence: IV.

9. Della Valle CJ, Momberger NG, Paprosky WG: Periprosthetic fractures of the acetabulum associated with a total hip arthroplasty. *Instr Course Lect* 2003;52:281-290.

10. Dubov A, Kim SY, Shah S, Schemitsch EH, Zdero R, Bougherara H: The biomechanics of plate repair of periprosthetic femur fractures near the tip of a total hip implant: The effect of cable-screw position. *Proc Inst Mech Eng H* 2011;225:857-865.

11. Dehghan N, McKee MD, Nauth A, Ristevski B, Schemitsch EH: Surgical fixation of Vancouver type B1 periprosthetic femur fractures: A systematic review. *J Orthop Trauma* 2014;28:721-727.

12. Froberg L, Troelsen A, Brix M: Periprosthetic Vancouver type B1 and C fractures treated by locking-plate osteosynthesis: Fracture union and reoperations in 60 consecutive fractures. *Acta Orthop* 2012;83:648-652.

13. Moore RE, Baldwin K, Austin MS, Mehta S: A systematic review of open reduction and internal fixation of periprosthetic femur fractures with or without allograft strut, cerclage, and locked plates. *J Arthroplasty* 2014;29:872-876.

14. Liporace FA, Donegan DJ, Langford JR, Haidukewych GJ: Contemporary internal fixation techniques for periprosthetic fractures of the hip and knee. *Instr Course Lect* 2013;62:317-332.

15. Fulkerson E, Koval K, Preston CF, Iesaka K, Kummer FJ, Egol KA: Fixation of periprosthetic femoral shaft fractures associated with cemented femoral stems: A biomechanical comparison of locked plating and conventional cable plates. *J Orthop Trauma* 2006;20:89-93.

16. Kubiak EN, Haller JM, Kemper DD, Presson AP, Higgins TF, Horwitz DS: Does the lateral plate need to overlap the stem to mitigate stress concentration when treating Vancouver C periprosthetic supracondylar femur fracture? *J Arthroplasty* 2015;30:104-108.

17. Zdero R, Walker R, Waddell JP, Schemitsch EH: Biomechanical evaluation of periprosthetic femoral fracture fixation. *J Bone Joint Surg Am* 2008;90:1068-1077.

18. Moloney GB, Westrick ER, Siska PA, Tarkin IS: Treatment of periprosthetic femur fractures around a well-fixed hip arthroplasty implant: Span the whole bone. *Arch Orthop Trauma Surg* 2014;134:9-14.

19. Yoon RS, Patel JN, Liporace FA: Nail and plate combination fixation for periprosthetic and interprosthetic fractures. *J Orthop Trauma* 2019;33(suppl 6):S18-S20.

    In this case-based technical series, the authors describe the use of nail-plate combination (NPC) technique for both Vancouver C periprosthetic fractures as well as interprosthetic fractures between THA and TKA. Benefits of NPC include moving the neutral axis more in line with the anatomic/mechanical axis, which allows for evenly distributed stress transfer during weight bearing and ambulation. Furthermore, linking the constructs together allow for an even more reliable construct for early weight bearing. Level of evidence: V.

20. Liporace FA, Yoon RS: Nail plate combination technique for native and periprosthetic distal femur fractures. *J Orthop Trauma* 2019;33:e64-e68.

    In this case-based technical series, the authors describe a step-by-step technique and rationale for NPC in stable, periprosthetic TKA fractures. Authors also prefer spanning the entire femur and prophylactic fixation of the femoral neck to remove any stress risers, lowering risk of future fracture. Level of evidence: V.

21. Laurer HL, Wutzler S, Possner S, et al: Outcome after operative treatment of Vancouver type B1 and C periprosthetic femoral fractures: Open reduction and internal fixation versus revision arthroplasty. *Arch Orthop Trauma Surg* 2011;131:983-989.

22. Su ET, Kubiak EN, Dewal H, Hiebert R, Di Cesare PE: A proposed classification of supracondylar femur fractures above total knee arthroplasties. *J Arthroplasty* 2006;21:405-408.

23. Abdel MP, Lewallen DG, Berry DJ: Periprosthetic femur fractures treated with modular fluted, tapered stems. *Clin Orthop Relat Res* 2014;472:599-603.

24. Amenabar T, Rahman WA, Avhad VV, Vera R, Gross AE, Kuzyk PR: Vancouver type B2 and B3 periprosthetic fractures treated with revision total hip arthroplasty. *Int Orthop* 2015;39:1927-1932.

25. Munro JT, Masri BA, Garbuz DS, Duncan CP: Tapered fluted modular titanium stems in the management of Vancouver B2 and B3 peri-prosthetic fractures. *Bone Joint J* 2013;95-B:17-20.

26. Klein GR, Parvizi J, Rapuri V, et al: Proximal femoral replacement for the treatment of periprosthetic fractures. *J Bone Joint Surg Am* 2005;87:1777-1781.

27. Kellett CF, Boscainos PJ, Maury AC, et al: Proximal femoral allograft treatment of Vancouver type-B3 periprosthetic femoral fractures after total hip arthroplasty. Surgical technique. *J Bone Joint Surg Am* 2007;89(2 suppl 1):68-79.

28. Rorabeck CH, Taylor JW: Classification of periprosthetic fractures complicating total knee arthroplasty. *Orthop Clin North Am* 1999;30:209-214.

29. Aldrian S, Schuster R, Haas N, et al: Fixation of supracondylar femoral fractures following total knee arthroplasty: Is there any difference comparing angular stable plate fixation versus rigid interlocking nail fixation? *Arch Orthop Trauma Surg* 2013;133:921-927.

30. Gliatis J, Megas P, Panagiotopoulos E, Lambiris E: Midterm results of treatment with a retrograde nail for supracondylar periprosthetic fractures of the femur following total knee arthroplasty. *J Orthop Trauma* 2005;19:164-170.

31. Jassim SS, McNamara I, Hopgood P: Distal femoral replacement in periprosthetic fracture around total knee arthroplasty. *Injury* 2014;45:550-553.

32. Abdel MP, Pagnano MW, Perry KI, Hanssen AD: Extensor mechanism reconstruction with use of Marlex mesh. *JBJS Essent Surg Tech* 2019;9:e21.

    In this technique description, the authors describe a step-by-step approach on the Marlex mesh technique for extensor mechanism reconstruction in revision TKA. Level of evidence: V.

33. Abdel MP, Salib CG, Mara KC, Pagnano MW, Perry KI, Hanssen AD: Extensor mechanism reconstruction with use of Marlex mesh: A series study of 77 total knee arthroplasties. *J Bone Joint Surg Am* 2018;100:1309-1318.

    In this retrospective series, authors describe outcomes following the use of Marlex mesh in extensor mechanism reconstruction in two-stage exchange. At 2 years, 75% reconstructions were in place and without evidence of infection; of note, all had improved function, without evidence of extensor lag. Level of evidence: V.

SECTION 2

Knee

Section Editor:
Michael A. Mont, MD, FAAOS

CHAPTER 17

Biomechanics of the Knee

WILLIAM A. JIRANEK, MD, FACS • JIBANANANDA SATPATHY, MD, MRCSEd
JENNIFER S. WAYNE, PhD

ABSTRACT

Key biomechanical characteristics of the knee joint include the tibiofemoral and patellofemoral articulations, their kinematics, and associated soft-tissue mechanics. Recent data report on alterations in biomechanics of the osteoarthritic knee and differences in biomechanics of various total knee arthroplasty designs. Surgeons will benefit from summaries of recent research on the biomechanics of patients after total knee arthroplasty.

Keywords: arthroplasty; biomechanics; knee; osteoarthritis

INTRODUCTION

Important parts of human knee anatomy relate to its biomechanical function, including the articular shape of all three knee compartments and soft-tissue mechanics, which contribute to normal and abnormal kinematics. The knowledge of biomechanical changes that occur in both an osteoarthritic knee and the knee following arthroplasty, including the mechanical differences between cruciate-sparing and cruciate-sacrificing total knee arthroplasty (TKA) designs, will be helpful to the orthopaedic surgeon.

Dr. Jiranek or an immediate family member has received royalties from DePuy, A Johnson & Johnson Company; serves as a paid consultant to or is an employee of DePuy, A Johnson & Johnson Company; has stock or stock options held in Biomech Holdings LLC; and serves as a board member, owner, officer, or committee member of the American Association of Hip and Knee Surgeons and the Hip Society. Dr. Wayne or an immediate family member serves as a board member, owner, officer, or committee member of ABET. Neither Dr. Satpathy nor any immediate family member has received anything of value from or has stock or stock options held in a commercial company or institution related directly or indirectly to the subject of this chapter.

KNEE ANATOMY AND ITS BIOMECHANICAL FUNCTION

Tibiofemoral Articulation and Kinematics

The convexity of the medial tibial plateau articular surface supplements the more extended dimensions of the medial femoral condyle, whereas the lateral tibial plateau has a more convex anterior-posterior surface. The tibiofemoral joint maintains its stability through a relationship among static and dynamic features. Dynamic features describe muscles acting on or across the knee joint. The quadriceps muscle group is the primary eccentric decelerator of the knee and reduces posterior subluxation. The hamstring muscles decrease anterior subluxation and capsular laxity through their insertion into the medial and lateral capsular ligaments. The gastrocnemius muscle heads and the iliotibial band supplement stability through attachments to capsular ligaments. Static stability is derived from a combination of tibiofemoral ligaments, the menisci, the anatomy of the articular surfaces, and the inherent intra-articular joint loads.[1]

Although the tibiofemoral articulation resembles a hinge joint, it actually possesses six degrees of freedom: three rotations and three translations about axes in three-dimensional space. Three of the primary motions include flexion-extension, internal-external rotation, and anterior-posterior translation.[2] The tibiofemoral joint has a passive range of motion up to 160° of flexion in the sagittal

This chapter is adapted from Tocks G, Jiranek WA, Satpathy J, Wayne JS: Biomechanics of the knee, in Mont MA, Tanzer M, eds: *Orthopaedic Knowledge Update®: Hip and Knee Reconstruction*, ed 5. Rosemont, IL, American Academy of Orthopaedic Surgeons, 2017, pp 85-93.

plane, with up to 130° of active flexion.[3] During flexion, there are coupled rotations in the other two planes causing incongruency between articulating surfaces across part of the range of motion. The knee achieves optimal weight support and stability in full extension. Flexion contractures are disabling and tiring because the quadriceps muscle force increases to maintain posture because the ground reaction force passes posterior to the knee joint.[4]

During gait, the knee flexes approximately 70° for the foot of the swinging leg to clear the ground. When the leg passes the contralateral leg before heel strike, the quadriceps muscles contract to bring the knee into full extension and to elevate the foot forward. As the knee extends from approximately 30° to 0° of flexion, the tibia externally rotates up to 30°. This refers to the screw-home mechanism (**Figure 1**). This tightens the soft-tissue structures and locks the knee before accommodating the weight-bearing impact load. After heel strike in midstance, the knee joint flexes up to 15°, and the quadriceps muscle absorbs energy. If locked in full extension, a rigid strut would be incapable of absorbing the impact load. After heel strike during knee flexion, the tibia internally rotates, and this couples with foot eversion, thus accommodating energy absorption.[4]

The circumference of the femoral condyles in the sagittal plane is greater than the anterior-posterior dimension of the tibial plateau. Hence, the femur would posteriorly roll off the tibial plateau at full flexion if this were only a rolling motion. During flexion, contact moves posteriorly, and the contact area with the tibial plateau is reduced as lesser radii of curvature of the femoral condyles are sequentially coming into contact (**Figure 2**). The center of contact on the medial side remains relatively stationary in the anterior-posterior position because of the tibia's medial concave surface. The lateral condyle rolls posteriorly toward the posterior horn of the mobile lateral meniscus until the meniscus starts resisting further translation. As the knee flexes, the anterior cruciate ligament comes under more tension and resists further posterior translation of the femur relative to the tibia. Consequently, the femur slides anteriorly while rolling posteriorly on the tibia during flexion.[1]

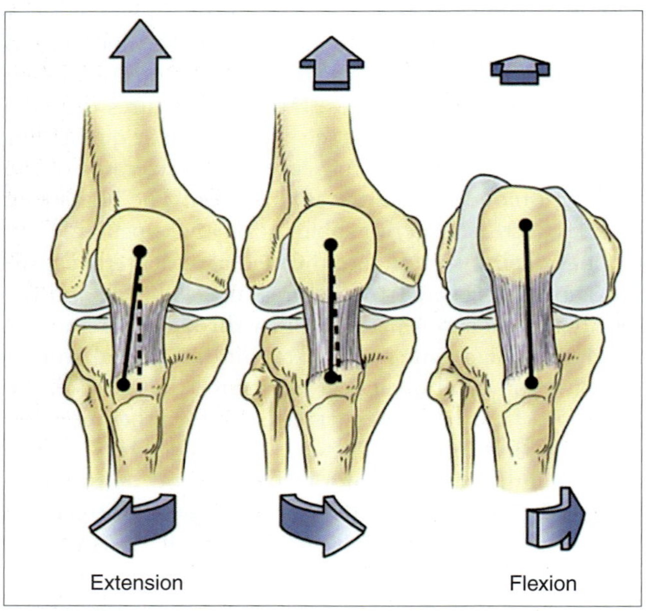

FIGURE 1 Illustration demonstrating the screw-home mechanism. The tibia externally rotates with extension and internally rotates with flexion. (Reproduced with permission from Scott WN: Anatomy, in Clarke HD, Kransdorf MJ, Conley CR, Scott WN, ed: *Insall & Scott Surgery of the Knee*, ed 6. Philadelphia, PA, Elsevier Churchill Livingstone, 2018, pp 2-49.)

Patellofemoral Articulation and Kinematics

The patella is the largest sesamoid bone in the body. Proximally, the patella attaches to the quadriceps tendon, and distally, it has attachments to the deeper layer of the patellar tendon. The convex articular surface contains a broader lateral facet, a medial facet, and a smaller, more medial odd facet. The patellar surface articulates with the femoral trochlea, which has a broader, higher lateral ridge than the medial portion to match the patella.[1]

The primary motor unit of the extensor mechanism is the quadriceps muscle group. The rectus femoris muscle courses parallel to the vastus intermedius muscle, but more superficially in the retinacular layer. The retinacular layer is an aponeurosis of the rectus femoris, vastus medialis obliquus, vastus medialis, vastus lateralis, and vastus lateralis obliquus muscles and unites into the anterior third-joint capsule. The vastus lateralis muscle is the largest of the quadriceps group and comprises approximately 50% of its mass.[1]

At full knee joint extension, the patellofemoral joint contact occurs at the distal end of the patella. The nearly colinear vectors of the patellar tendon and quadriceps muscle forces in the sagittal plane result in a small resultant joint contact force. During flexion, the patella articulates with the femoral trochlear groove, spreading the contact area and load across the width of the patella. The vector angle between the patellar tendon and the quadriceps increases, resulting in increasing patellofemoral joint force up to approximately 70° of flexion. In deep flexion, patella contact occurs only laterally and medially.[4]

Soft-tissue Mechanics

The motion of the knee joint is facilitated by ligaments, menisci, and retinacular structures, providing static stability by resisting excessive displacements between the femur, tibia, and fibula. The biomechanical functions of the menisci consist of load bearing, enlarging the area of contact, guiding rotation, and stabilizing translation.[2] The menisci elongate circumferentially and radially to accommodate the force as

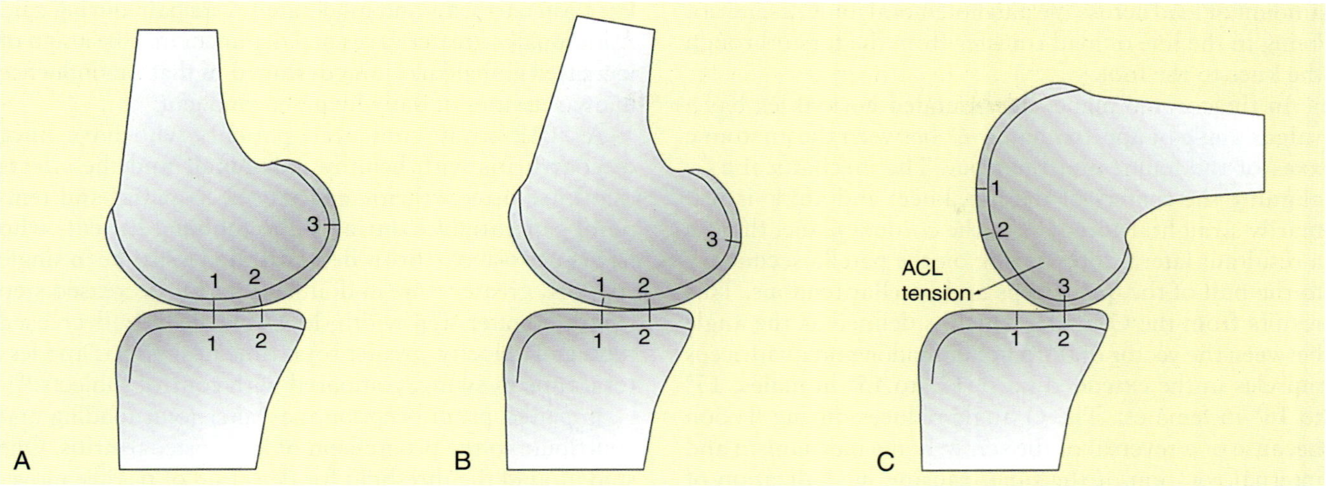

FIGURE 2 Illustration demonstrating sagittal plane knee joint kinematics. **A**, Extension: contact is located centrally. **B**, Early flexion: posterior rolling; contact continuously moves posteriorly. **C**, Deep flexion: femoral sliding; contact is located posteriorly; the unlocking of the ACL prevents further femoral roll back. ACL = anterior cruciate ligament. (Reprinted from *Orthop Trauma* 24[2]. Masouros SD, Bull AM, Amis AA: Biomechanics of the knee joint, 84-91. © 2010 Elsevier.)

the femur applies a pressure on the tibia. The menisci do not displace secondary to the insertional ligaments at the bone attachments, but the lateral meniscus is more mobile. Direct cartilage contact stress is decreased secondary to the increased contact area afforded by the menisci. The importance of the menisci increasing the contact area and reducing the contact stresses on the articular cartilage is supported by many experimental studies and the prevalence of osteoarthrosis after meniscectomy.[5]

The anterior cruciate ligament is the primary restraint to anterior tibial translation, prevents hyperextension, and functions as a secondary restraint to internal and valgus tibial rotations at full extension. The posterior cruciate ligament is the primary restraint to posterior tibial translation, primarily in mid to deep flexion. In extension, the posterior cruciate ligament relaxes, and the primary posterior restraint is supported by the posterolateral structures. Together, the anterior cruciate ligament and posterior cruciate ligament control the anterior-posterior rolling and sliding kinematics of the tibiofemoral joint during flexion-extension.[6]

The medial collateral ligament (MCL) is the primary restraint to valgus angulation and internal tibial rotation, specifically the superficial MCL portion. It functions as a secondary restraint to external tibial rotation and large anterior tibial translations. The posteromedial corner acts as a stabilizer to the extended knee, especially in the presence of concurrent internal tibial rotation and posterior drawer.[7] The lateral collateral ligament is the primary restraint to varus angulation in extension. It is a secondary restraint to large posterior translations. The lateral collateral ligament and posterolateral corner are primary restraints to external tibial rotation.[8]

The meniscus–meniscal ligament complex (ie, meniscus, meniscal insertional ligaments, meniscofemoral ligaments, and deep MCL) acts as primary restraint to tibial rotation. Specifically, the meniscofemoral ligaments are important restraints to posterior drawer, and the deep MCL is a secondary restraint to valgus at 60° to 90° of flexion.[9] The complex acts as a secondary restraint to anterior-posterior translation.

The lateral and medial retinacular structures are the passive stabilizers of the patellofemoral joint. The strong transverse attachment from the patella to the iliotibial tract is tightened as the knee flexes, whereas the capsular lateral patellofemoral ligament is tightest in extension.[10] The medial patellofemoral ligament acts as the primary passive restraint to lateral patellar displacements and supports guiding the patella into the trochlear groove in early knee flexion. The medial patellofemoral ligament is damaged with excessive lateral subluxation of the patella or any lateral dislocation.[10]

Articular Mechanics

The knee joint sustains external and muscular forces that create loading to enable posture and support body movement. Two studies estimated tibiofemoral joint forces at 3.4 times that of body weight when walking, 4.3 times that of body weight when ascending stairs, and 4.0 times that of body weight when descending a ramp.[11,12] A 1994 study reported tibiofemoral joint forces of up to 8.5 times that of body weight when walking downhill.[13] Rising from a seated position requires up to 100° of knee flexion, resulting in a tibiofemoral joint force of approximately 3.5 times body weight and a patellofemoral joint force of approximately 5.5 times body weight. This attests to the amount of load across the patellofemoral joint despite not being in the line of load transfer from the torso through the knee to the foot.

In the coronal plane, the extended normal leg has a valgus angle of approximately 6° between the anatomic axes of the femur and the tibia. The mechanical axis aligning the centers of the hip, knee, and ankle is primarily straight. Moreover, in the coronal plane, there is a resultant lateral force acting on the patella secondary to the pull of the quadriceps and patellar tendons. This results from the Q-angle, which is defined as the angle between the vector of the patellar tendon and quadriceps muscles in the extended knee (12° to 15° in males, 15° to 18° in females). The Q-angle reduces during flexion because of a reversal of the screw-home mechanism and internal rotation of the tibia, causing medialization of the tibial tubercle. The lateral pull of the patella from the Q-angle effect is resisted by the depth of the trochlear groove, with the sulcus angle being the single best predictor of symptoms of instability.[14] Before engaging the trochlear groove, the patella is most unstable at approximately 10° to 30° of knee flexion.[15]

ALTERATIONS IN BIOMECHANICS OF THE NATIVE OSTEOARTHRITIC KNEE

Differences in knee biomechanics between individuals with knee osteoarthritis and those with normal joints have been the subject of numerous experimental and clinical studies under various motion patterns such as simple gait, stair climbing, and stair descending. Focus on preventive measures for stabilization of the osteoarthritic knee may assist in postoperative TKA rehabilitation. During functional activities, knee instability may result from impaired proprioception and poor muscular stabilization in the frontal plane in individuals with medial knee osteoarthritis. A 2014 study found impaired varus proprioception acuity, decreased normalized varus muscle strength, and an impaired ability to actively stabilize the knee in the frontal plane. This demonstrates that the knee frontal plane sensorimotor control system is compromised in individuals with medial knee osteoarthritis.[16] A subsequent study showed that, compared with individuals without knee arthritis, individuals who have medial compartment osteoarthritis walked with less stance phase sagittal plane knee range of motion, less difference between peak knee flexion and extension moments, and greater knee adduction moment (KAM) as measured by the peak, impulse, and overall amplitude of an electromyogram wave form during gait analysis.[17] This study also shows that when controlled for the degree of arthritis, patient age had little effect on gait patterns. Another study demonstrated that greater knee flexion moment is present during the midstance phase of gait in patients who have knee osteoarthritis and moderate/severe pain during gait. Additionally, greater varus malalignment may be a sign of increased global knee joint dysfunction that can influence many activities of daily living beyond gait.[18]

A 2012 study compared patients who have knee osteoarthritis with healthy individuals and the effects that knee osteoarthritis had on select spatial and temporal gait variables during stair climbing. Patients who have knee osteoarthritis demonstrated less time in single support, greater time in double support, decreased step length, greater step width, less stride length, decreased total gait velocity, greater total time in support, and less total time in swing, compared with control subjects.[19]

Impaired proprioception may alter joint loading and contribute to the progression of knee osteoarthritis. One study found the threshold for detection of passive movement to be significantly higher in osteoarthritis patients in varus, valgus, flexion, and extension. This suggests a global, not a direction-specific, reduction in sensation in patients who have knee osteoarthritis.[20] Patients who have knee osteoarthritis are believed to walk with high loads at the knee. Another study showed patients who have osteoarthritis walked more slowly and had greater laxity and static and dynamic varus alignment, less flexion, greater KAM, and greater absolute medial loads when compared with healthy control subjects. They also maintained a greater percentage of total load on the medial compartment.[21]

As part of the kinetic chain, the position of the foot may alter knee biomechanics, in particular load on the medial tibiofemoral joint and the KAM. The KAM is an important surrogate measure for the mediolateral distribution of force across the knee joint in individuals who have knee osteoarthritis. A 2013 study investigated the relationship between tibia, rearfoot, and forefoot motion in the frontal and transverse planes as well as the KAM in patients who had medial compartment knee osteoarthritis. Increased rearfoot eversion, rearfoot internal rotation, and forefoot inversion are associated with reduced KAMs during the stance phase of gait, suggesting that medial knee joint loading could be reduced for those who walk with greater foot pronation. These findings have implications for the design of load-modifying interventions in patients who have medial knee osteoarthritis.[22]

Obesity has become a major epidemic in the United States. A 2013 study determined whether a reduction in body weight of 10% or greater induced by diet, with or without exercise, would improve knee compressive forces and clinical outcomes more than exercise alone.

This randomized clinical trial also analyzed intensive diet-induced weight loss plus exercise, intensive diet-induced weight loss, or exercise. Among overweight and obese adults who have knee osteoarthritis, after 18 months participants in the diet and exercise and diet groups had more weight loss than those in the exercise group; those in the diet group had greater reductions in knee compressive force than those in the exercise group.[23]

A higher KAM has been found in obese patients, which is improved with weight loss. The 2013 study used a subset of these participants to determine the influence of frontal plane knee alignment and obesity on knee joint loads in older, overweight, and obese adults with knee osteoarthritis.[23] Alignment was more closely associated with the asymmetry or imbalance of loads across the medial and lateral knee compartments as reflected by the frontal plane KAM, and body mass index was associated with the magnitude of total tibiofemoral force. In many cases of medial compartment knee osteoarthritis, the greater the varus moment at the knee, the more severe the symptoms. The authors used these data to suggest that lateral heel wedges as an intervention would be more effective in the obese.[24] These data may help select treatment options for patients who have knee osteoarthritis (eg, diet to reduce compression loads, or bracing treatment or wedges to change alignment).[25]

BIOMECHANICS OF SPECIFIC TKA DESIGNS

TKA systems are continually being developed by design engineers and surgeons in an effort to reproduce normal knee biomechanical patterns. These patterns can vary from normal after TKA and may be less predictable and reproducible particularly given the different design parameters among systems. In general, TKAs have provided good midterm to long-term survivorship.

Surgeons currently debate whether a cruciate-retaining or posterior-stabilized TKA provides the ideal biomechanics and postsurgical outcomes in patients. A 2015 study compared the maximum laxity of a cruciate-retaining and posterior-stabilized single-radius TKA. The laxity measured for the cruciate-retaining and posterior-stabilized TKAs revealed no significant differences across the studied flexion arc (0° to 110°; $P = 0.3$). Compared with the native knee, both TKAs exhibited slightly increased anterior drawer and decreased varus-valgus and internal-external rotational laxities.[26] A 2015 study evaluated the in vivo kinematics of stair climbing after posterior-stabilized and cruciate-retaining TKA. Cruciate-retaining TKAs were more sagittally stable in midflexion during stair climbing than posterior-stabilized TKAs. When using late cam-post–engaging posterior-stabilized TKA designs, attention must focus on minimizing posterior tibial slope to avoid unintended impingement of the anterior tibial post with knee extension.[27] Another 2015 study identified greater laxity with cruciate-retaining TKA compared with the native knee ($P = 0.006$) and bicruciate-retaining TKA ($P = 0.039$), but no differences in laxity were seen between the native and the bicruciate-retaining TKA.[28] Bicruciate-retaining TKAs may improve knee stability without using conforming geometry in the implant design.

Cruciate-retaining TKA designs also differ from posterior-stabilized designs in their degree of flexion as well. A 2010 study investigated the biomechanics of posterior-stabilized TKA patients during high flexion using dual-plane fluoroscopy. Initial cam-post engagement was observed at 100.3° ± 6.7° flexion, and five knees had cam-post disengagement before maximum flexion. Lateral femoral condylar liftoff was found in five of seven knees at maximum flexion.[29] Posterior-stabilized TKAs with different geometries can vary from one another and from native knees. Four current posterior-stabilized designs showed major differences in motion characteristics (symmetric mediolateral motion, susceptibility to excessive anterior-posterior medial laxity, and reduced laxity in high flexion) among themselves and with motion data from native knees determined in a previous study.[30] A 2015 study evaluated the effect of tibial posterior slope on posterior-stabilized TKAs and noticed anterior sliding of the tibial component and anterior impingement of the anterior aspect of the tibial post with tibial posterior slopes of at least 5° and 10°, respectively.[31] Tibial posterior slopes of less than 5° in posterior-stabilized TKAs were recommended.

Another TKA design feature is the rotating-platform mobile bearing and its comparison with fixed-bearing designs. A 2011 study assessed kinematics in fixed-bearing and rotating-platform mobile-bearing TKAs with femoral malrotation in a cadaver model tested in an Oxford-type knee rig. In a fixed-bearing TKA, femoral implant internal and external malrotation increased tibiofemoral rotation by 3.4° and 4°, respectively. Malrotation affected patellofemoral lateral shift by up to 2.5 mm. When the malrotated femoral implant was tested against a rotating bearing, the change in tibiofemoral rotation and patellofemoral lateral shift was less than 1° and 1 mm, respectively.[32] A 2013 study analyzed kinematic outcomes preoperatively and postoperatively in a subset of patients who had rotating-platform posterior-stabilized TKAs. These patients achieved an average posterior femoral roll back of the lateral condyle of −5.4 mm, and the average tibiofemoral axial rotation from full extension to maximum weight-bearing flexion was 3.9°.[33] A 2014 study examined the differences in weight-bearing knee kinematics in patients who had mobile-bearing and fixed-bearing TKAs performing step-up activities 1 year after surgery. Minimal kinematic differences were noted between the two TKAs.[34]

In addition to design differences, investigators have also questioned if there are sex-related difference in biomechanics of total knees.[35] Twenty-eight men and 24 women were studied the week before and 1 year after TKA. At follow-up, the authors found that men had decreased flexion moments compared with women, men had higher adduction moments than women, women had less internal and external rotation moments than men, and women had increased activation levels of the gastrocnemius in stance. The authors suggested that there was potential for design differences in sex-specific TKA implants.

LOWER LIMB BIOMECHANICS AFTER TKA

Multiple studies have analyzed the effects of TKA on knee kinematics postoperatively. The altered gait mechanics exhibited by patients after TKA may increase the loading on the nonsurgical knee, thus predisposing it to disease progression. A 2011 study examined the frontal plane kinetics and kinematics in unilateral TKAs during walking. The nonsurgical knees had higher adduction angles and higher dynamic loading, KAM, and impulse compared with the surgical knee. Measures of loading in the control knee did not differ from that of the nonsurgical knee in the TKA group.[36] A 2013 study investigated the biomechanical changes that occur in the lower limb before and at 12 months after TKA compared with control subjects. No significant changes ($P = 0.654$ and $P = 0.686$, respectively) in knee joint kinematics and kinetics after TKA were noted despite significant improvements in pain and function.[37] When data from 1 week before and 1 year following TKA were compared, a 2011 study reported increases in the early-stance knee flexion moment and the late-stance knee extension moment, indicating improved impact attenuation and function. Most changes moved toward an asymptomatic pattern and would be considered improvements in motion, function, and loading.[38]

A 2012 study investigated whether an abnormal flexor moment pattern at 12 months postoperatively could be predicted by using biomechanical gait measures assessed before surgery and at 4 months postoperatively. The gait pattern at 4 months was significantly associated with the 12-month postoperative gait pattern with more than one-half of those with a flexor moment pattern at 4 months retaining this pattern at 12 months.[39] A 2011 study compared the knee kinematics of patients after TKA with those of unimpaired control subjects during comfortable and fast walking speeds. For both speeds, the TKA group walked with significantly reduced cadence, reduced stride length, less knee flexion during stance and swing phases, and less knee extension during stance phase.[40]

A 2010 study compared neuromuscular activation patterns of the knee musculature during level walking 1 week before and 1 year after TKA and found significantly lower overall activation amplitudes for the quadriceps and hamstring muscles, with significant increases in gastrocnemius activity found in late stance.[41] In general, the postsurgical changes favored more typical asymptomatic patterns, supporting improved neuromuscular strategies during walking.[3]

A 2017 study suggested that improved patient outcomes could be correlated with improved biomechanical function of the TKA.[42] In this prospective study of 28 patients who had undergone TKA, the authors demonstrated modest but significant differences in flexion-extension range, as well as peak flexion moment, using the Knee Injury and Osteoarthritis Outcome Score to determine well-functioning from poorly functioning knees.

Although TKA improves functional mobility in patients with end-stage knee osteoarthritis, many subjects have reported continued difficulty with stair ascent and descent after surgery. One study found that when patients who have one total knee and one native knee were studied while climbing stairs, the peak extension moment was higher in the unreplaced knee and push-off knee and hip moments were higher in the replaced knees than in the unreplaced knee. These data suggest that in these patients, the loading response may be lower in the replaced knee than in a normal knee, and during stair climbing there are higher asymmetric loads on the replaced knee.[43] A 2010 study determined preoperative predictors of handrail use during stair ascent and descent after primary unilateral TKA. Before surgery, 63 of 105 subjects required a handrail. Two years after surgery, 60 required a handrail. At 2 years, the preoperative ability to ascend and descend stairs without a handrail was the best predictor of individuals who would not require a handrail after surgery.[44]

The need for high-flexion TKA designs has been investigated. A 2009 study documented the prevalence of knee flexion greater than 90° in 20 consecutive patients who received high-flexion TKAs, at a minimum of 2 years of follow-up. The knees flexed more than 90° for an average of 10 ± 3.8 minutes (0.5%) over a 35-hour period.[45] A 2014 study assessed kneeling and kinematics of TKAs and found tibial posterior translation and external rotation at all flexion angles. Moving from double-stance to single-stance kneeling tended to increase pressures in the cruciate-retaining group but decreased pressures in the posterior-stabilized group. The cruciate-retaining group had significantly larger contact areas than did the posterior-stabilized group, but no significant differences in pressures were reported between the two TKA designs.[46]

SUMMARY

The interaction of the tibiofemoral joint, the patellofemoral joint, and the soft-tissue environment contributes to the complex biomechanics of the knee joint. The articular geometry and soft-tissue restraints enable the specific kinematic movements for the knee during motion. These kinematics and loading conditions are markedly altered in arthritic conditions of the knee and are considerably improved in most cases following TKA. Debate continues on the optimal biomechanics for TKA designs, and further research is needed with randomized controlled studies to explore these concepts. Although current TKA systems do not replicate the kinematics of the normal native knee, they can improve biomechanics over the arthritic knee and allow long-term function.

KEY STUDY POINTS

- Understanding the mechanics of the three compartments of the knee as well as its static and dynamic restraints will help the surgeon understand its kinematics.
- Identification of the mechanical changes in osteoarthritis of the knee will help in the understanding of its biomechanical effects.
- Recent biomechanical studies assessing differences in TKA designs have helped explain their postoperative biomechanical effects.

ANNOTATED REFERENCES

1. Flandry F, Hommel G: Normal anatomy and biomechanics of the knee. *Sports Med Arthrosc Rev* 2011;19(2):82-92.
2. Blaha JD, Wojtys E: Motion and stability of the normal knee, in Scott WN, ed: *Insall & Scott Surgery of the Knee.* New York, NY, Churchill Livingstone, 2005, vol 1, pp 227-239.
3. Yildirim G, Walker PS, Sussman-Fort J, Aggarwal G, White B, Klein GR: The contact locations in the knee during high flexion. *Knee* 2007;14(5):379-384.
4. Masouros SD, Bull AM, Amis AA: Biomechanics of the knee joint. *Orthop Trauma* 2010;24(2):84-91.
5. McDermott ID, Amis AA: The consequences of meniscectomy. *J Bone Joint Surg Br* 2006;88(12):1549-1556.
6. Butler DL, Noyes FR, Grood ES: Ligamentous restraints to anterior-posterior drawer in the human knee: A biomechanical study. *J Bone Joint Surg Am* 1980;62(2):259-270.
7. Robinson JR, Bull AM, Thomas RR, Amis AA: The role of the medial collateral ligament and posteromedial capsule in controlling knee laxity. *Am J Sports Med* 2006;34(11): 1815-1823.
8. Davies H, Unwin A, Aichroth P: The posterolateral corner of the knee: Anatomy, biomechanics and management of injuries. *Injury* 2004;35(1):68-75.
9. Masouros SD, McDermott ID, Amis AA, Bull AM: Biomechanics of the meniscus-meniscal ligament construct of the knee. *Knee Surg Sports Traumatol Arthrosc* 2008;16(12):1121-1132.
10. Feller JA, Amis AA, Andrish JT, Arendt EA, Erasmus PJ, Powers CM: Surgical biomechanics of the patellofemoral joint. *Arthroscopy* 2007;23(5):542-553.
11. Morrison JB: Function of the knee joint in various activities. *Biomed Eng* 1969;4(12):573-580.
12. Morrison JB: Bioengineering analysis of force actions transmitted by the knee joint. *Biomed Eng* 1968;3:164-170.
13. Kuster M, Wood GA, Sakurai S, Blatter G: 1994 Nicola Cerulli Young Researchers Award. Downhill walking: A stressful task for the anterior cruciate ligament? A biomechanical study with clinical implications. *Knee Surg Sports Traumatol Arthrosc* 1994;2(1):2-7.
14. Davies AP, Costa ML, Shepstone L, Glasgow MM, Donell S: The sulcus angle and malalignment of the extensor mechanism of the knee. *J Bone Joint Surg Br* 2000;82:1162-1166.
15. Farahmand F, Senavongse W, Amis AA: Quantitative study of the quadriceps muscles and trochlear groove geometry related to instability of the patellofemoral joint. *J Orthop Res* 1998;16(1):136-143.
16. Chang AH, Lee SJ, Zhao H, Ren Y, Zhang LQ: Impaired varus-valgus proprioception and neuromuscular stabilization in medial knee osteoarthritis. *J Biomech* 2014;47(2):360-366.
17. Rutherford D, Baker M, Wong I, Stanish W: The effect of age and knee osteoarthritis on muscle activation patterns and knee joint biomechanics during dual belt treadmill gait. *J Electromyogr Kinesiol* 2017;34:58-64.

    This Level III study, a case controlled study, demonstrated that age had little effect on gait biomechanics, but the presence of knee osteoarthritis had substantial impact on gait biomechanics. Patients with medial knee osteoarthritis had less sagittal plane motion in the stance phase and a greater KAM. Level of evidence: III.
18. O'Connell M, Farrokhi S, Fitzgerald GK: The role of knee joint moments and knee impairments on self-reported knee pain during gait in patients with knee osteoarthritis. *Clin Biomech (Bristol, Avon)* 2016;31:40-46.
19. Hicks-Little CA, Peindl RD, Fehring TK, Odum SM, Hubbard TJ, Cordova ML: Temporal-spatial gait adaptations during stair ascent and descent in patients with knee osteoarthritis. *J Arthroplasty* 2012;27(6):1183-1189.
20. Cammarata ML, Schnitzer TJ, Dhaher YY: Does knee osteoarthritis differentially modulate proprioceptive acuity in the frontal and sagittal planes of the knee? *Arthritis Rheum* 2011;63(9):2681-2689.
21. Kumar D, Manal KT, Rudolph KS: Knee joint loading during gait in healthy controls and individuals with knee osteoarthritis. *Osteoarthritis Cartilage* 2013;21(2):298-305.
22. Levinger P, Menz HB, Morrow AD, Bartlett JR, Feller JA, Bergman NR: Relationship between foot function and medial knee joint loading in people with medial compartment knee osteoarthritis. *J Foot Ankle Res* 2013;6(1):33.
23. Messier SP, Mihalko SL, Legault C, et al: Effects of intensive diet and exercise on knee joint loads, inflammation, and clinical outcomes among overweight and obese adults with knee osteoarthritis: The IDEA randomized clinical trial. *J Am Med Assoc* 2013;310(12):1263-1273.

24. Russell EM, Miller RH, Umberger BR, Hamill J: Lateral wedges after mediolateral load distributions at the knee joint in obese individuals. *J Orthop Res* 2013;31(5):665-671.

25. Messier SP, Pater M, Beavers DP, et al: Influences of alignment and obesity on knee joint loading in osteoarthritic gait. *Osteoarthritis Cartilage* 2014;22(7):912-917.

26. Hunt NC, Ghosh KM, Blain AP, Rushton SP, Longstaff LM, Deehan DJ: No statistically significant kinematic difference found between a cruciate-retaining and posterior-stabilised Triathlon knee arthroplasty: A laboratory study involving eight cadavers examining soft-tissue laxity. *Bone Joint J* 2015;97-B(5):642-648.

27. Hamai S, Okazaki K, Shimoto T, Nakahara H, Higaki H, Iwamoto Y: Continuous sagittal radiological evaluation of stair-climbing in cruciate-retaining and posterior-stabilized total knee arthroplasties using image-matching techniques. *J Arthroplasty* 2015;30(5):864-869.

28. Halewood C, Traynor A, Bellemans J, Victor J, Amis AA: Anteroposterior laxity after bicruciate-retaining total knee arthroplasty is closer to the native knee than ACL-resecting TKA: A biomechanical cadaver study. *J Arthroplasty* 2015;30(12):2315-2319.

29. Moynihan AL, Varadarajan KM, Hanson GR, et al: In vivo knee kinematics during high flexion after a posterior-substituting total knee arthroplasty. *Int Orthop* 2010;34(4):497-503.

30. Walker PS, Lowry MT, Kumar A: The effect of geometric variations in posterior-stabilized knee designs on motion characteristics measured in a knee loading machine. *Clin Orthop Relat Res* 2014;472(1):238-247.

31. Okamoto S, Mizu-uchi H, Okazaki K, Hamai S, Nakahara H, Iwamoto Y: Effect of tibial posterior slope on knee kinematics, quadriceps force, and patellofemoral contact force after posterior-stabilized total knee arthroplasty. *J Arthroplasty* 2015;30(8):1439-1443.

32. Colwell CW Jr, Chen PC, D'Lima D: Extensor malalignment arising from femoral component malrotation in knee arthroplasty: Effect of rotating-bearing. *Clin Biomech (Bristol, Avon)* 2011;26(1):52-57.

33. Komistek RD, Murphy JA, O'Dell TL: Clinical and kinematic outcomes of a rotating platform posterior stabilized total knee system. *J Arthroplasty* 2013;28(4):624-630.

34. Okamoto N, Nakamura E, Nishioka H, Karasugi T, Okada T, Mizuta H: In vivo kinematic comparison between mobile-bearing and fixed-bearing total knee arthroplasty during step-up activity. *J Arthroplasty* 2014;29(1):2393-2396.

35. Ro DH, Kang T, Han DH, Lee DY, Han HS, Lee MC: Quantitative evaluation of gait features after total knee arthroplasty: Comparison with age and sex-matched controls. *Gait Posture* 2020;75:78-84.

    In this study, patients were studied after TKA and compared with age-matched and sex-matched control patients without TKA and showed a significant decrease in KAM in the stance phase of gait after TKA, and a significant improvement in stance phase alignment following TKA. Level of evidence: III.

36. Alnahdi AH, Zeni JA, Snyder-Mackler L: Gait after unilateral total knee arthroplasty: Frontal plane analysis. *J Orthop Res* 2011;29(5):647-652.

37. Levinger P, Menz HB, Morrow AD, Feller JA, Bartlett JR, Bergman NR: Lower limb biomechanics in individuals with knee osteoarthritis before and after total knee arthroplasty surgery. *J Arthroplasty* 2013;28(6):994-999.

38. Hatfield GL, Hubley-Kozey CL, Astephen Wilson JL, Dunbar MJ: The effect of total knee arthroplasty on knee joint kinematics and kinetics during gait. *J Arthroplasty* 2011;26(2):309-318.

39. Levinger P, Menz HB, Morrow AD, et al: Knee biomechanics early after knee replacement surgery predict abnormal gait patterns 12 months postoperatively. *J Orthop Res* 2012;30(3):371-376.

40. McClelland JA, Webster KE, Feller JA, Menz HB: Knee kinematics during walking at different speeds in people who have undergone total knee replacement. *Knee* 2011;18(3):151-155.

41. Hubley-Kozey CL, Hatfield GL, Astephen Wilson JL, Dunbar MJ: Alterations in neuromuscular patterns between pre and one-year post-total knee arthroplasty. *Clin Biomech (Bristol, Avon)* 2010;25(10):995-1002.

42. Naili JE, Wretenberg P, Lindgren V, Iversen MD, Hedström M, Broström EW: Improved knee biomechanics among patients reporting a good outcome in knee-related quality of life one year after total knee arthroplasty. *BMC Musculoskelet Disord* 2017;18(1):122.

    In this prospective study of 23 patients, 19 patients were classified as having a good outcome as defined by having Knee Injury and Osteoarthritis Outcome Scores greater than the minimally clinically important difference, which correlated with significant improvements in knee biomechanics, including increased knee flexion-extension range, reduced peak varus angle, increased peak flexion moment, and reduced peak valgus moment. These good-result patients also demonstrated significant increase in walking speed, a reduction of stance phase duration, and increased passive knee extension. Level of evidence: III.

43. Standifird TW, Saxton AM, Coe DP, Cates HE, Reinbolt JA, Zhang S: Influence of total knee arthroplasty on gait mechanics of the replaced and non-replaced limb during stair negotiation. *J Arthroplasty* 2016;31(1):278-283.

44. Zeni JA Jr, Snyder-Mackler L: Preoperative predictors of persistent impairments during stair ascent and descent after total knee arthroplasty. *J Bone Joint Surg Am* 2010;92(5):1130-1136.

45. Huddleston JI, Scarborough DM, Goldvasser D, Freiberg AA, Malchau H: 2009 Marshall Urist Young Investigator Award: How often do patients with high-flex total knee arthroplasty use high flexion? *Clin Orthop Relat Res* 2009;467(7):1898-1906.

46. Lee TQ: Biomechanics of hyperflexion and kneeling before and after total knee arthroplasty. *Clin Orthop Surg* 2014;6(2):117-126.

CHAPTER 18

Anatomy and Surgical Approaches to Knee Arthroplasty

GILES R. SCUDERI, MD • HENRY D. CLARKE, MD • CHRISTOPHER A. F. DODD, FRCS

ABSTRACT

Knee arthroplasty can be performed using a variety of different skin and arthrotomy incisions. Improving the early recovery of patients undergoing knee arthroplasty by using shorter skin incisions and reducing damage to the quadriceps muscle with minimally invasive surgical techniques was pioneered in unicondylar knee arthroplasty and then continued with primary total knee arthroplasty. Important work has been undertaken over the past decade to identify the optimal method for exposure in total knee arthroplasty. However, questions remain. Understanding the individual techniques is important for the surgeon performing knee arthroplasty. This is further challenging in revision total knee arthroplasty where adequate exposure is essential to performing the procedure. The decision to use any particular approach should be made by the surgeon performing the procedure after considering patient variables, the prosthesis system to be used, and the individual experience with the exposure options.

Keywords: minimally invasive surgery; revision total knee arthroplasty; surgical exposures; total knee arthroplasty; unicondylar knee arthroplasty

Dr. Scuderi or an immediate family member has received royalties from Biomet and Zimmer; is a member of a speakers' bureau or has made paid presentations on behalf of Biomet, Convatec, Medtronic, Pacira, and Zimmer; serves as a paid consultant to or is an employee of Acelity, Biomet, Medtronic, Pacira, and Zimmer; has stock or stock options held in Force Therapeutics; has received research or institutional support from Pacira; and serves as a board member, owner, officer, or committee member of the Operation Walk USA. Dr. Clarke or an immediate family member has received royalties from Biomet, ConforMIS, and Zimmer; is a member of a speakers' bureau or has made paid presentations on behalf of Biomet and Zimmer; serves as a paid consultant to or is an employee of Biomet, ConforMIS, Smith & Nephew, and Zimmer; serves as an unpaid consultant to Biomet, ConforMIS, OSSO VR, and Zimmer; has received research or institutional support from Stryker and Teleflex/Vidacare; and serves as a board member, owner, officer, or committee member of the American Academy of Orthopaedic Surgeons, the Association of Bone and Joint Surgeons, and ICJR. Dr. Dodd or an immediate family member has received royalties from Zimmer Biomet; is a member of a speakers' bureau or has made paid presentations on behalf of Zimmer; serves as a paid consultant to or is an employee of Zimmer; has received research or institutional support from Biomet, Stryker, and Zimmer; and serves as a board member, owner, officer, or committee member of the Knee Society.

INTRODUCTION

The goals in knee arthroplasty are to relieve pain and restore function in a joint that has been compromised by mechanical wear, trauma, or other etiologies. To accomplish these goals, accurate bony preparation and implantation of the prosthetic components is necessary with restoration of soft-tissue balance to the periarticular stabilizers. Historically, this has been accomplished through an extensile exposure using an anterior skin incision combined with a medial parapatellar arthrotomy.

In the early 2000s, a resurgence of unicondylar knee arthroplasty (UKA) performed through smaller skin and capsular incisions stimulated interest in performing total knee arthroplasty (TKA) using similar, minimally invasive concepts to improve recovery time and pain after surgery. Consequently, TKA performed through shorter skin incisions using various alternative arthrotomy incisions that were perceived to be less damaging to the quadriceps muscle and extensor mechanism was investigated and adopted. These so-called minimally invasive techniques broadly adhere to some or all of the following principles: a smaller skin incision, no eversion of the patella; avoidance of disruption of the suprapatellar pouch; and minimal or no incision of the quadriceps tendon.[1] After using these alternative exposures for more than a decade, no single technique has demonstrated unequivocal superiority. Instead, several different alternatives appear to be reasonable choices with relative risks and benefits afforded by each exposure. Indeed, the most appropriate exposure choice in a particular case may depend on patient characteristics, prosthesis and instrumentation variables, and the individual experience and skill of the surgeon performing the procedure. It is important to review the surgical techniques for each of the most widely used exposures for UKA and TKA, along with the relative advantages and disadvantages of each technique.

Despite the success of UKA and TKA, the incidence of revision TKA has been projected to grow. There are numerous causes of failure, but regardless of the etiology, safe and adequate exposure must be achieved. Surgeons should be familiar with the various extensile approaches for exposing the knee joint, safely removing the original components, and implanting the new prosthesis.

ANATOMY

The cutaneous blood supply over the anterior aspect of the knee is derived from an anastomosis of vessels that run superficial to the deep fascia and travels from deep to superficial fascia. Therefore, to avoid ischemia to the skin flaps, full-thickness subcutaneous flaps should be developed deep to the superficial fascia. This deep dissection will permit exposure of the extensor mechanism for the chosen arthrotomy.

In choosing the right approach to the knee, prior surgical incisions must be considered. Although a straight anterior midline incision is preferred, prior incisions may make that choice impossible. Knowing that the blood supply to the anterior aspect of the knee is predominately derived from the medial side, the lateral most prior skin incision should be used. Transverse incisions should be transected at a perpendicular angle. When trying to incorporate and extend prior oblique or curvilinear incisions, an angle of <60° to the previous incision should be avoided to avoid skin necrosis at the apex. If a longitudinal incision is made in the presence of a prior incision, the skin bridge should be >6 cm.

UNICOMPARTMENTAL KNEE ARTHROPLASTY

UKA and TKA were both developed in the early 1970s, and surgical exposure was critical. Initially, both procedures were performed via a long medial parapatellar incision, and the patella was everted laterally to aid exposure.

In 1992, UKAs were implanted via a shorter incision, and it was shown that patellar eversion was unnecessary, and that relative preservation of the extensor mechanism resulted in accelerated recovery and early discharge.[2] These early presentations stimulated great interest in minimally invasive surgery (MIS), not only for UKA, but also later resulted in the development of MIS TKA.

In 1998, the phase 3 mobile UKA introduced the technique for medial unicompartmental arthroplasty used with an MIS approach. The instruments were miniaturized for use via a small parapatellar arthrotomy. The functional results and the speed of recovery of phase 3 were found to be better than those of phase 2 mobile-bearing UKA. Since then, most surgeons now implant UKA using an MIS approach.

Medial Approach

For the medial approach, a paramedial skin incision is made from the medial pole of the patella to a point 3 cm distal to the joint line just medial to the tibial tubercle: two-thirds above the joint line to one-third below (**Figure 1**). The medial margin of the patella is identified. The retinacular incision is made along the medial side of the patella and patellar tendon. The anterior tibia is exposed. At its upper end, the retinacular incision is extended proximally for 2 to 3 cm into the vastus medialis obliquus (VMO) muscle. The direction is not critical, but most surgeons carry the incision proximally up toward the quadriceps tendon. Part of the retropatellar fat pad is excised and the anterior portion of the medial meniscus is removed. Self-retaining retractors are inserted into the synovial cavity. The anterior cruciate ligament (ACL), lateral side, and patellofemoral joint can now be inspected. If the ACL appears damaged, its integrity should be checked by pulling on the ligament with a tendon hook. Absence of a functioning ACL is a contraindication for a mobile-bearing UKA.

Lateral Approach

For a lateral approach, the incision is made over the junction of the central and lateral thirds of the patella and begins at the level of the superior pole of the patella and extends down and just lateral to the tibial tubercle. The retinacular incision is made on the lateral side of the patella and down beside the patellar tendon. The anterolateral portion of the tibia is exposed, and Gerdy tubercle and attachment of the iliotibial tract are identified. The incision is extended proximally around the patella and

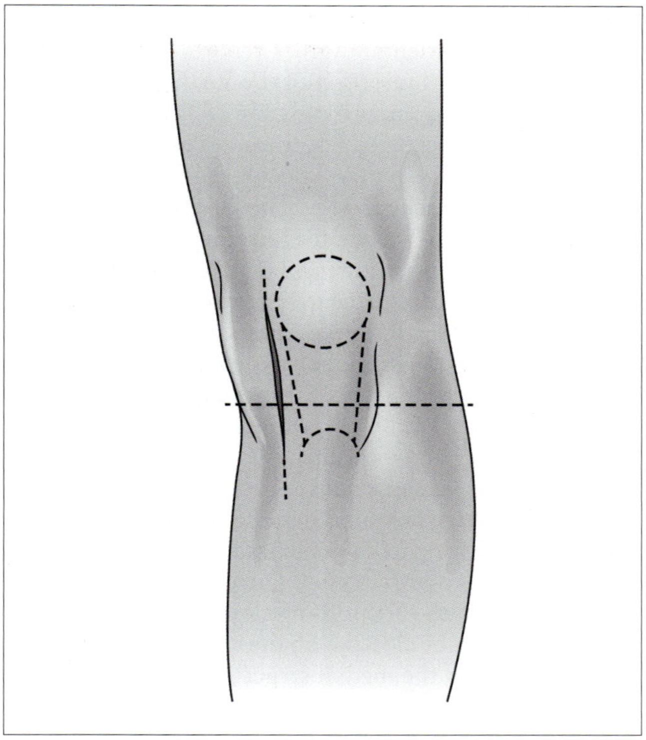

FIGURE 1 Illustration depicts planned medial skin incision for planned medial unicondylar arthroplasty.

up into the extensor mechanism. Generous excision of the fat pad is required. If concern exists about the ACL, pulling it with a tendon hook can assess its status. In general, the lateral MIS UKA incision is 2 to 3 cm longer than the medial incision.

CLINICAL RESULTS

In comparison with MIS TKA, few studies compare the effect of reduced incisions. Clearly, fewer UKAs are performed (10% of registered knee arthroplasties are UKAs), and surgical approaches are not as varied as in MIS TKA. In essence, the aforementioned medial approach has attained near-universal use.[3]

The only direct comparison describes the effect of the medial MIS approach.[4] This study compared the rate of recovery in 40 mobile-bearing UKAs performed via an MIS incision with modified instruments without patellar eversion with that in 20 mobile-bearing UKAs performed via an open approach with patellar eversion. Both groups were compared with 40 TKAs performed during the same period that were used as controls. The average rate of recovery after the MIS approach was twice as fast as that of open UKA and three times as fast as that of TKA. No study that assesses the effect of the lateral MIS UKA approach is known.[5]

TOTAL KNEE ARTHROPLASTY

The surgical approach for TKA has evolved over the past decade to less invasive exposures following the experience gained from MIS UKA. Several approaches have become popular, including the limited medial parapatellar approach, the subvastus approach, the midvastus approach, and the quadriceps-sparing approach.

The Medial Parapatellar Approach

The earliest description of the medial parapatellar approach has been credited to von Langenbeck, who described detachment of the VMO muscle from its insertion onto the quadriceps tendon and continuing the arthrotomy around the medial border of the patella and along the medial border of the patellar tendon.[6] This approach was modified by Insall with a straight incision along the medial border of the quadriceps tendon, over the medial border of the patella with a subperiosteal elevation of the medial retinaculum, and a straight incision along the medial border of the patellar tendon.[7] The limited medial patellar arthrotomy evolved from the Insall technique. Following a midline skin incision from the superior pole of the patella to the tibial tubercle, limited medial and lateral subcutaneous flaps are developed. The arthrotomy begins approximately 2 to 4 cm proximal to the superior pole of the patella and extends distally along the medial border of the quadriceps tendon.[8] The incision is continued in a straight manner, and the medial retinaculum is elevated from the medial border of the patella and along the medial border of the patellar tendon (**Figure 2, A** and **B**). This usually facilitates lateral subluxation of the patella and exposure to the joint. If necessary, the arthrotomy can be easily extended to a more traditional approach by gradual lengthening into the quadriceps tendon. This

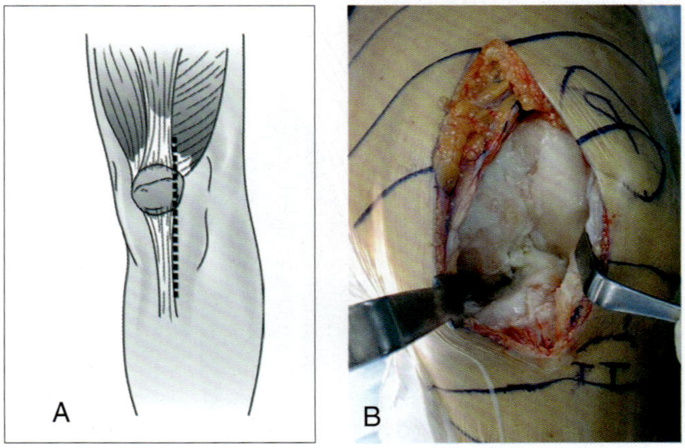

FIGURE 2 Images of a limited medial parapatellar arthrotomy. **A**, Illustration depicts planned arthrotomy. **B**, Intraoperative photograph demonstrates exposure.

approach is commonly used because of its familiarity, simplicity, and exposure of all knee joint compartments. Furthermore, this approach is extensile when needed, can be applied to all deformities, and is easily extended with a quadriceps snip when necessary.[9]

The Subvastus Approach

Originally, the subvastus approach was commonly used in TKA to preserve the attachment of the VMO muscle on the quadriceps tendon and follow the natural plane of dissection.[10] In the original description, this technique was performed through a standard-length anterior skin incision and the patella was typically everted. However, subsequent modifications allowed the exposure to be performed through a limited skin incision of 3 to 4 inches when preferred.[1] Following exposure of the extensor mechanism via a midline skin incision and development of limited medial and lateral subcutaneous flaps, an incision is made along the medial border of the patellar tendon and medial border of the patella to the attachment of the VMO tendon on the patella (**Figure 3**). The insertion of the VMO occurs at an angle of approximately 50° close to the midportion of the patella.[11] However, this insertion point varies among individuals, with three broad types described: type 1 has a high insertion of the VMO above the medial aspect of the patella, type 2 inserts at the superior medial border of the patella, and type 3 inserts as low as the middle of the patella and is usually seen in muscular male patients.[12] Other reports have described an even more distal insertion of the VMO tendon on the patella. In one study, approximately 25% of patients had an insertion that occurred distally in excess of 60% of the patellar length.[13] With this exposure, the insertion of the VMO remains attached to the patella, and the dissection proceeds transversely along the lower border of the VMO muscle belly. This procedure can often be performed with blunt finger dissection beneath the inferior border of the VMO and along the intermuscular septum. Care should be taken because the dissection extends above the adductor tubercle approaching the Hunter canal. This area has neurovascular structures at risk, including the descending geniculate artery and its branches, the intermuscular septal arteries, and the saphenous nerve. Following dissection of the VMO, the synovial fold in the suprapatellar pouch is released and the patella is subluxated laterally because the knee is moved into flexion. During closure, the horizontal portion of the arthrotomy along the inferior border of the VMO may be closed with the knee at 90° to prevent overtightening of the medial structures that could cause iatrogenic patella baja.[1]

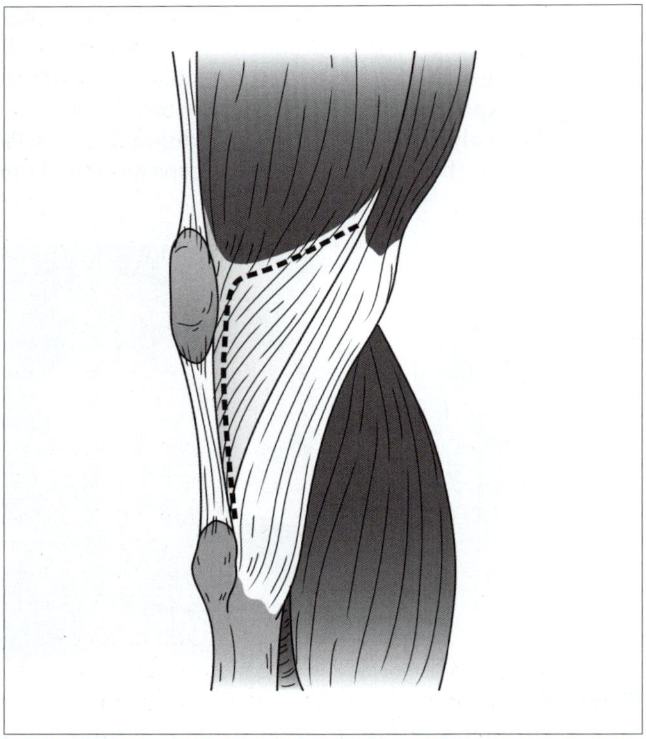

FIGURE 3 Illustration depicts the subvastus approach.

Proponents of the subvastus approach report exposure comparable with the medial parapatellar arthrotomy, with preservation of the extensor mechanism and minimization of patella instability. The major criticisms of the subvastus approach are poor exposure and difficulty with patellar mobilization. The contraindications for the subvastus approach include obesity, especially with a short femur; heavy, muscular thighs; hypertrophic osteoarthritis with limited range of motion, or substantial flexion contracture; prior high tibial osteotomy with patella baja; knees with excessive valgus; and revision TKA. In addition, when combined with a small skin incision, increased trauma to the skin can occur, especially with the stretching required to perform the proximal, medially directed portion of the arthrotomy; this can result in an increased risk of wound healing problems.

The Midvastus Approach

The midvastus approach was described as a compromise between the medial parapatellar and subvastus approaches.[14] Following exposure of the extensor mechanism via a midline skin incision and development of limited medial and lateral subcutaneous flaps, an incision is made along the medial border of the patellar tendon and the medial border of the patella to the attachment of the VMO on the superomedial border of the patella. With the knee in flexion to maintain tension in the extensor mechanism, the full thickness of the VMO is divided in line with its muscle fibers, starting at the superomedial border of the patella and extending proximally approximately 3 cm (**Figure 4**). The patella is subluxated laterally

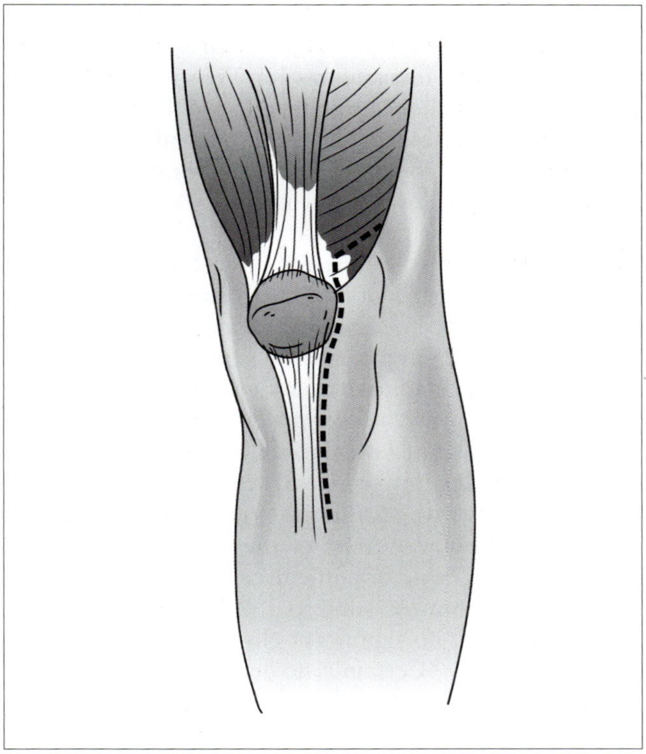

FIGURE 4 Illustration depicts the midvastus approach.

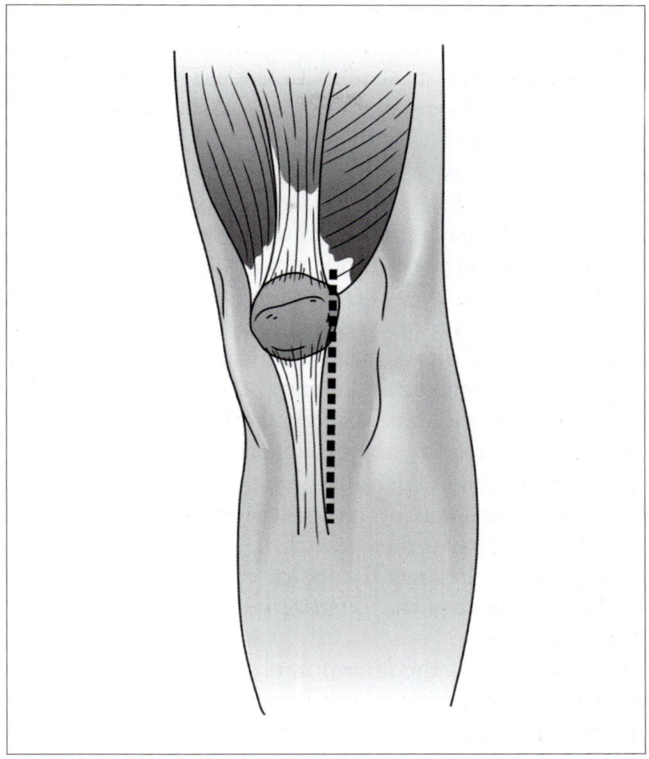

FIGURE 5 Illustration depicts the quadriceps-sparing approach.

to expose the knee joint. Inadvertent fascia or muscle fiber tears while exposing the joint have no adverse effects on the outcome.

Proponents of the midvastus approach report less postoperative pain, preservation of the patella vascularity, improved patellar tracking, better quadriceps strength, decreased blood loss, and more rapid recovery. Relative contraindications to this approach include obesity, hypertrophic osteoarthritis with limited range of motion or substantial flexion contracture, heavy muscular thigh, patella baja, and revision TKA.

Quadriceps-sparing Approach

The quadriceps-sparing approach for TKA was described based on experience with minimally invasive UKA.[15] The goal of this approach is to perform a TKA through a less invasive approach that permits more rapid recovery with less morbidity.

A curvilinear medial skin incision is made from the superior pole of the patella to the tibial joint line. The medial arthrotomy is in line with the skin incision and begins at the superior medial border of the patella at the insertion of the VMO. It ends approximately 2 cm distal to the tibial joint line just medial to the insertion of the patellar tendon at the tibial tubercle. The arthrotomy does not cut the quadriceps tendon or divide the fibers of the VMO (**Figure 5**). As noted in the discussion of the subvastus exposure, some variation exists in the insertion of the VMO along the medial border of the patella. For type 3, in which the insertion is at the midportion of patella or more distal, this surgical approach releases the VMO and is not truly quadriceps sparing.

When performing TKA using the quadriceps-sparing approach, specialized instruments that allow resection of the femur and tibia from the medial side of the knee joint are necessary. Complications following the quadriceps-sparing approach, including patellar tendon avulsion, rupture of the medial or lateral collateral ligaments, and cement retention, appear to decline with increased surgeon experience.[16]

Lateral Approach

The lateral approach to the knee was introduced in North America for use in patients undergoing TKA who had a preoperative valgus deformity.[17] When this approach was first described, a standard-length laterally based anterior incision was used, but the exposure has been subsequently modified for use with a small, minimally invasive skin incision.[18] The original technique follows the skin incision, and medial dissection is contraindicated.[17] A lateral arthrotomy is performed beginning proximally along the lateral border of the quadriceps tendon and continued distally 1 to 2 cm lateral to the border of the patella, through the medial edge of Gerdy tubercle, and extended into the lateral compartment fascia 1 to 2 cm lateral to the edge of the tibial tubercle (**Figure 6**). During exposure, incision through the fat pad should be avoided because mobilization of the vascularized fat pad is used at the end of the case to close the gap that will form in the lateral capsule as a result of valgus deformity correction. Instead, the fat pad is preserved with the transverse meniscal ligament and the anterior rim of the lateral meniscus by dissecting medially, deep to the patellar tendon. This soft-tissue mass is preserved as a laterally based flap with preserved blood supply from the inferior geniculate artery and should be protected during the subsequent surgery. The patella is subluxated medially during arthroplasty. At the time of closure, the vascularized, laterally attached fat pad with the meniscal remnant is mobilized. The fat pad is expanded with relaxing incisions made in line with the retained lateral meniscal rim. This soft-tissue mass is sutured to the lateral edge of the capsule that runs along the border of the extensor mechanism to close the capsular defect.

Proponents of the lateral approach note that valgus deformity correction is optimized with this exposure because the tight lateral structures are either released during the exposure or directly accessible for release after the lateral exposure has been performed.[17] The disadvantages of the technique include the relative lack of familiarity most surgeons have with a lateral perspective during TKA, instruments for TKA that are mostly designed for a medial approach, and problems with poor capsular closure, especially if the fat pad flap is damaged, which can contribute to postoperative drainage and infection, or slow rehabilitation.[17,18]

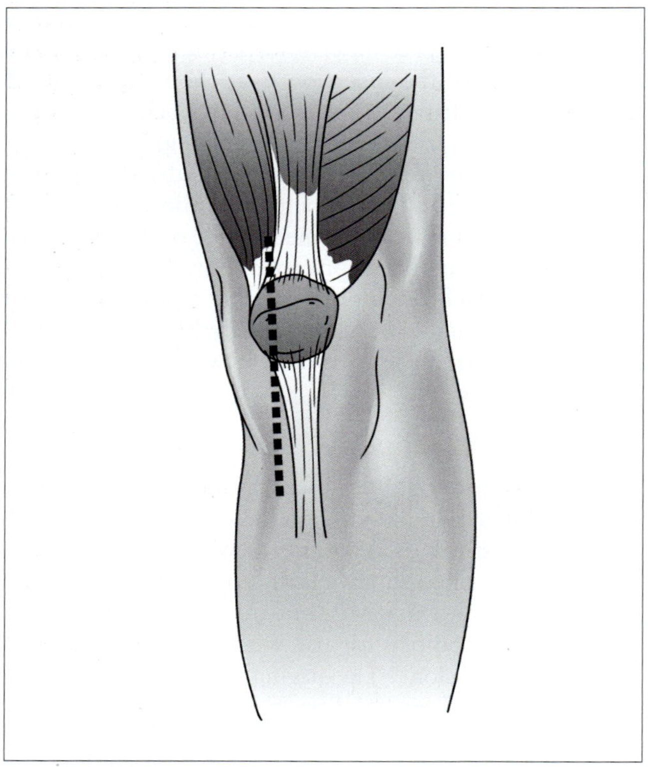

FIGURE 6 Illustration depicts the lateral arthrotomy.

Clinical Results

The clinical outcomes of TKA performed with different exposures have been compared in many trials to determine whether MIS exposures are superior to traditional approaches, and also to determine which MIS exposure is optimal. Even with the peer-reviewed publications from the past decade, limited conclusions can be drawn from the literature. Information from early reports that compared MIS techniques with traditional exposures demonstrated advantages; however, most of these were case-control studies using historic or contemporary control patients, instead of randomized subjects.[19-23] In more recent randomized studies, no significant clinical advantages have been identified.[24-29] Certainly, no definitive statements can be made that MIS approaches are superior in all ways to traditional exposures, nor does it appear that any single approach is superior to the others. Meta-analyses and systematic reviews have been performed on this topic over the past 5 years. However, the results of these studies are also equivocal with those that fail to identify any clinical advantages or problems[30,31] versus those that note small differences in early recovery or complications.[32,33]

A broad summary of the published literature suggests that small, early advantages in quadriceps strength, range of motion, and pain relief during the first few weeks after surgery may be possible with minimally invasive approaches versus traditional exposures. However, these benefits appear to be realized at the expense of a small but important increase in wound healing complications, increased surgical time, and potential concerns about long-term loosening resulting from less-accurate prosthesis alignment.[30-33]

Revision Total Knee Arthroplasty

Adequate surgical exposure can be challenging in revision TKA, but it is essential for the clinical success. Surgeons should be aware of the various surgical options. Once the extensor mechanism is identified, it is best to extend the exposure proximally and distally so that normal tissue and plans of dissection can be visualized. In most cases, a medial parapatellar arthrotomy can be performed. An extensive synovectomy is performed in the suprapatellar pouch. Clearing adhesions and scar tissue from the medial and lateral femoral gutters usually further assists exposure. The proximal medial tibia can also be exposed by a subperiosteal release of the deep medial collateral ligament and semimembranous attachment allowing external rotation of the tibia. With external rotation of the tibia, tension on the patella tendon at the tibial tubercle is reduced. To further facilitate exposure, fibrous tissue between the patella tendon and anterior tibia is excised. This will allow lateral subluxation of the patella.

In situations with limited motion or arthrofibrosis, there is a need for a more extensile exposure to avoid injury to the extensor mechanism at the patella tendon and tibial tubercle.

The Quadriceps Snip

The quadriceps snip is an easy next step when the aforementioned maneuvers are inadequate and exposure is difficult.[9] This approach is a superior lateral extension of the medial parapatellar arthrotomy (**Figure 7**). At the superior apex of the quadriceps tendon, an oblique incision at a 45° angle is made across the quadriceps tendon into the fibers of vastus lateralis. This releases the tension in the extensor mechanism and facilitates safe exposure. The arthrotomy closure is by a simple side-to-side repair. The advantage of the quadriceps snip is that it is technically easy, and the postoperative rehabilitation program does not need to be modified.

The Quadriceps V-Y Turndown

Following a medial parapatellar arthrotomy, the tendinous insertion of the vastus lateralis is divided at an angle of 45° extending inferiorly to the joint line detaching the musculotendinous of the vastus lateralis from the quadriceps tendon[34] (**Figure 8**). The entire extensor mechanism is then flipped distally exposing the joint. At the completion of the procedure, the medial arthrotomy and lateral musculotendinous release are repaired. Postoperatively, the knee is immobilized in extension and active motion is restricted for 6 weeks to allow healing of the arthrotomy.

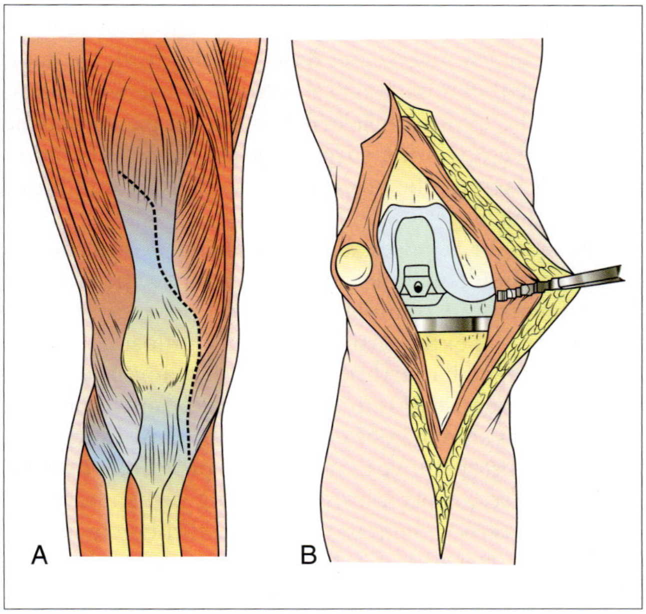

FIGURE 7 Illustration depicts the quadriceps snip: **A**, the planned incision; **B**, the expected exposure.

The Tibial Tubercle Osteotomy

For difficult exposures with limited motion, patella baja, or a well-cemented tibial stem extension, an osteotomy of the tibial tubercle may be required, allowing distal release of the extensor mechanism.[35] Exposure begins with a medial parapatellar arthrotomy and extends along the medial border of the tibial tubercle. The tibial tubercle osteotomy is 6 to 10 cm in length and begins with an osteotomy along the medial border of the tibial tubercle approximately 1 cm from the tubercle (**Figure 9**). The medial cortex is cut with an oscillating saw, to but not through the lateral tibial cortex. The distal tibial cut is tapered. The proximal osteotomy is made with an osteotome parallel to the joint line, trying to maintain a proximal bone bridge to prevent proximal migration of the osteotomy following closure at the conclusion of the procedure. To release the osteotomy, osteotomes are inserted through the medial cortex, cracking the lateral cortex and elevating the tibial tubercle, maintaining the lateral soft-tissue attachments. The knee is flexed and the osteotomy is hinged laterally, exposing the joint. At the conclusion of the procedure, the osteotomy is secured to the original anatomic location with the knee in extension with 16 gauge wires or screw fixation. With secure fixation, full weight bearing and range of motion is permitted.

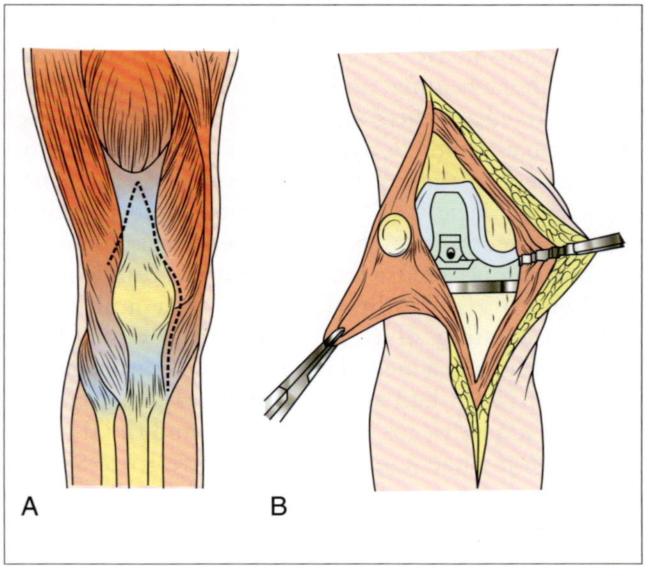

FIGURE 8 Illustration depicts the quadriceps V-Y turndown: **A**, the planned incision; **B**, the expected exposure.

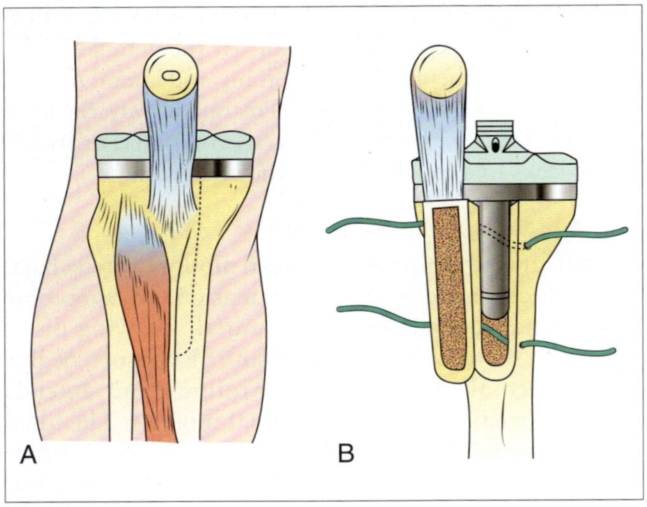

FIGURE 9 Illustration depicts the tibial tubercle osteotomy: **A**, the planned incision; **B**, the expected exposure.

Clinical Results

A well-planned surgical exposure is essential for the successful outcome following revision TKA. A stepwise approach toward exposure should provide safe extensile exposure. A medial parapatellar arthrotomy with synovectomy can be extended with a quadriceps snip when there is concern for risk of patella tendon injury. Studies have shown comparable clinical outcomes with similar isokinetic strength between the medial parapatellar arthrotomy and quadriceps snip.[9,36] Even with meticulous technique partial injury or avulsion of the patella tendon can occur. This observation highlights the benefit of the tibial tubercle osteotomy. This technique can provide excellent exposure in patients with limited motion or patella baja and preserves the extensor mechanism, avoids patella tendon injuries, permits bone-to-bone healing, and exposure of the tibial canal for well-fixed cemented stems.[35,37,38] Another advantage of the tibial tubercle osteotomy is that it allows for realignment of the extensor mechanism or correction of the patella height.[37,39] Complications following tibial tubercle osteotomy can be avoided with meticulous surgical technique, secure fixation, and carefully planned postoperative rehabilitation.[36,39,40] In a multicenter comparison study of all approaches in revision TKA, patients who had a medial parapatellar arthrotomy and quadriceps snip had similar outcomes. The patients who had a quadriceps V-Y turndown and tibial tubercle osteotomy had similar postoperative Knee Society scores, but they were significantly lower than those of the medial parapatellar arthrotomy and quadriceps snip. The quadriceps V-Y turndown had a significantly greater arc of motion than the tibial tubercle osteotomy, but a higher degree of extensor lag. The tibial tubercle osteotomy patients had greater difficulty with kneeling and stooping and reported more about return to daily activities.[36] These observations reveal the difficulties of surgical exposure and compromises in complex revision TKA with limited motion.

SUMMARY

The goal of knee arthroplasty is to restore function and eliminate pain in a knee joint that is compromised by mechanical damage or disease. Optimal surgical exposure is required to allow accurate preparation of the bones for implant placement and to perform soft-tissue balancing. Although most knee arthroplasties have been historically performed through a skin incision 20 cm or longer and a medial parapatellar arthrotomy, alternative surgical exposures using shorter incisions and more limited arthrotomies have been investigated to determine if less theoretical damage to the quadriceps muscle and periarticular soft tissue would result in better outcomes. In the setting of UKA, MIS approaches have become the standard exposure for the procedure. After studying the use of alternative techniques for almost 2 decades, including minimedial parapatellar arthrotomy, modified subvastus, midvastus, and quadriceps-sparing approaches, no conclusive evidence has demonstrated the superiority of any one technique in TKA. Although small, short-term advantages have been demonstrated by some authors with some techniques, the available literature instead suggests that each technique has relative minor advantages and disadvantages. Indeed, patient, instrumentation, prosthesis, and surgeon factors likely influence the most suitable exposure in any given case. Based on the available data, each surgical approach is reasonable for use with TKA. The specific exposure selected in each case should be made by the operating surgeon based on an evaluation of patient factors, the prosthetic system used, and his or her experience.

Revision TKA poses several challenges, and success begins with adequate exposure to remove the original components and reimplant new components without damage to the extensor mechanism. In most cases, the medial parapatellar arthrotomy with a synovectomy will provide adequate exposure. If further exposure is needed, a quadriceps snip may be considered because it does not affect the postoperative rehabilitation protocol. For more difficult cases, especially with a long cemented tibial stem that needs to be removed, a tibial tubercle osteotomy can be considered. The quadriceps V-Y turndown is performed less frequently and is mostly a historical exposure because of postoperative immobilization and reports of extensor lag.

KEY STUDY POINTS

- Exposure for knee arthroplasty was traditionally achieved with an anterior skin incision and a medial parapatellar arthrotomy.
- Less invasive exposures using short skin incisions and capsular arthrotomies were first used in UKA to reduce pain and speed rehabilitation and have become widely accepted.
- Similar concepts to improve early recovery generated significant interest in the 2000s in the so-called minimally invasive TKA using a variety of exposures performed through short skin incisions that theoretically caused less damage to the quadriceps muscle and extensor mechanism. These exposures included the mini-parapatellar, modified subvastus, mini-midvastus, and quadriceps-sparing approaches to the knee.
- After more than 2 decades of use in TKA, the published, randomized, prospective studies comparing both MIS techniques with a standard medial parapatellar arthrotomy, and different minimally invasive techniques to each other, have failed to identify a single approach that is clearly optimal.
- TKA can be successfully performed using a variety of surgical exposures that have relative advantages and disadvantages. The optimal technique in any case likely depends on several variables, including patient characteristics, implant and instrumentation design, and surgeon experience.
- A well-planned surgical exposure is essential for the successful outcome following revision TKA. A stepwise approach toward exposure should provide safe extensile exposure.
- Surgeons should be familiar with the various extensile approaches in revision TKA for exposing the knee joint, safely removing the original components, and implanting the new prosthesis.

ANNOTATED REFERENCES

1. Pagnano MW, Meneghini RM: Minimally invasive total knee arthroplasty with an optimized subvastus approach. *J Arthroplasty* 2006;21(4 suppl 1):22-26.
2. Repicci JA, Eberle RW: Minimally invasive surgical technique for unicondylar knee arthroplasty. *J South Orthop Assoc* 1999;8(1):20-27, discussion 27.
3. Pandit H, Jenkins C, Barker K, Dodd CA, Murray DW: The Oxford medial unicompartmental knee replacement using a minimally-invasive approach. *J Bone Joint Surg Br* 2006;88(1):54-60.
4. Price AJ, Webb J, Topf H, Dodd CA, Goodfellow JW, Murray DW, Oxford Hip and Knee Group: Rapid recovery after oxford unicompartmental arthroplasty through a short incision. *J Arthroplasty* 2001;16(8):970-976.
5. Weston-Simons JS, Pandit H, Kendrick BJ, et al: The mid-term outcomes of the Oxford Domed Lateral unicompartmental knee replacement. *Bone Joint J* 2014;96-B(1):59-64.
6. von Langenbeck B: Zur resection des kniegelenke. *Verh Dtsch En Geseuch F Chir* 1879;7:23.
7. Insall J: A midline approach to the knee. *J Bone Joint Surg Am* 1971;53(8):1584-1586.
8. Scuderi GR, Tenholder M, Capeci C: Surgical approaches in mini-incision total knee arthroplasty. *Clin Orthop Relat Res* 2004;428:61-67.
9. Garvin KL, Scuderi G, Insall JN: Evolution of the quadriceps snip. *Clin Orthop Relat Res* 1995;321:131-137.
10. Hofmann AA, Plaster RL, Murdock LE: Subvastus (Southern) approach for primary total knee arthroplasty. *Clin Orthop Relat Res* 1991;269:70-77.
11. Pagnano MW, Meneghini RM, Trousdale RT: Anatomy of the extensor mechanism in reference to quadriceps-sparing TKA. *Clin Orthop Relat Res* 2006;452(452):102-105.
12. Tria AJ Jr: Minimally invasive total knee arthroplasty using quadriceps-sparing approach, in Scuderi GR, Tria AJ Jr, Berger RA, eds: *MIS Techniques in Orthopaedics.* New York, NY, Springer, 2005, p 349.
13. Holt G, Nunn T, Allen RA, Forrester AW, Gregori A: Variation of the vastus medialis obliquus insertion and its relevance to minimally invasive total knee arthroplasty. *J Arthroplasty* 2008;23(4):600-604.
14. Engh GA, Holt BT, Parks NL: A midvastus muscle-splitting approach for total knee arthroplasty. *J Arthroplasty* 1997;12(3):322-331.
15. Tria AJ Jr, Coon TM: Minimal incision total knee arthroplasty: Early experience. *Clin Orthop Relat Res* 2003;416:185-190.
16. Jackson G, Waldman BJ, Schaftel EA: Complications following quadriceps-sparing total knee arthroplasty. *Orthopedics* 2008;31(6):547.
17. Keblish PA: The lateral approach to the valgus knee. Surgical technique and analysis of 53 cases with over two-year follow-up evaluation. *Clin Orthop Relat Res* 1991;271:52-62.
18. Seyler TM, Bonutti PM, Ulrich SD, Fatscher T, Marker DR, Mont MA: Minimally invasive lateral approach to total knee arthroplasty. *J Arthroplasty* 2007;22(7 suppl 3):21-26.
19. Chen AF, Alan RK, Redziniak DE, Tria AJ Jr: Quadriceps sparing total knee replacement. The initial experience with results at two to four years. *J Bone Joint Surg Br* 2006;88(11):1448-1453.
20. Dutton AQ, Yeo SJ, Yang KY, Lo NN, Chia KU, Chong HC: Computer-assisted minimally invasive total knee arthroplasty compared with standard total knee arthroplasty. A prospective, randomized study. *J Bone Joint Surg Am* 2008;90(1):2-9.

21. Haas SB, Cook S, Beksac B: Minimally invasive total knee replacement through a mini midvastus approach: A comparative study. *Clin Orthop Relat Res* 2004;428:68-73.
22. McAllister CM, Stepanian JD: The impact of minimally invasive surgical techniques on early range of motion after primary total knee arthroplasty. *J Arthroplasty* 2008;23(1):10-18.
23. Tashiro Y, Miura H, Matsuda S, Okazaki K, Iwamoto Y: Minimally invasive versus standard approach in total knee arthroplasty. *Clin Orthop Relat Res* 2007;463(463):144-150.
24. Aglietti P, Baldini A, Sensi L: Quadriceps-sparing versus mini-subvastus approach in total knee arthroplasty. *Clin Orthop Relat Res* 2006;452(452):106-111.
25. Bonutti PM, Zywiel MG, Ulrich SD, Stroh DA, Seyler TM, Mont MA: A comparison of subvastus and midvastus approaches in minimally invasive total knee arthroplasty. *J Bone Joint Surg Am* 2010;92(3):575-582.
26. Bourke MG, Jull GA, Buttrum PJ, Fitzpatrick PL, Dalton PA, Russell TG: Comparing outcomes of medial parapatellar and subvastus approaches in total knee arthroplasty: A randomized controlled trial. *J Arthroplasty* 2012;27(3):347-353.e1.
27. Heekin RD, Fokin AA: Mini-midvastus versus mini-medial parapatellar approach for minimally invasive total knee arthroplasty: Outcomes pendulum is at equilibrium. *J Arthroplasty* 2014;29(2):339-342.
28. Kim YH, Kim JS, Kim DY: Clinical outcome and rate of complications after primary total knee replacement performed with quadriceps-sparing or standard arthrotomy. *J Bone Joint Surg Br* 2007;89(4):467-470.
29. Nestor BJ, Toulson CE, Backus SI, Lyman SL, Foote KL, Windsor RE: Mini-midvastus vs standard medial parapatellar approach: A prospective, randomized, double-blinded study in patients undergoing bilateral total knee arthroplasty. *J Arthroplasty* 2010;25(6 suppl):5-11.
30. Bourke MG, Buttrum PJ, Fitzpatrick PL, Dalton PA, Jull GA, Russell TG: Systematic review of medial parapatellar and subvastus approaches in total knee arthroplasty. *J Arthroplasty* 2010;25(5):728-734.
31. Smith TO, King JJ, Hing CB: A meta-analysis of randomised controlled trials comparing the clinical and radiological outcomes following minimally invasive to conventional exposure for total knee arthroplasty. *Knee* 2012;19(1):1-7.
32. Cheng T, Liu T, Zhang G, Peng X, Zhang X: Does minimally invasive surgery improve short-term recovery in total knee arthroplasty? *Clin Orthop Relat Res* 2010;468(6):1635-1648.
33. Gandhi R, Smith H, Lefaivre KA, Davey JR, Mahomed NN: Complications after minimally invasive total knee arthroplasty as compared with traditional incision techniques: A meta-analysis. *J Arthroplasty* 2011;26(1):29-35.
34. Coonse K, Adams JD: A new operative approach to the knee joint. *Surg Gynecol Obstet* 1943;77:344-347.
35. Whiteside LA: Exposure in difficult total knee arthroplasty using tibial tubercle osteotomy. *Clin Orthop Relat Res* 1995;321:32-35.
36. Barrack RL, Smith P, Munn B, Engh G, Rorabeck C: The Ranawat Award: Comparison of surgical approaches in total knee arthroplasty. *Clin Orthop Relat Res* 1998;356:16-21.
37. Bruni D, Iacono F, Sharma B, Zaffagnini S, Maracci M: Tibial tubercle osteotomy or quadriceps snip in two-stage revision for prosthetic knee infection? A randomized prospective study. *Clin Orthop Relat Res* 2013;471(4):1305-1318.
38. Mendes MW, Caldwell P, Jiranek WA: The results of tibial tubercle osteotomy for revision total knee arthroplasty. *J Arthroplasty* 2004;19(2):167-174.
39. Sun Z, Patil A, Song EK, Kim HT, Seon JK: Comparison of quadriceps snip and tibial tubercle osteotomy in revision for infected total knee arthroplasty. *Int Orthop* 2015;39:879-885.
40. Ritter MA, Carr K, Keating EM, Faris PM, Meding JB: Tibial shaft fracture following tibial tubercle osteotomy. *J Arthroplasty* 1996;11(1):117-119.

CHAPTER 19

Kinematics in Total Knee Arthroplasty

WILLIAM M. MIHALKO, MD, PhD

ABSTRACT

Constant innovations in design and technique have improved functional results of total knee arthroplasty, but no clear consensus has been reached concerning the superiority of different designs. Implants that sacrifice, substitute, or retain the anterior and/or posterior cruciate ligament; implants with different positioning and shapes of the post and cam, and mobile-bearing or fixed-bearing designs all have advantages and disadvantages in the attempts to restore normal knee kinematics. No design to date has proven to consistently re-create normal knee kinematics, but bicruciate-sparing designs seem to have the greatest potential to do so, especially if the more demanding surgical technique can be simplified. Total knee kinematics can also be affected by surgical technique, about which debate continues (eg, mechanical or kinematic alignment, gap balancing, or matched resection), as well as patient-related factors (eg, age, body mass index, preexisting deformity, individual anatomy).

Dr. Mihalko or an immediate family member has received royalties from Aesculap/B.Braun; is a member of a speakers' bureau or has made paid presentations on behalf of Aesculap/B.Braun; serves as a paid consultant to or is an employee of Aesculap/B.Braun, Pacira, Inc., and Zimmer; has received research or institutional support from Aesculap/B. Braun, Department of Defense, Myoscience, Inc., National Institutes of Health (NIAMS & NICHD), and Stryker; and serves as a board member, owner, officer, or committee member of the American Academy of Orthopaedic Surgeons, the American Society for Testing Materials International, the Knee Society, and the Orthopaedic Research Society.

Keywords: arthroplasty; biomechanics; design; kinematics; knee

INTRODUCTION

Total knee arthroplasty (TKA) has seen many design changes over the last 4 decades, but the concept of total condylar arthroplasty remains largely unchanged. Some of these design changes include an increase in the number of sizes available, mobile bearings, bicruciate-substituting or bicruciate-retaining designs, and medial pivot–driven constraints. Many of these design rationales are derived from normal knee kinematic variables as well as the aim to improve patient satisfaction and function after surgery. In reality, the design variables used in a TKA implant often may not result in the desired motion that was aimed for by the designers. This has been proven in the literature by many in vivo studies showing kinematic profiles of TKAs, which do not follow conventional normal knee kinematic profiles.[1-7] These reported in vivo kinematics most likely rely on multiple variables, including patient anatomy, surgical technique, individual dynamic muscle forces and kinetics, and even excessive body mass index and joint loads.[8-14] In many cases, implant design also is dependent on surgical technique, about which there remains lively debate (ie, mechanical versus kinematic alignment, gap balancing versus matched resection).[15-18]

IMPLANT DESIGN AND EFFECTS ON KINEMATICS

A large degree of variability exists in the kinematics of the replaced knee, and there is no consensus on the definitive design that best reconstructs the joint to re-create the kinematics of the normal knee. This in part has to do with the fact that the arthritic knee, whether from inflammatory, posttraumatic, or osteoarthritic causes, has effects on more than just the surface geometry of the joint. Osteophytes and extra-articular deformities are just two such variables that can have an effect on the dynamics and kinematics of the knee joint over time. As osteophytes get larger, static (ligamentous) and dynamic (tendon) structures about the knee are effectively shorten, which in turn changes the kinetics and the kinematics of the knee joint over time.

Some designs have centered on the effect and importance of the posterior cruciate ligament (PCL). Functionally, the PCL provides most of the total restraining force against posterior translation of the tibia relative to the femur and supports stability of the knee and the joint space in flexion.[19] In the posterior cruciate-retaining (PCR) knee, the conservation of the PCL is designed to reduce the posterior translation of the tibia and contribute to femoral roll back in deep knee flexion.[20-22] Posterior cruciate retention theoretically enables roll back of the femur on the tibia with knee flexion, allowing more efficient use of the extensor mechanism and quadriceps musculature,[23] but debate continues in the literature regarding the benefits of retaining the PCL in TKA.[24-26] The design of a posterior-stabilized TKA differs in that it requires additional anterior-posterior stability effectively achieved by placement of a femoral cam and tibial post. The proponents of the posterior-stabilized designs argue that it offers a more reproducible kinematic profile and increased range of motion, whereas opponents point to increased femoral bone loss and added implant constraint that may increase the risk of aseptic loosening as downfalls of the design. Several studies report there is no difference in terms of functional outcome between patients receiving a posterior-stabilizing or cruciate-retaining TKA.[25,27,28] Opponents to posterior-stabilized implants also argue that the knee is more stable in flexion without affecting the flexion gap and retains important mechanoreceptors in the PCL that can affect function after surgery.[29] Recently, studies published for 10-year midterm survivorship reported cruciate-retaining TKAs having a better survivorship than posterior-stabilized TKAs. However, there have been reports within these studies showing patients who have better function with a posterior-stabilized TKA.[29-31]

Post and Cam Positioning in Posterior-stabilized Implant Design and Influence on Kinematics

The posterior-stabilized TKA implants afford stability to the knee by blocking posterior translation of the tibia on the femur through a post (on the polyethylene insert) and a cam (on the posterior femoral condyles or bridging a box between the condyles of the femur) (**Figure 1**). The design changes that affect the guided or constrained motion of the femur on the tibia are affected by the position and shape of the post and cam, as well as the amount of congruency in the tibial polyethylene.[32]

Starting with the Insall-Burstein design, the post and cam were symmetric in nature[31] (**Figure 2**). The post was positioned centrally within the tibial polyethylene insert, and the cam spanned the posterior femoral condyles. This design engaged the cam on the post around 60° and

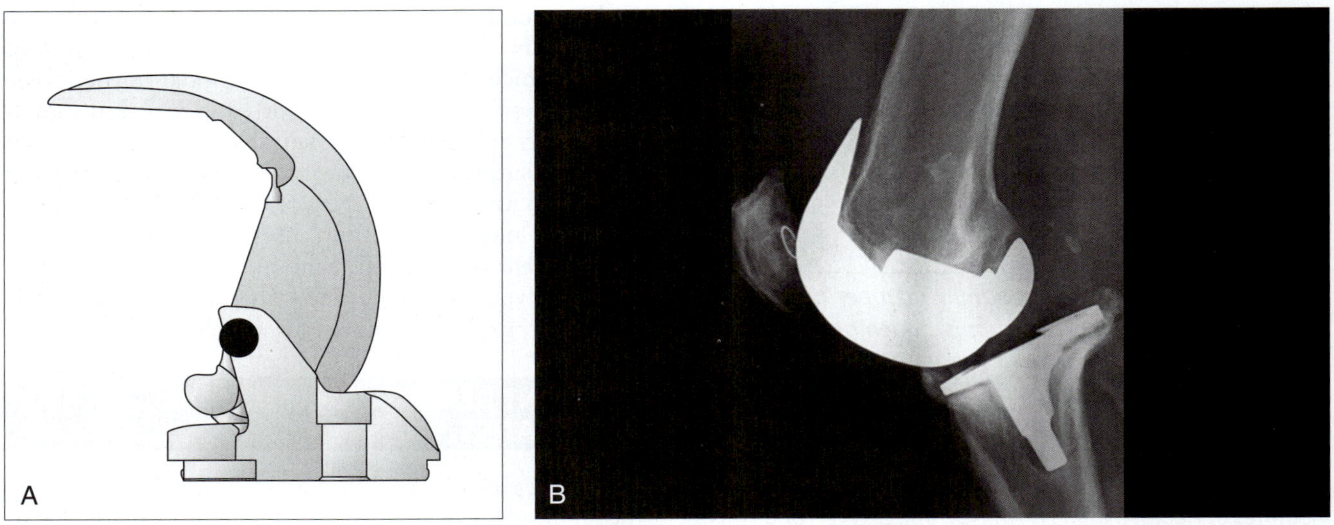

FIGURE 1 **A**, Illustration of a cam that is positioned at the top and most posterior aspect of the femoral posterior condyles, which tends to interact with the tibial post later in the flexion arc but will tend to remain at the base of the post in the extremes of flexion, thereby maximizing the jump height of the cam on the post. As the cam is moved anteriorly across the box (dark circle), the interaction will tend to occur earlier in flexion and will articulate higher on the post late in the flexion arc, thereby decreasing the jump height. **B**, Lateral radiograph of a patient who felt a pop while working under his vehicle and could not bend his knee. A jumped post in a posterior-stabilized design implant is one complication when the flexion space is greater than the jump height of the post.

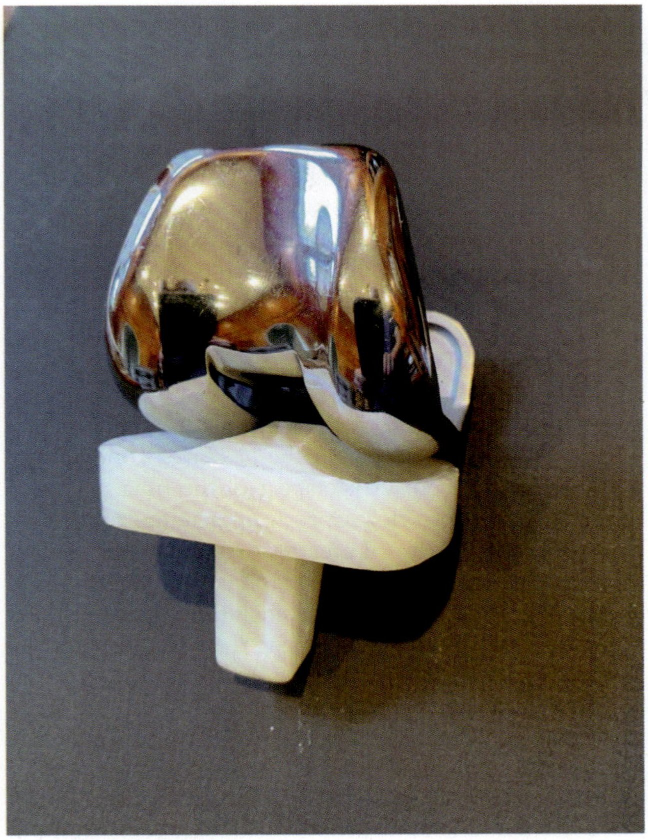

FIGURE 2 Photograph of Insall-Burstein total condylar implant, which was one of the first designs on the market. Symmetric condyles and trochlear flanges were bulky and have been updated in current modern-day designs.

then drove roll back of the posterior femoral condyles on the tibial polyethylene in a symmetric manner until edge loading of the posterior femoral condyles on the polyethylene insert occurred at around 120° of flexion. This was the basis of design for most posterior-stabilized TKA implants from this point forward.

If one examines how the post and cam positioning will affect when and how the interaction of the post and cam occurs, then a basic understanding of design attributes can be inferred. If the post is positioned centrally in the baseplate, how moving the cam will affect the interaction of the two and drive the motion of the femur with respect to the tibia can be determined. If the cam is positioned more anteriorly across the sides of the box, then the post will interact with the cam sooner during the flexion arc and once engaged will keep the contact of the cam in the midportion of the post. If the cam is moved more posterior on the femur or at the top of the femoral condyles, then the cam will contact the post later in the flexion arc and then move down the post and will remain at the base of the post even with extremes of flexion, thereby maximizing the jump height.[6,32,33] This is important to keep the knee stable in flexion and prevent a jumped post after surgery (**Figure 1**). Some implants have now incorporated an articulating area on the anterior aspect of the post with the anterior aspect of the box to guide motion in terminal extension. This type of dual-cam design adds another articulating surface but may guide motion in terminal extension more consistently.

Cam and post geometry in the transverse plane also will change the way the femur and tibia interacts. If the post has a rectangular cross section, it may constrain rotation of the femur on the tibia in the transverse plane depending on the overall width of the post. This design feature will cause edge loading of the post on the condylar edges of the femoral implant, as shown in a retrieved implant (**Figure 3**). This implant shows the square edges of the polyethylene post with a wear scar along the sides from overconstraint in the transverse plane. If the post has a rounded transverse plane geometry with less condylar constraint to internal and external rotation, less burnishing and edge wear may result[6,32,33] (**Figure 4**).

Post height and position also can affect flexion and kinematics in other ways. If the post is straight and too tall with a more anterior position, there is risk of impingement of the top of the post on the inferior aspect of the patellar button known as post patellar conflict. When this occurs, the patient typically feels a block to further flexion and pain as the post collides with patella.

Asymmetric cam designs in which one side of the cam has a larger diameter have now been introduced. The smaller diameter typically is placed on the medial side and

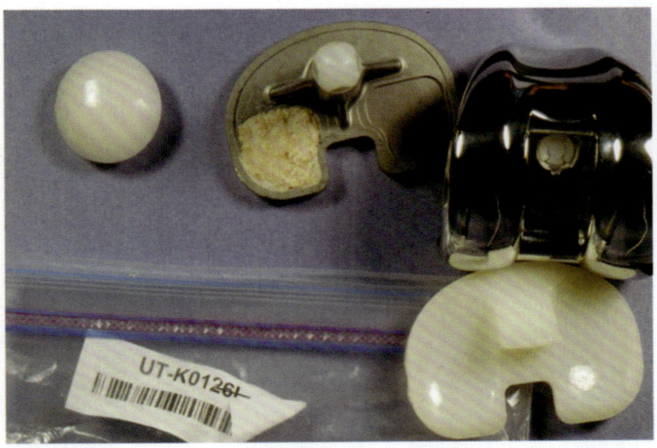

FIGURE 3 Photograph of a retrieved implant at the time of necropsy with more than 10 years of implantation, which shows an example of rectangular post cross section with sharp edges and a cam that is located midway along the height of the posterior condyles. This configuration gives contact sooner in the flexion arc and moves contact up the post after around 90° of flexion. The medial and lateral wear scars are symmetric and do not force as much roll back in this configuration with edge impingement seen in the posterior aspect of the polyethylene insert where it impinged on the posterior aspect of the femur in flexion.

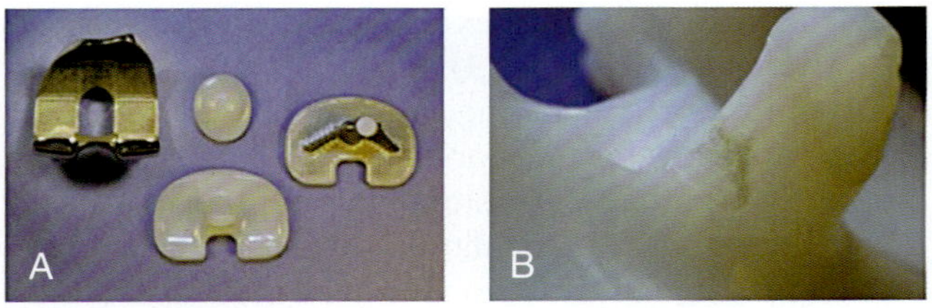

FIGURE 4 **A**, Photograph of a retrieved implant at the time of necropsy of a posterior-stabilized implant after over 10 years of implantation where the post has a more rounded cross section and the cam is more toward the base of the posterior femoral condyles. **B**, Photograph of the lateral aspect of the post that shows an impingement wear scar from the inner aspect of the lateral condyle of the femoral implant as well as impingement scar at the top of the straight post from where there was patellar button post conflict in flexion.

the varying larger diameter on the lateral side (**Figure 5**). This type of design feature is used with the intent to guide but not constrain a medial pivot. This occurs because the wider diameter of the cam on the lateral side with increasing flexion pushes the lateral femoral condyle (LFC) posteriorly to effect roll back, whereas the smaller diameter on the medial side tends to keep the medial femoral condyle (MFC) centrally located with more sliding motion.[34]

Cruciate-retaining TKA Implant Design Attributes and Influence on Kinematics

Cruciate-retaining designs have evolved from a flat-on-flat minimal constraint design (in the early 1990s) to ones that tend to balance the amount of implant constraint to aid in guiding femoral-tibial motion. To prevent the MFC from sliding forward, many designs incorporate a deep-dish or ultracongruent option for a tibial polyethylene insert. This design feature is used to make certain the MFC does not slide forward affording an anterior block to the MFC on the medial tibial polyethylene. Many designs, however, are still showing a tendency for the femoral articulation to slide forward with increasing flexion. A single-radius femoral condylar design can aid in keeping the MFC from sliding forward, but single-radius designs, though showing an improvement in roll back, have not showed improvements in axial rotation patterns and still do not approach normal knee kinematics.[28,29,34-36]

Range of motion after PCR TKA has been reported to be improved when the posterior condylar offset is re-established[8,9] (**Figure 6**). If the posterior condyles are overresected, the posterior aspect of the tibia may butt up against the posterior aspect of the femur and result in suboptimal flexion. Later reports have shown that measuring this variable radiographically is difficult and that a combination of variables, including implant design and tibial slope, also plays a role in the amount of flexion obtained and the function of the PCL after surgery.[8,34]

Most cruciate-retaining designs build posterior slope into the polyethylene insert to enhance roll-back and prevent the roll-forward anterior translation seen in fluorokinematic studies. Other design features to enhance a more normal kinematic profile include less constraint in the transverse plane to allow axial rotation throughout a range of motion. This design feature is accomplished by decreasing the constraint to rotation between the femoral condyles and polyethylene insert. Despite these

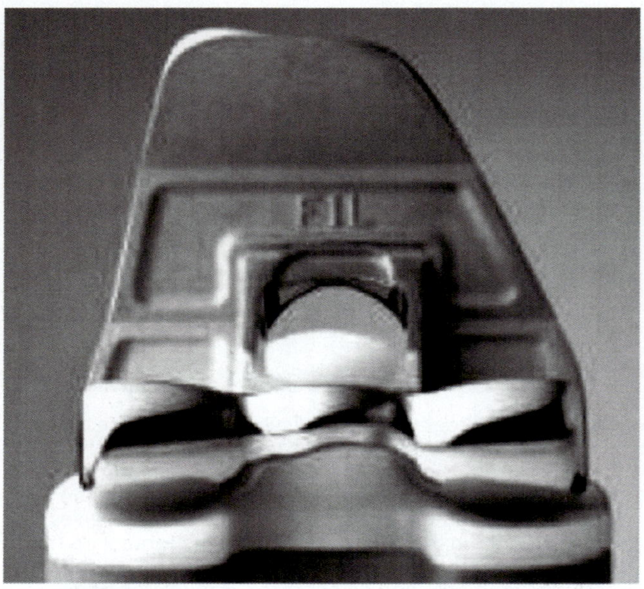

FIGURE 5 A photograph of asymmetric cam with a larger lateral diameter used to guide lateral roll back and a medial pivot.

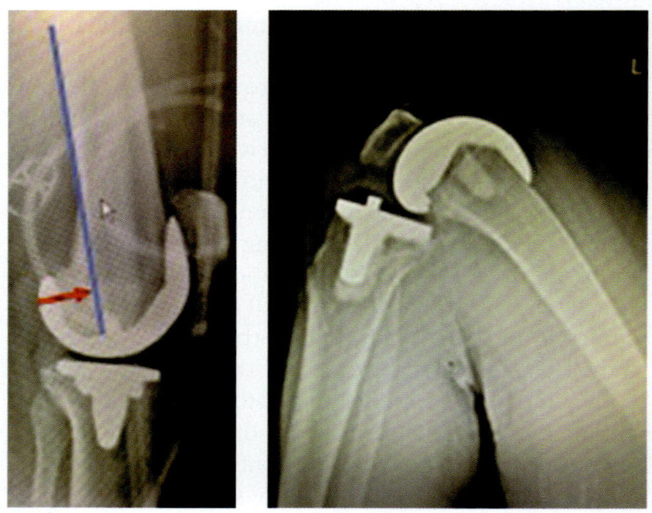

FIGURE 6 Lateral radiograph on the left depicts posterior condylar offset in cruciate-retaining total knee arthroplasty, which has been shown to be important to obtain optimal amounts of flexion after surgery. In many posterior-stabilized designs, thicker posterior condyles are used, as depicted on the lateral radiograph on the right, to obtain maximum flexion.

adaptations, cruciate-retaining knees have shown more variability in most fluorokinematic studies compared with other primary knee constraint designs.[35,36]

Bicruciate-substituting Total Knee Implant Design and Influence on Kinematics

An articulation of the anterior aspect of the post with the anterior aspect of the femoral box in posterior-stabilized designs also has been added to guide initial kinematics of the replaced knee in the first 30° of flexion. By designing this added articulation, a posterior-stabilized design becomes a bicruciate-substituting design because the anterior post/box articulation is meant to substitute for the anterior cruciate ligament (ACL). Although this is specific to one manufacturer, the benefits over posterior-stabilized designs have not been reported in general. The same basic concepts reviewed in the posterior-stabilized design section apply for the flexion effects on kinematics. This added articulation on the anterior aspect of the post means that it cannot sit as far posterior in the sagittal plane, so there tends to be a midflexion region where there is no guided motion from the post/cam articulations.[37]

Bicruciate-retaining TKA and Implant Kinematics

In the quest to reproduce normal kinematics, bicruciate-retaining (BCR) TKA designs have now emerged. The design rationale preserves both the anterior and the PCLs using a baseplate design that allows the preservation of both the ACL and PCL insertions. Proponents believe there is greater potential to restore normal posterior femoral roll back and joint kinematics in both the sagittal and transverse planes, but opponents point to the difficulty in obtaining proper soft-tissue balancing with intact cruciate ligaments. Others point to the fact that the ACL often is atrophied in advanced osteoarthritis of the knee as a reason not to advocate this design. Abnormal knee kinematics and paradoxical anterior femoral translation in more conventional/traditional TKA designs have been suggested as potential causes of patient dissatisfaction and a reason to aim for the preservation of the ACL. However, there are limited data on the in vivo kinematics and articular contact behavior of BCR TKA designs. Design variables of constraint can be more liberal in these designs because there is continued support of both cruciates, but adapting to patient anatomy can be difficult with a significant learning curve. Current clinical short-term and midterm outcomes of BCR are mixed in the literature.[35,38-40]

Mobile-bearing Design Rationale and Influence on Kinematics

Potential advantages of mobile-bearing knees include lower contact stresses at the articulating surfaces, rotational motion of the tibial polyethylene during gait, and self-alignment of the tibial polyethylene compensating for small rotational malalignment of the tibial baseplate during implantation. It should be identified that rotating-platform designs can be either cruciate-retaining or posterior-stabilized. Recent studies have found a higher revision rate in both the short-term and midterm follow-up period with a mobile-bearing insert compared with fixed-bearing TKA.[41,42] Whether mobile-bearing designs will outperform fixed-bearing designs is an ongoing debate and may be specific to individual manufacturer's design. Proponents point to lower tibial baseplate stresses and the ability of the soft-tissue sleeve to support rotation in the transverse plane and guide motion where fixed-bearing designs may constrain the knee's natural motion. Uncertainty about backside wear and the fact that in vivo fluorokinematic studies have not proven an advantage over fixed bearings to date have kept these designs from having a higher percentage of use in the United States. A recent meta-analysis found that there was moderate-quality to low-quality evidence that cruciate-retaining, mobile-bearing TKA was as good as fixed-bearing TKA.[43] A recent fluorokinematic study on stair-climbing activity with a popular rotating platform designed for patients with cruciate-retaining and posterior-stabilized TKA found negligible differences between the two implants. The rotating-platform cruciate-retaining (20 patients) and posterior-stabilized (10 patients) designs showed stable midrange flexion anterior-posterior translation, and both designs were consistent in the motion patterns. Isometric quadriceps forces also were compared and showed no significant differences.[44]

Medial Pivot Designs and Influence on Kinematics

Most medial pivot total knee implant designs will produce this movement by constraining the medial side of the knee. This is accomplished with a single-radius femoral condylar design in the sagittal plane and an asymmetric polyethylene insert where the medial side is ultraconforming (ball and socket) with a higher anterior and posterior lip to keep the medial condyle centered during flexion and the lateral side is less conforming to allow roll back of the LFC (**Figure 7**). Here one caveat is that constraining motion in the sagittal and transverse planes may force a knee to move in a way that may impart higher forces. Several fluorokinematic studies have reported a lateral pivot after TKA, and this amount of constraint may place higher forces on the posterior lip of the medial compartment polyethylene insert. The author has seen this in revisions of this type of implant where the posterior lip has worn away from edge loading of the MFC that rolls over the posterior lip causing excessive polyethylene wear. Adding a rotating platform aspect to this design may theoretically allow the insert to rotate and prevent this from occurring.[35,45-48]

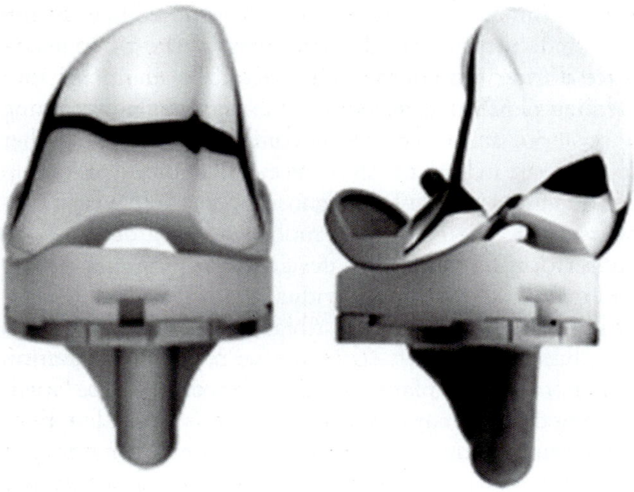

FIGURE 7 Photograph of medial pivot designs that use a ball-in-socket medial condylar constraint. In this example from Microport Orthopaedics, the medial side of the polyethylene has a more constraining conformity with higher anterior and posterior lips and the lateral side is less conforming, allowing more roll back. (Photograph from https://www.microportortho.com/products/knees/primary-total-knee-systems/evolution-knee-systems.)

IN VIVO TKA KINEMATICS

Regardless of the type of implant used for a primary TKA, gait differences compared with the normal knee remain. After a primary TKA in a patient who has a nonosteoarthritic contralateral knee, differences in gait symmetry are evident and have been reported.[35] The results of kinematic studies performed in a normal human knee have shown an increased posterior motion in the lateral condyle compared with the medial condyle throughout flexion, and these studies are typically used to compare the measured kinematics after TKA.[35,49] Although neither posterior-stabilized nor cruciate-retaining in vivo fluorokinematic or gait studies completely replicate normal knee kinematics, there are variations worth noting.

Numerous kinematic fluoroscopy studies have been conducted over the past 2 decades reporting the difference between implant designs. Recently, the authors of a 2019 study[35] published a review of fluorokinematic studies of different implant designs. Although many fluorokinematic studies have been reported during a lunge type of maneuver, there is some debate on whether this type of dynamic movement is applicable to clinical results because this kind of motion is seldom used during activities of daily living.

Cruciate-retaining In Vivo Kinematics

In the sagittal plane, cruciate-retaining designs have shown a forward sliding of the MFC in a lunge and/or squatting type of maneuver, but during gait, these motions have been less erratic.[35,50] Although the cruciate-retaining design has been used with great clinical success, the kinematics and flexion performance differ from those of a normal knee. In general, the sagittal movements of the cruciate-retaining TKA typically demonstrate similar motions to those of the ACL-deficient knee, which makes sense considering the design basis of these types of implants. Although many cruciate-retaining TKA designs exhibit a roll-forward pattern on the medial side of the implant, this tends to be improved in a single-radius design where the MFC tends to stay more centered. Designs that have a multiradius of curvature of the MFC tend to roll forward where the radius of curvature changes, and that is why after 40° of flexion most cruciate-retaining implants show no further roll-forward tendencies.[35,36]

In the transverse plane, cruciate-retaining TKA in vivo kinematics has shown that there is less overall rotation compared with the normal knee. The screw-home mechanism tends to be lost, and the cruciate-retaining TKA MFC starts more posterior on the tibial insert. This is also a reason why there have been reports of a lateral pivot during a deep knee bend or lunge type of dynamic loading.

Posterior-stabilized Fixed and Mobile Bearing

Posterior-stabilized designs have shown more consistent motion, but not one that is always comparable with the normal knee. Fluoroscopy also has been used to study cam-post interactions. One study investigated when the cam-post contact occurred throughout flexion and when contact occurs according to the location of the cam on the tibial post and the height of contact of the cam on the tibial post during deep knee bending for three types of implants: bicruciate-stabilized, fixed-bearing posterior-stabilized, and rotating-platform posterior-stabilized. The study found the location of contact on the tibial post remained centered in the rotating-platform posterior-stabilized designs, but in fixed-bearing posterior-stabilized designs, it moved from the medial aspect of the tibial post to the center of the tibial post during flexion.[2]

Another fluorokinematic study looked at how two different groups, one with greater than 15° of normal rotation and one with more than 3° of reverse rotation in the transverse plane, affected the maximal flexion angle. It was found that the group with reverse axial rotation had lower maximal flexion angles than those with normal rotation, indicating that axial rotation influences weight-bearing knee flexion. Knees with normal rotation obtained deeper flexion than those with reverse rotation, suggesting that the reverse rotation pattern may limit flexion and result in less patient satisfaction when this type of motion pattern occurs after TKA surgery.[3,4,11,13,35-37]

In vivo fluorokinematic studies of posterior-stabilized mobile-bearing designs have shown that the bearing rotation in the transverse plane may be nonphysiologic in some patients.[2,5,9] This internal transverse plane motion has been reported in all types of TKA bearings and does not seem to be specific to any one design. This described motion has not been completely explained, but it has been suggested that these patients tend to be less satisfied. One gait study in a sit-to-stand analysis, however, found patients who have this lateral pivot had excellent knee society scores and satisfaction.[51]

Bicruciate-substituting TKA Kinematics

Fluoroscopy also has been used to study cam-post interactions in bicruciate-substituting TKA. A study investigated when the cam-post occurred throughout flexion, the location of the cam on the tibial post when contact occurs, and the height of contact of the cam on the tibial post during deep knee bending for three types of implants: bicruciate-stabilized, fixed-bearing posterior-stabilized, and rotating-platform posterior-stabilized. The study found that the bicruciate-stabilized TKA had lower contact angles, lower cam-post distance throughout flexion, and a higher height of contact on the tibial post compared with both posterior-stabilized designs. It also found the location of contact on the tibial post remained centered in the rotating-platform posterior-stabilized designs, but in fixed-bearing posterior-stabilized designs, it moved from the medial aspect of the tibial post to the center of the tibial post during flexion.[2] Although a lunge type of movement is rarely used in daily activities, it does give a basis of comparison for TKA subjects under dynamic conditions. Some authors have analyzed more demanding activities, such as rising from a chair and kneeling.[1] Patients who have a posterior-stabilized design tend to have a neutral or anterior position of the femoral implant at full extension with progressive posterior femoral roll back being achieved with increasing knee flexion.

Another study that investigated a TKA with a dual-cam design tested the theory that this design would decrease intersurgeon variability in kinematics after surgery. Three different groups were created from three different surgeons. The overall motion patterns among the groups were similar, but intrasurgeon differences were found in in vivo kinematics. One group had a greater relative axial rotation than the other two groups. This difference shows that this type of implant does not function as a mechanically constrained system, and surgical technique and soft-tissue handling play a role in the outcome of implant function.[4]

Bicruciate-retaining TKA Implant Designs

With preservation of both the ACL and the PCL, BCR TKA has shown kinematic patterns most similar to the native knee. The kinematics recorded for a BCR TKA, whether during gait or a deep knee bend lunge maneuver, show similar roll back and transverse plane rotation. Currently, the number of BCR TKA implants used is far less than cruciate-retaining or posterior-stabilized TKA designs, but the roll back patterns in the sagittal plane are most similar to a native knee. The authors of a 2016 study[52] discussed the theoretic advantage of retaining proprioception with retention of the ACL and PCL over a posterior-stabilized TKA. The authors of a 2012 study showed that PCL proprioceptors are retained and maintained at similar levels to the numbers recorded in osteoarthritis native knees, suggesting that this may indeed be an advantage to this design of implant.[53] Even though the kinematics and possibly the proprioception of the knee are preserved with a BCR TKA, few studies have shown high patient satisfaction with the BCR TKA.[38,54] A systematic review by the authors of a 2017 study reported that, although preservation of both cruciates may allow for more normal knee kinematics, the surgery is more technically demanding. The authors found little difference in outcomes between the BCR and PCR designs and ultimately questioned the utility of the BCR design given equivocal outcomes.[39,55]

Medial Pivot TKA Implant Kinematics

The medial pivot TKA designs on the market were introduced because of reports of increased anterior-posterior translation being linked to poor patient-reported outcomes and feelings of instability.[56] The reports in the literature of in vivo kinematics of medial pivot TKA designs have proven that the knee seems to function as designed. There are far fewer variations of AP translation on the constrained medial aspect of these TKA designs. With fluoroscopic analysis, the authors of a 2003 study[57] reported that the medial pivot TKA had little anterior-posterior translation of the MFC, whereas the LFC moved posteriorly through flexion. Compared with PCR TKAs, the medial pivot design exhibited less variability with anterior-posterior motion. Patients who have a medial pivot kinematic pattern demonstrated greater excursion of the LFC compared with the PCR TKA. Other studies have confirmed medial pivot kinematics as the design as intended.[58-63]

SURGICAL TECHNIQUE EFFECTS ON KINEMATICS AFTER TKA

Mechanical Alignment Versus Kinematic Alignment Techniques

The debate continues as to whether mechanical axis alignment or kinematic alignment of the lower extremity is preferable during primary TKA. Whether one advocates for kinematic or mechanical alignment, the kinematics of the lower extremity seem to not be significantly different. A comparison during normal gait found better reproduction of normal gait parameters with kinematic alignment, whereas another study with higher power found no differences between the two. When the tibia is cut in varus and the femur in valgus, the theory is that, as the lower extremity is adducted at heel strike during the gait, the joint line would be parallel to the ground while with mechanical axis alignment keeps the joint line perpendicular to the lower extremity axis. Those who oppose kinematic alignment also point to the possibilities of inaccuracies in the tibial cut that may place the tibia in four or more degrees of varus, and this has been shown to be a major predictor of early tibial aseptic loosening.[64]

The authors of a 2019 study[65] compared 18 matched kinematic alignment and mechanical alignment TKAs and found better reproduction of kinematic parameters in the kinematic alignment group. The kinematic alignment group showed no significant knee kinematic differences compared with healthy knees in sagittal plane range of motion, maximal flexion, abduction-adduction curves, or knee external tibial rotation. Conversely, the mechanical alignment group displayed several significant knee kinematic differences compared with the healthy group: less sagittal plane range of motion (49.1° versus 54.0°, $P = 0.020$), decreased maximal flexion (52.3° versus 57.5°, $P = 0.002$), increased adduction angle (2.0° to 7.5° versus −2.8° to 3.0°, $P < 0.05$), and increased external tibial rotation (by a mean of 2.3° ± 0.7°, $P < 0.001$). The postoperative Knee Injury and Osteoarthritis Outcome Score was significantly higher in the kinematic alignment group compared with the mechanical alignment group (74.2 versus 60.7, $P = 0.034$). It should be noted, however, that the optical linkage used to perform the study is not as accurate as fluorokinematic analyses and even body habitus can affect the accuracy of the results.

Conversely, the authors f a 2019 study[66] reported no differences in 30 robotically performed mechanical alignment TKAs compared with 30 robotically performed kinematic alignment TKAs that were randomly assigned to a treatment group. Traditional three-dimensional gait analysis techniques were used to compare the two groups. The median follow-up duration of the mechanical alignment group was 8.7 (range 8.1 to 9.4) years and that of the kinematic alignment group was 8.4 (range 8.0 to 9.1) years. Clinical outcomes between the two groups showed no significant difference in Hospital for Special Surgery, Western Ontario and McMaster Universities Osteoarthritis Index, range of motion, Knee Society pain, or function score at the last follow-up. No significant difference in coronal plane laxity assessment, mechanical alignment of the lower limb, or perioperative complications was reported between the two groups. In gait analysis, no significant difference in kinematic or kinetic parameters was found except for varus angle ($P < 0.05$) and mediolateral ground reaction force ($P < 0.05$).

A meta-analysis of reports on differences in kinetics and kinematics after TKA in sit-to-stand activity showed the importance of quadriceps function after surgery and the fact that kinetics and kinematics do not return to normal.[67] It was also found that kinetic variables showed more adverse changes between kinematic alignment and control patients. Patients in the kinematic alignment group exhibited increased vertical ground reaction forces in the nonsurgical limb and hip extension moment in the surgical limb compared with control patients. In addition, the kinematic alignment group had decreased knee extension moment in the surgical limb compared with control patients. These changes in the early recovery (3 to 6 months post kinematic alignment) indicate that patients tend to avoid using the replaced knees while relying more on the ipsilateral hip to minimize knee loading of the surgical limb during sit to stand.

While the debate continues, there seems to be no clear indication of the superiority of one alignment technique over the other, but a recent meta-analysis of five randomized controlled trials comparing kinematic alignment with mechanical alignment TKAs found that kinematic alignment had better reported outcomes and lower revision rates than mechanical alignment TKAs.[68]

Tibial Slope

Increased tibial slope has been thought to aid cruciate-retaining TKA kinematics by reducing the tendency of the MFC to roll forward. Authors of a 2017 study analyzed 18 patients who underwent cruciate retaining TKA and had tibial slopes more than or less than 3°. The group that had less than 3° of posterior slope showed roll-forward motions from 20° to 90° flexion, whereas the group with tibial slope of more than 3° all showed a posterior rollback motion with flexion to 90°.[69]

A 2018 study analyzed the effects of a greater amount of tibial slope. The authors of this study analyzed 71 cruciate-retaining TKRs in 52 patients who had less than 7° of posterior tibial slope compared to those who had 8° or greater. No difference in transverse plane rotations between the two groups and no significant difference in anterior-posterior translations were reported. Greater flexion in the higher tibial slope group was found. This more conforming type of cruciate-retaining implant used in this study, however, may have negated the effects of the increased tibial slope that typically most surgeons do not advocate for the amount used in this study.[70]

It seems, in general, that increasing the tibial slope may decrease the variation of anterior-posterior translations in a cruciate-retaining TKA, but with an increased posterior slope, the integrity of the bony insertion of the PCL may be jeopardized and be detrimental to overall stability of the cruciate-retaining TKA. The individual implant attributes being used should be taken into consideration to determine the optimal surgical technique.

SUMMARY

Surgeons should understand how their surgical technique and implant design choices will affect their short-term and long-term choices when performing a primary TKA. In many instances, there still remains no clear evidence of kinematic and clinical superiority when comparing long-term results in the literature. There seems to be evidence now that higher constraint may lead to a lower long-term survivorship, but bicruciate retaining implant designs may be the exception.

KEY STUDY POINTS

- An understanding of normal knee kinematics and individual patient characteristics is necessary to demand match the appropriate implant design for each patient.
- TKA implant designs have evolved over the past 2 decades to include a number of modifications intended to improve knee kinematics after surgery; however, not all have been successful in improving functional outcomes.
- Several reports in the literature show no difference in functional outcomes between posterior-stabilizing and cruciate-retaining implants.
- Whether mobile-bearing designs will outperform fixed-bearing designs is yet to be determined, but studies have found a higher revision rate in both the early and midterm follow-up periods with a mobile-bearing insert compared with a fixed-bearing TKA.
- In addition to restoration of joint kinematics, outcomes can be affected by surgical technique, about which debate continues (eg, mechanical or kinematic alignment, gap balancing, or matched resection), as well as patient-related factors (eg, age, body mass index, preexisting deformity, individual anatomy).

ANNOTATED REFERENCES

1. Nakamura S, Sharma A, Kobayashi M, et al: 3D in vivo femoro-tibial kinematics of tri-condylar total knee arthroplasty during kneeling activities. *Knee* 2014;21(1):162-167.
2. Zingde SM, Leszko F, Sharma A, Mahfouz MR, Komistek RD, Dennis DA: In vivo determination of cam-post engagement in fixed and mobile-bearing TKA. *Clin Orthop Relat Res* 2014;472(1):254-262.
3. Meccia B, Komistek RD, Mahfouz M, Dennis D: Abnormal axial rotations in TKA contribute to reduced weightbearing flexion. *Clin Orthop Relat Res* 2014;472(1):248-253.
4. Victor J, Mueller JK, Komistek RD, Sharma A, Nadaud MC, Bellemans J: In vivo kinematics after a cruciate-substituting TKA. *Clin Orthop Relat Res* 2010;468(3):807-814.
5. Yamazaki T, Futai K, Tomita T, et al: 3D kinematics of mobile-bearing total knee arthroplasty using X-ray fluoroscopy. *Int J Comput Assist Radiol Surg* 2015;10(4):487-495.
6. Lin KJ, Huang CH, Liu YL, et al: Influence of post-cam design of posterior stabilized knee prosthesis on tibiofemoral motion during high knee flexion. *Clin Biomech (Bristol, Avon)* 2011;26(8):847-852.
7. Suzuki K, Hara N, Mikami S, et al: In vivo kinematic analysis of posterior-stabilized total knee arthroplasty for the valgus knee operated by the gap-balancing technique. *Knee* 2014;21(6):1124-1128.
8. Onodera T, Majima T, Nishiike O, Kasahara Y, Takahashi D: Posterior femoral condylar offset after total knee replacement in the risk of knee flexion contracture. *J Arthroplasty* 2013;28(7):1112-1116.
9. Hanratty BM, Thompson NW, Wilson RK, Beverland DE: The influence of posterior condylar offset on knee flexion after total knee replacement using a cruciate-sacrificing mobile-bearing implant. *J Bone Joint Surg Br* 2007;89(7):915-918.
10. Andrawis J, Akhavan S, Chan V, Lehil M, Pong D, Bozic KJ: Higher preoperative patient activation associated with better patient-reported outcomes after total joint arthroplasty. *Clin Orthop Relat Res* 2015;473(8):2688-2697.
11. Harman MK, Banks SA, Kirschner S, Lützner J: Prosthesis alignment affects axial rotation motion after total knee replacement: A prospective in vivo study combining computed tomography and fluoroscopic evaluations. *BMC Musculoskelet Disord* 2012;13:206.
12. Thompson JA, Hast MW, Granger JF, Piazza SJ, Siston RA: Biomechanical effects of total knee arthroplasty component malrotation: A computational simulation. *J Orthop Res* 2011;29(7):969-975.
13. Mihalko WM, Conner DJ, Benner R, Williams JL: How does TKA kinematics vary with transverse plane alignment changes in a contemporary implant? *Clin Orthop Relat Res* 2012;470(1):186-192.
14. Huffman KD, Sanford BA, Zucker-Levin AR, Williams JL, Mihalko WM: Increased hip abduction in high body mass index subjects during sit-to-stand. *Gait Posture* 2015;41(2):640-645.
15. Howell SM, Papadopoulos S, Kuznik K, Ghaly LR, Hull ML: Does varus alignment adversely affect implant survival and function six years after kinematically aligned total knee arthroplasty? *Int Orthop* 2015;39(11):2117-2124.
16. Ishikawa M, Kuriyama S, Ito H, Furu M, Nakamura S, Matsuda S: Kinematic alignment produces near-normal knee motion but increases contact stress after total knee arthroplasty: A case study on a single implant design. *Knee* 2015;22(3):206-212.
17. Roth JD, Howell SM, Hull ML: Native knee laxities at 0°, 45°, and 90° of flexion and their relationship to the goal of the gap-balancing alignment method of total knee arthroplasty. *J Bone Joint Surg Am* 2015;97(20):1678-1684.
18. Hommel H, Perka C: Gap-balancing technique combined with patient-specific instrumentation in TKA. *Arch Orthop Trauma Surg* 2015;135(11):1603-1608.

Section 2: Knee

19. Mihalko WM, Krackow KA: Posterior cruciate ligament effects on the flexion space in total knee arthroplasty. *Clin Orthop Relat Res* 1999;360:243-250.

20. DesJardings JD, Walker PS, Haider H, Perry J: The use of a force-controlled dynamic knee simulator to quantify the mechanical performance of total knee replacement designs during functional activity. *J Biomech* 2000;33(10):1231-1241.

21. Sessa P, Fioravanti G, Giannicola G, Cinotti G: The risk of sacrificing the PCL in cruciate retaining total knee arthroplasty and the relationship to the sagittal inclination of the tibial plateau. *Knee* 2015;22(1):51-55.

22. Fukubayashi T, Torzilli PA, Sherman MF, Warren RF: An in vitro biomechanical evaluation of anterior-posterior motion of the knee. Tibial displacement, rotation, and torque. *J Bone Joint Surg Am* 1982;64(2):258-264.

23. Bolanos AA, Colizza WA, McCann PD, et al: A comparison of isokinetic strength testing and gait analysis in patients with posterior cruciate-retaining and substituting knee arthroplasties. *J Arthroplasty* 1998;13(8):906-915.

24. Li G, Zayontz S, Most E, et al: Cruciate-retaining and cruciate-substituting total knee arthroplasty: An in vitro comparison of the kinematics under muscle loads. *J Arthroplasty* 2001;16(8 suppl 1):150-156.

25. Scott DF, Smith RR: A prospective, randomized comparison of posterior stabilized versus cruciate-substituting total knee arthroplasty: A preliminary report with minimum 2-year results. *J Arthroplasty* 2014;29(9 suppl):179-181.

26. Berend KR, Lombardi AV Jr, Adams JB: Which total knee replacement implant should I pick? Correcting the pathology: The role of knee bearing designs. *Bone Joint J* 2013;95-B(11 suppl A):129-132.

27. Lozano-Calderón SA, Shen J, Doumato DF, Greene DA, Zelicof SB: Cruciate-retaining vs posterior-substituting inserts in total knee arthroplasty: Functional outcome comparison. *J Arthroplasty* 2013;28(2):234-242.e1.

28. Joglekar S, Gioe TJ, Yoon P, Schwartz MH: Gait analysis comparison of cruciate retaining and substituting TKA following PCL sacrifice. *Knee* 2012;19(4):279-285.

29. Mayne A, Harshavardhan HP, Johnston LR, Wang W, Jariwala A: Cruciate retaining compared with Posterior Stabilised Nexgen total knee arthroplasty: Results at 10 years in a matched cohort. *Ann R Coll Surg Engl* 2017;99(8):602-606.

    In a matched-pair study comparing 107 Zimmer NexGen®-retaining knees with 107 NexGen posterior-stabilized knees matched for age, sex, BMI, and Knee Society score, no significant differences were found in functional score, range of motion, or patient satisfaction at 10-year follow-up. Level of evidence: III.

30. Vertullo CJ, Lewis PL, Lorimer M, Graves SE: The effect on long-term survivorship of surgeon preference for posterior-stabilized or minimally stabilized total knee replacement: An analysis of 63,416 prostheses from the Australian Orthopaedic Association National Joint Replacement Registry. *J Bone Joint Surg Am* 2017;99(13):1129-1139.

    Observational analysis from the Australian registry from 1999 to 2014 looking at revision rates of surgeons using posterior-stabilized or minimally stabilized implants found that surgeons who preferred posterior-stabilized implants had a higher revision rate irrespective of patient age. Level of evidence: IV.

31. Sando T, McCalden RW, Bourne RB, MacDonald SJ, Somerville LE: Ten-year results comparing posterior cruciate-retaining versus posterior cruciate-substituting total knee arthroplasty. *J Arthroplasty* 2015;30(2):210-215.

32. Mihalko WM, Lowell J, Higgs G, Kurtz S: Total knee post cam design variations and their effects on kinematics and wear patterns. *Orthopedics* 2016;39(3 suppl):S45-S49.

33. Indelli PF, Aglietti P, Buzzi R, Baldini A: The Insall-Burstein II prosthesis: A 5- to 9-year follow-up study in osteoarthritic knees. *J Arthroplasty* 2002;17(5):544-549.

34. Broberg JS, Ndoja S, MacDonald SJ, Lanting BA, Teeter MG: Comparison of contact kinematics in posterior-stabilized and cruciate-retaining total knee arthroplasty at long-term follow-up. *J Arthroplasty* 2020;35(1):272-277.

    Representational similarity analysis (RSA) of 21 cruciate-retaining and 21 posterior-stabilized TKAs was undertaken with evaluation at different flexion angles. Posterior-stabilized TKAs had larger posterior rollback on the lateral compartment and were found to have superior kinematics compared with cruciate-retaining TKAs that demonstrated PCL insufficiency. Level of evidence: III.

35. Angerame MR, Holst DC, Jennings JM, Komistek RD, Dennis DA: Total knee arthroplasty kinematics. *J Arthroplasty* 2019;34(10):2502-2510.

    This meta-analysis of fluorokinematic studies in the literature compiles the differences in kinematics recorded during gait and a lunge for normal knees and different implant designs.

36. Grieco TF, Sharma A, Komistek RD, Cates HE: Single versus multiple-radii cruciate-retaining total knee arthroplasty: An in vivo mobile fluoroscopy study. *J Arthroplasty* 2016;31(3):694-701.

37. Grieco TF, Sharma A, Dessinger GM, Cates HE, Komistek RD: In vivo kinematic comparison of a bicruciate stabilized total knee arthroplasty and the normal knee using fluoroscopy. *J Arthroplasty* 2018;33(2):565-571.

    This study analyzed 10 normal knees and 40 bicruciate-substituting TKAs using a mobile fluoroscopic analysis platform. Anterior translation was similar in the first 30 degrees of flexion, indicating that the anterior post-cam interaction supported native kinematic profiles in the replaced TKAs. Level of evidence: II.

38. Alnachoukati OK, Emerson RH, Diaz E, Ruchaud E, Ennin KA: Modern day bicruciate-retaining total knee arthroplasty: A short-term review of 146 knees. *J Arthroplasty* 2018;33(8):2485-2490.

    In this report of 146 bicruciate-retaining TKAs at 12-month follow-up, 91% of patients reported that their knee felt normal, with two revisions, one revision surgery, and one manipulation at 12 months. Level of evidence: III.

39. Scarvell JM, Perriman DM, Smith PN, Campbell DG, Bruce WJM, Nivbrant B: Total knee arthroplasty using bicruciate-stabilized or posterior-stabilized knee implants provided comparable outcomes at 2 years: A prospective, multicenter, randomized, controlled, clinical trial of patient outcomes. *J Arthroplasty* 2017;32(11):3356-3363.e1.

    This prospective randomized study evaluated 228 patients who were randomized to a bicruciate-stabilized (97 patients) or posterior-stabilized (98 patients) TKA. At 2 years, no difference in range of motion or Oxford Knee Scores existed between the two groups. Level of evidence: I.

40. Christensen JC, Brothers J, Stoddard GJ, et al: Higher frequency of reoperation with a new bicruciate-retaining total knee arthroplasty. *Clin Orthop Relat Res* 2017;475(1):62-69.

    Comparison of 78 bicruciate-retaining TKAs and 294 cruciate-retaining TKAs found that the BCR group had a higher frequency of revisions (5% versus 1.3%, P = 0.028) and a significantly lower short-term survivorship. Level of evidence: II.

41. Fransen B, Hoozemans MJ, Keijser LC, van Lent ME, Verheyen CC, Burger BJ: Does insert type affect clinical and functional outcome in total knee arthroplasty? A randomised controlled clinical trial with 5-year follow-up. *J Arthroplasty* 2015;30(11):1931-1937.

42. Namba R, Graves S, Robertsson O, et al: International comparative evaluation of knee replacement with fixed or mobile non-posterior-stabilized implants. *J Bone Joint Surg Am* 2014;96(suppl 1):52-58.

43. Hofstede SN, Nouta KA, Jacobs W, et al.Mobile bearing vs fixed bearing prostheses for posterior cruciate retaining total knee arthroplasty for postoperative functional status in patients with osteoarthritis and rheumatoid arthritis. *Cochrane Database Syst Rev* 2015;2:CD003130.

44. Murakami K, Hamai S, Okazaki K, et al: Kinematic analysis of stair climbing in rotating platform cruciate-retaining and posterior-stabilized mobile-bearing total knee arthroplasties. *Arch Orthop Trauma Surg* 2017;137(5):701-711.

    Analysis of 10 cruciate-retaining and 10 posterior-stabilized PFC Sigma rotating platform TKAs with lateral radiographic kinematic analysis found no difference in stair climbing between the two groups. Level of evidence: IV.

45. Katchky AM, Jones CW, Walter WL, Shimmin AJ: Medial ball and socket total knee arthroplasty: Five-year clinical results. *Bone Joint J* 2019;101-B(1 suppl A):59-65.

    Ninety-two patients with 100 medial constrained pivot TKAs were followed. A 5-year follow-up was reported for 81 knees, showing good range of motion, with two revision surgeries for lateral releases and a manipulation under anesthesia and seven major complications. Level of evidence: IV.

46. Nishitani K, Furu M, Nakamura S, et al: No differences in patient-reported outcomes between medial pivot insert and symmetrical insert in total knee arthroplasty: A randomized analysis. *Knee* 2018;25(6):1254-1261.

    Seventy patients were randomized into receiving a deep dish or a medial pivot insert. At 2 years, no differences in ROM or Knee Society Scores were reported. Level of evidence: I.

47. Benjamin B, Pietrzak JRT, Tahmassebi J, Haddad FS: A functional comparison of medial pivot and condylar knee designs based on patient outcomes and parameters of gait. *Bone Joint J* 2018;100-B(1 suppl A):76-82.

    This subset of patients from a larger study included 10 TKA with a single radius design and 10 TKA with a medial pivot design TKA. No differences in gait parameters, Knee Society Scores, or Oxford Knee Scores were found between the two groups up to 2 years after surgery. Level of evidence: III.

48. Karachalios T, Varitimidis S, Bargiotas K, Hantes M, Roidis N, Malizos KN: An 11- to 15-year clinical outcome study of the Advance Medial Pivot total knee arthroplasty: Pivot knee arthroplasty. *Bone Joint J* 2016;98-B(8):1050-1055.

49. Komistek RD, Dennis DA, Mahfouz MR: In vivo fluoroscopic analysis of the normal human knee. *Clin Orthop Relat Res* 2003;410:69-81.

50. Ploegmakers MJ, Ginsel B, Meijerink HJ, et al: Physical examination and in vivo kinematics in two posterior cruciate ligament retaining total knee arthroplasty designs. *Knee* 2010;17(3):204-209.

51. Sanford BA, Williams JL, Huffman KD, Zucker-Levin AR, Mihalko WM: Tibiofemoral rotation during sit-to-stand activity after TKA. *Orthopedics* 2016;39(3 suppl):S41-S44.

52. Baumann F, Bahadin €O, Krutsch W, et al: Proprioception after bicruciate-retaining total knee arthroplasty is comparable to unicompartmental knee arthroplasty. *Knee Surg Sports Traumatol Arthrosc* 2016;25:1697-1704.

53. Zhang K, Mihalko WM: Posterior cruciate mechanoreceptors in osteoarthritic and cruciate-retaining TKA retrievals: A pilot study. *Clin Orthop Relat Res* 2012;470(7):1855-1859.

54. Pritchett JW: Bicruciate-retaining total knee replacement provides satisfactory function and implant survivorship at 23 years. *Clin Orthop Relat Res* 2015;473(7):2327-2333.

55. Osmani FA, Thakkar SC, Collins K, Schwarzkopf R: The utility of bicruciate retaining total knee arthroplasty. *Arthroplast Today* 2017;3:61-66.

    This systematic review of four papers in the literature of bicruciate-retaining TKAs reported that all promoted more normal kinematics and proprioception, but, overall, no clear advantage in clinical outcomes was shown. Level of evidence: III.

56. Mochizuki T, Tanifuji O, Sato T, et al: Association between anteroposterior laxity in mid-range flexion and subjective healing of instability after total knee arthroplasty. *Knee Surg Sports Traumatol Arthrosc* 2016;25:3543-3548.

57. Schmidt R, Komistek RD, Blaha JD, Penenberg BL, Maloney WJ: Fluoroscopic analyses of cruciate-retaining and medial pivot knee implants. *Clin Orthop Relat Res* 2003;410:139-147.

58. Shimmin A, Martinez-Martos S, Owens J, Iorgulescu AD, Banks S: Fluoroscopic motion study confirming the stability of a medial pivot design total knee arthroplasty. *Knee* 2015;22:522-526.

59. Wautier D, Thienpont E: Changes in anteroposterior stability and proprioception after different types of knee arthroplasty. *Knee Surg Sports Traumatol Arthrosc* 2016;25:1792-1800.

60. Steinbrück A, Schröder C, Woiczinski M, et al: Femorotibial kinematics and load patterns after total knee arthroplasty: An in vitro comparison of posterior-stabilized versus medial-stabilized design. *Clin Biomech* 2016;33:42-48.

61. Moonot P, Shang M, Railton GT, Field RE, Banks SA: In vivo weight-bearing kinematics with medial rotation knee arthroplasty. *Knee* 2010;17:33-37.

62. Moonot P, Mu S, Railton GT, Field RE, Banks SA: Tibiofemoral kinematic analysis of knee flexion for a medial pivot knee. *Knee Surg Sports Traumatol Arthrosc* 2009;17:927-934.

63. Cho SH, Cho HL, Lee SH, Jin HK: Posterior femoral translation in medial pivot total knee arthroplasty of posterior cruciate ligament retaining type. *J Orthop* 2013;10:74-78.

64. Ritter MA, Davis KE, Meding JB, Pierson JL, Berend ME, Malinzak RA: The effect of alignment and BMI on failure of total knee replacement. *J Bone Joint Surg Am* 2011;93(17):1588-1596.

65. Blakeney W, Clément J, Desmeules F, Hagemeister N, Rivière C, Vendittoli PA: Kinematic alignment in total knee arthroplasty better reproduces normal gait than mechanical alignment. *Knee Surg Sports Traumatol Arthrosc* 2019;27(5):1410-1417.

This was a retrospective review of 18 kinematically aligned and 18 mechanically aligned TKA replacements in patients who underwent a gait and radiographic analysis for comparison with a group of healthy matched controls. The kinematically aligned group showed no differences in ROM or varus/valgus internal/external rotation curves through an arc of motion compared with the healthy control group, and KOOS scores were higher in the kinematically aligned group as well. Level of evidence: IV.

66. Yeo JH, Seon JK, Lee DH, Song EK: No difference in outcomes and gait analysis between mechanical and kinematic knee alignment methods using robotic total knee arthroplasty. *Knee Surg Sports Traumatol Arthrosc* 2019;27(4):1142-1147.

This prospective study randomized 60 patients into a robotically performed TKA using either kinematic or mechanical alignment. Each group was analyzed by 3D gait analysis for comparison at 8-year follow-up. No difference in HSS, WOMAC, or Knee Society pain scores resulted between the two groups. For gait analysis, results on the varus angle and mediolateral ground reaction forces were different. Level of evidence: II.

67. Li Y, Wang S, Wang Y, Yang M: Does kinematic alignment improve short-term functional outcomes after total knee arthroplasty compared with mechanical alignment? A systematic review and meta-analysis. *J Knee Surg* 2018;31(1):78-86.

This meta-analysis was performed to determine if kinematically aligned TKA improved short-term outcomes compared with mechanically aligned TKA and included six published trials with 561 patients combined. The kinematically aligned group walked a longer distance before discharge, and no differences in hip, knee, or ankle angles were found. Better short-term outcomes and flexion arcs were found in the kinematically aligned group. Level of evidence: II.

68. Takahashi T, Ansari J, Pandit HG: Kinematically aligned total knee arthroplasty or mechanically aligned total knee arthroplasty. *J Knee Surg* 2018;31(10):999-1006.

This systematic review was performed to determine if there were any clinical differences between kinematically and mechanically aligned TKAs. Five RCTs were included. WOMAC, Oxford, and Knee Society Scores and postoperative ROM were all improved in the kinematically aligned group. Level of evidence: I.

69. Pan XQ, Peng AQ, Wang F, et al: Effect of tibial slope changes on femorotibial contact kinematics after cruciate-retaining total knee arthroplasty. *Knee Surg Sports Traumatol Arthrosc* 2017;25(11):3549-3555.

Eighteen TKAs in nine patients were reviewed for tibial slope change on preoperative to postoperative radiographs at 2-year follow-up. Those with less than 3 degrees of change were found to have paradoxical anterior translation of the medial femoral condyle. Level of evidence: III.

70. Fujito T, Tomita T, Yamazaki T, Oda K, Yoshikawa H, Sugamoto K: Influence of posterior tibial slope on kinematics after cruciate-retaining total knee arthroplasty. *J Arthroplasty* 2018;33(12):3778-3782.e1.

Seventy-one TKAs with a high conforming medial implant design were analyzed in 52 patients according to either having less than 7 degrees of posterior tibial slope or more than 8 degrees posterior slope. In vivo kinematics were used to analyze the patients during a deep knee bend. The higher slope group had better flexion and ROM, but no other parameters were found to be different. Level of evidence: IV.

CHAPTER 20

Implant Designs of Total Knee Arthroplasty

KARTIK MANGUDI VARADARAJAN, PhD • DANIEL HOLTZMAN, MD
GUOAN LI, PhD • JEFFREY K. LANGE, MD • BRIAN P. CHALMERS, MD
STEVEN B. HAAS, MD • HARRY E. RUBASH, MD, FAOA • ANDREW A. FREIBERG, MD

ABSTRACT

The continued development of implant geometries and materials used in total knee arthroplasty (TKA) is motivated by the recognition of patient dissatisfaction, increased use in young and active patients, and concerns regarding metal hypersensitivity. One of the overarching goals is to restore native patient anatomy and knee kinematics in hopes of improving patient satisfaction. Single-radius and multiradius femoral designs appear to be associated with equivalent clinical outcomes. Anatomic tibial trays can reduce the likelihood of internal rotation if tibial coverage is maximized to guide placement. Recent meta-analyses and registry studies suggest equivalent outcomes for all-polyethylene and metal-backed tibial components. Anatomic or biomimetic articular surfaces together with anterior cruciate ligament retention or substitution may be key to restoring normal kinematics following TKA. Restoration of the native joint line through surgical technique or the use of asymmetric polyethylene thickness may also play an important role in improving function following TKA. Several materials have shown promise as alternatives to cobalt-chromium-molybdenum alloys. Bulk ceramics and oxidized zirconia have shown particularly excellent midterm to long-term outcomes and may be viable options for patients with suspected metal hypersensitivity.

Dr. Varadarajan or an immediate family member has received royalties from Stryker; has stock or stock options held in Orthopaedic Technology Group; has received research or institutional support from Evonik, Heraeus Medical, and Johnson & Johnson; and serves as a board member, owner, officer, or committee member of the Orthopaedic Research Society. Dr. Li or an immediate family member serves as a paid consultant to or is an employee of Mako Medical, Inc. Dr. Haas or an immediate family member has received royalties from Smith & Nephew; is a member of a speakers' bureau or has made paid presentations on behalf of Smith & Nephew; serves as a paid consultant to or is an employee of OrthAlign and Smith & Nephew; has stock or stock options held in OrthoSecure; and has received research or institutional support from Smith & Nephew. Dr. Rubash or an immediate family member has received royalties from Ceramtec and Stryker; serves as a paid consultant to or is an employee of BioDirection, Clozex, Flexion, GLG Consulting, and Stryker; and has stock or stock options held in Orthopaedic Technology Group. Dr. Freiberg or an immediate family member serves as a paid consultant to or is an employee of Biomet and Zimmer and has stock or stock options held in ArthroSurface, Orthopaedic Technology Group, and Zimmer. None of the following authors or any immediate family member has received anything of value from or has stock or stock options held in a commercial company or institution related directly or indirectly to the subject of this chapter: Dr. Holtzman, Dr. Lange, and Dr. Chalmers.

Keywords: ACL function; all-polyethylene tibial component; anatomic articular surface; anatomic joint line; anterior cruciate ligament; ceramics

INTRODUCTION

There continue to be 20 to 30% of patients not fully satisfied after primary total knee arthroplasty (TKA). Further, the incidence of TKA is growing in patients <65 years with higher activity and longevity expectations. However, TKA implant designs continue to evolve. New implant technologies, together with improvements in technique and instrumentation, can hopefully result in a more normal-feeling knee postoperatively, with longevity extending to the second and third decade. It is important for the orthopaedic surgeon to be aware of the considerations and developments related to implant geometry and implant materials, with a focus on new technologies that are being explored.

IMPLANT GEOMETRY

The implant geometry directly influences joint biomechanics, including function of the native soft tissues, tibiofemoral kinematics, and patellar tracking. Previously, sex-specific implants were proposed to better fit male or female knee anatomy. Subsequent research has not supported the need for sex-specific designs, but instead has shown a need for size-specific aspect ratios and/or provisions for sufficient implant sizes. Similarly, although high-flexion designs reduce tibiofemoral contact stresses in deep flexion, they do not provide increased range of motion (ROM). In addition, these newer designs do not treat the underlying kinematic limitations of contemporary implants, which have been associated with functional limitations and patient dissatisfaction.[1-7] One study reported that patients who underwent TKA have greater difficulty performing activities such as kneeling, carrying loads, playing tennis, dancing, and gardening compared with their age-matched peers; only 40% of the functional deficit seemed attributable to the normal effects of aging.[1] Research and development efforts are ongoing to create implant designs that can provide more normal kinematics via modifications of the femoral and tibial articular surfaces, the provision of asymmetric components to reduce rotational malpositioning, and the restoration of anterior cruciate ligament (ACL) and posterior cruciate ligament (PCL) function via retention or substitution.

Femoral Implant

Single-radius Versus Multiradius Designs

Both single-radius and multiradius femoral implant designs are commercially available (**Figure 1**). Multiradius designs use a changing radius of curvature with increased knee flexion that results in a center of rotation that shifts through the ROM. Single-radius designs have a consistent radius of curvature throughout the flexion-extension arc and a more posterior center of rotation. Theoretically this creates more consistent soft-tissue/collateral ligament tension to minimize instability in midflexion and increases quadriceps muscle strength. A 2015 study examined three cohorts of patients (16 patients after single-radius TKA, 16 patients after multiradius TKA, and 16 healthy control patients) in a gait analysis laboratory.[2] Preoperatively, no significant differences in gait cycle parameters existed between patients in the single-radius and multiradius groups. Postoperatively, several significant differences were noted between the patients in the multiradius cohort and control patients in several gait parameters, including increased knee extension and decreased power absorption in the multiradius cohort. No significant differences between the single-radius cohort and control patients were detected. Despite these findings, no functional differences were observed in patient-reported outcome measures.[1-4]

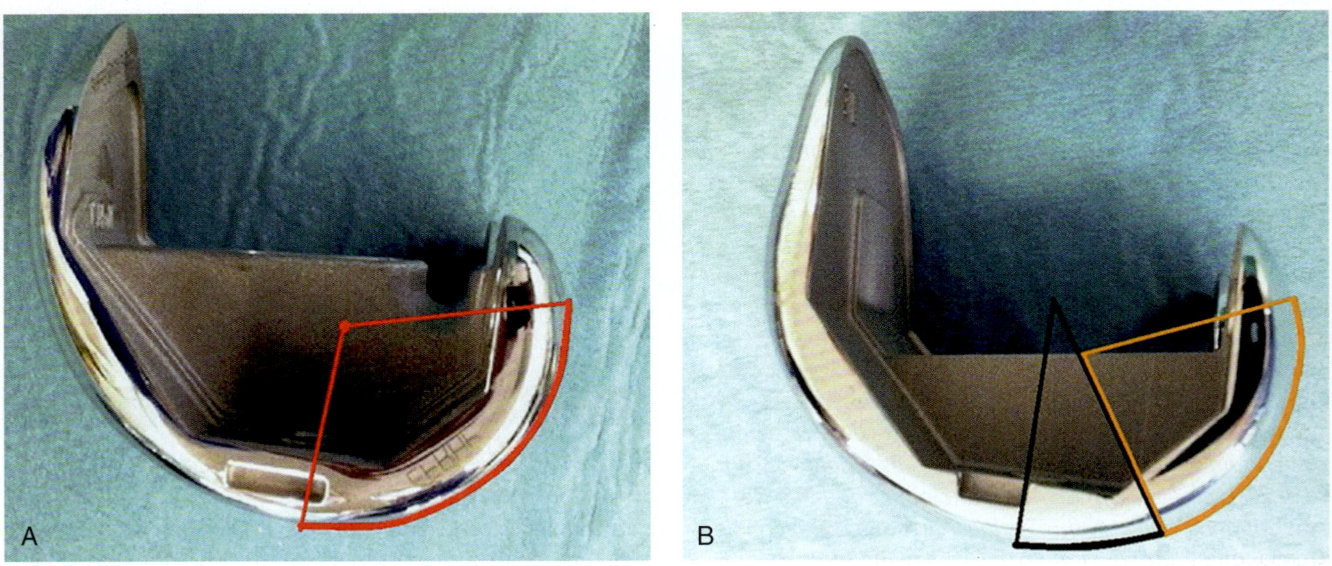

FIGURE 1 Photographs of a single-radius total knee arthroplasty femoral implant (Triathlon®, Stryker) (**A**) with a constant radius over 10° to 110° of flexion (red outline) and a multiradius femoral implant (GENUTECH®, Surgival) (**B**) with one radius from 0° to 45° of flexion (black outline) and a different radius from 45° to 130° of flexion (orange outline). (Reprinted by permission from Springer Nature: *Knee Surg Sports Traumatol Arthrosc*. Hinarejos P, Puig-Verdie L, Leal J, et al: No differences in functional results and quality of life after single-radius or multiradius TKA, 24:2634–2640. Copyright © 2015.)

Similarly, a prospective cohort study with a standardized surgical and rehabilitation protocol reported on 250 patients who underwent single-radius TKA and 224 patients who underwent multiradius TKA with 5-year follow-up.[3] No significant differences existed between the single-radius and multiradius groups at 1 and 5 years following surgery in Knee Society Scores, Medical Outcomes Study 36-Item Short Form physical scores, postoperative ROM, or patient satisfaction. In addition, a recent meta-analysis of 15 studies compared single-radius and multiradius TKA designs and found no difference in Knee Society Scores, knee flexion, complications, isometric peak torque of the knee, or implant survival rates.[4] Thus, the theoretical advantages of a single-radius design are not supported by available clinical data. This finding may be because the actual geometric difference between single-radius and multiradius femoral designs for most of the active flexion range (10° to 110°) is small. Implant systems with single-radius versus multiradius designs also vary substantially in the geometry of other components, such as the tibial articular geometry. Therefore, it may be difficult to ascertain the effects of femoral design alone from clinical data.

Restoration of the Anatomic Joint Line

Historically, the two primary approaches to coronal plane positioning of the joint line were anatomic and functional alignment. Anatomic alignment, along with its modern iteration termed kinematic alignment, aims to restore the natural joint line orientation to promote natural knee mechanics. Functional alignment, also termed mechanical alignment, is the prevailing convention and aims to create a joint line perpendicular to the overall mechanical axis of the lower limb. This approach is thought to load each compartment equally, avoiding an overload of the tibial component medially.[5]

Although mechanical alignment has produced excellent results in millions of patients, natural knee kinematics are not maintained when this method is used. This is, in part, because although the implants generally have equal medial and lateral femoral condylar thicknesses, the corresponding bone cuts have asymmetric thicknesses. For example, in a typical varus knee, approximately 9 mm of bone is removed from the distal medial femoral condyle, which equals the implant thickness, and approximately 7 mm of bone is removed from the distal lateral femoral condyle, which is less than the thickness of the implant. In this situation, the medial joint line will remain anatomic, but the lateral joint line will be displaced distally by approximately 2 mm with standard femoral implants (**Figure 2**). Joint line depression is not ideal, because it is linked to patellofemoral pain, subluxation, and diminished functional gains at deviations as small as 3 mm of depression.[6] Alternatively, if distal femoral resection increases by 2 mm, the lateral joint line will remain anatomic and the medial joint line will be elevated. Joint line elevation also is not ideal, because it is linked to patellar impingement on the tibial component, midflexion instability, and patellofemoral pain at deviations as small as 5 mm of elevation.[6] Furthermore, because mechanical alignment does not re-create natural knee kinematics, collateral ligament tension and strain are significantly altered during knee ROM.[7]

One approach to restoration of the anatomic joint line is to use standard nonanatomic implants positioned parallel to the native joint line. However, placing nonanatomic implants in an anatomic coronal position can be problematic. Placing the tibial component in varus has been associated with high failure rates in many studies.[8] In addition, placing the tibial component in varus necessitates internal rotation of the femoral implant to create a symmetric flexion gap, which elevates the lateral anterior femoral flange and rotates the trochlear groove medially. Furthermore, by placing the femoral implant in relative valgus, the proximal trochlear groove is shifted medially, which potentially predisposes the patella to tilt and maltracking.[9] Despite these issues, proponents of kinematic alignment report reasonable midterm results.[10] Long-term studies are necessary to clarify the role of this method in TKA.

Instead of placing components in anatomic position, another option is to restore the anatomic joint line using the implant design. This restoration is achieved in some designs by using the concept of anatomic contour matching to match the thickness of the bone removed to the thickness of the bone replaced. To restore an anatomic varus joint line orientation of 3°, the lateral side of the tibial insert is thicker than the medial side. Concomitantly, the distal medial side of the femoral implant is thicker than the distal lateral side. Using asymmetric implant thicknesses allows these designs to more closely match the normal anatomy of the typical femur and tibia while using standard mechanical alignment bone cuts (**Figure 3**). Thus, an anatomic joint line can be achieved while maintaining a tibial cut perpendicular to the tibial mechanical axis, thereby minimizing shear forces and the potential for mechanical failure at the tibial interface. Restoration of the anatomic joint line in conjunction with other design features, such as anatomic tibial articular geometry and bicruciate substitution, may contribute to the reproduction of near-normal knee kinematics.

Tibial Tray

Symmetric/Asymmetric Versus Anatomic Design

Tibial tray design has the potential to influence tibial coverage and rotational alignment. In practice, coverage and rotation may be conflicting, prompting reduction of the tibial component size and coverage to optimize

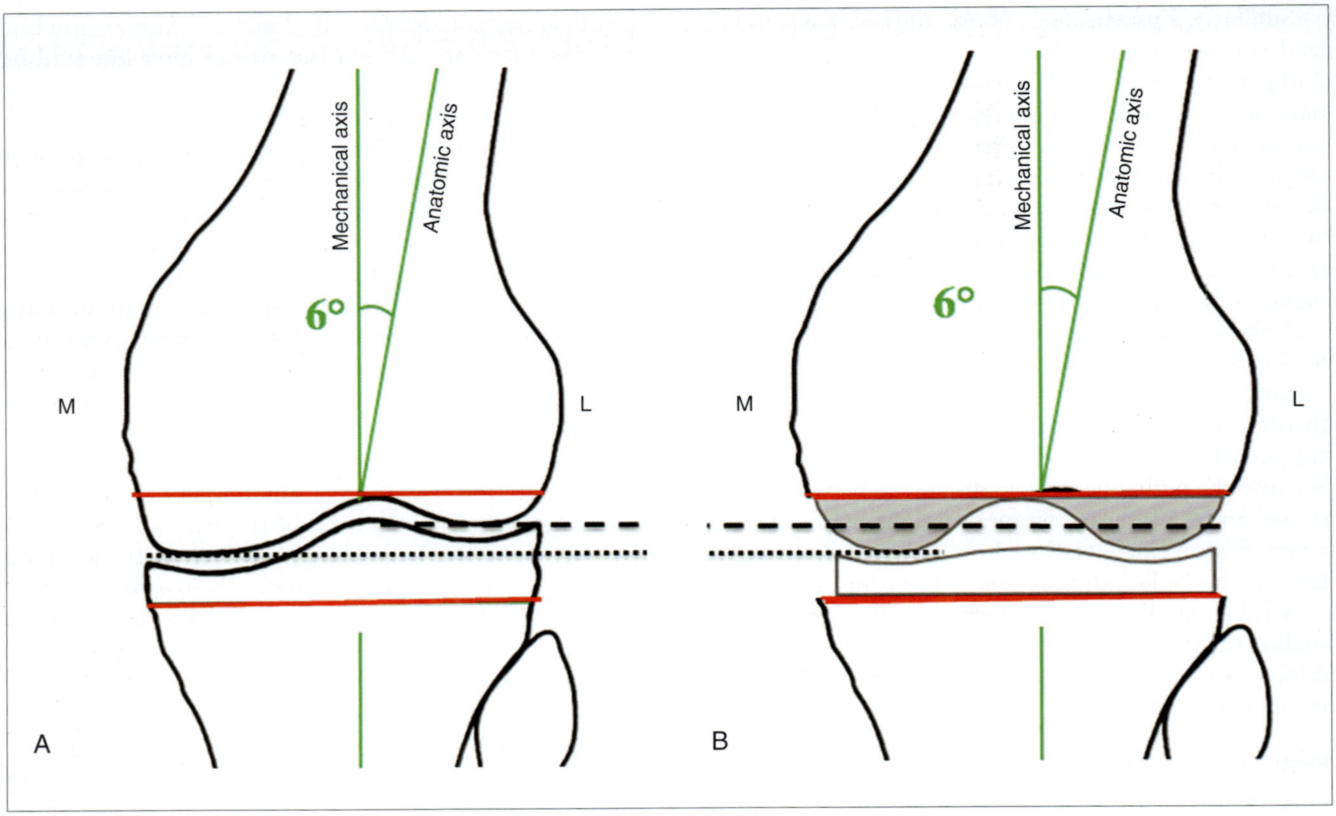

FIGURE 2 Illustrations of the distal femur and proximal tibia in the coronal plane demonstrate symmetric distal femoral condylar resurfacing, which causes depression of the lateral joint line. **A**, The area of planned resection for a standard total knee arthroplasty (TKA) is between the two red lines. **B**, The area of planned resection noted in (**A**) has been replaced by a schematic of a TKA (shaded area). Note the medial joint line remains in its anatomic location, and the lateral joint line is translated distal to its anatomic location. Lines parallel to the cut proximal tibial surface clarify the relationship between the native and resurfaced joint line positions medially (dotted line) and laterally (dashed line). L = lateral, M = medial.

rotational alignment. Increased recognition of population and ethnic differences in proximal tibial morphology has resulted in more tibial tray implant design options. Currently, symmetric, asymmetric, and anatomic designs are commercially available (**Figure 4**). A 2014 study compared proximal tibial morphology obtained from the CT scans of Caucasian cadavers and living Indian, Korean, Chinese, and Japanese subjects with six contemporary TKA designs.[11] Compared with asymmetric and symmetric designs, the anatomic design demonstrated better conformity to tibial size, shape, and tibial coverage (92% versus 85% to 87%, respectively) and a lower incidence of downsizing (3% versus 39% to 60%, respectively) to ensure rotational alignment. An MRI-based study of symmetric, asymmetric, and anatomic tibial trays from a single manufacturer showed significantly higher proximal tibial coverage with the anatomic design (80.8%) compared with the symmetric (76.3%) and asymmetric (75.8%) designs when rotational alignment was constrained to the anterior-posterior axis.[12] In contrast, another 2014 study found similar tibial coverage for symmetric, asymmetric, and anatomic trays aligned to the tibial anterior-posterior axis,[13] as well as similar variations in rotational position when maximizing tibial coverage. However, in that study, symmetric and asymmetric designs were biased toward internal rotation and the anatomic design was biased toward external rotation, which indicates that anatomic designs may provide only a slight advantage regarding tibial coverage. However, anatomic designs may reduce the incidence of internal tibial rotation if maximal tibial coverage is used to guide tray placement.[12,13]

All-polyethylene Versus Modular Tibial Components

All-polyethylene tibial components have been used since the earliest tibial component designs were developed. However, most knee implants currently use modular metal-backed tibial components because of advantages such as intraoperative flexibility, the potential for isolated bearing exchange, and the availability of a press-fit fixation option. Modular metal-backed tibial components also are proposed to diminish stress and strain at the implant-cement interface.

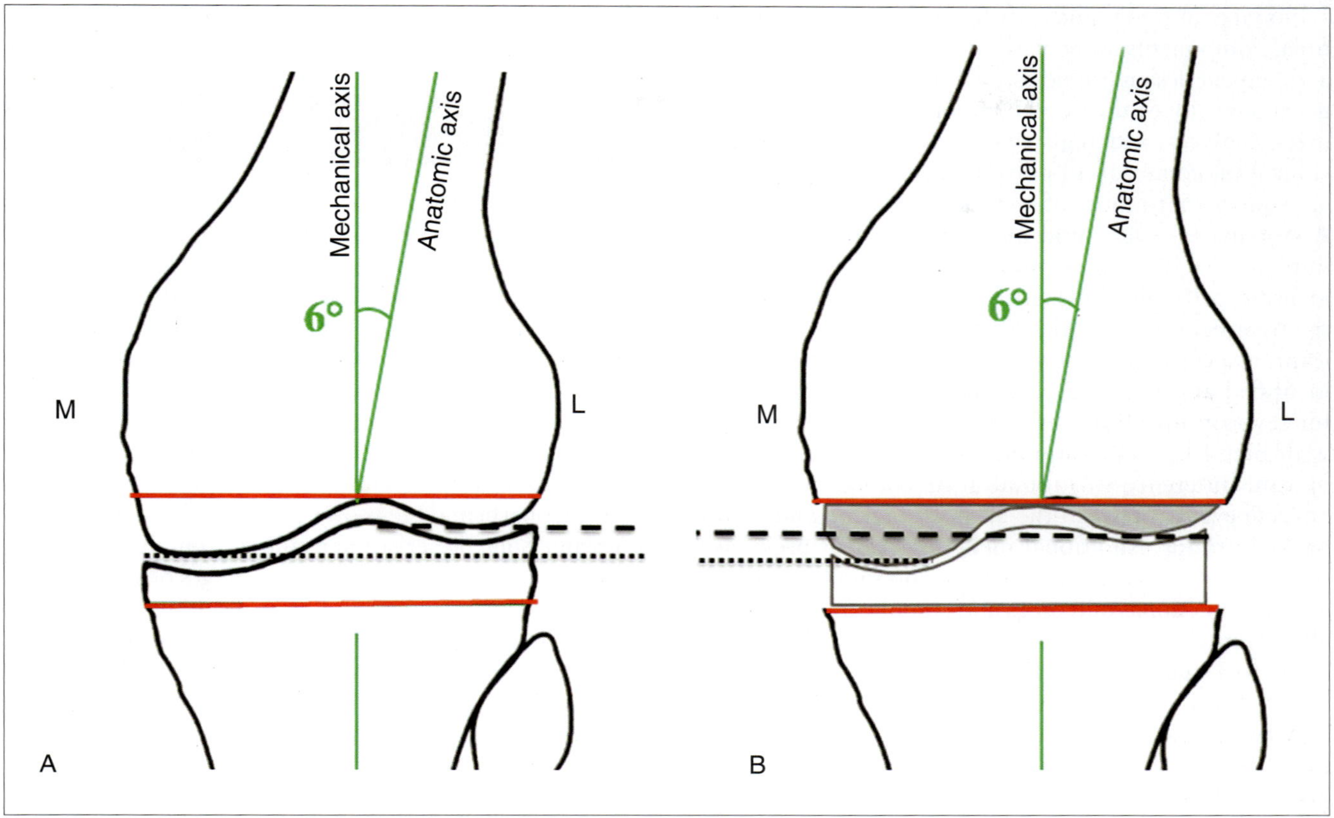

FIGURE 3 Illustrations of the distal femur and proximal tibia in the coronal plane demonstrate asymmetric distal femoral condylar morphology matched using implant design. **A**, The area of planned resection for a standard total knee arthroplasty (TKA) is located between the two red lines. **B**, The area of planned resection as noted in (**A**) has been replaced by a schematic of a TKA with asymmetric distal femoral condylar surfaces (shaded area). Asymmetry of the femoral implant is matched by asymmetry of the tibial component, restoring both the medial and lateral joint lines to their anatomic locations. Lines parallel to the cut proximal tibial surface clarify the relationship between the native and resurfaced joint line positions medially (dotted line) and laterally (dashed line). L = lateral, M = medial.

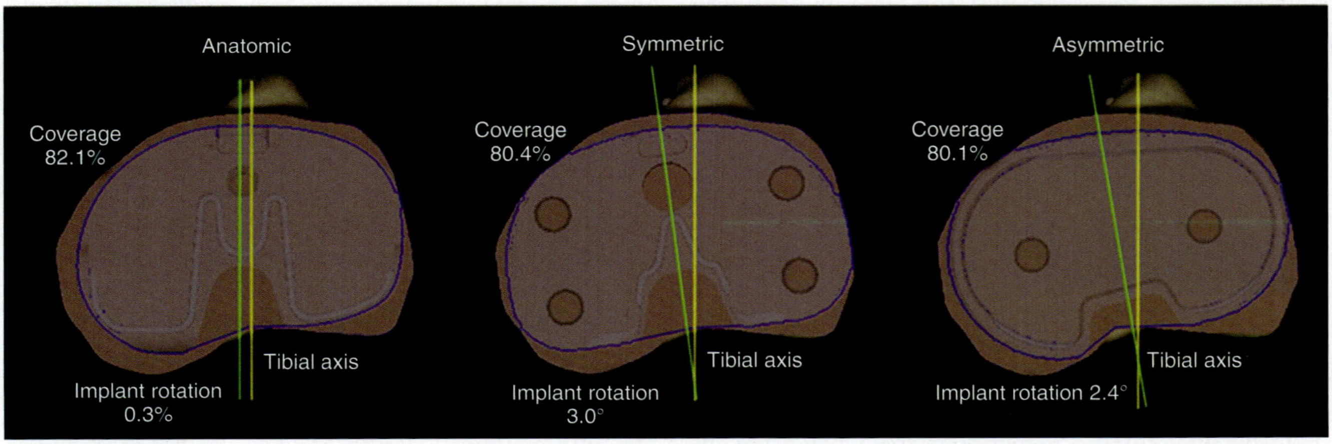

FIGURE 4 Illustration depicts anatomic, symmetric, and asymmetric tibial trays overlaid on a proximal tibial surface. The maximum tibial coverage and resulting rotation for each tray design are also indicated. (Reprinted from *J Arthroplasty* 30[10]. Stulberg SD, Goyal N: Which tibial tray design achieves maximum coverage and ideal rotation: Anatomic, symmetric, or asymmetric? An MRI-based study, 1839-1841. Copyright © 2015, with permission from Elsevier.)

Initial poor results and early failures for all-polyethylene tibial components were attributed to surgical technique and implant design problems, specifically, the lack of articular congruity of the tibial component. However, recent meta-analyses and registry-level studies suggest that clinical outcomes of all-polyethylene tibial components are equivalent to those of metal-backed components.[14,15] A systematic review and meta-analysis of 1,798 TKA implants in 12 studies published from 1990 to 2011 identified all-polyethylene tibial components as one of the treatment arms.[14] Although no findings were significant, respective risk reductions of 29% and 14% were identified at 10 and 15 years after the index procedure for revision for all-polyethylene components compared with metal-backed components. Furthermore, no significant difference was found in functional outcome or adverse events between the all-polyethylene and metal-backed groups. Additional meta-analyses of previously published studies also demonstrated no significant differences in functional outcomes and complications between all-polyethylene and metal-backed tibial components.[15]

A 2013 study published data from a large community-based total joint registry of 27,657 patients who underwent TKA with the same implant (91.7% in the metal-backed group and 8.3% in the all-polyethylene group).[16] The surface geometry of the tibial implant was the same for both the metal-backed and all-polyethylene tibial components. The revision rate was lower for all etiologies in the all-polyethylene group than in the metal-backed group (1.95% versus 2.17%, $P < 0.001$). After adjusting for age and sex, the risk of revision for all etiologies of an all-polyethylene tibial component was 0.51 times higher than the risk of revision for a metal-backed component (95% confidence interval: 0.33 to 0.78). A 2014 study published the comparative revision rates of cruciate-retaining all-polyethylene and metal-backed tibial components performed with the same implant with identical surface geometry in 27,733 patients from the Swedish Knee Arthroplasty Register (median follow-up, 4.5 years; 57.7% metal-backed components, 42.3% all-polyethylene components).[17] Unadjusted 10-year survival was 96.6% for the metal-backed tibial component and 97.2% for the all-polyethylene tibial component ($P = 0.002$). Cox multiple regression analysis demonstrated that all-polyethylene tibial components had a lower risk of revision for any reason, with an adjusted relative risk of 0.75 (95% confidence interval: 0.64 to 0.89), compared with metal-backed tibial components.

In addition, all-polyethylene tibial components may provide the added benefit of reduced costs. One study showed a 20% to 30% reduction in cost when using all-polyethylene components compared with metal-backed components; another study calculated $95,000 in savings on implant costs for every 100 patients who received an all-polyethylene component instead of a metal-backed component.[18,19]

PCL FUNCTION: RETENTION, SUBSTITUTION, OR SACRIFICE

The debate regarding the merits of PCL retention in cruciate-retaining designs versus PCL substitution in posterior-stabilized designs has been long-standing. However, multiple prior studies and a 2018 systematic review did not find any clinically relevant differences in pain, clinical, or radiologic outcomes for cruciate-retaining versus posterior-stabilized designs.[20] In a cruciate-substituting or ultracongruent design, the PCL is sacrificed, with no cam-post mechanism (unlike posterior-stabilized designs) to substitute its function. One potential advantage of ultracongruent designs over posterior-stabilized designs is greater bone preservation resulting from the absence of a femoral box cut. Potential disadvantages of ultracongruent designs include increased wear resulting from greater contact area and reduced ROM because of reduced roll back or greater paradoxical anterior sliding. These designs generally share the same tibial articular geometries as their cruciate-retaining counterparts, except for a higher anterior lip (and often a higher posterior lip), which is designed to minimize anterior femoral sliding in flexion. However, some studies show greater anterior femoral translation in flexion and less intraoperative ROM for ultracongruent designs compared with posterior-stabilized and cruciate-retaining designs,[21-25] indicating that the anterior lip may not fully compensate for the stability provided by the PCL or the post-cam mechanism. Therefore, although there are concerns about anterior-posterior knee stability with ultracongruent designs,[25] no significant differences in clinical outcomes, including ROM, function scores, and radiographic evaluation, have been noted for ultracongruent versus cruciate-retaining or posterior-stabilized designs.[22-24] Similarly, a multicenter study found no difference in 10-year survivorship for ultracongruent, cruciate-retaining, or posterior-stabilized TKA designs.[26] A 2018 prospective randomized controlled trial of 101 patients reported no significant differences in clinical outcome scores, ROM, pain, or radiographic results of posterior-stabilized (n = 56) compared with an anterior-lipped congruent design.[27]

The similar outcomes among ultracongruent, cruciate-retaining, and posterior-stabilized designs may partly be explained by their relatively similar kinematics, compared with their kinematic differences from the preoperative or normal condition. Two separate studies both found paradoxical anterior translation approximately 2 mm greater for ultracongruent designs than for posterior-stabilized and cruciate-retaining designs.[21,22] In contrast, another study measured the intraoperative kinematics of patients receiving ultracongruent implants and reported 8 mm of anterior translation of the medial condyle and 20 mm of anterior translation of the lateral condyle relative to the preoperative condition.[24]

TIBIAL ARTICULAR SURFACE

One important factor responsible for kinematic limitations of contemporary implants is the nonanatomic tibial articular geometry.[28] In the native knee, the medial tibial plateau has a shallow dish profile, and the lateral plateau is convex. This geometry, coupled with the differential stability of the medial versus lateral menisci, results in differential anterior-posterior excursion of the medial and lateral femoral condyles during flexion. However, the ball-in-socket analogy commonly used to describe the medial condyle is only partially true because its motion is not completely restricted. During activities of limited flexion such as walking or stair climbing, the anterior-posterior motion of the medial and lateral condyles can be similar, resulting in lateral or variable pivot patterns.[29,30] Nevertheless, for its full ROM and during high-flexion activities, the knee shows an overall medial pivot with greater roll back of the lateral femoral condyle.[30]

In contrast to asymmetric native tibial anatomy, most contemporary implants (eg, cruciate-retaining and posterior-stabilized implants) have identical medial and lateral articular geometries.[31] A notable exception is the ball-in-socket medial pivot concept that was first introduced in the mid 1990s. Several newer versions of these designs that maintain this original philosophy have been introduced in recent years. In vivo and in vitro studies show that the design objectives of minimizing medial condyle motion and paradoxical anterior sliding are achieved via these ball-in-socket implants.[31,32] However, the extent of medial pivot rotation and lateral condyle roll back are smaller in magnitude compared with normal knees.[31,32] This feature may be a result of the prominent posterior lip or the absence of normal lateral convexity, which limits lateral condyle roll back. Other concerns with the strict ball-in-socket concept are the inability to accommodate normal pivot center variations during low-flexion activities and conflicts with the PCL if used in the cruciate-retaining setting.[29,33,34] The conflict with native PCL may explain why ball-in-socket implants are generally indicated for use with a PCL-sacrificing technique.[31,32] Thus, development continues of advanced articular surfaces that allow restoration of activity-dependent kinematics of the knee.

In 2015, a new biomimetic technique was described to create articular surfaces directly from the in vivo kinematics of healthy knees, which was achieved by moving the femoral implant in virtual space along the in vivo kinematics to carve a compatible biomimetic tibial articular surface.[28] Theoretically, this method accounts for normal anatomy and kinematics, allows hand-in-hand design of femoral and tibial articular surfaces, and incorporates the effect of surgical placement. The resulting biomimetic surface has an anatomic profile, including a shallow medial surface similar to some conventional implants, and a convex lateral plateau with a relatively low anterior and minimal posterior lip. Progressive deviations from the biomimetic geometry resulted in increasingly abnormal kinematics during a simulated knee bend.[28] In another study, a biomimetic cruciate-retaining implant was found to more closely mimic normal kinematic patterns than contemporary cruciate-retaining implants during various simulated activities[35] (**Figure 5**). The biomimetic cruciate-retaining implant particularly showed medial pivot motion during the deep knee bend and chair sit while accommodating pivot center variations during stair ascent. This concept has not been evaluated in vivo.

In contrast, an ACL-/PCL-substituting (bicruciate-substituting) implant with anatomic tibial articular surfaces has been available since 2005, and a cruciate-retaining version of the same design was recently introduced (**Figure 6**). Positive results regarding the restoration of normal kinematic patterns have been reported for the bicruciate-substituting design.[36,37] One study reported profiles of the patellar tendon angle and patellar flexion for the bicruciate-substituting knee to be more normal than other TKA designs.[36] During a deep knee bend activity, another study measured medial and lateral condyle roll back of 14 and 23 mm, respectively, in bicruciate-substituting knees. Average axial rotation patterns were similar but lower in magnitude than in normal knees[37] (**Figure 6**).

ACL FUNCTION

Currently, three strategies are being explored to incorporate ACL function in TKA: native ACL and PCL retention, ACL substitution and native PCL retention, and ACL and PCL substitution.

ACL and PCL Retention

Retention of the ACL and PCL during TKA is a concept that was introduced in the 1970s. However, ACL and PCL retention did not attain widespread acceptance because of perceived difficulties in balancing both the ACL and PCL, concerns regarding the viability of the ACL in the arthritic knee, fracture of the tibial bony eminence, polyethylene wear, and the strength of the tibial baseplate.[38] Many of these challenges were specific to a few designs as well as older generation polyethylene, which was susceptible to oxidative degradation. Avoiding keels in the tibial baseplate that can weaken the tibial bone island, minimizing the removal of cortical bone anterior to the tibial eminence, and avoiding eminence undercutting can

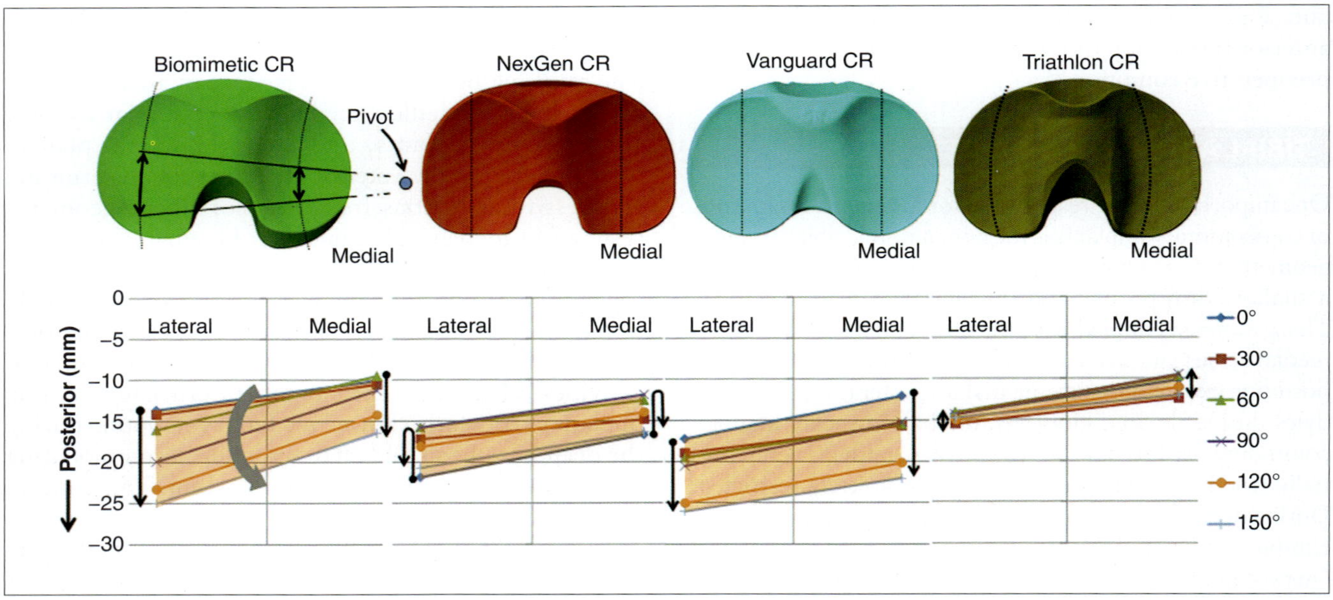

FIGURE 5 Illustration depicts simulated deep knee bend kinematics of a biomimetic cruciate-retaining implant (Biomimetic CR) and three contemporary cruciate-retaining implants (NexGen® CR, Zimmer Biomet; Vanguard® CR, Zimmer Biomet; and Triathlon® CR, Stryker). The biomimetic cruciate-retaining implant exhibited an overall medial pivot with greater lateral roll back compared with medial roll back, and no paradoxical anterior sliding. Contemporary cruciate-retaining implants exhibited no medial pivot, the NexGen cruciate-retaining implant exhibited paradoxical anterior sliding, and the Triathlon cruciate-retaining implant exhibited minimal roll back. (Reprinted from *J Arthroplasty* 30[12]. Varadarajan KMM, Zumbrunn T, Rubash HE, Malchau H, Li G, Muratoglu OK: Cruciate retaining implant with biomimetic articular surface to reproduce activity dependent kinematics of the normal knee, 2149-2153. Copyright © 2015, with permission from Elsevier.)

help reduce the risk of bone island failure.[38-41] Despite the aforementioned challenges, some clinical series have shown excellent long-term outcomes.[38-41] The clinical aspects of ACL retention are beyond the scope of this chapter.

Patients who have bicruciate-retaining implants generally have been reported to exhibit more normal kinematics than patients who have ACL-sacrificing implants.[38-40] However, a 2015 study noted that the analysis of available kinematic data shows that contemporary bicruciate-retaining implants do not fully restore normal kinematics.[38] Furthermore, a 2018 cadaver study showed that the retained ACL in bicruciate-retaining TKAs has different kinematics and in situ force compared with native ACLs during passive flexion-extension movements.[39] Abnormal early posterior femoral shift and subsequent paradoxical anterior sliding, which are observed with ACL-sacrificing implants, are generally not observed with contemporary bicruciate-retaining implants.[38-40] However, as with ACL-sacrificing implants, contemporary bicruciate-retaining implants also show symmetric medial/lateral condylar roll back, and, thus, minimal axial rotation.[38-40] The 2015 study used dynamic computer simulations to compare the kinematics of a biomimetic bicruciate-retaining design with an anatomic tibial articular surface with that of contemporary bicruciate-retaining and cruciate-retaining implants[38] (**Figure 7**). The biomimetic bicruciate-retaining implant exhibited kinematics most similar to healthy knees. Another study compared biomimetic bicruciate-retaining and biomimetic cruciate-retaining implants and reported that the absence of the ACL in the cruciate-retaining design resulted in a more posterior location of the femur and reduced femoral roll back.[28] However, restoration of the native articular geometry in the biomimetic cruciate-retaining implant preserved medial rotation features, which may indicate that restoration of the native anatomy together with ACL preservation is required to achieve kinematics close to those of the native knee.[28]

Early studies of modern bicruciate-retaining designs show mixed results.[41-43] In the largest series of 146 consecutive bicruciate-retaining knees, a 2018 study reported a 6% patient dissatisfaction rate and a >90% rate of patients feeling that they have a normal knee at least some of the time.[41] However, another recent study of 141 consecutive bicruciate-retaining knees showed a higher revision rate than expected, with an 88% revision-free survival at 3 years.[42] The main indications for revision were tibial loosening and ACL impingement.[42] Kinematic studies suggest that native knee rotational kinematics are restored with bicruciate-retaining knee implants.[43] Longer term follow-up and more patients are necessary to continue to follow the clinical outcome of bicruciate-retaining designs.

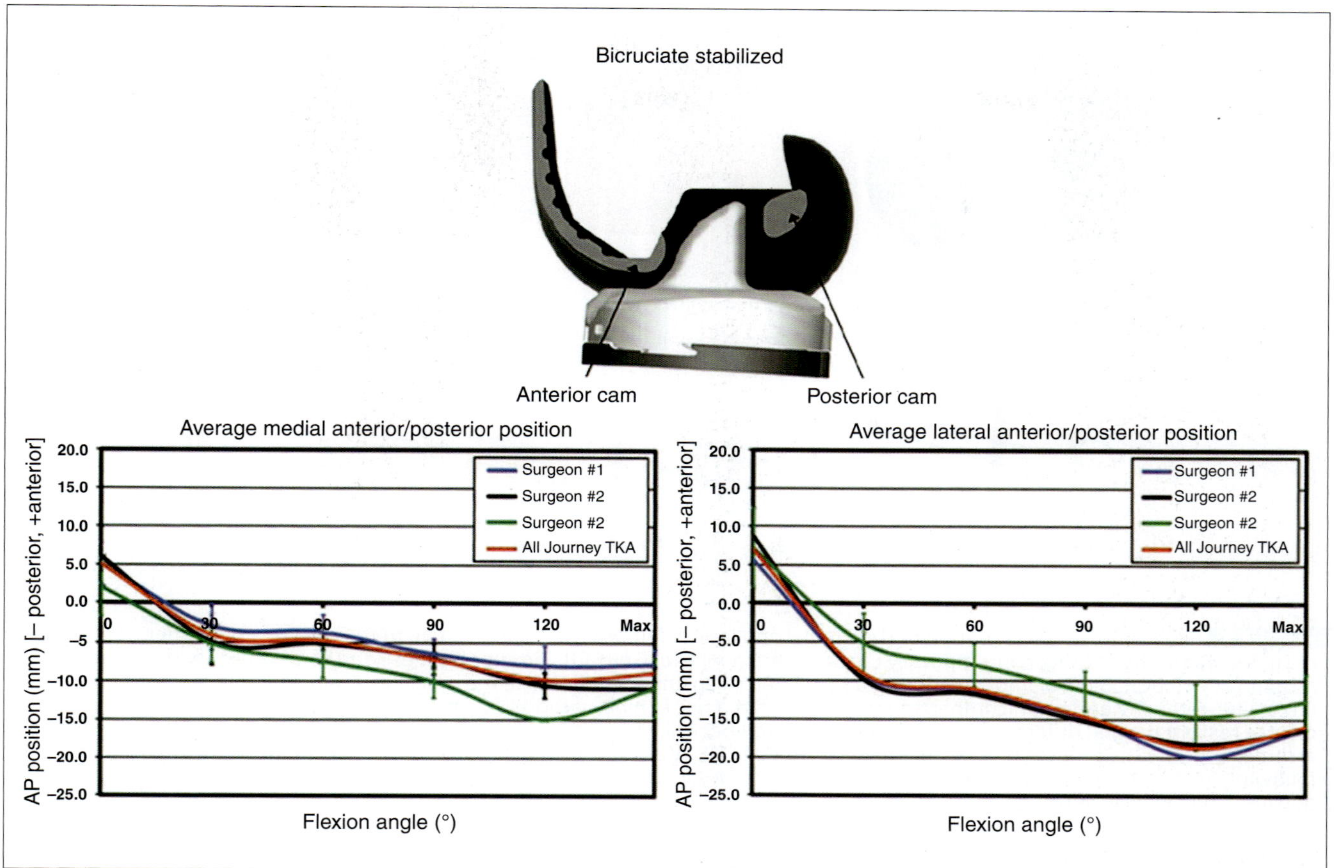

FIGURE 6 Illustration depicts in vivo medial and lateral condyle motion in patients who have a bicruciate-substituting implant (JOURNEY II, Smith & Nephew, Inc.) during deep knee bend activity. Although the surgical technique affected the kinematics, the characteristic motion patterns of normal knees, including greater lateral condyle roll back and absence of anterior sliding, were typically observed. (Reproduced with permission from Victor J, Mueller JK, Komistek RD, Sharma A, Nadaud MC, Bellemans J: In vivo kinematics after a cruciate-substituting TKA. *Clin Orthop Relat Res* 2010;468[3]:807-814.)

ACL Substitution

ACL Substitution and PCL Retention

An alternative to native ACL retention is to substitute its function to avoid the potential challenges discussed previously and to provide an option for patients who have an absent or nonfunctional ACL at surgery (approximately 14% to 75% of patients).[44] The concept of an ACL-substituting and PCL-retaining implant (ASCR) has been proposed recently as an evolution of the cruciate-retaining implant in which the ACL is sacrificed with no mechanism to substitute for its function.[39] In the ASCR implant, the anterior surface of a post on the tibia engages with the femoral intercondylar notch in low flexion to substitute for the absent ACL (**Figure 8**). The tibial post also is designed to accommodate the native PCL. A 2016 study used dynamic simulations to compare the kinematics of the ASCR design with ACL-retaining and ACL-sacrificing (ie, cruciate-retaining) implants during deep knee bend, chair sit, stair ascent, and walking.[45] As with ACL-retaining implants, the ASCR design provides kinematic improvements over contemporary ACL-sacrificing implants by reducing abnormal early posterior femoral shift and avoiding paradoxical anterior sliding. However, this concept has not been evaluated clinically.

ACL and PCL Substitution

In a bicruciate-substituting design, ACL and PCL function are substituted using anterior and posterior cam-post interaction, respectively. The bicruciate-substituting concept can be considered as an extension of the posterior-stabilized philosophy that substitutes not only for the missing PCL but also for the ACL. First-generation bicruciate-substituting designs were introduced in 2005 and showed promising kinematic results. Several in vivo studies showed more normal kinematics than contemporary TKA, including the magnitude of internal tibial rotation and posterior femoral roll back as well as the absence of paradoxical anterior sliding[37,38] (**Figure 6**). A 2018 study reported decreased varus-valgus laxity in midflexion and deep flexion in patients who have bicruciate-substituting

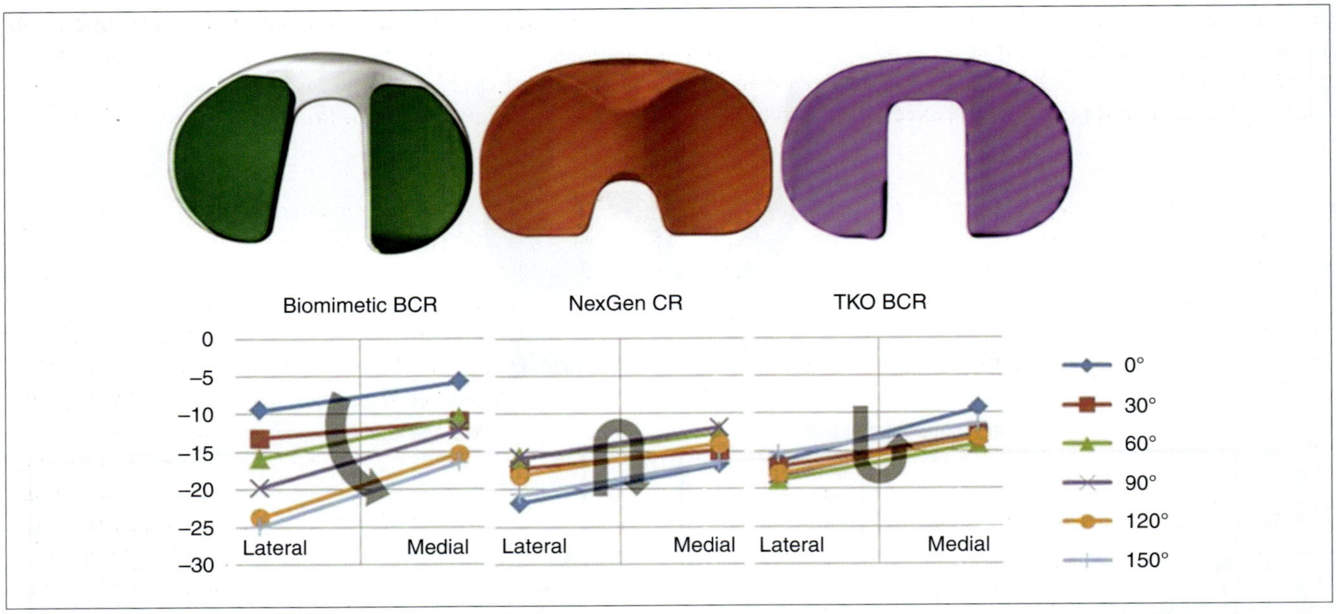

FIGURE 7 Illustration depicts motion of the medial and lateral femoral condyles relative to the tibia of a biomimetic bicruciate-retaining (Biomimetic BCR), contemporary cruciate-retaining (NexGen® CR, Zimmer Biomet), and contemporary bicruciate-retaining (TKO BCR, BioPro) implants during a simulated deep knee bend. Unlike the cruciate-retaining implant, contemporary bicruciate-retaining and bi-unicompartmental implants did not exhibit paradoxical anterior sliding. However, these implants did not restore normal differential medial and lateral roll back like the biomimetic bicruciate-retaining implant. (Adapted from *J Arthroplasty* 30[12]. Zumbrunn T, Varadarajan KM, Rubash HE, Malchau H, Li G, Muratoglu OK: Regaining native knee kinematics following joint arthroplasty: A novel biomimetic design with ACL and PCL preservation, 2143-2148. Copyright © 2015, with permission from Elsevier.)

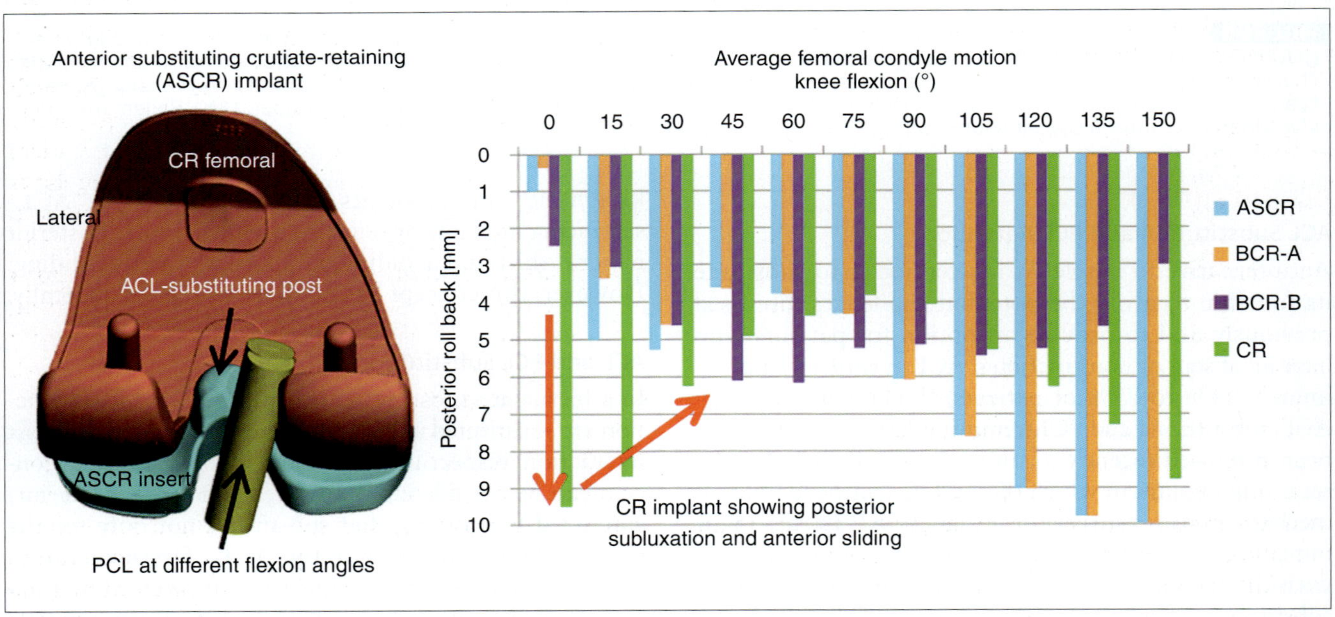

FIGURE 8 Illustration depicts mean femoral roll back of the medial and lateral condyles during a simulated deep knee bend for an anterior cruciate ligament (ACL)–substituting and posterior cruciate ligament (PCL)–retaining (ASCR), two ACL-retaining (BCR-A, BCR-B), and a contemporary cruciate-retaining (CR) total knee arthroplasty. Both the ASCR and ACL-retaining designs avoided the abnormal early posterior shift and subsequent paradoxical anterior slide that were observed in the CR implant. BCR = bicruciate-retaining. (Reproduced with permission from Varadarajan KM, Zumbrunn T, Duffy MP, Rubash HE, Malchau H, Muratoglu OK: *Poster No. 1885. Is retention of native ACL the only option for addressing abnormal anteroposterior kinematics of cruciate retaining TKA? Proceedings of the 62nd Annual Meeting of the Orthopaedic Research Society*. Rosemont, IL, Orthopaedic Research Society, 2016, p 146.)

designs.[46] Reported rates of clinical complications were higher than expected, including dislocation and iliotibial band syndrome.[47,48] These complications seem to be related to insufficient jump height, excessively forced roll back by posterior cam, and a prominent anterior femoral flange.[49] However, no complications were reported regarding fracture of the bicruciate-substituting tibial post or wear of the anatomic tibial articular surface. Second-generation bicruciate-substituting designs have been introduced to address these design issues and have shown good early results. Two-year results show mean Knee Society Score of 96.2 with high satisfaction scores (35.22 of 40).[49]

IMPLANT MATERIALS

The most commonly used materials in TKA implants are cobalt-chromium-molybdenum alloy for the femoral implant, conventional (minimally cross-linked or non–cross-linked) ultra-high–molecular-weight polyethylene for the tibial insert, and titanium alloy for the tibial baseplate. However, the pursuit of improved implant survivorship via the reduction of polyethylene damage and concerns regarding metal hypersensitivity have motivated the exploration of alternative materials. Clinical and registry studies continue to monitor the long-term performance of highly cross-linked ultra-high–molecular-weight polyethylene, which was introduced in the early 2000s, and newer antioxidant-stabilized polyethylene, which was introduced in 2008.

Bulk Ceramics

Ceramics have several advantages, including reduced coefficient of friction, increased lubricity owing to reduced wetting angle, high hardness and abrasion resistance, and excellent biocompatibility. In the past 5 years, mid- to long-term clinical data have been published for several ceramic TKA implants. One study reported 5-year survivorship of 98.6% with no revisions for aseptic loosening, osteolysis, or ceramic fractures for an alumina medial-pivot TKA.[50] Another study published 10-year clinical results for an alumina ceramic implant that has been used in Japan since 1992.[51] At a mean follow-up of 11.7 years, the mean Knee Society Score was 93.3, survivorship with any revision surgery or radiographic failure as an end point was 95.9%, and no fractures of the ceramic femoral implant occurred. Another study reported on the clinical outcomes of a ceramic TKA with an alumina matrix composite femoral implant that was strengthened with yttria-stabilized tetragonal zirconia particles.[52] At 5-year follow-up, implant survivorship was 96.0%, with no implant migration or loosening. In one case, a midline longitudinal crack was noted on the ceramic femoral implant following a traumatic event, and two fractures of the femoral implant that occurred during intraoperative impaction were reported. Subsequent analysis showed hard impaction at high velocity and the femoral resection angle to be likely causes of failure.[53]

Ceramicized Metals

TKA implants with various ceramic coatings are currently in clinical use, including titanium nitride (TiN) on Ti6Al4V (a grade 5 titanium alloy), TiN on cobalt-chromium (CoCr), zirconium nitride (ZrN)–coated CoCr, and titanium niobium nitride (TiNbN)–coated CoCr. Although many preclinical studies indicate favorable tribologic properties (eg, high scratch resistance, low coefficient of friction, less ultra-high–molecular-weight polyethylene wear) of these ceramic coatings (Reference), other studies have not replicated these findings and concerns have been noted regarding loss of coating and increased wear.[54] However, the coating process may have a substantial effect on coating performance (Reference). One particular ZrN coating technology uses a top coat of ZrN, five layers of chromium nitride–chromium carbonitride (CrN-CrCN), and a thin chromium bond coat on top of a standard CoCr alloy (overall thickness, 3.5 to 5.0 µm).[55] The multilayer coating provides a gradient between the hard coating and the relatively soft substrate to improve the mechanical integrity of the coating. A 2011 study reported no scratches, pitting, or coating damage during a 3-million-cycle knee simulator study of a mobile-bearing implant with ZrN-coated metallic components created with this coating technology.[55] A few recent studies have published clinical performance data for such ceramic-coated knee implants. A 2015 retrospective study compared short-term (mean follow-up, 2 years) clinical results for a TiNbN-coated implant with CoCr implants of the same design. This study found no differences in clinical, radiographic, or patient-reported outcomes, and no patients underwent revision in either group.[56] A 2014 retrospective study of 305 TiN-coated mobile-bearing implants reported 10-year survivorship of 95.1% with revision for any reason as the end point and 99.1% with revision for aseptic loosening as the end point.[57]

Oxidized zirconium (OxZr) knee implants were introduced in 1997.[58] Unlike the ceramic coating applied to a metal substrate, OxZr is created via thermal diffusion, which transforms the surface of wrought zirconium-niobium (2.5% niobium) alloy to a ZrO_2 (monoclinic) layer approximately 5 µm thick. Although numerous laboratory wear studies have demonstrated a reduction in polyethylene wear with OxZr versus CoCr femoral components (range, 42% to 85%), until recently, in vivo data have been lacking.[58] That recent retrieval study found significantly lower femoral implant roughness as well as lower damage scores for both femoral components and polyethylene inlays with OxZr compared

Section 2: Knee

with matched paired CoCr TKAs.[58] Furthermore, a 2017 study that performed three-dimensional laser scanning of retrieved polyethylene inserts reported a substantially lower polyethylene volume loss related to in vivo wear rather than creep for OxZr bearing surfaces compared with cobalt alloys.[59] A 2011 study published results of a randomized controlled trial with patients who underwent bilateral TKA with a CoCr femoral implant in one knee and an OxZr implant in the contralateral knee.[60] At 5-year follow-up, no significant differences were reported between the two groups regarding mean Knee Injury and Osteoarthritis Outcome Scores or radiologic evaluation findings. In a retrospective review of 109 OxZr TKAs performed in 82 patients with a mean follow-up of 5.9 years, no revisions were performed for wear, loosening, osteolysis, or infection.[61] The mean Knee Society Score was 92 points (range, 49 to 100 points) and the mean function score was 81 points (range, 30 to 100 points). A 2014 study reported 10-year results of a prospective study for 84 patients at final follow-up.[62] Overall survivorship was 97.8%; two knees needed revision for femoral implant loosening. The mean knee score was 84 points (range, 64 to 100 points) and the mean function score was 83 points (range, 55 to 100 points).

SUMMARY

Implant design has a major influence on both short- and long-term outcomes following TKA. Important issues pertaining to implant geometry and materials are currently being debated, and new technologies are under investigation.

Available evidence does not indicate superiority of single-radius or multiradius femoral designs in relation to clinical outcomes. Anatomic tibial trays may offer only a slight advantage for increased tibial coverage; however, they could reduce the probability of internal rotation if attainment of maximal tibial coverage is used to guide tray placement. Cost advantages coupled with equivalent outcomes to metal-backed components could increase the use of all-polyethylene tibial components. PCL-retaining (cruciate-retaining), PCL-substituting (posterior-stabilized), and PCL-sacrificing (ultracongruent) designs seem to have similar clinical outcomes and long-term survivorship. However, the high anterior tibial lips in ultracongruent designs may not fully compensate for PCL function, resulting in increased anterior femoral sliding and potential anterior-posterior instability.

Contemporary implants show significant kinematic alterations relative to the preoperative and native knee, which may partly explain the similar patient outcomes observed with cruciate-retaining, posterior-stabilized, and ultracongruent designs. Provision of anatomic or biomimetic articular surfaces together with ACL retention or substitution may be key to restoring normal kinematics following TKA. However, such new implant designs do not preclude the importance of surgical technique. Techniques designed to facilitate more normal collateral ligament function via anatomic joint line restoration may play a crucial role in achieving normal knee function following TKA.

Several materials continue to be evaluated as an alternative to cobalt-chromium-molybdenum alloy. Bulk ceramics and oxidized zirconia have demonstrated excellent midterm to long-term outcomes and may be viable options for patients who have suspected metal hypersensitivity. Early clinical results of ceramic-coated metal seem to be positive, but more clinical data are needed to determine whether ceramic-coated metals are a cost-effective alternative.

KEY STUDY POINTS

- Both anatomic articular geometry and ACL function (via retention or substitution) may be required to restore normal knee kinematics following TKA.
- Anatomic joint line restoration via the appropriate positioning of standard implants or implants with asymmetric thicknesses may facilitate more normal soft-tissue function.
- All-polyethylene tibial components have been shown to have long-term clinical outcomes equivalent to those of metal-backed components.
- OxZr and bulk ceramics are alternatives to CoCr that have excellent midterm to long-term survivorship, potentially lower wear properties, and favorable clinical outcomes.

ANNOTATED REFERENCES

1. Noble PC, Gordon MJ, Weiss JM, Reddix RN, Conditt MA, Mathis KB: Does total knee replacement restore normal knee function? *Clin Orthop Relat Res* 2005;431:157-165.
2. Larsen B, Jacofsky MC, Jacofsky DJ: Quantitative, comparative assessment of gait between single-radius and multi-radius total knee arthroplasty designs. *J Arthroplasty* 2015;30(6):1062-1067.
3. Hinarejos P, Puig-Verdie L, Leal J, et al: No differences in functional results and quality of life after single-radius or multiradius TKA. *Knee Surg Sports Traumatol Arthrosc* 2016;24(8):2634-2640.
4. Liu S, Long H, Zhang Y, Ma B, Li Z: Meta-analysis of outcomes of a single-radius versus multi-radius femoral design in total knee arthroplasty. *J Arthroplasty* 2016;31(3):646-654.
5. Cherian JJ, Kapadia BH, Banerjee S, Jauregui JJ, Issa K, Mont MA: Mechanical, anatomical, and kinematic axis in TKA: Concepts and practical applications. *Curr Rev Musculoskelet Med* 2014;7(2):89-95.

6. Babazadeh S, Dowsey MM, Swan JD, Stoney JD, Choong PF: Joint line position correlates with function after primary total knee replacement: A randomised controlled trial comparing conventional and computer-assisted surgery. *J Bone Joint Surg Br* 2011;93(9):1223-1231.
7. Delport H, Labey L, De Corte R, Innocenti B, Vander Sloten J, Bellemans J: Collateral ligament strains during knee joint laxity evaluation before and after TKA. *Clin Biomech (Bristol, Avon)* 2013;28(7):777-782.
8. Gromov K, Korchi M, Thomsen MG, Husted H, Troelsen A: What is the optimal alignment of the tibial and femoral components in knee arthroplasty? *Acta Orthop* 2014;85(5):480-487.
9. Matsuda S, Miura H, Nagamine R, Urabe K, Hirata G, Iwamoto Y: Effect of femoral and tibial component position on patellar tracking following total knee arthroplasty: 10-year follow-up of Miller-Galante I knees. *Am J Knee Surg* 2001;14(3):152-156.
10. Dossett HG, Estrada NA, Swartz GJ, LeFevre GW, Kwasman BG: A randomised controlled trial of kinematically and mechanically aligned total knee replacements: Two-year clinical results. *Bone Joint J* 2014;96-B(7):907-913.
11. Dai Y, Scuderi GR, Bischoff JE, Bertin K, Tarabichi S, Rajgopal A: Anatomic tibial component design can increase tibial coverage and rotational alignment accuracy: A comparison of six contemporary designs. *Knee Surg Sports Traumatol Arthrosc* 2014;22(12):2911-2923.
12. Stulberg SD, Goyal N: Which tibial tray design achieves maximum coverage and ideal rotation: Anatomic, symmetric, or asymmetric? An MRI-based study. *J Arthroplasty* 2015;30(10):1839-1841.
13. Clary C, Aram L, Deffenbaugh D, Heldreth M: Tibial base design and patient morphology affecting tibial coverage and rotational alignment after total knee arthroplasty. *Knee Surg Sports Traumatol Arthrosc* 2014;22(12):3012-3018.
14. Voigt J, Mosier M: Cemented all-polyethylene and metal-backed polyethylene tibial components used for primary total knee arthroplasty: A systematic review of the literature and meta-analysis of randomized controlled trials involving 1798 primary total knee implants. *J Bone Joint Surg Am* 2011;93(19):1790-1798.
15. Nouta KA, Verra WC, Pijls BG, Schoones JW, Nelissen RG: All-polyethylene tibial components are equal to metal-backed components: Systematic review and meta-regression. *Clin Orthop Relat Res* 2012;470(12):3549-3559.
16. Mohan V, Inacio MC, Namba RS, Sheth D, Paxton EW: Monoblock all-polyethylene tibial components have a lower risk of early revision than metal-backed modular components. *Acta Orthop* 2013;84(6):530-536.
17. Gudnason A, Hailer NP, W-Dahl A, Sundberg M, Robertsson O: All-polyethylene versus metal-backed tibial components—An analysis of 27,733 cruciate-retaining total knee replacements from the Swedish Knee Arthroplasty Register. *J Bone Joint Surg Am* 2014;96(12):994-999.
18. Gioe TJ, Sinner P, Mehle S, Ma W, Killeen KK: Excellent survival of all-polyethylene tibial components in a community joint registry. *Clin Orthop Relat Res* 2007;464:88-92.
19. Pomeroy DL, Schaper LA, Badenhausen WE, et al: Results of all-polyethylene tibial components as a cost-saving technique. *Clin Orthop Relat Res* 2000;380:140-143.
20. Longo UG, Ciuffreda M, Mannering N, et al: Outcomes of posterior-stabilized compared with cruciate-retaining total knee arthroplasty. *J Knee Surg* 2018;31(4): 321-340.

    This study is a systematic review and meta-analysis of 37 studies including nearly 10,000 knees analyzing clinical outcomes from cruciate-retaining and posterior-stabilized designs. There were similar results for nearly all clinical outcome measures and complication rates between the two implant designs. Level of evidence: II.
21. Iwamoto K, Tomita T, Yamazaki T, et al: Comparison of in vivo kinematics of total knee arthroplasty between cruciate retaining and condylar stabilized insert. *Orthop Proc* 2014;96-B(suppl 11):167.
22. Kim TW, Lee SM, Seong SC, Lee S, Jang J, Lee MC: Different intraoperative kinematics with comparable clinical outcomes of ultracongruent and posterior stabilized mobile-bearing total knee arthroplasty. *Knee Surg Sports Traumatol Arthrosc* 2016;24(9):3036-3043.
23. Lützner J, Firmbach FP, Lützner C, Dexel J, Kirschner S: Similar stability and range of motion between cruciate-retaining and cruciate-substituting ultracongruent insert total knee arthroplasty. *Knee Surg Sports Traumatol Arthrosc* 2015;23(6):1638-1643.
24. Massin P, Boyer P, Sabourin M: Less femorotibial rotation and AP translation in deep-dished total knee arthroplasty. An intraoperative kinematic study using navigation. *Knee Surg Sports Traumatol Arthrosc* 2012;20(9): 1714-1719.
25. Fritzsche H, Beyer F, Postler A, Lützner J: Different intraoperative kinematics, stability, and range of motion between cruciate-substituting ultracongruent and posterior-stabilized total knee arthroplasty. *Knee Surg Sports Traumatol Arthrosc* 2018;26(5):1465-1470.

    This study measured intraoperative kinematics, stability, and ROM in 40 patients before bone cuts and soft-tissue releases and after implantation of components. Both cruciate-substituting ultracongruent and posterior-stabilized designs were included. Ultracongruent designs had significantly more paradoxical anterior translation and increased anterior-posterior translation in 60° and 90° of flexion compared with posterior-stabilized designs. Level of evidence: II.
26. Argenson JN, Boisgard S, Parratte S, et al, French Society of Orthopedic and Traumatologic Surgery (SOFCOT): Survival analysis of total knee arthroplasty at a minimum 10 years' follow-up: A multicenter French nationwide study including 846 cases. *Orthop Traumatol Surg Res* 2013;99(4): 385-390.
27. Scott DF. Prospective randomized comparison of posterior-stabilized versus condylar-stabilized total knee arthroplasty: Final report of a five-year study. *J Arthroplasty* 2018;33(5):1384-1388.

This prospective randomized trial included 56 posterior-stabilized knees and 55 cruciate substituting, anterior lipped designs at a minimum follow-up of 5 years. There were no significant differences in clinical outcomes, ROM, complications, or revision rates. Level of evidence: I.

28. Varadarajan KM, Zumbrunn T, Rubash HE, Malchau H, Muratoglu OK, Li G: Reverse engineering nature to design biomimetic total knee implants. *J Knee Surg* 2015;28(5):363-369.
29. Li JS, Hosseini A, Cancre L, Ryan N, Rubash HE, Li G: Kinematic characteristics of the tibiofemoral joint during a step-up activity. *Gait Posture* 2013;38(4):712-716.
30. Johal P, Williams A, Wragg P, Hunt D, Gedroyc W: Tibio-femoral movement in the living knee. A study of weight bearing and non-weight bearing knee kinematics using 'interventional' MRI. *J Biomech* 2005;38(2):269-276.
31. Shimmin A, Martinez-Martos S, Owens J, Iorgulescu AD, Banks S: Fluoroscopic motion study confirming the stability of a medial pivot design total knee arthroplasty. *Knee* 2015;22(6):522-526.
32. Barnes CL, Blaha JD, DeBoer D, Stemniski P, Obert R, Carroll M: Assessment of a medial pivot total knee arthroplasty design in a cadaveric knee extension test model. *J Arthroplasty* 2012;27(8):1460-1468.
33. Koo S, Andriacchi TP: The knee joint center of rotation is predominantly on the lateral side during normal walking. *J Biomech* 2008;41(6):1269-1273.
34. Lew WD, Lewis JL: The effect of knee-prosthesis geometry on cruciate ligament mechanics during flexion. *J Bone Joint Surg Am* 1982;64(5):734-739.
35. Varadarajan KM, Zumbrunn T, Rubash HE, Malchau H, Li G, Muratoglu OK: Cruciate retaining implant with biomimetic articular surface to reproduce activity dependent kinematics of the normal knee. *J Arthroplasty* 2015;30(12): 2149-2153.
36. van Duren BH, Pandit H, Price M, et al: Bicruciate substituting total knee replacement: How effective are the added kinematic constraints in vivo? *Knee Surg Sports Traumatol Arthrosc* 2012;20(10):2002-2010.
37. Victor J, Mueller JK, Komistek RD, Sharma A, Nadaud MC, Bellemans J: In vivo kinematics after a cruciate-substituting TKA. *Clin Orthop Relat Res* 2010;468(3):807-814.
38. Zumbrunn T, Varadarajan KM, Rubash HE, Malchau H, Li G, Muratoglu OK: Regaining native knee kinematics following joint arthroplasty: A novel biomimetic design with ACL and PCL preservation. *J Arthroplasty* 2015;30(12): 2143-2148.
39. Okada Y, Teramoto A, Takagi T, et al: ACL function in bicruciate-retaining total knee arthroplasty. *J Bone Joint Surg Am* 2018;100(17):e114.

    This cadaver study investigated knee kinematics during flexion and extension motion of native knees, bicruciate-retaining implants, and bicruciate-retaining implants with the ACL transected. The authors found that the ACL in situ force in the bicruciate-retaining knees was twofold to sixfold higher than that of intact knees. Level of evidence: III.

40. Stiehl JB, Komistek RD, Cloutier JM, Dennis DA: The cruciate ligaments in total knee arthroplasty: A kinematic analysis of 2 total knee arthroplasties. *J Arthroplasty* 2000;15(5):545-550.
41. Alnachoukati OK, Emerson RH, Diaz E, Ruchaud E, Ennin KA: Modern day bicruciate-retaining total knee arthroplasty: A short-term review of 146 knees. *J Arthroplasty* 2018;33(8):2485-2490.

    This study reviewed the outcomes of 146 bicruciate retaining consecutive TKAs with minimum 1-year follow-up. They reported that 91% of patients reported their knee always or sometimes felt normal and that 6% of patients were dissatisfied. There was a 1.4% revision rate at an average follow-up of 12 months. Level of evidence: IV.

42. Pelt CE, Sandifer PA, Gililland JM, Anderson MB, Peters CL: Mean three-year survivorship of a new bicruciate-retaining total knee arthroplasty: Are revisions still higher than expected? *J Arthroplasty* 2019;34(9):1957-1962.

    In this study of 141 bicruciate-retaining TKAs at a single institution, the survivorship free of revision was 88% at 3 years. Overall, 19 knees were revised; primary failure modes included tibial loosening ($n = 5$), ACL impingement ($n = 3$), and ACL deficiency ($n = 1$). Level of evidence: IV.

43. Wada K, Hamada D, Takasago T, et al: The medial constrained insert restores native knee rotational kinematics after bicruciate-retaining total knee arthroplasty. *Knee Surg Sports Traumatol Arthrosc* 2019;27(5):1621-1627.

    This study analyzed the rotation angle of the tibia in six cadavers with bicruciate-retaining implants with a flat insert, bicruciate-retaining implants with a medial concave insert, and native knees. They found that only the medially congruent bicruciate-retaining design reestablished normal knee kinematics while the flat surface did not. Level of evidence: III.

44. Johnson AJ, Howell SM, Costa CR, Mont MA: The ACL in the arthritic knee: How often is it present and can preoperative tests predict its presence? *Clin Orthop Relat Res* 2013;471(1):181-188.
45. Varadarajan KM, Zumbrunn T, Duffy MP, Rubash HE, Malchau H, Muratoglu OK: *Poster No. 1885. Is retention of native ACL the only option for addressing abnormal anteroposterior kinematics of cruciate retaining TKA? Proceedings of the 62nd Annual Meeting of the Orthopaedic Research Society*. Rosemont, IL, Orthopaedic Research Society, 2016, p 146.
46. Hino K, Kutsuna T, Watamori K, et al: Bi-cruciate substituting total knee arthroplasty provides varus-valgus stability throughout the midflexion range. *Knee* 2018;25(5):897-902.

    Preoperative and postoperative varus-valgus laxity was analyzed in 51 osteoarthritic knees replaced with a bicruciate-substituting TKA. They found that postoperative varus-valgus laxity significantly decreased from preoperative levels at 20° to 120° of flexion. Level of evidence: IV.

47. Christen B, Neukamp M, Aghayev E: Consecutive series of 226 journey bicruciate substituting total knee replacements: Early complication and revision rates. *BMC Musculoskelet Disord* 2014;15:395.

48. Arnout N, Vandenneucker H, Bellemans J: Posterior dislocation in total knee replacement: A price for deep flexion? *Knee Surg Sports Traumatol Arthrosc* 2011;19(6):911-913.

49. Harris AI, Luo TD, Lang JE, Kopjar B: Short-term safety and effectiveness of a second-generation motion-guided total knee system. *Arthroplast Today* 2018;4:240-243.

This study is a prospective evaluation of 209 primary second-generation bicruciate-substituting knee arthroplasty. The results showed mean Knee Society Score of 96.2 and with mean function score of 81.49. There were no revisions for instability or aseptic loosening. Level of evidence: IV.

50. Iida T, Minoda Y, Kadoya Y, et al: Mid-term clinical results of alumina medial pivot total knee arthroplasty. *Knee Surg Sports Traumatol Arthrosc* 2012;20(8):1514-1519.

51. Nakamura S, Kobayashi M, Ito H, Nakamura K, Ueo T, Nakamura T: The Bi-Surface total knee arthroplasty: Minimum 10-year follow-up study. *Knee* 2010;17(4):274-278.

52. Bergschmidt P, Bader R, Ganzer D, et al: Prospective multicentre study on a composite ceramic femoral component in total knee arthroplasty: Five-year clinical and radiological outcomes. *Knee* 2015;22(3):186-191.

53. Kluess D, Bergschmidt P, Mueller I, Mittelmeier W, Bader R: Influence of the distal femoral resection angle on the principal stresses in ceramic total knee components. *Knee* 2012;19(6):846-850.

54. van Hove RP, Sierevelt IN, van Royen BJ, Nolte PA: Titanium-nitride coating of orthopaedic implants: A review of the literature. *Biomed Res Int* 2015;2015:485975.

55. Affatato S, Spinelli M, Lopomo N, Grupp TM, Marcacci M, Toni A: Can the method of fixation influence the wear behaviour of ZrN coated unicompartmental mobile knee prostheses? *Clin Biomech (Bristol, Avon)* 2011;26(2):152-158.

56. Thienpont E: Titanium niobium nitride knee implants are not inferior to chrome cobalt components for primary total knee arthroplasty. *Arch Orthop Trauma Surg* 2015;135(12):1749-1754.

57. Mohammed A, Metcalfe A, Woodnutt D: Medium-term outcome of titanium nitride, mobile bearing total knee replacement. *Acta Orthop Belg* 2014;80(2):269-275.

58. Schüttler KF, Efe T, Heyse TJ, Haas SB: Oxidized zirconium bearing surfaces in total knee arthroplasty: Lessons learned. *J Knee Surg* 2015;28(5):376-381.

59. Anderson FL, Koch CN, Elpers ME, Wright TM, Haas SB, Heyse TJ: Oxidised zirconium versus cobalt alloy bearing surfaces in total knee arthroplasty: 3D laser scanning of retrieved polyethylene inserts. *Bone Joint J* 2017;99-B(6):793-798.

Twenty retrieved tibial inserts that had articulated with oxidized zirconium were matched with 20 retrieved inserts that had articulated with cobalt alloy. Changes in dimensions of the polyethylene were analyzed with a laser scanner. There was substantially more polyethylene volume loss in the cobalt alloy group compared with the oxinium group that could not be explained by creep. Level of evidence: III.

60. Hui C, Salmon L, Maeno S, Roe J, Walsh W, Pinczewski L: Five-year comparison of oxidized zirconium and cobalt-chromium femoral components in total knee arthroplasty: A randomized controlled trial. *J Bone Joint Surg Am* 2011;93(7):624-630.

61. Hofer JK, Ezzet KA: A minimum 5-year follow-up of an oxidized zirconium femoral prosthesis used for total knee arthroplasty. *Knee* 2014;21(1):168-171.

62. Innocenti M, Matassi F, Carulli C, Nistri L, Civinini R: Oxidized zirconium femoral component for TKA: A follow-up note of a previous report at a minimum of 10 years. *Knee* 2014;21(4):858-861.

Special Considerations in Primary Total Knee Arthroplasty

SIMON GREENBAUM, MD • ANDREW B. OLD, MD • WILLIAM J. LONG, MD, FRCSC
RAN SCHWARZKOPF, MD, MSc • W. NORMAN SCOTT, MD, FACS

ABSTRACT

The number of total knee arthroplasties is projected to increase annually. Two patient groups, young patients (age 55 years and younger) and obese patients, will contribute most to that increased number. Both groups have unique surgical challenges and should be given special consideration when total knee arthroplasty is performed. Proper implant positioning and fixation are essential for a successful outcome. Concerns regarding early failure secondary to aseptic loosening, infection, and implant positioning should prompt the surgeon to counsel patients preoperatively and maximize outcomes in the operating room by means of thorough planning.

Keywords: aseptic loosening; infection; malalignment; obesity; total knee arthroplasty; young patient

INTRODUCTION

Total knee arthroplasty (TKA) is routinely performed across the United States in a range of hospital settings, including large academic institutions, small community hospitals, and, increasingly, outpatient surgical centers. A large percentage of TKAs are performed by practitioners who are not fellowship trained in adult reconstruction. Despite being commonplace, TKA in certain patient cohorts requires special consideration. Young patients and obese patients are susceptible to higher rates of complications such as early aseptic loosening and infection. Technical tips are available to maximize results in these challenging patient cohorts.

TKA IN YOUNG PATIENTS

The rate of TKAs is expected to increase dramatically, and a higher percentage of these patients will be categorized as young, usually defined as aged 55 years or younger. By 2030, primary TKAs in the United States are projected to increase by 637% and revisions by 601% compared

Dr. Long or an immediate family member has received royalties from OrthoDevelopment; is a member of a speakers' bureau or has made paid presentations on behalf of Convatec, Pacira, and Think Surgical; serves as a paid consultant to or is an employee of DePuy, A Johnson & Johnson Company, Pacira, Think Surgical, and TJO; and serves as a board member, owner, officer, or committee member of the American Academy of Orthopaedic Surgeons. Dr. Schwarzkopf or an immediate family member has received royalties from Smith & Nephew; serves as a paid consultant to or is an employee of Intelijoint and Smith & Nephew; has stock or stock options held in Gauss Surgical and Intelijoint; has received research or institutional support from Smith & Nephew; and serves as a board member, owner, officer, or committee member of the American Academy of Orthopaedic Surgeons and the American Association of Hip and Knee Surgeons. Dr. Scott or an immediate family member serves as a paid consultant to or is an employee of OrthoDevelopment Medical Advisor to Board of Directors and serves as a board member, owner, officer, or committee member of President & CEO ICJR (International Congress for Joint Reconstruction). Neither of the following authors nor any immediate family member has received anything of value from or has stock or stock options held in a commercial company or institution related directly or indirectly to the subject of this chapter: Dr. Greenbaum and Dr. Old.

with numbers reported in 2005.[1] Similar trends have been observed in the United Kingdom and New Zealand, suggesting that this is an international phenomenon.[2,3] With these staggering projections and the financial burden to the healthcare system, the young patient undergoing TKA requires special consideration.

Young patients generally will place higher physical demands on their implants. Although constant improvements have been made in prosthetics and implants overall, the same implants initially designed for low-demand, somewhat frail community ambulators are now expected to withstand the high demands of the younger patient. Expectations are much higher than simply pain relief and the renewed ability to complete activities of daily living such as walk on level ground, climb stairs, and perhaps engage in light activity. The original Knee Society scoring system assessed only the patient's ability to walk and climb stairs and was later modified to accommodate patients' expanded expectations.[4] The young patient's expectations now include strenuous activity and higher impact sports and recreation, and they are reflected in the updated Knee Society scoring system.[5]

Despite these higher expectations, young patients may report greater residual symptoms following TKA. A national multicenter study[6] assessed 661 young patients (mean age, 54 years) regarding residual symptoms and daily functional deficits. Although 89% of young patients were satisfied with their ability to perform activities of daily living, 33% reported pain, 41% reported stiffness, 33% reported swelling, and 38% and 31% reported difficulties getting in and out of a car and a chair, respectively. More than one-half of young patients reported difficulty navigating stairs. Given this outcome, the surgeon must manage patients' expectations preoperatively and counsel them appropriately regarding the goals of care.

Along with higher expectations and greater residual symptoms, the young patient also requires the implant to last longer to avoid revision arthroplasty. Currently, the likelihood is much greater that the implant will not outlive the recipient,[7] so the primary TKA should last for as long as possible. At 10-year follow-up, researchers found that patients younger than 47 years at the time of their index TKA were twice as likely to require a revision as they were to die. Patients approximately 58 years old at the time of their index TKA had a 50:50 likelihood of requiring revision versus dying. Patients approximately 62 years or older at the time of their index TKA were more likely to die within 10 years before requiring revision.[7] A large national registry found that the rate of revision for patients younger than 55 years was six times greater than that for patients older than 75 years at 10 years.[8]

Given the increased demands on the TKA prosthesis, the young patient population may experience increased rates of aseptic loosening of their implants over time; however, prostheses seem to be failing even earlier than would be expected.[9] Generally, osteolysis resulting from polyethylene wear particles would cause loosening, but evidence suggests that TKAs performed in young patients are failing before obvious polyethylene wear occurs. One study retrospectively compared a cohort of patients younger than 50 years with a matched cohort of patients aged 60 to 70 years[10] and determined the etiology of failure for the index procedure and any subsequent revisions that were performed. The mean time from the initial TKA to the first revision in the younger cohort was 36 months (range, 1 to 210 months) compared with 59 months (range, 1 to 230 months) in the older cohort. Essentially, TKA failure occurred in a shorter time frame in younger patients.

Young patients also may present technical challenges to performing TKA. Early joint degeneration requiring arthroplasty may be secondary to trauma, which can leave the limb with retained hardware, angular deformity, or previous traumatic or surgical incisions. Obese patients present their own challenges to TKA, as discussed later. Obese patients are more likely to require knee arthroplasty at a younger age than those patients who have normal body mass indexes (BMIs).[11] Arthroplasty surgeons may therefore be faced with the surgical and rehabilitation challenges and risk profiles that accompany both youth and obesity in the same patient.

Infection

Infection has been reported as the second major cause of early revision TKA in the young patient population (after aseptic loosening),[10] comprising 23% of failures. A 2014 study[12] evaluated the increased revision rate for TKA secondary to infection in young patients and reported that patients younger than 50 years underwent revision TKA because of infection at approximately twice the rate of patients aged 65 years or older (1.36% versus 0.73% incidence). This result excludes patients with inflammatory arthritis, who have a higher rate of infection. The study also noted male sex and African American race as independent risk factors for infection. Congestive heart failure, obesity, psychosis, and diabetes were all comorbidities that independently increased the risk of periprosthetic infections. Reasons for increased rates of infection in young patients can be a result of patients in this group having a higher percentage of posttraumatic arthritis or more surgical attempts at joint preservation (such as multiple injections, arthroscopies, ligament reconstructions, or meniscal allografts).[7]

Aseptic Loosening

The literature has shown that young patients also have a higher rate of aseptic loosening. A 2014 study reported that revision for aseptic mechanical failure was 1.15%, but increased to 3.49% for those younger than 50 years and decreased to 0.75% for those aged 65 years or older.[10] Aseptic loosening has been reported to account for 27% of early failures. Early aseptic revisions have been performed for loosening, continued pain, poor range of motion, and instability.[7] Given the poor performance of revision procedures in the young patient cohort, the surgeon must clearly delineate the diagnosis and the reason a revision will resolve the patient's problem. Persistent pain without a clear cause is a poor indication for revision TKA and will likely result in patient dissatisfaction after the revision procedure.

Success in the Young Cohort

Some investigators have documented good success rates and longevity with their younger patient cohorts.[13,14] The findings of an ongoing longitudinal outcome study showed that overall survivorship without revision for any cause after 30 years was 70.1%, and the survivorship for tibial or femoral loosening was 82.5%.[13] The mean Hospital for Special Surgery score improved from 57.9 points preoperatively to 85.3 points at 30-year follow-up. The mean Knee Society score was 87.4, and the mean functional Knee Society score was 62.1 points. The mean Tegner and Lysholm activity score improved from 1.5 points preoperatively to 3.0 points postoperatively.

A literature review that included 908 TKAs in 671 patients[14] reported that implant survivorship was between 90.6% and 99.0% during the first decade in patients younger than 55 years. This decreased to between 85.0% and 96.5% during the second decade. Patients showed functional improvement, with the mean Knee Society clinical and functional scores improving by 47 and 37 points, respectively.

TKA IN PATIENTS WITH OBESITY

Obesity has now reached epidemic proportions, with slightly more than one-third of adults in the United States classified as obese.[15] Patients presenting to an orthopaedic clinic for osteoarthritis are more likely to be obese relative to the general population.[16] The consequences of obesity to a person's general health are well documented, as are the subsequent increases in healthcare costs.[17-20] In addition, improvement in BMI may not return these patients to baseline risk levels.[21] Studies show that obese patients are at higher risk for overall complications,[22] including infection,[20,23,24] respiratory complications, poor wound healing,[19] implant malalignment, and suboptimal implant positioning,[18] and that obesity is an independent risk factor for revision TKA.[8,25] In patients who had already undergone revision TKA, those who have a BMI higher than 40 kg/m² were reported to have a 2.9-fold increased likelihood of requiring a second revision.[10] A 2016 study showed a significant increase in obesity (from 31.5% to 38.1%) for women between 60 and 65 years of age ($P = 0.006$), a population subset that commonly undergoes TKA.[26] The population that undergoes TKA is expanding, and given that obesity is considered an independent risk factor for knee osteoarthritis and more than one-half of those undergoing TKA are obese,[26] surgeons must give special consideration to these challenging cases.

Patients who have obesity are those who have BMI greater than 30 kg/m² (**Table 1**). Obesity is then categorized into three classes: I (obese), BMI 30 to 35 kg/m²; II (severely obese), BMI 35 to 40 kg/m²; and III (morbidly obese), BMI higher than 40 kg/m². A patient is considered morbidly obese if he or she satisfies one of the following criteria: a BMI greater than 40 kg/m² (class III), weight in excess of 100 lb (45.5 kg) more than his or her ideal body weight, or a BMI higher than 35 kg/m² and obesity-related health problems such as hypertension, diabetes, sleep apnea, or coronary artery disease. Patients who have a BMI of 50 kg/m² or higher are considered super obese. Obesity has an *International Classification of Diseases, 10th Revision* (ICD-10) code that allows it to be added to TKA procedure codes.

Surgeons must be willing to accept the unique challenges that accompany performing TKA in patients who have obesity. Special consideration should be given to preoperative counseling regarding the surgical risks: soft-tissue handling, surgical exposure, implant alignment, and postoperative rehabilitation.

TABLE 1

Body Mass Index Classification

Classification	Body Mass Index (kg/m²)
Underweight	<18
Normal weight	18.0-24.9
Overweight	25.0-29.9
Obesity class I: Obese	30.0-34.9
Obesity class II: Severely obese	35.0-39.9
Obesity class III: Morbidly obese	40.0-49.9
Super obese	≥50

Infection

Patients who have obesity are at higher risk for the development of infection[23] because of several factors: increased complexity of the surgical procedure, poor wound healing because of poor nutrition, decreased tissue oxygen supply, inappropriate dosing of antibiotics,[27] and increased comorbidities. Patients who have obesity must be informed about the increased risk of infection and wound healing problems and the consequences of infection. It is not uncommon for patients undergoing arthroplasty to be obese; however, no consensus on BMI or weight exists that clearly denotes the increased risk of infection. Researchers have investigated for a BMI that should be used as a threshold for safely performing TKA. One study's findings showed that for patients who have a BMI of 35.0 to 39.9 kg/m², the risk of prosthetic joint infection was twice as high as for those with a BMI of less than 35 kg/m², and the risk was four times as high for those with a BMI of 40 kg/m² or higher.[26] The study also identified 100 kg as an absolute weight threshold for safely performing TKA. A 2016 study[28] found all-cause (not just infection-related) revision arthroplasty to be increased in those with a BMI higher than 35 kg/m². The revision rate was more than twofold greater for those with a BMI of 35 kg/m² as for those with a BMI of less than 35 kg/m². For patients who had a BMI of 35 kg/m² or higher and those with BMI less than 35 kg/m², survivorship at 5 years was 96.4% and 98.3%, respectively, and at 10 years was 93.7% and 97.2%, respectively.

Although increased BMI is an independent risk factor for revision TKA,[10] several potential reasons exist. The complexity of the case can result in increased surgical time in patients who have obesity, which has been associated with an increased rate of infection. For every additional 15 minutes of surgical time, the infection risk increases by 9%.[23] Patients who have obesity may require longer surgical time for exposure, correct implant position, and complex, multilayer closure, all secondary to excessive adipose tissue. During arthroplasty, the knee needs to bend at least 75° to 90° for implant placement; therefore, it is also important to consider not only the overall BMI but also the local soft-tissue envelope, which can be measured with a calf-to-thigh ratio.[29] This ratio representing the depth of the soft tissues about the knee may be more predictive of complications than BMI. From a technical standpoint, if the knee cannot bend because the posterior calf meets the thigh and prevents it from flexing, surgical exposure becomes much more difficult.

Implant Position

Adipose tissue that creates a large soft-tissue envelope can make implant positioning a challenge. It can be argued that implant positioning is even more critical in the patient who had obesity because of the increased mechanical loads applied to the joint.[30] Excessive effort required to sufficiently externally rotate the tibial implant or lateralize the femoral implant can result in implant malposition, increased mechanical strain on the bearing surfaces, and eventual premature implant failure. Increased BMI was associated with an increased risk of postoperative malalignment ($P = 0.076$), and the surgeon should aim for a deviation of ±3° from neutral of the mechanical axis. This is supported by a 2011 study[31] that reported that patients who had a BMI greater than 41 kg/m² had a higher failure rate than did those with a BMI between 23 and 26 kg/m². The rate increased from 0.7% to 2.6% ($P = 0.0046$) in well-aligned knees, from 1.6% to 2.9% ($P = 0.0180$) in varus-aligned knees, and from 1.0% to 7.1% ($P = 0.0260$) in valgus-aligned knees. In addition, a 10.8% increased risk of failure was reported for those who had a BMI greater than 41 kg/m². The data showed that for implant longevity, it is vital to ensure that the tibia is not cut in varus for those with a BMI greater than 41 kg/m². A failure rate of 21.9% was reported for a varus tibial cut in patients who have a BMI greater than 41 kg/m².

Accurate placement of standard cutting guides can be difficult in obese patients, and advanced technologies such as patient-specific cutting guides (or patient-specific instrumentation), navigation, and robotic-assisted surgery have been developed to help address this issue. Authors have reported satisfactory results with patient-specific instrumentation,[32] navigation,[33] and robotics.[34] Although these technologies are based on imaging studies (patient-specific instrumentation, some robotics and imaging-based navigation) or a digitally constructed model (imageless navigation and other robotics) specific to the patient, the bony cuts must be double-checked, as with standard instrumentation, to ensure that appropriate cuts are made. Although an experienced surgeon may think that he or she is able to align the joint within a 3° range of neutral, evidence suggests that the use of these technologies can limit the outliers of implant malpositioning.[32-35] Although there is some evidence that robotic-assisted unicompartmental knee arthroplasty in the obese has no worse clinical outcomes at mean 2-year follow-up,[36] there is no literature on robotic-assisted TKA for this group.

Although fewer alignment outliers can be expected when using these technologies, large well-designed studies will be needed to determine if they also improve implant longevity and long-term clinical outcomes in the obese population. However, acknowledging that there is increased risk to obese patients who have malaligned implants,[31] it is reasonable to add some adjunctive technology.

Preoperative Counseling

Because TKA is a purely elective procedure, it is in the patient's best interest to postpone surgery until preoperative health is optimized. Optimization should include more than a simple medical "clearance," and evidence demonstrates decreased readmissions and decreased costs with a program designed to screen and optimize both medical and psychosocial risk factors.[37] Despite minimal evidence that suggests preoperative weight loss in isolation will improve the patient's outcome,[38,39] its role in improving the patient's overall health will be beneficial. Weight loss can be achieved by diet, exercise, or even surgical intervention, as well as by addressing any nutritional deficits.[40,41]

SURGICAL RECOMMENDATIONS

The approach to TKA for both young and obese patients requires special consideration and planning on the surgeon's behalf. Neither case should be considered typical; therefore, surgeons experienced in adult reconstruction should handle these challenging cases. Both young and obese patients have higher-than-normal rates of revision surgery because of infection or aseptic loosening, which compromise implant longevity. These complications can be minimized by limiting handling of soft tissues, distalizing the surgical incision, proper implant positioning, resurfacing the patella, obtaining adequate fixation, and appropriate wound management.

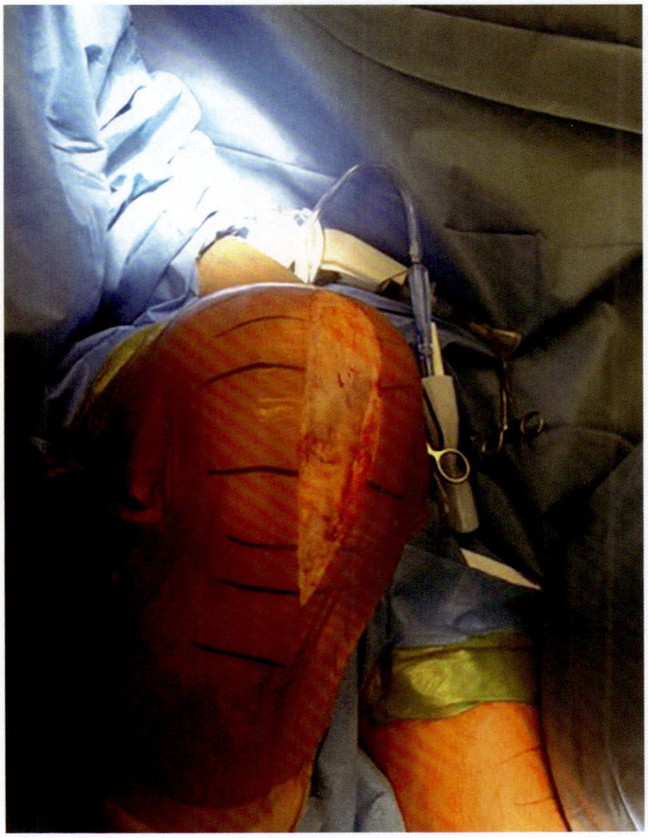

FIGURE 1 Intraoperative photograph demonstrates the no-hands skin incision with the knee in hyperflexion to minimize additional trauma to the peri-incisional soft-tissue.

No-hands Technique for Incision

Wound complications after an otherwise successful TKA are frustrating and may lead to infection. Infection is responsible for a large percentage of TKA revisions[7,10] in both obese and young patient cohorts; therefore, attention to the soft tissues is paramount. To optimize wound healing, handling of the soft tissues should be minimized. The surgeon can perform the skin incision with the knee in deep flexion with a no-hands technique during which no assistants are required to hold skin retractors (**Figure 1**). Sharp dissection is performed through skin and subcutaneous tissue down to the level of the vastus medialis obliquus muscle. A medial parapatellar arthrotomy can be performed, but either a midvastus or a subvastus approach can be used. The surgeon can avoid undermining the soft tissues by making thick soft-tissue flaps. Delaminating the subcutaneous adipose tissue from the fascia creates dead space for fluid to occupy and compromises the blood supply, which can result in incision-related complications.[42,43]

Assuming the location of the skin incision is correct, the arthrotomy will require no additional soft-tissue dissection. The soft tissue is left attached to the patella, and resurfacing is performed as the last of the three steps. Usually, additional tissue dissection is not needed to place the patellar clamp because at the end of the procedure, the tissue has been manipulated enough to allow correct placement of the patellar clamp.

The arthrotomy should be performed with the knee in deep flexion and should be as straight as possible to avoid the creation of acute angles around the patella. The surgeon can bring the arthrotomy as close to the patellar tendon as possible and not be concerned if a few fibers of the patellar tendon are included on the medial aspect of the arthrotomy. This reduces the amount of tissue to mobilize laterally when placing a retractor in the lateral aspect of the knee to expose the entire tibia. This facilitates the surgeon's access to the knee in the obese patient, for whom exposure can be challenging because of a substantial fat pad. After the arthrotomy is performed, the knee is moved out of flexion and a medial exposure is performed. This is the first time a retractor will be required.

Incision Location

Although it is important to obtain adequate visualization, the incision can be limited to only the necessary length. Instead of centering the incision over the patella, it should

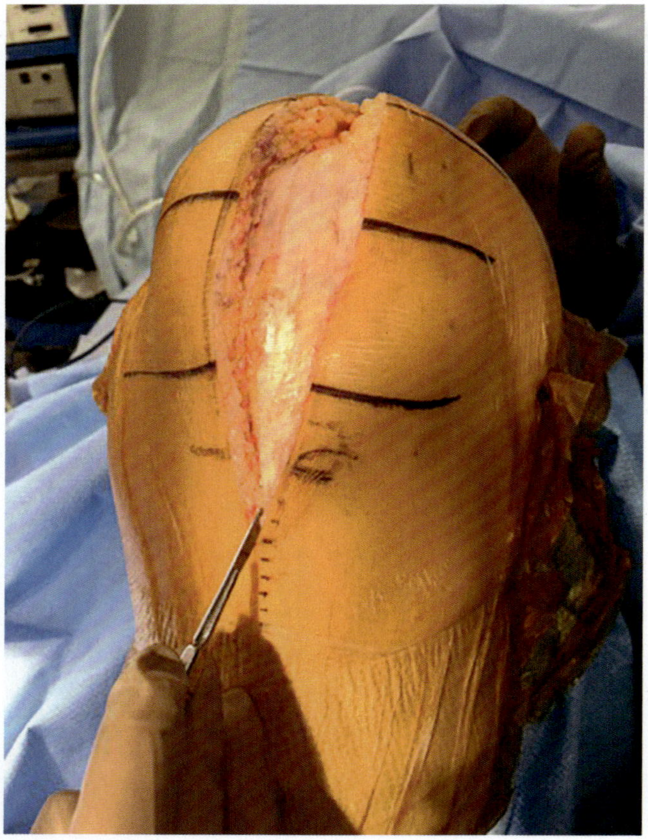

FIGURE 2 Intraoperative photograph shows the skin incision used during exposure for total knee arthroplasty. The distalized incision allows good visualization of the joint without unnecessary length.

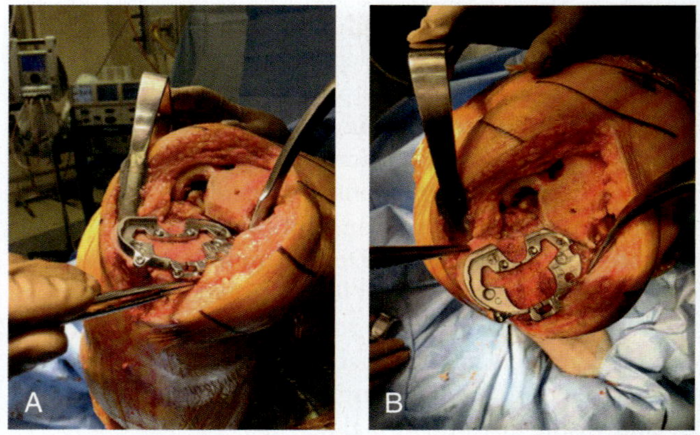

FIGURE 3 Intraoperative photographs obtained during total knee arthroplasty show external rotation of the tibial implant (**A**) and a superior view that shows a lateralized tibial implant with some uncovered medial tibia (**B**).

be biased slightly more distal so that less of the incision length is proximal to the superior pole of the patella and more length is distal to the inferior pole of the patella (**Figure 2**). Generally, any extension of the incision for exposure will be required distally. To perform a satisfactory medial release, the incision likely will have to extend past the tibial tubercle.

Implant Positioning: External Rotation of the Tibial Implant

External rotation of both the femoral and tibial implants is well documented to optimize flexion gaps and patellar tracking. Conventionally, the center of the tibial implant should align with the medial one-third of the tibial tubercle. Poor exposure of the posterolateral corner can result in malpositioning of the tibial implant into relative internal rotation if care is not taken to externally rotate the tibial implant appropriately (**Figure 3**). Slightly more external rotation should result in optimal tracking and reduce the need for a lateral retinacular release.

Resurface the Patella

Although no definitive evidence suggests that the patella should be resurfaced,[44,45] the rate of revision surgery is higher in patients whose patellae are not resurfaced during the index TKA. This may occur because patients still reporting anterior knee pain after arthroplasty without patellar resurfacing provide the surgeon with a potential reason for their continued discomfort and therefore may undergo a secondary patellar resurfacing. Meta-analyses have not been able to establish a superior technique.

It is important to ensure the implant is well positioned, which is achieved by placing the implant on the superomedial edge of the patella. After partial lateral facetectomy, if indicated, a symmetric or oval, domed, all-polyethylene three-peg button can be used to ensure the implant is fully seated on bone with no overlap into the soft tissues.

Obtain Adequate Fixation

Metaphyseal fixation is necessary to counteract the shear forces placed across the tibial implant. For younger or obese patients, every attempt should be made to maximize tibial fixation.[46] Several manufacturers provide a stem extension to the tibial baseplate keel to support the primary implants without adding a large stem that would be more commonly used in a revision setting. Although the literature has failed to demonstrate a clear benefit,[46-48] some still recommend[49] a stemmed implant be used in patients whose BMI is higher than 35 kg/m^2 (**Figure 4**) as it provides additional fixation and aids with alignment.

A more liberal approach to the use of metaphyseal fixation by using trabecular metal cones that provide excellent fixation and bony ingrowth can be implemented, although their use rarely is required in the primary setting (**Figure 5**). Studies have reported good results with metaphyseal sleeves to provide metaphyseal

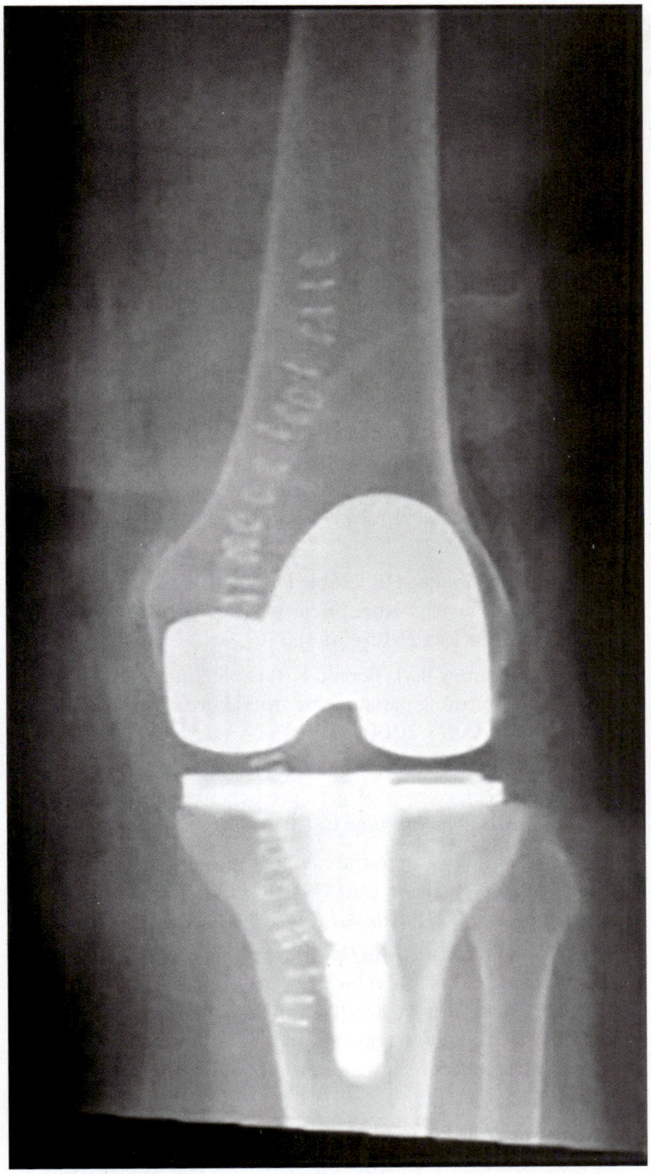

FIGURE 4 AP radiograph of the knee obtained following total knee arthroplasty shows the tibial implant with stem extension used for additional fixation of the tibial implant in patients who have a body mass index higher than 35 kg/m^2.

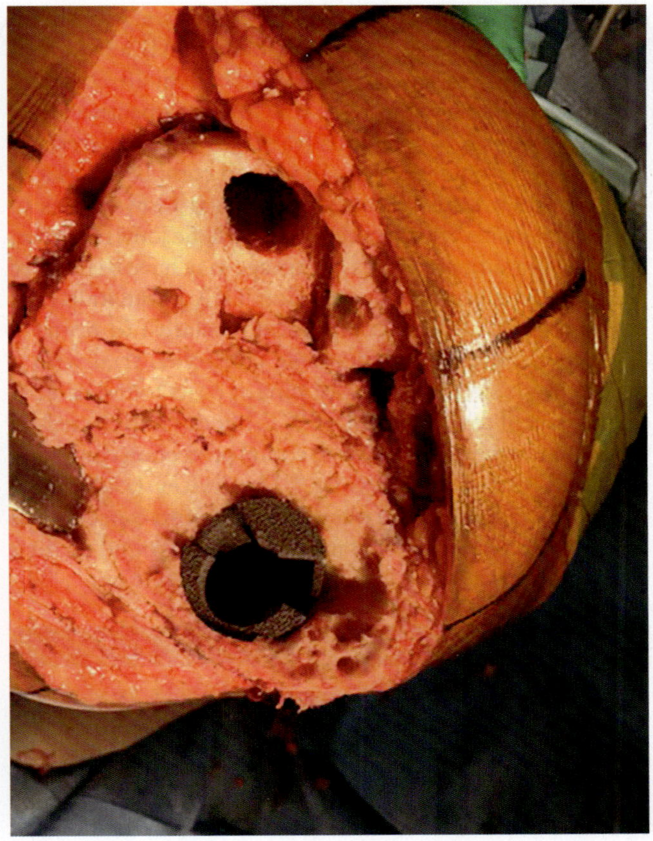

FIGURE 5 Intraoperative photograph shows the insertion of a tibial trabecular metal cone to obtain metaphyseal fixation during total knee arthroplasty and thus minimize the likelihood of loosening. This technique can be applied to both young patients and obese patients.

fixation.[50,51] However, cones can be placed independently of the tibial implant, which allows for optimal orientation, depending on where the metaphyseal region requires supplementation.

One of the disadvantages of placing a metaphyseal cone or sleeve is the amount of bone that has to be removed for placement. Although removal of bone is generally discouraged, it may be necessary, and bone should be sacrificed if the surgeon thinks the extra fixation will secure the implant and increase longevity. Aseptic loosening is the primary reason for revision of TKA in those younger than 55 years, and so secure fixation must be obtained in the primary TKA.[10] Cementless implants have been advocated as a solution to this problem: biologic metaphyseal fixation without excessive bony resection. Although at least one study concluded that cementless implants had improved survival in the obese population,[52] there were significant differences between the experimental groups in age, BMI, prosthesis design, and follow-up. Other studies have failed to demonstrate a difference between cemented and cementless fixation in obese[53,54] or young patients.[55]

Wound Management

Appropriate incision length and position, as well as soft-tissue handling as described earlier, are the first steps to avoiding wound problems. Despite the surgeon's best efforts, many obese patients still end up with wound problems. One technique for managing the wound in obese patients is the use of an incisional negative pressure wound therapy (iNPWT) device. These have been shown

Section 2: Knee

to improve short-term wound complications after hip and knee arthroplasty.[56] Obese patients (BMI >35 kg/m^2) undergoing TKA saw the greatest benefit in reducing wound complications in this study. A retrospective study (of revision TKAs) found an advantage to iNPWT relative to an antimicrobial dressing in wound complications and surgical site infections, and trends toward lower rates of superficial wound dehiscence, periprosthetic joint infection, and revision surgery.[57] This advantage may have been more pronounced given that the revision TKA population is at increased risk of these complications relative to primary TKA. A prospective randomized controlled trial with a small sample size primarily looking at costs found no economic benefit to the use of iNPWT, but did find decreased wound drainage and improved wound protection compared with conventional dry dressing.[58] The devices should therefore be considered in the obese TKA patient, especially in those with additional risk factors for poor wound healing such as diabetes, smoking, or in a revision setting.

SUMMARY

With the increase in the number of people requiring TKA, the surgeon performing arthroplasty will be expected to take the lead for challenging patient cohorts: both the young patient and the obese patient require special considerations. Both groups are at risk for experiencing early failure secondary to aseptic loosening and infection. Unique challenges include correct implant positioning and obtaining adequate fixation. Arthroplasty performed in either of these two patient populations should not be regarded as routine, and greater care must be taken to reduce the number of revisions performed in these groups. Meticulous surgical technique when handling the tissues, adequate exposure to allow optimal implant orientation, and satisfactory implant fixation are key to success in these demanding cases.

KEY STUDY POINTS

- Young patients are at increased risk for requiring revision surgery or even revision arthroplasty because of infection or aseptic loosening.
- Obesity is an independent risk factor for knee arthritis. A large percentage of the US population is considered overweight or obese; therefore, the expected number of arthroplasties in obese patients is expected to increase, and these individuals are at increased risk for the development of perioperative complications.
- Obese patients need to be counseled preoperatively regarding their risk of requiring revision secondary to infection, loosening, implant positioning, and wound complications.

ANNOTATED REFERENCES

1. Kurtz S, Ong K, Lau E, Mowat F, Halpern M: Projections of primary and revision hip and knee arthroplasty in the United States from 2005 to 2030. *J Bone Joint Surg Am* 2007;89(4):780-785.
2. Patel A, Pavlou G, Mújica-Mota RE, Toms AD: The epidemiology of revision total knee and hip arthroplasty in England and Wales: A comparative analysis with projections for the United States. A study using the National Joint Registry dataset. *Bone Joint J* 2015;97-B(8):1076-1081.
3. Hooper G, Lee AJ, Rothwell A, Frampton C: Current trends and projections in the utilisation rates of hip and knee replacement in New Zealand from 2001 to 2026. *NZ Med J* 2014;127(1401):82-93.
4. Insall JN, Dorr LD, Scott RD, Scott WN: Rationale of the Knee Society clinical rating system. *Clin Orthop Relat Res* 1989;248:13-14.
5. Scuderi GR, Bourne RB, Noble PC, Benjamin JB, Lonner JH, Scott WN: The new Knee Society Knee Scoring System. *Clin Orthop Relat Res* 2012;470(1):3-19.
6. Parvizi J, Nunley RM, Berend KR, et al: High level of residual symptoms in young patients after total knee arthroplasty. *Clin Orthop Relat Res* 2014;472(1):133-137.
7. Wainwright C, Theis JC, Garneti N, Melloh M: Age at hip or knee joint replacement surgery predicts likelihood of revision surgery. *J Bone Joint Surg Br* 2011;93(10):1411-1415.
8. Australian Orthopaedic Association National Joint Replacement Registry (AOANJRR): *Hip, Knee & Shoulder Arthroplasty: 2019 Annual Report*. Adelaide, AOA, 2019.

   This is the 20th annual publication of the Australian Orthopaedic Association National Joint Replacement Registry, including nearly 1.5 million arthroplasties. This is a large national registry with analysis of outcomes focusing on adverse outcomes, implant survivorship, and revision rates.
9. Vince KG: You can do arthroplasty in a young patient, but...: Commentary on articles by John P. Meehan, MD, et al: "Younger age is associated with a higher risk of early periprosthetic joint infection and aseptic mechanical failure after total knee arthroplasty," and Vinay K. Aggarwal, et al: "Revision total knee arthroplasty in the young patient. Is there trouble on the horizon?" *J Bone Joint Surg Am* 2014;96(7):e58.
10. Aggarwal VK, Goyal N, Deirmengian G, Rangavajulla A, Parvizi J, Austin MS: Revision total knee arthroplasty in the young patient: Is there trouble on the horizon? *J Bone Joint Surg Am* 2014;96(7):536-542.
11. Clement ND, Deehan DJ: Overweight and obese patients require total hip and total knee arthroplasty at a younger age. *J Orthop Res* 2020;38(2):348-355.

    This retrospective study looked at both total hip arthroplasty and TKA. There were 4,740 primary TKAs performed. Linear regression analysis was performed and, after controlling for confounders, indicated that patients with increased BMI underwent TKA at an earlier age. Compared to normal weight patients, TKA was performed at a significantly earlier age that became progressively earlier for patients in the overweight and class I, II, and III obesity groups. Levels of evidence: III.

12. Meehan JP, Danielsen B, Kim SH, Jamali AA, White RH: Younger age is associated with a higher risk of early periprosthetic joint infection and aseptic mechanical failure after total knee arthroplasty. *J Bone Joint Surg Am* 2014;96(7):529-535.
13. Long WJ, Bryce CD, Hollenbeak CS, Benner RW, Scott WN: Total knee replacement in young, active patients: Long-term follow-up and functional outcome. A concise follow-up of a previous report. *J Bone Joint Surg Am* 2014;96(18):e159.
14. Keeney JA, Eunice S, Pashos G, Wright RW, Clohisy JC: What is the evidence for total knee arthroplasty in young patients? A systematic review of the literature. *Clin Orthop Relat Res* 2011;469(2):574-583.
15. Ogden CL, Carroll MD, Kit BK, Flegal KM: Prevalence of childhood and adult obesity in the United States, 2011-2012. *J Am Med Assoc* 2014;311(8):806-814.
16. Welton KL, Gagnier JJ, Urquhart AG: Proportion of obese patients presenting to orthopedic total joint arthroplasty clinics. *Orthopedics* 2016;39(1):e127-e133.
17. Cawley J, Meyerhoefer C: The medical care costs of obesity: An instrumental variables approach. *J Health Econ* 2012;31(1):219-230.
18. Workgroup of the American Association of Hip and Knee Surgeons Evidence Based Committee: Obesity and total joint arthroplasty: A literature based review. *J Arthroplasty* 2013;28(5):714-721.
19. D'Apuzzo MR, Novicoff WM, Browne JA: The John Insall Award: Morbid obesity independently impacts complications, mortality, and resource use after TKA. *Clin Orthop Relat Res* 2015;473(1):57-63.
20. Kerkhoffs GM, Servien E, Dunn W, Dahm D, Bramer JA, Haverkamp D: The influence of obesity on the complication rate and outcome of total knee arthroplasty: A meta-analysis and systematic literature review. *J Bone Joint Surg Am* 2012;94(20):1839-1844.
21. Inacio MC, Paxton EW, Fisher D, Li RA, Barber TC, Singh JA: Bariatric surgery prior to total joint arthroplasty may not provide dramatic improvements in post-arthroplasty surgical outcomes. *J Arthroplasty* 2014;29(7):1359-1364.
22. Issa K, Pivec R, Kapadia BH, et al: Does obesity affect the outcomes of primary total knee arthroplasty? *J Knee Surg* 2013;26(2):89-94.
23. Namba RS, Inacio MC, Paxton EW: Risk factors associated with deep surgical site infections after primary total knee arthroplasty: An analysis of 56,216 knees. *J Bone Joint Surg Am* 2013;95(9):775-782.
24. Jämsen E, Nevalainen P, Eskelinen A, Huotari K, Kalliovalkama J, Moilanen T: Obesity, diabetes, and preoperative hyperglycemia as predictors of periprosthetic joint infection: A single-center analysis of 7181 primary hip and knee replacements for osteoarthritis. *J Bone Joint Surg Am* 2012;94(14):e101.
25. Paxton EW, Inacio MC, Khatod M, Yue E, Funahashi T, Barber T: Risk calculators predict failures of knee and hip arthroplasties: Findings from a large health maintenance organization. *Clin Orthop Relat Res* 2015;473(12):3965-3973.
26. Lübbeke A, Zingg M, Vu D, et al: Body mass and weight thresholds for increased prosthetic joint infection rates after primary total joint arthroplasty. *Acta Orthop* 2016;87(2):132-138.
27. Brill MJ, Houwink AP, Schmidt S, et al: Reduced subcutaneous tissue distribution of cefazolin in morbidly obese versus non-obese patients determined using clinical microdialysis. *J Antimicrob Chemother* 2014;69(3):715-723.
28. Zingg M, Miozzari HH, Fritschy D, Hoffmeyer P, Lübbeke A: Influence of body mass index on revision rates after primary total knee arthroplasty. *Int Orthop* 2016;40(4):723-729.
29. Yu S, Siow M, Odeh K, Long WJ, Schwarzkopf R, Iorio R: Periarticular soft tissue envelope size and postoperative wound complications following total knee arthroplasty. *J Arthroplasty* 2018;33:S249-S252.

    Finding BMI to be an inaccurate predictor of the size of the leg and surgical difficulty, the authors come up with the Periarticular Soft Tissue Index. They find it to be better correlated with the rate of minor complications and a nonsignificant trend for major complications than BMI. Levels of evidence: III.
30. Estes CS, Schmidt KJ, McLemore R, Spangehl MJ, Clarke HD: Effect of body mass index on limb alignment after total knee arthroplasty. *J Arthroplasty* 2013;28(8 suppl):101-105.
31. Ritter MA, Davis KE, Meding JB, Pierson JL, Berend ME, Malinzak RA: The effect of alignment and BMI on failure of total knee replacement. *J Bone Joint Surg Am* 2011;93(17):1588-1596.
32. Anwar R, Kini SG, Sait S, Bruce WJ: Early clinical and radiological results of total knee arthroplasty using patient-specific guides in obese patients. *Arch Orthop Trauma Surg* 2016;136(2):265-270.
33. Shetty GM, Mullaji AB, Bhayde S, Lingaraju AP: No effect of obesity on limb and component alignment after computer-assisted total knee arthroplasty. *Knee* 2014;21(4):862-865.
34. Mannan A, Vun J, Lodge C, Eyre-Brook A, Jones S: Increased precision of coronal plane outcomes in robotic-assisted total knee arthroplasty: A systematic review and meta-analysis. *Surgeon* 2018;16(4):237-244.

    This study did not specifically look at obese patients. This systematic review and meta-analysis assembled five studies (402 TKAs). Robotic-assisted TKAs had just 1/181 (0.006%) with a mechanical axis deviation greater than 3°, whereas in the conventional instrumentation group 42/159 (26.4%) were found to deviate greater than 3°. Their reported meta-analysis odds ratio was 0.04 (95% CI 0.01 to 0.14), with $P < 0.00001$. Levels of evidence: II.
35. Heyse TJ, Tibesku CO: Improved tibial component rotation in TKA using patient-specific instrumentation. *Arch Orthop Trauma Surg* 2015;135(5):697-701.
36. Plate JF, Augart MA, Seyler TM, et al: Obesity has no effect on outcomes following unicompartmental knee arthroplasty. *Knee Surg Sports Traumatol Arthrosc* 2017;25:645-651.

In this retrospective review of over 700 robotic arm-assisted medial unicompartmental knee arthroplasties (UKAs) with a minimum of 24-month follow-up (average BMI 32 kg/m^2), the authors looked at BMI and determined that it did not influence the rate of revision to TKA (5.8%) or 90-day readmission. It did, however, correlate with increased opioid requirements and increased number of physical therapy sessions to achieve discharge criteria. The authors suggest that some surgeons' use of BMI >30 kg/m^2 as a contraindication for UKA is outdated in the era of modern UKA techniques and technology. Level of evidence: IV.

37. Kim KY, Anoushiravani AA, Chen KK, et al: Perioperative orthopedic surgical home: Optimizing total joint arthroplasty candidates and preventing readmission. *J Arthroplasty* 2019;34:S91-S96.

    This retrospective study looked at nearly 4,200 elective total joint arthroplasties and identified the patients at highest preoperative risk for readmissions (Readmission Risk Assessment Tool score >3). Two hundred sixteen patients were identified who had been through the POSH preoperative optimization protocol that delays surgery until modifiable social and medical issues are optimized, and 978 patients were identified who proceeded to surgery without POSH optimization (they still had standard medical preoperative clearance). Participating patients experienced lower 30-day (1.6% versus 5.3%, $P = 0.03$) and 90-day (3.2% versus 7.4%, $P < 0.05$) readmissions and discharged to rehab at lower rates (15.3% versus 23.4%, $P = 0.01$). Level of evidence: I

38. Lui M, Jones CA, Westby MD: Effect of non-surgical, non-pharmacological weight loss interventions in patients who are obese prior to hip and knee arthroplasty surgery: A rapid review. *Syst Rev* 2015;4:121.
39. Severson EP, Singh JA, Browne JA, Trousdale RT, Sarr MG, Lewallen DG: Total knee arthroplasty in morbidly obese patients treated with bariatric surgery: A comparative study. *J Arthroplasty* 2012;27(9):1696-1700.
40. Nelson CL, Elkassabany NM, Kamath AF, Liu J: Low albumin levels, more than morbid obesity, are associated with complications after TKA. *Clin Orthop Relat Res* 2015;473(10):3163-3172.
41. Huang R, Greenky M, Kerr GJ, Austin MS, Parvizi J: The effect of malnutrition on patients undergoing elective joint arthroplasty. *J Arthroplasty* 2013;28(8 suppl):21-24.
42. Vince KG, Abdeen A: Wound problems in total knee arthroplasty. *Clin Orthop Relat Res* 2006;452:88-90.
43. Vince K, Chivas D, Droll KP: Wound complications after total knee arthroplasty. *J Arthroplasty* 2007;22(4 suppl 1):39-44.
44. Pilling RW, Moulder E, Allgar V, Messner J, Sun Z, Mohsen A: Patellar resurfacing in primary total knee replacement: A meta-analysis. *J Bone Joint Surg Am* 2012;94(24):2270-2278.
45. Pavlou G, Meyer C, Leonidou A, As-Sultany M, West R, Tsiridis E: Patellar resurfacing in total knee arthroplasty: Does design matter? A meta-analysis of 7075 cases. *J Bone Joint Surg Am* 2011;93(14):1301-1309.
46. Abdel MP, Bonadurer GF III, Jennings MT, Hanssen AD: Increased aseptic tibial failures in patients with a BMI ≥35 and well-aligned total knee arthroplasties. *J Arthroplasty* 2015;30(12):2181-2184.
47. Parratte S, Ollivier M, Lunebourg A, Verdier N, Argenson JN: Do stemmed tibial components in total knee arthroplasty improve outcomes in patients with obesity? *Clin Orthop Relat Res* 2017;475(1):137-145.

    A prospective randomized controlled trial investigated the functional outcomes scores, quality of life score, and mechanical complications or premature revisions in obese patients receiving either standard or short-stemmed tibial implants in 120 patients. Although there were small differences in functional outcomes scores favoring the stemmed tibias, the authors felt it was not likely to be clinically significant and concluded that they did not have evidence to support the use of stemmed implants. Level of evidence: I.

48. Steere JT, Sobieraj MC, DeFrancesco CJ, Israelite CL, Nelson CL, Kamath AF: Prophylactic tibial stem fixation in the obese: Comparative early results in primary total knee arthroplasty. *Knee Surg Relat Res* 2018;30(3):227-233.

    In the early-term (24 to 46 months follow-up) comparison of 178 consecutive primary TKAs in obese patients (BMI >35 kg/m^2), 50 of had stem extensions (30 mm stubby stem) implanted. There were no difference between the stemmed and standard tibial implant groups in terms of aseptic loosening or radiolucent lines, despite the stemmed group having a significantly higher average BMI (44 versus 40 kg/m^2). Levels of evidence: III.

49. Martin JR, Jennings JM, Dennis DA: Morbid obesity and total knee arthroplasty: A growing problem. *J Am Acad Orthop Surg* 2017;25:188-194.

    This review article covers many of the challenges of performing TKA in obese patients. Despite citing a lack of evidence, the authors suggest using stemmed tibial implants in obese patients.

50. Bugler KE, Maheshwari R, Ahmed I, Brenkel IJ, Walmsley PJ: Metaphyseal sleeves for revision total knee arthroplasty: Good short-term outcomes. *J Arthroplasty* 2015;30(11):1990-1994.
51. Graichen H, Scior W, Strauch M: Direct, cementless, metaphyseal fixation in knee revision arthroplasty with sleeves: Short-term results. *J Arthroplasty* 2015;30(12):2256-2259.
52. Bagsby DT, Issa K, Smith LS, et al: Cemented vs cementless total knee arthroplasty in morbidly obese patients. *J Arthroplasty* 2016;31(8):1727-1731.
53. Boyle KK, Nodzo SR, Ferraro JT, Augenblick DJ, Pavlesen S, Phillips MJ: Uncemented vs cemented cruciate retaining total knee arthroplasty in patients with body mass index greater than 30. *J Arthroplasty* 2018;33(4):1082-1088.

    This retrospective study looked at 325 TKAs performed in obese patients. One hundred fifty-four patients had uncemented cruciate-retaining (CR) TKAs implanted, and 171 had cemented CR TKAs implanted. The authors found similar rates of aseptic loosening and revision. Levels of evidence: III.

54. Lizaur-Utrilla A, Miralles-Muñoz FA, Sanz-Reig J, Collados-Maestre I: Cementless total knee arthroplasty in obese patients: A prospective matched study with follow-up of 5-10 years. *J Arthroplasty* 2014;29:1192-1196.
55. Kim YH, Park JW, Lim HM, Park ES: Cementless and cemented total knee arthroplasty in patients younger than fifty five years. Which is better? *Int Orthop* 2014;38:297-303.

56. Keeney JA, Cook JL, Clawson SW, Aggarwal A, Stannard JP: Incisional negative pressure wound therapy devices improve short-term wound complications, but not long-term infection rate following hip and knee arthroplasty. *J Arthroplasty* 2019;34:723-728.

This prospective randomized controlled trial included 398 patients (185 iNPWT and 203 standard dry dressing) and found no difference in superficial or deep infection. They did find that obese patients (BMI > 35 kg/m^2) undergoing TKA experienced significantly fewer complications (1.3% versus 21.6%, $P < 0.01$) when iNPWT was used instead of conventional dry dressing. Levels of evidence: II.

57. Cooper HJ, Bas MA: Closed-incision negative-pressure therapy versus antimicrobial dressings after revision hip and knee surgery: A comparative study. *J Arthroplasty* 2016;31:1047-1052.

58. Manoharan V, Grant AL, Harris AC, Hazratwala K, Wilkinson MPR, McEwen PJC: Closed incision negative pressure wound therapy vs conventional dry dressings after primary knee arthroplasty: A randomized controlled study. *J Arthroplasty* 2016;31:2487-2494.

CHAPTER 22

Unicondylar, Patellofemoral, Bicompartmental, and Bicruciate-Retaining Knee Arthroplasty

MOHAMAD J. HALAWI, MD • JORDAN LEBOVIC, MD, MBA • ANIL S. RANAWAT, MD
ANTONIO CUSANO, MD • JIBANANANDA SATPATHY, MD, MRCSEd
GREGORY J. GOLLADAY, MD • SAMIK BANERJEE, MD • JESS H. LONNER, MD
CHRISTOPHER E. PELT, MD • CHRISTOPHER L. PETERS, MD • WAEL K. BARSOUM, MD

ABSTRACT

Evolving indications, improved implant designs, growing availability of longer term results, and increased interest among both patients and surgeons in kinematic preservation and rapid recovery have expanded the use of unicondylar, patellofemoral, bicompartmental, and bicruciate-retaining total knee arthroplasties. Considering the projected increase in the prevalence of knee osteoarthritis, the merits of partial knee arthroplasty can be realized by a larger segment of the population with focal disease using appropriate indications and surgical techniques. In addition, if retaining the cruciate ligaments during total knee arthroplasty has the potential to re-create normal kinematics and a knee that feels more natural, it is possible that patients could be more satisfied with total knee arthroplasty.

Keywords: arthroplasty; bicompartmental; bicruciate-retaining TKA; patellofemoral; unicompartmental

INTRODUCTION

Among patients who have tibiofemoral osteoarthritis, the prevalence of medial, lateral, and bicompartmental involvement has been reported at 29.5%, 8.2%, and 14.9%, respectively.[1] In addition, among patients who have symptomatic knee osteoarthritis and are older than 20 years, 11% of men and 24% of women have isolated patellofemoral osteoarthritis.[2] Considering the projected increase in the prevalence of knee osteoarthritis, the merits of partial knee arthroplasty can be realized by a larger segment of the population with focal disease using appropriate indications and surgical technique. For patients who do not undergo partial knee arthroplasty, recent interest has been developed regarding the potential for retention of the anterior and posterior cruciate ligaments to potentially improve outcomes and optimize patient satisfaction.[3-6] The anterior cruciate ligament (ACL) is often intact in patients undergoing conventional total knee arthroplasty (TKA).[7] Retention of native soft tissues for knee stability, as opposed to traditional reliance on metal against plastic, could also

This chapter is adapted from Brother JG, Peters CL: Bicruciate-retaining total knee arthroplasty, in Mont MA, Tanzer M, eds: *Orthopaedic Knowledge Update®: Hip and Knee Reconstruction*, ed 5. Rosemont, IL, American Academy of Orthopaedic Surgeons, 2017, pp 143-148 and Halawi MJ, Yellin JL, Ranawat A, et al: Unicompartmental, patellofemoral, and bicompartmental knee arthroplasty, in Mont MA, Tanzer M, eds: *Orthopaedic Knowledge Update®: Hip and Knee Reconstruction*, ed 5. Rosemont, IL, American Academy of Orthopaedic Surgeons, 2017, pp 149-162.

potentially lead to decreased mechanical wear of the implant. If in doing so decreased prosthetic constraint and more normal sensation and kinematics are achieved, the advocated benefits of bicruciate-retaining (BCR) TKA could potentially help address issues of dissatisfaction and even implant survivorship. The ultimate goals of unicondylar, patellofemoral, bicompartmental, and BCR TKAs are to alleviate knee pain and restore motion while also preserving normal knee kinematics.

MEDIAL UNICONDYLAR KNEE ARTHROPLASTY

Indications and Contraindications

The indications for medial unicondylar knee arthroplasty (UKA) are not universally agreed on, but stringent criteria[8] have continued to provide a fundamentally sound and broadly accepted framework. These indications include osteoarthritis isolated to the medial compartment, age older than 60 years, weight less than 82 kg, low activity level, minimal pain at rest (noninflammatory etiology), intact ACL, flexion arc of at least 90°, and minimal fixed deformities (<5° flexion contracture and <10° varus angulation).[8]

Although contraindications to UKA are considered violations of the aforementioned criteria, a couple of studies have called these into question, especially with regard to activity level, obesity, age, ACL insufficiency, and the presence of anterior pain or patellofemoral degenerative disease. One study demonstrated a 94% UKA survival rate in a cohort of 62 patients aged 60 years or younger (mean age 54 years) at 12 years postoperatively, with more than 80% of the patients returning to sport activities.[9] The authors of a 2017 study found that the aforementioned indications would have failed in 68% of the 1,000 patients who underwent UKA.[10] When comparing UKA patients who have contraindications versus the ideal candidates, no differences were noted in pain or functional scores at 10 years. Furthermore, the ideal candidates had a higher rate of poor functional scores after 10 years.

Dr. Ranawat or an immediate family member has received royalties from DePuy, a Johnson & Johnson Company and Stryker Mako; is a member of a speakers' bureau or has made paid presentations on behalf of Ceramtec, Medtronic, Smith & Nephew, and Stryker Mako; serves as a paid consultant to or is an employee of Ceramtec, Medtronic, Moximed, Smith & Nephew, and Stryker Mako; has stock or stock options held in ConforMIS, Inc. and Enhatch; has received research or institutional support from DePuy Mitek-Synthes and Stryker; and serves as a board member, owner, officer, or committee member of the American Orthopaedic Society for Sports Medicine and EOA. Dr. Golladay or an immediate family member has received royalties from Orthosensor, Inc.; is a member of a speakers' bureau or has made paid presentations on behalf of Orthosensor, Inc.; serves as a paid consultant to or is an employee of Orthosensor; has stock or stock options held in Orthosensor, Inc.; has received research or institutional support from KCI and Orthosensor; and serves as a board member, owner, officer, or committee member of the American Association of Hip and the Knee Surgeons and Virginia Orthopaedic Society. Dr. Lonner or an immediate family member has received royalties from Biomet, Smith & Nephew, and Zimmer; is a member of a speakers' bureau or has made paid presentations on behalf of Biomet, Smith & Nephew, and Zimmer; serves as a paid consultant to or is an employee of Force Therapeutics, Muvr Labs, Smith & Nephew, and Zimmer Biomet; has stock or stock options held in Force Therapeutics, Muvr Labs, and Proteonova; has received research or institutional support from Force Therapeutics, Muvr Labs, Smith & Nephew, and Zimmer Biomet; and serves as a board member, owner, officer, or committee member of the American Association of Hip and Knee Surgeons. Dr. Pelt or an immediate family member has received royalties from TJO (Total Joint Orthopedics); is a member of a speakers' bureau or has made paid presentations on behalf of KCI, Smith & Nephew, TJO (Total Joint Orthopedics), and Zimmer Biomet; serves as a paid consultant to or is an employee of KCI, Smith & Nephew, TJO (Total Joint Orthopedics), and Zimmer Biomet; has received research or institutional support from Zimmer Biomet; and serves as a board member, owner, officer, or committee member of the American Academy of Orthopaedic Surgeons and the American Association of Hip and Knee Surgeons. Dr. Peters or an immediate family member has received royalties from Biomet; is a member of a speakers' bureau or has made paid presentations on behalf of Biomet; serves as a paid consultant to or is an employee of Biomet; has stock or stock options held in CoNextions Medical and Muve Health; has received research or institutional support from Biomet; and serves as a board member, owner, officer, or committee member of the American Association of Hip and Knee Surgeons and the Knee Society. Dr. Barsoum or an immediate family member has received royalties from Custom Orthopaedic Solutions, Exactech, Inc., Stryker, and Zimmer; is a member of a speakers' bureau or has made paid presentations on behalf of Stryker; serves as a paid consultant to or is an employee of Stryker; has stock or stock options held in Beyond Limits, Capsico Health, Custom Orthopaedic Solutions, Health XL, PeerWell, PT Genie, and Sight Medical; and has received research or institutional support from DJO, Inc., NIH, Orthosensor, Stryker, Third Frontier, and Zimmer. None of the following authors or any immediate family member has received anything of value from or has stock or stock options held in a commercial company or institution related directly or indirectly to the subject of this chapter: Dr. Halawi, Dr. Lebovic, Dr. Cusano, Dr. Satpathy, and Dr. Banerjee.

UKA in obese patients also continues to lack consensus in the literature. In a 2016 meta-analysis of clinical studies and national registries, it was concluded that patients who had a body mass index (BMI) greater than 30 kg/m^2 had no increased risk for poor outcomes.[11] Interestingly, the authors of a 2018 study reported that, in patients who had a BMI greater than 35 kg/m^2, UKA was associated with lower infection rates (zero versus 0.5%), fewer manipulations under anesthesia (0.5% versus 6.5%), and fewer returns to the operating room for any reason (3.7% versus 9.2%) compared with TKA.[12]

ACL deficiency has traditionally been a contraindication to medial UKA, particularly for mobile-bearing implants. Because the ACL primarily restrains anterior tibial translation relative to the femur, patients who have deficient ACLs have altered biomechanics that result in posterior contact loading and increased strain at the anterior tibial bone-cement interface that may result in tibial loosening.[13] However, a 2014 study reported no significant difference in the survivorship of fixed-bearing UKA (primarily medial UKA) between patients with and without intact ACLs in the absence of clinical instability at 6-year follow-up.[14] Patients undergoing UKA who had a deficient ACL were compared with those undergoing UKA who had simultaneous ACL reconstruction.[15] Increased implant survival was found in the ACL reconstruction group. Furthermore, fixed-bearing implants were found to have lower revision rates than mobile-bearing implants. The primary reason for revision in the mobile-bearing implants was tibial implant loosening. Therefore, it is reasonable to perform a fixed-bearing UKA in an ACL-deficient knee, as long as there is no functional instability and the tibial chondral wear pattern is in the anterior half of the plateau; however, longer follow-up studies are needed to determine whether ACL reconstruction improves long-term implant survival.

Another traditional contraindication to medial UKA is the presence of anterior knee pain and/or degeneration of the patellofemoral joint. It has been suggested that patellofemoral joint arthritis is caused by improper knee alignment, which may be potentially corrected through UKA. In a meta-analysis of the literature, no significant differences were found in the revision rates or functional outcomes in patients undergoing UKA stratified by presence or absence of patellofemoral joint arthritis.[11] Similarly, equivalent functional outcomes were found in patients who had mobile-bearing implants, regardless of the presence of patellofemoral joint arthritis.[10]

The primary indication for medial UKA should be isolated, end-stage medial compartment osteoarthritis in a knee with at least 90° flexion arc, <5° flexion contracture, and <10° coronal angulation. Data continue to be presented from obese patients, younger patients, and those who have high activity levels. Inflammatory arthritis and the presence of severe pain or advanced osteoarthritis in another compartment are contradictions to isolated medial UKA. The requirement of an intact ACL is controversial, and longer term studies are needed to ascertain the validity of performing fixed-bearing UKA in ACL-deficient knees.

Preoperative Evaluation

A thorough preoperative history and physical examination must be performed, in addition to the evaluation of appropriate radiographic studies, to ensure the aforementioned indications and contraindications for medial UKA have been addressed. A surgical candidate's history should reveal progressive medial knee pain that has markedly affected the patient's quality of life and/or has interfered with normal daily activities. A history of inflammatory arthritis should be ruled out as the etiology. Physical examination should not reveal erythema because this may indicate an infectious or systemic etiology. Range of motion (ROM) should be greater than 90°. A flexion contracture, if present, should not exceed 5° to 10°. The lateral compartment should be evaluated, with no lateral pathology evident on McMurray test or palpation of lateral joint line. The integrity of the ACL should be assessed with both the Lachman and pivot-shift tests. Varus deformities should be partially or completely correctable on valgus stressing in 20° of flexion or under 10° of flexion if fixed, although accurate determination of correctability is not possible until osteophytes are removed.[16]

On radiographic assessment, only the medial compartment should demonstrate signs of osteoarthritis. Standing AP, bilateral PA in flexion, and lateral views are used to assess the degree of osteoarthritis and may reveal osteophytes, sclerosis, joint space narrowing, subchondral cysts, and signs of bone loss (**Figure 1**). Minimal tibiofemoral subluxation is acceptable. On the lateral view, identification of posteromedial tibial wear can be a sign of chronic ACL insufficiency. A sunrise view can help assess degeneration of the patellofemoral joint. Long leg radiographs are useful in assessing overall alignment. MRI may be obtained if there is concern for ligamentous, chondral, or meniscal injury in the other compartments.

Surgery should be recommended only after nonsurgical treatment options have failed. The preoperative evaluation should include a description of the intended surgical procedure and its common risks and benefits, including the potential conversion to a TKA if deemed necessary.

Surgical Technique

In medial UKA, the two prevailing bearing designs are fixed and mobile bearing. In the fixed-bearing design, stability is mildly restricted by its nonconforming articulating

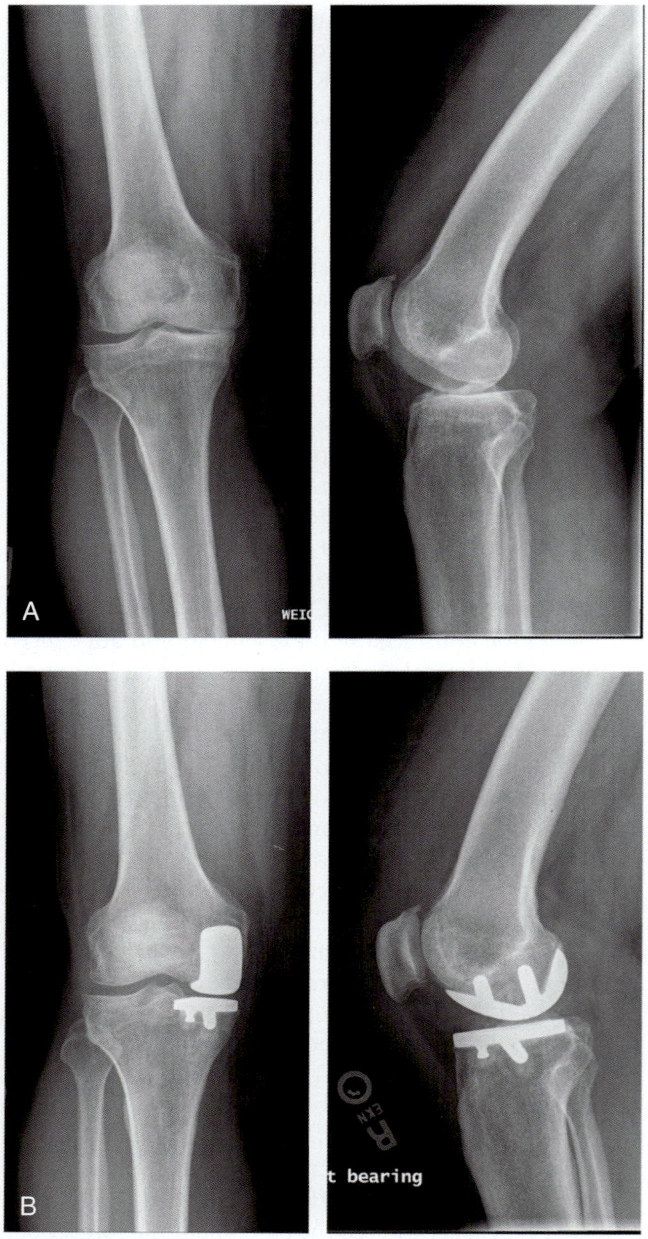

FIGURE 1 Weight-bearing AP and lateral radiographs of a 59-year-old man with a 3-year history of right knee pain (**A**) before and (**B**) at 1-year follow-up after medial unicompartmental knee arthroplasty.

surface, thus predisposing the implants to peripheral wear and repetitive edge loading.[17] However, proponents of fixed-bearing UKA favor its relative technical ease of implantation, specifically regarding ligamentous balancing, and its decreased risk of implant dislocation, when compared with mobile-bearing UKA.[18]

Regardless of implant type used, the key predictors of successful outcomes with medial UKA procedures include restoration of limb mechanical axis, accurate implant positioning, and proper ligament balancing.[19] Earlier surgical techniques relied on standard jigs, based on techniques used in TKA, to produce accurate intraoperative alignment. This so-called conventional UKA uses either extramedullary or intramedullary instrumentation to make appropriately angled tibial and femoral osteotomies.[20] However, the literature has demonstrated that many conventional systems are inherently limited and possibly inaccurate (conceivably because of the limited visibility/exposure of a UKA compared with TKA), thus requiring a great deal of surgical judgment both preoperatively and intraoperatively.[19] An alternative technique is computer-assisted or robotic-assisted UKA. In computer-assisted UKA, infrared stereoscopic cameras are linked to position sensors attached to a patient's femur or tibia, and surgical instruments are used to create a digital model of the joint. Real-time visualization of this model is then used throughout the case, especially during implant positioning to ensure proper alignment. However, in a study comparing mechanical axis, hip-knee-ankle angle, coronal plane alignment, and tibial slope between conventional and navigated UKAs, a statistically significant difference favoring computer navigation was only noted in the posterior tibial slope.[21] Robotic-assisted UKA uses a robotic arm guided by tactile feedback and a preoperative computer interface to allow the surgeon to resurface only the degenerative knee surfaces, thereby preserving healthy bony and soft-tissue structures while insuring optimal alignment.[22] In a study comparing 44 conventional with 33 robotic-assisted UKAs, there was greater implant positioning accuracy in the sagittal and coronal planes for robotic-assisted cohort.[23] Newer image-free robotic technology using a free-hand sculpting tool has shown equivalent precision and an ability to quantify soft-tissue balance without the need for preoperative CT scans. Registration and mapping are performed entirely intraoperatively and protection against inadvertent bone removal is achieved by modulating the exposure or speed of the sculpting burr.[24,25] Additionally, by eliminating the CT scan required for preoperative planning, this robotic device minimizes exposure to unnecessary radiation. In a recent study, it was reported that the learning curve associated with robotic UKA was six cases.[26] In terms of the revision rate, the authors of a 2018 study found that the 2-year revision rate in the manually instrumented group was 3.6% compared with zero in the robotic-assisted group.[27]

Outcomes

When examining outcomes of medial UKA, useful information can be gleaned through comparisons between fixed-bearing versus mobile-bearing implants, metal-backed versus all-polyethylene tibial implants, cemented versus cementless bearings, and medial UKA versus TKA.

Fixed Versus Mobile Bearings

No consensus currently exists as to whether fixed-bearing or mobile-bearing UKA provides better overall long-term results. A systematic review that included only comparative studies between fixed-bearing and mobile-bearing implants, focusing on complications, was performed.[18] The most common reason for revision surgery in mobile-bearing UKA was progression of arthritis followed by aseptic loosening and bearing dislocation. In the fixed-bearing group, the most common reason for revision surgery was polyethylene wear, followed by progression of arthritis, aseptic loosening, and persistent unexplained pain. However, the overall rate of revision surgery between the two groups was almost identical.

Metal-backed Versus All-polyethylene Implants

A total of 160 metal-backed, fixed-bearing medial UKA were analyzed at mean 20-year follow-up (range, 0 to 20 years); 74% implant survival and excellent clinical outcomes as measured by Knee Society Score knee and function scores were reported at most recent follow-up.[28] Similar improvements were demonstrated in Knee Society Score knee and function scores using all-polyethylene tibial implant in 53 medial UKAs.[29] However, there have been no effective head-to-head trials comparing metal-backed to all-polyethylene UKA. A randomized trial comparing metal-backed and all-polyethylene implants found higher 7-year survivorship for metal-backed implants (93.8% versus 56.5%).[30]

Cemented Versus Cementless Fixation

Aseptic loosening is the primary cause of revision UKA, and high failure rates are associated with earlier cementless implants. However, cemented UKA implants have proved challenging because of smaller surface areas and limited visibility. This has led to increased interest in cementless fixation with improved implant designs. In a randomized controlled trial of 43 patients who underwent cemented versus cementless UKA with a mobile-bearing design, a higher rate of complete radiolucencies with cemented implants was noted at 2-year follow-up (zero versus 25%).[31] Cemented and cementless UKA implants have comparable survival rates after 10 years.[32]

Medial UKA Versus TKA

UKA survival rates have been consistently reported as inferior to those of TKA.[33] Intermediate data from the Kaiser Permanente Total Joint Registry found a higher rate of aseptic revision in UKA compared with TKA (2.0% versus 1.4%).[34] Large-scale national registry data, based on patient-reported outcome scores, demonstrated no advantage in satisfaction or functional improvement in UKA when compared with TKA.[35] It should be noted, however, that several advantages for UKA over TKA have been reported, particularly in regard to decreased morbidly, hospital length of stay, readmission, and mortality.[36] The authors of a 2017 study differentiated causes of failure of UKA in the Norwegian database between 1992 to 2004 and 2005 to 2015.[37] An increased proportion of failures in UKA is now caused by osteoarthritis progression, whereas fewer failures in UKA are due to periprosthetic fractures, aseptic loosening, and polyethylene wear. Notably, TKA demonstrated increased improvement in 10-year implant survival (91% to 94%), whereas UKA implant survival rates remained similar (80% to 81%). Although the revision rates tend to be higher in UKA, it is worth noting that higher UKA revision rates may be due to UKA revision generally being a far less complicated and time-intensive procedure, thus potentially lowering the threshold for revision surgery.[38]

Cost Effectiveness of UKA Versus TKA

A cost-effectiveness study comparing UKA and TKA was performed.[39] The study found decreased lifetime costs and increased quality-adjusted life-years associated with UKA compared with TKA in all patients older than 65 years. This finding was largely contingent on the rehabilitation costs associated with TKA. In cases when either TKA rehabilitation costs decreased or UKA rehabilitation costs increased, UKA was no longer cost effective relative to TKA.

LATERAL UKA

Indications and Contraindications

Isolated lateral compartment arthritis is seen in about 5% to 10% of patients who have knee osteoarthritis.[39] Accordingly, lateral UKA accounts for only a small proportion of partial knee arthroplasty procedures. Ideal candidates for lateral UKA are similar to those described for medial UKA. Patients should have exhausted all nonsurgical management and experience pain and functional deficits that affect the daily quality of life. Primary osteoarthritis, traumatic arthropathy, and osteonecrosis are the most frequent diagnoses. Inflammatory arthropathy is generally considered a relative contraindication. Comorbid conditions need to be optimized as for any elective surgery, and patient expectations need to be set appropriately relative to expected outcomes, risks, and benefits.

Preoperative Evaluation

Patients who have isolated lateral compartment arthrosis will have pain localized exclusively laterally. Physical examination should confirm ROM greater than 90° with less than 10° of flexion contracture, less than 10° of fixed valgus deformity, and intact collateral and cruciate ligaments.[2] Radiographic imaging should include

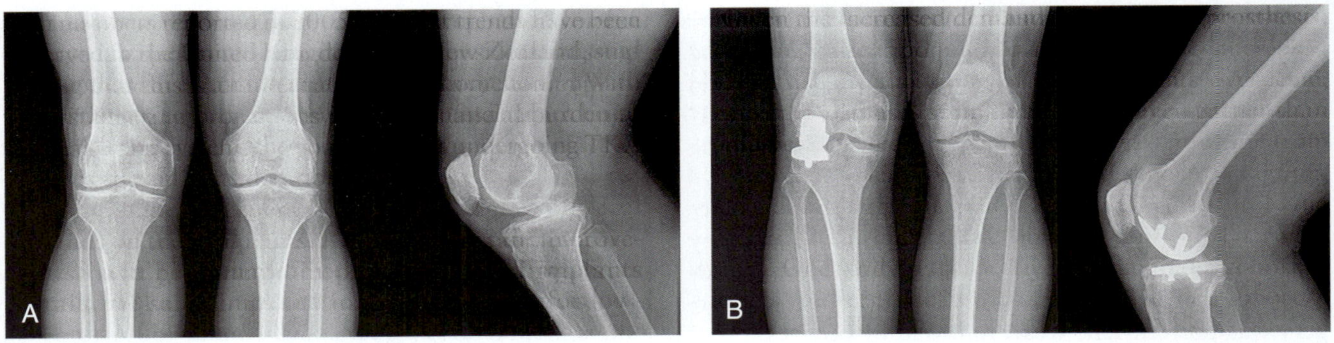

FIGURE 2 **A**, Preoperative AP (left) and lateral (right) radiographs obtained from a 61-year-old man with right knee pain for approximately 10 years following a skiing accident. **B**, AP (left) and lateral (right) views for this patient 4 weeks after lateral unicompartmental knee arthroplasty.

weight-bearing AP, lateral, PA flexion, sunrise, and long leg alignment radiographs (**Figure 2**). The deformity should be passively correctable. A history of anterior knee pain, patellofemoral crepitus/apprehension, or radiographic findings of degenerative joint disease in other compartments are relative contraindications to lateral UKA. If patellofemoral arthrosis is present, lateral facet changes are more likely well tolerated than medial disease because deformity correction will tend to shift patellar contact medially.

Surgical Technique

The surgical approach can be either a medial or lateral parapatellar depending on the surgeon's preference. A lateral parapatellar incision is a less-invasive technique that allows easier soft-tissue balancing and has been suggested to afford a greater degree of improvement in postoperative flexion.[40] Exposure is facilitated with figure-of-4 positioning of the leg. Extension tightness can be alleviated with release of the posterolateral capsule and arcuate ligament. Care should be taken to avoid damage to the intermeniscal ligament to preserve the functional integrity of the medial meniscus. Some surgeons prefer a medial parapatellar approach for all cases in the event that intraoperative conversion to TKA is necessary.[41] There are also concerns that less-invasive approaches may adversely affect implant positioning[42] and risk loosening or revision surgery.[43]

Bony preparation is performed through a variety of techniques including standard instrumentation with or without navigation, patient-specific instrumentation (PSI), or robotic assistance. Although computer-assisted and robotic-assisted procedures improve radiographic alignment especially in the sagittal plane,[44,45] there is paucity of robust long-term data to suggest superiority over conventional instrumentation. With regard to PSI, the authors of a 2017 study demonstrated a trend toward more precise measurements with narrower standard deviations when using PSI even in the hands of novice operators.[46] A total of 12 orthopaedic trainees naïve to lateral UKA were instructed to perform the procedure on sawbones using conventional instrumentation alone and separately using PSI. The primary outcome was the ability to perform the procedure according to a preoperative plan. Overall, PSI was associated with more precise values in the mean translational alignment of the femoral implant and mean rotational alignment of the femoral and tibial implants. More accurate implant positioning may result in improved long-term outcomes that not only affect the lateral compartment itself but also prevent disease progression in the medial compartment.[47] The femoral implant should be sized appropriately to avoid encroachment on the trochlea that can result in patellar impingement. Minimal femoral resection is recommended to avoid joint line elevation. The femoral implant should be externally rotated and lateralized to fill the flexion gap, minimize impingement on the lateral patellar facet, and promote congruent articulation with the tibia in terminal extension. Conversely, care should be taken to internally rotate the tibial implant to aid in tibiofemoral congruency in terminal extension.[48] In addition, 10° to 15° of internal rotation of the tibial implant[28] and residual valgus alignment of 3° to 7° appear to favorably affect survivorship.[49] It is important not to overload the medial compartment. Typically, lateral UKAs feel slightly looser compared with medial UKAs. Natural tibial slope should be reproduced. Maintaining a tibial slope of less than 7° results in lower loosening rates.[50] Undercutting or damaging the ACL insertion should be carefully avoided.

Outcomes

There has traditionally been a higher risk of bearing dislocation in mobile-bearing lateral UKAs, with rates as high as 8.5% at 5 years irrespective of surgeon's learning curve.[51] Recent literature, however, has shown improved short-term outcomes for mobile-bearing lateral UKA using a newly developed domed tibial implant.[52]

In a retrospective review of 41 patients undergoing lateral UKA at a single institution using this dome-shaped design, there was only 1 of 41 bearing dislocations (2.4%) at a minimum 2-year follow-up.[52] Similar findings were observed in two other groups. In a retrospective review of 61 lateral UKAs in 58 patients using the same domed mobile-bearing design, only one patient (1.72%) experienced bearing dislocation at a median follow-up of 84 months.[53] In another series of 265 consecutive lateral UKAs, the authors reported a dislocation rate of 1.5% at a mean follow-up of 4 years.[54] Therefore, technical and implant design modifications appear to have reduced the incidence of bearing dislocation in mobile-bearing lateral UKAs.[55]

Fixed-bearing design is particularly preferred in lateral UKA, primarily driven by higher technical demands and concerns of bearing dislocation in the mobile-bearing design. In a retrospective review of 52 consecutive fixed-bearing lateral UKAs with a minimum follow-up of 3 years, the authors noted an implant survival rate of 98% with only one revision secondary to progression of medial compartment osteoarthritis.[56] In another retrospective review of 101 fixed-bearing lateral UKAs in 100 patients, implant survivorship was 95.5% at 5 years.[57] One case was revised for subsidence of the tibial implant and another for progression of medial compartment osteoarthritis.

Midterm to long-term follow-up data show lateral UKA to be an effective treatment for isolated valgus osteoarthritis with survivorship equivalent to that of medial UKA and TKA, even in patients younger than 60 years. Currently, most revisions of lateral UKA are due to progression of arthritis, aseptic loosening, wear, or unexplained pain.[58] Conversion of a failed UKA to TKA may be accomplished with similar results to primary TKA, although need for revision components may limit the clinical outcomes.[59]

Medial Versus Lateral UKA

In a recent cadaver study using computer navigation to compare joint kinematics of medial and lateral UKAs before and after surgery, the authors found that only lateral UKA preserved native rotational kinematics.[60] Interestingly, in a recent retrospective review using serial radiographic evaluations of lateral versus medial UKAs performed by a single surgeon over an 11-year period, the rate of tibiofemoral osteoarthritis was significantly higher for lateral UKA compared with medial UKA.[61]

PATELLOFEMORAL ARTHROPLASTY

Indications and Contraindications

The primary indication for patellofemoral arthroplasty (PFA) is isolated patellofemoral degenerative disease with the goal of preserving native joint kinematics, joint stability, and healthy tissues in the medial and lateral tibiofemoral compartments. Pain should be restricted to the retropatellar and/or peripatellar areas and usually exacerbated with activities, such as stair or hill ambulation, squatting, lunging, kneeling, or prolonged sitting. Typically, patients who have isolated patellofemoral degenerative disease report less pain when standing or while walking on level ground. Characteristically, patients who have undergone PFA for primary patellofemoral osteoarthritis may have a higher incidence of progression to tibiofemoral osteoarthritis compared with those with patellofemoral osteoarthritis secondary to trochlear dysplasia, patellar maltracking, or posttraumatic patellofemoral arthritis.[62]

Moderate patellar tilt or subluxation observed on preoperative tangential radiographs or at the time of surgery can easily be corrected with a lateral retinacular recession or release, medialization of the patellar component, or lateral partial facetectomy. However, patients who have excessive Q angles should undergo tibial tubercle realignment before or concurrent with PFA (although some trochlear prosthesis contours and shapes may accommodate a slightly increased Q angle). There are no upper age criteria for PFA, provided the other criteria are met.[63]

Contraindications to PFA include considerable uncorrectable patellar maltracking or malalignment, coexisting coronal or sagittal plane deformity, inflammatory arthritis, active infection, chondrocalcinosis, and advanced degenerative changes (Kellgren-Lawrence grade III or higher) in the tibiofemoral compartments. There should be no symptoms of tibiofemoral arthritis including pain with ambulation on level ground. The presence of medial or lateral joint line pain suggests more diffuse chondral disease and should be considered a contraindication to isolated PFA. Patients who have inappropriate expectations and those with unusually excessive or disproportionate pain requiring narcotics may not be suitable candidates. Severe quadriceps atrophy/weakness, flexion contracture, and limited ROM are also contraindications to PFA. Despite intuitive concerns, currently there are no data on whether obesity or cruciate ligament insufficiency places PFA at higher risk for failure. Severe patella baja with patellar tendon scarring or patella alta may affect the results of PFA in terms of patellar tracking and/or predisposing to residual peripatellar pain. However, these are relative contraindications to PFA depending on individual circumstances, implant designs, and surgeon experience. Although PFA is useful for some patients who have Kellgren-Lawrence grade IV chondromalacia of the lateral patellar facet and/or lateral trochlea, no specific recommendation could be made to perform PFA in patients who have isolated advanced chondromalacia of the medial patellar facet and/or medial trochlea because medial-sided patellofemoral chondral wear typically should not be very painful. However, when it is, other sources of anterior pain should be ruled out and nonsurgical options pursued.

Intuitively, because of the increased patellofemoral stresses associated with increased weight, obese patients are thought to be at increased risk of failure after PFA.[64] Obese patients are more likely to have subtle or overt tibiofemoral disease that can compromise the results of PFA. Previous studies have demonstrated that obese patients (BMI >30 kg/m^2) are at higher risk for revision surgery for a variety of reasons.[65,66] However, to date, there is no accepted BMI cutoff for PFA. Similarly, there is currently no consensus regarding optimal age for patients undergoing PFA, although studies generally have advocated for a younger patient population (30 to 60 years of age) compared with that undergoing TKA.[67] Nevertheless, excellent outcomes are achievable even in octogenarians who have isolated patellofemoral arthritis.[68]

Also, the association between psychological distress or psychiatric disease and suboptimal postoperative outcomes is being recognized.[68] Accordingly, it is important to determine the mental status of patients before proceeding with PFA and set appropriate and realistic expectations. **Table 1** summarizes the indications and contraindications of PFA.

Preoperative Evaluation

A detailed history and physical examination are usually sufficient to localize pain to the anterior compartment of the knee. Several key components of the history include determining whether there was previous trauma, a history of subluxation or dislocation, or previous treatments that failed or succeeded in relieving the pain. The pain associated with patellofemoral chondromalacia or osteoarthritis is almost always directly retropatellar or just medial or lateral to the patella. Typically, patellofemoral pain worsens when descending stairs or hills, squatting, sitting for a long time, and rising from a seated position. Patellofemoral crepitus is often present. Other causes of anterior knee pain must be ruled out, including patellar tendinitis, quadriceps tendinitis, prepatellar or pes anserine bursitis, medial or lateral meniscal tear, and concomitant tibiofemoral arthritis.

The physical examination should assess lower extremity coronal and sagittal alignment, muscle strength, and patellar tracking. It should also determine whether the pain is localized to the patellofemoral compartment. Patellar inhibition and/or compression should produce pain and crepitus. Any associated tenderness along the medial or lateral joint lines should raise the suspicion of more diffuse chondral injury and meniscal pathology, which are contraindications to isolated PFA. Careful assessment of patellar tracking, including the presence of the J sign and evaluation of the Q angle, is important. If there appears to be associated malalignment or evidence of subluxation, then patellar realignment may be needed before or during PFA. ROM should typically demonstrate full extension and reasonable amount of flexion. ROM assessment should also focus on the location of pain and its relation to the degree of flexion.

TABLE 1

Indications and Contraindications for PFA

Indications	Contraindications	Relative Contraindications
Advanced primary isolated patellofemoral osteoarthritis	Tibiofemoral osteoarthritis or ≥ grade III tibiofemoral chondromalacia	BMI >40 kg/m^2
Posttraumatic patellofemoral osteoarthritis	Tibiofemoral subchondral bone edema	Isolated grade IV chondromalacia of medial patellar facet and/or medial trochlea
Patellofemoral osteoarthritis secondary to patellar maltracking ± trochlear dysplasia	Inflammatory arthritis or chondrocalcinosis	Preoperative opioid dependence
Mild patellar subluxation or tilt	Knee instability	Disproportionate pain
Grade IV chondromalacia of lateral patellar facet and/or lateral trochlea	Limb malalignment (valgus > 8°, varus > 5°)	Anterior pain during level ground walking equivalent to pain with descending stairs, kneeling, or squatting
Retropatellar/peripatellar pain worsened by descending stairs, kneeling, squatting	Flexion contracture	Age < 30 yr
—	Uncorrectable patellar malalignment	Tibiofemoral tenderness

BMI = body mass index, PFA = patellofemoral arthroplasty

Pain occurring predominantly beyond 30° to 40° and persisting throughout the ROM to full flexion may be associated with patellofemoral disease. More proximal patellar lesions present with pain in initial flexion, whereas more distal lesions present with pain in deep knee flexion. Evaluation for the presence and location of any scars around the knee, neurovascular status, and examination of the hip and the lumbar spine is a part of the comprehensive evaluation of a patient who has presumed patellofemoral osteoarthritis.

Radiographic evaluation with weight-bearing AP and midflexion PA views is important to rule out tibiofemoral arthritis (**Figure 3**). Mild squaring of the femoral condyles and small marginal osteophytes are acceptable, provided there is no tibiofemoral joint line pain or greater than grade III chondromalacia (based on MRI and clinical assessment). Lateral radiographs may show patellofemoral osteophytes, joint space narrowing, and the presence of patella alta or baja (**Figure 3**). Axial radiographs (eg, sunrise projection at 30° of knee flexion) can demonstrate

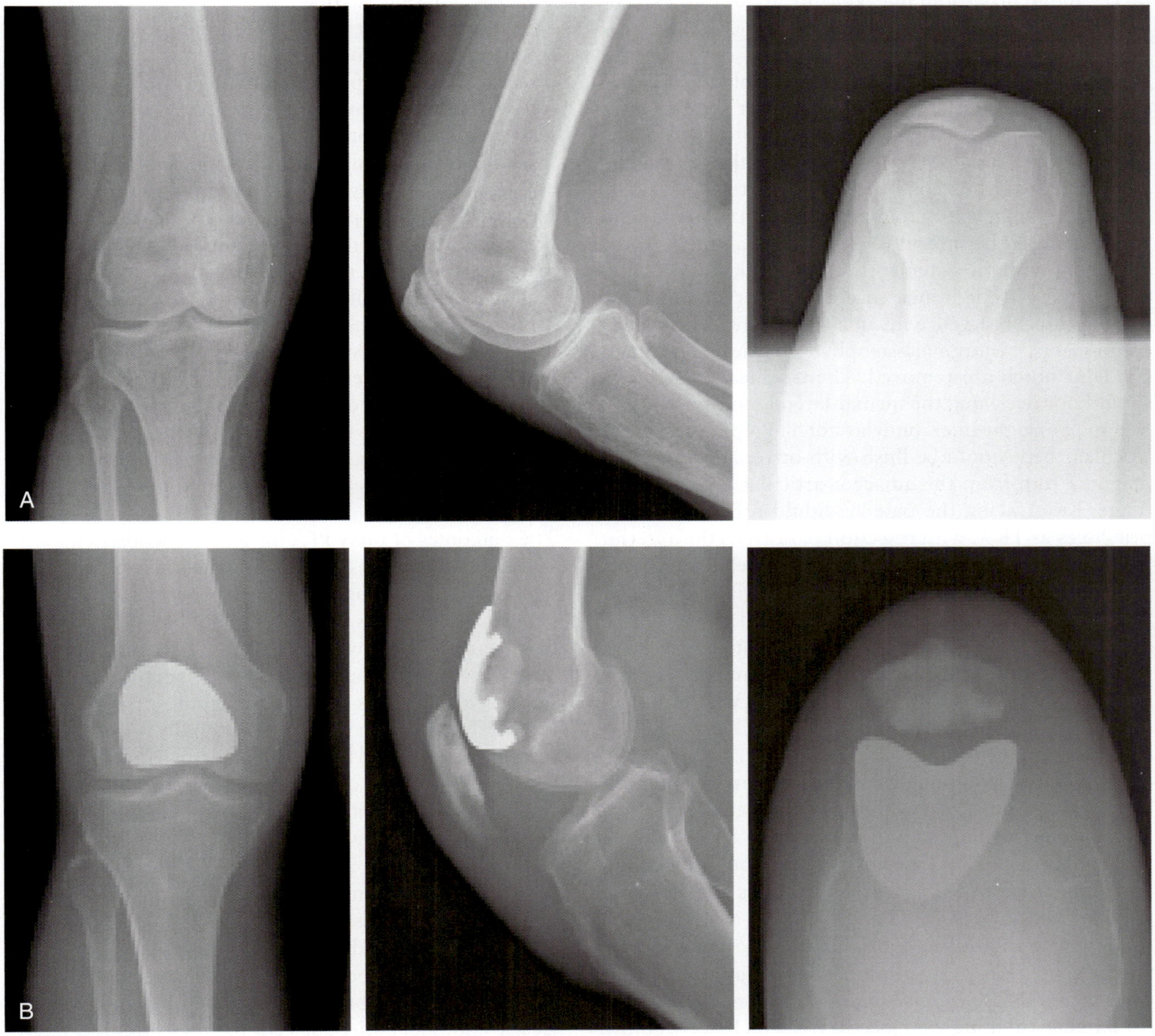

FIGURE 3 **A**, Weight-bearing AP, lateral, and sunrise radiographs demonstrating patellofemoral arthritis. **B**, Postoperative AP, lateral, and sunrise radiographs for a patient after patellofemoral arthroplasty. (Reproduced from Newman MT, Lonner JH, Ries M: Unicompartmental, patellofemoral, and bicompartmental arthroplasty, in Glassman AH, Lachiewicz PF, Tanzer M, eds: *Orthopaedic Knowledge Update®: Hip and Knee Reconstruction*, ed 4. Rosemont, IL, American Academy of Orthopaedic Surgeons, 2011, pp 107-118.)

the position of the patella in the trochlear groove and whether there is any trochlear dysplasia, patellar tilt, or subluxation (**Figure 3**). MRI can help determine whether there is cartilage loss in the tibiofemoral compartments or condylar edema (which would contraindicate isolated PFA), and status of the menisci and ligaments. If applicable, previous arthroscopy images should be reviewed to confirm isolated patellofemoral arthritis and rule out associated tibiofemoral pathology. CT scans may be used occasionally for evaluation of trochlear dysplasia, bone stock, measuring tibial tubercle–trochlear groove distance, and malrotation, but typically are not necessary.

Surgical Technique

Several key steps in the procedure will enhance surgical outcomes. The first step is ensuring that the trochlear component is externally rotated so that it is perpendicular to the AP axis of the femur (or parallel to the epicondylar axis), thus ensuring proper patellar tracking. This prerequisite is often impossible with inlay designs, which tend to be internally rotated as a result of the alignment with the anterior trochlear peaks[69,70] accounting for the very high incidence of patellar catching and subluxation observed with inlay compared with onlay components.[71] Marginal osteophytes bordering the intercondylar notch are removed. The trochlear component should not overhang the medial-lateral femoral margins or impinge on the intercondylar notch. Preparation of the trochlear bed should be flush with or recessed approximately 1 mm from the adjacent articular condylar cartilage. Resurfacing the patella should follow the same principles as TKA, with resection parallel to the anterior patellar cortex, restoration of proper patellar thickness, and medialization of the component. The lateral patellar facet and osteophytes should be removed or beveled to avoid lateral impingement and enhance patellar tracking.

With the trial components in place, patellar tracking is assessed. Additionally, checking for ACL impingement from the distal aspect of the trochlear implant is essential at this stage. If patellar tilt, subluxation, or catching of components is present, proper component position must be ensured and any deficiencies corrected. A lateral retinacular recession or release can be performed. In severe cases of subluxation, a proximal realignment with vastus medialis obliquus advancement may be necessary. If the Q angle is high, tibial tubercle realignment should be considered. Postoperative care is similar to TKA protocols with immediate full weight bearing and ROM exercises unless additional procedures for patellar tracking were necessary, which may require a more cautious approach to rehabilitation. Most cases are safely performed on an outpatient basis with standard risk-stratified prophylaxis protocols for venous thromboembolism.[72]

The critical distinction between early success and failure after PFA is determined by whether the patellar prosthesis tracks well in the trochlear prosthesis.[71] Several trochlear design features, including sagittal radius of curvature, proximal extension, width, thickness, tracking angle, asymmetry, constraint, and perhaps most importantly, whether it is inlay-style or onlay-style prosthesis, can affect patellar tracking.[73] Most inlay designs, with narrow trochlear flange widths, replaced only the trochlear cartilage, thus preserving the subchondral bone and resulting in the trochlear implant positioned flush with the adjacent cartilage. Inherently, this resulted in the femoral implant being placed parallel to the native trochlear inclination leading to internal rotation of the prosthesis, causing patellar tracking problems, instability, and subluxation. On the contrary, onlay designs, with broader anterior trochlear flange widths and valgus-trochlear tracking angles, replace both subchondral bone and cartilage. Onlay designs require the same anterior femoral bone cuts, perpendicular to Whiteside line, as performed in conventional TKA. These morphometric features, including narrowed distal trochlear widths, facilitate better patellar tracking and patellofemoral congruity during flexion with minimal impingements during extension from narrowed distal trochlear widths. Some newer generation designs have asymmetrical trochlear designs with elevated lateral flanges to resist lateral displacement forces, whereas others have lateralized and deepened trochlear grooves to improve patellar tracking.

Outcomes

The outcomes of inlay PFA have been inconsistent, with high rates of failures caused by patellar instability and maltracking, resulting in the need for secondary surgeries or revision.[71] This is primarily related to the inlay-style trochlear implants, which as a result of being positioned flush with the articular cartilage surface of the native anterior trochlea with its rotational alignment parallel to the trochlear inclination tend to be internally rotated. This is further compounded by the often narrower medial-lateral coverage and more obtuse radius of curvature of inlay trochlear components. This often results in component flexion and proximal step-off from the prepared bone leading to catching and instability in the initial arc of flexion.[74] This common problem led to the development of onlay trochlear designs, which have markedly improved patellar tracking and functional outcomes.[75-77]

Recently, improved short-term and midterm outcomes have been reported because of further refinements in surgical technique, patient selection, and optimized onlay-style trochlear implant designs.[73,78] Improvements in onlay trochlear designs include more anatomic trochlear tracking angles, better valgus trochlear groove orientations, smaller and more physiologic radii of curvatures, broader medial-lateral size ranges, increased proximal trochlear extension, and lateral facet thicknesses less than 5 mm. In addition, the trochlear components have near-perfect congruity with the patellar implants during the initial 60° of flexion, keeping the patella engaged until it transitions onto the native femoral condyles in deeper flexion. By optimizing patellar tracking, onlay-style trochlear components have minimized the need for secondary surgeries and rates of revision or conversion to TKA compared with inlay designs[71] (**Figure 4**). Moreover, onlay-type PFAs are versatile and can be used in all patients regardless of the native trochlear morphology or dysplasia. With the current generation of onlay prostheses, progression of tibiofemoral osteoarthritis is considered the main cause for PFA failures in multiple studies.[79] Component loosening and wear are rare with cemented onlay designs, with more than 90% survivorship at midterm follow-up.[76,79] In a meta-analysis of 22 studies on PFA involving more than 1,100 patients, significantly higher odds of revision (odds ratio 4.9) and revision surgery (odds ratio 4.3) were found with first-generation compared with second-generation PFA implants.[80] Although PFA may potentially improve patellofemoral congruence by correcting trochlear dysplasia,[81] patients with mild patellofemoral arthritis on radiographs demonstrate less functional improvement after PFA than do those with end-stage arthritis.[82]

In the absence of tibiofemoral osteoarthritis, revision of inlay-style PFA to onlay designs to correct patellar maltracking or instability secondary to internal rotation of the trochlear component has been shown to be effective.[83] However, conversion to TKA can provide predictable outcomes for treating patients with failed or malpositioned PFA, with results comparable with those of primary TKA if revision of the patella can be avoided.[84] In the event that conversion to TKA is necessary, retaining a well-positioned and unworn all-polyethylene patellar component is recommended.

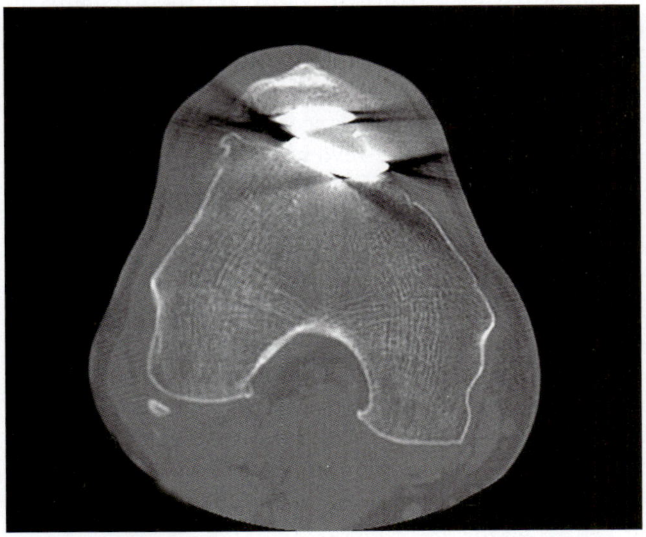

FIGURE 4 Axial CT scan showing internal rotation of inlay-style trochlear component relative to the AP axis of the femur, resulting in lateral patellar subluxation. (Reproduced from Newman MT, Lonner JH, Ries M: Unicompartmental, patellofemoral, and bicompartmental arthroplasty, in Glassman AH, Lachiewicz PF, Tanzer M, eds: *Orthopaedic Knowledge Update®: Hip and Knee Reconstruction*, ed 4. Rosemont, IL, American Academy of Orthopaedic Surgeons, 2011, pp 107-118.)

BICOMPARTMENTAL ARTHROPLASTY

Indications and Contraindications

Bicompartmental arthroplasty (BCA) is an alternative to TKA that addresses bicompartmental degenerative disease, usually in the patellofemoral joint and either the medial or lateral tibiofemoral compartments. Among patients undergoing knee arthroplasty in the United States, it has been reported that 28% of them have bicompartmental arthritis.[85] Given the growing demand for knee arthroplasty in younger patients who have bicompartmental disease pattern, BCA is an appealing bone-preserving and bicruciate-preserving procedure, especially given the increased risk of future revision surgery in this patient population and the desire for more normal kinematics and function.

The indications for BCA are evolving. Current indications are similar to UKA, except that changes of any extent in the patellofemoral joint are permitted. Coronal and sagittal deformities should not exceed 10°, all ligaments should be clinically intact,[85] and there should be at least 90° arc of motion.[86] Contraindications include global knee pain, advanced tricompartmental degenerative joint disease, inflammatory arthritis, and previous ligamentous reconstruction or periarticular osteotomies.[45]

Preoperative Evaluation

Appropriate patient selection is important. History should elicit pain location, duration of symptoms, and presence of inflammatory arthropathy, as well as prior injuries and treatment. Tenderness on examination must be limited to the patellofemoral joint and one tibiofemoral compartment. Assessment of ROM, coronal alignment, ligamentous stability, and fixed flexion contracture is necessary. Preoperative imaging studies should include weight-bearing AP, 45° flexion PA, lateral, and patellofemoral axial views (**Figure 5**). A stress view may be obtained if the coronal deformity does not correct on clinical examination, although complete correction is not a requirement.[87] MRI may aid in evaluating the quality of articular cartilage but is not routinely indicated.

Surgical Technique

A standard midline incision is often used. A medial parapatellar, lateral parapatellar, or subvastus arthrotomy is

Section 2: Knee

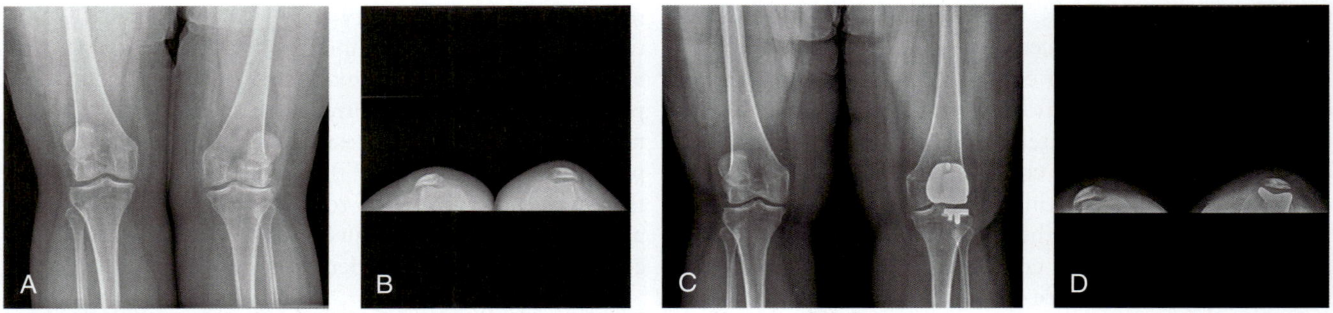

FIGURE 5 Preoperative AP (**A**) and Merchant (**B**) radiographs obtained from a 36-year-old woman with a history of patellar dislocations in the left knee, a medical history indicative of Ehlers-Danlos syndrome hypermobility type, and patellar realignment surgery. AP (**C**) and Merchant (**D**) views obtained 6 weeks after patellofemoral and lateral unicompartmental arthroplasty.

performed depending on the involved compartments or extent of exposure required. Two implant designs are available: a monolithic (single piece) or modular (separate implants for each compartment). The complexity of surgery depends on the implant type with higher technical demands involved with the use of the monolithic design. In a single-surgeon retrospective study, the learning curve for this design was 40 cases, which correlated with a reduction in surgical time from 114 to 65 minutes.[85] The primary challenge with the monolithic design is that coronal alignment is dictated by the opposition of the lateral edge of the trochlear component on the unresurfaced lateral femoral condyle.[88] With high variability in the morphology of the distal femur, relying on implant fit in one compartment may lead to a sizing and alignment mismatch in the other linked compartment. A custom-made monolithic or modular implant along with PSI based on CT scan of the affected knee is available and may allow more accurate positioning.[89] Preparation of the proximal tibia is usually performed first in a similar manner to UKA. The tibia is cut perpendicular to the anatomic axis. The femoral condyle is then prepared next. The flexion-extension gaps are assessed with spacer blocks to ensure equal gaps after preparation, usually with the goal of 2° of undercorrection. The patella is resurfaced in a manner similar to TKA. Robotic arm assistance is also available, which can optimize component position and alignment.[88] In a retrospective review of 30 robotic-assisted unlinked, modular BCAs in 29 patients at a mean follow-up of 27 months (range, 12 to 54 months), 24 of 29 (84%) had good to excellent outcomes using the Oxford Knee Score.[90]

Outcomes

The outcomes of BCA are widely variable, with most long-term studies reporting unacceptable results.[49] The monolithic design has been particularly associated with higher incidence of patellofemoral complications. In a midterm follow-up of 40 patients who had BCA using this design, the rate of persistent anterior knee pain was 24%.[87] In a prospective randomized trial, it was found that despite higher improvement in patient-reported outcomes among patients undergoing BCA compared with TKA, this advantage did not persist after 1 year, and there was a significantly increased complication rate in this group.[91]

In contrast with the limited success of the monolithic design, excellent short-term and midterm outcomes have been reported with use of modular, unlinked implants. These designs allow independent sizing and alignments of each implant, thereby eliminating the technical problems of monolithic implants. In a retrospective review of 29 consecutive modular BCAs with a minimum follow-up of 2 years, there was significant improvement in functional scores with no cases of patellar instability, implant loosening, or progressive arthritis.[87] However, there remains no clear advantage of modular BCA over conventional TKA. In a prospective, randomized clinical trial comparing TKA with modular BCA, there were no differences in ROM, pain scores, or knee-specific scores at 5-year follow-up.[92] In another prospective review comparing 15 BCAs in 11 patients to 16 TKAs in 13 patients followed up to 12 months postoperatively, there were no differences in knee muscle strength and physical function, although the TKA group performed better in stair climbing.[93] In a systematic review with meta-analysis of patients undergoing modular BCA versus TKA, the authors found no differences in terms of patient-reported outcomes, length of stay, or rates of complication and revision surgery at a minimum of 2-year follow-up (range, 2 to 5 years). There was reduction in intraoperative blood loss in the BCA group at the expense of increased surgical time.[94]

BICRUCIATE-RETAINING TOTAL KNEE ARTHROPLASTY

Indications/Contraindications

In contrast to UKA, for which the unresurfaced compartments pose a concern for existing or later degeneration, BCR TKA manages disease in all three knee compartments. Furthermore, without retained cartilage, progression of inflammatory disease is not a concern. The most essential requirement to perform a BCR TKA is the presence of functionally intact cruciate ligaments. Most current designs have little constraint and therefore require the native stability of these ligaments. Partial ACL degeneration is a controversial contraindication, but at least two studies have shown good results in this subset of patients.[5,12] Although late failure of the ACL may not cause catastrophic failure, patients who have a BCR TKA and subsequent ACL tear demonstrate more abnormal kinematics, which may lead to instability.[16] ACL competency can be determined intraoperatively using direct visualization or preoperatively using MRI, physical examination, or radiography. It is estimated that 78% of patients undergoing TKA have an intact ACL.[5] The Lachman test performed with the patient under anesthesia has poor sensitivity when used alone (33%), which increases to 90% when combined with an MRI. Sagittal wear on plain radiographs is another indicator of the ACL status. Anterior wear of the medial tibial plateau indicates an intact ACL, whereas posterior medial tibial wear indicates an incompetent ACL.

BCR TKA does not have the capability to correct severe malalignment because of the internal constraint of the cruciate ligaments. The following deformity parameters should be considered as relative contraindications: greater than 10° of varus or valgus joint deformity, less than 90° of flexion, and greater than 10° of flexion contracture, and recurvatum deformity.[7] Of interest, when both cruciate ligaments are preserved, most knees will not incur significant flexion contracture or coronal plane deformity because of maintained posterior roll back, intact posteromedial cartilage, and preserved native soft-tissue tension.[95]

Except for the aforementioned requirement of having functionally intact cruciate ligaments and avoidance in cases of excessive deformity, the same indications and contraindications for traditional TKA also apply to BCR TKA.

Surgical Technique

Bicruciate TKA is performed in much the same way as traditional TKA (**Figure 6**). However, variations in alignment, ligament balancing, joint line restoration, and fixation remain areas of ongoing investigation. Surgery is often performed through a medial parapatellar approach. The femoral cuts are made first using a measured resection technique, with 5° of valgus and rotation set to match the epicondylar axis. Departure from the traditional TKA technique occurs on the tibial side with the goal of achieving a minimal resection to allow for the thinnest bearing/baseplate couple that re-creates the native joint line (meniscal remnant line can be used as a reference). This depth of resection, which is forced by the need to maintain the appropriate tension on the retained cruciate ligaments, is often more than most surgeons may typically take in the setting of traditional cruciate-retaining or posterior-stabilized TKA. The tibial rotation is set in line with the

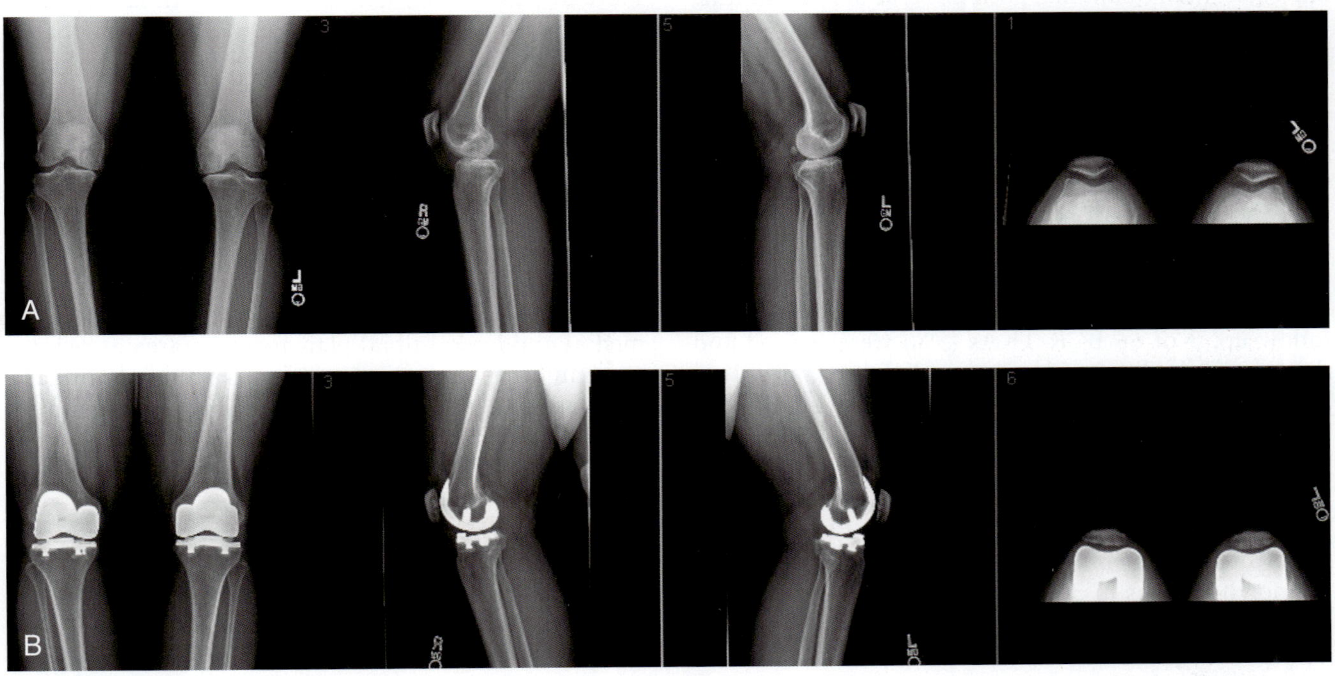

FIGURE 6 AP, lateral, and sunrise radiographs in a 47-year-old woman with bilateral knee osteoarthritis (**A**) before and (**B**) at 5-year follow-up after bilateral bicruciate-retaining total knee arthroplasty.

axis of the PCL/ACL island and the native proximal tibial rotation. The tibial resection should also match the native tibial slope without exceeding a maximum of 7°, over which there is concern for increased risk of tibial subsidence. Given the inherent lack of significant ligament contracture due to the indications for BCR TKA, ligamentous balancing is either rarely performed or minimal. The cruciate ligaments are protected and undermining is avoided. Careful cementation is performed with perforation of any sclerotic bone with a drill bit and/or use of a multispiked bone punch. The bony surfaces are thoroughly irrigated with pulse-lavage irrigation and dried. The implants are then cemented, the tibial component first followed by the femoral implant. The trial bearing is inserted and the knee is taken to extension and held still with slight constant pressure until the cement had fully cured. Only then is the knee moved, inspected, and cleaned of any residual extruded cement. Trial bearing is exchanged for the final polyethylene bearing. Differential bearing thicknesses or types could be used depending on surgeon discretion to achieve optimum soft-tissue balance.

Clinical Outcomes

The outcomes of earlier BCR TKA designs showed promising features, including increased patient preference compared with traditional TKA designs, improved proprioception, more natural kinematics, and good survivorship (excluding failures related to polyethylene wear).[96] During assessment of the Forgotten Joint Score, the outcomes of BCR TKA were found to be similar to UKA and better than traditional posterior cruciate-substituting TKA.[97,98] To date, few other studies have been able to demonstrate superior patient-reported outcomes with the use of BCR TKA compared with traditional TKA designs.

In a series of 146 BCR TKAs followed up to 12 months postoperatively, the authors found a 94% rate of neutral to high patient satisfaction with only two revisions (1.4%) and one manipulation under anesthesia.[6] In another study[5] using the same implant design and similar surgical technique, the authors found less favorable results when assessing 66 of the first 78 BCR TKAs. At 12-month follow-up, 3 of 66 BCR TKAs (5%) were revised and there was a higher incidence of radiolucent lines. In a more recent retrospective review of 175 BCR TKAs using a different implant design, a survivorship of 88% (82% to 93%) was reported at a mean follow-up of 3 years (range, 0.34 to 4.9 years).[99] The reasons for the revisions in 19 patients were isolated tibial implant loosening in 5 patients, ACL impingement in 3, persistent pain in 4, unknown reasons in 3, femoral and tibial components loosening in 2, and ACL deficiency and arthrofibrosis in 1 patient each. There was no clustering of revisions in the early experience. There was also no change in the rate of revision over time, suggesting no correlation between revisions and the learning curve. It should be noted, however, that in addition to its retrospective nature, the study was limited by the fact that 34 knees (19%) were excluded because of lack of follow-up data.

To address some unique failure patterns and challenges that are introduced when using BCR TKA, modern designs have added various adaptations including cross-linked polyethylene to address the concern of increased wear seen with earlier implant designs,[96] although the long-term outcomes of this change are unknown. In addition, because restoration of the normal joint line is of importance to appropriately balance all four retained ligaments in the setting of BCR TKA, increased tibial bone resection is often required compared with posterior-stabilized and cruciate-retaining TKA. If not adequately resected, joint line elevation may occur. Altering the joint line (primarily joint line elevation or overstuffing) can lead to increased ACL tension in extension, intraoperative and late ligament failure, and bone island fractures.[3,5,6] Furthermore, the ACL must be protected throughout the duration of the surgical procedure to prevent iatrogenic injury and often requires the use of additional cutting jigs, smaller saw blades, and protective guides. The central bone block at the ACL insertion determines tibial implant rotation and becomes another possible step to introduce error into the surgical technique. Tibial fixation, with a dominant mode of failure being tibial implant loosening, is another concern.[5] Tibial loosening may be influenced by the cementing technique, which may be more difficult in the setting of reduced tibial exposure and reduced tibial fixation given the challenge of adding a central keel while preserving a central tibial bone block.[100] Clinical studies of a recently introduced BCR TKA design containing a tibial keel are not yet available to tell if the addition of such a keel, among other modifications, is successful at addressing the issues of tibial fixation. Furthermore, although attempting to couple the medial and lateral tibial resections using with a single baseplate design as widely adopted by most modern BCR TKA designs, the connection between the medial and lateral tibial plateaus is an area at risk for mechanical fatigue fracture of the tibial implant. Last, postoperative arthrofibrosis in patients suffering from preoperative stiffness has been described to be more common in BCR TKA than posterior-stabilized TKA.[101]

SUMMARY

The demographic demands and expectations of patients undergoing knee arthroplasty are changing and dissatisfaction continues to be an issue. With the belief that improved proprioception and more natural kinematics could improve on this issue, partial knee arthroplasty and BCR TKA have seen a resurgence in interest and utilization. With appropriate patient selection and technique, UKA, PFA, and BCA can be successful, less-invasive options for localized degenerative knee disease. Surgical indications, especially for UKA, continue to evolve and are primarily driven by bearing design. As for BCR TKA, despite the introduction of modern designs that aim to improve on the shortcomings of previous implant materials and designs, several technical complexities unique to BCR TKA along with few studies showing significant differences in patient-reported outcomes between BCR and traditional TKA may ultimately limit its widespread adoption.

KEY STUDY POINTS

- With appropriate patient selection and technique, UKA is a successful and less-invasive option for tibiofemoral osteoarthritis limited to one compartment. Improvement in alignment in one tibiofemoral compartment may facilitate normalization of the joint space and, consequently, prevent or slow down the progression of degenerative changes in the other compartment. Surgical indications continue to evolve and are primarily driven by the bearing design.
- Current evidence suggests that PFA has excellent functional outcomes and survivorship of more than 90% with modern generation onlay designs at midterm follow-up. Using current generation onlay designs, avoiding anterior femoral notching, obtaining correct rotational alignment perpendicular to Whiteside line or parallel to the transepicondylar axis, lateral translating the femoral implants, partial lateral patellar facetectomy, medializing the patellar component, and performing lateral retinacular release to optimize patellar tracking if necessary are all key steps to improve the outcomes of PFA.
- Modular, unlinked BCA appears to be a promising alternative to TKA, with equivalent preliminary outcomes. However, larger long-term prospective studies are needed to clearly establish the utility, cost effectiveness, and survival of BCA.
- Although the prospect of retaining both cruciate ligaments during TKA seems to offer some potential benefits in terms of proprioception, patient satisfaction, and constraint afforded by native soft tissues, there appears to be increased rates of failure and revision. At this time, given outcome scores that do not seem to differ markedly enough from traditional TKA and the increased potential mechanisms of failure, caution was made against the widespread adoption of BCR TKA until further study and refinement of implants or surgical technique.

ANNOTATED REFERENCES

1. Wise BL, Niu J, Yang M, et al: Patterns of compartment involvement in tibiofemoral osteoarthritis in men and women and in whites and African Americans. *Arthritis Care Res (Hoboken)* 2012;64(6):847-852.
2. Davies AP, Vince AS, Shepstone L, Donell ST, Glasgow MM: The radiologic prevalence of patellofemoral osteoarthritis. *Clin Orthop Relat Res* 2002;402:206-212.
3. Lombardi AV: The bi-cruciate retaining TKA: "A thing of beauty is a joy forever" – Affirms. *Bone Joint J* 2015;97-B(suppl 1):69.
4. Lombardi AV: The bi-cruciate retaining knee: A bridge too far – Opposes. *J Bone Joint Surg Br* 2017;99-B(suppl 7):87.

   In this point-counterpoint debate on BCR TKA, the author provides argument in favor of the use of BCR TKA implants. Levels of evidence: IV.
5. Christensen JC, Brothers J, Stoddard GJ, et al: Higher frequency of reoperation with a new bicruciate-retaining total knee arthroplasty. *Clin Orthop Relat Res* 2017;475(1):62-69.

   This is a short-term follow-up of a modern BCR TKA design demonstrating higher rates of radiolucent lines, revision surgeries, and all-cause revisions compared with a cruciate-retaining control group. Most revision surgeries were due to wound issues and débridements, but the trend was concerning and the authors concluded that further prospective studies were warranted to understand the findings. Level of evidence: III.
6. Alnachoukati OK, Emerson RH, Diaz E, Ruchaud E, Ennin KA: Modern day bicruciate-retaining total knee arthroplasty: A short-term review of 146 knees. *J Arthroplasty* 2018;33(8):2485-2490.

   In contrast to the aforementioned study, 1-year follow-up of the same modern BCR TKA found that 91% of respondents reported the knees always or sometimes feel normal, with only 9% of respondents reporting the knees never feel normal. About 94% of patients reported neutral satisfaction or higher, with only 6% of patients reporting dissatisfaction and 1% reported being very dissatisfied. At short-term follow-up, of all the 146 BCR TKAs implanted, there were only 2 revisions (1.4%) and 1 revision surgery (0.7%), a manipulation under anesthesia. Levels of evidence: IV.
7. Cushner FD, La Rosa DF, Vigorita VJ, Scuderi GR, Scott WN, Insall JN: A quantitative histologic comparison: ACL degeneration in the osteoarthritic knee. *J Arthroplasty* 2003;18(6):687-692.
8. Kozinn SC, Scott R: Unicondylar knee arthroplasty. *J Bone Joint Surg Am* 1989;71(1):145-150.
9. Felts E, Parratte S, Pauly V, Aubaniac JM, Argenson JN: Function and quality of life following medial unicompartmental knee arthroplasty in patients 60 years of age or younger. *Orthop Traumatol Surg Res* 2010;96(8):861-867.
10. Hamilton TW, Pandit HG, Jenkins C, Mellon SJ, Dodd CAF, Murray DW: Evidence-based indications for mobile-bearing unicompartmental knee arthroplasty in a consecutive cohort of thousand knees. *J Arthroplasty* 2017;32(6):1779-1785.

The authors analyzed a prospective series of 1,000 consecutive medial UKAs and found that 68% of 1,000 patients who underwent UKA would have failed the indications proposed by Kozinn and Scott in 1989. When comparing UKA patients who were traditionally contraindicated versus the ideal candidates, no differences were noted in pain or functional scores at 10 years. Furthermore, the ideal candidates had a higher rate of poor functional scores after 10 years. The authors found no significant difference in the 15-year implant survival for patients younger than 60 years compared with patients older than 60 years. Furthermore, equivalent functional outcomes were found in patients with mobile-bearing implants, regardless of the presence of patellofemoral joint arthritis. Levels of evidence: II.

11. van der List JP, Chawla H, Zuiderbaan HA, Pearle AD: The role of preoperative patient characteristics on outcomes of unicompartmental knee arthroplasty: A meta-analysis critique. *J Arthroplasty* 2016;31(11):2617-2627.

12. Lum ZC, Crawford DA, Lombardi AV Jr, et al: Early comparative outcomes of unicompartmental and total knee arthroplasty in severely obese patients. *Knee* 2018;25(1):161-166.

    This retrospective review of patients with BMI greater than 35 kg/m^2 undergoing TKA showed lower infection rates (zero versus 0.5%), fewer manipulations under anesthesia (0.5% versus 6.5%), and fewer returns to the operating room for any reason (3.7% versus 9.2%) compared with patients undergoing TKA. Levels of evidence: III.

13. Chen L, Liang W, Zhang X, Cheng B: Indications, outcomes, and complications of unicompartmental knee arthroplasty. *Front Biosci (Landmark Ed)* 2015;20:689-704.

14. Engh GA, Ammeen DJ: Unicondylar arthroplasty in knees with deficient anterior cruciate ligaments. *Clin Orthop Relat Res* 2014;472(1):73-77.

15. Mancuso F, Dodd CA, Murray DW, Pandit H: Medial unicompartmental knee arthroplasty in the ACL-deficient knee. *J Orthop Traumatol* 2016;17(3):267-275.

16. Kreitz TM, Maltenfort MG, Lonner JH: The valgus stress radiograph does not determine the full extent of correction of deformity prior to medial unicompartmental knee arthroplasty. *J Arthroplasty* 2015;30(7):1233-1236.

17. Scott RD: Mobile- versus fixed-bearing unicompartmental knee arthroplasty. *Instr Course Lect* 2010;59:57-60.

18. Ko YB, Gujarathi MR, Oh KJ: Outcome of unicompartmental knee arthroplasty: A systematic review of comparative studies between fixed and mobile bearings focusing on complications. *Knee Surg Relat Res* 2015;27(3):141-148.

19. Cossey AJ, Spriggins AJ: The use of computer-assisted surgical navigation to prevent malalignment in unicompartmental knee arthroplasty. *J Arthroplasty* 2005;20(1):29-34.

20. Song EK, Mohite N, Lee SH, Na BR, Seon JK: Comparison of outcome and survival after unicompartmental knee arthroplasty between navigation and conventional techniques with an average 9-year follow-up. *J Arthroplasty* 2016;31(2):395-400.

21. Valenzuela GA, Jacobson NA, Geist DJ, Valenzuela RG, Teitge RA: Implant and limb alignment outcomes for conventional and navigated unicompartmental knee arthroplasty. *J Arthroplasty* 2013;28(3):463-468.

22. Roche M: Robotic-assisted unicompartmental knee arthroplasty: The MAKO experience. *Orthop Clin North Am* 2015;46(1):125-131.

23. Coon TM, Driscoll MD, Conditt MA: Robotically assisted UKA is more accurate than manually instrumented UKA. *J Bone Joint Surg Br* 2010;92(suppl 1):157.

24. Lonner JH: Robotically assisted unicompartmental knee arthroplasty with a handheld image-free sculpting tool. *Orthop Clin North Am* 2016;47(1):29-40.

25. Lonner JH, Smith JR, Picard F, Hamlin B, Rowe PJ, Riches PE: High degree of accuracy of a novel image-free handheld robot for unicondylar knee arthroplasty in a cadaveric study. *Clin Orthop Relat Res* 2015;473(1):206-212.

26. Kayani B, Konan S, Pietrzak JRT, Huq SS, Tahmassebi J, Haddad FS: The learning curve associated with robotic-arm assisted unicompartmental knee arthroplasty: A prospective cohort study. *Bone Joint J* 2018;100-B(8):1033-1042.

    This prospective single-surgeon cohort study assessed the learning curve associated with robotic UKA and found that it was six cases. Levels of evidence: II.

27. Gilmour A, MacLean AD, Rowe PJ, et al: Robotic-arm-assisted vs conventional unicompartmental knee arthroplasty. The 2-year clinical outcomes of a randomized controlled trial. *J Arthroplasty* 2018;33(7 suppl):S109-S115.

    This single-center, prospective, randomized controlled trial compared robotic-assisted UKA with conventional surgery. The authors found that the 2-year revision rate in the conventional group was 3.6% compared with zero in the robot group. Levels of evidence: I.

28. Argenson JN, Blanc G, Aubaniac JM, Parratte S: Modern unicompartmental knee arthroplasty with cement: A concise follow-up, at a mean of twenty years, of a previous report. *J Bone Joint Surg Am* 2013;95(10):905-909.

29. Manzotti A, Cerveri P, Pullen C, Confalonieri N: A flat all-polyethylene tibial component in medial unicompartmental knee arthroplasty: A long-term study. *Knee* 2014;21(suppl 1):S20-S25.

30. Hutt JR, Farhadnia P, Masse V, LaVigne M, Vendittoli PA: A randomised trial of all-polyethylene and metal-backed tibial components in unicompartmental arthroplasty of the knee. *Bone Joint J* 2015;97-B(6):786-792.

31. Kendrick BJ, Kaptein BL, Valstar ER, et al: Cemented versus cementless Oxford unicompartmental knee arthroplasty using radiostereometric analysis: A randomised controlled trial. *Bone Joint J* 2015;97-B(2):185-191.

32. Schlueter-Brust K, Kugland K, Stein G, et al: Ten year survivorship after cemented and uncemented medial Uniglide(R) unicompartmental knee arthroplasties. *Knee* 2014;21(5):964-970.

33. Niinimaki T, Eskelinen A, Makela K, Ohtonen P, Puhto AP, Remes V: Unicompartmental knee arthroplasty survivorship is lower than TKA survivorship: A 27-year Finnish registry study. *Clin Orthop Relat Res* 2014;472(5):1496-1501.

34. Bini SA, Cafri G, Khatod M: Midterm-adjusted survival comparing the best performing unicompartmental and total knee arthroplasties in a registry. *J Arthroplasty* 2017;32(11):3352-3355.

Prospectively collected data from the Kaiser Permanente Total Joint Registry found the revision rate in UKA was lower than TKA (2.1% versus 2.4%), yet the rate of aseptic revision was higher (2.0% versus 1.4%) at midterm follow-up. Levels of evidence: III.

35. Robertsson O, Dunbar M, Pehrsson T, Knutson K, Lidgren L: Patient satisfaction after knee arthroplasty: A report on 27,372 knees operated on between 1981 and 1995 in Sweden. *Acta Orthop Scand* 2000;71(3):262-267.

36. Liddle AD, Judge A, Pandit H, Murray DW: Adverse outcomes after total and unicompartmental knee replacement in 101,330 matched patients: A study of data from the National Joint Registry for England and Wales. *Lancet* 2014;384(9952):1437-1445.

37. Dyrhovden GS, Lygre SHL, Badawy M, Gothesen O, Furnes O: Have the causes of revision for total and unicompartmental knee arthroplasties changed during the past two decades? *Clin Orthop Relat Res* 2017;475(7):1874-1886.

The authors retrospectively reviewed 60,623 TKAs (2,426 revisions) and 7,648 UKAs (725 revisions) from the Norwegian Arthroplasty Register. Causes of failure of UKA were differentiated between 1992 to 2004 and 2005 to 2015. An increased proportion of failures in UKA is now caused by osteoarthritis progression, whereas fewer failures in UKA are due to periprosthetic fractures, aseptic loosening, and polyethylene wear. Notably, TKA experienced improvements in 10-year survival (91% to 94%), whereas UKA survival rates remained similar (80% to 81%). Level of evidence: III.

38. Murray DW, Liddle A, Dodd CA, Pandit H: Unicompartmental knee arthroplasty: Is the glass half full or half empty? *Bone Joint J* 2015;97-B(10 suppl A):3-8.

39. Ghomrawi HM, Eggman AA, Pearle AD: Effect of age on cost-effectiveness of unicompartmental knee arthroplasty compared with total knee arthroplasty in the U.S. *J Bone Joint Surg Am* 2015;97(5):396-402.

40. Edmiston TA, Manista GC, Courtney PM, Sporer SM, Della Valle CJ, Levine BR: Clinical outcomes and survivorship of lateral unicompartmental knee arthroplasty: Does surgical approach matter? *J Arthroplasty* 2018;33(2): 362-365.

This is a retrospective review of a consecutive series of 65 patients who underwent lateral UKA via either a medial or lateral parapatellar approach with a minimum of 2-year follow-up. Of the 65 patients, 52 (80%) underwent lateral UKA via a lateral parapatellar approach and 13 (20%) medial parapatellar. At a mean follow-up of 82 months, the overall survivorship was 94%. No differences were observed in Knee Society Scores or revision to TKA (5% versus 7%). However, greater postoperative flexion (123.6° versus 116.5°) and greater overall improvement in flexion from baseline (3° versus −8°) were associated with the lateral parapatellar approach. Levels of evidence: IV.

41. Berend KR, Kolczun MC II, George JW Jr, Lombardi AV Jr: Lateral unicompartmental knee arthroplasty through a lateral parapatellar approach has high early survivorship. *Clin Orthop Relat Res* 2012;470(1):77-83.

42. O'Rourke MR, Gardner JJ, Callaghan JJ, et al: The John Insall Award: Unicompartmental knee replacement. A minimum twenty-one-year followup, end-result study. *Clin Orthop Relat Res* 2005;440:27-37.

43. Fisher DA, Watts M, Davis KE: Implant position in knee surgery: A comparison of minimally invasive, open unicompartmental, and total knee arthroplasty. *J Arthroplasty* 2003;18(7 suppl 1):2-8.

44. Hamilton WG, Collier MB, Tarabee E, McAuley JP, Engh CA Jr, Engh GA: Incidence and reasons for reoperation after minimally invasive unicompartmental knee arthroplasty. *J Arthroplasty* 2006;21(6 suppl 2):98-107.

45. Canetti R, Batailler C, Bankhead C, Neyret P, Servien E, Lustig S: Faster return to sport after robotic-assisted lateral unicompartmental knee arthroplasty: A comparative study. *Arch Orthop Trauma Surg* 2018;138(12): 1765-1771.

Twenty-five patients who underwent 28 lateral UKAs between 2012 and 2016, of which 11 were robotically assisted, were retrospectively reviewed. Primary outcome was return to sport activities, which was assessed using the University of California at Los Angeles Scale activity rating scale and direct patient questioning. Robotic-assisted procedures were associated with a statistically quicker return to sports activities compared with conventional instrumentation (4.2 ± 1.8 months, range 1 to 6 months versus 10.5 ± 6.7 months, range 3 to 24 months). Patients primarily returned to low-impact and mid impact sports, such as hiking, cycling, skiing, and swimming, with comparable overall rates of return to sports noted between the two groups (100% versus 94%) at most recent follow-up. Level of evidence: III.

46. Ng CTJ, Newman S, Harris S, Clarke S, Cobb J: Patient-specific instrumentation improves alignment of lateral unicompartmental knee replacements by novice surgeons. *Int Orthop* 2017;41(7):1379-1385.

Twelve orthopaedic trainees naïve to lateral UKA were chosen and instructed to perform the procedure on sawbones using conventional instrumentation alone and separately with help of PSI. Adherence to a preoperative plan was assessed. There was a trend toward higher precision with narrower standard deviations in the mean translational displacement of the femoral implant and mean rotational displacement of both implants in the PSI group. Levels of evidence: IV.

47. Zuiderbaan HA, Khamaisy S, Thein R, Nawabi DH, Pearle AD: Congruence and joint space width alterations of the medial compartment following lateral unicompartmental knee arthroplasty. *Bone Joint J* 2015;97-B(1): 50-55.

48. Scott RD: Lateral unicompartmental replacement: A road less traveled. *Orthopedics* 2005;28(9):983-984.

49. Hernigou P, Deschamps G: Posterior slope of the tibial implant and the outcome of unicompartmental knee arthroplasty. *J Bone Joint Surg Am* 2004;86-A(3):506-511.

50. Lonner JH, John TK, Conditt MA: Robotic arm-assisted UKA improves tibial component alignment: A pilot study. *Clin Orthop Relat Res* 2010;468(1):141-146.

Section 2: Knee

51. Walker T, Zahn N, Bruckner T, et al: Mid-term results of lateral unicondylar mobile bearing knee arthroplasty: A multicentre study of 363 cases. *Bone Joint J* 2018;100-B(1):42-49.

This multicenter study retrospectively evaluated 363 consecutive lateral UKAs (346 patients) using the Oxford domed lateral UKA prosthesis between 2006 and 2014. Midterm results, including implant survival rate, dislocation events, revision rates, and patient-reported outcomes, were assessed. Of 346 patients, 36 (10.5%) underwent revision surgery. The overall 3- and 5-year survival rates were 90.1% (95% confidence interval (CI): 86.1 to 93.1) and 85% (95% CI: 77.9 to 89.9), respectively. Of 346 patients, 18 (5.6%) and 20 (8.5%) sustained a bearing dislocation event at 3 and 5 years, respectively. Good to excellent clinical outcomes were shown, with a mean Tegner activity score of 3.2 (95% CI: 3.1 to 3.3), mean Oxford Knee Score of 40.3 (95% CI: 39.4 to 41.2), and mean University of California at Los Angeles activity rating scale of 5.7 (95% CI: 5.5 to 5.9). Still, despite good functional outcomes at most recent follow-up, the authors ultimately recommended the discontinuation of the mobile-bearing lateral UKA in favor of a fixed-bearing implant for future use because of the observed high revision rates. Levels of evidence: IV.

52. Kim KT, Lee S, Kim J, Kim JW, Kang MS: Clinical results of lateral unicompartmental knee arthroplasty: Minimum 2-year follow-up. *Clin Orthop Surg* 2016;8(4):386-392.

53. Newman SDS, Altuntas A, Alsop H, Cobb JP: Up to 10 year follow-up of the Oxford Domed Lateral Partial Knee Replacement from an independent centre. *Knee* 2017;24(6):1414-1421.

Fifty eight patients (64 knees) who underwent Oxford Domed UKA by a single surgeon between 2005 and 2009 were identified. Medium-term outcomes, in terms of revision surgery, reoperation, and Oxford Knee Score were assessed. Sixty-one knees had confirmed follow-up at a median of 84 months. One patient sustained two bearing dislocations ultimately requiring elective bearing exchange, two knees underwent conversion to TKR, and five patients required further revision surgeries to the affected knee. Median Oxford Knee Score improved from 26 (9 to 36) preoperatively to 42 (10 to 48) at final follow-up. Levels of evidence: IV.

54. Weston-Simons JS, Pandit H, Kendrick BJ, et al: The midterm outcomes of the Oxford Domed Lateral unicompartmental knee replacement. *Bone Joint J* 2014;96-B(1):59-64.

55. Robinson BJ, Rees JL, Price AJ, et al: Dislocation of the bearing of the Oxford lateral unicompartmental arthroplasty. A radiological assessment. *J Bone Joint Surg Br* 2002;84(5):653-657.

56. Greco NJ, Cook GJE, Lombardi AV Jr, Adams JB, Berend KR: Lateral unicompartmental knee arthroplasty utilizing a modified surgical technique and specifically adapted fixed-bearing implant. *Surg Technol Int* 2019;34:371-378.

Fifty-two patients who underwent consecutive lateral UKAs (56 knees) between January 2013 and May 2016 at a single practice with a minimum of 2-year follow-up were retrospectively reviewed. At a mean follow-up of nearly 3 years, Knee Society clinical and functional scores improved by 41 and 21 points, respectively. The failure rate was 1.78%, with two cases requiring revision surgery—one for medial osteoarthritis progression treated with medial UKA and one for superficial wound débridement. Levels of evidence: IV.

57. Smith JR, Robinson JR, Porteous AJ, et al: Fixed bearing lateral unicompartmental knee arthroplasty – short to midterm survivorship and knee scores for 101 prostheses. *Knee* 2014;21(4):843-847.

58. Deroche E, Batailler C, Lording T, Neyret P, Servien E, Lustig S: High survival rate and very low wear of lateral unicompartmental arthroplasty at long term: A case series of 54 cases at a mean follow-up of 17 years. *J Arthroplasty* 2019;34(6):1097-1104.

Over a 15-year period from January 1988 to October 2003, 54 lateral UKAs (52 patients) were performed at a single center via an extensive lateral approach with a tibial tubercle osteotomy. Thirty-nine knees (30 alive, 9 deceased at time of analysis) had greater than 15 years of follow-up data available. Of the 39 knees, 8 knees (20.5%) required surgical revision, with the most common indication being progression of osteoarthritis (87.5%) followed by aseptic loosening of the tibial component (12.5%). At a mean follow-up of 17.9 years, the mean polyethylene wear was 0.061 mm/yr. There was no radiographic evidence of loosening in the surviving implants and no revisions required for wear. Mean function and objective International Knee Society scores at latest follow-up were 66.5 ± 26.8 and 84.4 ± 13.2, respectively. Levels of evidence: IV.

59. Thienpont E: Conversion of a unicompartmental knee arthroplasty to a total knee arthroplasty: Can we achieve a primary result? *Bone Joint J* 2017;99-B(1 suppl A):65-69.

A systematic review was carried out looking for English-language articles published between 2006 and 2016 on UKA revisions and failures. Thirty-nine articles were deemed clinically relevant and included in the meta-analysis. Failures most commonly occurred because of liner dislocation, aseptic loosening, disease progression in other compartments, or unexplained pain. Various revision scenarios, including revision of UKA to UKA, surgery with addition of another UKA, conversion to a primary TKA, and conversion to a TKA using revision components, were analyzed and outcomes assessed. Conversion of a failed UKA to TKA may be accomplished with similar results to primary TKA, although a third of revision cases may require the use of revision TKA components, usually on the tibial side with augment and stem supplementation required.

60. Wada K, Hamada D, Takasago T, et al: Native rotational knee kinematics is restored after lateral UKA but not after medial UKA. *Knee Surg Sports Traumatol Arthrosc* 2018;26(11):3438-3443.

Navigation-assisted UKA was carried out on six fresh-frozen cadaver specimens (medial UKAs on all right knees and lateral UKAs on all left knees) using a standard medial parapatellar approach. The tibial rotation angles in early flexion within the medial UKA arm were significantly larger than those of native knees, yet were preserved in lateral UKAs. There were no significant differences in varus/valgus kinematics between native and UKA knees. Levels of evidence: III.

61. Kinsey TL, Anderson DN, Phillips VM, Mahoney OM: Disease progression after lateral and medial unicondylar knee arthroplasty. *J Arthroplasty* 2018;33(11):3441-3447.

    Serial radiographic evaluations of 20 lateral UKAs and 114 medial UKAs performed by a single surgeon were carried out between January 2007 and December 2018. Radiographs were obtained preoperatively and 1 and 5+ years postoperatively (mean 5.3 years, range 5.1 to 6.4 years). Radiographs were independently graded by two radiologists for the degree of tibiofemoral and patellofemoral compartment arthritis according to the Kellgren, Ahlback, and Altman scoring systems. All mean disease grades for both tibiofemoral and patellofemoral compartments worsened over time. Specifically, the rate of progression as the radiologists pertain to the Kellgren grade for tibiofemoral and patellofemoral compartments and the Ahlback score for tibiofemoral osteoarthritis degenerated quickly for lateral UKA compared with medial UKA. Levels of evidence: IV.

62. Argenson JN, Flecher X, Parratte S, Aubaniac JM: Patellofemoral arthroplasty: An update. *Clin Orthop Relat Res* 2005;440:50-53.

63. McAlindon TE, Snow S, Cooper C, Dieppe PA: Radiographic patterns of osteoarthritis of the knee joint in the community: The importance of the patellofemoral joint. *Ann Rheum Dis* 1992;51(7):844-849.

64. Kim N, Browning RC, Lerner ZF: The effects of pediatric obesity on patellofemoral joint contact force during walking. *Gait Posture* 2019;73:209-214.

    In this study, the authors evaluated patellofemoral joint forces in 10 obese children compared with 10 healthy-weight children during treadmill walking. The authors concluded that obese children had 1.98 times greater absolute ($P = 0.002$) and 1.81 times greater patellar-area-normalized ($P = 0.008$) patellofemoral joint contact forces compared with the healthy-weight children. The author concluded that increased patellofemoral loads contribute to the increased risk of knee pain in this population. Levels of evidence: III.

65. Liow MH, Goh GS, Tay DK, Chia SL, Lo NN, Yeo SJ: Obesity and the absence of trochlear dysplasia increase the risk of revision in patellofemoral arthroplasty. *Knee* 2016;23(2):331-337.

66. van Jonbergen HP, Werkman DM, Barnaart LF, van Kampen A: Long-term outcomes of patellofemoral arthroplasty. *J Arthroplasty* 2010;25(7):1066-1071.

67. Leadbetter WB: Patellofemoral arthroplasty in the treatment of patellofemoral arthritis: Rationale and outcomes in younger patients. *Orthop Clin North Am* 2008;39(3):363-380, vii.

68. Kazarian GS, Tarity TD, Hansen EN, Cai J, Lonner JH: Significant functional improvement at 2 years after isolated patellofemoral arthroplasty with an onlay trochlear implant, but low mental health scores predispose to dissatisfaction. *J Arthroplasty* 2016;31(2):389-394.

69. Kamath AF, Slattery TR, Levack AE, Wu CH, Kneeland JB, Lonner JH: Trochlear inclination angles in normal and dysplastic knees. *J Arthroplasty* 2013;28(2):214-219.

70. Dejour D, Saffarini M, Malemo Y, et al: Early outcomes of an anatomic trochlear-cutting patellofemoral arthroplasty: Patient selection is key. *Knee Surg Sports Traumatol Arthrosc* 2019;27(7):2297-2302.

    This study reported the outcomes of a recently introduced anatomic trochlear-cutting PFA system with dome patellar button and systematic lateral facetectomy in 28 patients at a minimum follow-up of 3 years. Mean age was 63 years with 82% of patients having trochlear dysplasia. Three patients (11%) required conversion to TKA for progression of tibiofemoral osteoarthritis. The authors concluded that patient selection is critical and PFA should be restricted to patients with trochlear dysplasia. Levels of evidence: III.

71. Leadbetter WB, Seyler TM, Ragland PS, Mont MA: Indications, contraindications, and pitfalls of patellofemoral arthroplasty. *J Bone Joint Surg Am* 2006;88(suppl 4):122-137.

72. Levack A, Kamath AF, Lonner JH: Incidence of symptomatic thromboembolic disease after patellofemoral arthroplasty. *Am J Orthop (Belle Mead NJ)* 2012;41(10):456-460.

73. Lonner JH: Patellofemoral arthroplasty: The impact of design on outcomes. *Orthop Clin North Am* 2008;39(3):347-354, vi.

74. Lonner JH, Bloomfield MR: The clinical outcome of patellofemoral arthroplasty. *Orthop Clin North Am* 2013;44(3):271-280, vii.

75. Bohu Y, Klouche S, Sezer HB, Gerometta A, Lefevre N, Herman S: Hermes patellofemoral arthroplasty: Annual revision rate and clinical results after two to 20 years of follow-up. *Knee* 2019;26(2):484-491.

    In this review, the authors summarized the outcomes of PFA. The authors reported that PFA has a long record of use in the management of isolated patellofemoral arthritis, with outcomes influenced by patient selection, surgical technique, and trochlear implant design. The trochlear components have evolved from inlay-style to onlay-style designs, which have reduced the incidence of patellar instability. Minimizing the risk of patellar instability with onlay-design PFA has enhanced midterm and long-term results, leaving progressive tibiofemoral arthritis as the primary failure mechanism beyond 10 to 15 years. Levels of evidence: IV.

76. Metcalfe AJ, Ahearn N, Hassaballa MA, et al: The avon patellofemoral joint arthroplasty: Two- to 18-year results of a large single-centre cohort. *Bone Joint J* 2018;100-B(9):1162-1167.

    In this study of 558 PFAs in 431 patients, the authors reported on the clinical outcomes and implant survivorship at a follow-up of 18 years. There were significant improvements in Oxford Knee Score and Western Ontario and McMaster Universities Osteoarthritis Index scores at 2 years. There were 105 revisions with 61 (58%) for progression of tibiofemoral arthritis with conversion to standard primary TKA in all patients. The implant survival rate was 77.3% at 10 years and 67.4% at 15 years. Regression analysis found that cases performed in the last 9 years of the study had improved survival compared with the first 9 years. The individual operating surgeon had the strongest effect on survivorship. The authors concluded that satisfactory long-term results can be obtained with PFA with maintenance of patient-reported outcome measures, satisfactory survival, and low rates of loosening and wear. Levels of evidence: IV.

77. Odgaard A, Madsen F, Kristensen PW, Kappel A, Fabrin J: The Mark Coventry Award: Patellofemoral arthroplasty results in better range of movement and early patient-reported outcomes than TKA. *Clin Orthop Relat Res* 2018;476(1):87-100.

In a blinded RCT, the authors compared the outcomes of PFA with those of TKA in 100 patients with mean age of 64 years. There were significant higher improvements in the SF-36 physical functioning, Knee Injury and Osteoarthritis Outcome Score, and Oxford Knee Score up to 2 years for PFA compared with TKA. The authors concluded that PFA patients recover faster and regain ROM quicker, and the functional outcomes are better up to 9 months than in patients undergoing TKA. Level of evidence: I.

78. Osarumwense D, Syed F, Nzeako O, Akilapa S, Zubair O, Waite J: Patellofemoral joint arthroplasty: Early results and functional outcome of the Zimmer Gender Solutions Patello-Femoral Joint system. *Clin Orthop Surg* 2017;9(3):295-302.

The authors evaluated the early results and outcomes of 50 PFAs for the treatment of isolated patellofemoral osteoarthritis. At a minimum follow-up of 2 years, the authors reported significant improvements in Oxford Knee Score. There were no significant differences in the Oxford Knee Score between unilateral and bilateral procedures and between obese and nonobese patients. Two knees (4%) were revised for progression of osteoarthritis, which led the authors to conclude that PFA in obese patients and bilateral procedures can produce good results. Levels of evidence: IV.

79. Ahearn N, Metcalfe AJ, Hassaballa MA, et al: The journey patellofemoral joint arthroplasty: A minimum 5 year follow-up study. *Knee* 2016;23(5):900-904.

80. Dy CJ, Franco N, Ma Y, Mazumdar M, McCarthy MM, Gonzalez Della Valle A: Complications after patellofemoral versus total knee replacement in the treatment of isolated patello-femoral osteoarthritis. A meta-analysis. *Knee Surg Sports Traumatol Arthrosc* 2012;20(11):2174-2190.

81. Valoroso M, Saffarini M, La Barbera G, et al: Correction of patellofemoral malalignment with patellofemoral arthroplasty. *J Arthroplasty* 2017;32(12):3598-3602.

The authors evaluated the modified patellar heights, tilts, and tibial tuberosity–trochlear groove distances in a series of 16 patients who received PFAs. Mean age of the study cohort was 65 years. Preoperative to postoperative change in the median patellar tilt without quadriceps contraction was 17.5° to 0.3° and with quadriceps contraction was 19.8° to 6.1°. Similarly, the change in median Caton-Deschamps index was 0.91 to 1.11, and the median tibial tuberosity–trochlear groove distance was 14.5 to 10.1 mm. Trochlear-cutting PFA improves patellofemoral congruence by correcting trochlear dysplasia and standardizing radiologic measurements such as patellar tilt and tibial tuberosity–trochlear groove distance. The addition of lateral patellar facetectomy improves patellar tracking by reducing the patellar tilt. Levels of evidence: IV.

82. deDeugd CM, Pareek A, Krych AJ, Cummings NM, Dahm DL: Outcomes of patellofemoral arthroplasty based on radiographic severity. *J Arthroplasty* 2017;32(4):1137-1142.

The authors evaluated the 75 PFAs performed between 2002 and 2013 and stratified the outcomes based on preoperative Iwano grading of radiographic severity of patellofemoral arthritis. Mean age of the study cohort was 51 years. There was significantly more improvement in Knee Society Score pain, Knee Society Score function, University of California at Los Angeles score, Tegner score, and pain quality in the Iwano grade II-IV group versus the Iwano grade I group. The authors concluded that caution should be exercised when considering PFA for patients with minimal radiographic evidence of patellofemoral arthritis.

83. Hendrix MR, Ackroyd CE, Lonner JH: Revision patellofemoral arthroplasty: Three- to seven-year follow-up. *J Arthroplasty* 2008;23(7):977-983.

84. Lonner JH, Jasko JG, Booth RE Jr: Revision of a failed patellofemoral arthroplasty to a total knee arthroplasty. *J Bone Joint Surg Am* 2006;88(11):2337-2342.

85. Heekin RD, Fokin AA: Incidence of bicompartmental osteoarthritis in patients undergoing total and unicompartmental knee arthroplasty: Is the time ripe for a less radical treatment? *J knee Surg* 2014;27(1):77-81.

86. Tria AJ Jr: Bicompartmental arthroplasty of the knee. *Instr Course Lect* 2010;59:61-73.

87. Kamath AF, Levack A, John T, Thomas BS, Lonner JH: Minimum two-year outcomes of modular bicompartmental knee arthroplasty. *J Arthroplasty* 2014;29(1):75-79.

88. Tria AJ Jr: Bicompartmental knee arthroplasty: The clinical outcomes. *Orthop Clin North Am* 2013;44(3):281-286, vii.

89. Ogura T, Le K, Merkely G, Bryant T, Minas T: A high level of satisfaction after bicompartmental individualized knee arthroplasty with patient-specific implants and instruments. *Knee Surg Sports Traumatol Arthrosc* 2019;27(5):1487-1496.

This is a retrospective review of 59 BCAs in 55 patients performed using custom-made implants and PSI based on preoperative CT scan. All BCAs included PFAs and either medial (41/59) or lateral (18/59) UKAs. There was high level of patient satisfaction (91%), despite a third of the BCAs requiring subsequent surgical procedures. The mean follow-up was 3.8 years (range 1 to 6 years). Levels of evidence: IV.

90. Tamam C, Plate JF, Augart M, Poehling GG, Jinnah RH: Retrospective clinical and radiological outcomes after robotic assisted bicompartmental knee arthroplasty. *Adv Orthop* 2015;2015:747309.

91. Engh GA, Parks NL, Whitney CE: A prospective randomized study of bicompartmental vs. total knee arthroplasty with functional testing and short term outcome. *J Arthroplasty* 2014;29(9):1790-1794.

92. Yeo NE, Chen JY, Yew A, Chia SL, Lo NN, Yeo SJ: Prospective randomised trial comparing unlinked, modular bicompartmental knee arthroplasty and total knee arthroplasty: A five years follow-up. *Knee* 2015;22(4):321-327.

93. Chung JY, Min BH: Is bicompartmental knee arthroplasty more favourable to knee muscle strength and physical performance compared to total knee arthroplasty? *Knee Surg Sports Traumatol Arthrosc* 2013;21(11):2532-2541.

94. Kooner S, Johal H, Clark M: Bicompartmental knee arthroplasty vs total knee arthroplasty for the treatment of medial compartment and patellofemoral osteoarthritis. *Arthroplast Today* 2017;3(4):309-314.

This is a systematic review with meta-analysis of four prospective studies and two retrospective cohort studies consisting of 277 knees in 274 patients undergoing either BCA or TKA. The authors found no differences in terms of patient-reported outcomes, length of stay, or rates of complication and revision surgery at a minimum of 2-year follow-up (range 2 to 5 years) with analyzing modular, unlinked BCA. There was reduction in intraoperative blood loss in the BCA group at the expense of increased surgical time because of increased technical demands. In contrast, there were high revision and failure rates with use of monolithic BCA. Levels of evidence: III.

95. White SH, Ludkowski PF, Goodfellow JW: Anteromedial osteoarthritis of the knee. *J Bone Joint Surg Br* 1991;73(4):582-586.

96. Pritchett JW: Patients prefer a bicruciate-retaining or the medial pivot total knee prosthesis. *J Arthroplasty* 2011;26(2):224-228.

97. Pritchett JW: Bicruciate-retaining total knee replacement provides satisfactory function and implant survivorship at 23 years. *Clin Orthop Relat Res* 2015;473(7):2327-2333.

98. Baumann F, Bahadin O, Krutsch W, et al: Proprioception after bicruciate-retaining total knee arthroplasty is comparable to unicompartmental knee arthroplasty. *Knee Surg Sports Traumatol Arthrosc* 2017;25(6):1697-1704.

This study found superior static balance after preservation of both cruciate ligaments in arthroplasty of the knee, indicating superior proprioceptive function. Hence, BCR implants could provide improved functional properties. Superior proprioceptive function of BCR implants can be an important factor in implant selection. The authors conclude, though, that prospective, randomized studies are needed to investigate the kinematics and long-term survivorship of BCR implants. Levels of evidence: II.

99. Pelt CE, Sandifer PA, Gililland JM, Anderson MB, Peters CL: Mean three-year survivorship of a new bicruciate-retaining total knee arthroplasty: Are revisions still higher than expected? *J Arthroplasty* 2019;34(9):1957-1962.

The study attempted to determine the 3-year survivorship and patient-reported outcomes of a contemporary BCR TKA design. Revision-free survival of 88% was lower than traditional TKA designs. The primary failure mechanisms were tibial loosening, ACL impingement, and pain. In the setting of higher-than-anticipated revision rates, despite patient-reported outcomes that are not different than seen in the general population, it is possible that further refinement in implant design or surgical technique may be needed before widespread use of BCR implants. Levels of evidence: IV.

100. Saxena V, Anari JB, Ruutiainen AT, Voleti PB, Stephenson JW, Lee GC: Tibial component considerations in bicruciate-retaining total knee arthroplasty: A 3D MRI evaluation of proximal tibial anatomy. *Knee* 2016;23(4):593-599.

101. Lavoie F, Al-Shakfa F, Moore JR, Mychaltchouk L, Iguer K: Postoperative stiffening after bicruciate-retaining total knee arthroplasty. *J Knee Surg* 2018;31(5):453-458.

This retrospective comparative cohort study of 100 BCR TKAs (90 patients) and 100 postoperative stiffening (PS) TKAs (88 patients) demonstrated that knees with a BCR design lost significantly more flexion than PS TKA in the early postoperative period when the preoperative flexion was less than 130° (loss of 40° versus loss of 24°). Postoperative stiffening seems to be more frequent and of greater magnitude after BCR TKA, compared with PS TKA, in patients suffering from preoperative flexion stiffness. It is suggested that further investigation on the causes of this phenomenon is warranted. Levels of evidence: III.

CHAPTER 23

Robotic-Assisted and Computer-Assisted Knee Arthroplasty

MICHAEL J. DUNBAR, MD, FRCSC, PhD, FCAHS • ALEXANDER R. MELDRUM, MD, FRCSC
PIERRE P. ZAHARIA, MD, FRCSC

ABSTRACT

Computer-assisted surgery and robotic-assisted knee arthroplasty are increasingly used by joint arthroplasty surgeons in the surgical management of knee arthritis. Numerous computer navigation and robotic devices are now available and are FDA approved for unicompartmental, patellofemoral, bicompartmental, and total knee arthroplasty. As the trend for increased adoption is likely to continue, it is important to be knowledgeable about the available navigation devices, robotic devices, the intraoperative applications and indications, and the evidence for use.

Keywords: arthroplasty; computer-assisted knee arthroplasty; knee; replacement; robotic

Dr. Dunbar or an immediate family member has received royalties from Stryker; serves as a paid consultant to or is an employee of Stryker; has received research or institutional support from DePuy, Stryker, and Zimmer; and serves as a board member, owner, officer, or committee member of the Canadian Arthroplasty Society – President, the Canadian Joint Replacement Registry – Co-chair, the Canadian Orthopaedic Association, and the Canadian RSA Network – Chair. Neither of the following authors nor any immediate family member has received anything of value from or has stock or stock options held in a commercial company or institution related directly or indirectly to the subject of this chapter: Dr. Meldrum and Dr. Zaharia.

INTRODUCTION

One of the basic tenets of knee arthroplasty is that clinical outcomes are related, in an important way, to the accuracy and precision with which the procedure is performed. Conventional implant systems provide manual instruments to prepare the bone surfaces and to assist in achieving appropriate alignment, with a specific focus on the coronal plane.[1] Registry and outcome data have shown that technical issues now account for up to 30% of knee revisions and poor patient outcomes.[2,3] Computer-assisted surgery (CAS) techniques were developed in the 1990s to address the inherent limitations of mechanical instrumentation, mostly around the precision of bone cuts and the accuracy of obtaining the desired implant position and overall limb alignment. The goal of computer-assisted knee arthroplasty devices is to provide the surgeon with reliable and precise real-time surgical feedback regarding the alignment of the extremity and placement of instruments, cutting guides, resection planes, implant positioning, and alignment.

Robotics has been used for decades in automotive, industrial, and aerospace applications for consistency, reproducibility, and efficiency. The integration of robotics into knee arthroplasty procedures began in the early 2000s,[4] building off the concept of CAS and integrating robotic arms/devices to improve precision and accuracy. Robotic-assisted knee arthroplasty (RKA) has seen significant adoption in the past several years with near exponential growth in the number of cases performed each year. The accuracy and precision of robotics allows

This chapter is adapted from Roche M: Robotic-assisted knee arthroplasty, in Mont MA, Tanzer M, eds: *Orthopaedic Knowledge Update®: Hip and Knee Reconstruction*, ed 5. Rosemont, IL, American Academy of Orthopaedic Surgeons, 2017, pp 163-172 and Stullberg SD, Dunbar M, Lee GC: Computer-assisted knee arthroplasty, in Mont MA, Tanzer M, eds: *Orthopaedic Knowledge Update®: Hip and Knee Reconstruction*, ed 5. Rosemont, IL, American Academy of Orthopaedic Surgeons, 2017, pp 173-181.

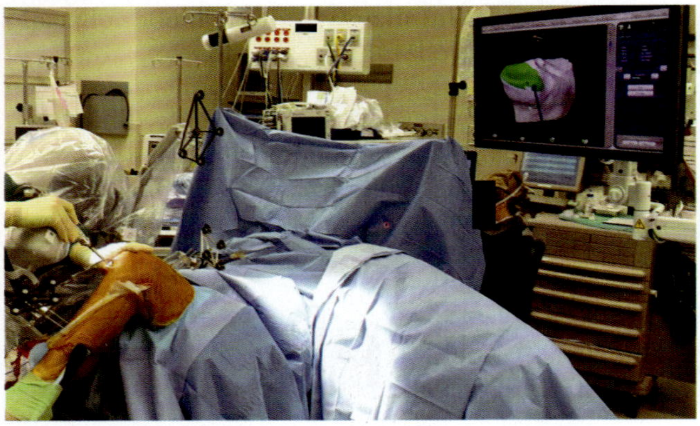

FIGURE 1 Intraoperative photograph shows a semiactive robotic arm with computer display used during unicompartmental knee arthroplasty.

the surgeon to reliably implant unicompartmental knee arthroplasties (UKAs) and total knee arthroplasties (TKAs) in the prescribed position and alignment. This has implications for a move to a patient-specific alignment and implant position target.

Patient and surgeon expectations motivate an increased interest in an enhanced understanding of a patient's specific knee pathology, and subsequently, enabled through CAS/RKA, prescribing a patient-specific target. CSA/RKA integrates preoperative and intraoperative planning with computer modeling and assists the surgeon in executing the surgical plan in a precise, accurate, and efficient manner[5] (**Figure 1**). The improved accuracy of the procedure, with customization to the patient's specific knee pathology, improves implant congruency, limb alignment, gap balancing, and potential errors that may cause failure and poor outcomes (**Figures 2** and **3**). The benefits of potentially minimizing bone resection, and soft-tissue injury, through RKA lead to improved outcomes.[6]

SURGICAL INDICATIONS

The indications for CAS/RKA utilization are broad, and the technology can also be used in cases where traditional techniques are not possible. The primary driver is the patient's clinical presentation, combined with the surgeon's preference for the technologic benefits of CAS/RKA surgery. FDA clearance for device applications defines its specific use in the continuum of knee arthroplasty. CAS/TKA allows a surgeon to define the patient-specific approach for procedures, including UKAs (medial, lateral, patellofemoral), bicompartmental knee arthroplasty (medial/lateral unicompartmental with a patellofemoral arthroplasty), and TKA.

Preoperative level of disability, physical findings, and patient expectations determine the suitability of a candidate for CAS/RKA. Similarly, for the conventional

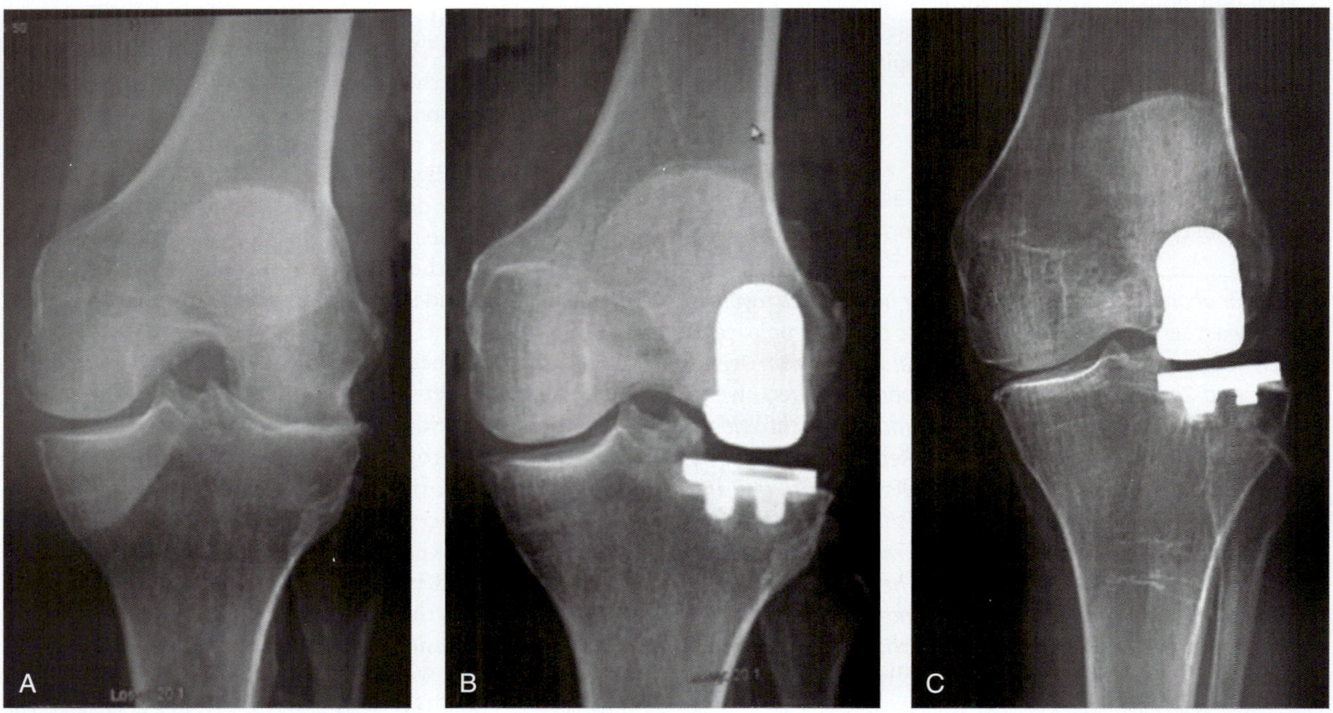

FIGURE 2 Radiographs show a preoperative arthritic lateral joint (**A**) that underwent robotic-assisted lateral unicompartmental knee arthroplasty (UKA, **B**). **C**, Radiograph shows conventional lateral UKA. The tibia is positioned in varus and overcorrected alignment.

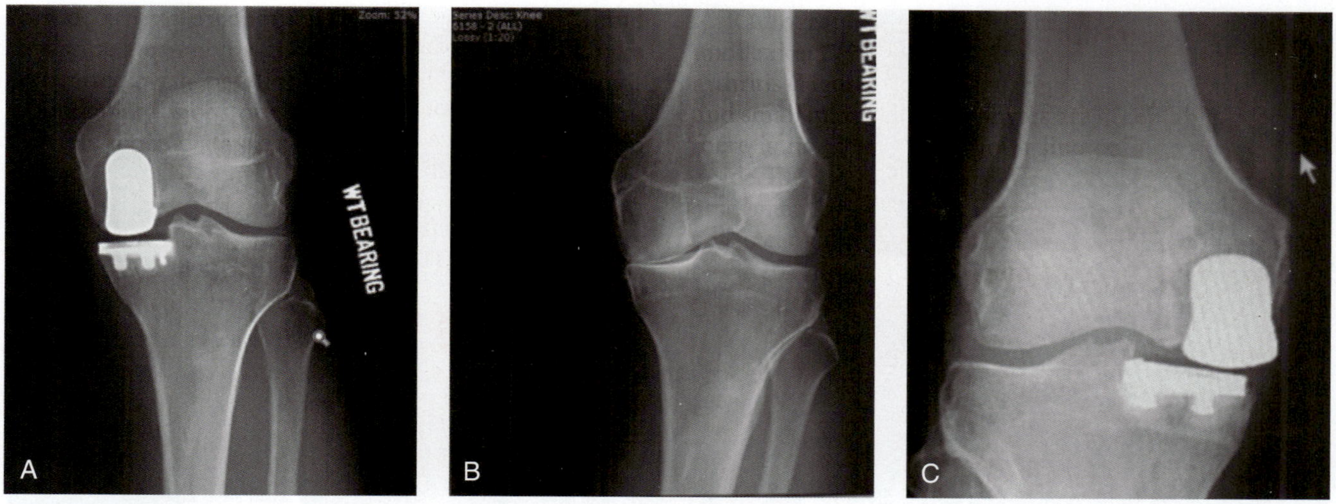

FIGURE 3 Radiographs show a robotic-assisted medial unicompartmental knee arthroplasty (UKA) (**A**), a preoperative medial arthritic joint (**B**), and a manual UKA with coronal implant incongruency (**C**).

approach, gait, alignment, knee motion and stability, skin integrity, neurovascular status, and the patient's hip and ankle are evaluated to rule out fixed deformities or ligamentous instability that would interfere with a consistent surgical outcome. Preoperative films should include standard weight-bearing and long limb films. CT/MRI or fluoroscopy is used for several CAS/RKA systems and can aid in surgical registration as well as in preoperative bone density and subchondral bone evaluation. Contraindications are similar to those for conventional knee arthroplasty surgery but would include poor bone stock if concerns about navigation pin stability are present.

The specific surgical procedure and risks should be discussed with the patient. Postoperative protocols and expectations need to be defined. With a modular robotic approach, surgeons have the ability to modify the plans intraoperatively based on intraoperative findings. In a UKA plan, the need to resurface the patellofemoral joint in the presence of advanced arthritic findings is currently debated.[7]

CAS SYSTEM TYPES

The three types of navigated computer-assisted techniques used in knee arthroplasty are preoperative image-based (eg, CT or MRI), intraoperative image-based (such as, fluoroscopy), and imageless techniques. These techniques can be used to acquire anatomic information to be used for presurgical or intraoperative surgical planning. With image-based systems, the presurgical or intraoperative surgical plan helps with intraoperative placement of cutting tools and to establish knee alignment and stability.[8]

Imageless CAS Systems

Imageless systems use a combination of kinematic and surface registration techniques to create a virtual bone map. Kinematic registration is used to characterize important anatomic landmarks outside the incision.[9] The center of the femoral head can be located by circumducting the femur around the hip with the pelvis stabilized (**Figure 4**). Surface registration involves directly contacting multiple points on the surface of the distal femur and proximal tibia with a digitizing device that communicates with the computer. The information is processed by the computer to extrapolate the shape, surface contour, and relative size of the distal femur and proximal tibia[10] (**Figure 5**). Cardinal axes of alignment and rotation are also imputed, such as the transepicondylar axis, anterior-posterior axis of the distal femur, and relative rotation of the tibia. The accuracy of the information collected by using surface registration requires that the surgeon correctly identifies specific points. All conventional imageless systems use a combination of surface and kinematic registration to identify the mechanical axis of the limb.

Optical Navigation Systems

Optical navigation systems, which have been used to assist with knee arthroplasty since the late 1990s, commonly use optical localization to communicate between the surgical extremity and the computer. Two types of optical tracking are used: active and passive. Active tracking systems use markers (also called trackers or rigid bodies) that have light-emitting diodes (LEDs) that emit light pulses to a camera (optical localizer). Three or more, for redundancy, of these LEDs are attached to screws or pins that are rigidly attached to the femur and tibia. The camera system to which the light is transmitted consists of two planar or three linear charge-coupled devices rigidly mounted onto a solid. Passive systems use reflecting spheres placed on tracking markers that are attached to screws or pins rigidly implanted in the femur and

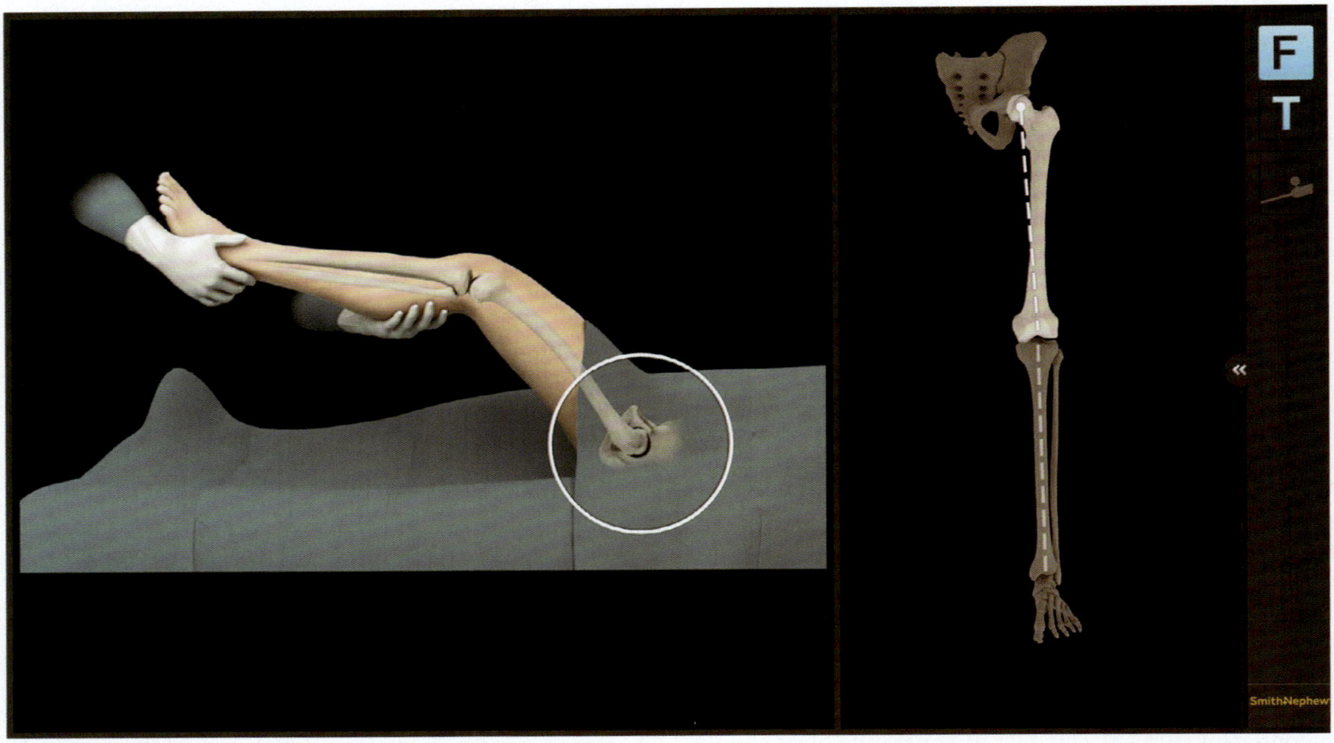

FIGURE 4 Computer-generated illustration demonstrates kinematic referencing of the center of the femoral head that involves circumducting the hip joint. The center of the femoral head is identified as the point of a cone (the base of the cone is the circumference of rotation of the knee). (Copyright Smith+Nephew.)

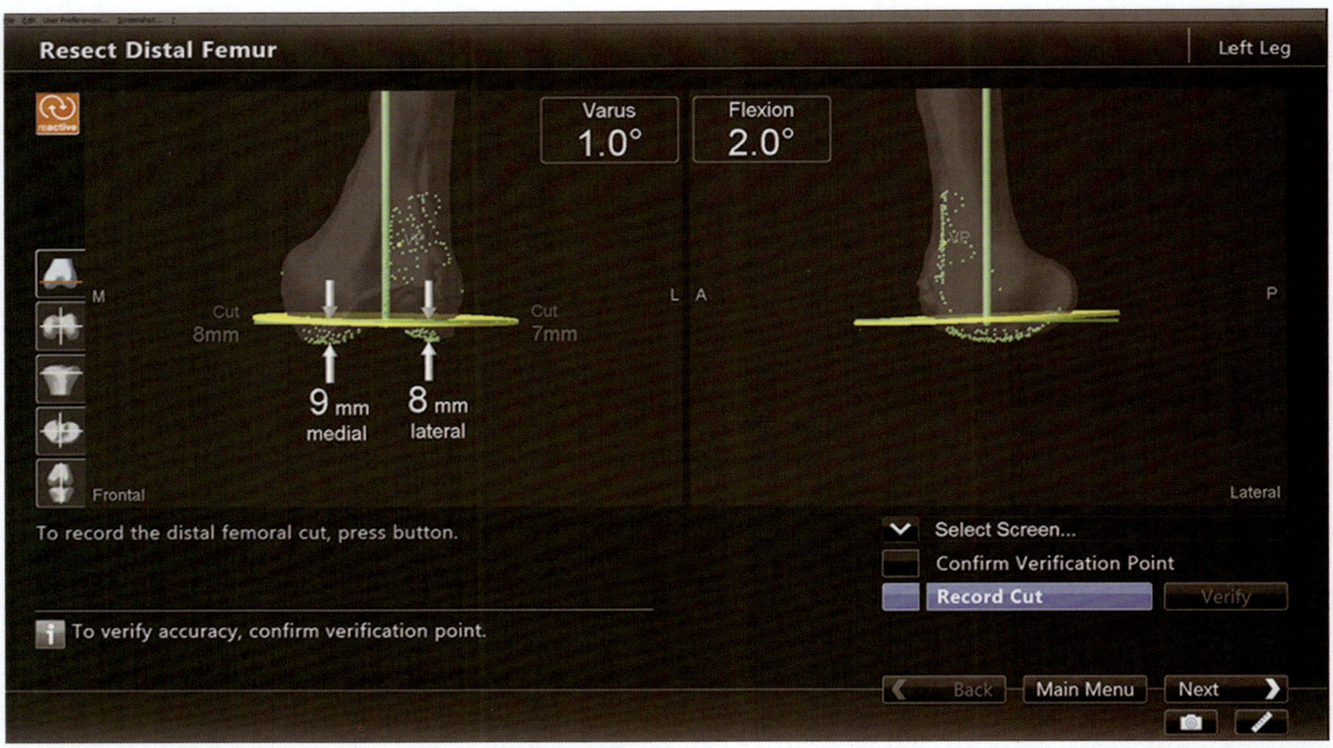

FIGURE 5 Image shows digitized points (green dots) that create a point cloud and allow the computer software to create a virtual image of the bone (bone morphing). (Used with permission from Stryker® OrthoMap® Precision Knee Navigation Software User Manual Version 5.0, 2012. © Stryker, Kalamazoo, MI.)

tibia. Infrared flashes sent by LED arrays on the camera housing illuminate the spheres. The two planar or three linear charge-coupled devices detect the reflections and interpolate the spatial location of each light source. It is important for surgeons and staff to realize that the arrays on the tracking markers, whether active or passive, are specific to each CAS system. The advantages of optical localizing systems are that these systems are reliable, flexible, highly accurate, and have good operating room compatibility. A disadvantage of these systems is that a free line of sight is necessary between the LED/spheres and the charge-coupled device arrays in the camera.

Limited Optical Navigation Systems

Limited optical navigation systems use a similar technique to that used by accelerometer-based systems. In place of an accelerometer, an infrared emitter or reflective ball transmits the position of the cutting guide to a stand-alone optical localizer (camera).

The surgeon registers points on the distal femur and proximal tibia. The system then calculates the position in the coronal and sagittal planes of bone resection.[10] Resection depth is incorporated into the bony cuts, and implant rotation can be calculated but not used to position the cutting guide. Conventional posterior referencing cutting guides are used to position the cutting blocks for correct femoral rotation.

Because the same tracking device is used for the femur and the tibia, the relative position of the femur to the tibia (the limb alignment axis) cannot be calculated. Moreover, these systems cannot provide information regarding ligament balance or limb alignment through a range of motion.

Because these systems use a less cumbersome registration process than do conventional navigation systems, the surgical times associated with the systems's use is often shorter. However, as with conventional navigation systems, these limited systems depend on precise surface registration of anatomic landmarks for accuracy.

Comprehensive Optical Navigation Systems

Most prosthesis companies offer a comprehensive CAS system for TKA. The kinematic and surface registration processes are similar to those used with the limited optical systems. Differentially, data collected during the procedure are available throughout the procedure. Data collection is achieved by utilization of two trackers rigidly fixed to the distal femur and proximal tibia, either within the incision or through separate stab incisions. Information regarding prosthesis position, including femoral and tibial rotation, implant size, and gap balancing, can then be displayed. Comprehensive optical systems can link the mechanical axis of the femur and tibia to compute the alignment of the limb.[9,10] The alignment of the limb throughout range of motion can also be analyzed as an alignment curve[10] (**Figure 6**).

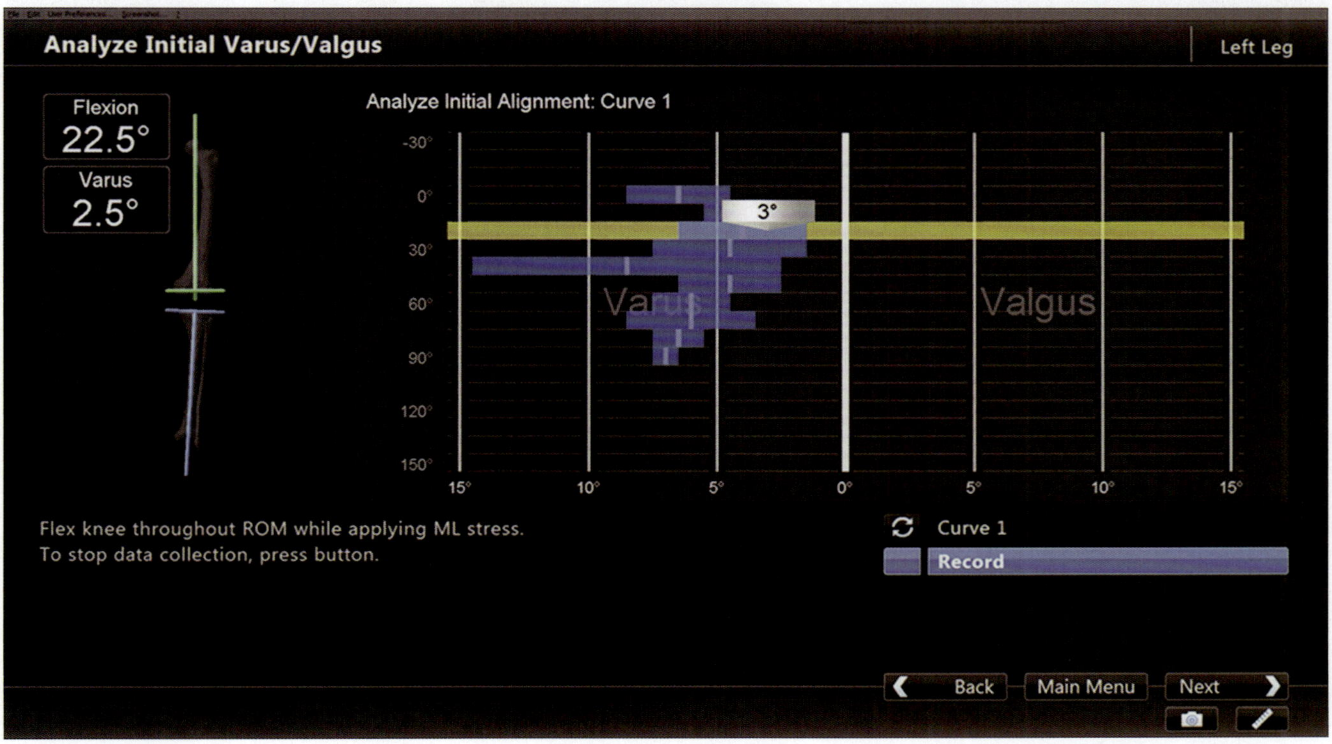

FIGURE 6 Image shows comprehensive optical navigation, which displays information regarding alignment throughout range of motion. (Used with permission from Stryker® OrthoMap® Precision Knee Navigation Software User Manual Version 5.0, 2012. © Stryker, Kalamazoo, MI.)

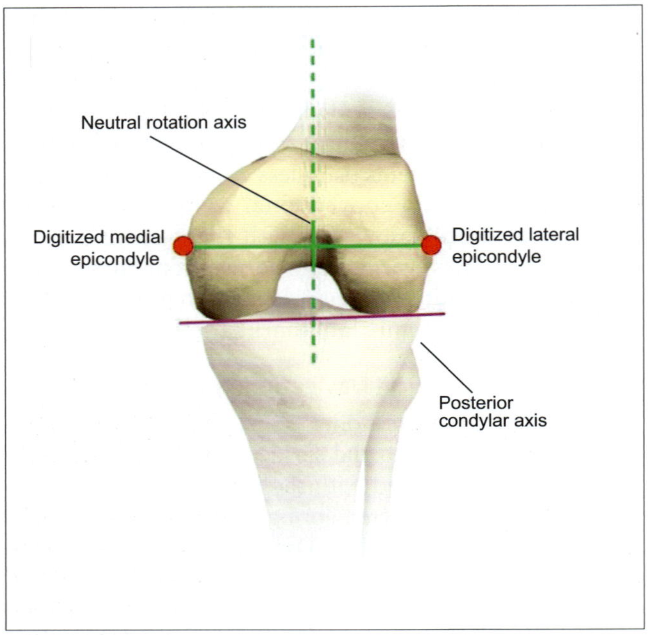

FIGURE 7 Illustration shows the rotational axes of the limb digitized for the surgeon. Correct identification of these landmarks is critical to maximize precision. (Used with permission from Stryker® OrthoMap® Precision Knee Navigation Software User Manual Version 5.0, 2012. © Stryker, Kalamazoo, MI.)

Femoral implant rotation can be established relative to any of the conventionally used axes (transepicondylar, posterior condylar, or Whiteside line)[9,10] (**Figure 7**). All axes are digitized by the surgeon using a pointer. Precise identification of landmarks is imperative. For example, a large potential for error exists in detecting the transepicondylar axis, with combined errors reported as high as 13.5 mm.[10,11]

Comprehensive optical navigation systems also provide information on implant size and can be modified by using either anterior or posterior referencing according to surgeon preference. Adjustments to implant size or position may have implications for notching and medial and lateral overhang, as well as posterior condylar offset, which can also be displayed. The distance between the planned femoral and tibial cuts can be shown, allowing for a gap balancing technique. The surgeon can use a planning screen (**Figure 8**) that will show the real-time effect of any potential changes to the surgical plan, such as changing implant size or resection level.

This type of system offers the most detailed intraoperative information currently available to the surgeon. All digitized points are stored on the navigation unit and can be reviewed during the surgical procedure. As a result, the validity of the points can be assessed during

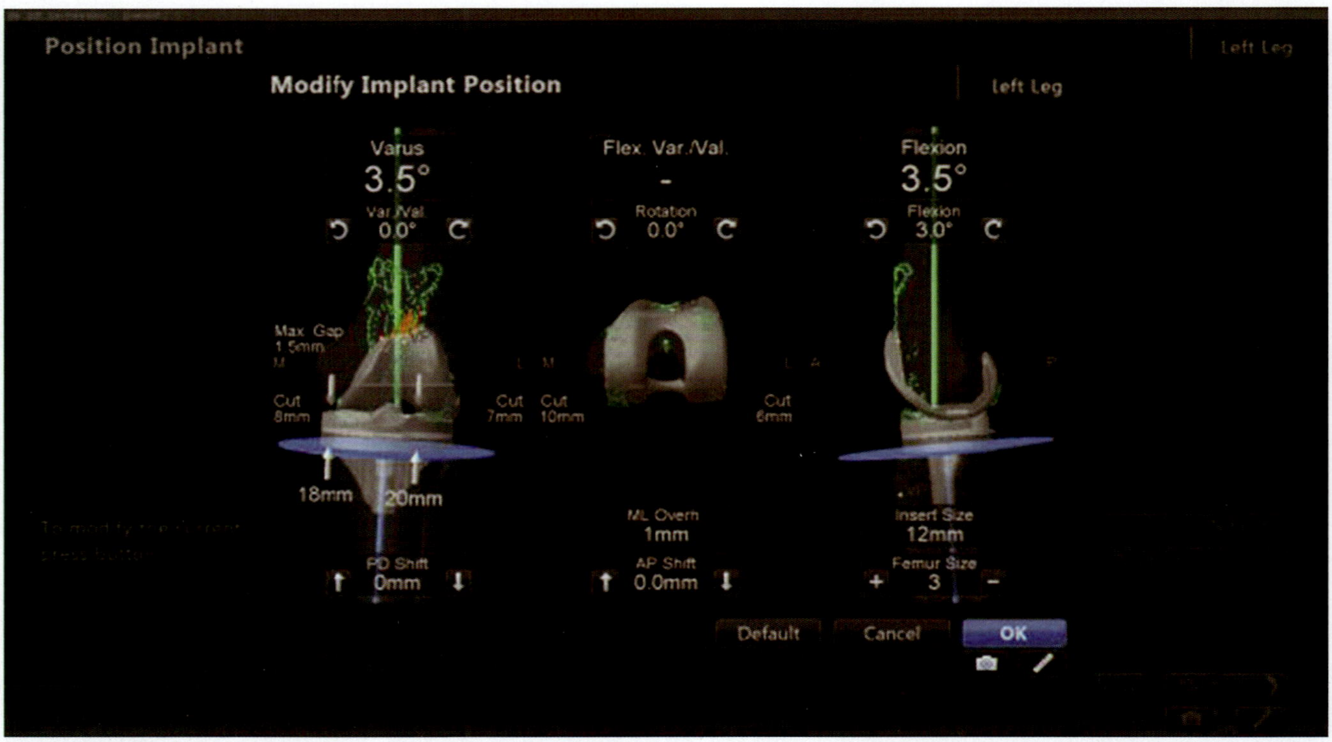

FIGURE 8 Image shows comprehensive optical navigation system, which allows sophisticated intraoperative planning before bone resection. (Used with permission from Stryker® OrthoMap® Precision Knee Navigation Software User Manual Version 5.0, 2012. © Stryker, Kalamazoo, MI.)

the procedure. The surgeon is also able to alter bone cuts and assess the effect of this change on ligament balance and overall limb alignment.

Drawbacks to comprehensive optical navigation systems include increased surgical time, the need to maintain a direct line of sight from the trackers to the sensors on the navigation unit, and the need for additional drill holes in the distal femur and proximal tibia (for the trackers) that may result in fracture and increase infection risk, both at very low rates. Key features of the accelerometer, limited optical, and comprehensive optical systems are summarized in **Table 1**.

Accelerometer-based Systems

Although the technology has been used in other fields (such as aviation) for decades, accelerometer-based CAS systems are relatively recent additions to the arthroplasty surgeon's CAS armamentarium. The systems use two components: an accelerometer attached to bone, which identifies the mechanical axis of the limb, and a sensor attached to the cutting guide, which identifies the position of the cutting guide relative to the accelerometer.[12] This information is displayed within the surgical field, either on a digital display or via a LED display system.

Unlike conventional optical navigation systems, accelerometer-based CAS TKA systems do not require that a clear line of sight be maintained between the surgical extremity and the computer system. All computer hardware is contained within the sterile surgical field. However, the information provided to the surgeon is limited to the distal femoral and proximal tibial resections. Conventional instruments are required to set the depth and rotation of the femoral and tibial cuts and to determine the size of the implants.

TYPES OF ROBOTIC-ASSISTED KNEE ARTHROPLASTY SYSTEM

RKA technologies include three systems: active, semiactive, and passive. All three robotic applications are FDA approved for use in knee arthroplasty. Active systems have a robotic arm automated to perform a function as prescribed by the surgeon. With semiactive systems, the robot augments the surgeon's ability to control resections

TABLE 1

Features of Currently Available Navigation Technologies in Total Knee Arthroplasty

Feature	Accelerometer	Limited Optical System	Comprehensive Optical System
Provides real-time surgical feedback	Y	Y	Y
Provides information for placement of guides for bone cuts	Y	Y	Y
Preoperative radiographic image necessary	N	N	N
Requires precise digitization of multiple anatomic points	N	Y	Y
Calculates coronal alignment of the limb	N	N	Y
Calculates sagittal alignment of the limb	N	N	Y
Requires separate trackers rigidly fixed to bones	N	N	Y
Requires stand-alone tower in operating room	N	Y	Y
Displays implant rotation	N	N	Y
Calculates implant size	N	N	Y
Calculates flexion/extension gaps	N	N	Y
Displays femoral implant notching and mediolateral overhang	N	N	Y
Displays alignment curve of limb throughout range of movement	N	N	Y
Facilitates measured resection technique	Y	Y	Y
Facilitates gap balancing technique	N	N	Y
Permits real-time digital manipulation of implant position to aid surgical planning	N	N	Y

N = no, Y = yes

by guiding and physically constraining the surgeon within a three-dimensional space, but it does not autonomously perform bone resection. With passive systems, the robot positions a cutting guide at a computer-navigated position, but does not perform surgical manipulation of the patient and does not constrain the surgeon.[13]

Image-based and Imageless RKA Systems

RKA is an extension of standard CAS and uses either an image-based or imageless user interface. Image-based RKA systems use preoperative CT, MRI, or radiography for intraoperative referencing with surgical tracking technologies for surgical execution. Imageless RKA systems use intraoperative acquisition of the patient's anatomy and landmarks to integrate into the surgical plan and execution. Intraoperative acquisition of the patient's anatomy is through technology and techniques as described previously for navigation systems.

Although imageless RKA systems may reduce costs and minimize radiation, preoperative image-based planning enables anatomic implant matching and potentially improves operating room efficiency. Image-based systems provide information regarding osteophytes and hip-to-ankle bone pathology, and in the case of CT-based systems, these systems are able to provide information on bone cysts and bone density evaluation. Three-dimensional bone models are created from a CT scan, MRI, or special biplanar two-dimensional radiography, depending on the system used. The three-dimensional model enables patient matching and millimetric intraoperative registration and tracking accuracy. The surgeon can position the implant on the three-dimensional model in the preferred angulation, depth, and rotation. The joint line can be defined, and the personalized fit to the cortical boundaries can be obtained. A virtual model of the surgical plan is presented for review.

Implant placement accounts for anatomic fit and can be adjusted based on the patient's intraoperative kinematics (**Figure 9**). The parameters that will adjust the initial plan are the preferred mechanical alignment, the implant gap distances, and an optimized implant articulation through a full range of motion. It is common to adjust the implants after kinematic inputs in unicompartmental knee surgery because balance and alignment are modified via bone resection and implant position.

A number of different RKA systems are available and use either a burr or saw to perform resections. The patient is positioned in a standard supine fashion, and an articulating leg holder is used. The robotic arms are sterilely draped, positioned for access into the knee, and registered to the navigation tracking system. The navigation camera system, if required, is positioned to prevent tracking interference. In all systems, the patient's anatomy is registered using tracking devices and sensors as reference points.

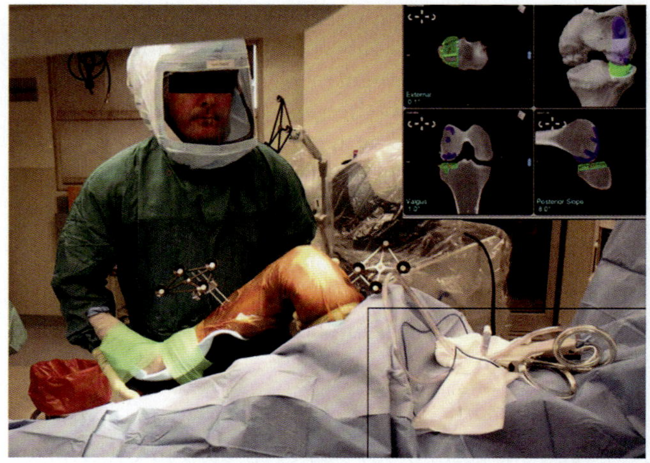

FIGURE 9 Photograph shows a surgeon evaluating the kinematic tracking before bone resection.

The reference points are registered and referenced to the robotic device and are then tracked by using either direct attachment between the robot and the bone or through an optical tracking system. The surgeon modifies the implant placement based on preresection inputs to optimize alignment, gap distance, and implant congruity.

Using kinematic inputs, a surgeon can balance a robotic-assisted UKA preresection, by modifying the depth of angular resection. In an RKA, the accuracy of the robotic arm allows the surgeon to use intraoperative sensors to define the patient's specific kinetic signature and achieve balance through bone and angular adjustments instead of soft-tissue releases.[14,15] With an active RKA system, the robotic arm performs all prescribed cuts autonomously, whereas the surgeon protects soft tissues and monitors the robotic arm for safety. In a semiactive system, the surgeon then maneuvers the robotic device while visualizing the execution on a computer screen. Semiactive systems use a combination of visual, audible, and haptic feedback, along with speed control of the burr/saw to keep the cutting instrument within predefined margins. In a passive system, the robotic arm places the cutting guide at the predefined location and the surgeon then uses a saw/burr to perform the cuts in a traditional manner. The system uses independent tracking probes to confirm implant placement. Implants are either cemented or noncemented and are unique to each system (**Figure 10**).

Robotic Utilization in UKA

The first clinical robotic-assisted medial UKA case was performed in 2006.[16] Indications have expanded to include bicompartmental[17] and TKA applications.[6] The systems integrate preoperative planning with a robotic device that executes the defined surgical plan. The value of RKA applications focuses on patient customization

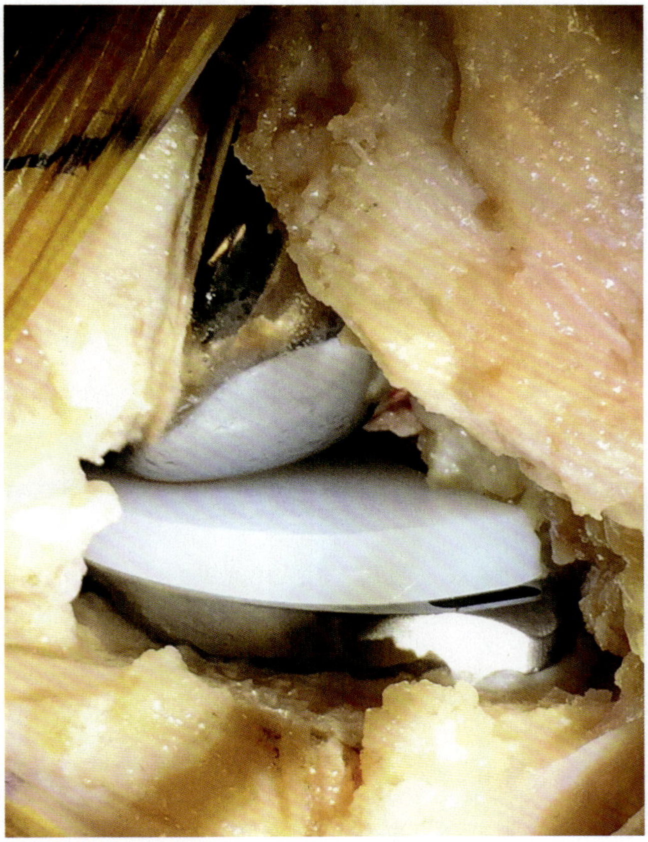

FIGURE 10 Intraoperative photograph shows a cemented unicompartmental knee arthroplasty.

and an efficient, accurate execution of the surgical plan. With traditional techniques, early failure of UKAs often results from poor bone preparation, implant malposition, overcorrection of alignment, and poor cement technique. This can lead to either aseptic loosening of the tibial and femoral implant or overloading of the contralateral compartment and development of arthritis.

Intraoperative data and precision bone preparation minimizes outliers. The ability to obtain accurate implant placement includes avoiding independent as well as combined potential errors.[18,19] The sagittal, coronal, and axial planes on each prepared condyle, as well as the preservation of the joint line and limb alignment, are critical to obtain a successful outcome. The bone resection depth, mechanical alignment, cortical rim coverage, rotation, and slope are defined before bone resection. The surgeon performs a standard approach, inspects the knee pathology, and assesses the ligament stability. The surgeon can modify the plan to include resurfacing of other compartments if required. The surgeon attaches the navigation trackers/pins and registers the limb and knee anatomy as per the process defined by the device manufacturer. Probes are used to collect bony and cartilage registration points, which are referenced to preoperative imaging if applicable. The registration is now verified to be within the submillimeter accuracy required by the system specifications to allow progression to the next steps. Cartilage mapping in bicompartmental knee arthroplasty can be performed to provide a smooth transition for the patella across the trochlear groove because it articulates on the femoral implant in early flexion.[20]

The surgeon removes osteophytes and moves corrected limb positions through a full range of motion to capture the patient's baseline limb alignment and ligament balance. The surgeon uses the navigation to obtain a corrected position and ensures that the mechanical axis is within acceptable parameters. As the knee is taken through a range of motion, the surgeon inspects the femorotibial tracking on the computer to define implant-to-implant articulation and gap balancing. The femoral and tibial implants can now be adjusted to obtain a centered tracking path, corrected alignment, and an appropriate gap distance of 1 to 2 mm through a full range of motion.[15] The implants can be rotated, flexed, extended, translated, or adjusted in the coronal and sagittal planes on the computer screen to obtain the appropriate preresection positions. Before surgical bone preparation, the surgeon can modify and adjust the surgical plan to define the mechanical alignment, implant tracking, bone resection depths, joint line, and gap distances in millimeters. The surgical plan is then executed with the robotic-controlled instrument.

The surgical leg is controlled in a modular leg holder, and soft-tissue retractors are positioned. The robotic arm activates when it enters the volume of bone resection to be prepared. In active/semiactive systems, the safety elements include deactivation of the burr/saw if the planned resection levels are breached on any plane. Passive systems rely on the surgeon to control the burr/saw within and outside the planned resection.

After the bone has been prepared, residual meniscus and/or osteophytes are removed (**Figure 11**). The trial implants then allow a kinematic assessment, and the executed plan is confirmed. The final implants are implanted, the navigation pins are removed, and standard closure is performed.

Robotic-assisted TKA Applications

The first robotic-assisted TKA surgery was performed in 1988. Despite this, RKA usage in TKA has only become popularized in the last decade and has been built off platforms designed for UKAs. There are now numerous FDA-approved TKA robots. The principles/techniques of robotic-assisted TKA follow those that were previously described for robotic-assisted UKAs. The surgical approach is surgeon specific, and initial registration defines the limb alignment and knee

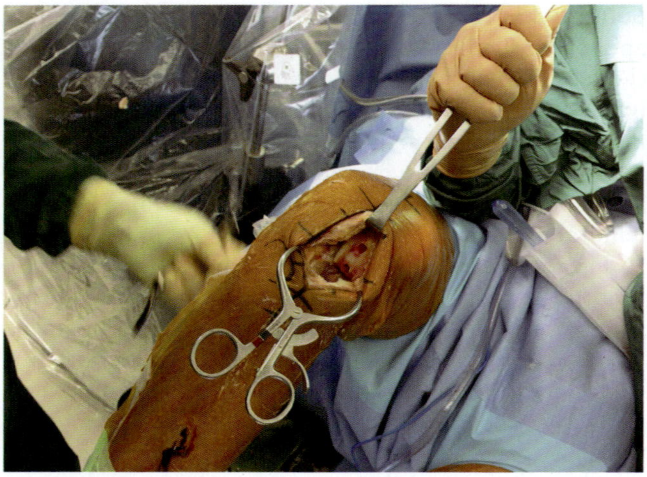

FIGURE 11 Clinical photograph shows a unicompartmental knee prepared for final implantation.

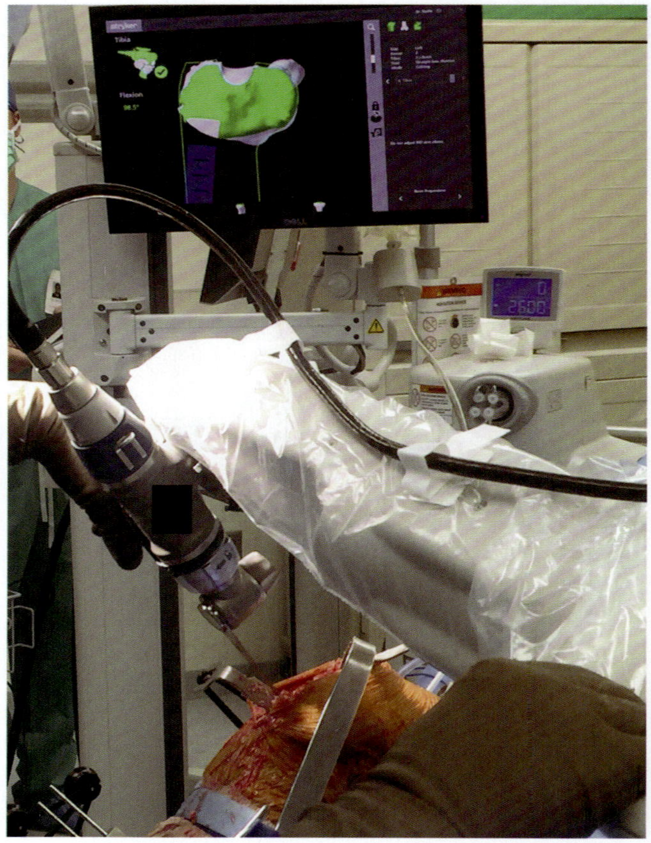

FIGURE 12 Intraoperative photograph of a robotic-assisted total knee arthroplasty demonstrates the surgeon resecting the tibia under haptic control using the interactive computer screen.

kinematics to which the surgical plan is adjusted. Soft-tissue balancing is performed by using navigation input and surgical preference. Cemented and noncemented TKA are available (**Figure 12**).

Surgical Efficiencies

As with any new technology, a dedicated, experienced surgical team will improve efficiency and shorten the overall learning curve. Surgeon learning curve has been well documented with RKA; after approximately seven cases, steady-state surgical times can be reached and complications are minimal during the learning curve.[21] The surgeon, if not accustomed to navigation and robotic technology, should slowly integrate the systems into the surgical day, to accommodate for increased surgical times.

Preoperative imaging has the potential advantages of defining implant choice preoperatively and minimizing the required instrumentation during surgery, thus improving efficiency. Efficiencies are gained with RKA systems as these systems do not use multiple cutting guides as required by traditional instrument systems.

Robotic Safety Checks

Although the robotic arm ensures accurate implant placement, many additional factors are required for a successful surgical outcome.[5,16,22] There are several safety systems in place throughout the procedure to ensure that accuracy is achieved. Tibial and femoral checkpoints must be verified before each section of bone is prepared. At any point throughout the procedure, the robotic arm and mechanical burr/saw can be removed from the surgical zone, and bony references and resections can be verified with the computer display.

The navigation pins must be placed so that there is no interference with the robotic arm during knee motion. The pins should be placed in a standard fashion to minimize risk of bone fractures. Checkpoints should be placed in an accessible area but away from cortical margins to avoid stress risers. Care must be taken to avoid water, debris, or lights directly on the reflective disks for camera-based systems. Care must also be taken not to knock or move the arrays after registration. When adjusting the knee's flexion angle, it is important to do so in a stable manner. The robotic platform will identify velocity and rapid movements and will halt burr/saw activation.

The integration of haptics in some semiactive systems has advanced the safety and efficiency of TKA. Robotic arm assistance allows a surgeon to have a controlled, highly accurate system that is integrated into the surgical workflow.[16] Haptics is the science of applying touch or tactile sensation and control to interactions with computer applications. The surgeon receives a tactile sensation of the arm physically resisting a surgeon's applied force when the haptic boundary is approached. The saw/burr is shut off if the haptic boundary is breached. Boundaries are specified to match the implant shape, size, and placement based on surgical planning. Compared with passive RKA systems that position cutting jigs for use with a handheld saw, haptic robots may better protect periarticular soft tissues from harm, by more effectively constraining the cutting tool within a specified working field.

The current active and semiactive systems provide irrigation to keep the burr tips cool and avoid thermal bone injury. In passive systems, the surgeon visualizes the burr/saw blade and irrigates the area in a standard manner. The risk of malfunction of the RKA system is minimal in current systems,[23] but the surgeon should understand the surgical plan and have access to conventional instruments if desired.

Active and semiactive systems are designed to not cut outside of the planned resection of bone, but it is the responsibility of the surgeon to use retractors and positioning to protect soft tissues from damage. Passive systems rely on the surgeon to control the burr/saw to avoid cutting outside of the planned resection, in addition to protecting soft tissues with retractors and positioning. RKA has been shown to have less damage to soft tissues than conventional UKAs and TKAs,[24] but there has been concern about an increase in infections in robotic-assisted UKA compared with conventional UKAs.[25]

Economic Issues

As with any new technology in a healthcare environment, value must be proved before widespread acceptance. Currently, without a reimbursement for RKA, the hospital system or ambulatory surgery center must make a significant investment in this technology. The hospital determines the initial return on investment by looking at the orthopaedic product line and marketing potential. Surgeons are required to invest time and evaluate clinical data to ensure this approach improves patient outcomes. A 2019 economic analysis has shown that RKA systems are highly cost effective.[26] RKA systems will potentially take cost out of the system by minimizing surgical errors that can lead to revisions. As RKA systems evolve, surgical efficiency should improve, and earlier discharges will be supported. Substantial cost benefits could be realized if long-term outcomes of CAS/RKA continue to show reduced revision rates.

CLINICAL STUDIES FOR COMPUTER-ASSISTED NAVIGATION

Proposed advantages of CAS include increased accuracy in implant position, decreased blood loss, potentially fewer complications, and better clinical function and implant survivorship secondary to improved implant position.[9]

Several studies have shown similar accuracy with fewer outliers from the traditional mechanical axis between CAS and conventional instrumentation in terms of alignment.[27,28] A meta-analysis of all 23 randomized controlled trials (RCTs) in the literature from 1986 to 2009 reported that patients undergoing CAS TKA had a significantly lower risk of implant malalignment in both coronal and sagittal planes for both implants.[29] This finding was supported by a 2019 meta-analysis showing improved sagittal alignment of the femoral implant and improved coronal alignment of the tibial implant when compared with conventional instrumentation.[30] Studies focused on implant rotation have also highlighted the potential benefits of computer navigation in TKA. Femoral implant rotation has been found to be significantly more accurate when using CAS compared with conventional instrumentation.[31] Consequently, CAS is successful in improving implant position accuracy in primary TKA.

An advantage of CAS compared with conventional instrumentation is the elimination of the need to violate the medullary canal, thus potentially reducing blood loss and thromboembolic complications. A 2012 study compared total blood loss in patients undergoing TKA by using CAS versus conventional instruments and found that patients in the CAS group had significantly lower total blood loss (1,137 versus 1,362 mL; $P = 0.016$) compared with control patients.[28] A review of 47 studies involving 7,151 TKAs reported that imageless navigation provided lower blood loss compared with that of traditional TKA.[32] Furthermore, a retrospective study compared a group of 100 patients undergoing TKA by using an abbreviated CAS protocol with traditional intramedullary instrumentation and found that navigation resulted in less hourly drain output, hemoglobin change, and estimated blood loss.[27] However, despite a clinical advantage in blood loss reduction, comparative studies have not shown a significant decrease in overall complications between the two techniques.[27,32] A systematic review that included 21 comparative studies and 2,333 TKAs showed similar rates of early postoperative complications in patients undergoing TKA by using navigation compared with conventional instrumentation.[33,34] In addition, navigation can be associated, although rarely, with pin-site fractures and infections. Therefore, CAS does not markedly reduce postoperative complications compared with conventional instrumentation, and the immediate clinical benefits of CAS remain unclear.

The principal argument for the use of CAS in TKA centers on the premise that improved implant position will lead to improved clinical ratings (such as the Knee Society Score and the Western Ontario and McMaster Universities Osteoarthritis Index) and increased implant survivorship. Several recent comparative studies have not shown significant differences in terms of clinical rating scores between the two techniques. One retrospective study reported that, in a group of patients who have valgus arthritic knees, CAS TKA resulted in fewer implant position outliers and lower lateral release rates compared with traditional instrumentation, but there were no significant differences in survivorship, Hospital for Special Surgery, and International Knee Society scores between the two groups at a mean follow-up of 46 months.[35] A trial of 108 patients was randomly assigned to CAS or conventional TKA; at 9 years, no significant differences in survivorship, radiographic analysis, and clinical functional scores were found.[36] A 2017 RCT confirmed these findings in 296 patients undergoing same-day bilateral TKA. One knee was randomized to CAS, whereas the other underwent conventional instrumentation. At a mean follow-up of 15 years, no difference was found in functional outcome scores, radiographic parameters, or complications.[37] These observations have also been confirmed at the registry level. A 2020 study analyzed 19,221 CAS TKA from the New Zealand National Joint Registry with a mean follow-up of 4.5 years and found no difference in revision rates and Oxford Knee Score when compared with conventional instrumentation.[38] A 2018 RCT did, however, show improved Knee Injury and Osteoarthritis Outcome Score in the subscales of symptoms and sports and recreation as well as improved stiffness when compared with conventional instrumentation at 2-year follow-up.[39] However, navigation in TKA may be of benefit in younger patients undergoing TKA. A recent analysis of the Australian Orthopaedic Association National Joint Arthroplasty Registry showed that, although overall implant survivorship was not significantly different between patients undergoing TKA using CAS, patients younger than 65 years undergoing TKA using CAS had significantly lowered risks for revision for aseptic loosening and lysis compared with knees not undergoing CAS.[40] The reasons for these findings are unclear, but the study emphasizes the importance of reasonable implant position on implant survivorship in the younger and more active patient.

CLINICAL STUDIES FOR HANDHELD NAVIGATION (ACCELEROMETERS)

Handheld or portable navigation devices have been shown effective in improving bone resection accuracy without adding significant cost or time to the procedure. A 2013 study compared a portable accelerometer-based navigation to an imageless, large-console navigation system in primary TKA, and the accelerometer-based navigation was found to be equally accurate in restoring alignment within the traditional mechanical axis target with a significant decrease in surgical time.[41] Another study found that the portable accelerometer was more accurate in restoring tibial alignment compared with conventional extramedullary tibial cutting guides.[42] These findings may force a recalculation of the cost-benefit equation for the use of navigation in primary TKA. As newer generations of navigation systems become more compact, portable, accurate, and less costly, the application and use of this technology may broaden and increase over time.

CLINICAL STUDIES FOR RKA SYSTEMS

Initial data have shown that robotic-assisted UKAs are two to three times more accurate and three times more reproducible than conventionally performed manual UKAs.

Results from a clinical RCT performed in 2013 revealed lower visual analog scale pain scores during the first 8 weeks postoperatively compared with manual surgery, with improved alignment as assessed by CT scans.[43] Two-year follow-up of these patients showed greater improvement in robotic-assisted UKAs than traditional UKAs for patient reported outcome measures among patients who have higher preoperative activity scores.[44] A 2013 study of 701 RIO (Stryker Mako) robotic-assisted UKAs from a multicenter trial revealed a 1.1% revision rate at 2-year follow-up,[22] lower than the 3.4% to 4.8% rates for revision 2 years after conventional UKA in international registry data.[25,45] Midterm outcomes are now available for cemented robotic-assisted UKA and reveal a revision rate of 2.2% for medial UKAs in a study of 802 medial UKAs at 5-year follow-up,[46] which is lower than the 6.1% to 8.0% revision rate seen in international registries.[25,45]

Early registry data from the Australian registry is beginning to show a trend toward an overall reduction in revision of robotic-assisted UKA compared with conventional technique UKAs, with statistical significance between 9 and 18 months. Robotic-assisted UKAs were found to have fewer revisions for loosening, progression of disease, fracture, and pain than traditional UKAs, but more revisions were undertaken for infection of robotic-assisted UKAs.[25]

Emerging evidence is currently available for robotic-assisted TKAs. Current evidence from a 2018 study of 40 consecutive conventional TKAs, followed by 40 robotic-assisted TKAs, showed minimal learning curve, early functional recovery, decreased blood loss, and decreased time to discharge for the robotic-assisted TKAs.[6] A systematic review from 2018 showed only 1/181 robotic-assisted TKA had a malalignment of >3°, compared with a rate of 42/159 in conventional TKA.[47] A 2018 study has shown this increased accuracy has been maintained at 10-year follow-up, although no improvement in survival or clinical outcomes was found.[48] An RCT from 2014 has shown increased accuracy of the joint line position and fewer incidences of notching and alignment outliers.[49]

There is an epistemological argument the reader should consider regarding the literature around CAS and RKA. Most studies in the literature report outcomes when aiming for a target of neutral mechanical alignment. Paradoxically, CAS and RKA have driven the recent increased adoption of a patient-specific target that may not be limited to neutral mechanical alignment. It is hypothesized that the ability to precisely and accurately achieve the desired patient-specific target of implant position and limb alignment will further improve clinical outcomes and survivorship.

FUTURE APPLICATIONS

RKA enables engineers and surgeons to design future implants that may change geometries and articular bearings as bone resection techniques advance. Enabling accurate bone resection will increase the use of bone ingrowth implants (**Figure 13**), fixation options, and the potential kinematic advantages.[50]

RKA will enable a surgeon to define the initial bone resections, implant positions, and alignment. These variables can be precisely adjusted intraoperatively based on an individual's soft-tissue balance. Integrated sensors will provide real-time data on the individual's soft-tissue tension, enabling the surgeon to optimize the knee balance based on implant or axis adjustments.[51] These data will allow evaluation of the short-term and long-term effects on mechanical and kinematic constitutional approaches in all three planes.[50,52,53] RKA will likely facilitate the increased acceptance and adoption of a patient-specific target regarding the shapes and positioning of the implants as well as overall limb alignment.[54] RKA clearly increases precision and accuracy in consideration of a patient-specific target.

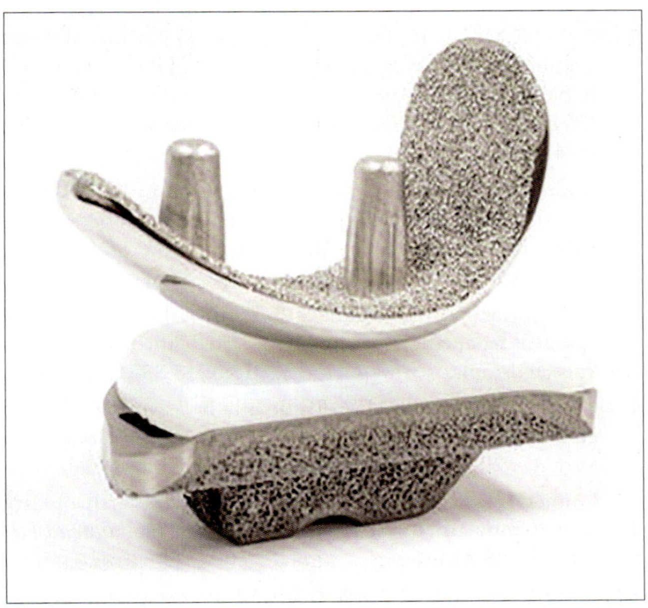

FIGURE 13 Photograph shows a press-fit unicompartmental implant.

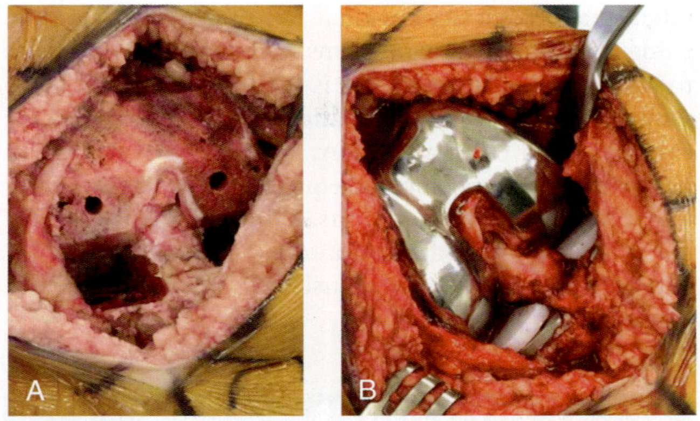

FIGURE 14 Intraoperative photographs show (**A**) a prepared bicruciate-retaining knee and (**B**) the final implant with independent tibial implants.

The potential benefits of an ACL-preserved TKA have been reevaluated recently with a manual approach.[55] The potential to achieve appropriate intercompartmental alignment, slope, joint line, and optimal tension on the cruciate and collateral ligaments should allow a more consistent surgical result in which outcome data can be evaluated (**Figure 14**). Promising results have been reported with no postoperative complications and more accurate joint line reconstruction in a group of modular bicompartmental arthroplasties using the RIO platform.[56]

SUMMARY

Computer navigation and computer-assisted technologies can improve accuracy and minimize outliers in TKA. Although CAS is more reliable and reproducible in achieving the planned targets compared with conventional instrumentation, clinical outcomes have not been consistently shown to be significantly different when the traditional mechanical axis target is used. Additionally, cost and time considerations currently place navigation at a disadvantage for routine use in TKA.

The use of passive, semiactive, and active RKA platforms continues to increase. RKA systems incorporate specific patient planning with accurate execution of the surgical plan. This precision and consistency can be documented and then tracked to evaluate these variables on patient outcomes.[57] Integration of alignment, implant rotation, and soft-tissue balance are the cornerstones of successful knee arthroplasty outcomes.[58] To date, imprecise manual instruments and subjective decisions are used to assess these variables. Robotic technologies create an efficient approach to individual arthritic presentations by using modular implant systems that extend from UKAs to TKAs. Emerging evidence is showing increased accuracy of implant positioning, and improved outcomes for robot-assisted UKA and TKA. The future of RKA will be driven by the consumer's request, surgeon acceptance, and economic considerations. Long-term studies will allow the orthopaedic community to assess the data, compare approaches, and translate this into efficient and safe surgical procedures.

KEY STUDY POINTS

- RKA and CAS technology are evolving in the care of symptomatic knee arthritis. Integrating patient-specific data with intraoperative flexibility and improved accuracy will enable a patient-specific approach to address the continuum of knee pathologies.
- Current RKA devices are active, semiactive, or passive, all of which require surgeon input to maintain efficient, accurate, and safe execution of the surgical plan.
- RKA has shown promising early results to minimize surgical errors that result in a significant number of revisions and poor patient satisfaction. Further long-term studies are required to support the capital investment and sustained improvement in patient outcomes.
- CAS technologies have been shown to be more accurate in mechanically aligned primary TKA than conventional instrumentation; however, comparative studies have shown minimal improvement in outcomes.
- RKA will likely evolve to become the standard of care in the future because RKA allows for an accurate and precise approach to a patient-specific TKA plan.

ANNOTATED REFERENCES

1. Mihalko WM, Boyle J, Clark LD, Krackow KA: The variability of intramedullary alignment of the femoral component during total knee arthroplasty. *J Arthroplasty* 2005;20:25-28.
2. Sharkey PF, Hozack WJ, Rothman RH, Shastri S, Jacoby SM: Insall Award paper: Why are total knee arthroplasties failing today? *Clin Orthop Relat Res* 2002;404:7-13.
3. Babazadeh S, Stoney JD, Lim K, Choong PF: The relevance of ligament balancing in total knee arthroplasty: How important is it? A systematic review of the literature. *Orthop Rev (Pavia)* 2009;1:e26.
4. Cobb J, Henckel J, Gomes P, et al: Hands-on robotic unicompartmental knee replacement: A prospective, randomised controlled study of the acrobot system. *J Bone Joint Surg Br* 2006;88:188-197.
5. Roche M, O'Loughlin PF, Kendoff D, Musahl V, Pearle AD: Robotic arm-assisted unicompartmental knee arthroplasty: Preoperative planning and surgical technique. *Am J Orthop (Belle Mead NJ)* 2009;38:10-15.
6. Kayani B, Konan S, Tahmassebi J, Pietrzak JRT, Haddad FS: Robotic-arm assisted total knee arthroplasty is associated with improved early functional recovery and reduced time to hospital discharge compared with conventional jig-based total knee arthroplasty. *Bone Joint J* 2018;100-B(7): 930-937.

   This is a prospective cohort study of 40 robotic TKAs and 40 manual TKAs, which showed improved early functional recovery and time to discharge for robotic TKAs.
7. Beard DJ, Pandit H, Gill HS, Hollinghurst D, Dodd CA, Murray DW: The influence of the presence and severity of pre-existing patellofemoral degenerative changes on the outcome of the Oxford medial unicompartmental knee replacement. *J Bone Joint Surg Br* 2007;89:1597-1601.
8. da Mota e Albuquerque RF: Navigation in total knee arthroplasty. *Rev Bras Ortop* 2015;46:18-22.
9. Bae DK, Song SJ: Computer assisted navigation in knee arthroplasty. *Clin Orthop Surg* 2011;3:259-267.
10. OrthoMap Precision Knee Navigation: *Surgical Technique Manual for the OrthoMap Express Knee Navigation Software. Kalamazoo, MI, Stryker*, 2012. Available at: https://www.strykermeded.com/media/2007/navigation-orthomap-precision-knee-surgical-technique.pdf. Accessed May 15, 2020.
11. Pitto RP, Graydon AJ, Bradley L, Malak SF, Walker CG, Anderson IA: Accuracy of a computer-assisted navigation system for total knee replacement. *J Bone Joint Surg Br* 2006;88:601-605.
12. KneeAlign 2 System: *Surgical Technique Manual, Tibial and Distal Femur Navigation*. Aliso Viejo, CA, OrthAlign, 2012.
13. Picard F, Moody JE, DiGioia AM, Jaramaz B: Clinical classification of CAOS systems, in DiGioia AM, Jaramaz B, Picard F, Nolte LP, eds: *Computer and Robotic Assisted Hip and Knee Surgery*. New York, NY, Oxford University Press, 2004, pp 43-48.
14. Anderson C, Roche M, Golladay G, Elson L: Bony cuts or soft-tissue release? Using intra-operative sensors to refine balancing techniques in TKA. *Bone Joint J* 2016;98-B (suppl 1):16.
15. Plate JF, Mofidi A, Mannava S, et al: Achieving accurate ligament balancing using robotic-assisted unicompartmental knee arthroplasty. *Adv Orthop* 2013;2013:837167.
16. Conditt MA, Roche MW: Minimally invasive robotic-arm-guided unicompartmental knee arthroplasty. *J Bone Joint Surg Am* 2009;91:63-68.
17. Lonner JH: Modular bicompartmental knee arthroplasty with robotic arm assistance. *Am J Orthop (Belle Mead NJ)* 2009;38:28-31.
18. Citak M, Suero EM, Citak M, et al: Unicompartmental knee arthroplasty: Is robotic technology more accurate than conventional technique? *Knee* 2013;20:268-271.

19. Dunbar NJ, Roche MW, Park BH, Branch SH, Conditt MA, Banks SA: Accuracy of dynamic tactile-guided unicompartmental knee arthroplasty. *J Arthroplasty* 2012;27(5):803-808.e1.

20. *Mako Partial Knee Medial Unicondylar Resurfacing Surgical Reference Guide*. Mahwah, NJ, Stryker, 2016. Available at: https://www.strykermeded.com/media/2238/mako-partial-knee_medial-unicondylar-resurfacing_surgical-reference-guide.pdf. Accessed May 15, 2020.

21. Kayani B, Konan S, Huq S, et al: Robotic-arm assisted total knee arthroplasty has a learning curve of seven cases for integration into the surgical workflow but no learning curve effect for accuracy of implant positioning. *Knee Surg Sports Traumatol Arthrosc* 2019;27:1132-1141.

    This study of 60 consecutive traditional TKAs and robotic-assisted TKAs showed a seven-case learning curve for surgical time and stress, with no learning curve for implant positioning. There were no increased complications during the learning curve. Level of evidence: II.

22. Conditt M, Coon T, Roche M, et al: Two year survivorship of robotically guided unicompartmental knee arthroplasty. *Bone Joint J* 2013;95-B(suppl 34):294.

23. Lonner JH, Kerr GJ: Robotically assisted unicompartmental knee arthroplasty. *Oper Tech Orthop* 2012;22(4):182-188.

24. Khlopas A, Chughtai M, Hamp EL, et al: Robotic-arm assisted total knee arthroplasty demonstrated soft tissue protection. *Surg Technol Int* 2017;30:441-446.

    Cadaveric study of 6 RTKA and 7 manual TKA controls. There was decreased tibial subluxation and patella eversion found in the RTKA group. Two of seven MTKA had slight PCL damage versus none in the RTKA group. Level of evidence: III.

25. Australian Orthopaedic Association National Joint Replacement Registry: *Annual Report 2013*. Available at: https://aoanjrr.sahmri.com/documents/10180/668596/Hip%2C+Knee+%26+Shoulder+Arthroplasty/c287d2a3-22df-a3bb-37a2-91e6c00bfcf0. Accessed May 15, 2020.

26. Clement ND, Deehan DJ, Patton JT: Robot-assisted unicompartmental knee arthroplasty for patients with isolated medial compartment osteoarthritis is cost-effective: A Markov decision analysis. *Bone Joint J* 2019;101-B(9):1063-1070.

    An economic analysis of robotic UKAs versus manual UKAs and TKAs, which uses a Markov decision analysis to show robotic UKAs are highly cost-effective per quality-adjusted life-year gained.

27. Licini DJ, Meneghini RM: Modern abbreviated computer navigation of the femur reduces blood loss in total knee arthroplasty. *J Arthroplasty* 2015;30:1729-1732.

28. McConnell J, Dillon J, Kinninmonth A, Sarungi M, Picard F: Blood loss following total knee replacement is reduced when using computer-assisted versus standard methods. *Acta Orthop Belg* 2012;78:75-79.

29. Hetaimish BM, Khan MM, Simunovic N, Al-Harbi HH, Bhandari M, Zalzal PK: Meta-analysis of navigation vs conventional total knee arthroplasty. *J Arthroplasty* 2012;27:1177-1182.

30. Rhee SJ, Kim HJ, Lee CR, Kim CW, Gwak HC, Kim JH: A comparison of long-term outcomes of computer-navigated and conventional total knee arthroplasty: A meta-analysis of randomized controlled trials. *J Bone Joint Surg Am* 2019;101(20):1875-1885.

    This meta-analysis of nine RCTs comparing CAS and conventional TKA showed improved sagittal alignment of the femoral implant and improved coronal alignment of the tibial implant in the CAS group. Level of evidence: I.

31. Hernandez-Vaquero D, Noriega-Fernandez A, Fernandez-Carreira JM, Fernandez-Simon JM, Llorens de los Rios J: Computer-assisted surgery improves rotational positioning of the femoral component but not the tibial component in total knee arthroplasty. *Knee Surg Sports Traumatol Arthrosc* 2014;22:3127-3134.

32. Moskal JT, Capps SG, Mann JW, Scanelli JA: Navigated versus conventional total knee arthroplasty. *J Knee Surg* 2014;27:235-248.

33. Cheng T, Pan XY, Mao X, Zhang GY, Zhang XL: Little clinical advantage of computer-assisted navigation over conventional instrumentation in primary total knee arthroplasty at early follow-up. *Knee* 2012;19:237-245.

34. Cheng T, Zhao S, Peng X, Zhang X: Does computer-assisted surgery improve postoperative leg alignment and implant positioning following total knee arthroplasty? A meta-analysis of randomized controlled trials? *Knee Surg Sports Traumatol Arthrosc* 2012;20:1307-1322.

35. Huang TW, Kuo LT, Peng KT, Lee MS, Hsu RW: Computed tomography evaluation in total knee arthroplasty: Computer-assisted navigation versus conventional instrumentation in patients with advanced valgus arthritic knees. *J Arthroplasty* 2014;29:2363-2368.

36. Zhu M, Ang CL, Yeo SJ, Lo NN, Chia SL, Chong HC: Minimally invasive computer-assisted total knee arthroplasty compared with conventional total knee arthroplasty: A prospective 9-year follow-up. *J Arthroplasty* 2016;31:1000-1004.

37. Kim YH, Park JW, Kim JS: 2017 Chitranjan S. Ranawat Award: Does computer navigation in knee arthroplasty improve functional outcomes in young patients? A randomized study. *Clin Orthop Relat Res* 2018;476(1):6-15.

    This is an RCT of patients undergoing same-day bilateral TKA with one knee being randomized to CAS and the other undergoing conventional technique. No difference was found in regard to function, radiographic parameters, or complications. Level of evidence: I.

38. Roberts TD, Frampton CM, Young SW: Outcomes of computer-assisted surgery compared with conventional instrumentation in 19,221 total knee arthroplasties. *J Bone Joint Surg* 2020;102(7):550-556.

    An analysis of the New Zealand Joint Registry comparing CAS and conventional instrumentation showed no difference in revision rates or outcome scores. Level of evidence: III.

39. Petursson G, Fenstad AM, Gøthesen Ø, et al: Computer-assisted compared with conventional total knee replacement: A multicenter parallel-group randomized controlled trial. *J Bone Joint Surg Am* 2018;100(15):1265-1274.

This is an RCT that compared CAS and conventional instrumentation. At 2-year follow-up, there was improved outcome score in symptoms, sports/recreation, and stiffness in the CAS group. Level of evidence: I.

40. de Steiger RN, Liu YL, Graves SE: Computer navigation for total knee arthroplasty reduces revision rate for patients less than sixty-five years of age. *J Bone Joint Surg Am* 2015;97:635-642.

41. Nam D, Weeks KD, Reinhardt KR, Nawabi DH, Cross MB, Mayman DJ: Accelerometer-based, portable navigation vs imageless, large-console computer-assisted navigation in total knee arthroplasty: A comparison of radiographic results. *J Arthroplasty* 2013;28:255-261.

42. Nam D, Cody EA, Nguyen JT, Figgie MP, Mayman DJ: Extramedullary guides versus portable, accelerometer-based navigation for tibial alignment in total knee arthroplasty. A randomized, controlled trial: Winner of the 2013 HAP Paul Award. *J Arthroplasty* 2014;29:288-294.

43. Bell SW, Anthony I, Jones B, MacLean A, Rowe P, Blyth M: Improved accuracy of component positioning with robotic-assisted unicompartmental knee arthroplasty: Data from a prospective, randomized controlled study. *J Bone Joint Surg Am* 2016;98(8):627-635.

44. Gilmour A, MacLean AD, Rowe PJ, et al: Robotic-arm–assisted vs conventional unicompartmental knee arthroplasty. The 2-year clinical outcomes of a randomized controlled trial. *J Arthroplasty* 2018;33(7):S109-S115.

A 2-year follow-up of an RCT of robotic UKAs versus manual UKAs showed similar outcome scores and survivorship. Subgroup analysis showed more improvement for robotic UKAs with a higher preoperative activity score. Level of evidence: I.

45. Canadian Institute for Health Information: *Hip and Knee Replacements in Canada–Canadian Joint Replacement Registry (CJRR) 2017-2018 Annual Report*, 2019. Available at: https://www.cihi.ca/sites/default/files/document/cjrr-update-summer-2019-en.pdf. Accessed May 15, 2020.

An overview of the 2019 annual report is presented, with an analysis of findings.

46. Burger JA, Kleeblad LJ, Laas N, et al: Mid-term survivorship and patient-reported outcomes of robotic-arm assisted partial knee arthroplasty: A single-surgeon study of 1,018 knees. *Bone Joint J* 2020;102(1):108-116.

Midterm outcomes for robotic-assisted partial knee arthroplasty are presented. This single-surgeon study had revision rates for medial UKAs of 2.2%, lateral UKAs 2.3%, and patellofemoral/bicompartmental knee arthroplasties of 6.7%. Level of evidence: III.

47. D Mannan A, Vun J, Lodge C, Eyre-Brook A, Jones S: Increased precision of coronal plane outcomes in robotic-assisted total knee arthroplasty: A systematic review and meta-analysis. *Surgeon* 2018;16(4):237-244.

This is a meta-analysis of studies comparing robotic TKAs with manual instrument TKA. Findings were that robotic TKAs were highly accurate compared with manual TKAs. Level of evidence: II.

48. Cho KJ, Seon JK, Jang WY, Park CG, Song EK: Robotic versus conventional primary total knee arthroplasty: Clinical and radiological long-term results with a minimum follow-up of ten years. *Int Orthop* 2019;43(6):1345-1354.

Evaluation of 390 RTKA and conventional TKA. There was no difference in clinical outcomes or survivorship, but there were decreased alignment outliers in the RTKA group. Level of evidence: III.

49. Liow MH, Xia Z, Wong MK, Tay KJ, Yeo SJ, Chin PL: Robot-assisted total knee arthroplasty accurately restores the joint line and mechanical axis. A prospective randomised study. *J Arthroplasty* 2014;29(12):2373-2377.

50. Koenig JH, Hepinstall MS: Available robotic platforms in partial and total knee arthroplasty. *Oper Tech Orthop* 2015;25(2):85-94.

51. Gustke KA: Soft-tissue and alignment correction: The use of smart trials in total knee replacement. *Bone Joint J* 2014;96-B:78-83.

52. Bellemans J, Colyn W, Vandenneucker H, Victor J: The Chitranjan Ranawat Award: Is neutral mechanical alignment normal for all patients? The concept of constitutional varus. *Clin Orthop Relat Res* 2012;470:45-53.

53. Howell SM, Howell SJ, Kuznik KT, Cohen J, Hull ML: Does a kinematically aligned total knee arthroplasty restore function without failure regardless of alignment category? *Clin Orthop Relat Res* 2013;471:1000-1007.

54. Scalise J, Dunbar M, Jacofsky D: Evolving beyond craft surgery is both inevitable and essential.*J Knee Surg* 2017;30(1):3-6.

This editorial discusses orthopaedic surgery utilizing technology such as computer assisted surgery and robotics to improve patient outcomes. Level of evidence: V.

55. Sabouret P, Lavoie F, Cloutier JM: Total knee replacement with retention of both cruciate ligaments: A 22-year follow-up study. *Bone Joint J* 2013;95-B(7):917-922.

56. Pourmoghaddam A, Kreuzer SW, Freedhand A: Early clinical outcomes in robotic assisted bi-unicompartmental total knee replacement compared to unicompartmental and conventional knee arthroplasty. *Bone Joint J* 2013;95-B(suppl 34):381.

57. Bourne RB, Chesworth BM, Davis AM, Mahomed NN, Charron KD: Patient satisfaction after total knee arthroplasty: Who is satisfied and who is not? *Clin Orthop Relat Res* 2010;468:57-63.

58. Kim YH, Park JW, Kim JS, Park SD: The relationship between the survival of total knee arthroplasty and postoperative coronal, sagittal and rotational alignment of knee prosthesis. *Int Orthop* 2014;38:379-385.

CHAPTER 24

The Difficult Primary Total Knee Arthroplasty

WAYNE A. WILKIE, DO, MHSA • NEQUESHA S. MOHAMED, MD
ETHAN A. REMILY, DO • SCOTT McDERMOTT, MD • JORDAN BONIER, DO, MS
JAMES NACE, DO, MPT • RONALD E. DELANOIS, MD

ABSTRACT

The efficacy of primary total knee arthroplasty for the management of knee arthritis in noncomplicated patients has been well established. The evolution of surgical techniques and implant design has expanded the indications of total knee arthroplasty to include more complex cases. However, patients who have large deformities, severe knee stiffness, or posttraumatic arthritis may have difficult surgical exposures and worse outcomes. Furthermore, surgical optimization is necessary for patients who have certain comorbidities such as cardiovascular disease, obesity, inflammatory arthritis, and Charcot arthropathy. By understanding general principles, orthopaedic surgeons may avoid complications while improving outcomes of difficult primary total knee arthroplasties.

Keywords: charcot arthropathy; comorbidity; inflammatory arthritis; posttraumatic arthritis; valgus/varus deformity

Dr. Nace or an immediate family member serves as a paid consultant to or is an employee of Microport; has received research or institutional support from Microport, Stryker, and United Orthopedics; and serves as a board member, owner, officer, or committee member of the Arthritis Foundation. Dr. Delanois or an immediate family member has received research or institutional support from Flexion Therapeutics, Orthofix, Stryker, Tissue Gene, and United Orthopedics; serves as a board member, owner, officer, or committee member of the Baltimore City Medical Society. None of the following authors or any immediate family member has received anything of value from or has stock or stock options held in a commercial company or institution related directly or indirectly to the subject of this chapter: Dr. Wilkie, Dr. Mohamed, Dr. Remily, Dr. McDermott, and Dr. Bonier.

INTRODUCTION

The majority of total knee arthroplasties (TKAs) are performed in patients who possess minimal deformities using standard instrumentation through a medial parapatellar arthrotomy. However, patients who have various deformities, diseases, and comorbidities may pose a challenge for reconstruction surgeons, requiring extra attention during preoperative management and modification of surgical techniques to optimize the postoperative results. This may include more advanced surgical approaches, the use of different instrumentation or navigation, and greater soft-tissue releases about the knee. Additionally, one must be prepared with an assortment of components with varying constraint options when performing a difficult TKA.

KNEE-SPECIFIC CONDITIONS

Large Intra-articular Varus/Valgus Deformities at the Knee

Patients who have a preoperative varus/valgus deformity greater than 8° of varus or 11° of valgus have an increased risk of failure after TKA, independent of postoperative

This chapter is adapted from Mistry JB, Sayeed SA, Chughtai M, Elmallah RK, Mont MM, Delanois RE: The difficult primary total knee arthroplasty, in Mont MA, Tanzer M, eds: *Orthopaedic Knowledge Update®: Hip and Knee Reconstruction*, ed 5. Rosemont, IL, American Academy of Orthopaedic Surgeons, 2017, pp 183-196.

alignment.[1] This higher failure rate may be attributed to increased tibial surface strain or ligamentous instability. However, the achievement of sufficient soft-tissue balance and restoration of neutral limb alignment can significantly improve outcomes after TKA, as overcorrection or undercorrection of the deformity may result in joint instability and polyethylene overload. Thus, surgeons should manage large preoperative varus or valgus deformities by restoring neutral alignment and using a stepwise progression of releases to appropriately balance the knee.

Severe Varus Deformity

Varus knees are characterized by a mechanical axis less than 180°. Because 24% of the population possess constitutionally varus knees,[2] and constitutional varus is associated with increased risk of knee arthritis,[3] there is no surprise that varus alignment is the most common angular deformity in patients undergoing primary TKA. Varus deformity is associated with medial joint space narrowing, flexion and medial soft-tissue contractures, lateral soft-tissue elongation, varus proximal tibial deformity, and loss of tibial bone and/or cartilage in the medial compartment. Severe deformities with medial subluxation of the femur on the tibia represent less than 10% of cases, but require more complex reconstruction.[4]

Patients in 0° to 3° of varus are considered normal or well aligned, whereas those knees in 4° to 10° of varus may be classified as having a common deformity.[5] These knees are usually correctable with minimal releases. However, patients in greater than 10° of varus often have a rigid, noncorrectable varus deformity that requires more extensive medial releases to achieve proper balance and alignment.[4,5] Knees in greater than 20° of varus often have extra-articular involvement such as femoral bowing or proximal tibial varus deformity, which makes neutral correction difficult with conventional surgical techniques.

An examination under anesthesia should be performed to determine if the knee is correctable or has a fixed deformity. After a standard medial parapatellar exposure, the anteromedial capsule and deep medial collateral ligament (MCL) should be released to the semimembranosus bursa with subsequent removal of osteophytes from the medial femoral and tibial condyles. Patients who have flexion contractures may require release of the semimembranosus tendon if the deformity persists after bony preparation. By placing the leg in a figure-four position and externally rotating the foot (Randall maneuver), the tendon can be adequately exposed.

The standard valgus correction angle (VCA), or distal femoral resection, of 5° to 7° of valgus may be used in most cases; however, the appropriate VCA in patients who have severe deformities may vary from 2° to 12°.[6] Therefore, the most accurate VCA is achieved by examination of the hip-knee-ankle angle on full-length standing radiographs. In varus knees, the more normal condyle is often the lateral condyle; therefore, the amount of bone resected from the medial condyle should be equal to or slightly less than the thickness of the implant. However, this resection may be adjusted based on the amount of wear and degeneration present within the joint. The degree of external rotation of the femur can be guided by assessment of the anterior-posterior axis (Whiteside line), transepicondylar axis, posterior condylar axis, and medial-lateral flexion gap asymmetry. Excessive external rotation may result in posteromedial laxity with flexion and tightness of lateral structure, whereas internal rotation may present with posterolateral laxity with flexion and tightness of the medial structures.

The lateral tibial plateau, which is the unaffected side when compared with the medial plateau, can be referenced to guide tibial resection. By referencing approximately two-thirds of the lateral plateau in an anterior-to-posterior manner, the extent of proximal tibial resection can be determined to accommodate the implant. When trial components are in place, medial-lateral stability should be assessed throughout the range of motion (ROM), including medial-lateral stress testing to tension the medial soft-tissue sleeve.

Soft-tissue release of the medial structures may be necessary if the compartment is deemed too tight throughout the arc of motion. The release should be performed in a sequential manner. First, the deep MCL should be released from the proximal tibia. If medial tightness persists, the MCL can be released from the distal tibia. Another described technique uses an 18-gauge needle. In this technique, the MCL is first identified and palpated. Then, an 18-gauge needle is used to place five punctures in the tightest fibers of the MCL.[7] Medial asymmetric tightness in extension requires multiple needle punctures of the posterior aspect of the MCL with the knee in extension, whereas medial asymmetric tightness in flexion can be addressed with multiple punctures of the anterior aspect of the superficial MCL with the knee in flexion. Each series of five needle punctures should be followed with serial stress examinations until the medial compartment opens 1 to 2 mm during extension and 2 to 3 mm in flexion. Surgeons should be cautious because these techniques may place the MCL at increased risk of iatrogenic transection or over release. If the MCL is completely released or is not sufficient to affect balancing, a constrained condylar implant should be used.

Different techniques for management of the varus knee have shown promising results. One study reported on 34 knees that underwent TKA with a preoperative fixed-varus deformity and flexion contracture.[8] These knees required the use of the inside-out technique, which involves a posteromedial capsulotomy at the level of the tibial cut along with pie-crusting of the superficial MCL.

Coronal alignment was corrected from 21.1° of varus preoperatively to 4.5° of valgus postoperatively, and there were no cases of instability at a mean follow-up of 3.1 years. Another report examined a multiple-needle-puncture technique used to balance the MCL in 35 knees with a mean of 12.5° of varus (range, 9° to 23°) before TKA.[9] Thirty-four knees (97%) were successfully corrected with 2 to 4 mm of maximum opening during extension, and 2 to 6 mm of maximum opening during flexion. Similar results were seen in another study in which 62 of 65 varus knees (95%) were successfully corrected by multiple needle punctures of the MCL, based on 2 to 4 mm of joint opening during extension and 2 to 6 mm of opening during flexion.[9] Despite these findings, controversy still remains as to whether leaving a patient in some residual or constitutional varus may actually help with gap balancing and potentially improve patient outcomes.

Severe Valgus Deformity

Approximately 10% of patients who undergo TKA present with a valgus deformity. This can be a result of bone loss from the lateral femoral condyle, lateral femoral condyle hypoplasia, and/or central and posterior tibial bone loss.[10] Additionally, this deformity is often associated with contracted soft tissues laterally and elongated soft tissues medially. Soft-tissue releases will involve both static and dynamic stabilizers in the lateral compartment, including the popliteus tendon, the lateral collateral ligament (LCL), the iliotibial band (ITB), and the posterolateral capsule. Although cadaver studies have demonstrated involvement of the popliteus tendon and LCL throughout the ROM, they contribute more to stability in knee flexion rather than extension. Alternatively, the ITB and posterolateral capsule provide stability primarily during extension.[11] Knees in less than 10° of valgus, which represent 80% of valgus deformity cases, are usually correctable as contractures may occur in lateral tissues without elongation of the MCL.[10] In 15% of cases, the knee is in between 10° and 20° of valgus, with contracture of lateral tissues and an elongated but functional MCL. The final 5% of patients have valgus deformities greater than 20° with tight lateral tissues and medial stabilizers that are no longer functional.

As with varus knees, a preoperative examination under anesthesia should be performed to determine if the knee has a correctable or fixed deformity. Fixed-valgus deformities will likely require substantial soft-tissue balancing, whereas correctable deformities may require few, if any, releases. A standard medial parapatellar approach may be used; however, this approach may lead to poor access to the lateral compartment for extensive lateral tissue release.[10] Although a tibial tuberosity osteotomy (TTO) may alleviate this problem, this technique has been associated with patellar devascularization after a medial parapatellar approach and lateral release. Alternatively, a lateral parapatellar approach may be used, which involves an incision along the lateral border of the patella. The patella may then be dislocated medially with or without a TTO. There is less concern for patellar devascularization in this approach, as the medial blood supply is left intact. However, this approach has been associated with a difficult closure, as a correction of a severe deformity may lead to a gap in the lateral capsule. A two-step process may be used to alleviate this problem. Inferiorly, the infrapatellar fat pad can be pulled laterally and sutured directly into the lateral retinaculum. Superiorly, the superficial and deep layers from the medial and lateral flaps, respectively, of the incised lateral retinaculum may be sutured together.[12]

Although forceful flexion and external rotation of the tibia can help provide exposure in varus knees, this technique may stretch the already compromised medial structures in valgus knees, and therefore should be limited or even avoided. Osteophytes in the lateral compartment should be removed, and any soft-tissue releases should be addressed after bony preparation. Posterior cruciate ligament (PCL) contractures may require balancing or releasing during TKA. If the PCL is to be released, a cruciate-substituting implant is necessary. Severe valgus deformities may also present with patellar maltracking. This may necessitate a lateral retinacular release and/or medial imbrication during TKA. If maltracking issues are noted after trial components have been tested, release the tourniquet because of its tethering effect on the extensor mechanism and reevaluate overall component alignment.

When the distal femur is prepared, the initial intramedullary entry hole should be made in the notch medial to the anterior-posterior axis and anterior to the PCL attachment. This positioning accounts for the lateral bowing of the distal femur in a valgus knee. This starting point should also be confirmed with preoperative templating. A 3° to 5° resection of the distal femur can help prevent undercorrection in a valgus knee while reducing stress on the compromised medial structures. The amount of bone resected from the medial condyle, which is usually more normal, should be equal to the thickness of the metallic medial condyle of the implant. Patients who have severe lateral condyle deformities should not have this area of bone resected because it can create flexion-extension balancing difficulties and raise the joint line, resulting in midflexion instability. Rotational alignment should be derived from the anterior-posterior and transepicondylar axes. Posterior referencing to determine femoral implant rotation should be used with caution because of the higher incidence of hypoplastic lateral femoral condyle, which may result in falsely internally rotating the femoral implant. When preparing the tibia for resection, the extramedullary alignment guides should be placed at a 90° angle to the longitudinal axis of the tibia. In severely valgus knees, intramedullary alignment should be used with caution because of the valgus bowing of the tibial shaft. The degree of posterior slope is dependent on the implant design and the status of the PCL. In general, a posterior slope of 0° can be used in posterior cruciate-substituting and cruciate-sacrificing designs. If the PCL is to be retained, the slope can vary between 3° and 5°, based on implant specifications.

Flexion gaps may be balanced with adjustment of polyethylene insert thickness. The knee should be extended, and balance should be checked medially and laterally. If lateral tightness exists only in flexion, assessment should be performed for possible errors in femoral rotation. If rotation is determined to be satisfactory, the LCL can be released via pie-crusting or incremental release from the femur. Additionally, the popliteus tendon can be released if there is an internal rotation contracture associated with lateral tightness during flexion. Knees with lateral tightness in both flexion and extension can be addressed with release of the popliteus tendon, the LCL, or both. Any remaining lateral tightness during extension can be addressed with release of the posterolateral capsule or pie-crusting of the ITB. Serial examinations and stress testing should be performed until the knee opens 2 to 4 mm laterally and 2 to 3 mm medially in flexion and 1 to 3 mm laterally and 1 to 2 mm medially in extension. If instability persists even after these releases, a more constrained implant should be used.

One study investigated TKA in valgus knees and reported 91% survival of 60 knees (46 patients) at 13-year follow-up; however, their technique for lateral release led to an instability rate of 24%.[13] Another report examining 78 valgus knees (53 patients) after TKA described significant improvement in mean Hospital for Special Surgery knee scores (48 to 91 points; $P < 0.001$), mean tibiofemoral alignment (valgus 20° to 5°; $P < 0.001$), and mean ROM (65° to 110°; $P < 0.001$) at a mean follow-up of 10 years (range, 8 to 14 years).[6] These studies highlight the importance of adequate soft-tissue release and implant selection when performing TKA in knees with severe valgus deformity.

Knee Stiffness

Knee stiffness occurs in 1.3% to 5.3% of patients after TKA.[14] Stiffness can be defined as a decrease in postoperative ROM less than 110°, persistent pain, and functional compromise. This may be a product of contractures, posttraumatic or septic arthritis, heterotopic ossification, or patella baja. Limitations in knee ROM are often functionally debilitating. For example, basic activities such as walking (95°), ascending stairs (105°), descending stairs (107°), and picking up objects off the floor (117°) require a greater ROM.[15,16] The most important predictor of ROM after TKA is preoperative ROM,[10] as one study demonstrated a direct correlation between preoperative and postoperative flexion at 6 months, 1 year, 3 years, and 5 years postoperatively (Pearson correlation coefficient, 0.363, 0.403, 0.406, 0.359, respectively; $P < 0.0001$ for all).[17] Flexion contractures, which frequently occur in patients who have osteoarthritis, place patients at greater risk of a residual flexion deformity. As a general rule, if the knee is unable to obtain full extension in the operating room when the patient is anesthetized, it will not obtain full extension postoperatively. This poses a problem for patients because knees that cannot attain full extension during ambulation require increased energy expenditure for quadriceps contraction to maintain stability.[18] Additionally, these deformities may cause a limb-length discrepancy or affect gait kinematics. It is recommended that objective preoperative ROM be assessed with a goniometer. Furthermore, documentation of intraoperative ROM after the final components have been placed can be of value in the postoperative course in determining if a manipulation under anesthesia would be beneficial. It also is imperative to rule out other etiologies of knee stiffness such as structural deformities, infections, or ankylosis.[18]

Preoperative planning should include assessing ROM, presence of deformities, neurovascular status, and the prosthesis design that will be used. Full-length weight-bearing radiographs of the limb can provide information on bony landmarks and any existing structural deformity or ankylosis. In cases of stiff knees with particularly difficult surgical exposure, it may be necessary to use a standard medial parapatellar approach, an additional proximal extension of the quadriceps tendon, and a lateral retinacular release. After a medial arthrotomy, adhesions of the suprapatellar pouch and lateral and medial gutters should be cleared. To enhance patellar mobilization, it may be necessary to carefully elevate the subperiosteum of the deep MCL along the proximal tibia from the posteromedial corner (just anterior to the semimembranosus insertion) and place the tibia in external rotation. If 90° of knee flexion still cannot be achieved, other extensile approaches may be required. These approaches include the quadriceps snip, tibial tubercle osteotomy, and the V-Y turndown.

Quadriceps Snip

The quadriceps snip involves the proximal extension of the arthrotomy along the quadriceps tendon directed in the proximal-lateral direction approximately 30° to 45° in line with the fibers of the vastus lateralis muscle (**Figure 1**). This approach allows preservation of both the tendinous insertion of the vastus lateralis and lateral superior genicular blood flow to the patella. Additionally, performing the quadriceps snip does not result in a change to postoperative protocol. Taken together, these benefits suggest the quadriceps snip should be used as the first option if additional exposure is required.[19,20] One study compared 31 patients who underwent a quadriceps snip with 63

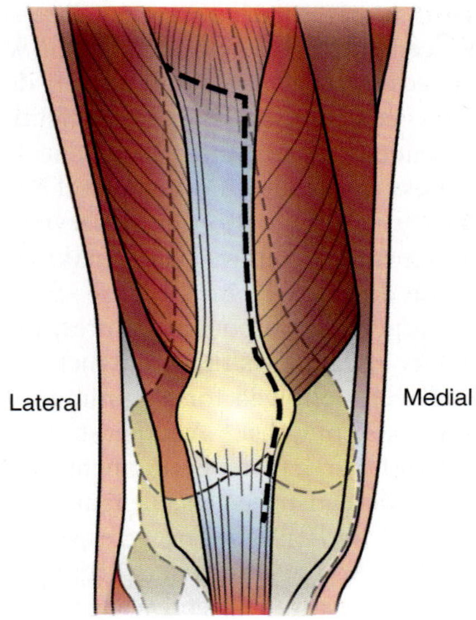

FIGURE 1 Illustration shows a planned quadriceps snip.

patients who underwent the standard medial parapatellar incision and demonstrated equivalent objective and functional outcomes, total Knee Society Scores (KSSs), ROM, patient satisfaction, and incidence of extension lag and patellofemoral pain.[21] Another study compared Western Ontario and McMaster Universities Osteoarthritis Index function, pain, stiffness, and satisfaction scores between 50 patients who underwent a quadriceps snip and 57 patients who underwent a standard medial parapatellar approach and reported that no negative effect was associated with the quadriceps snip at a mean follow-up of 41 months.[22]

Tibial Tubercle Osteotomy

The tibial tubercle osteotomy (TTO) may be used when further exposure of the stiff knee is necessary, but the quadriceps snip approach is not sufficient. Most would agree that a TTO is rarely needed for exposure but may be helpful in difficult stem extraction, tibial tubercle malposition, and patellar ligament contracture.[19,20] A 2016 study compared 106 patients who underwent TTO with 474 patients who underwent the standard medial parapatellar approach and demonstrated no significant difference in clinical outcomes (Western Ontario and McMaster Universities Osteoarthritis Index, KSS knee and function scores, and knee flexion ROM) after 1 year following TKA (P = 0.337, 0.278, 0.269, 0.318, respectively).[23] A 2011 study compared 22 patients who underwent TTO with 22 patients who underwent the standard medial parapatellar approach and found no significant difference in postoperative International Knee Society System Scores at 7-year follow-up ($P < 0.05$).[24]

V-Y Quadriceps Turndown

The V-Y quadriceps turndown may be used when a quadriceps snip would not provide sufficient exposure, a TTO is contraindicated secondary to osteoporotic bone or poor distal skin quality, or a true lengthening of the extensor mechanism is desired.[25] The medial parapatellar approach is used with a diverging incision that starts at the proximal apex and runs distally and laterally through both the quadriceps tendon and the insertion of the vastus lateralis tendon. The incision is then extended inferolaterally at a 45° angle over the lateral retinaculum (**Figure 2**). Although this approach provides excellent exposure by allowing the entire patella to be everted distally, it should be used with caution because damage to the superior lateral geniculate artery may interrupt the blood supply to the patella, potentially resulting in necrosis of the extensor mechanism. Postoperatively, the knee may be kept immobilized in full extension for a minimum of 2 weeks to minimize the degree of extensor lag.[20] One study assessing this approach in 29 revision TKAs (27 patients) noted postoperative radiographic evidence of osteonecrosis in eight patellae.[26] At 6 weeks postoperatively, all patients had significant extensor lag, with recovery of quadriceps strength occurring gradually up to 1 year after surgery. Another study used bone scanning to demonstrate reduced patellar isotope uptake in 56.4% of knees that underwent a lateral release concomitantly with the V-Y quadriceps turndown, compared with 15% of knees that did not undergo a lateral release.[27] This finding was attributed to the compromised blood supply of the patella associated with this approach. Given these complications, the V-Y quadriceps turndown should be reserved as a last resort.

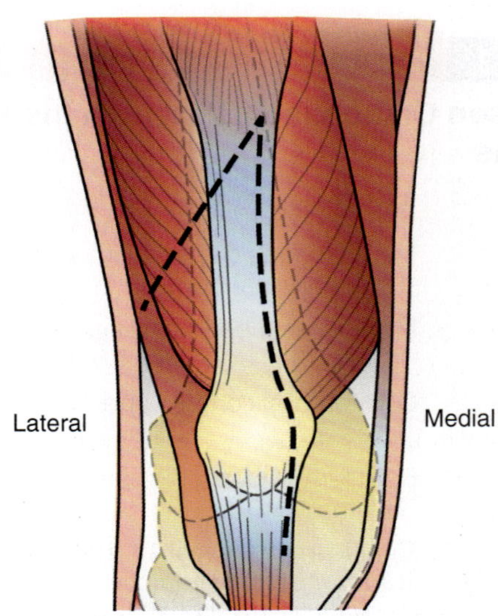

FIGURE 2 Illustration shows a planned V-Y turndown.

Posttraumatic Arthritis

Posttraumatic arthritis can be difficult to manage in the setting of intra-articular bony defects, malunion, limb malalignment, retained hardware, and stiffness. Careful preoperative planning should be performed before TKA is undertaken. This includes assessment of the degree of intra-articular bone loss, prosthetic choice regarding constraint, the need for hardware removal if it is in the way of the prosthesis, and possible osteotomy for extra-articular deformity. The goal of achieving an anatomic joint line will optimize ligamentous stability and restore joint kinematics.

Evaluation of intra-articular bone defects may include CT to evaluate the extent of intra-articular bone defects. Three-dimensional CT may be beneficial to characterize the degree of bone loss. Several classification systems have been developed to describe the extent of bone loss. The widely used Anderson Orthopaedic Research Institute (AORI) classification system helps categorize the degree of bone loss and predict the most appropriate method for bone reconstruction[28] (**Table 1**).

Instability of the knee in the setting of bone loss should be treated with a posterior stabilized implant or a more constrained prosthesis. Patients who have AORI type 2 or smaller type 3 bone defects will have improved outcomes by using prostheses with lesser degrees of constraint.[29] Conversely, in cases with high degrees of type 3 bone loss and loss of ligamentous stability, a hinged knee prosthesis is more appropriate.[30]

Small contained defects of 5 mm or less may be reconstructed with bone cement. When this method is used, screws may be added to enhance the biomechanical properties of the construct.[31] However, in vitro studies have shown that metal wedge augments are superior to either bone cement alone or bone cement with screw fixation for reconstruction of these smaller defects.[32] In general, if the defect is the size of the metal augment, it is recommended to use a metal augment; however, if the defect is less than the size of the metal augment, the surgeon must weigh the option of preserving bone and filling with cement and screws versus making a step-cut and filling the defect with metal. One study reported no revision surgeries, component failures, or loose tibial components in 22 TKAs that used metal wedges (20 patients) and were followed for a minimum of 2 years (mean follow-up, 37 months).[32] Another study of 24 TKAs (21 patients) with a metal wedge augmentation for tibial bone deficiency demonstrated excellent and good clinical outcomes in 67% and 29% of knees, respectively, at 5.6-year follow-up.[33] At 4.8 years after surgery, radiolucent lines were seen beneath the metal wedge at the cement-bone interface in 13 knees: 11 were less than 1 mm wide and 2 were between 1 and 3 mm wide. No radiolucencies were progressive.

Type 2 and 3 defects are typically managed with metal augments such as modular blocks and wedges, porous cones, and metal sleeves. The use of structural allograft has declined in the past several years with the advent of porous cones and metallic sleeves, and long-term data have shown a revision surgery rate of up to 23% with allograft failure.[34-38] Metal augmentation using modular blocks or wedges can be used to reconstruct areas of small to moderate-size uncontained segmental femoral and tibial defects of 5 to 20 mm deep.[39] Most TKA systems offer varied sizes of augments that

TABLE 1

Anderson Orthopaedic Research Institute Classification of Bone Defects and Treatment Options

Type	Description	Treatment Options
Type 1	Minimal bone defects with stable, intact metaphyseal bone	Bone cement ± screws; impact autograft/allograft
Type 2	Metaphyseal bone damage with loss of cancellous bone that involves:	
A	One femoral condyle and/or one tibial plateau	Bone cement ± screws; impact autograft/allograft; metal wedge augments
B	Both femoral condyles and/or both tibial plateaux	Impact autograft/allograft; metal wedge augments; porous cones; metal sleeves; custom-made implants
Type 3	Significant bone loss of the femoral condyles and/or tibial plateaux with possible collateral or patellar ligament detachment	Bulk allograft; porous cones; metal sleeves; custom implants; modular endoprosthesis; megaprosthesis

attach directly to the components. In one study evaluating type 2 defects treated with modular augments and stems, successful long-term survivorship of 92% was reported at 11 years.[40] Porous cones and metal sleeves are advantageous because they offer improved mechanical support to the prosthesis and allow for osseous integration. Additionally, they obviate the risk of disease transmission and graft resorption leading to failure and revision surgery and allow immediate weight bearing postoperatively. One study examined 15 knees with porous metaphyseal cones and demonstrated improved KSS scores from 52 points preoperatively to 85 points at short-term follow-up of 34 months.[41] Additionally, all cones showed evidence of osseointegration with reactive osseous trabeculation at contact points with the tibia without loosening or migration of these components at the time of follow-up. The only study providing midterm results of tibial cone implantation, which had a mean follow-up of 5.8 years, has shown revision-free survival greater than 95%.[42] Of 66 tibial cones implanted for AORI type 2 or 3 defects, only three were revised: one for aseptic loosening, one for periprosthetic fracture, and one for infection.[42]

ADDITIONAL CONSIDERATIONS

Patients Who Have Cardiovascular Pathology

Patients who undergo TKA may have cardiovascular, peripheral vascular, and cerebrovascular diseases, which are associated with a variety of surgical risks and complications. Thorough evaluation of a patient's cardiac history is necessary before performing TKA, including determination of arrhythmias; fluid shifts; oxygen saturation; smoking status; effects of anesthesia; history of cardiovascular surgery; and history of hematologic and pulmonary disease. It is also critical to check if vascular calcifications are seen on the preoperative radiographs and to ask if the patient has had any vascular surgeries on the surgical limb. In these cases, vascular surgery consultation should be obtained. Furthermore, the surgeon should consider limiting tourniquet time to implant cementation or performing the surgery entirely without a tourniquet. Additionally, these patients can be more challenging to treat if they are receiving anticoagulants such as clopidogrel. Although guidelines recommend cessation of clopidogrel for 5 days before surgery, there is an increased risk of cardiovascular and thromboembolic events if it is discontinued for an extended period.[43] The decision of withholding anticoagulation therapy preoperatively and resuming anticoagulation therapy postoperatively remains controversial and is best determined on a case-by-case basis with input from the patient's cardiologist.

Studies have shown varying outcomes after TKA in patients who have cardiovascular pathology. A 2011 study reported that 16.7% of patients who had a previous cardiac event (n = 514) and 2% of patients who have no history of cardiac event (n = 1,094) experienced a cardiac event (eg, congestive heart failure, myocardial infarction, arrhythmia) after TKA.[44] Moreover, 20.7% of patients who have and 3.6% of patients without a history of thromboembolism experienced a thromboembolic event (deep vein thrombosis [DVT] or pulmonary embolism) after TKA. Conversely, a 2014 study reported no increased risk of mortality after TKA in patients who have a history of cardiac disease.[45] However, it should be noted that these patients had an increased risk of minor local complications (P = 0.01), including superficial wound infection and wound dehiscence. Thorough assessment of a patient's cardiovascular history is necessary before performing TKA. It is vital that surgeons identify these potentially high-risk patients to ensure sufficient preoperative management and education.

Obese Patients

The incidence of obesity (body mass index [BMI] greater than 30 kg/m^2) has reached an epidemic proportion, with nearly 38% of the American population meeting this definition. Patients who have obesity have a greater risk of developing early osteoarthritis compared with nonobese patients. Subsequently, the rate of obesity among TKA patients has increased dramatically; a concern with the projected increase in the total number of TKAs that will be performed over the next decade.[46,47] Thus, orthopaedic surgeons should be familiar with the risks obese patients may experience when undergoing TKA.

Following TKA, obese patients are at greater risk of delayed wound healing, infection, prolonged wound drainage, poor mobilization, and reduced tolerance for rehabilitation.[48] Although the risk of complications increases with increasing BMI, no definitive cutoff exists that places patients at a substantially higher risk.[49,50] Because morbidly obese patients (BMI greater than 40 kg/m^2) have a greater risk of wound dehiscence and postoperative infection, this BMI threshold may be used as a cutoff to reassess treatment options as well as provide patient education.[51] However, the use of a cutoff to avoid short-term complications may lead to decreased access to a procedure with proven long-term benefits. A cost-effective analysis of TKA versus nonsurgical management in 2018 demonstrated that TKA would be cost effective across all BMI categories, suggesting a BMI cutoff may unjustly restrict access.[52] Regardless of the decision to operate or pursue nonsurgical management, obese patients may benefit from bariatric surgery consultation and evaluation of the patient's overall nutritional status as these patients are oftentimes malnourished.

Nonobese patients (BMI less than 30 kg/m^2) have demonstrated greater implant survivorship compared with their obese or morbidly obese counterparts.[53] One study reported that 5-year implant survivorship (with revision as the end point) was significantly lower in morbidly obese patients compared with nonobese patients.[53] Another study demonstrated significantly lower implant survivorship in morbidly obese patients compared with obese patients and nonobese patients at a mean 5-year follow-up (88% versus 95% versus 97%, respectively; $P < 0.05$). However, a 2013 study noted no difference in implant survivorship between nonobese patients and superobese (greater than 50 kg/m^2) patients (98% versus 94%) at a mean 5-year follow-up.[54]

Patients Who Have Other Comorbidities

Diabetes Mellitus

The prevalence of diabetes mellitus is rising in the United States and is becoming an increasingly common comorbidity in patients undergoing TKA. Diabetes mellitus is known to delay collagen synthesis and impair wound healing, which may lead to poor recovery and increased risk of infection.[55] Some studies have demonstrated altered bone metabolism in patients who have this disease,[56] potentially delaying fracture healing and contributing to component loosening in TKA. Additionally, diabetes mellitus is associated with poorer outcomes[57] and increased risk of DVT.[58] It is imperative that these patients receive thorough perioperative management, as tight control of blood glucose levels may help reduce postoperative morbidity.

In a 2015 study of 462 patients who have diabetes (714 TKAs), those who have hemoglobin A_{1c} levels greater than 8% had an increased likelihood of having superficial surgical site infections (odds ratio [OR], 6.1; 95% confidence interval [CI], 1.6 to 23.4; $P = 0.008$).[59] This association also was seen in patients who had a fasting blood glucose of 200 mg/dL or higher (OR, 9.2; 95% CI, 2.2 to 38.2; $P = 0.038$). In another study, patients who have diabetes mellitus had a significantly higher rate of revision compared with patients without diabetes mellitus (3.6% versus 0.4%; $P < 0.05$).[60] A 2013 retrospective analysis of 245 patients undergoing TKA, 53 of whom had diabetes mellitus, showed that patients who have diabetes mellitus were 2.76 times more likely to have DVT.[61] Moreover, a 2012 study examining functional outcomes after TKA in 367 patients who have diabetes mellitus and a cohort without diabetes mellitus matched for age, sex, BMI, and baseline functional movement showed worse outcomes in those who have diabetes.[62] At 1-year follow-up, the cohort with diabetes mellitus had significantly lower total ROM ($P < 0.001$), KSS ($P = 0.034$), and maximal flexion ($P < 0.001$). Similar results were seen at 5-year (except for KSS) and 10-year follow-up. Given the rising prevalence of diabetes, orthopaedic surgeons must be prepared to treat an increasing number of surgical patients who have this disease. Adequate glycemic control in patients who have diabetes may help reduce the risk of perioperative complications and improve functional outcomes.

Metabolic Syndrome

Metabolic syndrome is a series of risk factors that place patients at an increased risk of developing type 2 diabetes mellitus and cardiovascular disease.[63] Patients must have three of the following five components to meet the criteria for diagnosis of metabolic syndrome: hypertension, elevated fasting blood glucose levels, elevated triglyceride levels, low levels of high-density lipoprotein, and increased abdominal circumference.[64] Patients who have metabolic syndrome require special consideration, because they have an increased risk of complications after total joint arthroplasty (TJA).

A 2013 study investigated the association between control of metabolic syndrome components and incidence of perioperative complications (including but not limited to DVT, pulmonary embolism, wound infection, periprosthetic infection, and acute renal failure) after TJA.[65] One hundred thirty-three patients undergoing TJA with all components of metabolic syndrome were matched with patients who did not have metabolic syndrome. Within the metabolic syndrome cohort, 35 patients (26%) were found to have at least one uncontrolled component. The complication rates for patients who have uncontrolled, controlled, and no metabolic syndrome were 49%, 8%, and 8%, respectively. Additionally, the metabolic syndrome cohort had significantly greater length of hospital stay (5.1 days versus 4.0 days; $P < 0.001$) and higher complication rate (18.3% versus 8.3%; $P = 0.018$) compared with patients without metabolic syndrome. In a 2013 study examining the incidence of pulmonary embolism after THA or TKA, patients who have metabolic syndrome had a significantly greater likelihood of this complication compared with patients without metabolic syndrome (OR, 1.6; 95% CI, 1.01 to 2.56; $P = 0.043$).[66] Moreover, the odds of pulmonary embolism increased 1.23 times (95% CI, 1.02 to 1.48; $P = 0.028$) per each additional component of metabolic syndrome. Another study evaluated 1,460 TKA patients to determine the relationship between metabolic syndrome and the incidence of DVT.[67] Of the 65 patients diagnosed with DVT (4.4%, n = 1,460), 21 had metabolic syndrome (15.5%, n = 135) while 45 did not (3.4%, $n = 1{,}325$; $P < 0.001$ for all). In addition, this analysis demonstrated that DVT risk in patients who have metabolic syndrome was 3.2 times the risk in patients without metabolic syndrome (95% CI, 1.0 to 15.4; $P = 0.04$). Because of their worse outcomes after TKA, it is crucial for orthopaedic surgeons to identify these high-risk patients to ensure appropriate preoperative education, management, and counseling of these patients regarding expectations for postoperative outcomes.

Inflammatory Arthropathies

Patients who have inflammatory arthropathies who have bone damaged from either their disease or their associated medications are often considered challenging candidates for TKA because of concerns regarding implant ingrowth, stability, and infection. However, as both medical and surgical management of these patients have evolved, better postoperative outcomes have been observed after TKA. There has been a substantial increase in the amount of medications that can be given to these patients who have inflammatory arthropathies. As such, special guidelines have been agreed on between the American College of Rheumatology and the American Association of Hip and Knee Surgeons with regard to when a specific medication should be held and resumed in the those undergoing arthroplasty.[68] The following details the more common inflammatory arthropathies encountered in an orthopaedic surgeon's practice.

Rheumatoid Arthritis

Rheumatoid arthritis is a systemic, progressive inflammatory process that can result in joint destruction and instability. Medical management of rheumatoid arthritis typically includes a combination of glucocorticoids, NSAIDs, and disease-modifying antirheumatic drugs. Although NSAIDs are effective in symptomatic management, they should be withheld for 1 week before surgery to minimize the risk of bleeding.[69] Additionally, patients who have rheumatoid arthritis who have undergone chronic treatment with corticosteroids are at risk of poor wound healing, weakening of the immune system, and reduced bone quality. These patients are also susceptible to adrenal insufficiency secondary to prolonged suppression of corticotrophin-releasing hormones from the hypothalamus.[70] Moreover, the cervical spine is often affected in patients who have rheumatoid arthritis who may present with atlantoaxial subluxation.[71] This involvement is often asymptomatic; therefore, patients scheduled to receive general anesthesia should undergo a comprehensive radiographic assessment of the cervical spine. Patients who have substantial atlantoaxial instability should be considered for alternative methods of anesthetic management, such as fiberoptic intubation or epidural/spinal anesthesia.

Intraoperatively, orthopaedic surgeons must be aware of the poor quality of bone and soft-tissue in patients who have rheumatoid arthritis. Chronic use of corticosteroids, as well as the autoimmune nature of the disease, can lead to inferior subchondral bone stock and osteopenia.[57] These deficiencies may contribute to inadequate implant fixation, reduced implant longevity, and the formation of bone cysts. Small bone cysts may be filled during cementation; however, larger cysts may require filling with allograft from morcellized femoral head or autologous graft from prior bone cuts. Additionally, the ligamentous laxity seen in these patients may require the use of components with increased constraint.[70] However, prostheses with greater constraint can impart increased rotational and shear forces on the bone-cement interface, potentially resulting in early failure.

Numerous reports have described higher complication rates in patients who have rheumatoid arthritis compared with patients who have osteoarthritis. A meta-analysis[72] comparing complications in lower extremity TJA between rheumatoid arthritis and osteoarthritis demonstrated an increased risk of infection and early revision in rheumatoid arthritis patients (OR, 1.24; 95% CI, 1.1 to 1.4). In a 2015 study, a Nationwide Inpatient Sample database was used to examine acute postoperative outcomes in patients who have TKA with various types of inflammatory arthropathies compared with patients who have osteoarthritis.[73] The authors noted a significantly greater likelihood of hematoma/seroma (OR, 1.3; 95% CI, 1.2 to 1.3), infection (OR, 1.1; 95% CI, 1.0 to 1.2), and periprosthetic fracture (OR, 1.6; 95% CI, 1.4 to 1.9) in patients who have rheumatoid arthritis compared with patients who have osteoarthritis ($P < 0.05$ for all). Additionally, a 2016 study described a significantly greater incidence of pneumonia in patients who have rheumatoid arthritis within 30 days postoperatively (2.1% versus 0.4%; $P = 0.003$).[74] Despite these complications, favorable long-term results also have been shown after TKA in patients who have rheumatoid arthritis. At a mean follow-up of 10.5 years, one study reported good or excellent results in 95% of 46 knees with rheumatoid arthritis treated with a cruciate-retaining component.[62] Furthermore, a 2013 study evaluating 47 patients who have rheumatoid arthritis demonstrated a 10- and 15-year implant survivorship of 88% and 78%, respectively.[75]

Juvenile Rheumatoid Arthritis

Juvenile rheumatoid arthritis (JRA) is a conglomerate of disorders with a common presentation of persistent arthritis in at least one joint that typically presents within the first 2 decades of life. As the leading cause of childhood disability, it has an estimated incidence of 6 cases per 10,000 children, or 294,000 total cases in the United States.[76] In addition to flexion contractures and poor bone quality, patients who have JRA often have complex deformities such as valgus alignment as well as trumpet-shaped femurs and tibias as a result of prematurely closed growth plates.[77] Nonetheless, TKA in patients who have JRA can restore function and provide pain relief with appropriate medical and surgical management.

Patients who have JRA are managed with similar medications as those used in rheumatoid arthritis, including corticosteroids, disease-modifying antirheumatic drugs, and biologic agents. As such, they also are at risk of impaired wound healing, compromise of the immune system, and adrenal crises.[77] JRA presents with multiple joint involvement, especially in the lower extremities. Because flexion contracture of the hip complicates rehabilitation by making full knee extension difficult, THA should be performed before TKA.

The recommendation for otherwise healthy patients who have contractures in both knees is to undergo simultaneous bilateral TKA.[77] Severe deformities can make the initial exposure more difficult and therefore may require more extensive exposures. Osteotomies of the tibial tubercle are not recommended, particularly in the setting of osteopenia.[77] Moreover, the proximal tibia may be dysplastic and present with rapid tapering of the metaphysis, which necessitates careful placement of retractors to avoid compression fractures. If the patella is ankylosed to the femur, patellar resurfacing is recommended.[78] Complications experienced by these patients include fractures, arthrofibrosis, periprosthetic infection, and sciatic nerve injury. Despite the potential setbacks, TKA has shown success in patients who have JRA. A study examining 349 TKAs in patients who have JRA reported 10- and 20-year implant survivorship at 95% and 82%, respectively.[79] However, other studies have shown long-term failure rates ranging from 6% to 42% in patients who have JRA.[80,81]

Systemic Lupus Erythematosus

Systemic lupus erythematosus (SLE) is a chronic, multisystem, autoimmune disease that commonly occurs in young women, most prevalently among African Americans. Patients typically present with a wide spectrum of symptoms, including rash, fever, and polyarthralgia. Patients who have a diagnosis of SLE are twice as likely to require TKA compared with the general population.[82] Furthermore, the incidence of lower extremity TJA in patients who have SLE increased from 0.17 to 0.83 per 100,000 people in the United States from 1991 to 2005.[83] Because of the complexity of SLE, these patients often require involvement of several medical specialties to ensure they are adequately treated.

Patients who have SLE who undergo TKA tend to be younger than patients without SLE;[82] however, good postoperative outcomes are possible. A 2016 study comparing a cohort of patients who have SLE who underwent TKA with a matched cohort that did not have the disease revealed similar outcomes with respect to implant survivorship, complication rates, functional outcomes, physical and mental scores, and activity scores at midterm follow-up of 6 years.[84] Another study demonstrated similar outcomes between patients who have SLE and patients who have osteoarthritis who underwent TKA with respect to pain, function, activity, and quality of life.[84] As TKA continues to demonstrate favorable outcomes, it should be presented as an option to patients who have SLE.

Charcot Arthropathy

Charcot arthropathy, also known as neuropathic arthropathy, is caused by the deterioration of periarticular sensation resulting in joint destruction and fragmentation. This degenerative condition is associated with nerve damage, decreased proprioception, and periarticular insensitivity. Clinically, this disorder presents with joint effusion, crepitus, lack of proprioception, and instability.[85] Furthermore, patients are often unaware of pain in the affected joint, potentially contributing to the substantial destruction of the articular surfaces.

It is believed that the knee joint is the most frequently affected large joint in the setting of neuropathic disease; therefore, early detection and treatment of patients who have Charcot arthropathy is crucial to joint preservation. Immobilization with casts or non–weight-bearing devices may inhibit osteolytic processes within the joint. Moreover, joint destruction may be delayed with joint aspiration, NSAID use, supportive orthoses, exercise, and gait training.[86] However, definitive guidelines for bracing treatment and casting for the neuropathic knee have not been firmly established.

Orthopaedic surgeons encounter several challenges with these patients, including bone loss, instability, and deformity. In the past, Charcot arthropathy of the knee joint was managed with arthrodesis or bracing treatment. However, as implant designs and surgical techniques have advanced, more favorable postoperative outcomes have been achieved.[85] It is important to understand the staging of Charcot arthropathy as this helps determine the most appropriate time for surgical intervention. Patients whose disease process is in the early inflammatory or fragmentation stages should have their TKA postponed until the reconstruction or coalescence stages.[87,88]

In 2012, the successful use of porous tantalum cones has been reported at short-term follow-up.[88] These implants are thought to aid in reconstruction of bony defects while simultaneously providing an anchor for the fragmented proximal tibia.[85] Other commonly used reconstruction methods to address these technical challenges include bone grafting, hinged or semiconstrained implants, and stem extensions.[89] One study described results after TKA in 10 patients (19 knees) who have Charcot arthropathy.[90] A cemented condylar, constrained prosthesis was used in all but two knees. At a mean follow-up of 5.2 years (range, 5 to 6 years), the mean Hospital for Special Surgery knee score improved from 36.5 points preoperatively to 76 points after TKA. However, at final follow-up, three knees (16%) had aseptic loosening requiring arthrodesis, six knees (31%) were described as poorly functioning, and 10 knees (53%) were described as satisfactory.[90] Another series reported significant improvements in KSS pain and function scores and ROM at 7.9-year follow-up in 29 patients who underwent TKA for Charcot arthropathy.[87] Bony defects and ligamentous instability were reinforced with metal wedge augments, bone grafts, stem extensions, and hinged or semiconstrained implants. Patients in this study experienced complications, including aseptic loosening, instability, and periprosthetic fracture. As surgical technique and implant design continue to evolve, patients who have Charcot arthropathy may experience better outcomes after TKA.

SUMMARY

Primary TKA in the setting of various deformities, conditions, and comorbidities remains challenging for orthopaedic surgeons. Thorough preoperative management of these diseases and comorbidities is necessary for postoperative success. As such, preoperative planning should include assessment of the soft tissues, bony deformity, surgical approach, and implant selection. Special consideration should be placed on patients who have comorbidities that may affect postoperative outcomes. With appropriate assessment, planning, and treatment of these complex cases, orthopaedic surgeons can appropriately manage difficult TKAs. As newer reconstructive modalities become available, orthopaedic surgeons may be able to customize TKAs for unique cases to optimize outcomes.

KEY STUDY POINTS

- Bony deformities about the knee joint can complicate TKA. In addition to osteotomies, various soft-tissue releases are available to help achieve successful component implantation.
- Preoperative planning should include assessment of ROM, presence of deformities, neurovascular status, radiographic evaluation, and selection of appropriate prosthesis design. In complex cases, advanced surgical approaches can be used to attain sufficient exposure intraoperatively.
- Patients who have other nonsurgical comorbidities may require extra considerations. Orthopaedic surgeons should take care to ensure these conditions are managed in the preoperative setting.

ANNOTATED REFERENCES

1. Ritter MA, Davis KE, Davis P, et al: Preoperative malalignment increases risk of failure after total knee arthroplasty. *J Bone Joint Surg Am* 2013;95(2):126-131.

2. Victor JM, Bassens D, Bellemans J, Gürsu S, Dhollander AA, Verdonk PC: Constitutional varus does not affect joint line orientation in the coronal plane. *Clin Orthop Relat Res* 2014;472(1):98-104.

3. Vandekerckhove PTK, Matlovich N, Teeter MG, MacDonald SJ, Howard JL, Lanting BA: The relationship between constitutional alignment and varus osteoarthritis of the knee. *Knee Surg Sports Traumatol Arthrosc* 2017;25: 2873-2879.

   This study describes the correlation between the constitutional alignment of a knee and end-stage varus osteoarthritis. They found a constitutional varus knee is likely to contribute to medial compartment arthritis and varus deformities. Level of evidence: III.

4. Rossi R, Cottino U, Bruzzone M, Dettoni F, Bonasia DE, Rosso F: Total knee arthroplasty in the varus knee: Tips and tricks. *Int Orthop* 2019;43(1):151-158.

   This review describes the difficulties of TKA in varus knees and the methods that can be used to improve outcomes. This review highlights ligamentous balancing, appropriate implant selection, approaches, and osteotomies. Level of evidence: III.

5. De Muylder J, Victor J, Cornu O, Kaminski L, Thienpont E: Total knee arthroplasty in patients with substantial deformities using primary knee components. *Knee Surg Sports Traumatol Arthrosc* 2015;23(12):3653-3659.

6. Mullaji AB, Shetty GM: Correcting deformity in total knee arthroplasty: Techniques to avoid the release of collateral ligaments in severely deformed knees. *Bone Joint J* 2016;98-B(1 suppl A):101-104.

7. Bellemans J: Multiple needle puncturing: Balancing the varus knee. *Orthopedics* 2011;34(9):e510-e512.
8. Ranawat CS, Meftah M, Ranawat AS: The "inside-out" technique for correcting a fixed varus deformity with flexion contracture in total knee arthroplasty. *JBJS Essent Surg Tech* 2012;2(3):e16.
9. Bellemans J, Vandenneucker H, Van Lauwe J, Victor J: A new surgical technique for medial collateral ligament balancing: Multiple needle puncturing. *J Arthroplasty* 2010;25(7):1151-1156.
10. Rossi R, Rosso F, Cottino U, Dettoni F, Bonasia DE, Bruzzone M: Total knee arthroplasty in the valgus knee. *Int Orthop* 2014;38(2):273-283.
11. Rajgopal A, Dahiya V, Vasdev A, Kochhar H, Tyagi V: Long-term results of total knee arthroplasty for valgus knees: Soft-tissue release technique and implant selection. *J Orthop Surg (Hong Kong)* 2011;19(1):60-63.
12. Aurich M, Lenz M, Best N: A modified lateral approach for total knee replacement in type 2 valgus deformity. *Orthopedics* 2017;40(5):313-316.

    A medial parapatellar approach on a severely valgus knee may not provide sufficient exposure. These researchers describe a lateral parapatellar approach, the benefits of performing this on a severely valgus knee, and some difficulties encountered. Level of evidence: IV.
13. Miyasaka KC, Ranawat CS, Mullaji A: 10- to 20-year followup of total knee arthroplasty for valgus deformities. *Clin Orthop Relat Res* 1997;345:29-37. Available at: http://www.ncbi.nlm.nih.gov/pubmed/9418618. Accessed September 8, 2019.
14. Manrique J, Gomez MM, Parvizi J: Stiffness after total knee arthroplasty. *J Knee Surg* 2015;28:119-126.
15. Stamos VP, Bono JV: *Management of the Stiff Total Knee Arthroplasty*. New York, NY, Springer, 1997.
16. Ebert JR, Munsie C, Joss B: Guidelines for the early restoration of active knee flexion after total knee arthroplasty: Implications for rehabilitation and early intervention. *Arch Phys Med Rehabil* 2014;95(6):1135-1140.
17. Ritter MA, Harty LD, Davis KE, Meding JB, Berend ME: Predicting range of motion after total knee arthroplasty: Clustering, log-linear regression, and regression tree analysis. *J Bone Joint Surg Am* 2003;85(7):1278-1285.
18. Ritter MA, Lutgring JD, Davis KE, Berend ME, Pierson JL, Meneghini RM: The role of flexion contracture on outcomes in primary total knee arthroplasty. *J Arthroplasty* 2007;22(8):1092-1096.
19. Della Valle CJ, Berger RA, Rosenberg AG: Surgical exposures in revision total knee arthroplasty. *Clin Orthop Relat Res* 2006;446:59-68.
20. Abdel MP, Della Valle CJ: The surgical approach for revision total knee arthroplasty. *Bone Joint J* 2016;98-B(1 suppl A):113-115.
21. Barrack R: Surgical exposure of the stiff knee. *Acta Orthop Scand* 2009;71(1):85-89.
22. Meek RMD, Greidanus NV, McGraw RW, Masri BA: The extensile rectus snip exposure in revision of total knee arthroplasty. *J Bone Joint Surg Br* 2003;85(8):1120-1122. Available at: http://www.ncbi.nlm.nih.gov/pubmed/14653591. Accessed September 17, 2019.
23. Langen S, Gaber S, Zdravkovic V, Giesinger K, Jost B, Behrend H: Lateral subvastus approach with tibial tubercle osteotomy for primary total knee arthroplasty: Clinical outcome and complications compared to medial parapatellar approach. *Eur J Orthop Surg Traumatol* 2016;26(2):215-222.
24. Nikolopoulos DD, Polyzois I, Apostolopoulos AP, Rossas C, Moutsios-Rentzos A, Michos IV: Total knee arthroplasty in severe valgus knee deformity: Comparison of a standard medial parapatellar approach combined with tibial tubercle osteotomy. *Knee Surg Sports Traumatol Arthrosc* 2011;19(11):1834-1842.
25. Annunziata CC, Archibeck MJ, Arsht SJ, et al: Modified V-Y quadriceps turndown, in Cushner FD, Scott N, Scuderi GR, eds: *Surgical Techniques for the Knee*. New York, NY, Thieme Clinical Collections, 2005, pp 35-40. Available at: https://www.thieme-connect.de/products/ebooks/pdf/10.1055/b-0034-82890.pdf#.
26. Smith PN, Parker DA, Gelinas J, Rorabeck CH, Bourne RB: Radiographic changes in the patella following quadriceps turndown for revision total knee arthroplasty. *J Arthroplasty* 2004;19(6):714-719.
27. Scuderi G, Scharf SC, Meltzer LP, Scott WN: The relationship of lateral releases to patella viability in total knee arthroplasty. *J Arthroplasty* 1987;2(3):209-214.
28. Engh GA, Ammeen DJ: Bone loss with revision total knee arthroplasty: Defect classification and alternatives for reconstruction. *Instr Course Lect* 1999;48:167-175. Available at: http://www.ncbi.nlm.nih.gov/pubmed/10098042. Accessed September 17, 2019.
29. Shen C, Lichstein PM, Austin MS, Sharkey PF, Parvizi J: Revision knee arthroplasty for bone loss: Choosing the right degree of constraint. *J Arthroplasty* 2014;29(1):127-131.
30. Daines BK, Dennis DA: Management of bone defects in revision total knee arthroplasty. *J Bone Joint Surg Am* 2012;94(12):1131-1139.
31. Ritter MA, Harty LD: Medial screws and cement: A possible mechanical augmentation in total knee arthroplasty. *J Arthroplasty* 2004;19(5):587-589.
32. Brand MG, Daley RJ, Ewald FC, Scott RD: Tibial tray augmentation with modular metal wedges for tibial bone stock deficiency. *Clin Orthop Relat Res* 1989;248:71-79. Available at: http://www.ncbi.nlm.nih.gov/pubmed/2805499. Accessed September 17, 2019.
33. Pagnano MW, Trousdale RT, Rand JA: Tibial wedge augmentation for bone deficiency in total knee arthroplasty. A followup study. *Clin Orthop Relat Res* 1995;321:151-155. Available at: http://www.ncbi.nlm.nih.gov/pubmed/7497661. Accessed September 17, 2019.

34. Backstein D, Safir O, Gross A: Management of bone loss: Structural grafts in revision total knee arthroplasty. *Clin Orthop Relat Res* 2006;446:104-112.

35. Bauman RD, Lewallen DG, Hanssen AD: Limitations of structural allograft in revision total knee Arthroplasty. *Clin Orthop Relat Res* 2009;467(3):818-824.

36. Clatworthy MG, Ballance J, Brick GW, Chandler HP, Gross AE: The use of structural allograft for uncontained defects in revision total knee arthroplasty: A minimum five-year review. *J Bone Joint Surg Am* 2001;83(3):404-411.

37. Engh GA, Ammeen DJ: Use of structural allograft in revision total knee arthroplasty in knees with severe tibial bone loss. *J Bone Joint Surg Am* 2007;89(12):2640-2647.

38. Lachiewicz PF, Bolognesi MP, Henderson RA, Soileau ES, Vail TP: Can tantalum cones provide fixation in complex revision knee arthroplasty? *Clin Orthop Relat Res* 2012;470: 199-204.

39. Mabry TM, Hanssen AD: The role of stems and augments for bone loss in revision knee arthroplasty. *J Arthroplasty* 2007;22(4 suppl 1):56-60.

40. Patel JV, Masonis JL, Guerin J, Bourne RB, Rorabeck CH: The fate of augments to treat type-2 bone defects in revision knee arthroplasty. *J Bone Joint Surg Br* 2004;86(2):195-199. Available at: http://www.ncbi.nlm.nih.gov/pubmed/15046432. Accessed September 17, 2019.

41. Meneghini RM, Lewallen DG, Hanssen AD: Use of porous tantalum metaphyseal cones for severe tibial bone loss during revision total knee replacement. Surgical technique. *J Bone Joint Surg Am* 2009;91(2 suppl 1):131-138.

42. Kamath AF, Lewallen DG, Hanssen AD: Porous tantalum metaphyseal cones for severe tibial bone loss in revision knee arthroplasty: A five to nine-year follow-up. *J Bone Joint Surg Am* 2015;97(3):216-223.

43. Nandi S, Aghazadeh M, Talmo C, Robbins C, Bono J: Perioperative clopidogrel and postoperative events after hip and knee arthroplasties. *Clin Orthop Relat Res* 2012;470(5):1436-1441.

44. Singh JA, Jensen MR, Harmsen WS, Gabriel SE, Lewallen DG: Cardiac and thromboembolic complications and mortality in patients undergoing total hip and total knee arthroplasty. *Ann Rheum Dis* 2011;70(12):2082-2088.

45. Belmont PJ, Goodman GP, Waterman BR, Bader JO, Schoenfeld AJ: Thirty-day postoperative complications and mortality following total knee arthroplasty: Incidence and risk factors among a national sample of 15,321 patients. *J Bone Joint Surg Am* 2014;96(1):20-26.

46. Flegal KM, Kruszon-Moran D, Carroll MD, Fryar CD, Ogden CL: Trends in obesity among adults in the United States, 2005 to 2014. *J Am Med Assoc* 2016;315(21): 2284-2291.

47. George J, Klika AK, Navale SM, Newman JM, Barsoum WK, Higuera CA: Obesity epidemic: Is its impact on total joint arthroplasty underestimated? An analysis of national trends. *Clin Orthop Relat Res* 2017;475(7):1798-1806.

    This study asked, if the prevalence of obesity is growing in the general population, is it also growing in the TKA population? They concluded the proportion of patients undergoing TKA who were obese increased 52% between 1998 and 2011. Level of evidence: II.

48. Mokdad AH, Ford ES, Bowman BA, et al: Prevalence of obesity, diabetes, and obesity-related health risk factors, 2001. *J Am Med Assoc* 2003;289(1):76-79.

49. Samson AJ, Mercer GE, Campbell DG: Total knee replacement in the morbidly obese: A literature review. *ANZ J Surg* 2010;80(9):595-599.

50. Martin JR, Jennings JM, Dennis DA: Morbid obesity and total knee arthroplasty: A growing problem. *J Am Acad Orthop Surg* 2017;25(3):188-194.

    This study reported the preoperative considerations to optimize patients before TKA, including nutritional status, weight loss, and bariatric surgery. They also discussed postoperative issues, such as tibial loosening, wound complications, and cardiovascular issues. Level of evidence: III.

51. D'Apuzzo MR, Novicoff WM, Browne JA: The John Insall Award: Morbid obesity independently impacts complications, mortality, and resource use after TKA. *Clin Orthop Relat Res* 2015;473(1):57-63.

52. Ponnusamy KE, Vasarhelyi EM, Somerville L, McCalden RW, Marsh JD: Cost-effectiveness of total knee arthroplasty vs nonoperative management in normal, overweight, obese, severely obese, morbidly obese, and super-obese patients: A Markov model. *J Arthroplasty* 2018;33(7):S32-S38.

    This cost-effectiveness analysis used a Markov model to determine the effectiveness of TKA in multiple BMI categories. They concluded that TKA would be cost effective in patients of all BMI categories. Level of evidence: II.

53. Patton JT, Gaston M, Cook RE, Brenkel IJ, Amin AK, Clayton RAE: Total knee replacement in morbidly obese patients. Results of a prospective, matched study. *J Bone Joint Surg Br* 2006;88-B(10):1321-1326.

54. Naziri Q, Issa K, Malkani AL, Bonutti PM, Harwin SF, Mont MA: Bariatric orthopaedics: Total knee arthroplasty in super-obese patients (BMI > 50 kg/m2). Survivorship and complications. *Clin Orthop Relat Res* 2013;471(11):3523-3530.

55. Han HS, Kang SB: Relations between long-term glycemic control and postoperative wound and infectious complications after total knee arthroplasty in type 2 diabetics. *Clin Orthop Surg* 2013;5(2):118-123.

56. Einhorn TA, Boskey AL, Gundberg CM, Vigorita VJ, Devlin VJ, Beyer MM: The mineral and mechanical properties of bone in chronic experimental diabetes. *J Orthop Res* 1988;6(3):317-323.

57. Singh JA, Lewallen DG: Diabetes: A risk factor for poor functional outcome after total knee arthroplasty. *PLoS One* 2013;8(11):e78991.

58. Zhao Z, Wang S, Ma W, et al: Diabetes mellitus increases the incidence of deep vein thrombosis after total knee arthroplasty. *Arch Orthop Trauma Surg* 2014;134(1):79-83.

59. Hwang JS, Kim SJ, Bamne AB, Na YG, Kim TK: Do glycemic markers predict occurrence of complications after total knee arthroplasty in patients with diabetes? *Clin Orthop Relat Res* 2015;473(5):1726-1731.

60. Meding JB, Reddleman K, Keating ME, et al: Total knee replacement in patients with diabetes mellitus. *Clin Orthop Relat Res* 2003;416:208-216.

61. Wang S, Zhao Y: Diabetes mellitus and the incidence of deep vein thrombosis after total knee arthroplasty: A retrospective study. *J Arthroplasty* 2013;28(4):595-597.

62. Robertson F, Geddes J, Ridley D, McLeod G, Cheng K: Patients with type 2 diabetes mellitus have a worse functional outcome post knee arthroplasty: A matched cohort study. *Knee* 2012;19(4):286-289.

63. Isomaa B, Henricsson M, Almgren P, Tuomi T, Taskinen MR, Groop L: The metabolic syndrome influences the risk of chronic complications in patients with type II diabetes. *Diabetologia* 2001;44(9):1148-1154.

64. Grundy SM, Becker D, Clark LT, et al: Detection, evaluation, and treatment of high blood cholesterol in adults (Adult Treatment Panel III). *Circulation* 2002;106(25):3143-3421.

65. Zmistowski B, Dizdarevic I, Jacovides CL, Radcliff KE, Mraovic B, Parvizi J: Patients with uncontrolled components of metabolic syndrome have increased risk of complications following total joint arthroplasty. *J Arthroplasty* 2013;28(6):904-907.

66. Mraovic B, Hipszer BR, Epstein RH, et al: Metabolic syndrome increases risk for pulmonary embolism after hip and knee arthroplasty. *Croat Med J* 2013;54(4):355-361.

67. Gandhi R, Razak F, Tso P, Davey JR, Mahomed NN: Metabolic syndrome and the incidence of symptomatic deep vein thrombosis following total knee arthroplasty. *J Rheumatol* 2009;36(10):2298-2301.

68. Goodman SM, Springer B, Guyatt G, et al: American College of Rheumatology/American Association of Hip and Knee Surgeons guideline for the perioperative management of antirheumatic medication in patients with rheumatic diseases undergoing elective total hip or total knee arthroplasty. *J Arthroplasty* 2017;32(9):2628-2638.

This is a collaboration between the American College of Rheumatology and the American Association of Hip and Knee Surgeons to develop an evidence-based guideline for the perioperative management of drug therapies in patients with inflammatory arthropathies who are undergoing TKA. Level of evidence: V.

69. Lee JK, Choi CH: Total knee arthroplasty in rheumatoid arthritis. *Knee Surg Relat Res* 2012;24(1):1-6.

70. Danoff JR, Moss G, Liabaud B, Geller JA: Total knee arthroplasty considerations in rheumatoid arthritis. *Autoimmune Dis* 2013;2013:185340.

71. Neva M, Häkkinen A, Mäkinen H, Hannonen P, Kauppi M, Sokka T: High prevalence of asymptomatic cervical spine subluxation in patients with rheumatoid arthritis waiting for orthopaedic surgery. *Ann Rheum Dis* 2006;65(7):884-888.

72. Ravi B, Escott B, Shah PS, et al: A systematic review and meta-analysis comparing complications following total joint arthroplasty for rheumatoid arthritis versus for osteoarthritis. *Arthritis Rheum* 2012;64(12):3839-3849.

73. Schnaser EA, Browne JA, Padgett DE, Figgie MP, D'Apuzzo MR: Perioperative complications in patients with inflammatory arthropathy undergoing total knee arthroplasty. *J Arthroplasty* 2015;30(9 suppl):76-80.

74. Jauregui JJ, Kapadia BH, Dixit A, et al: Thirty-day complications in rheumatoid patients following total knee arthroplasty. *Clin Rheumatol* 2016;35(3):595-600.

75. Feng B, Weng X, Lin J, Jin J, Wang W, Qiu G: Long-term follow-up of cemented fixed-bearing total knee arthroplasty in a Chinese population: A survival analysis of more than 10 years. *J Arthroplasty* 2013;28(10):1701-1706.

76. Behrens EM, Beukelman T, Gallo L, et al: Evaluation of the presentation of systemic onset juvenile rheumatoid arthritis: Data from the Pennsylvania Systemic Onset Juvenile Arthritis Registry (PASOJAR). *J Rheumatol* 2008;35(2):343-348. Available at: http://www.ncbi.nlm.nih.gov/pubmed/18085728. Accessed September17, 2019.

77. Abdel MP, Figgie MP: Surgical management of the juvenile idiopathic arthritis patient with multiple joint involvement. *Orthop Clin North Am* 2014;45(4):435-442.

78. Parvizi J, Lajam CM, Trousdale RT, Shaughnessy WJ, Cabanela ME: Total knee arthroplasty in young patients with juvenile rheumatoid arthritis. *J Bone Joint Surg Am* 2003;85(6):1090-1094.

79. Heyse TJ, Ries MD, Bellemans J, et al: Total knee arthroplasty in patients with juvenile idiopathic arthritis. *Clin Orthop Relat Res* 2014;472(1):147-154.

80. Thomas A, Rojer D, Imrie S, Goodman SB: Cemented total knee arthroplasty in patients with juvenile rheumatoid arthritis. *Clin Orthop Relat Res* 2005;433:140-146.

81. Malviya A, Foster HE, Avery P, Weir DJ, Deehan DJ: Long term outcome following knee replacement in patients with juvenile idiopathic arthritis. *Knee* 2010;17(5):340-344.

82. Mukherjee S, Culliford D, Arden N, Edwards C: What is the risk of having a total hip or knee replacement for patients with lupus? *Lupus* 2015;24(2):198-202.

83. Mertelsmann-Voss C, Lyman S, Pan TJ, Goodman S, Figgie MP, Mandl LA: Arthroplasty rates are increased among us patients with systemic lupus erythematosus: 1991-2005. *J Rheumatol* 2014;41(5):867-874.

84. Issa K, Pierce TP, Scillia AJ, Festa A, Harwin SF, Mont MA: Midterm outcomes following total knee arthroplasty in lupus patients. *J Arthroplasty* 2016;31(3):655-657.

85. Troyer J, Levine BR: Proximal tibia reconstruction with a porous tantalum cone in a patient with Charcot arthropathy. *Orthopedics* 2009;32(5):358. Available at: http://www.ncbi.nlm.nih.gov/pubmed/19472957. Accessed September 17, 2019.

86. Fullerton BD, Browngoehl LA: Total knee arthroplasty in a patient with bilateral Charcot knees. *Arch Phys Med Rehabil* 1997;78(7):780-782.

87. Parvizi J, Marrs J, Morrey BF: Total knee arthroplasty for neuropathic (Charcot) joints. *Clin Orthop Relat Res* 2003;416:145-150.

88. Sugitani K, Arai Y, Takamiya H, Minami G, Higuchi T, Kubo T: Total knee arthroplasty for neuropathic joint disease after severe bone destruction eroded the tibial tuberosity. *Orthopedics* 2012;35(7):e1108-e1111.

89. Long WJ, Scuderi GR: Porous tantalum cones for large metaphyseal tibial defects in revision total knee arthroplasty. A minimum 2-year follow-up. *J Arthroplasty* 2009;24(7):1086-1092.

90. Kim YH, Kim JS, Oh SW: Total knee arthroplasty in neuropathic arthropathy. *J Bone Joint Surg Br* 2002;84(2):216-219.

CHAPTER 25

Outcomes of Primary Total Knee Arthroplasty

DAVID C. AYERS, MD • PATRICIA D. FRANKLIN, MD, MBA, MPH
MATTHEW E. DEREN, MD

ABSTRACT

Total knee arthroplasty (TKA) can relieve arthritic pain and improve quality of life in patients who have debilitating arthritis. Currently, long-term survivorship rates of TKAs have been demonstrated through multiple registry-based studies and clinical studies. Studies comparing survivorship rates of various knee arthroplasty designs and systems combined with patient-reported outcome measures (PROMs) have provided guidance for optimizing the results of surgery. PROMs have historically been used in clinical research and have become increasingly prevalent in clinical practice. These instruments provide patient-centered benchmarks for measuring the success of TKAs by comparing patient-reported pain and function both before and after TKA; PROMs are therefore able to document patient improvement and affect quality of life. Patient satisfaction has historically lagged behind the pain relief provided by TKA and represents an area of continued opportunity for optimization.

Keywords: patient satisfaction; patient-reported outcome measures; scoring systems; survivorship

Dr. Ayers or an immediate family member has received nonincome support (such as equipment or services), commercially derived honoraria, or other non–research-related funding (such as paid travel) from resTORbio and serves as a board member, owner, officer, or committee member of the American Academy of Orthopaedic Surgeons and the American Orthopaedic Association. Dr. Franklin or an immediate family member has received research or institutional support from Zimmer. Dr. Deren or an immediate family member has received nonincome support (such as equipment or services), commercially derived honoraria, or other non–research-related funding (such as paid travel) from Stryker.

INTRODUCTION

Total knee arthroplasty (TKA) has proved to be a major success, with long-term survivorship rates exceeding 90% in most studies. It has also provided marked and consistent quality-of-life improvements for recipients. The parameters governing success rates in TKA, including implant design, bearing surface material, fixation techniques, alignment strategies, and patient-related factors, have been studied extensively over the past few decades. In 2020, there is the benefit of decades of experience with multiple TKA strategies. Many registries and clinical studies provide a large amount of high-quality data that can inform current strategies and drive future optimization of total TKA. Multiple tools exist to allow evaluation of the success of these surgeries. It is important to review the current landscape regarding objective and subjective outcomes following TKA, as well as some of the tools used to track outcomes.

This chapter is adapted from Ayers DC, Franklin PD, Gandhi R, et al: Outcomes of primary total knee arthroplasty, in Mont MA, Tanzer M, eds: *Orthopaedic Knowledge Update®: Hip and Knee Reconstruction*, ed 5. Rosemont, IL, American Academy of Orthopaedic Surgeons, 2017, pp 207-222.

SURVIVORSHIP ASSESSMENTS

Annual Registry Reports

The increasing utilization of research registries has improved the ability to analyze outcomes following TKA. Currently, multiple registries provide detailed information regarding longitudinal outcomes after TKA. The outcome measures collected in many registries encompass patient demographics, implant details, and patient-reported outcomes. The following summarizes some of the patient-specific and implant-specific data reported by two national total joint arthroplasty registries with long-term follow-up. Information regarding patient-reported outcomes is detailed subsequently.

The 2018 annual report of the Australian National Joint Arthroplasty Registry[1] notes an overall range of 3.0% to 13.3% cumulative revision rates at 10-year follow-up for all tracked primary TKA femoral and tibial implant combinations. A total of 60 component combinations with 350 or more procedures recorded per year were included in this analysis. Of the 60 combinations, 18 (30.0%) demonstrated revision rates less than 5% at 10 years. These 18 combinations included cruciate-retaining (CR) and cruciate-sacrificing (CS) designs. When analyzed by primary diagnosis, findings for osteoarthritis and rheumatoid arthritis continued to be similar at 10- and 14-year follow-up with 5% to 7% revision rates. For other inflammatory arthritis diagnoses, osteonecrosis, and other diagnoses, the revision rates were higher at 10 years. When comparing outcomes of cemented versus cementless TKA at 15 and 17 years, rates of revision were higher for cementless TKA. The 15-year cumulative revision rate for total knee prostheses ranged from 4.4% to 14.3%. Only two combinations of prostheses had a revision rate of less than 5% at 15 years.

The 2019 British National Joint Registry Annual Report[2] demonstrates an overall revision rate following primary TKA of 6.41%, with a rate of 4.74% for cemented constructs, 6.16% for cementless constructs, and 4.37% for hybrid constructs at 15-year follow-up. Revision rate is inversely correlated with increasing age (**Figure 1**). For patients younger than 55 years, the revision rate at 15 years was 17.48% for males and 15.54% for females. For patients aged 75 years and older, the revision rate at 15 years was 2.63% for men and 2.62% for women. For cemented, cementless, and hybrid constructs in male patients younger than 55 years, the revision rates at 15 years were 13.64%, 15.08%, and 10.31%, respectively. In female patients younger than 55 years, the revision rates were 10.31%, 10.80%, and 10.58%, respectively. For cemented, cementless, and hybrid constructs in male patients aged 75 years and older, the revision rates at 10 years were 2.26%, 2.33%, and 1.99%, respectively, compared with 2.18%, 3.30%, and 2.12%, respectively, for females.

Registries are also able to track which implant types have performed poorly compared with their counterparts; these analyses are important applications of registry data. However, the most accurate assessment of

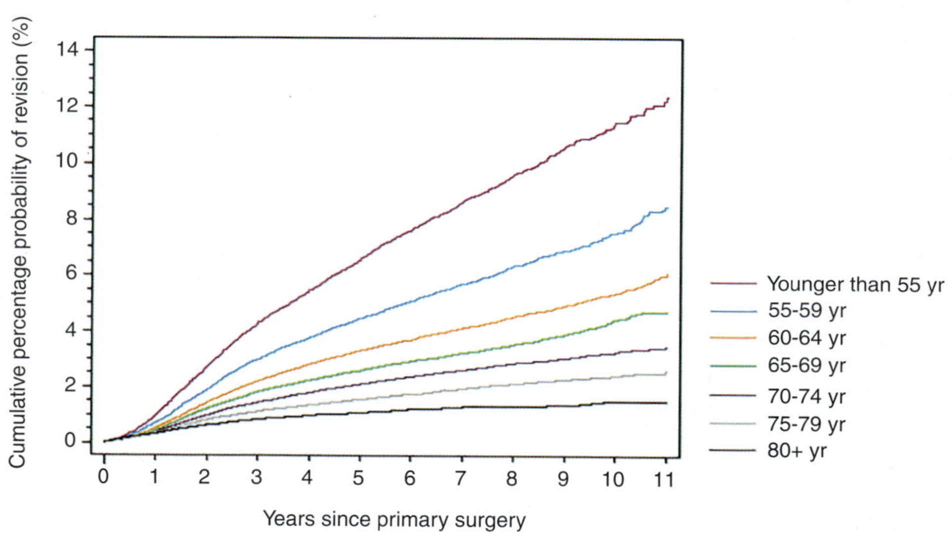

FIGURE 1 Graph shows revision rates following primary total knee arthroplasty, stratified by age. (Reproduced with permission from the National Joint Registry for England, Wales, Northern Ireland and the Isle of Man: *12th Annual Report*. Available at: http://www.njrcentre.org.uk/njrcentre/. Accessed July 6, 2016.)

outcomes over time requires longitudinal monitoring. Furthermore, it is important to note that summary results reported through national registries cannot be generalized to all patients. It is the combination of both clinical studies aimed at evaluating the results of TKA in specific patient populations and registry reports that can inform the management of specific patient populations.

Peer-Reviewed Studies

Peer-reviewed clinical and registry-based studies continue to corroborate the high survivorship rates of TKAs. A multicenter nationwide study followed 846 TKA recipients for at least 10 years and reported an overall survivorship rate of 92%. When subcategorized by implant type, the range in survivorship was 90% to 95%, without any significant differences among implant types. These results were comparable to those of multiple contemporary single-center studies[3] (**Table 1**). A study of 117 consecutive CS mobile-bearing TKAs at a mean follow-up of 10 years demonstrated a survivorship rate of 97.7%.[4] A systematic review of studies analyzing outcomes after primary TKA using one device reported survivorship based on 15 peer-reviewed studies comprising 4,025 TKAs in addition to 233,843 knee arthroplasties identified among five national joint arthroplasty registries.[5] Based on peer-reviewed literature alone, survivorship was found to be 97% at 13 years postoperatively, and pooled registry data showed a 10-year survivorship rate of 95.7%.[5] A comparison between data from Norway's National Joint Arthroplasty Registry and Kaiser Permanente's Total Joint Arthroplasty Registry (United States) reported survivorship at midterm follow-up of TKAs at 94.8% and 96.3%, respectively.[6] A review of survivorship of TKAs across multiple national registries and clinical studies reported the overall survivorship rate to be 93.8% at 10 years.[7] Thus, in studies spanning multiple follow-up intervals, implant types, and patient demographics, TKA has proven to exhibit high survivorship rates.

TABLE 1

Ten-Year Survivorship Rates of Total Knee Arthroplasty Designs

Clinical Study	No. of Patients[a]	Implant	Mean Patient Age (yr)	Clinical Score (Knee/Function)	10-Yr Overall Survivorship (95% Confidence Interval)
Fixed-bearing TKAs					
Hoffman et al	176/300	Natural Knee CR	65	—	95.1% (93.2-98.0)
Barrington et al	87/127	Nexgen PS	70	94/75 (KSS)	97% (94-100)
Schwartz et al	126/179	Nexgen PS	62.4	85.4 (HSS)	97.7% (96.3-99.0)
Nakamura et al	309/507	Bisurface PS	68.5	93.3/52.7 (KSS)	97.4% (95.8-99.0)
Moutet et al	80/117	Europ CR	73	88/80 (KSS)	97.8% (91.5-99.5)
Present series	846/942	Multiple PS + CR	71	83/74 (KSS)	92% (90-94)
Mobile-bearing TKAs					
Callaghan et al	82/114	LCS PS	70	90/75	100%
Buechel	309/309	LCS CR	71	—	97.4% (95-100)
Vogt and Saarbach	59/101	LCS PS	70	78/66 (KSS)	95%
Metsovitis et al	326	Rotaglide UC	66.7	92.6/66.7 (KSS)	96% (93-98)
Meftah et al	106/138	LCS PS	69.2	94 (HSS)	98.3% (97.1-99.5)
Argenson et al	108/116	Nexgen Flex PS	69	94/88 (KSS)	98.3% (97.1-99.5)
Current series	846/942	Multiple PS + CR	71	83/74 (KSS)	92% (90-94)

CR = cruciate (posterior cruciate ligament) retention, HSS = Hospital for Special Surgery score, KSS = Knee Society Score, PS = posterior-stabilized, TKA = total knee arthroplasty, UC = ultracongruent

[a]Data are the number of patients followed up/total number of patients.

Adapted from *Orthop Traumatol Surg Res* 99[4]. Argenson J-N, Boisgard S, Parratte S, et al; French Society of Orthopedic and Traumatologic Surgery (SOFCOT): Survival analysis of total knee arthroplasty at a minimum 10 years' follow-up: A multicenter French nationwide study including 846 cases, 385-390. Copyright © 2013, with permission from Elsevier Masson SAS.

CR Versus CS Designs

Over the past decades, multiple studies have evaluated the relative efficacy of CR versus CS TKA implant designs. Most studies found similar survivorship and clinical outcomes. A systematic review of 17 randomized controlled trials comparing the results of CR and CS implants at short-term to midterm follow-up showed no clinically relevant differences in outcomes after TKA with respect to range of motion, pain, and clinical and radiographic outcome measures.[8] A 2014 meta-analysis of eight randomized controlled trials comparing the outcomes of CR and CS implants in 963 primary TKAs found no significant differences in survivorship or clinical outcomes, with the exception of a modest improvement in range-of-motion scores with CS constructs at short-term to midterm follow-up.[9] The clinical relevance of this statistically significant finding was not assessed.

International registry data demonstrate similar survivorship rates between CR and CS TKAs. At 15 years postoperatively, the 2018 Australian National Joint Arthroplasty Annual Report[1] notes revision rates of 7.2% (95% confidence interval [CI]: 7.0 to 7.3) and 8.2% (95% CI: 7.9 to 8.6) for CR and CS constructs, respectively. The 2019 British National Joint Registry Annual Report[2] demonstrates a similar pattern but separates its results by sex and age. At 15 years postoperatively, cumulative revision rates of fixed-bearing cemented CR versus CS constructs are as follows: 13.20% (95% CI: 11.03 to 15.74) and 14.07% (95% CI: 11.93 to 16.55) in males younger than 55 years; 9.88% (95% CI: 8.71 to 11.19) and 12.01% (95% CI: 10.48 to 13.74) in females younger than 55 years; 1.99% (95% CI: 1.83 to 2.17) and 2.96% (95% CI: 2.20 to 3.99) in men aged 75 years and older; and 1.92% (95% CI: 1.79 to 2.07) and 2.63% (95% CI: 2.16 to 3.19) in women aged 75 years and older.

Mobile-Bearing Versus Fixed-Bearing Designs

Mobile-bearing TKA implant designs were developed in an effort to reduce polyethylene wear by decreasing the degree of constraint in the implant system. Multiple investigators have reported satisfactory results using these implants, with similar survivorship of mobile-bearing designs compared with fixed-bearing designs. A prospective randomized trial evaluating rotating-platform versus fixed-bearing designs, using a single implant type, in 444 patients who had simultaneous bilateral TKA (mobile bearing on one side, fixed bearing on the other) demonstrated no significant differences in survivorship or radiographic outcomes at a minimum 10-year follow-up (mean, 12.1 years).[10] Another prospective randomized trial compared mobile-bearing to fixed-bearing cruciate-substituting primary TKAs (PFC Sigma PS) with and without patellar resurfacing;[11] no single combination of bearing type and patellar surface showed a significant benefit, and all constructs resulted in clinical improvement at 2-year follow-up. These findings corroborate multiple earlier studies.[12] No data are yet available to demonstrate reduced wear in mobile-bearing designs, as longer follow-up is needed.

Registry data also reflect these relationships. The 2018 Australian registry report demonstrates a slightly lower revision rate in fixed-bearing versus mobile-bearing designs, which are of three types: rotating, sliding, and rotating-sliding.[1] The revision rates reported at 15 years postoperatively are 7.2% (95% CI: 7.0 to 7.4) for fixed-bearing designs, 8.2% (95% CI: 7.9 to 8.5) for rotating designs, 10.3% (95% CI: 9.2 to 11.5) for rotating-sliding designs, and 8.1% (95% CI: 6.4 to 10.1) for sliding designs. The 2019 British registry report separates results by sex, age, and stability.[2] At 10 years postoperatively, cumulative revision rates for fixed-bearing versus mobile-bearing designs show no significant differences: 7.79% (95% CI: 7.18 to 8.46) and 8.85% (95% CI: 7.24 to 10.79) for CR constructs in males younger than 55 years; 6.63% (95% CI: 6.15 to 7.14) and 7.80% (95% CI: 6.40 to 9.50) for CR constructs in females younger than 55 years; 10.37% (95% CI: 9.26 to 11.60) and 8.71% (95% CI: 46.57 to 11.51) for CS constructs in males younger than 55 years; and 9.02% (95% CI: 8.14 to 10.00) and 8.78% (95% CI: 6.74 to 11.40) for CS constructs in females younger than 55 years, respectively.

Cemented Versus Cementless Constructs

Over the past few decades, many investigators have assessed the survivorship of cementless and cemented primary TKAs. Conflicting reports exist. Reported survivorship rates have ranged from 85% to 98% and 76% to 99% at 10- to 20-years' follow-up for cemented and cementless constructs, respectively.[13] These reports reflect varying levels of evidence. A meta-analysis of 15 randomized controlled trials or observational studies demonstrated likelihood of revision that was 4.2 times greater after cementless fixation (95% CI: 2.7 to 6.5).[14] Follow-up for studies included in this meta-analysis ranged from 2 to 11 years. The 2018 Australian registry report[1] notes a hazard ratio of 1.25 for revision of cementless versus cemented primary TKAs at 17-year follow-up ($P < 0.001$) (**Figure 2**). This reflects an average revision rate of 9.4% (95% CI: 8.8 to 10.0) for cementless constructs and 7.6% (95% CI: 7.0 to 8.2) for cemented constructs. The 2019 annual report of the British registry[2] notes 15-year revision rates of 4.74% (95% CI: 4.61 to 4.88) and 6.16% (95% CI: 5.60 to 6.78) for cemented versus cementless primary TKAs, respectively.

Furthermore, most reports indicate that most primary TKAs being performed worldwide use cement. In 2018, the Australian registry reported a continued decrease in

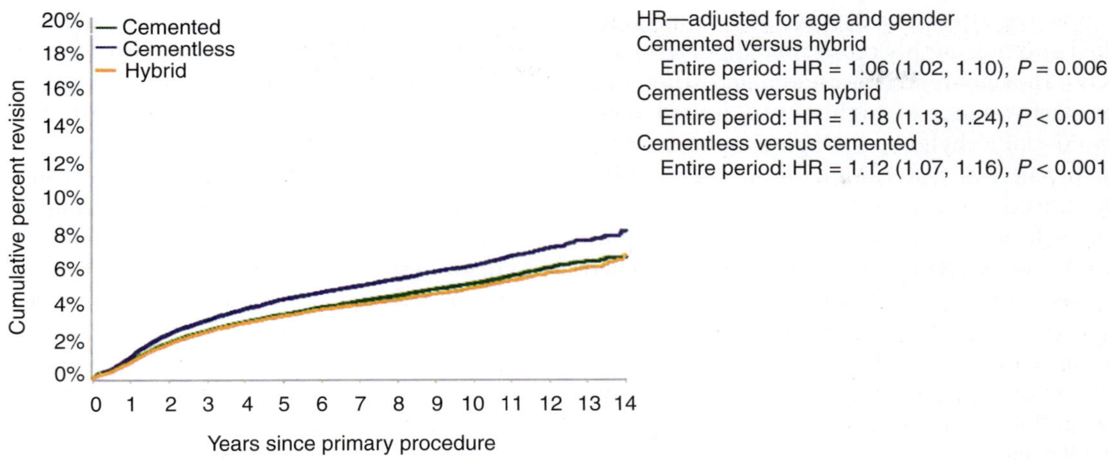

FIGURE 2 Graph shows Kaplan-Meier estimates of the cumulative percentage probability of a first revision of primary total knee arthroplasty by age and at increasing years after primary surgery. HR = hazard ratio. (Adapted with permission from the Australian Orthopaedic Association: *National Joint Arthroplasty Registry Annual Report 2015*. 2015. Available at: https://aoanjrr.sahmri.com/annual-reports-2015. Accessed July 13, 2020.)

cementless technique in 10.9% of all primary TKAs.[1] The British registry demonstrated an even more dramatic trend, with cementless TKA constructs comprising 1.8% of all knee arthroplasty procedures in 2018, which had decreased from 2.5% in 2014.[2] This registry data show a trend of decreased utilization in cementless knee technology. Some reports suggest reasonable outcomes after cementless TKA in specific situations; many large-scale reports suggest that cemented primary TKA remains the benchmark and, on average, confers superior survivorship.

IMPROVING SURVIVORSHIP

New Technologies

Despite its excellent track record, TKA is not a perfect intervention. Approximately 20% of patients may experience dissatisfaction after surgery.[15] In addition to patient dissatisfaction, a certain percentage of primary TKAs fail, requiring revision surgery. A United States multicenter retrospective review of 844 failed TKAs requiring revision documented the incidence of failure mechanisms,[16] with aseptic loosening, instability, infection, and polyethylene wear among the most common mechanisms affecting the original implant longevity. In an effort to optimize TKA surgery outcomes, many investigators continue to develop new strategies to tackle these challenges. Two current areas of focus have been fixation methods and alternative bearing surfaces.

As noted previously, cemented TKA constructs have been considered the benchmark for use in primary TKA. With the introduction of highly porous metal technology, however, short-term radiographic survivorship is promising. For instance, a randomized controlled trial compared traditional modular cemented tibial components with highly porous metal tibial components, either cemented or cementless, in primary TKA.[17] The all-cause revision rates were equivalent among constructs at a mean of 5 years. A retrospective review of 115 TKAs using porous tantalum implants noted a 95.7% cumulative survivorship at a mean of 7 years' follow-up, with no evidence of aseptic loosening as cause for revision.[18] Another study reported on a prospectively collected cohort of 105 consecutive porous tantalum TKAs, demonstrating no aseptic loosening at a minimum 3 years' follow-up and an overall revision rate of 1%.[19] A recent randomized controlled trial found no difference in clinical outcome scores of loosening when comparing cemented and cementless versions of the same design at 2-year follow-up.[20] Longer term studies are necessary to clarify the role of using highly porous metal surfaces in the setting of primary TKA.

The advent of highly cross-linked polyethylene has provided the potential for improved wear characteristics of TKA designs. Multiple investigators have assessed wear rates at midterm and long-term follow-up, and the results are not yet clear. The Australian Orthopaedic Association National Joint Arthroplasty Registry was assessed regarding differential wear rates between highly cross-linked and conventional polyethylene bearing TKAs over a 15-year period.[21] The revision rate for highly cross-linked polyethylene was 5.0% whereas for non-highly cross-linked polyethylene it was 7.9%.[1] When comparing patients younger than 65 years, the revision rate was 7.2% and 12.1% for highly cross-linked and non-highly cross-linked polyethylene, respectively.[1] In a prospective randomized study evaluating the performance of highly cross-linked versus conventional polyethylene, a single implant system was used in patients undergoing simultaneous bilateral TKA.[22] Study results indicated no radiographic or clinical differences between knees at a minimum follow-up of 5 years. Although there may be a benefit to highly cross-linked polyethylene in primary TKA in younger patients, more long-term follow-up is needed to clarify the role of this new technology.

The Australian Registry noted an increase in computer navigation in TKA, increasing from 2.4% in 2003 to 33.5% of TKA in 2017.[1] A recent meta-analysis of randomized controlled trials comparing computer-navigated with conventional TKA demonstrated a significantly better outcome in femoral sagittal alignment and tibial coronal alignment with computer-navigated TKA, but no difference in functional outcomes, revision rates, or aseptic loosening.[23] Robotic-assisted TKA has become more widespread in its utilization. Robotic-assisted TKA has also increased recently, with one prospective cohort study showing better short-term range of motion, earlier discharge from the hospital, and decreased analgesia requirements postoperatively when compared with conventional TKA technique.[24] The development of new technologies, such as porous metal components, and robotic-assisted surgery has the potential to improve survivorship of primary TKAs going forward, although current data do not demonstrate that these technologies confer survivorship benefits. Therefore, routine use of these new technologies in general orthopaedic practice is not yet supported.

SCORING SYSTEMS

Scoring systems provide a numerical rating of each patient's outcome after TKA. The scores generated through administration of outcome instruments (typically validated patient questionnaires) provide the most concise, clear measure, especially when comparing large groups of patients and treatments. In the past, outcome scores were generated by the treating surgeon during systematic assessment of the patient. Recent focus has shifted toward the patient's own assessment of his or her pain and function before and after TKA, as well as the extent to which his or her expectations have been fulfilled by the procedure. Patient-reported outcome measures (PROMs), traditionally used in clinical research, have now moved into routine clinical practice. These scoring systems are generally measures of the patient's global or disease-specific health. Global scoring systems consist of one or more domains relating to a particular facet of health (such as pain, function, satisfaction, or mental health). Summary global scores may be calculated by combining related domain scores that reflect the patients' overall physical health (physical composite score) or emotional health (mental composite score); physical composite score and mental composite score have proven to be very useful measures in TKA patients. Despite methodologic differences, scoring systems that have undergone formal validation have broad applicability and are generally accepted for measurement of outcomes after joint arthroplasty.[25] When developing or selecting a scoring system for quantification of outcomes, it must be recognized that every outcome score will be affected by the multidimensional facets of each patient's experience. Thus, all outcome measures are subject to the attitudes, abilities, and expectations of patients as well as to their motivations to undergo surgery.

Generic and Disease-Specific Outcome Measures

One approach to assessing the outcome of knee arthroplasty is through evaluation of the general health of the patient before and after treatment. This approach assumes that the value of medical intervention is reflected in a measurable improvement in patients' health-related quality of life. Thus, items that assess a patient's physical health, physiologic function, emotional health, and social function are expected to provide insight into the effect of a given treatment on the overall outcome of a broad demographic of patients.

One of the most frequently cited instruments for measurement of generic health outcomes is the Medical Outcomes Study 36-Item Short Form (SF-36), which was developed to measure the effect of interventions, including TKA, on the overall health and quality of life of patients[25,26] (**Table 2**). Demand resulted in the development and validation of a shorter version, the 10-Item Short Form (SF-10) or the 12-Item Short Form (SF-12), which consists of either 10 or 12 items from the functional status and well-being sections of the SF-36 that were found to be most predictive of the original outcome score.[3] The SF-36, SF-10, and SF-12 have been used extensively to evaluate patients before and after treatment of a wide variety of disease and surgical procedures, including TKA. Although scores generated by the SF-36, SF-10, and SF-12 instruments demonstrate that the patient's quality of life dramatically improves after TKA, these instruments are not highly sensitive or responsive to subtle changes among individual subjects with varied severity of knee problems or levels of recovery.[27] They are also affected by the patients' medical and musculoskeletal comorbid conditions.

To provide a more comprehensive assessment of patient outcomes, both a generic and a specific outcome measure are often administered. Disease-specific outcome measures in TKA patients focus all questions on the knee to specifically assess symptoms and function of that individual joint.[28] Because disease-specific scales have a narrower focus, they are often more responsive than generic health measures. The most commonly used disease-specific outcome measures are the Western Ontario and McMaster Universities Arthritis Index (WOMAC), the Knee Injury and Osteoarthritis Outcome Score (KOOS), and the Oxford Knee Score.[29]

The KOOS was developed as an extension of the WOMAC, using some of its subscales to measure the condition of the knee in younger, more active patients who have early-stage osteoarthritis or knee symptoms[30] (**Table 2**). Five scores are generated from the subscales of the KOOS (pain [9 items]; symptoms [7 items]; activities of daily living function [17 items]; sport and recreation function [5 items]; and quality of life [4 items]) using item responses on a five-point Likert scale. The KOOS has been demonstrated as a valid, reliable, and responsive assessment instrument, especially for patients who have expectations of physical activity or for those investigating physical function as a primary outcome.[31,32] A computer adaptive technology version of the KOOS that is under development will minimize the number of questions a patient answers while improving the accuracy of the score by using an item bank of questions. Attempts to decrease the number of questions asked in the KOOS and WOMAC have led to the development of shorter versions of specific outcome measures. The KOOS for Joint Replacement (KOOS JR) shortened the number of questions to 10 but lost the ability to determine separate

TABLE 2

Generic and Disease-Specific Outcome Measurement Instruments

Scoring System	Section	Subsection	Deductions
Medical Outcomes Study 36-Item Short Form	Functional status	Physical functioning Social functioning Role limitations attributed to physical problems	—
Well-being	Mental health Energy/fatigue Pain	—	—
	Overall evaluation of health	—	—
Knee Society Score	Objective score (100 points)	Pain (50 points) Range of motion (25 points) Stability (25 points)	Flexion contracture Extension lag Malalignment
	Function score (100 points)	Walking (50 points) Stair climbing (50 points)	Reliance on walking aids
The New Knee Society Score	Objective knee score (100 points)	Anterior-posterior alignment (25 points) Stability/instability (25 points) Range of motion (25 points) Symptoms (25 points)	Flexion contracture Extension lag Malalignment
	Satisfaction score (40 points)	Pain level while sitting (8 points) Pain level while lying in bed (8 points) Knee function while getting out of bed (8 points) Knee function while performing light household duties (8 points) Knee function while performing recreational activities (8 points)	—
	Expectations score (15 points)	Pain relief (5 points) Ability to perform ADL (5 points) Ability to perform leisure, recreational, or sports activities (5 points)	—

(continued)

TABLE 2

Generic and Disease-Specific Outcome Measurement Instruments—(continued)

Scoring System	Section	Subsection	Deductions
	Functional activity score (100 points)	Walking and standing (30 points) Standard activities (30 points) Advanced activities (25 points) Discretionary activities (15 points)	—
Knee Society Score Short Form	Symptoms (3 items)	—	—
	Satisfaction (1 item)	Satisfaction while performing light household activities	—
	Functional score (100 points)	How long can you walk? (20 points) Walking on an uneven surface (15 points) Climbing and descending stairs (15 points) Getting up from low couch or chair without arms (15 points) Running (20 points) Discretionary activities (15 points)	—
The Oxford 12-Item Knee Score	Pain	—	—
	Physical function	—	—
	Limitations	—	—
Knee Injury and Osteoarthritis Outcome Score	Self-administered queries	Pain (9 items) Symptoms (7 items) Function during ADL (17 items) Sport and recreation function (5 items) Quality of life (4 items)	—
Total Knee Function Questionnaire	Symptoms and activities	ADL (17 items) Movement and lifestyle activities (8 items) Recreational activities (8 items)	—
	Additional items	Walking and running (5 items) Satisfaction (1 item) Activity level and expectations (3 items) Pain and other symptoms (4 items) Patient information (9 items)	—
Knee Replacement Expectations Survey	Patient expectations	Pain (1 item) Psychologic well-being (1 item) Physical functions (15 items)	—

ADL = activities of daily living

pain and function subscores in addition to the composite score. The full KOOS, the KOOS-12, and the KOOS JR were compared in over 8,000 TKA patients. The TKAs were performed by over 200 surgeons in 28 states in the United States as part of the Function and Outcomes Research for Comparative Effectiveness in Total Joint Replacement (FORCE-TJR) registry. Patients completed a preoperative assessment of demographics, clinical risk factors, and PROMs. Postoperatively, PROMs collected at 1 year and 83% of patients completed the postoperative assessment at 1 year. KOOS-12 summary scores and KOOS JR floor and ceiling effects were compared. Outcomes for composite scores and subscores were compared between the full KOOS, KOOS-12, and KOOS JR in the same patient population. The results showed that the KOOS-12 summary score had the lowest percentage at the ceiling indicating that the KOOS-12 summary score was better able to distinguish between patients at higher levels of knee health than the other summary measures (KOOS JR). Tests of construct validity supported convergent and discriminant validity of the KOOS-12 at pre-TKR and post-TKR. Correlation between KOOS-12 pain and full KOOS pain subscores had an $r > 9.0$ as did correlation of KOOS-12 function scores with full KOOS function scores. KOOS-12 quality-of-life score and full KOOS quality-of-life scores are identical (as they use the same questions). In summary, the KOOS-12 is the only specific outcome measure that provides the ability to look at outcomes of pain, function, and quality of life separately while minimizing the number of questions asked of the patient. The KOOS-12 is currently available on the KOOS website and may be used free of charge. It will likely become the routinely used PROM for TKA in the near future.[33]

The 12-Item Oxford Knee Score (Oxford-12) was developed to assess the health outcomes of TKA patients on the basis of responses to 12 items that query pain, physical function, and limitations associated with the knee, each scored on a five-point scale[29] (**Table 2**). The scoring system expresses the status of the knee in terms of a single score, rather than as separate subscores, and has demonstrated reliability and validity. The Oxford-12 has been considered a simple and reliable tool for assessment of outcome. However, because there is only one score, the ability to evaluate improvement in pain relief or improvement in function as discrete scores is not possible. This limitation is significant, because pain relief and functional improvement after TKA may be different.

Functional Rating Systems

Although knee arthroplasty primarily aims to relieve the pain of joint degeneration, an important goal for most patients is maximum restoration of function. The functional outcome of the procedure is often linked to the patient's satisfaction with the procedure and has assumed greater importance as increasingly younger and more active patients have undergone the procedure. Functional rating systems have been designed with a primary focus on the ability of patients to participate in activities related to daily living, sports, and recreation. Thus, the ability of PROM to provide separate scores for function is considered very important. Another tool that may be used to measure knee function is the Total Knee Function Questionnaire, which is a self-administered instrument that collects information relating to physical activities in terms of their importance to each patient, the frequency with which each patient performs the activity, and the occurrence of symptoms when the patient performs the activity[34] (**Table 2**). The Total Knee Function Questionnaire queries participation in 33 different activities, ranging from least demanding (walking and standing) to most demanding (running, downhill skiing); these are condensed from a larger battery of activities considered in pilot studies. Additional items ask patients about satisfaction with TKA outcome and the extent to which the outcome has fulfilled expectations.

Applications of PROM in Clinical Practice

Routine use of PROM in clinical practice is in keeping with the Institute of Medicine's vision for medicine in the 21st century: to use information technology to support patient-centered evidence-based decisions. PROMs have moved into clinical practice for TKA patients.[35,36] Orthopaedic surgeon reimbursement in the United States is currently increased by reporting PROM through a qualified clinical data repository in the Physician Quality Reporting System of the Centers for Medicare & Medicaid Services program. Commercial insurance programs are expected to follow the lead of Centers for Medicare & Medicaid Services. In Massachusetts, for example, there is a pilot pay-for-performance quality-reporting program offered by a commercial insurer, and patient-reported outcomes are increasingly being used as a measure of quality. As health care moves from a volume-based to a value-based reimbursement system, PROMs are being used as the numerator of the value equation.[37-39]

PROM can be collected in a busy practice on a routine basis with data that are more than 85% complete at 1-year follow-up.[35] Data collection should be invisible to the surgeon and be efficient enough not to affect/delay the flow of the patient visit. To accomplish this, Internet-based electronic platforms have been developed so data can be entered before the office visit (either in the waiting room or at home before the visit); real-time scoring, using computer adaptive technology, allows scores to be used for decision making during the same office visit. PROM brings value to the visit by showing both the surgeon and the patient how the patient's function and pain compare with that of age-matched control patients as well as how they have changed after treatment prescribed at the previous visit.[35] The measures are increasingly used for shared decision making, including when to proceed with elective TKA and to gather objective data about a patient's recovery after TKA.[39] The addition of PROM to risk-adjustment models significantly increases the accuracy of models used to predict the risk of readmission after total joint arthroplasty.[40,41] PROMs have also been used to assess patient selection and timing of TKA surgery across the United States and have been added to modern joint arthroplasty registries.[42] The combination of PROM with demographic data and information relating to implant selection and survivorship now enables registries to provide valuable feedback regarding factors associated with pain and function after TKA.[41]

Performance-Based Measures

Performance-based tools, such as the Timed Up and Go test[43] and the 6-minute walk test,[44] examine changes in physical function after TKA and capture objective information about patients' actual function that is not evaluated by patient-reported measures. Unlike patient-reported measures, performance-based measures are derived from objective measures of function rather than from the patient's perceived function and are not body-part or body-function specific.[45] One study of TKA patients has shown poor correlation between preoperative patient-reported measures (WOMAC and SF-36) and a performance-based measure (Timed Up and Go test), highlighting the importance of both types of tests for a comprehensive assessment of disability.[46] An expert group of 138 clinicians and researchers from 16 countries was commissioned to recommend a set of performance-based tests for use following TKA. The Osteoarthritis Research Society International consensus group suggested five tools: 30-second chair stand test, 40-m fast-paced walk test, stair-climb test, timed up-and-go test, and 6-minute walk test. The first three were suggested as the minimal core set of performance-based tests for knee osteoarthritis.[47] Further research is required to fully assess the psychometric properties of these measures (reliability and validity) and to define the minimally clinically important difference for relevant time points following TKA.

Global Knee Rating Systems

A global knee rating system has been operationally defined as an outcome instrument that includes, at a minimum, assessments of pain, function, and range of motion and summarizes these outcomes as a single score on a global scale.

The American Knee Society Clinical Rating System, or Knee Society Score (KSS), recognized some of the limitations of the earlier Hospital for Special Surgery Score and implemented a scoring method that has been widely adopted and supported.[48] The KSS consists of two separate subscores, each on a 100-point scale (**Table 2**): the clinician-administered "Objective Knee Score" and the "Function Score." This separation enables surgeons to assess patients' knee conditions independent of any functional deterioration due to comorbidities. Psychometric testing has shown that the KSS Objective component has poor reliability with acceptable responsiveness, whereas the KSS Functional component has good reliability with questionable responsiveness.[49] In view of these deficiencies, both of these KSS subscores are often administered to assess outcome, a practice that had previously been widely accepted in clinical use.[48]

Given that the KSS functional component is only based on the patient's ability to walk and climb stairs, the KSS is not indicative of a patient's ability to perform functional tasks that are more demanding (such as running, cycling, and yoga). Thus, the KSS functional component has a marked ceiling effect, with many patients receiving the maximum possible score. This deficiency has become increasingly apparent in assessing contemporary TKA patients, approximately one-third of whom are 55 years or younger and who frequently participate in sporting and workout activities.[50] In recognition of this deficiency, a new KSS System was developed and formally validated in 2011 to account for the preoperative patient expectations, satisfaction, and physical activities of the younger, more diverse population of contemporary TKA patients.[51] This new KSS preserves the original objective and functional subscores and includes items relating to patient satisfaction; it also surveys the patient's ability to participate in a broad range of activities, both preoperatively and at follow-up (**Table 2**). The functional activity score in the new KSS places greater emphasis on the patient's assessment of the importance of specific activities by allowing him or her to select some of the activities forming the basis of the assessment of outcome; in addition, a wide variety of activities, ranging from walking to running, are included.

Despite the advantages of the new KSS, a deficiency revealed in initial trials was a higher-than-expected incidence of incomplete responses during self-administration.[51] This resulted in the development and validation of a short-form version of the new KSS to increase the usefulness of the instrument for routine follow-up of patients after TKA[52] (**Table 2**). During validation, the short form still provided acceptable discrimination between clinically different groups of patients before and after TKA, with virtually the same estimated effect size as the original functional activities subscale of the new KSS. This resulted in the conclusion that the short-form version of the KSS was practical, valid, reliable, and responsive for assessing functional outcome of TKA. It was recommended that the long-form version of the new KSS be used for research studies and for more sensitive measurement of the outcomes of individual patients. In addition, it was recommended that the short-form version be adopted in general clinical practice for use with large patient populations based on expected improvement in the rate of patient completion and ease of administration.[52]

SUMMARY

TKA is a highly successful surgery, providing sustainable relief and improved quality of life to its recipients. Many factors affect the success of TKA, some of which have been elucidated and some of which remain obscure.

Outcomes instruments exist to help in the understanding of the objective and subjective patient experience following TKA. Continued monitoring of long-term results following TKA is advocated, along with continued study of new technologies and incorporation of outcomes instruments in the study of TKA to optimize this already highly successful intervention.

KEY STUDY POINTS

- Overall survivorship rates of primary TKA are 90% or higher in most long-term follow-up studies, including clinical and registry-based studies.
- Many TKA designs and strategies have high success rates, although not all designs and strategies have comparable success rates.
- Recent focus has shifted from surgeon-reported to patient-reported outcomes to assess a patient-centered concept of success following TKA.
- Patient satisfaction following TKA is multifactorial and includes factors intrinsic and extrinsic to patients.
- Patient satisfaction rates following TKA have been determined to be 85% or lower in multiple studies.

ANNOTATED REFERENCES

1. Australian Orthopaedic Association: *National Joint Arthroplasty Registry—Annual Report 2018*. 2018. Available at: https://aoanjrr.sahmri.com/annual-reports-2015. Accessed December 9, 2019.

   This report summarizes the results of a large number of TKAs performed in Australia over more than 1 decade. Level of evidence: II.

2. National Joint Registry for England, Wales, Northern Ireland and the Isle of Man: *16th Annual Report*. Available at: http://www.njrcentre.org.uk/njrcentre/. Accessed December 10, 2019.

   Revision rates for primary TKA are summarized.

3. Argenson JN, Boisgard S, Parratte S, et al, French Society of Orthopedic and Traumatologic Surgery (SOFCOT): Survival analysis of total knee arthroplasty at a minimum 10 years' follow-up: A multicenter French nationwide study including 846 cases. *Orthop Traumatol Surg Res* 2013;99(4):385-390.
4. Meftah M, Ranawat AS, Ranawat CS: Ten-year follow-up of a rotating-platform, posterior-stabilized total knee arthroplasty. *J Bone Joint Surg Am* 2012;94(5):426-432.
5. Hopley CD, Dalury DF: A systematic review of clinical outcomes and survivorship after total knee arthroplasty with a contemporary modular knee system. *J Arthroplasty* 2014;29(7):1398-1411.
6. Paxton EW, Furnes O, Namba RS, Inacio MC, Fenstad AM, Havelin LI: Comparison of the Norwegian knee arthroplasty register and a United States arthroplasty registry. *J Bone Joint Surg Am* 2011;93(suppl 3):20-30.
7. Pabinger C, Berghold A, Boehler N, Labek G: Revision rates after knee replacement. Cumulative results from worldwide clinical studies versus joint registers. *Osteoarthr Cartil* 2013;21(2):263-268.
8. Verra WC, van den Boom LG, Jacobs W, Clement DJ, Wymenga AA, Nelissen RG: Retention versus sacrifice of the posterior cruciate ligament in total knee arthroplasty for treating osteoarthritis. *Cochrane Database Syst Rev* 2013;2013(10):CD004803.
9. Li N, Tan Y, Deng Y, Chen L: Posterior cruciate-retaining versus posterior stabilized total knee arthroplasty: A meta-analysis of randomized controlled trials. *Knee Surg Sports Traumatol Arthrosc* 2014;22(3):556-564.
10. Kim YH, Park JW, Kim JS, Kulkarni SS, Kim YH: Long-term clinical outcomes and survivorship of press-fit condylar sigma fixed-bearing and mobile-bearing total knee prostheses in the same patients. *J Bone Joint Surg Am* 2014;96(19):e168.
11. Ferguson KB, Bailey O, Anthony I, James PJ, Stother IG, Blyth MJG: A prospective randomised study comparing rotating platform and fixed bearing total knee arthroplasty in a cruciate substituting design: Outcomes at two year follow-up. *Knee* 2014;21(1):151-155.
12. Smith H, Jan M, Mahomed NN, Davey JR, Gandhi R: Meta-analysis and systematic review of clinical outcomes comparing mobile bearing and fixed bearing total knee arthroplasty. *J Arthroplasty* 2011;26(8):1205-1213.
13. Ranawat CS, Meftah M, Windsor EN, Ranawat AS: Cementless fixation in total knee arthroplasty: Down the boulevard of broken dreams – Affirms. *J Bone Joint Surg Br* 2012;94(11 suppl A):82-84.
14. Gandhi R, Tsvetkov D, Davey JR, Mahomed NN: Survival and clinical function of cemented and uncemented prostheses in total knee replacement: A meta-analysis. *J Bone Joint Surg Br* 2009;91(7):889-895.
15. Bourne RB, Chesworth BM, Davis AM, Mahomed NN, Charron KD: Patient satisfaction after total knee arthroplasty: Who is satisfied and who is not? *Clin Orthop Relat Res* 2010;468(1):57-63.
16. Schroer WC, Berend KR, Lombardi AV, et al: Why are total knees failing today? Etiology of total knee revision in 2010 and 2011. *J Arthroplasty* 2013;28(8 suppl):116-119.
17. Pulido L, Abdel MP, Lewallen DG, et al: The Mark Coventry Award: Trabecular metal tibial components were durable and reliable in primary total knee arthroplasty. A randomized clinical trial. *Clin Orthop Relat Res* 2015;473(1):34-42.
18. Kwong LM, Nielsen ES, Ruiz DR, Hsu AH, Dines MD, Mellano CM: Cementless total knee replacement fixation: A contemporary durable solution – Affirms. *Bone Joint J* 2014;96-B(11 suppl A):87-92.
19. Helm AT, Kerin C, Ghalayini SR, McLauchlan GJ: Preliminary results of an uncemented trabecular metal tibial component in total knee arthroplasty. *J Arthroplasty* 2009;24(6):941-944.

20. Nam D, Lawrie CM, Salih R, Nahhas CR, Barrack RL, Nunley RM: Cemented versus cementless total knee arthroplasty of the same modern design: A prospective, randomized trial. *J Bone Joint Surg Am* 2019;101(13):1185-1192.

The authors compared clinical outcomes of cemented and cementless TKAs with the same design 2 years after surgery, and found that the cementless TKA had results similar to that of the cemented TKA, with no aseptic failure of either implant. Level of evidence: I.

21. de Steiger RN, Muratoglu O, Lorimer M, Cuthbert AR, Graves SE: Lower prosthesis-specific 10-year revision rate with crosslinked than with non-crosslinked polyethylene in primary total knee arthroplasty. *Acta Orthop* 2015;86(6):721-727.

22. Kim YH, Park JW: Comparison of highly cross-linked and conventional polyethylene in posterior cruciate-substituting total knee arthroplasty in the same patients. *J Bone Joint Surg Am* 2014;96(21):1807-1813.

23. Rhee SJ, Kim HJ, Lee CR, Cim CW, Gwak HC, Kim JH: A comparison of long-term outcomes of computer-navigated and conventional total knee arthroplasty: A meta-analysis of randomized controlled trials. *J Bone Joint Surg Am* 2019;101(20):1875-1885.

The authors found that computer-navigated TKA had better outcomes in postoperative component alignment than conventional TKA. No significant differences in survivorship and long-term functional outcomes were found between the two techniques. Level of evidence: I.

24. Kayani B, Konan S, Thmassebi J, Pietrzak JRT, Haddad FS: Robotic-arm assisted total knee arthroplasty is associated with improved early functional recovery and reduced time to hospital discharge compared with conventional jig-based total knee arthroplasty. *Bone Joint J* 2018;100-B(7):930-937.

Robotic arm-assisted TKA was compared with conventional jig-based TKA; decreased pain, improved early recovery of function, and reduced time to hospital discharge were noted with robotic arm-assisted TKA. Level of evidence: II.

25. Ramkumar PN, Harris JD, Noble PC: Patient-reported outcome measures after total knee arthroplasty: A systematic review. *Bone Joint Res* 2015;4(7):120-127.

26. Ware JE Jr, Gandek B: Overview of the SF-36 Health Survey and the International Quality of Life Assessment (IQOLA) project. *J Clin Epidemiol* 1998;51(11):903-912.

27. Ware J Jr, Kosinski M, Keller SD: A 12-Item Short-Form Health Survey: Construction of scales and preliminary tests of reliability and validity. *Med Care* 1996;34(3):220-233.

28. Ko Y, Lo NN, Yeo SJ, et al: Comparison of the responsiveness of the SF-36, the Oxford Knee Score, and the Knee Society Clinical Rating System in patients undergoing total knee replacement. *Qual Life Res* 2013;22(9):2455-2459.

29. Dawson J, Fitzpatrick R, Murray D, Carr A: Questionnaire on the perceptions of patients about total knee replacement. *J Bone Joint Surg Br* 1998;80(1):63-69.

30. Jenny JY, Diesinger Y: The Oxford Knee Score: Compared performance before and after knee replacement. *Orthop Traumatol Surg Res* 2012;98(4):409-412.

31. Roos EM, Roos HP, Lohmander LS, Ekdahl C, Beynnon BD: Knee injury and Osteoarthritis Outcome Score (KOOS): Development of a self-administered outcome measure. *J Orthop Sports Phys Ther* 1998;28(2):88-96.

32. Peer MA, Lane J: The Knee injury and Osteoarthritis Outcome Score (KOOS): A review of its psychometric properties in people undergoing total knee arthroplasty. *J Orthop Sports Phys Ther* 2013;43(1):20-28.

33. Gandek B, Roos EM, Franklin PD, Ware JE Jr: A 12-item short form of the Knee injury and Osteoarthritis Outcome Score (KOOS-12): Tests of reliability, validity and responsiveness. *Osteoarthr Cartil* 2019;27(5):762-770.

The KOOS-12 test was found to be a good alternative to KOOS, providing three domain-specific and summary knee impact scores with lower burden to respondents. Level of evidence: III.

34. Weiss JM, Noble PC, Conditt MA, et al: What functional activities are important to patients with knee replacements? *Clin Orthop Relat Res* 2002;404:172-188.

35. Ayers DC, Zheng H, Franklin PD: Integrating patient-reported outcomes into orthopaedic clinical practice: Proof of concept from FORCE-TJR. *Clin Orthop Relat Res* 2013;471(11):3419-3425.

36. Ayers DC, Bozic KJ: The importance of outcome measurement in orthopaedics. *Clin Orthop Relat Res* 2013;471(11):3409-3411.

37. Franklin PD, Lewallen D, Bozic K, Hallstrom B, Jiranek W, Ayers DC: Implementation of patient-reported outcome measures in U.S. total joint replacement registries: Rationale, status, and plans. *J Bone Joint Surg Am* 2014;96(suppl 1):104-109.

38. Franklin PD, Allison J, Ayers DC: Beyond joint implant registries: A patient-centered research consortium for comparative effectiveness in total joint replacement. *J Am Med Assoc* 2012;308(12):1217-1218.

39. Ayers DC, Franklin PD: Joint replacement registries in the United States: A new paradigm. *J Bone Joint Surg Am* 2014;96(18):1567-1569.

40. Ayers DC, Li W, Oatis C, Rosal MC, Franklin PD: Patient-reported outcomes after total knee replacement vary on the basis of preoperative coexisting disease in the lumbar spine and other nonoperatively treated joints: The need for a musculoskeletal comorbidity index. *J Bone Joint Surg Am* 2013;95(20):1833-1837.

41. Ayers DC, Fehring T, Odum S, Franklin PD: Using joint registry data from FORCE-TJR to improve the accuracy of risk-adjustment prediction models for thirty-day readmission after total hip replacement and total knee replacement. *J Bone Joint Surg Am* 2015;97(8):668-671.

42. Ayers DC, Li W, Harrold L, Allison J, Franklin PD: Preoperative pain and function profiles reflect consistent TKA patient selection among US surgeons. *Clin Orthop Relat Res* 2015;473(1):76-81.

43. Podsiadlo D, Richardson S: The timed "Up & Go": A test of basic functional mobility for frail elderly persons. *J Am Geriatr Soc* 1991;39(2):142-148.

44. Guyatt GH, Sullivan MJ, Thompson PJ, et al: The 6-minute walk: A new measure of exercise capacity in patients with chronic heart failure. *Can Med Assoc J* 1985;132(8):919-923.
45. Dobson F, Hinman RS, Hall M, Terwee CB, Roos EM, Bennell KL: Measurement properties of performance-based measures to assess physical function in hip and knee osteoarthritis: A systematic review. *Osteoarthr Cartil* 2012;20(12):1548-1562.
46. Gandhi R, Tsvetkov D, Davey JR, Syed KA, Mahomed NN: Relationship between self-reported and performance-based tests in a hip and knee joint replacement population. *Clin Rheumatol* 2009;28(3):253-257.
47. Dobson F, Hinman RS, Roos EM, et al: OARSI recommended performance-based tests to assess physical function in people diagnosed with hip or knee osteoarthritis. *Osteoarthr Cartil* 2013;21(8):1042-1052.
48. Insall JN, Dorr LD, Scott RD, Scott WN: Rationale of the Knee Society Clinical Rating System. *Clin Orthop Relat Res* 1989;248:13-14.
49. Lingard EA, Katz JN, Wright RJ, Wright EA, Sledge CB, Kinemax Outcomes Group: Validity and responsiveness of the Knee Society Clinical Rating System in comparison with the SF-36 and WOMAC. *J Bone Joint Surg Am* 2001;83(12):1856-1864.
50. Dahm DL, Barnes SA, Harrington JR, Sayeed SA, Berry DJ: Patient-reported activity level after total knee arthroplasty. *J Arthroplasty* 2008;23(3):401-407.
51. Noble PC, Scuderi GR, Brekke AC, et al: Development of a new Knee Society Scoring System. *Clin Orthop Relat Res* 2012;470(1):20-32.
52. Scuderi GR, Sikorskii A, Bourne RB, Lonner JH, Benjamin JB, Noble PC: The Knee Society short form reduces respondent burden in the assessment of patient-reported outcomes. *Clin Orthop Relat Res* 2016;474(1):134-142.

Complications of Total Knee Arthroplasty

CHRISTIAN J. ECCLES, MD • JAMES F. BAKER, MD • ARTHUR L. MALKANI, MD

ABSTRACT

Total knee arthroplasty (TKA) has been one of the most successful procedures for the management of end-stage knee arthritis, with survival rates reported as high as 90% at 20 years. Despite outstanding results, complications following primary TKA do occur and can lead to readmissions, poor clinical outcomes, patient dissatisfaction, and increased healthcare costs. There has been a substantial increase in the number of patients, both elderly and young, undergoing primary TKA over the past decade because of multiple factors including increased life expectancy along with increased number of morbidly obese and younger active individuals presenting with end-stage knee arthritis. Given the increased volume of patients choosing TKAs, it would be helpful for surgeons to define modifiable patient risk factors, provide concepts for continuous practice improvement, and outline successful methods to decrease complications and improve patient-reported outcomes, and which would help decrease overall healthcare costs related to the management of complications following primary TKA.

Dr. Malkani or an immediate family member has received royalties from Stryker; is a member of a speakers' bureau or has made paid presentations on behalf of Stryker; serves as a paid consultant to or is an employee of Stryker; and has received research or institutional support from Stryker. Neither of the following authors nor any immediate family member has received anything of value from or has stock or stock options held in a commercial company or institution related directly or indirectly to the subject of this chapter: Dr. Eccles and Dr. Baker.

Keywords: arthrofibrosis; complications; extensor mechanism; instability; patellofemoral; polyethylene wear; total knee arthroplasty

INTRODUCTION

The number of total knee arthroplasty (TKA) cases performed continues to increase, and continued improvements in various aspects of these procedures are required to improve long-term survivorship to decrease costs and revision incidence.[1] The most common etiology of failure following primary TKA continues to be periprosthetic joint infection (PJI). Other causes of failure include instability, aseptic loosening, polyethylene wear and osteolysis, arthrofibrosis, and neurovascular injury. Complications following primary TKA can be divided into early versus late. Despite patient optimization before surgery, postoperative medical complications can occur because of the patient's underlying comorbid condition, which may require comanagement with the consultant colleagues. Polyethylene wear, instability, arthrofibrosis, patellofemoral issues, extensor mechanism, and neurovascular complications are discussed. It is important to be knowledgeable about the most up-to-date research and currently accepted guidelines for the assessment, diagnosis, and management of these complications following TKA.

POLYETHYLENE WEAR AND ASSOCIATED COMPLICATIONS

First-generation polyethylene used in primary TKA is known for its compromised wear properties. Wear and subsequent particle-induced osteolysis leading to aseptic loosening remains an important cause of mid to late failure following primary TKA (**Figure 1**). However, with

This chapter is adapted from Krebs VE, Malkani AL, Ulrich SD, Backstein D: Complications of knee arthroplasty, in Mont MA, Tanzer M, eds: *Orthopaedic Knowledge Update®: Hip and Knee Reconstruction*, ed 5. Rosemont, IL, American Academy of Orthopaedic Surgeons, 2017, pp 233-266.

technologic advancements in manufacturing, studies have demonstrated a decline in wear-related aseptic revisions.[2-5] One study reported the number of late revisions for polyethylene wear decreased from more than 40% in 2002 to 4.3% in 2012.[5] Another study also showed a decrease in the incidence of polyethylene wear to 7% compared with failure rates of 10% to 25% in earlier studies.[4] Polyethylene wear was responsible for 18.5% of late TKA failures. The etiology of polyethylene wear is multifactorial and related to polyethylene manufacturing, implant design, patient factors (eg, body mass index), surgical technique, and implant alignment. As the volume of TKA procedures continue to rise along with the increased longevity and younger and more active patient populations opting for TKA, surgeons and the industry need to continue to evolve and find means to reduce polyethylene wear and osteolysis by advancing the science of polyethylene manufacturing, implant design, implant positioning/alignment, and patient-related factors to further improve implant survival and durability.

Evolution of Polyethylene

The science and manufacturing of polyethylene have undergone considerable advancement in the past few decades. Improvements in polyethylene wear characteristics have contributed to decreased TKA failure rates related to wear and osteolysis.[2-5] Issues related to wear with polyethylene were initially much larger in total hip arthroplasty (THA) failure, which led to scientific efforts to improve the overall wear characteristics of polyethylene, which also benefited TKA. The bearing surface in TKA, with its sliding, rolling, and rotational behavior, is not as conforming as THA, leading to increased contact stresses. The shift away from polyethylene irradiation in air is considered by many to be the most important improvement in reducing free-radical formation that ultimately results in osteolysis. Considerable research has focused on sterilization, packaging, cross-linking, and manufacturing techniques, with contemporary polyethylene knee bearings currently being gamma irradiated or ethylene oxide sterilized and packaged in an inert environment.

Many proprietary manufacturing processes have also been developed, and each company has published data defining advantages and improved wear resistance that generally fall into one of two categories: highly cross-linked polyethylene (HXLPE) or vitamin E-infused polyethylene (VEPE). HXLPE is already in its second generation, with thermal stabilization added to the manufacturing process by remelting or annealing the polyethylene to minimize oxidation and maximize cross-linking. Remelting is a process undertaken at a higher temperature to convert the crystalline structure of polyethylene back to an amorphous state that releases free radicals. Free-radical elimination by this method is nearly complete, but it reduces the crystallinity of the polyethylene and makes the material potentially more brittle and less resistant to fatigue-crack propagation. Despite promising results of sequentially irradiated and annealed second-generation HXLPE in the literature on THA, there are concerns about its benefits in TKA. The knee bearing surface has a wear mechanism different from that of the hip, in which wear is abrasive and adhesive unlike

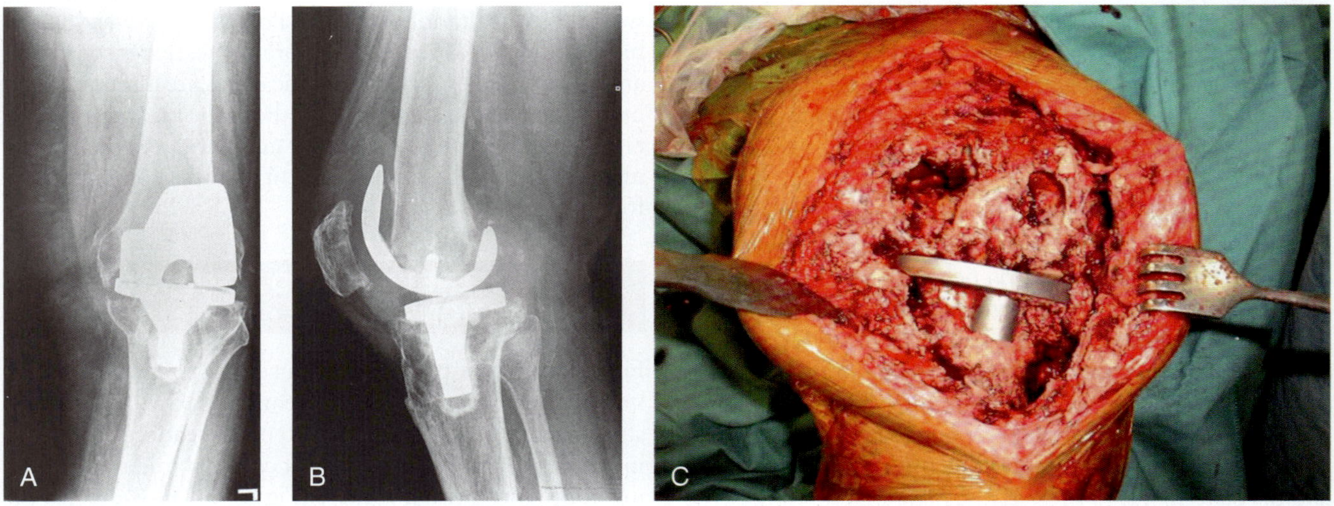

FIGURE 1 AP (**A**) and lateral (**B**) radiographs of extensive osteolysis around the femoral and tibial implant of total knee arthroplasty 11 years postoperatively. **C**, Intraoperative view on the size of bone defects after removal of the failed femoral implant and débridement of the osteolytic cavity. (Reprinted from *Acta Biomater* 9[9]. Gallo J, Goodman SB, Konttinen YT, et. al. Osteolysis around total knee arthroplasty: a review of pathogenetic mechanisms, 8046-8058. Copyright © 2013 Acta Materialia Inc.)

TKA where pitting and delamination predominate. One study proposes that the reduction of mechanical properties by newer generations of polyethylene and resistance to fatigue and crack propagation may lead to breakage and failure of the insert over time.[6] Recent studies, however, have demonstrated the safety of first-generation and second-generation HXLPE in the setting of TKA. A multicenter minimum 5-year follow-up study of second-generation HXLPE versus conventional polyethylene did not demonstrate any osteolysis or insert failure in either group.[7] Another study compared two first-generation HXLPEs with conventional polyethylene, and no revisions were noted as a direct result of polyethylene failure.[8]

Antioxidant vitamin–infused polyethylene with vitamin E is another method developed to improve on earlier-generation polyethylene. Synthetically derived vitamin E is either added to the polyethylene powder before cross-linking or diffused into irradiated polyethylene to stabilize free radicals.[9] Knee simulator studies have attempted to answer the question of whether VEPE is a viable alternative to conventional polyethylene. Conventional polyethylene laced with vitamin E was compared with plain conventional polyethylene with both samples undergoing the same postprocessing sterilization.[10] The VEPE showed no signs of oxidation or reduction in mechanical properties compared with conventional polyethylene. Concerns with VEPE lie mainly with the intra-articular and systemic effects of vitamin E.[6] The natural form of vitamin E, α-tocopherol, is nontoxic to humans; however, the effects of steps in the VEPE manufacturing process on the structure of vitamin E, such as irradiation, are unknown.[9]

The use of newer generations of polyethylene in TKA is still controversial because conventional polyethylene has good long-term clinical outcomes and is cost effective compared with HXLPE and VEPE. In a study, the cost of conventional polyethylene at two different institutions was found to be approximately US $150 less compared with the newer polyethylene.[11] Some recent studies show promising short-term results with newer polyethylene, but additional studies and longer follow-up is necessary to determine if newer generations of polyethylene are beneficial. Surface damage and oxidation were reduced on an HXLPE at a midterm follow-up of at least 2.5 years compared with a patient-matched direct compression-molded polyethylene.[12] A retrieval analysis demonstrated vitamin E–stabilized HXLPE tibial inserts had less surface damage and oxidation compared with remelted HXLPE controls.[13] On the other hand, another retrieval study found that despite their stabilization treatment, sequentially annealed HXLPE tibial inserts had similar oxidation levels when compared with gamma inert sterilized controls.[14]

Etiology and Risk Factors

The true incidence of polyethylene wear and osteolysis in functioning TKAs is difficult to quantify, because information published is primarily related to failures and revisions in retrieval analysis. As an isolated cause of failure, rates of wear and osteolysis range from 4.3% to 7.0% in recent literature.[3,5] The true incidence is likely much higher because wear and osteolysis always occur in conjunction with all other failure mechanisms, and a patient can remain asymptomatic up to the point of implant failure. Numerous studies suggest that polyethylene wear–induced periprosthetic osteolysis is a time-related progression that is closely associated with mechanical and biologic dynamics.[15] The wear particle accumulation in TKA results from a combination of delamination, pitting, adhesion, abrasion, and burnishing backside wear.[16] Decreasing wear and bioactive particle generation has been the prime strategy for elimination of osteolysis and aseptic loosening. Unfortunately, these causes of failure are multifactorial and involve the inseparable aspects of TKA: biology, implant design, patient factors, and surgical technique (**Table 1**).

Advances in the basic science of particle-induced osteolysis are becoming relevant because an understanding of this process can lead to the development of clinically relevant interventions. Polyethylene particles accumulating in the joint space activate several cell lines of innate and adaptive immunity. The activation of macrophages into an M1 phenotype is accountable for the triggering and maintenance of chronic inflammation, which enables growth of the interface membrane. In addition, polarized M2 macrophages produce anti-inflammatory cytokines (such as CCL2, CCL5, CXCL12, and CX3CL1) and homeostatic repair molecules.[17,18] The predominant feature of periprosthetic osteolysis is an overactivation of the receptor activator nuclear factor-κB ligand (RANKL)–induced osteoclastogenesis caused by an interaction of the RANKL/RANK/osteoprotegerin axis.[19] Elevated RANKL expression leads to osteolysis and, subsequently, to bone loss. However, osteoprotegerin blocks the activation of osteoclasts and thereby decreases bone resorption. In the future, pharmacologic interventions may be able to target chronic inflammation and osteoclast maturation in a local or systemic application. Comparable studies are available for other osteolysis-targeted therapies including anticytokine (such as anti–tumor necrosis factor and anti-interleukin-1/interleukin-6), antienzyme (such as inhibition of matrix metalloproteinase-9), hormonal (such as parathyroid hormone and calcitonin), and pharmacologic (such as simvastatin and diphosphonate).

Polyethylene quality, sterilization, processing, and thickness have been shown to have the greatest effect on debris generation and osteolysis. Polyethylene inserts

TABLE 1

Factors That Affect Polyethylene Wear and Osteolysis in Total Knee Arthroplasty

Implant Design
Bearing conformity, congruity, and constraint
Locking mechanisms
Fixed versus mobile bearing
Materials and finish
Patient Factors
Body mass index/weight
Activity level
Age
Surgical Technique
Alignment
Balance and stability
Kinematics

at least 8 mm in thickness are recommended in mobile bearings and obese patients.[20] The introduction of tibial tray modularity is a very important etiology of wear debris because high-volume submicron particles that are generated with modular tibial trays play a major role in osteolysis. In one study, the backside wear rate in modular tibial trays was lower for fixed-bearing inserts mated to polished cobalt-chromium trays than for inserts from rough titanium trays.[21] Another study showed that wear rates were lower for rotating-platform inserts than for fixed-bearing inserts. However, two groups of researchers showed that rotating-platform and fixed-bearing inserts had similar tibiofemoral damage.[22] In a large registry study from Australia and Norway that evaluated over 100,000 TKAs, the authors demonstrated that a rotating-platform design showed a higher risk of revision for aseptic loosening than fixed-bearing TKAs.[23] The level of constraint also influences wear patterns. One study compared 18 varus-valgus constrained liners to a matched group of posterior-stabilized liners in a retrieval analysis and showed statistically more damage in the posts of the varus-valgus constrained group (13.0 ± 5.0, compared with 4.7 ± 1.9 in the posterior-stabilized group; $P < 0.001$).[24]

The polyethylene wear patterns are influenced by patient factors such as age, body mass index (BMI), and activity level. As indications have expanded, younger patients are undergoing TKA in the anticipation of returning to their high activity lifestyle. In one study, the following definitions of high activity in arthroplasty patients were proposed: more than 3 million cycles/yr; 1 hr/d in high-activity mode; 40% of cycles in high-activity mode.[25] The Finnish Arthroplasty Registry revealed that patients younger than 55 years had worse 5-year implant survival rates (92%) compared with those between ages 56 and 65 years (95%) and those older than 65 years (97%; $P < 0.001$). In a retrospective cohort study of 1,291 revisions for aseptic loosening, patients with morbid obesity had an increased risk of repeat revision, revision surgery, and infection. The implant survival rates were significantly different for morbidly obese and nonmorbidly obese patients, 96% and 100% at 5 years, and 81% and 93% at 10 years, respectively.[26] However, a literature search of 209 knee revisions identified no host factors associated with aseptic loosening. They found that obesity (BMI of 30 kg/m^2 or greater) was not associated with aseptic loosening.[27]

Surgical technique and factors are becoming the most important modifiable aspects of knee arthroplasty surgery to decrease implant wear and failure. Deviations from the optimal alignment of the mechanical axis can lead to a localized increase in surface contact pressures. Alterations also lead to subtle instability, and a combination of the two can lead to increased polyethylene wear and mechanical overload of the underlying bone. Mechanical axis alignment of the tibial implant in 3° of varus leads to almost double the polyethylene volumetric penetration rate.[28] This malalignment and instability permutation results in wear debris, direct bone damage, synovial fluid access to the implant bone interface, and osteolysis.[24,29] Increasing the level of constraint to balance a poorly aligned knee also affects joint wear. One study showed significantly more damage in the posts of the varus-valgus constrained inserts versus posterior-stabilized inserts ($P < 0.001$). In addition, within the varus-valgus constrained group, the total damage score and cold flow damage were significantly higher with excessive joint line changes (5 mm or greater; $P = 0.01$). Damage scores were increased with femoral implant malposition ($P = 0.04$), anterior tibial slope ($P = 0.04$), and tibial implant malposition ($P = 0.04$).[24]

One study assessed the effect of limb alignment, implant position, and joint line position on the pattern of wear in a retrieval analysis of 83 posterior-stabilized tibial inserts. The total damage score was significantly higher in knees with postoperative varus alignment greater than 3° ($P = 0.03$). In addition, the total damage score to the post was significantly more in knees with joint line elevation greater than 9.7 ± 3.9 mm, compared with 6.5 ± 3.7 mm in knees with less joint line elevation ($P = 0.05$).[30] In another retrieval study of 17 inserts that were implanted with a tibial varus angle of greater than 3°, twice the medial compartment wear was observed.[28] In contrast, previous studies have reported that mechanical alignment outliers with a radiographic axis of 0° ± 3°

had a lower revision rate than those that were mechanically aligned within ±3° of anatomic alignment resulting from aseptic loosening, mechanical failure, or wear.

Diagnosis

Wear-induced osteolysis is often asymptomatic, and the lesions are frequently identified incidentally on routine follow-up radiographs or CT and MRI scans obtained for other reasons. Symptomatic osteolysis should be evaluated like all painful knee arthroplasties, with infection ruled out first, as the radiographic findings can be similar. The use of CT or MRI is highly effective for assessing osteolysis and wear and has been shown to be superior to radiographs in sensitivity and accuracy.[31] There is no currently accepted or validated classification system to evaluate patients or guide treatment of wear and osteolysis in TKA.

Treatment and Results

Radiographic observation may be reasonable management for focal asymptomatic and nonprogressive tibial and femoral lesions. In the absence of clinical symptoms, stable osteolytic lesions less than 1 cm can be closely monitored with serial radiographic follow-up and referral to a metabolic bone specialist versed in the use of osteolysis-targeted therapies.[32] There is no real consensus on a lesion size that warrants surgery. The decision tree is multifactorial and is based on the location of the lesion, the level of progression, the frailty of the patient, and the symptoms. Surgical indications are based on the risk of failure or periprosthetic fracture with continued observation. Surgical management of a periosteolytic lesion in a well-fixed tibial and femoral implant is guided by the size of the lesion, any progressive change in that size, and the presence of any associated symptoms.

Focal defects can be treated with intralesional débridement and impaction grafting along with polyethylene liner exchange when the existing implants are well-fixed and appropriately aligned in all planes and the joint is well-balanced with intact ligaments.[32] This treatment requires that the defects be peripherally accessible through a cortical window. One study of 10 knees with a mean follow-up of approximately 5 years after window bone grafting and polyethylene exchange showed total incorporation of the graft material into previously lytic regions on radiographs at final follow-up; no revisions were required. The indications included lytic lesions that could potentially compromise mechanical stability and smaller lesions that showed expansion on serial radiographs. The lesion size in this study ranged from 2 to 6 cm on standard radiographs.[33]

Revision options are limited and are more challenging in larger, symptomatic, or progressive lesions that are at risk for fracture or catastrophic loosening. These defects require more complex reconstruction techniques. Metaphyseal bone defects that preserve the peripheral cortical rim with a thin shell and larger contained defects require distal stem fixation, structural allograft, or newer-generation porous metal sleeves or cones (**Figure 2**). The use of a structural allograft has decreased in recent years because of the high failure rates with long-term follow-up as well as with the advent of highly porous metal augments, cones, and sleeves that accentuate biologic metaphyseal fixation.[34] Several midterm clinical studies (range, 1.0 to 8.8 years) with porous tantalum cones for bone loss in the revision setting have shown promising results, with a cumulative mean revision rate for aseptic cone loosening of 1.1%.[35,36] In addition, the clinical outcomes of titanium sleeves at short-term follow-up (range, 2.0 to 5.3 years) have been excellent, with a 2.6% revision rate for aseptic loosening.[37-39] Surgical goals include suitable management of bone loss and a strategy to restore or maintain implant stability and limb alignment. In addition, it is crucial to assess the status of the epicondyles to best determine the patency of the collateral ligaments. In the absence of functional collateral ligaments, a more constrained or hinged prostheses is suggested to maintain coronal stability and to prevent failure.

INSTABILITY

Instability continues to be a major topic and is a common cause of failure following TKA accounting for up to 20% of revision TKAs. It can occur in the coronal or sagittal plane because of mismatching of extension and flexion gaps respectively. Reports show that 1% to 2% of TKA patients are symptomatic, but the true incidence is likely much higher.[40] A meta-analysis demonstrated that instability is reported more frequently in a younger patient population and approximately 16.4% more females underwent revision surgery because of instability.[41] They also found that the average time between the primary and revision surgery was 44.7 months (95% CI [33.8, 55.7]).

Diagnosis

A patient will typically present with pain, recurrent joint effusions, and decreased function such as difficulty with ascending and descending stairs. Patients who have mild effusions and a negative workup for infection should be evaluated for instability.[42] Etiology of instability is multifactorial and include implant malposition in the coronal, axial, sagittal planes; ligamentous insufficiency or rupture; an incompetent posterior cruciate

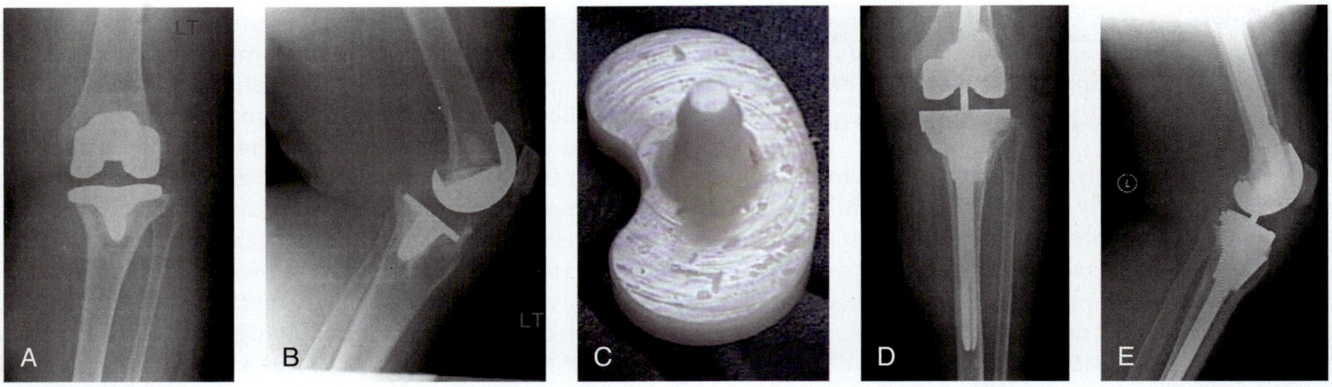

FIGURE 2 AP (**A**) and lateral (**B**) radiographs of failed left total knee arthroplasty (TKA) in a 65-year-old woman with tibial baseplate subsidence and a large osteolytic lesion along the anterior tibial metaphysis. **C**, Intraoperative photograph of the explanted rotating-platform polyethylene liner shows delamination and pitting. AP (**D**) and lateral (**E**) radiographs obtained following revision TKA with a cementless tibial cone for reconstruction of the metaphyseal defect. (Reproduced with permission from Mont MA, Tanzer M: Chapter 20: Complications of knee arthroplasty, in *Orthopaedic Knowledge Update®: Hip and Knee Reconstruction 5*. Rosemont, IL, American Academy of Orthopaedic Surgeons, 2017, p 254.)

ligament; extensor mechanism deficiency; or a mismatch between the medial and lateral gaps and/or between the flexion and extension gaps. Timing of a patient's complaints, which usually consists of giving way, buckling, and pain with activity, can help in determining the cause of instability. In the immediate postoperative period, the instability can be related to asymmetric ligament balance, implant malalignment, ligamentous injury, or an incompetent posterior cruciate ligament. If a patient had a previously well-functioning TKA from months to years since the index procedure, the instability could be due to asymmetric polyethylene wear or true laxity secondary to attrition of the collateral or posterior cruciate ligaments.[5]

Extension instability occurs when the extension gap is greater than the flexion gap and typically results in varus and valgus imbalance with potential hyperextension. Flexion instability occurs when the flexion gap is greater than the extension gap. This can be diagnosed when the knee is flexed to approximately 90° and an anterior drawer test shows laxity greater than 1 cm or by the posterior sag sign of the tibia[43] (**Figures 3** and **4**). A recent topic in arthroplasty is the concept of midflexion instability. The idea is that a patient's knee replacement can theoretically be balanced and stabile in extension and 90° of flexion yet have instability between approximately 40° and 70° during the swing phase. Although difficult to assess clinically, a computational analysis of various TKA implant designs and position showed that elevation of the joint line and anteriorizing the femoral implant can cause the knee to be loose at midflexion.[44] A review article on midflexion instability demonstrated multiple factors as an etiology including multiradius implant design, posterior-stabilized femoral prostheses, surgical technique with joint line elevation, and excessive medial soft-tissue release, but concluded it is difficult to ascertain if midflexion instability has any clinical importance.[45]

Treatment

If instability is symmetric in both flexion and extension, then a thicker tibial polyethylene liner may be used as this can address both flexion and extension gaps simultaneously. If the instability is asymmetric, then implant revision is usually required. Intraoperatively, extension instability can be either symmetrical caused by joint line elevation or asymmetrical with failure to achieve medial and lateral extension gap balancing. Treatment of symmetrical extension instability includes tightening the extension gap with distal femoral augments. Asymmetrical extension instability can be corrected by balancing the medial and lateral gaps in the coronal plane. Flexion instability can sometimes be addressed by revising the femoral implant to a larger size or adding posterior femoral augments. In all situations, especially those with ligament incompetence, a more constrained prosthesis may be required.[46]

ARTHROFIBROSIS

Excessive formation of fibrous scar tissue caused by an exaggerated inflammatory response postoperatively can lead to pain and decreased range of motion and functional outcome after TKA. Patients typically need 70° of knee flexion to walk normally, 90° to ascend stairs, 100° to descend stairs, and 105° to arise from a seated position without using arm support.[47]

A meta-analysis that included 48,873 TKAs demonstrated an incidence of 4% for arthrofibrosis.[48] Postoperative stiffness has been demonstrated

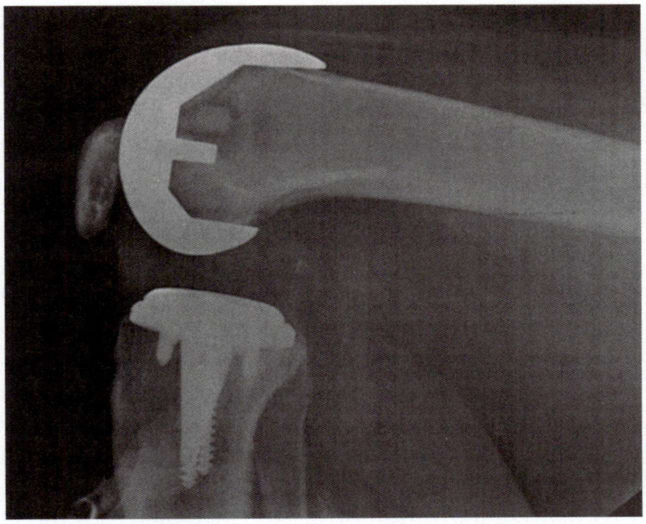

FIGURE 3 Lateral radiograph of a primary posterior cruciate-retaining total knee arthroplasty. This radiograph shows marked posterior translation of the tibia on the femur during posterior drawer testing most likely due to an incompetent posterior cruciate ligament or excessive tibial slope. This knee otherwise was well aligned and well-fixed, but the patient reported having persistent pain and a sense of instability. The knee replacement subsequently was revised to a posterior-stabilized implant. (Reproduced with permission from Pagnano MW, Hanssen AD, Lewallen DG, Stuart MJ: Flexion instability after primary posterior cruciate retaining total knee arthroplasty. *Clin Orthop Relat Res* 1998;356:39-46.)

to be one of the most common causes of readmission within the first 90 days after surgery, and it is one of the common reasons for revision TKA.[49] One study identified stiffness as the third leading cause of TKA revision (18%) within the first 2 years postoperatively behind infection and instability.[50]

Risk Factors

Preoperative range of motion is the strongest predictor of postoperative stiffness.[5] Female sex and a BMI ≥30 kg/m^2 have been shown to contribute as well.[48] Other causes are multifactorial, ranging from surgical technique or complexity, postoperative rehabilitation delay or inadequacy, genetic predisposition, and prior surgeries.[51]

Diagnosis

Historically, there has been a lack of agreement regarding the terms stiffness and arthrofibrosis after TKA. An international consensus has defined postoperative arthrofibrosis of the knee as a limited range of movement in flexion and/or extension, which is not attributable to an osseous or prosthetic block to movement from malaligned, malpositioned, or incorrectly sized implants; metal hardware; ligament reconstruction; infection (septic arthritis); pain; chronic regional pain syndrome; or other specific causes, but because of soft-tissue fibrosis that was not present preoperatively. The group also classified the limitation of movement as mild, moderate, or severe according to the range of flexion (90° to 100°, 70° to 89°, <70°) or extension deficit (5° to 10°, 11° to 20°, >20°).[52] Patient education, perioperative NSAID administration, and early range of motion and mobilization have all been shown to decrease the formation postoperative arthrofibrosis.[53,54]

Treatment

It is estimated that approximately 25% of arthrofibrosis cases require additional surgery to improve motion.[55] An initial conservative approach with aggressive physical therapy and potential manipulation under anesthesia is typically chosen if the patient is within 2 to 3 months from surgery. This is performed in the operating room with the

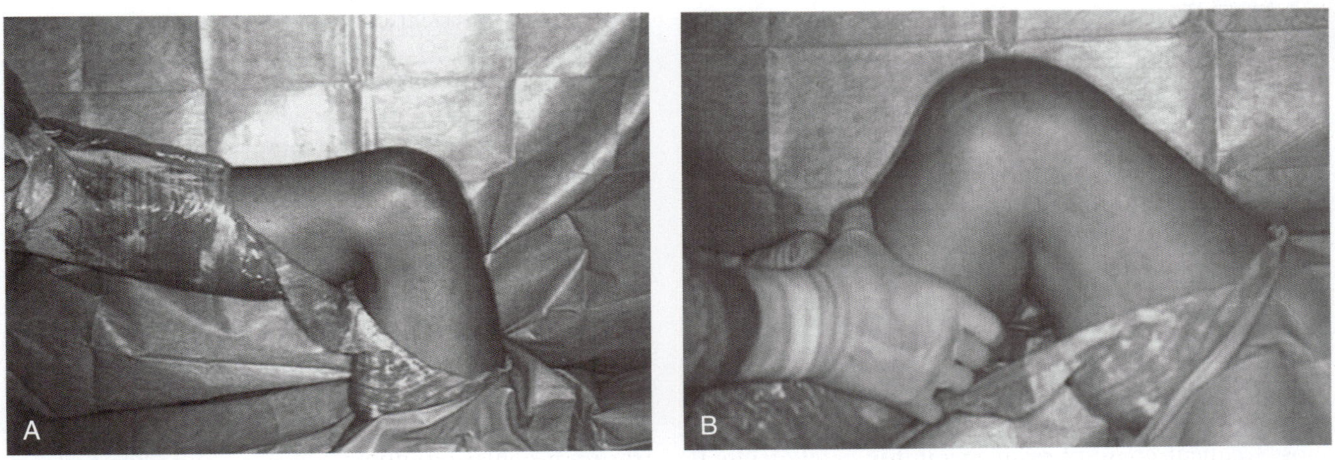

FIGURE 4 **A**, Clinical photograph showing marked posterior sag present at 90° knee flexion in this patient who had undergone a primary cruciate ligament-retaining total knee arthroplasty. **B**, Clinical photograph showing a marked posterior drawer in the same patient. (Reproduced with permission from Pagnano MW, Hanssen AD, Lewallen DG, Stuart MJ: Flexion instability after primary posterior cruciate retaining total knee arthroplasty. *Clin Orthop Relat Res* 1998;356:39-46.)

patient sedated while the surgeon flexes the ipsilateral hip to 90° while slowly flexing the proximal tibia to break up adhesions. This has been shown to typically gain over 30° of flexion.[53]

Arthroscopic or open lysis of adhesions can be considered if the patient is outside the 2- to 3-month postoperative window. Revision TKA may be necessary if the stiffness is due to implant sizing or position issues or improper soft-tissue balance; however, caution is advised given high rates of complications and revision surgeries.[56]

In a recent study, 34 patients underwent revision TKA for arthrofibrosis and received rotating-hinge implants.[57] The rotating-hinge cohort had a 20° increase in the mean arc of motion (74° to 94°) compared with a 12° (87° to 99°) increase in a matched cohort that underwent a revision TKA without a rotating-hinge ($P = 0.048$). However, survivorship free of any revision at 10 years was 54% in the rotating-hinge group compared with 90% in the non–rotating-hinge group.

PATELLOFEMORAL COMPLICATIONS

Patella complications account for approximately 10% of all TKA complications.[58] They are associated with poor outcomes and may require multiple surgical procedures or revision arthroplasty to address these complications. Preoperative risk factors for patellofemoral complications following primary TKA include greater than 10° of valgus deformity, prior patella maltracking issues, BMI greater than 30 kg/m^2, and a native patella thickness less than 18 mm. Intraoperative risk factors for increased likelihood for patellofemoral complications include an asymmetric bone cut, lateral retinacular release, femoral or tibial implant malrotation, implant with a single central peg, and a patella remnant less than 12 mm.[59-65] Patella fracture occurs in about 1.2% of all TKAs and is correlated with patellar resurfacing.

Patellofemoral Instability

The stability of the patellofemoral joint in TKA can be influenced by multiple factors including positioning of the patella, femoral and tibial implants and overall alignment, implant design, patellar preparation, and soft-tissue balancing. Patellar implant instability and malalignment is an important etiology of most patellar-related complications including implant subluxation, dislocation, loosening, and catastrophic wear.[66] Malrotation of either the femoral or tibial implant has been recognized as the most frequent cause of problems in the patellofemoral joint.[61,66] Understanding the etiology and management of the unstable patella in TKA allows for minimization of complications.

Internal rotation and medialization of the femoral implant results in medialization of the trochlear grove. This results in lateralization of the patella in relation to the femur and increased tension on the lateral soft tissues and increases chance of patella subluxation/dislocation laterally.[61,67-69] Internal rotation of the femoral implant usually arises from using instrumentation that references from the posterior femoral condyles when the lateral posterior condyle is deficient. This commonly arises with a valgus knee when deficiencies of the posterior lateral femoral condyle are not recognized. When these deficiencies are recognized, utilization of the transepicondylar axis has been shown to be more reliable.[70] Internal rotation and medialization of the tibial implant may also result in patella maltracking by causing the tibia to rotate externally during knee flexion, driving the tubercle laterally. Lateralization of the tubercle increases the Q angle and leads to lateral patellar tracking and subluxation. A 1998 study demonstrated that the severity of maltracking is directly related to the combined amount of internal rotation of the tibial and femoral implants.[61] Lateralization of the patellar implant also increases the tension on the lateral soft tissues and the risk of dislocation.[66,71] Soft-tissue structures surrounding the knee can also lead to lateral patellar maltracking. This frequently occurs in patients with severe valgus deformities. Lateral maltracking can also be the result of disruption of the capsular repair. The disruption is often multifactorial but can be caused by suture failure, overly intensive physical therapy, or traumatic rupture.[66]

Clinical evaluation begins with a thorough history and physical examination. Patients may describe sensations of subluxation/dislocation, which may not be obvious clinically. They may complain only of peripatellar pain and limited knee flexion. The limited flexion is due to subluxation of the patella and impingement before full flexion. On physical examination, the surgeon should assess alignment, Q angle, patellar tracking, and implant rotation. Increased hip internal rotation with both hips and knees flexed to 90° is suggestive of femoral implant internal rotation. External rotation of the foot in the same position is indicative of internal rotation of the tibia implants.[66] Radiographic examination begins with standard AP, lateral, and merchant views. The merchant view will demonstrate subluxation of the patella if present, patellar tilt, and the angle of patellar resection. The varus/valgus positioning of the femoral implant can be assessed on the AP view, and the size of and flexion/extension of the femoral implant can be seen on the lateral view. Multiple techniques have been investigated to determine the rotational position of the femoral and tibia implants. Recent studies suggest the use of three-dimensional CT reconstruction is superior to both two-dimensional CT reconstruction and plain radiographs[72,73] (**Figure 5**).

Measurement of the femoral rotation can be reliably measured by comparing the posterior condylar axis with the epicondylar axis.[73,74] This can be directly compared with the contralateral side, or it can be compared with the native rotation value for the posterior condylar angle. The normal has been shown to be 0.3° (±1.2°) of internal rotation for women and 3.5° (±1.2°) of internal rotation for men relative to the epicondylar axis.[75] A commonly used technique to evaluate tibia rotation is to compare the posterior axis of the tibial implant with the posterior tibial condylar axis.[72]

To provide a stable patellofemoral joint, surgeons must confirm appropriate positioning of implants. This can be accomplished by using the guidelines. To obtain a rectangular and balanced flexion gap and central patellar tracking, the femoral implant should be externally rotated on the femur relative to the posterior condyles. A number of landmarks have been developed to allow this: anterior-posterior axis (Whiteside line), the transepicondylar axis, and the posterior condylar axis.[66] The transepicondylar axis is a line connecting the lateral epicondylar prominence and the medial sulcus on the medial epicondyle.[75] The posterior condylar axis is defined as a line that crosses both posterior femoral condyles. This will be ~3° to 5° of internal rotation compared with transepicondylar axis. Whiteside line is a line through the deepest part of the patellar groove anteriorly and the center of the intercondylar notch posteriorly.[76] The anterior and posterior femoral cuts should be made parallel to the transepicondylar axis, perpendicular to Whiteside line, or 3° to 5° externally rotated from the posterior condylar axis. In a valgus knee, the posterior condylar axis should not be referenced because it will result in an internally rotated femoral implant because of lateral condyle hypoplasia. The femoral implant should be lateralized to reduce tension on the lateral soft tissues and to move the trochlea more laterally. The midportion of the tibial tray should be aligned with the attachment of the patellar tendon. Landmarks for appropriate alignment are the crest of the tibia or the medial third of the tibial tubercle. The patellar implant should be medialized to improve patellar tracking and lateral soft-tissue tension. A 2010 study suggested medializing the implant 2.5 mm to reduce patellofemoral contact forces, lateral tilt of the patella, and lateral soft-tissue tension.[77] Multiple studies have shown decreased incidence of lateral release with medialization of the patellar implant.[78,79] A symmetric patella cut should be made with equal bone remaining in all four quadrants of the patella, and the overall thickness of the patellofemoral joint should be maintained.[67] This involves appropriate sizing and positioning of implants and reproducing

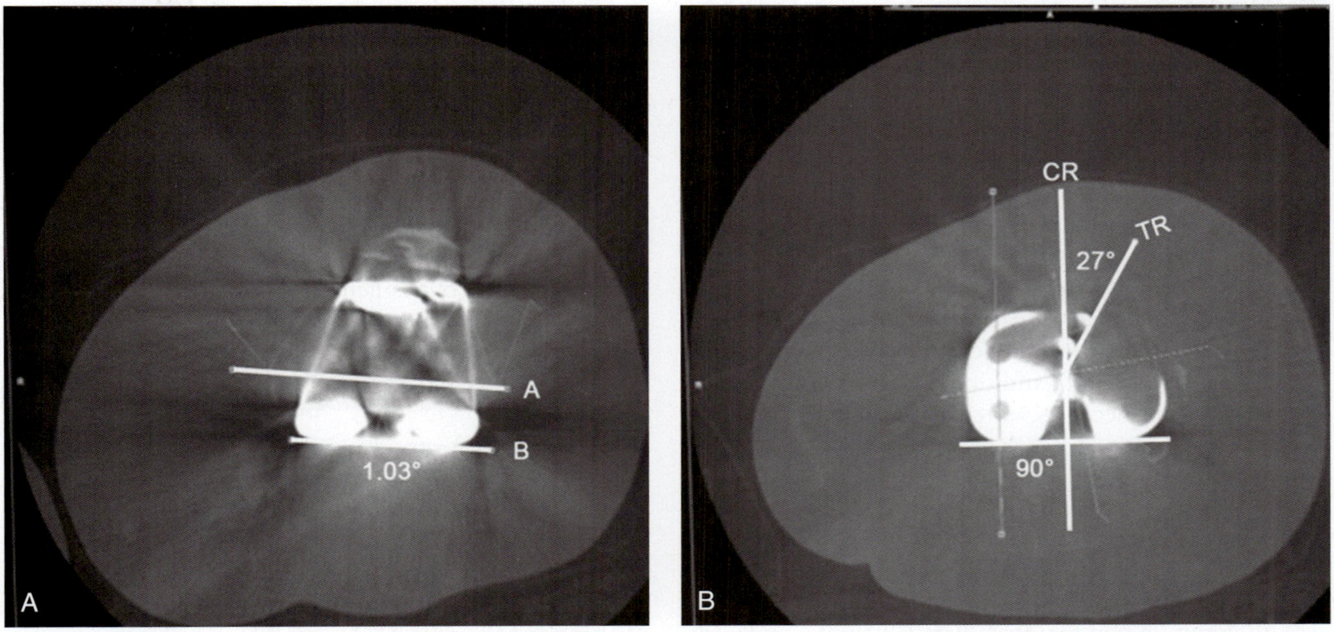

FIGURE 5 Determination of tibial and femoral total knee arthroplasty (TKA) implant rotation for patellofemoral instability. **A**, CT scan at the level of the femoral epicondyles. Line A represents the epicondylar axis of the femur and line B represents the femoral implant posterior condylar surface and the implant rotational axis. In this patient, the femoral implant is 1.03° internally rotated. **B**, The lines for the tibial implant axis (condylar reference) and the tibial anatomic axis (tubercle reference), the line from the geometric center to the center of the tibial tubercle, are drawn. The angle between the two lines is the rotation of the tibial implant. In this patient, the tibial implant was in 27° of internal rotation. (Reproduced with permission from Konigsberg B, Hess R, Hartman C, Smith L, Garvin KL: Inter- and intraobserver reliability of two-dimensional CT scan for total knee arthroplasty component malrotation. *Clin Orthop Relat Res* 2014;472[1]:212-217.)

the native patellar thickness. A caliper should be used before resecting the patellar and compared with the thickness of the resurfaced patella.[66] Sufficient thickness of bone should be left to anchor the patellar implant and to prevent fracture.[62] Patellar tracking should be assessed intraoperatively. Tracking can be tested using the single-suture technique. The surgeon reapproximates the medial retinaculum at the superior pole of the patella with a single suture or a towel clip.[78,80] Utilization of the single suture test to evaluate patellar tracking results in a lower incidence of lateral release and thus avoids its potential complications.[65,78,80] Evaluation of patellar tracking intraoperatively cannot account for the dynamic forces that act on the patella.

The management of patellofemoral maltracking is based on its etiology. The precise cause of the instability should be identified and corrected. Nonsurgical management with bracing treatment and strengthening do not address the cause of instability and have high rates of failure. If the etiology of the patellofemoral instability is implant malalignment, then revision TKA is required. Lateral releases are only indicated when correct implant alignment has been confirmed. Lateral release can be done via an outside-in or inside-out incision. The release should extend from the tibial bone to the fibers of the vastus lateralis center 2 cm from the lateral border of the patella.[81] The lateral superior geniculate artery should be preserved to prevent consequences of compromised blood supply to the patella such as osteonecrosis and patella fracture.[59] A 2016 study described medial patellofemoral ligament augmentation using hamstring tendons. In this study of six patients at an average follow-up of 23 months, the authors reported no recurrent dislocations.[82] The use of a quadriceps tendon strip to augment the medial patellofemoral ligament has also been described to avoid the need for patellar fixation.[83] A tibial tuberosity osteotomy can be used alone or in combination with medial patellofemoral ligament reconstruction. However, the presence of the prosthetic stem is a complicating factor. In addition, complications include hematoma, skin necrosis, extensor mechanism disruption, and nonunion.[84]

Patellar Clunk Syndrome and Crepitus

Posterior-stabilized TKAs have been shown to have excellent long-term clinical outcomes.[85,86] Despite these results, anterior knee pain and patellofemoral issues remain common complaints.[87] Patellar clunk syndrome was first coined in 1989, and although it is primarily a complication of posterior-stabilized TKAs, it has been reported with patellofemoral arthroplasty and cruciate-retaining TKA as well.[88-90] It has been shown to occur in 3% patients undergoing TKA with posterior-stabilized femoral implants.[91] This syndrome is one of the leading reasons for non–revision surgery in TKA.[92] Patellar clunk syndrome and crepitus share a common pathophysiology: peripatellar fibrosynovial hyperplasia at the junction of the superior pole of the patella and the distal quadriceps tendon (**Figure 6**). In patellar clunk syndrome, this hyperplastic tissue develops into a nodule that will engage within the intercondylar box. During extension, this tissue is forced from the intercondylar box and results in an often-audible clunk and pain.[93]

The hyperplastic tissue in patella crepitus does not develop into a nodule and does not engage the intercondylar box. Patients tend to experience symptoms when climbing stairs or when rising from a seated position and typically present 7 to 11 months after TKA. In patellar crepitus, no audible clunk is present. These patients will generally complain of anterior knee pain and a sensation of grinding with 30° to 60° of knee flexion.[93] A 2014 study evaluated 60 patients who had either patellar clunk or crepitus. The study identified a reduced preoperative or postoperative patellar tendon length, a thinner postoperative composite patellar implant thickness, a reduced patellar implant size, an increased posterior femoral condylar offset, and a history of previous knee surgery as risk factors.[93] The management of patellar clunk and crepitus begins with simply conservative management including quadriceps and hamstrings strengthening. A 2017 study showed that about 60% of patients can be treated solely with conservative management. Of those patients in whom nonsurgical management failed, 85% were treated successfully with arthroscopic débridement. The remaining 15% of patients underwent a successful repeat débridement.[94] A 2014 study demonstrated that patients who underwent arthroscopic treatment had no significant reduction in functional outcomes compared with patients without patella clunk or crepitus.[91] Open treatment of patella clunk or crepitus has also been described but is generally reserved for failures of arthroscopic treatment.[94,95]

EXTENSOR TENDON COMPLICATIONS

Extensor tendon rupture is a rare but serious complication following TKA. Rupture occurs in 0.1% to 2.5% of TKAs and results in a lack of active knee extension and severely impaired knee function.[96] Disruption of the extensor mechanism during or after TKA is a technically challenging problem. The etiology of extensor mechanism disruption following TKA is multifactorial, and given the suboptimal results with these complications the importance of prevention needs to be emphasized. Although a variety of surgical options exist, treatment options are based on the quality of the host tissue and the patient's functional demands. Extensor mechanism ruptures can be classified into either quadriceps tendon rupture or

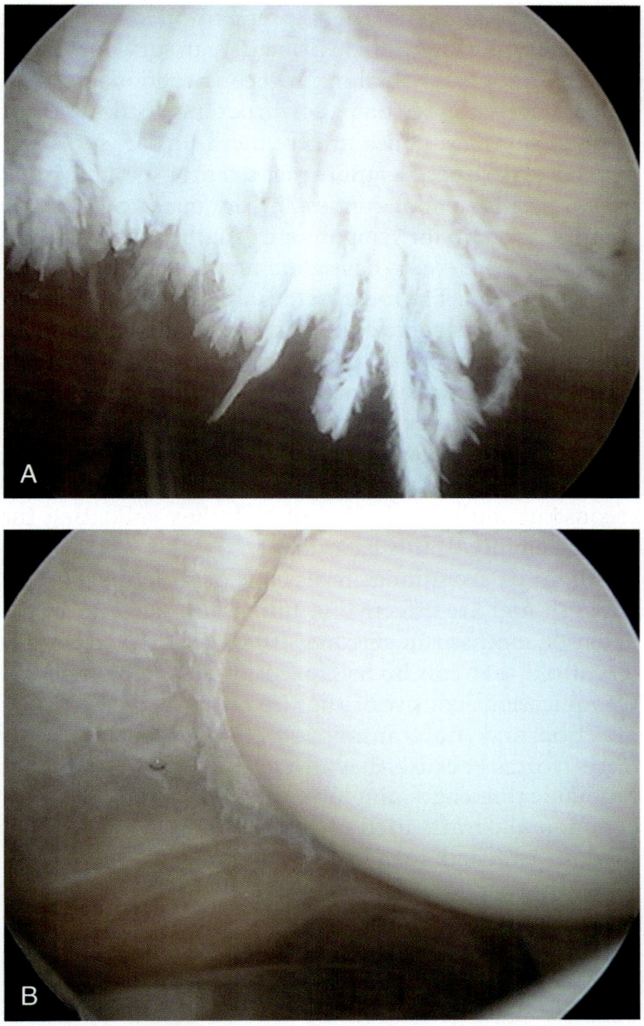

FIGURE 6 **A**, An arthroscopic photograph of the fibrous nodule at the proximal pole of the patella. **B**, Subsequent photograph after arthroscopic débridement. (Reprinted from *J Arthroplasty* 29[9 Suppl]. Costanzo JA, Aynardi MC, Peters JD, Kopolovich DM, Purtill JJ: Patellar clunk syndrome after total knee arthroplasty; risk factors and functional outcomes of arthroscopic treatment, 201-204. Copyright © 2014, with permission from Elsevier.)

patella tendon rupture. Distal rupture or avulsion of the patella tendon is the most common disruption encountered following TKA.[97]

Risk Factors

Quadriceps tendon rupture is associated with incomplete healing after extended surgical approaches, overresection of the patella, and injury to the vascular supply along with trauma. Patella tendon rupture has been associated with obesity, diabetes mellitus, rheumatoid arthritis, systemic lupus erythematosus, chronic renal failure, and trauma. Multiple prior surgical procedures may result in increased scar tissue and contribute to the reduction in blood supply and weakening of the surrounding tissue. Patella tendon rupture has also been associated with malalignment of the tibial or femoral implants, patellofemoral instability, joint line elevation, and hinged implants. Delayed knee manipulation can also result in disruption of the extensor mechanism.

Diagnosis

Acute rupture secondary to trauma may be diagnosed by an inability to lock the knee while walking or complete loss of active knee extension, and a palpable gap in the quadriceps or patellar tendon. Chronic ruptures may present as a feeling of insecurity or instability with loss of knee extension strength, extension lag, and hyperextending to lock the knee while walking. Diagnostic imaging can be useful when the diagnosis is in question. MRIs can be used, but metal artifact may hinder the interpretation and limit the diagnostic utility. Ultrasonography is a powerful diagnostic tool for partial extensor mechanism rupture and allows for evaluation of tissue quality.[98]

Treatment

Surgical treatment can be separated into four categories: simple repair, repair with autograft augmentation, allograft or mesh reconstruction, and salvage procedures.[99] Simple repair of the patella tendon has been shown to have poor outcomes but does have a limited role in the treatment of quadriceps tendon repairs. The complication rate after repair of patellar tendons (63.16%) was significantly higher than the complication rate after repair of quadriceps tendons (25.37%).[100] Repair with autograft augmentation generally consists of direct repair with either semitendinosus tendon autograft or quadriceps tendon turndown flap. The semitendinosus tendon autograft consists of the semitendinosus tendon passed through a transverse tunnel in the patella and the free end being sutured back to its insertion on the tibia (**Figure 7**). For patients with a thin or fragile patella, the tendon is passed through the quadriceps tendon instead of through a patellar tunnel.[101]

A 2016 study reported on nine patients undergoing this procedure and final follow-up at 4 years. All patients were able to walk without brace or aids, were satisfied with the procedure, and had a median of extension lag of 5°.[101] A quadriceps tendon turndown flap can be used to augment the repair of the tendon repair (**Figure 8**). This surgical procedure consists of repairing the tendon ends along the quadriceps tendon rupture and the associated medial and lateral retinacular tears with the knee in full extension. A modified full-thickness, long triangular V-Y turndown flap is made and prepared for augmentation of the primary repair. After flap transfer, the quadriceps tendon is closed by advancing and suturing the vastus medialis and lateralis muscles together to form the remaining tendon proper. A 2019 study of 24 patients

Section 2: Knee

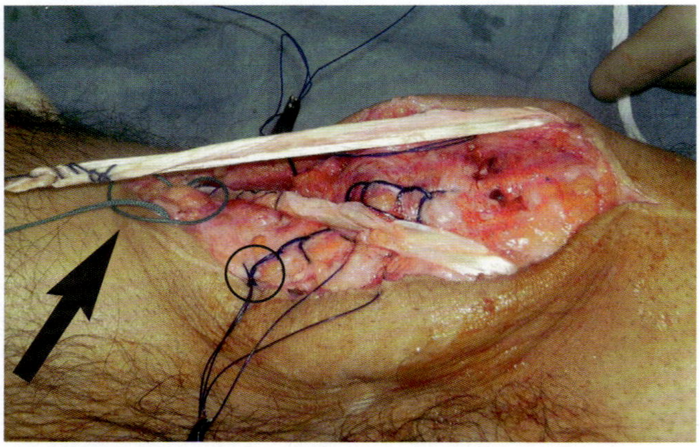

FIGURE 7 Intraoperative photograph showing a hamstring autograft. The free end of the tendon has been passed through a patellar tunnel. The free end will then be sutured to itself at its insertion. Arrow showing sutures placed into the residual patella tendon insertion. (Reproduced with permission from Maffulli N, Del Buono A, Loppini M, Denaro V: Ipsilateral hamstring tendon graft reconstruction for chronic patellar tendon ruptures: Average 5.8-year follow-up. *J Bone Joint Surg Am* 2013;95[17]:e1231-e1236.)

showed excellent outcome following quadriceps tendon turndown flap. Patients had significant improvements in mean Knee Society knee score and mean strength, and all were able to walk without assistive devices. In this study, one patient had a residual extensor lag of >35° and four patients had lag of >5°.[102]

Multiple mesh options exist for the surgical reconstruction of anatomic defects. Historically, knitted monofilament polypropylene mesh (Marlex, C.R. Bard) has been used in hernia repairs and gynecologic procedures, but its use is declining because of the propensity to form dense adhesions.[103,104] In general surgery, excessive scar formation may be unappealing, but the increased scar-tissue formation may enhance integration of the mesh to the host soft-tissue to provide a more durable reconstruction.[103] The surgical technique using the Marlex mesh reconstruction (**Figure 9**) starts with a 10 × 14-in sheet of Marlex mesh rolling onto itself 8 to 10 times and sewing together with one to two heavy, nonabsorbable sutures in a running-locked closure. If the tibial implant is not being revised, a trough is created in the proximal-anterior aspect of the tibia for the Marlex mesh to be cemented in place. After the cement cures, a lag screw is placed across the mesh and cement into the host bone for additional fixation. If the tibial implant is being revised, the mesh is cemented in the canal during the cementation of the tibial implant. The mesh is then passed through a distal tunnel and incorporated with the remaining aspects of the host patellar tendon. The vastus medialis and vastus lateralis are mobilized, the mesh is sutured to the vastus lateralis, and then the vastus medialis is closed over the mesh.[103] A 2018 study evaluating 77 patients undergoing reconstruction using the aforementioned technique showed promising results with a 2-year survivorship of 86% for patients with no prior reconstruction and 95% for patients with previous reconstructions of the extensor mechanism that did not involve mesh. In this series, 12 patients experienced a failure that required mesh revision: five for patellar tendon rupture, five for quadriceps tendon rupture, and two for symptomatic lengthening. Of the 12 patients, 10 went on to have good functional outcome following revision. The mean extensor lag improved by 26° with 46 patients achieving full or near-full extension.[103] This study suggests that mesh reconstruction provides substantial functional benefit with excellent survivorship for patients who have extensor mechanism disruption. These results are consistent with a 2011 study showing a similar improvement in extensor lag, with a mean post-reconstruction extensor lag of 10°, thus validating the reproducibility of this technique.[105]

Allograft techniques have considerable mechanical strength and are effective in filling large defects in the extensor mechanism (**Figures 10** and **11**). They provide a scaffold that can be colonized by host fibrous tissue. Complications consist of rupture or gradual distension, infection, and viral transmission. Allografts are generally fresh frozen because they are characterized by higher mechanical strength and lower antigenicity.[106] The most common allografts used for reconstruction are Achilles tendon attached to a calcaneal bone block, partial allografts, and total allografts. Achilles allograft is most commonly used for patellar tendon rupture with an intact patella that can be displaced downward but can also be used for quadriceps tendon ruptures.[107] A 2018 study evaluated 17 patients undergoing reconstruction. At 2-year follow-up, the average extensor lag was 8.4° and quadriceps strength maintained at an average of 4 out of 5. One patient in the series suffered a rerupture.[107] Multiple surgical techniques have been described for Achilles allograft. A 2002 study showed an increased proximal migration of the patella using a single-bundle only technique.[108] A 2014 study of five patients showed improved outcomes when a double-bundle technique was used.[109]

Partial extensor mechanism allograft has also been described to reconstruct an extensor mechanism when little to no residual patellar tendon is viable and the patella has not been resurfaced or has minimal bony defect (**Figure 12**). A 2008 study described a patella-patellar tendon-tibial tubercle allograft that was used in four patients who had minimal residual extensor lag.[110] Total extensor mechanism allograft reconstruction has also been described for the management of extensor mechanism rupture with damage to the patella. A 1994 study and a 1999 study demonstrated mediocre to poor outcomes following extensor mechanism allograft reconstruction.[111,112] A 2004 study postulated that these poor

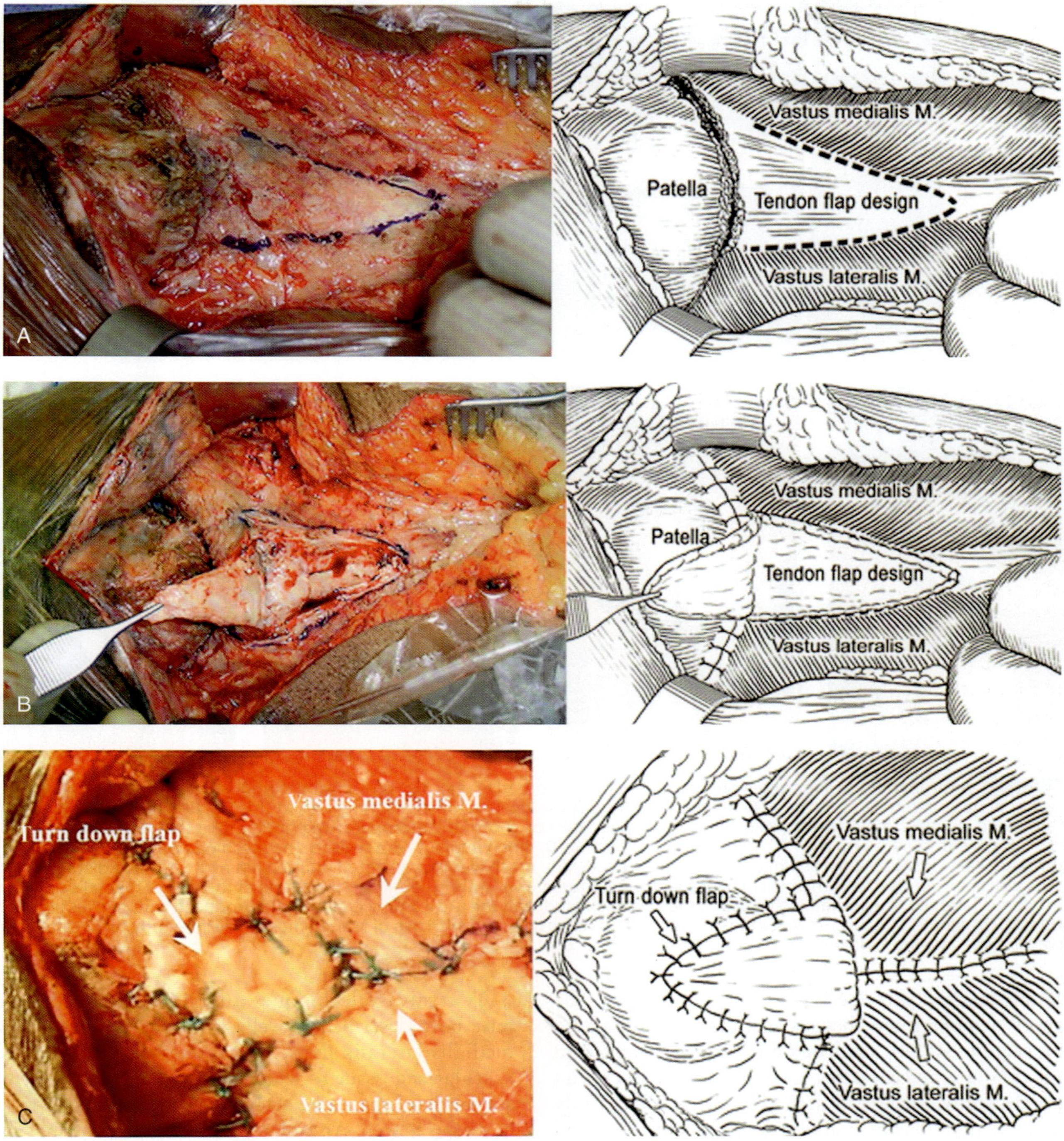

FIGURE 8 **A**, Intraoperative photograph and illustration showing the V-Y turndown flap design. **B**, Intraoperative photograph and illustration showing the V-Y flap in use as a full-thickness tendon graft, preserving the joint capsule. **C**, Intraoperative photograph and illustration showing the completed and reinforced V-Y turndown flap. (Reproduced with permission from Shi S-M, Shi GG, Laurent EM, et al.: Modified V-Y turndown flap augmentation for quadriceps tendon rupture following total knee arthroplasty: A retrospective study. *J Bone Joint Surg Am* 2019;101[11]:1010-1015.)

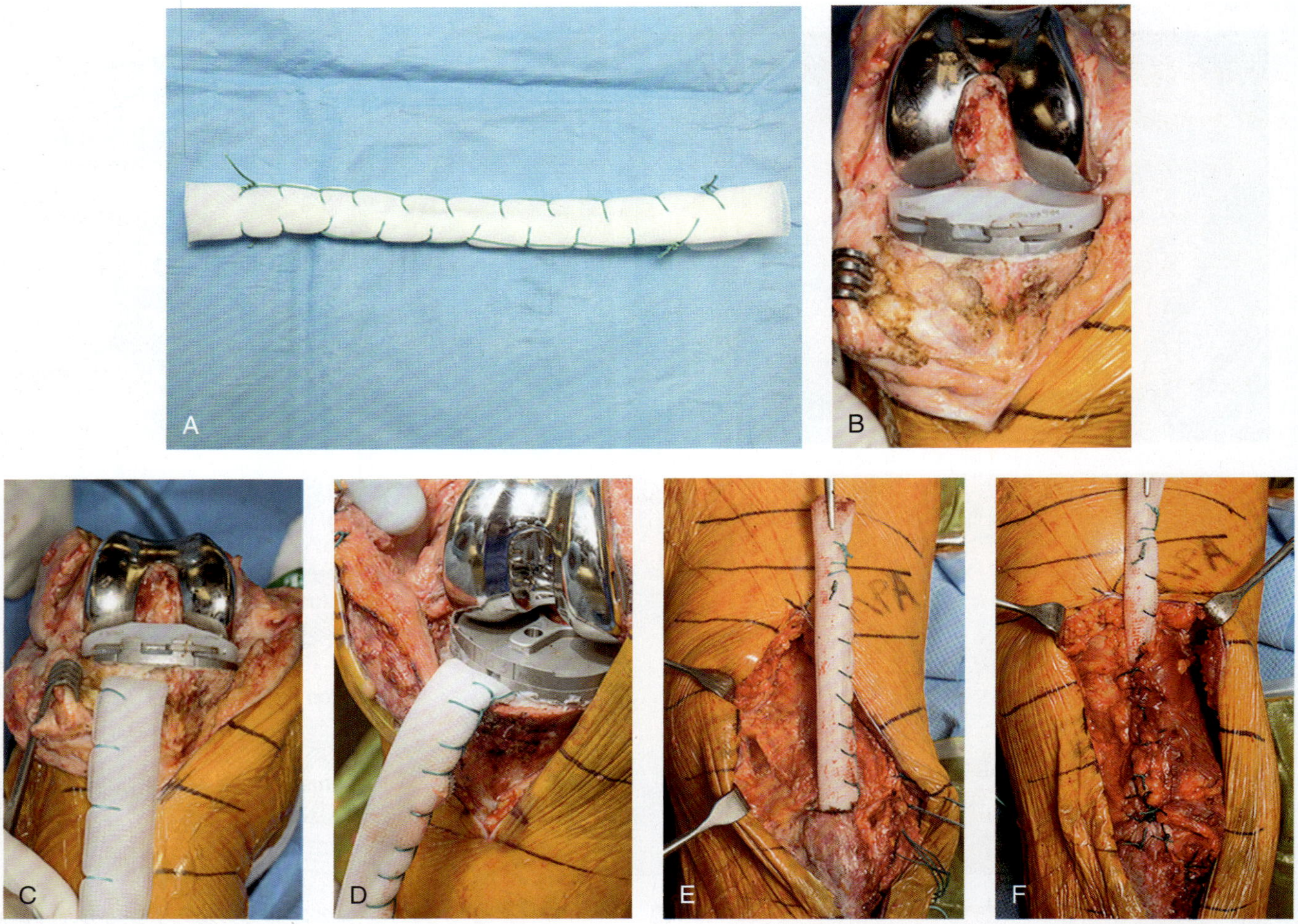

FIGURE 9 **A** through **F**, Intraoperative photographs. **A**, Intraoperative photograph showing the 10 × 14-in sheet of Marlex mesh that has been rolled onto itself 8-10 times and then sewn together with a running-locked closure. **B**, When implants are maintained, a tibial trough was created with a high-speed burr as shown. **C**, Intraoperative photographs show the cementation of the mesh into the trough, with the mesh reflected distally. **D**, When implants are revised, the mesh was cemented in an intramedullary position with the tibial implant and stem. **E**, The mesh was incorporated into remaining host tissue distally. **F**, The mesh was incorporated with the proximal tissue after aggressive ventral and dorsal mobilization of the vastus medialis obliquus and vastus lateralis. The remaining proximal mesh was excised, and the arthrotomy is closed. (Reproduced with permission from Abdel MP, Salib CG, Mara KC, et al.: Extensor mechanism reconstruction with use of Marlex mesh: A series study of 77 total knee arthroplasties. *J Bone Joint Surg Am* 2018;100[15]:1309-1318.)

outcomes were in part due to inadequate tensioning. The authors demonstrated that all cases tensioned using a prior technique with inadequate tensioning resulted in clinical failure and all cases tensioned in full extension were clinically successful at 2 years.[113] A 2015 study evaluated the 10-year outcomes with these improved tensioning techniques and demonstrated a 38% failure rate and a 10-year allograft survival rate of 56.2%.[114] In a 2019 study, the authors compared mesh reconstruction with extensor mechanism allograft reconstruction and concluded that synthetic reconstruction for extensor mechanism disruption demonstrated improved results with respect to extensor lag, graft failure, revision surgery, and cost when compared with extensor mechanism allograft.[115]

Two salvage techniques after failed reconstruction have been described as well: gastrocnemius and vastus medialis/lateralis flaps. Gastrocnemius flaps provide vascularized tissue to which the remnants of the extensor mechanism can be attached and provide soft-tissue coverage as well. An isolated medial gastrocnemius flap is used if the patella is present or a medial/lateral gastrocnemius flap extended to the Achilles tendon in the absence of the patella[116,117] (**Figure 13**). Following failed extensor mechanism allograft resulting in large defects, gastrocnemius flaps may not be able to provide sufficient coverage. In these cases, vastus medialis/lateralis flaps alone or in combination with a gastrocnemius flap have been described. The vastus medialis or lateralis muscle is detached from its distal insertions, then transferred

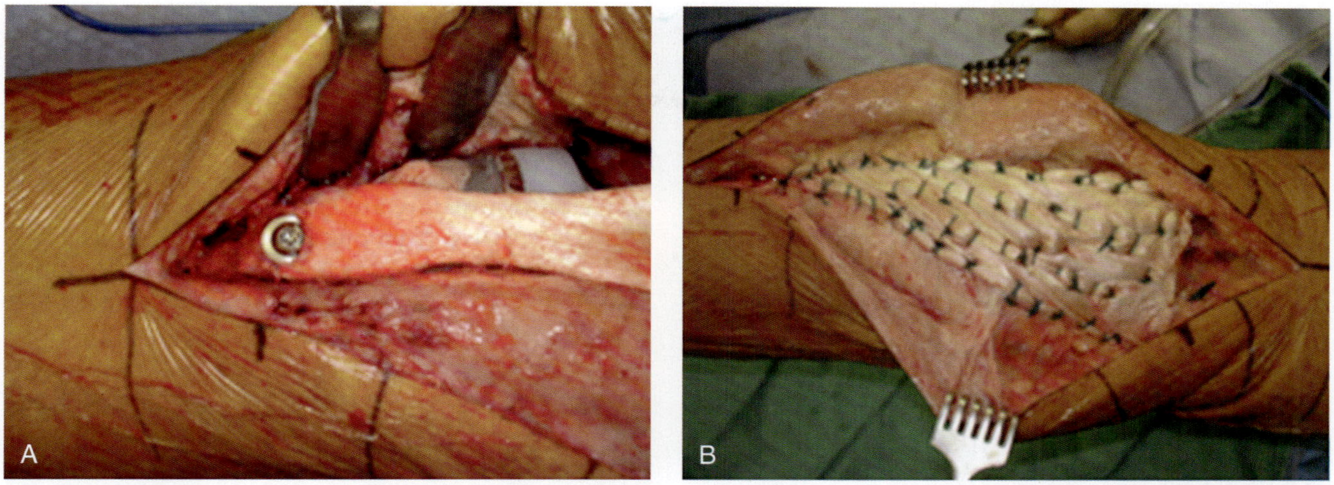

FIGURE 10 **A**, Intraoperative photograph showing Achilles tendon allograft bone block secured with a screw. **B**, Intraoperative photograph showing a completed extensor mechanism repair using Achilles tendon allograft. (Reprinted by permission from Springer Nature: *Int Orthop*. Wise BT, Erens G, Pour AE, Bradbury TL, Roberson JR. Long-term results of extensor mechanism reconstruction using Achilles tendon allograft after total knee arthroplasty, 42[10]:2367-2373. Copyright © 2018.)

anteriorly and sutured using transosseous sutures to the anterior tibial tuberosity. Both muscles can be used, in which case the vastus lateralis is placed under the vastus medialis. Two studies evaluating vastus medialis/lateralis flaps showed mean extensor lags of 12° at 1-year follow-up with improved lag in those knees that included gastrocnemius or soleus muscle transfer. None of the flaps developed necrosis following surgery.[118,119]

A 2019 meta-analysis evaluated 28 reports, concerning extensor mechanism rupture. The complication rate following repair of patellar tendon (64%) was higher than complications following repair of quadriceps tendon (25%). The complication rate for patellar and quadriceps tendon tears following reconstruction was 19%. Extension lag of 30° or greater occurred in 45% of patients after extensor mechanism repair or reconstruction, and the risk or rerupture and infection was 25% and 23%, respectively. These authors recommended patellar tendon reconstruction in both the early and late presentation stages. Quadriceps rupture can be treated with repair in early ruptures or with reconstruction in the late rupture or in the case of revision surgery.[100] It should be noted that these recommendations are based solely on level IV evidence.

NEUROVASCULAR INJURY

It is essential to document a thorough preoperative and postoperative neurovascular assessment in patients undergoing primary TKA. The incidence of vascular injury

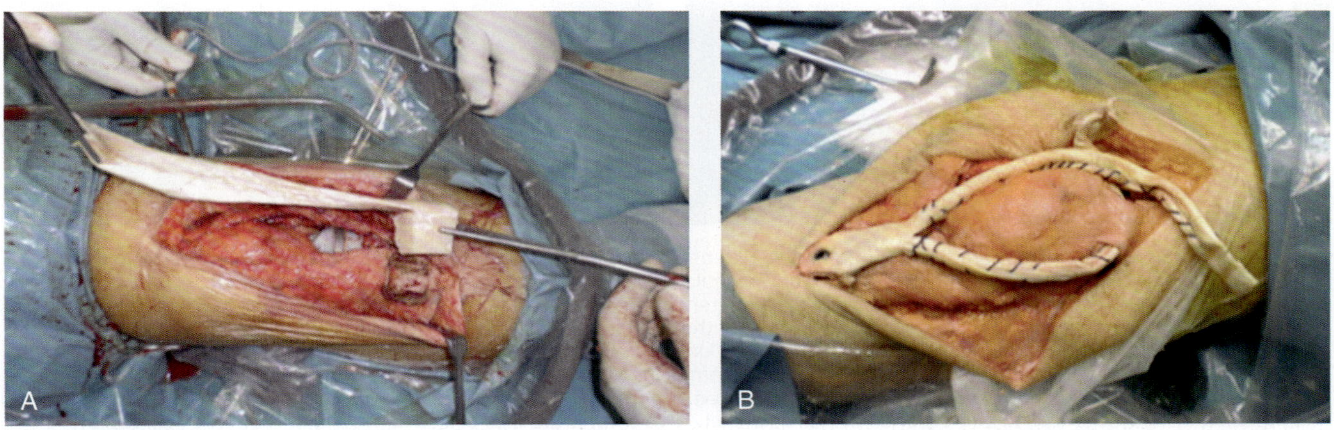

FIGURE 11 **A**, Intraoperative photograph showing Achilles tendon allograft with bone block shaped to fit the proximal tibia trough. **B**, Intraoperative photograph showing completed Achilles tendon allograft technique with crossover of the bundles. (Reprinted by permission from Springer Nature: *Arch Orthop Trauma Surg*. Ares O, Lozano LM, Medrano-Najera C, et al. New modified Achilles tendon allograft for treatment of chronic patellar tendon ruptures following total knee arthroplasty, 134[5]:713-717. Copyright © 2014.)

during a TKA is rare with a reported incidence from 0.003% to 0.23%.[120] The popliteal artery has been shown to lie 9 mm posterior to the posterior cortex of the tibia at 90° of knee flexion and just lateral to midline.[121] If an arterial injury is suspected, the tourniquet should be deflated before closure to identify and repair any vascular injury. Arterial injury at this level can result in ischemia, compartment syndrome, and potential amputation.

Various risk factors exist for postoperative neurologic injury following TKA (**Table 2**). The incidence of nerve injury following TKA has been reported to be 0.3% to 1.3%.[122] Damage to a nerve during TKA typically occurs by means of traction of the surrounding tissue leading to neural ischemia, direct traction on the nerve itself, or direct pressure from postoperative dressing.[123] Patients who have a valgus deformity and a flexion contracture are at the highest risk for peroneal nerve palsy. If peroneal nerve palsy is suspected following TKA, the patient's knee should be immediately flexed, and all compressive dressings should

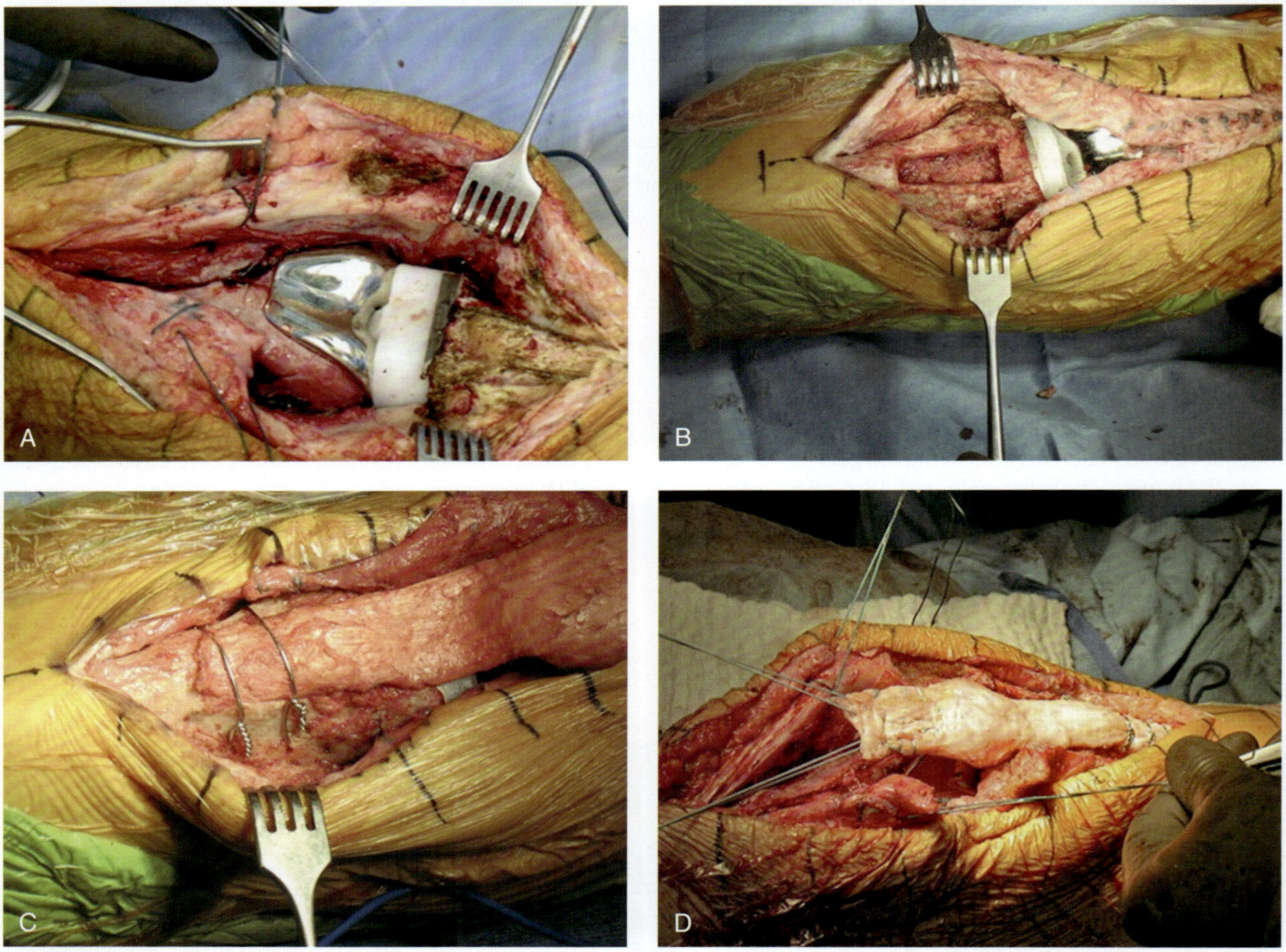

FIGURE 12 **A** through **F**, Intraoperative photographs. **A**, Extensor mechanism allograft. The patella has been removed and medial and lateral sleeves created, allowing direct exposure to the implants and the anterior aspect of the tibia and tubercle. **B**, Completed anterior tibial trough, which is ready to accept the allograft extensor mechanism. The host proximal tibial trough was marked with careful attention to the location of this trough in the region of the tibial tubercle or slightly medial to it will allow for improved patellar tracking. The trough has been beveled under to allow for a locking fit of the allograft tibial block. **C**, The allograft tibial block is press-fit into the host tibial trough. Fixation of the tibial allograft is accomplished with stainless steel wires, which are drilled through the tibia, beneath the allograft. **D**, Two running, locked sutures are placed into the medial and lateral host quadriceps retinaculum allowing the host extensor mechanism to be tensioned by pulling distally. Two sutures are also placed in the allograft quadriceps to allow the allograft to be tensioned proximally. The extensor mechanism and allograft are tensioned by pulling the knee into an extension position. **E**, The sutures in the allograft quadriceps are pulled under the host quadriceps and out proximally through the host extensor mechanism. **F**, The medial and lateral sleeves of retinaculum cover the allograft completely, reducing the exposure of the allograft to the subcutaneous tissues. (Reproduced with permission from Burnett RS, Berger RA, Della Valle CJ, Sporer S, et al: Extensor mechanism allograft reconstruction after total knee arthroplasty. *J Bone Joint Surg Am* 2005;87[1 suppl 2]:175-194.)

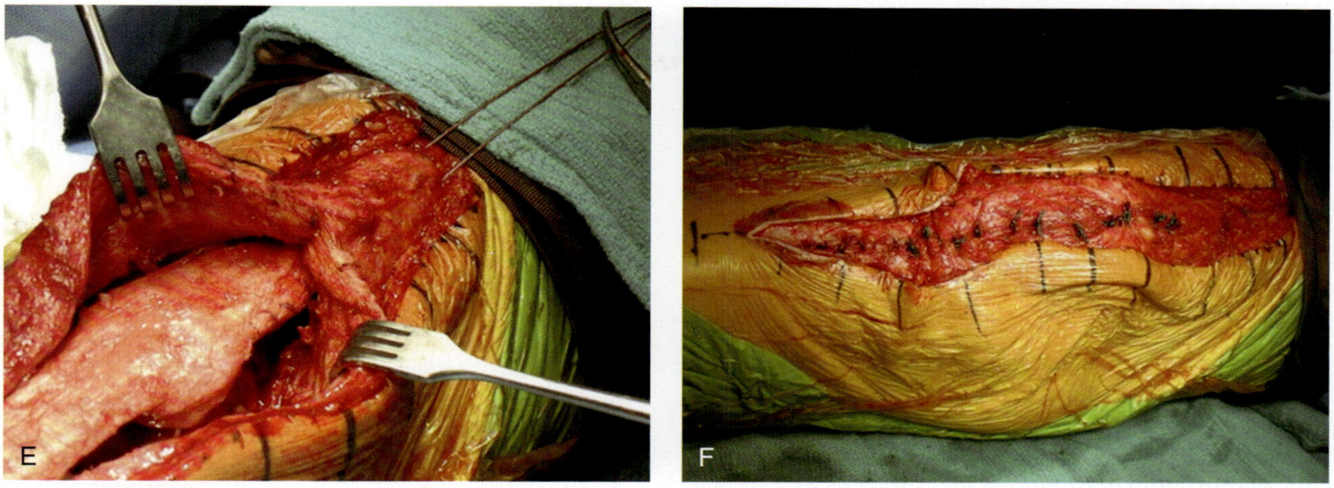

FIGURE 12 Cont'd

be removed. Initial management for footdrop should include using an ankle-foot orthosis. If dorsiflexion does not recover, a late decompression of the nerve or muscle transfer can be considered. It has been recommended that at least 3 months of observation be trialed prior surgical intervention for footdrop and that peroneal nerve decompression has led to successful outcomes in up to 97% of cases in one study.[124]

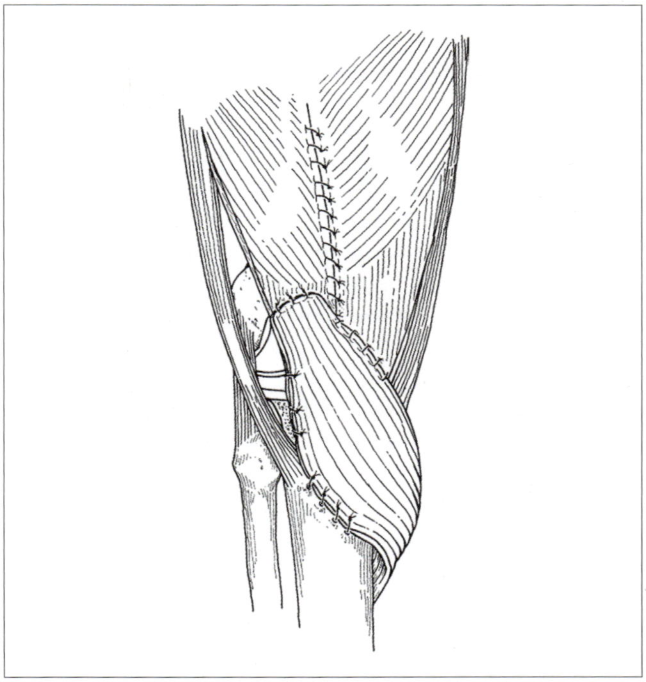

FIGURE 13 Illustration showing the medial gastrocnemius flap sutured to the distal fibrous portions of the transferred vastus flaps. (Reproduced with permission from Whiteside LA: Surgical technique: Vastus medialis and vastus lateralis as flap transfer for knee extensor mechanism deficiency. *Clin Orthop Relat Res* 2013;471[1]:221-230.)

READMISSION AFTER TKA

With modern-day bundle payment models and the importance of overall patient satisfaction, it is ideal to try to minimize hospital readmissions and minimize healthcare costs. In a national database of almost 190,000 patients who underwent TKA, the incidence of overall 30-day readmission was 3.19%.[125] The top five causes of readmission included superficial surgical site infection (SSI; 9.7%), non-SSI (9.5%), cardiovascular complications (9.3%), gastrointestinal complications (8.8%), and venous thromboemboli (8.8%). The authors also quantified the most common cause of readmission with various postoperative weeks: week 1 was cardiovascular complications (12.2%), week 2 was superficial SSI (11.6%), week 3 was deep SSI (11.4%), and week 4 was deep SSI (12.4%). Another study showed that the majority of readmissions were due to medical-related issues (79.1%) compared with reasons that required surgical intervention (20.9%),

TABLE 2

Factors Affecting Neurovascular Injury Following Total Knee Arthroplasty

Severe valgus and flexion deformities
Preoperative neuropathy
Tourniquet use longer than 120 min
Postoperative bleeding complications
Epidural anesthesia

Reproduced from Scuderi GR, Trousdale RT: Complications after total knee arthroplasty, in Barrack RL, Booth RE, Lonner JH, McCarthy JC, Mont MA, Rubash HE, eds: *Orthopaedic Knowledge Update®: Hip and Knee Reconstruction*, ed 3. Rosemont, IL, American Academy of Orthopaedic Surgeons, 2006, pp 147-156.

Section 2: Knee

and the mean additional cost was $8,588 per readmission.[126] Interestingly, in their cohort of patients, half were readmitted to a different facility than their index surgery hospital. Risk factors for postoperative readmission included age >75 years, BMI >35 kg/m^2, history of congestive heart failure, diabetes mellitus, and renal disease.

SUMMARY

The demographics of the patient population undergoing primary TKA is changing to include younger, more active patients, the morbidly obese, greater number of patients who have posttraumatic arthritis, along with increased number of elderly patients who have multiple comorbidities and poor bone stock. Surgeons performing knee arthroplasty must scrupulously select and optimize patients preoperatively to minimize complications and to achieve lasting durable results. It is important to educate patients on the risks and explain that certain risks cannot be eliminated, but only modified. Industry partners have helped develop, study, and refine knee implants to a point at which wear and durability is no longer the leading cause of failure. Surgeons need to be aware of the aspects such as polyethylene wear, instability, arthrofibrosis, patellofemoral subluxation, extensor mechanism disruption, and neurovascular complications; identify the at-risk patient; and learn how to manage these complications when they occur. Patients presenting with a painful TKA or dissatisfaction require a thorough evaluation to identify the etiology of the failed TKA. Emphasis should be placed on the need to support a global implant registry, standardize clinical data collection, and establish large-scale prospective clinical trials to evaluate the multitude of factors that influence knee arthroplasty complications, function, and longevity.

KEY STUDY POINTS

- Complications following primary TKA include infection, fracture, polyethylene wear, instability, postoperative stiffness, patellofemoral subluxation, extensor mechanism disruption, neurovascular, and unplanned hospital readmission.
- Patients at risk for specific complications should be identified preoperatively, and steps should be taken to minimize complications and readmission incidence following primary TKA.
- Surgeons need to adhere to meticulous surgical technique to assure balanced gaps and achieve the target limb and implant alignment, and patellofemoral stability.

ANNOTATED REFERENCES

1. Kurtz SM, Ong KL, Lau E, Bozic KJ: Impact of the economic downturn on total joint replacement demand in the United States: Updated projections to 2021. *J Bone Joint Surg Am* 2014;96(8):624-630.
2. Khan M, Osman K, Green G, Haddad FS: The epidemiology of failure in total knee arthroplasty: Avoiding your next revision. *Bone Joint J* 2016;98-B(1 suppl A):105-112.
3. Schroer WC, Berend KR, Lombardi AV, et al: Why are total knees failing today? Etiology of total knee revision in 2010 and 2011. *J Arthroplasty* 2013;28(8 suppl):116-119.
4. Thiele K, Perka C, Matziolis G, Mayr HO, Sostheim M, Hube R: Current failure mechanisms after knee arthroplasty have changed: Polyethylene wear is less common in revision surgery. *J Bone Joint Surg Am* 2015;97(9):715-720.
5. Sharkey PF, Lichstein PM, Shen C, Tokarski AT, Parvizi J: Why are total knee arthroplasties failing today – Has anything changed after 10 years? *J Arthroplasty* 2014;29(9):1774-1778.
6. Sakellariou VI, Sculco P, Poultsides L, Wright T, Sculco TP: Highly cross-linked polyethylene may not have an advantage in total knee arthroplasty. *HSS J* 2013;9(3):264-269.
7. Meneghini RM, Lovro LR, Smits SA, Ireland PH: Highly cross-linked versus conventional polyethylene in posterior-stabilized total knee arthroplasty at a mean 5-year follow-up. *J Arthroplasty* 2015;30(10):1736-1739.
8. Paxton EW, Inacio MC, Kurtz S, Love R, Cafri G, Namba RS: Is there a difference in total knee arthroplasty risk of revision in highly crosslinked versus conventional polyethylene? *Clin Orthop Relat Res* 2015;473(3):999-1008.
9. Gigante A, Bottegoni C, Ragone V, Banci L: Effectiveness of vitamin-E-doped polyethylene in joint replacement: A literature review. *J Funct Biomater* 2015;6(3):889-900.
10. Haider H, Weisenburger JN, Kurtz SM, et al: Does vitamin E-stabilized ultrahigh-molecular-weight polyethylene address concerns of cross-linked polyethylene in total knee arthroplasty? *J Arthroplasty* 2012;27(3):461-469.
11. Lachiewicz PF, Soileau ES: Is there a benefit to highly crosslinked polyethylene in posterior-stabilized total knee arthroplasty? A randomized trial. *Clin Orthop Relat Res* 2016;474(1):88-95.
12. Stavrakis A, Weitzler L, Wright T, Padgett DE: Less midterm damage and oxidation are seen in retrieved highly cross-linked ultrahigh-molecular-weight polyethylene tibial inserts than in direct compression molded polyethylene inserts. *HSS J* 2018;14(2):159-165.

   The authors identified 19 highly cross-linked ultrahigh–molecular-weight tibial inserts with at least 30 months in vivo and compared them with patient-matched direct compression-molded inserts. The direct compression inserts showed more surface damage and oxidation. Level of evidence: III.

13. Spece H, Schachtner JT, MacDonald DW, et al: Reasons for revision, oxidation, and damage mechanisms of retrieved vitamin E-stabilized highly crosslinked polyethylene in total knee arthroplasty. *J Arthroplasty* 2019;34(12): 3088-3093.

    This retrieval study compares 103 vitamin E-stabilized HXLPE and 67 HXLPE without vitamin E. They concluded that the vitamin E cohort demonstrated less surface damage and less oxidation using spectroscopy. Level of evidence: III.

14. MacDonald DW, Higgs GB, Chen AF, Malkani AL, Mont MA, Kurtz SM: Oxidation, damage mechanisms, and reasons for revision of sequentially annealed highly crosslinked polyethylene in total knee arthroplasty. *J Arthroplasty* 2018;33(4):1235-1241.

    This multicenter retrieval project between 2000 and 2016 compared 456 revised tibial inserts that were either sequentially annealed HXLPE or conventional polyethylene. Loosening, infection, and instability were the main reasons for revision. They used a semiquantitative scoring method to assess surface damage and spectroscopy to measure oxidation. The authors concluded that there was similar surface damage and oxidation between the two liners. Level of evidence: III.

15. Gallo J, Goodman SB, Konttinen YT, Wimmer MA, Holinka M: Osteolysis around total knee arthroplasty: A review of pathogenetic mechanisms. *Acta Biomater* 2013;9(9):8046-8058.

16. Goldvasser D, Marchie A, Bragdon LK, Bragdon CR, Weidenhielm L, Malchau H: Incidence of osteolysis in total knee arthroplasty: Comparison between radiographic and retrieval analysis. *J Arthroplasty* 2013;28(2):201-206.

17. Gibon E, Ma T, Ren PG, et al: Selective inhibition of the MCP-1-CCR2 ligand-receptor axis decreases systemic trafficking of macrophages in the presence of UHMWPE particles. *J Orthop Res* 2012;30(4):547-553.

18. Fritton K, Ren PG, Gibon E, et al: Exogenous MC3T3 preosteoblasts migrate systemically and mitigate the adverse effects of wear particles. *Tissue Eng Part A* 2012;18(23-24):2559-2567.

19. Nich C, Goodman SB: Role of macrophages in the biological reaction to wear debris from joint replacements. *J Long Term Eff Med Implants* 2014;24(4):259-265.

20. Pijls BG, Van der Linden-Van der Zwaag HM, Nelissen RG: Polyethylene thickness is a risk factor for wear necessitating insert exchange. *Int Orthop* 2012;36(6):1175-1180.

21. Berry DJ, Currier JH, Mayor MB, Collier JP: Knee wear measured in retrievals: A polished tray reduces insert wear. *Clin Orthop Relat Res* 2012;470(7):1860-1868.

22. Stoner K, Jerabek SA, Tow S, Wright TM, Padgett DE: Rotating-platform has no surface damage advantage over fixed-bearing TKA. *Clin Orthop Relat Res* 2013;471(1):76-85.

23. Gothesen O, Lygre SHL, Lorimer M, Graves S, Furnes O: Increased risk of aseptic loosening for 43,525 rotating-platform vs. fixed-bearing total knee replacements. *Acta Orthop* 2017;88(6):649-656.

    The authors in this study looked at the Norwegian and Australian joint registries between 2003 and 2013 and analyzed rotating-platform and fixed-bearing total knee arthroplasties. They used aseptic loosening as their primary end point and all revisions as secondary end point. They found that the rotating-platform knee arthroplasties had an increased risk of revision for aseptic loosening compared with the fixed-bearing implants in both Norway (RR = 6, 95% CI 4 to 8) and Australia (RR = 2.1, 95% CI 1.8 to 2.5). Level of evidence: III.

24. Pang HN, Bin Abd Razak HR, Jamieson P, Teeter MG, Naudie DDR, MacDonald SJ: Factors affecting wear of constrained polyethylene tibial inserts in total knee arthroplasty. *J Arthroplasty* 2016;31(6):1340-1345.

25. Robertson NB, Battenberg AK, Kertzner M, Schmalzried TP: Defining high activity in arthroplasty patients. *Bone Joint J* 2016;98-B(1 suppl A):95-97.

26. Watts CD, Wagner ER, Houdek MT, Lewallen DG, Mabry TM: Morbid obesity: Increased risk of failure after aseptic revision TKA. *Clin Orthop Relat Res* 2015;473(8):2621-2627.

27. Cherian JJ, Jauregui JJ, Banerjee S, Pierce T, Mont MA: What host factors affect aseptic loosening after THA and TKA? *Clin Orthop Relat Res* 2015;473(8):2700-2709.

28. Srivastava A, Lee GY, Steklov N, Colwell CW Jr, Ezzet KA, D'Lima DD: Effect of tibial component varus on wear in total knee arthroplasty. *Knee* 2012;19(5):560-563.

29. Ritter MA, Davis KE, Davis P, et al: Preoperative malalignment increases risk of failure after total knee arthroplasty. *J Bone Joint Surg Am* 2013;95(2):126-131.

30. Pang HN, Jamieson P, Teeter MG, McCalden RW, Naudie DD, MacDonald SJ: Retrieval analysis of posterior stabilized polyethylene tibial inserts and its clinical relevance. *J Arthroplasty* 2014;29(2):365-368.

31. Solomon LB, Stamenkov RB, MacDonald AJ, et al: Imaging periprosthetic osteolysis around total knee arthroplasties using a human cadaver model. *J Arthroplasty* 2012;27(6):1069-1074.

32. Dalling JG, Math K, Scuderi GR: Evaluating the progression of osteolysis after total knee arthroplasty. *J Am Acad Orthop Surg* 2015;23(3):173-180.

33. Nunez L, Broome B, Pace T, Harman M: Treatment for wear and osteolysis in well-fixed uncemented TKR. *ISRN Orthop* 2013;2013:398298.

34. Sculco PK, Abdel MP, Hanssen AD, Lewallen DG: The management of bone loss in revision total knee arthroplasty: Rebuild, reinforce, and augment. *Bone Joint J* 2016;98-B(1 suppl A):120-124.

35. Derome P, Sternheim A, Backstein D, Malo M: Treatment of large bone defects with trabecular metal cones in revision total knee arthroplasty: Short term clinical and radiographic outcomes. *J Arthroplasty* 2014;29(1):122-126.

36. Kamath AF, Lewallen DG, Hanssen AD: Porous tantalum metaphyseal cones for severe tibial bone loss in revision knee arthroplasty: A five to nine-year follow-up. *J Bone Joint Surg Am* 2015;97(3):216-223.

37. Alexander GE, Bernasek TL, Crank RL, Haidukewych GJ: Cementless metaphyseal sleeves used for large tibial defects in revision total knee arthroplasty. *J Arthroplasty* 2013;28(4):604-607.

38. Huang R, Barrazueta G, Ong A, et al: Revision total knee arthroplasty using metaphyseal sleeves at short-term follow-up. *Orthopedics* 2014;37(9):e804-e809.

39. Barnett SL, Mayer RR, Gondusky JS, Choi L, Patel JJ, Gorab RS: Use of stepped porous titanium metaphyseal sleeves for tibial defects in revision total knee arthroplasty: Short term results. *J Arthroplasty* 2014;29(6):1219-1224.

40. Wellman SS, Bolognesi MP: *AAOS Comprehensive Orthopaedic Review*, ed 2. Rosemont, IL, American Academy of Orthopaedic Surgeons, 2014, vol 2.

41. Wilson CJ, Theodoulou A, Damarell RA, Krishnan J: Knee instability as the primary cause of failure following total knee arthroplasty (TKA): A systematic review on the patient, surgical and implant characteristics of revised TKA patients. *Knee* 2017;24(6):1271-1281.

This meta-analysis evaluated publications of knee instability between 2005 and 2015. The mean time to failure between primary and revision TKA was 44.6 months (95% CI [33.8, 55.7]). Their results demonstrate that instability was reported more frequently in a younger patient population and 16.4% more females underwent revision surgery because of instability. Level of evidence: I.

42. Park CN, White PB, Meftah M, Ranawat AS, Ranawat CS: Diagnostic algorithm for residual pain after total knee arthroplasty. *Orthopedics* 2016;39(2):e246-e252.

43. Can A, Erdogan F, Erdogan AO: Tibiofemoral instability after primary total knee arthroplasty: Posterior-stabilized implants for obese patients. *Orthopedics* 2017;40(5):e812-e819.

In this study, 13 knees with tibiofemoral instability after cruciate ligament–retaining TKA were identified, which required revision surgery at an average of 23.4 months (range, 9 to 45 months). The main cause of instability was posterior cruciate ligament rupture and incompetence. Of note, all patients affected were obese and female. Level of evidence: IV.

44. Evangelista PJ, Laster SK, Lenz NM, Sheth NP, Schwarzkopf R: A computer model of mid-flexion instability in a balanced total knee arthroplasty. *J Arthroplasty* 2018;33(7 suppl):S265-S269.

This study aimed to evaluate TKA stability while changing the femoral implant size and position. They measured ligamentous forces in both posterior-stabilized and cruciate-retaining implants through knee midflexion ranges of 15° to 75°. Their computational analysis showed that elevation of the joint line and anteriorizing the femoral implant can cause the knee to be loose at midflexion. Level of evidence: IV.

45. Nagle M, Glynn A: Midflexion instability in primary total knee arthroplasty: A review article. *J Knee Surg* 2020;33(5):459-465.

The authors review current literature regarding midflexion instability and identify the best available evidence and prevention methods regarding this concept. Level of evidence: III.

46. Su EP: Instability in total knee replacement: Causes and management. *Semin Arthroplasty* 2015;26(4):246-250.

47. Scott RD: *Total Knee Arthroplasty*, ed 2. Philadelphia, PA, Elsevier/Saunders, 2015.

48. Tibbo ME, Limberg AK, Salib CG, et al: Acquired idiopathic stiffness after total knee arthroplasty: A systematic review and meta-analysis. *J Bone Joint Surg Am* 2019;101(14):1320-1330.

This is a meta-analysis of studies from 2002 to 2017 regarding arthrofibrosis after TKA. They found that the prevalence of acquired idiopathic stiffness was significantly lower in males (1%, $I = 85\%$) than females (3%, $I = 95\%$) ($P < 0.0001$) as well as in patients with a BMI of <30 kg/m^2 (2%, $I = 94\%$) compared with those with a BMI of ≥30 kg/m^2 (5%, $I = 97\%$) ($P = 0.027$). Level of evidence: IV.

49. Zmistowski B, Restrepo C, Hess J, Adibi D, Cangoz S, Parvizi J: Unplanned readmission after total joint arthroplasty: Rates, reasons, and risk factors. *J Bone Joint Surg Am* 2013;95(20):1869-1876.

50. Le DH, Goodman SB, Maloney WJ, Huddleston JI: Current modes of failure in TKA: Infection, instability, and stiffness predominate. *Clin Orthop Relat Res* 2014;472(7):2197-2200.

51. Cheuy VA, Foran JRH, Paxton RJ, Bade MJ, Zeni JA, Stevens-Lapsley JE: Arthrofibrosis associated with total knee arthroplasty. *J Arthroplasty* 2017;32(8):2604-2611.

This is a narrative review of the literature regarding the etiology, risk factors, economic burden, treatment strategies, and future research directions of arthrofibrosis after TKA. Level of evidence: III.

52. Kalson NS, Borthwick LA, Mann DA, et al: International consensus on the definition and classification of fibrosis of the knee joint. *Bone Joint J* 2016;98-B(11):1479-1488.

53. Thompson R, Novikov D, Cizmic Z, et al: Arthrofibrosis after total knee arthroplasty: Pathophysiology, diagnosis, and management. *Orthop Clin North Am* 2019;50(3):269-279.

This review article outlines arthrofibrosis diagnosis, management, and prevention after TKA. Level of evidence: III.

54. Manrique J, Gomez MM, Parvizi J: Stiffness after total knee arthroplasty. *J Knee Surg* 2015;28(2):119-126.

55. Stephenson JJ, Quimbo RA, Gu T: Knee-attributable medical costs and risk of re-surgery among patients utilizing non-surgical treatment options for knee arthrofibrosis in a managed care population. *Curr Med Res Opin* 2010;26(5):1109-1118.

56. Rutherford RW, Jennings JM, Levy DL, Parisi TJ, Martin JR, Dennis DA: Revision total knee arthroplasty for arthrofibrosis. *J Arthroplasty* 2018;33(7 suppl):S177-S181.

This is a retrospective review of 46 TKAs that were revised because of arthrofibrosis and had a minimum of 2-year follow-up. The mean postoperative flexion improved from 88° to 103° and extension improved from 11° to 3° ($P < 0.001$); however, 30% of patients had a net decrease in arc of motion. The authors caution that the rate of complications was 28.2% with a 17.4% revision surgery rate. Level of evidence: IV.

57. Bingham JS, Bukowski BR, Wyles CC, Pareek A, Berry DJ, Abdel MP: Rotating-hinge revision total knee arthroplasty for treatment of severe arthrofibrosis. *J Arthroplasty* 2019;34(7 suppl):S271-S276.

This study evaluated the 10-year survivorship of 34 patients who underwent revision TKA because of arthrofibrosis with a rotating-hinge compared with 68 matched patients who underwent revision to a non–rotating-hinge knee. Although mean arc of motion improved in the rotating-hinge group, there was a significant increase in the rate of revision in the rotating-hinge group, 40% of which were related to the insert and bushing exchanges. Level of evidence: III.

58. Maheshwari AV, Tsailas PG, Ranawat AS, Ranawat CS: How to address the patella in revision total knee arthroplasty. *Knee* 2009;16(2):92-97.

59. Chalidis BE, Tsiridis E, Tragas AA, Stavrou Z, Giannoudis PV: Management of periprosthetic patellar fractures. A systematic review of literature. *Injury* 2007;38(6):714-724.

60. Abadie P, Galaud B, Michaut M, Fallet L, Boisrenoult P, Beaufils P: Distal femur rotational alignment and patellar subluxation: A CT scan in vivo assessment. *Orthop Traumatol Surg Res* 2009;95(4):267-271.

61. Berger RA, Crossett LS, Jacobs JJ, Rubash HE: Malrotation causing patellofemoral complications after total knee arthroplasty. *Clin Orthop Relat Res* 1998;356:144-153.

62. Hamilton WG, Ammeen DJ, Parks NL, Goyal N, Engh GA, Engh CA Jr: Patellar cut and composite thickness: The influence on postoperative motion and complications in total knee arthroplasty. *J Arthroplasty* 2017;32(6):1803-1807.

This is a retrospective review of 3,655 TKAs, which had caliper measurement of patellar thickness before the patellar cut, after implantation of the implant, and postoperative motion recorded. The study did not show a strong correlation of losing motion with increased thickness, and authors recommended avoiding compromise of the patellar bone stock and tendon insertion. When native patellar bone is thin (<18 mm), we recommend maintaining 12 mm of patellar bone stock and accept the increase in composite thickness. Level of evidence: IV.

63. Meding JB, Fish MD, Berend ME, Ritter MA, Keating EM: Predicting patellar failure after total knee arthroplasty. *Clin Orthop Relat Res* 2008;466(11):2769-2774.

64. Pagnano MW, Trousdale RT: Asymmetric patella resurfacing in total knee arthroplasty. *Am J Knee Surg* 2000;13(4):228-233.

65. Putman S, Boureau F, Girard J, Migaud H, Pasquier G: Patellar complications after total knee arthroplasty. *Orthop Traumatol Surg Res* 2019;105(1 suppl):S43-S51.

This is a systematic review of patellar complications and management options. Level of evidence: V.

66. Malo M, Vince KG: The unstable patella after total knee arthroplasty: Etiology, prevention, and management. *J Am Acad Orthop Surg* 2003;11(5):364-371.

67. Briard JL, Hungerford DS: Patellofemoral instability in total knee arthroplasty. *J Arthroplasty* 1989;(4 suppl):S87-S97.

68. Rhoads DD, Noble PC, Reuben JD, Mahoney OM, Tullos HS: The effect of femoral component position on patellar tracking after total knee arthroplasty. *Clin Orthop Relat Res* 1990;260:43-51.

69. Anouchi YS, Whiteside LA, Kaiser AD, Milliano MT: The effects of axial rotational alignment of the femoral component on knee stability and patellar tracking in total knee arthroplasty demonstrated on autopsy specimens. *Clin Orthop Relat Res* 1993;287:170-177.

70. Franceschini V, Nodzo SR, Gonzalez Della Valle A: Femoral component rotation in total knee arthroplasty: A comparison between transepicondylar axis and posterior condylar line referencing. *J Arthroplasty* 2016;31(12):2917-2921.

71. Yoshii I, Whiteside LA, Anouchi YS: The effect of patellar button placement and femoral component design on patellar tracking in total knee arthroplasty. *Clin Orthop Relat Res* 1992;275:211-219.

72. Hirschmann MT, Konala P, Amsler F, Iranpour F, Friederich NF, Cobb JP: The position and orientation of total knee replacement components: A comparison of conventional radiographs, transverse 2D-CT slices and 3D-CT reconstruction. *J Bone Joint Surg Br* 2011;93(5):629-633.

73. De Valk EJ, Noorduyn JC, Mutsaerts EL: How to assess femoral and tibial component rotation after total knee arthroplasty with computed tomography: A systematic review. *Knee Surg Sports Traumatol Arthrosc* 2016;24(11):3517-3528.

74. Berger RA, Rubash HE: Rotational instability and malrotation after total knee arthroplasty. *Orthop Clin North Am* 2001;32(4):639-647.

75. Berger RA, Rubash HE, Seel MJ, Thompson WH, Crossett LS: Determining the rotational alignment of the femoral component in total knee arthroplasty using the epicondylar axis. *Clin Orthop Relat Res* 1993;286:40-47.

76. Whiteside LA, Arima J: The anteroposterior axis for femoral rotational alignment in valgus total knee arthroplasty. *Clin Orthop Relat Res* 1995;321:168-172.

77. Anglin C, Brimacombe JM, Wilson DR, et al: Biomechanical consequences of patellar component medialization in total knee arthroplasty. *J Arthroplasty* 2010;25(5):793-802.

78. Lewonowski K, Dorr LD, McPherson EJ, Huber G, Wan Z: Medialization of the patella in total knee arthroplasty. *J Arthroplasty* 1997;12(2):161-167.

79. Hofmann AA, Tkach TK, Evanich CJ, Camargo MP, Zhang Y: Patellar component medialization in total knee arthroplasty. *J Arthroplasty* 1997;12(2):155-160.

80. Bindelglass DF, Vince KG: Patellar tilt and subluxation following subvastus and parapatellar approach in total knee arthroplasty. Implication for surgical technique. *J Arthroplasty* 1996;11(5):507-511.

81. Maniar RN, Singhi T, Rathi SS, Baviskar JV, Nayak RM: Surgical technique: Lateral retinaculum release in knee arthroplasty using a stepwise, outside-in technique. *Clin Orthop Relat Res* 2012;470(10):2854-2863.

82. Lamotte A, Neri T, Kawaye A, Boyer B, Farizon F, Philippot R: Medial patellofemoral ligament reconstruction for patellar instability following total knee arthroplasty: A review of 6 cases. *Orthop Traumatol Surg Res* 2016;102(5):607-610.

83. van Gennip S, Schimmel JJ, van Hellemondt GG, Defoort KC, Wymenga AB: Medial patellofemoral ligament reconstruction for patellar maltracking following total knee arthroplasty is effective. *Knee Surg Sports Traumatol Arthrosc* 2014;22(10):2569-2573.

84. Piedade SR, Pinaroli A, Servien E, Neyret P: Tibial tubercle osteotomy in primary total knee arthroplasty: A safe procedure or not? *Knee* 2008;15(6):439-446.

85. Wing CK, Kwok-Hing C: Sixteen years' result of posterior-stabilized TKA. *J Knee Surg* 2012;25(3):245-248.

86. Meftah M, White PB, Ranawat AS, Ranawat CS: Long-term results of total knee arthroplasty in young and active patients with posterior stabilized design. *Knee* 2016;23(2):318-321.

87. Meftah M, Ranawat AS, Ranawat CS: The natural history of anterior knee pain in 2 posterior-stabilized, modular total knee arthroplasty designs. *J Arthroplasty* 2011;26(8):1145-1148.

88. Hozack WJ, Rothman RH, Booth RE Jr, Balderston RA: The patellar clunk syndrome. A complication of posterior stabilized total knee arthroplasty. *Clin Orthop Relat Res* 1989;241:203-208.

89. Niikura T, Tsumura N, Tsujimoto K, Yoshiya S, Kurosaka M, Shiba R: Patellar clunk syndrome after TKA with cruciate retaining design: A report of two cases. *Orthopedics* 2008;31(1):90.

90. Sringari T, Maheswaran SS: Patellar clunk syndrome in patellofemoral arthroplasty – A case report. *Knee* 2005;12(6):456-457.

91. Costanzo JA, Aynardi MC, Peters JD, Kopolovich DM, Purtill JJ: Patellar clunk syndrome after total knee arthroplasty; Risk factors and functional outcomes of arthroscopic treatment. *J Arthroplasty* 2014;29(9 suppl):201-204.

92. Zmistowski B, Restrepo C, Kahl LK, Parvizi J, Sharkey PF: Incidence and reasons for nonrevision reoperation after total knee arthroplasty. *Clin Orthop Relat Res* 2011;469(1):138-145.

93. Conrad DN, Dennis DA: Patellofemoral crepitus after total knee arthroplasty: Etiology and preventive measures. *Clin Orthop Surg* 2014;6(1):9-19.

94. Gholson JJ, Goetz DD, Westermann RW, Hart J, Callaghan JJ: Management of painful patellar clunk and crepitance: Results at a mean follow-up of five years. *Iowa Orthop J* 2017;37:171-175.

The authors reviewed 1,488 TKA cases, and 46 patients (3.1%) were identified to have clinical signs and symptoms of patellar clunk or crepitus during postoperative clinical follow-up. Eighteen patients underwent arthroscopic excision of the suprapatellar lesion after failing conservative management. Three cases had recurrence of patellar clunk or crepitus after arthroscopy (16.7%), and each of these patients was successfully treated with a second arthroscopic excision procedure. Patient satisfaction after arthroscopic excision was rated extremely satisfied or very satisfied in 79% of patients and moderately satisfied in 21% of patients. Level of evidence: IV.

95. Messieh M: Management of patellar clunk under local anesthesia. *J Arthroplasty* 1996;11(2):202-203.

96. Schoderbek RJ Jr, Brown TE, Mulhall KJ, et al: Extensor mechanism disruption after total knee arthroplasty. *Clin Orthop Relat Res* 2006;446:176-185.

97. Papalia R, Vasta S, D'Adamio S, Albo E, Maffulli N, Denaro V: Complications involving the extensor mechanism after total knee arthroplasty. *Knee Surg Sports Traumatol Arthrosc* 2015;23(12):3501-3515.

98. Nam D, Abdel MP, Cross MB, et al: The management of extensor mechanism complications in total knee arthroplasty. AAOS Exhibit selection. *J Bone Joint Surg Am* 2014;96(6):e47.

99. Bonnin M, Lustig S, Huten D: Extensor tendon ruptures after total knee arthroplasty. *Orthop Traumatol Surg Res* 2016;102(1 suppl):S21-S31.

100. Vajapey SP, Blackwell RE, Maki AJ, Miller TL: Treatment of extensor tendon disruption after total knee arthroplasty: A systematic review. *J Arthroplasty* 2019;34(6):1279-1286.

This is a systematic review of 28 articles. The complication rate after repair of patellar tendon (63.16%) was higher than the complication rate after repair of quadriceps tendon (25.37%). However, the complication rate for patellar and quadriceps tendon tears after autograft, allograft, or mesh reconstruction was similar (18.8% versus 19.2%, respectively). The most common complication after extensor mechanism repair or reconstruction was extension lag of 30° or greater (45.33%). This was followed by rerupture and infection (25.33% and 22.67%, respectively). Early ruptures had a higher overall complication rate than late injuries. Quadriceps rupture can be treated with repair in early ruptures or with reconstruction in the late rupture or in the case of revision surgery. Level of evidence: III.

101. Spoliti M, Giai Via A, Padulo J, Oliva F, Del Buono A, Maffulli N: Surgical repair of chronic patellar tendon rupture in total knee replacement with ipsilateral hamstring tendons. *Knee Surg Sports Traumatol Arthrosc* 2016;24(10):3183-3190.

102. Shi SM, Shi GG, Laurent EM, Ninomiya JT: Modified V-Y turndown flap augmentation for quadriceps tendon rupture following total knee arthroplasty: A retrospective study. *J Bone Joint Surg Am* 2019;101(11):1010-1015.

In this retrospective review, 24 quadriceps tendon ruptures in 23 patients who underwent TKA, including 1 tendon rerupture, were treated with use of a modified V-Y turndown. Before repair with the V-Y flap, none of the patients was able to walk independently, requiring either a wheelchair or a walker. No patient had quadriceps strength greater than 3 (of 5), although all had full passive extension. Following the repair procedure, patients had significant improvements in mean Knee Society knee score and mean strength, and all were able to walk without assistive devices. Major adverse events were limited to a single hematoma and an unacceptable extensor lag (35°) after repair. The modified V-Y quadriceps tendon turndown flap was a reliable alternative treatment for achieving restoration of the extensor mechanism after complete quadriceps tendon rupture following TKA. Level of evidence: IV.

103. Abdel MP, Salib CG, Mara KC, Pagnano MW, Perry KI, Hanssen AD: Extensor mechanism reconstruction with use of Marlex mesh: A series study of 77 total knee arthroplasties. *J Bone Joint Surg Am* 2018;100(15): 1309-1318.

This is a retrospective review of 77 TKAs that underwent reconstruction with the use of Marlex mesh for an extensor mechanism disruption. Eighteen of the patients (23%) underwent mesh reconstruction with the primary TKA in place, and 59 (77%) had mesh reconstruction at the time of revision TKA. The mean time between disruption and reconstruction was 7 months. Twelve patients experienced a failure that required mesh revision: five for patellar tendon rupture, five for quadriceps tendon rupture, and two for symptomatic lengthening. Four additional patients with mesh failure were treated nonsurgically with bracing. The 2-year survivorship free of mesh revision was 86% for patients with no prior reconstruction and 95% for patients with previous reconstructions of the extensor mechanism that did not involve Marlex mesh. Extensor lag improved by a mean of 26°, with mean postoperative extensor lag measuring 9° ($P < 0.001$). Level of evidence: IV.

104. Junge K, Binnebosel M, von Trotha KT, et al: Mesh biocompatibility: Effects of cellular inflammation and tissue remodelling. *Langenbecks Arch Surg* 2012;397(2): 255-270.

105. Browne JA, Hanssen AD: Reconstruction of patellar tendon disruption after total knee arthroplasty: Results of a new technique utilizing synthetic mesh. *J Bone Joint Surg Am* 2011;93(12):1137-1143.

106. Smith CW, Young IS, Kearney JN: Mechanical properties of tendons: Changes with sterilization and preservation. *J Biomech Eng* 1996;118(1):56-61.

107. Wise BT, Erens G, Pour AE, Bradbury TL, Roberson JR: Long-term results of extensor mechanism reconstruction using Achilles tendon allograft after total knee arthroplasty. *Int Orthop* 2018;42(10):2367-2373.

Sixteen patients who underwent extensor mechanism reconstruction (10 patellar tendons, 7 quadriceps tendons) with Achilles tendon allograft were retrospectively studied. After reconstruction, the average extensor lag was 6.6° and average knee flexion was 105.1°. Quadriceps strength was maintained at an average of 4/5. Achilles tendon allograft reconstruction is a reliable and durable treatment for patients who sustain not only patellar tendon ruptures but also quadriceps tendon ruptures following TKA. Despite the success of this technique, the injury and procedure have a profound effect on overall function Level of evidence: IV.

108. Crossett LS, Sinha RK, Sechriest VF, Rubash HE: Reconstruction of a ruptured patellar tendon with Achilles tendon allograft following total knee arthroplasty. *J Bone Joint Surg Am* 2002;84(8):1354-1361.

109. Ares O, Lozano LM, Medrano-Najera C, et al: New modified Achilles tendon allograft for treatment of chronic patellar tendon ruptures following total knee arthroplasty. *Arch Orthop Trauma Surg* 2014;134(5):713-717.

110. Malhotra R, Garg B, Logani V, Bhan S: Management of extensor mechanism deficit as a consequence of patellar tendon loss in total knee arthroplasty: A new surgical technique. *J Arthroplasty* 2008;23(8):1146-1151.

111. Emerson RH Jr, Head WC, Malinin TI: Extensor mechanism reconstruction with an allograft after total knee arthroplasty. *Clin Orthop Relat Res* 1994;303:79-85.

112. Leopold SS, Greidanus N, Paprosky WG, Berger RA, Rosenberg AG: High rate of failure of allograft reconstruction of the extensor mechanism after total knee arthroplasty. *J Bone Joint Surg Am* 1999;81(11):1574-1579.

113. Burnett RS, Berger RA, Paprosky WG, Della Valle CJ, Jacobs JJ, Rosenberg AG: Extensor mechanism allograft reconstruction after total knee arthroplasty. A comparison of two techniques. *J Bone Joint Surg Am* 2004;86(12):2694-2699.

114. Brown NM, Murray T, Sporer SM, Wetters N, Berger RA, Della Valle CJ: Extensor mechanism allograft reconstruction for extensor mechanism failure following total knee arthroplasty. *J Bone Joint Surg Am* 2015;97(4):279-283.

115. Wood TJ, Leighton J, Backstein DJ, et al: Synthetic graft compared with allograft reconstruction for extensor mechanism disruption in total knee arthroplasty: A multicenter cohort study. *J Am Acad Orthop Surg* 2019;27(12):451-457.

The authors retrospectively reviewed 27 patients who underwent extensor mechanism reconstruction using either allograft or synthetic graft. A significantly greater postoperative extensor lag was found in the allograft group ($P = 0.05$). Graft failure after synthetic reconstruction was zero, with an overall revision surgery rate of 15%. Graft failure was 21%, and the revision surgery rate was 43% after allograft reconstruction. The allograft cost was significantly higher compared with the synthetic graft cost. The mean total cost was 4,733.08 CAD for the synthetic group and 24,050.40 CAD for the allograft group. Synthetic reconstruction for extensor mechanism disruption shows benefit in postoperative extensor lag, graft failure, revision surgery, and cost when compared with allograft. Level of evidence: III.

116. Chiou HM, Chang MC, Lo WH: One-stage reconstruction of skin defect and patellar tendon rupture after total knee arthroplasty. A new technique. *J Arthroplasty* 1997;12(5):575-579.

117. Jaureguito JW, Dubois CM, Smith SR, Gottlieb LJ, Finn HA: Medial gastrocnemius transposition flap for the treatment of disruption of the extensor mechanism after total knee arthroplasty. *J Bone Joint Surg Am* 1997;79(6):866-873.

118. Whiteside LA: Surgical technique: Vastus medialis and vastus lateralis as flap transfer for knee extensor mechanism deficiency. *Clin Orthop Relat Res* 2013;471(1):221-230.

119. Whiteside LA: Surgical technique: Muscle transfer restores extensor function after failed patella-patellar tendon allograft. *Clin Orthop Relat Res* 2014;472(1):218-226.

120. Papadopoulos DV, Koulouvaris P, Lykissas MG, Giannoulis D, Georgios A, Mavrodontidis A: Popliteal artery damage during total knee arthroplasty. *Arthroplast Today* 2015;1(3):53-57.

121. Ninomiya JT, Dean JC, Goldberg VM: Injury to the popliteal artery and its anatomic location in total knee arthroplasty. *J Arthroplasty* 1999;14(7):803-809.

122. Shetty T, Nguyen JT, Sasaki M, et al: Risk factors for acute nerve injury after total knee arthroplasty. *Muscle Nerve* 2018;57(6):946-950.

The authors retrospectively reviewed a database of patients with nerve injury after TKA from 1998 to 2013. They used multivariable logistic regression models to assess for potential risk factors. In their data of almost 40,000 TKAs, females (OR 3.28, P = 0.003) and patients with a history of lumbar pathology (OR 6.12, P = 0.026) were associated with the most risk of postoperative nerve damage. Level of evidence: IV.

123. Park JH, Restrepo C, Norton R, Mandel S, Sharkey PF, Parvizi J: Common peroneal nerve palsy following total knee arthroplasty: Prognostic factors and course of recovery. *J Arthroplasty* 2013;28(9):1538-1542.

124. Poage C, Roth C, Scott B: Peroneal nerve palsy: Evaluation and management. *J Am Acad Orthop Surg* 2016;24(1):1-10.

125. Curtis GL, Jawad M, Samuel LT, et al: Incidence, causes, and timing of 30-day readmission following total knee arthroplasty. *J Arthroplasty* 2019;34(11):2632-2636.

This is a national database study of incidence and causes of readmissions after primary TKA from 2012 to 2016. The authors showed that the 30-day readmission rate was 3.19% (6,014/188,251) and that this has significantly declined from 2012 to 2016. The most common causes of readmission changed from week to week postoperatively. Level of evidence: IV.

126. Phillips JLH, Rondon AJ, Vannello C, Fillingham YA, Austin MS, Courtney PM: How much does a readmission cost the bundle following primary hip and knee arthroplasty? *J Arthroplasty* 2019;34(5):819-823.

This review from a high-volume institution from 2015 to 2016 evaluated claims data of 4,704 patients following primary hip and knee arthroplasty. There were 325 readmissions in 286 patients (6.1%). They review cost per readmission (average $8,588) and risk factors. Level of evidence: IV.

CHAPTER 27

Revision Total Knee Arthroplasty

KELLY G. VINCE, MD, FRCSC • BRADFORD S. WADDELL, MD
GEOFFREY WESTRICH, MD

ABSTRACT

The technical, emotional, legal, and financial challenges of revision knee arthroplasty are daunting. Success with revision means nothing less than a satisfied patient, which requires realistic expectations, astute indications for surgery, superior surgical technique, and an appropriate implant. The evaluation of the patient and the problem arthroplasty should be systematic (following the same method for each patient) and comprehensive (all modes of failure to be considered for each patient). In the absence of an identifiable explanation for problems, revision is best deferred. The most common problems leading to revision surgery are prosthetic joint infection and aseptic loosening. These are also the most common reasons that revision surgeries fail. Aseptic causes of failure may be characterized as structural (loosening, periprosthetic fracture, or implant breakage) or kinematic (extensor insufficiency, stiffness, or patellar complications including malrotation and tibiofemoral instability). Surgical techniques adapted to the mode of failure are more likely to ensure that the causes are eliminated by the revision. The literature on revision is relatively low quality. There is a frequent assumption that the results of revision are poor, yet the literature probably reflects an unrealistically optimistic view of revision surgery as surgeons are less likely to submit poor results for publication. In short, more questions than answers emerge from careful reading of existing literature.

Keywords: arthroplasty; complications; failure; knee; prosthetic joint infection; revision

Dr. Vince or an immediate family member has received royalties from Zimmer; is a member of a speakers' bureau or has made paid presentations on behalf of Zimmer; and serves as a paid consultant to or is an employee of Zimmer. Dr. Waddell or an immediate family member serves as a paid consultant to or is an employee of OrthAlign and Smith & Nephew. Dr. Westrich or an immediate family member has received royalties from Exactech, Inc. and Stryker; is a member of a speakers' bureau or has made paid presentations on behalf of Exactech, Inc., Mallinckrodt Pharmaceuticals, and Stryker; serves as a paid consultant to or is an employee of Exactech, Inc. and Stryker; has received research or institutional support from Exactech, Inc. and Stryker; and serves as a board member, owner, officer, or committee member of the Eastern Orthopedic Association and the Knee Society.

INTRODUCTION

Revision of the failed total knee arthroplasty (TKA) is distinctly different from a primary procedure; most attempts to make the case resemble a primary procedure actually make it more difficult. The same diagnostic protocols should be applied to each patient, with full consideration of all possible causes of failure. Revision arthroplasty is not one surgical procedure, but rather at least eight procedures depending on the cause of failure. The essence of the procedure is to position implants inside the soft-tissue envelope of the failed knee to restore functional tension no matter how the muscles, tendons, and ligaments may have been altered by the failure. The previous osseous anatomy of the knee may or may not be a reliable guide,

This chapter is adapted from Meneghini RM, Vince KG, Waddell BS, Westrich G: Revision total knee arthroplasty, in Mont MA, Tanzer M, eds: *Orthopaedic Knowledge Update®: Hip and Knee Reconstruction*, ed 5. Rosemont, IL, American Academy of Orthopaedic Surgeons, 2017, pp 267-277.

despite current preoccupation with the joint line. The single most important recent advance to revision TKA is the organized approach to the diagnosis of prosthetic joint infection (PJI). New materials and implants have made the procedure potentially more successful than ever; however, they did not compensate for a lack of diagnostic accuracy or surgical technique.

THE CHALLENGE OF FAILED TKA

According to a 2017 study, infection and aseptic loosening are the major reasons for repeat TKA.[1] This squares with data from major registries and identifies unsolved problems that occur during TKA.

Infection may be the more challenging of the two problems. In a 2017 study of 11,134 knees that combined registry data and multi-institution chart reviews, the risk of revision or revision surgery by 15 years was 2.0% for infection and 1.2% for aseptic loosening. About half of the PJIs occurred within 2 years of the TKA, whereas half the cases of loosening occurred more than 8 years after the primary procedure, showing that infected cases experienced less service before failing.[2]

The emotional and financial costs of a revision surgery to patients, their families, health care providers, and society are formidable, compounded by the numbers of patients who will require revision knee arthroplasty in the future. The incidence of revision TKA is projected to increase by 78% to 182%, from 2014 to 2030; this is more than double the rate for revision total hip arthroplasties. Infection and aseptic loosening are still expected to be the main indications for revision in the future. The incidence is expected to increase for patients aged 55 to 74 years, yet it decreases in patients older than 74 years.[3]

In a 2017 study to determine whether higher volume hospitals provided better value in revision arthroplasty surgery, the conclusions were complex and complicated by selection bias: higher volume hospitals treated more complex cases. High-volume hospitals comprised 178 of the 789 institutions (23%) studied, but performed 51% of the revisions, including 91% of the most complex cases. The mean Medicare expenditures to these hospitals were higher, but these were less likely to be cost outliers (less likely to be in the upper quartile for expenditures).[4]

In a 2020 study of 23,644 aseptic revision TKAs, a higher risk for re-revision in hospitals performing fewer than 25 revision procedures per year was observed. Furthermore, higher volume hospitals performed more revisions of failed revisions and revisions of stemmed prostheses.[5] This highlights the complexity of revision arthroplasty surgery and the need for expertise.

The prospect for a quality result is highest with the first revision procedure. The overall societal cost of revision surgery is best reduced by improving results of primary TKA.[6] Ensuring successful revision surgery is essential to lowering cost. Second revisions, and specifically infected revisions, are distinctly more expensive and are associated with worse outcomes.[7]

New Zealand registry data were evaluated to identify risk factors for 12.1% of 1,720 aseptic revision surgeries that failed. Younger age and male sex predicted re-revision, implicating activity level as a risk factor for failure, but raising the question that some older patients with problematic failures may not be offered second revision surgery for numerous reasons. Isolated femoral implant revision predicted failure as distinct from isolated tibial implant and complete revision surgery, raising questions about the definition of a revision procedure.[8] A coherent argument can be made because the tibia is common to both flexion and extension gaps, and it is the femur that enables the surgeon to manipulate gap balance. In addition, if both implants are not revised, there is usually no option for the constrained implants that are often necessary in revision surgery.

Clinical series that ask why TKAs fail usually review the revision experience of one institution or practitioner.[9] This represents a strong patient selection bias, as there can be no way to know what cases are revised at other institutions. A review of world registries concluded that aseptic loosening was the most common indication for revision (29.8%) followed by infection (14.8%) and pain (9.5%).[10] There is consensus that pain is not a reasonable indication for revision and that PJI is widely underdiagnosed. Whether revised or not, kinematic failures (stiffness, instability, and maltracking) are usually associated with poor surgical technique and are underrepresented in registries.

The literature on revision knee arthroplasty is abundant and interesting, but with notable exceptions, it is of poor quality and inconclusive. Any update to the current knowledge about revision TKA identifies more questions than answers. Bias, most frequently due to skewed patient selection, is ubiquitous. Many reports of specific products, for example, are biased by inclusion of only the patients deemed appropriate for the implant under consideration. The same is true of surgical protocols for PJI.

There is undoubtedly a bias against publishing poor results because of the disincentive to showcase failure, except perhaps if the failure originated elsewhere.[11] The good results of published series generally outshine the hard reality of registry data. Even registries can have a bias toward better results: to qualify as a failure, a revision must be re-revised, something that may be avoided in many cases because of technical challenge or patient frailty. Few registries track amputations or fusions, so these failures may not contribute to the results. Accordingly, in the absence of reliable data, and faced with pressing clinical problems, biomechanical principles and clear thinking can reasonably drive clinical decisions.

PATIENT SATISFACTION: REASONABLE EXPECTATIONS

Patient satisfaction requires expectations for function and pain relief that can be achieved; astute and highly specific indications for surgery; superior surgical technique and a sound reconstruction that addresses the individual cause of failure; and an appropriate implant.

Patient expectations of surgery can be modified by preoperative education and rank with patient selection and surgical technique as a major determinant of outcome, specifically satisfaction. Empathetic counseling may ensure that the patient and surgeon are clear about expectations (what the patient thinks will occur) for revision surgery as distinct from desires (what the patient wishes might occur). A TKA outcomes checklist significantly improved patient satisfaction after primary TKA across multiple dimensions, emphasizing the advantages of plain communication before surgery. The major advantage was improved satisfaction with the *experience* of surgery; satisfaction with relief from pain and return to function were not, however, significantly improved.[12] A modified checklist might help manage the expectations of revision surgery, especially if the ultimate outcome is discussed.

The complex relationship between mental state and results of arthroplasty cannot be reduced to the prejudiced view that depressed or anxious individuals always have worse results. In a 2020 study, total hip and knee data were sourced from two prospective international multicenter studies with the goal of assessing the degree to which patient satisfaction changes between 1 and 3 years after arthroplasty and the factors associated with those changes.[13] Patients who had undergone TKA and who had preoperative anxiety or depression improved in satisfaction between the first and third years. Lower preoperative health states did correlate with lower satisfaction in hip and knee patients across the study period.[13] The findings regarding a low health state suggest possible continued frustration with ill health despite arthroplasty or the unrealistic expectation that arthroplasty would permit activities never really feasible because of comorbidities.

Most studies of satisfaction after knee arthroplasty identify dissatisfaction rates of about 20% as confirmed by a 2015 systematic review of 19 studies[14] and a 2018 review of 208 studies.[15]

Satisfaction With Septic Versus Aseptic Revision

Revision for PJI is perhaps the most challenging of all knee arthroplasties, requiring eradication of infection and restoration of function. More than one surgery is required for two-stage protocols, and many patients will have undergone prior failed procedures. Because patients with comorbidities and complex arthropathies are predisposed to PJI, the population facing revision is a higher risk group.

A 2007 study followed up 93 patients for 2 years after septic and aseptic revisions. Although the infected patients had (nonsignificantly) lower mental health scores before revision, postrevision scores were (nonsignificantly) higher. It can be argued that patients with PJI can benefit from revision surgery and have results similar to those of patients without infection.[16] In another study, in which an antibiotic-loaded articulating spacer system had been developed, 47 septic revisions performed with their product were compared with 55 revisions for aseptic failure. Similar postoperative mental status scores were noted between the two groups.[17] There are typical and recurrent problems outlined in articles on satisfaction (and indeed outcome) after revision for PJI. Mental health status is an important metric, but it is not identical to patient satisfaction. In addition, by only quantifying the results of patients who have PJI, who were accepted for two-stage treatment, and who then made it to a specified clinical follow-up postrevision, numerous problem cases are excluded: patients who die from PJI, those who never qualified for surgical treatment of infection, or those whose prostheses could not be reimplanted, in short, all individuals with a PJI who did not make it to the 2-year mark with a prosthesis that could be evaluated.[18] When a commitment exists to a product, it is never clear which patients might not have been considered appropriate for treatment with that device. This represents significant selection bias.[19,20]

Satisfaction After Revision Unicompartmental Knee Arthroplasty

Some types of revision, such as conversion of a failed unicompartmental knee arthroplasty (UKA) to a TKA, might be expected to have satisfactory results. However, revision of a UKA to another UKA has been abandoned.[21] In a 2016 study of failed aseptic revisions, 768 revised TKAs were compared with 578 revised UKAs. The 10-year survival rate of both revisions was similar: 82% UKA versus 81% TKA. Perhaps surprisingly, 25% of the patients with UKA revisions were dissatisfied compared with 22% of those who underwent TKA revisions.[22] It was concluded that failure of a UKA is not to be taken lightly and that it may be as difficult to achieve satisfaction as when a TKA has failed. The TKA-to-TKA revisions were more complex, included many more difficult cases (such a stiffness), and required more sophisticated implants.

Central Sensitization

Constitutional or physiologic factors outside of the knee joint clearly play a role in outcomes after TKA, including revision surgery. Central sensitization is how nociceptor inputs can trigger a prolonged but reversible increase in the excitability and synaptic efficacy of neurons in central nociceptive pathways. Central sensitization has been described as a heightened response of central nervous system neurons to nociceptive stimuli. It manifests as a reduced threshold to pain (allodynia), with an increased responsiveness and prolonged aftereffects to noxious stimuli (hyperalgesia), and a receptive field expansion that leads noninjured tissue to produce pain (secondary hyperalgesia). This is a clear, hypothetical model of the physiology of pain perception.[23]

A diagnostic questionnaire was developed to identify central sensitization and predict pain experience in patients who have undergone primary TKA. Patients with higher scores on this inventory sustained persistently higher pain scores (more pain) and significantly lower satisfaction scores after TKA.[24]

A 2019 prospective, randomized controlled trial of 464 patients who had undergone TKA identified 80 patients who met the criteria for central sensitization. Half of these received duloxetine (a selective serotonin and norepinephrine reuptake inhibitor antidepressant medication). Reduced pain and improved quality of recovery after TKA were noted in the central sensitization group treated with duloxetine.[25]

The central sensitization questionnaire was later applied to 68 patients who had undergone revision knee arthroplasty. Twenty patients (29%) could be assigned to the central sensitization group by the scores on the Central Sensitization Inventory. These patients had higher prerevision Western Ontario and McMaster Universities Osteoarthritis Index and visual analog scale pain scores that persisted after surgery. Overall satisfaction in the group without central sensitization was 91.7%; it was 15% among patients with central sensitization. Odds of dissatisfaction with revision TKA increased 39 times when patients had a diagnosis of central sensitization. The indications for revision were comparable in both groups, but the criteria for making the diagnoses were not reported[26] (**Figure 1**).

Central sensitization seems to be a patient attribute that can be identified by questionnaire, with consequences for satisfaction after surgery ostensibly independent of mode of failure, surgical technique, or implant. The implications regarding patient selection for revision surgery are important, especially in the absence of a mechanical or biologic diagnosis. If a patient is dissatisfied for reasons extrinsic to the arthroplasty, revision can only cause harm.

Satisfaction With TKA, Severity of Arthritis, and Selection for Revision

A 2020 study has confirmed that less severe arthritis before arthroplasty was associated uniformly with lower levels of satisfaction after surgery.[13] Several phenomena may explain this. Some patients may have had pain referred from other sources, such as the hip or spine, which was misinterpreted as significant knee pathology that arthroplasty would obviously not relieve. Other patients may have been trying to function, perhaps athletically, at a level that modest arthritis precluded but which arthroplasty could not support. Tolerance to pain may have been low and expectations may have been high in these patients—a recipe for dissatisfaction. The implications for patient selection before revision are profound. The patient with minimal arthropathy before knee replacement, whose problem TKA has been submitted to a systematic and comprehensive evaluation that did not explain symptoms, will not achieve satisfaction after revision. Even if problems are identified with the TKA, when minimal osteoarthritis is apparent on radiographs obtained before the primary surgery, the prospect for a successful revision is guarded.

Satisfaction With Revision: Severity of Failure and Mode of Failure

There will be a parallel to revision surgeries: less severe failures and tenuous objective evidence of failure are likely to produce poor outcomes. This is modulated by the varying levels of difficulty of resolving certain causes of failure. A study of prospectively collected patient-reported outcome measures from 23,393 primary TKAs and 797 aseptic revision surgeries at 6 to 12 months after surgery reported smaller improvements in the Oxford Knee Score and EuroQol 5-dimensional questionnaire score after revision procedures. The percentage of satisfied patients who had undergone revision surgery (66%) was lower than that of patients who had undergone primary surgery (83%). Among revisions, there were more satisfied patients when loosening or osteolysis was the cause (72%) and the fewest patients when revision was performed for stiffness (47%).[27] Even the best revision group did not approach the levels of function and satisfaction observed after primary TKA at a mean of 7 months postoperatively. Overall, 83% of those undergoing primary TKA were satisfied; 66% of the patients reported being satisfied following revision TKA.

If patients are to be informed about the outcome of revision, the diagnosis must be understood in depth. How a problem TKA is evaluated will be important. Out of necessity with such a large database in this study, only diagnosis could be considered as a variable, quality of surgery could not.

PATIENT SELECTION FOR REVISION

Evaluation of the Problem TKA

A meaningful diagnosis must be defined by specific criteria. Consensus on a process for collecting and interpreting essential information is also required. Those fundamentals

1. I feel tired and unrefreshed when I wake from sleeping.	Never	Rarely	Sometimes	Often	Always
2. My muscles feel stiff and achy.	Never	Rarely	Sometimes	Often	Always
3. I have anxiety attacks.	Never	Rarely	Sometimes	Often	Always
4. I grind or clench my teeth.	Never	Rarely	Sometimes	Often	Always
5. I have problems with diarrhea and/or constipation.	Never	Rarely	Sometimes	Often	Always
6. I need help in performing my daily activities.	Never	Rarely	Sometimes	Often	Always
7. I am sensitive to bright lights.	Never	Rarely	Sometimes	Often	Always
8. I get tired very easily when I am physically active.	Never	Rarely	Sometimes	Often	Always
9. I feel pain all over my body.	Never	Rarely	Sometimes	Often	Always
10. I have headaches.	Never	Rarely	Sometimes	Often	Always
11. I feel discomfort in my bladder and/or burning when I urinate.	Never	Rarely	Sometimes	Often	Always
12. I do not sleep well.	Never	Rarely	Sometimes	Often	Always
13. I have difficulty concentrating.	Never	Rarely	Sometimes	Often	Always
14. I have skin problems such as dryness, itchiness, or rashes.	Never	Rarely	Sometimes	Often	Always
15. Stress make my physical symptoms get worse.	Never	Rarely	Sometimes	Often	Always
16. I feel sad or depressed.	Never	Rarely	Sometimes	Often	Always
17. I have low energy.	Never	Rarely	Sometimes	Often	Always
18. I have muscle tension in my neck and shoulders.	Never	Rarely	Sometimes	Often	Always
19. I have pain in my jaw.	Never	Rarely	Sometimes	Often	Always
20. Certain smells, such as perfumes, make me feel dizzy and nauseated.	Never	Rarely	Sometimes	Often	Always
21. I have to urinate frequently.	Never	Rarely	Sometimes	Often	Always
22. My legs feel uncomfortable and restless when I am trying to go to sleep at night.	Never	Rarely	Sometimes	Often	Always
23. I have difficulty remembering things.	Never	Rarely	Sometimes	Often	Always
24. I suffered trauma as a child.	Never	Rarely	Sometimes	Often	Always
25. I have pain in my pelvic area.	Never	Rarely	Sometimes	Often	Always

FIGURE 1 A questionnaire for patients, used to diagnose central sensitization. The extent to which this differs from generalized increased anxiety is unclear. (Reprinted with permission from Mayer TG, Neblett R, Cohen H, Howard KJ, Choi YH, Williams MJ, et al. The development and psychometric validation of the central sensitization inventory. *Pain Pract* 2012;12:276e85.)

are missing with respect to the problem knee arthroplasty. Most current discussions or publications that refer to a diagnosis, such as instability, assume there is agreement on what constitutes the unstable knee replacement. However, instability in wobbly joints is often seen as secondary to loosening and bone loss; it also can be considered a case of aseptic loosening, where the causes of the problem and the solution are distinctly different from those for tibial femoral instability from ligament incompetence.

Despite the importance of modes of failure and their causes, currently no study that describes and validates a comprehensive system of modes of failure, much less the process required to assign a diagnosis, with the exception of PJI, which has been discussed extensively in the literature, exists. The most current criteria for PJI are discussed in a 2018 study.[28] These criteria, based on common clinical and laboratory data, will undoubtedly be refined (**Figure 2**).

The process by which a diagnosis of PJI might be established or excluded has been outlined in an American Academy of Orthopaedic Surgeons Clinical Practice Guideline.[29] The practicable protocol begins with establishing clinical suspicion of PJI by history and physical examination and measurement of serum inflammatory markers. According to a recent study, the alpha defensin level in synovial fluid is considered a reliable means to diagnose PJI.[30] The key messages are that PJI may be present in any problem arthroplasty and should be diagnosed before revision. It is likely that a high proportion

Major criteria (at least one of the following)	Decision
Two positive cultures of the same organism	Infected
Sinus tract with evidence of communication to the joint or visualization of the prosthesis	

Preoperative diagnosis		Minor criteria	Score	Decision
	Serum	Elevated CRP *or* D-dimer	2	≥6 Infected
		Elevated ESR	1	
	Synovial	Elevated synovial *WBC count or* leukocyte esterase	3	2-5 Possibly infected [a]
		Positive alpha defensin	3	
		Elevated synovial PMN (%)	2	0-1 Not infected
		Elevated synovial CRP	1	

Intraoperative diagnosis	Inconclusive preoperative score *or* dry tap [a]	Score	Decision
	Preoperative score	-	≥6 Infected
	Positive histology ?frozen section?	3	4-5 Inconclusive [b]
	Positive purulence	3	
	Single positive culture	2	≤3 Not infected

FIGURE 2 Current scoring system used to diagnose prosthetic joint infection. [a]For patients with inconclusive minor criteria, operative criteria can also be used to fulfill definition for PJI. [b]Consider further molecular diagnostics such as next-generation sequencing. CRP = C-reactive protein, ESR = erythrocyte sedimentation rate, PMN = polymorphonuclear leukocyte, WBC = white blood cell. (Reprinted from *J Arthroplasty* 33[5]. Parvizi J, Tan TL, Goswami K, et al. The 2018 Definition of Periprosthetic Hip and Knee Infection: An Evidence-Based and Validated Criteria, 1309-1314e2. © 2018, with permission from Elsevier Inc.)

of undiagnosed infections were revised as aseptic failures in the past, wasting the expensive revision procedure.

In the absence of similarly rigorous definitions for mechanical modes of failure and a uniform protocol for investigation, discussion by experts can be helpful.[31] Studies have focused on the problem of pain in knee arthroplasty.[32] One scheme includes a prerevision data collection worksheet, focusing on standard information from history, clinical examination, laboratory findings, and imaging studies (**Figure 3**) to assign failures to eight diagnostic categories that cover most problem arthroplasties. The emphasis is on a systematic (the same algorithm for each patient) and comprehensive (consideration of all modes of failure even if one is established) evaluation as there may be more than one problem in any arthroplasty. The stiff TKA, for example, may also be infected.[33] A conservative, nonsurgical approach to evaluation is recommended when a detailed explanation for the patient's experience is missing.[34]

Radiographs

The standard radiographic evaluation of the problem TKA includes a single-leg weight-bearing AP view, lateral projection, patellofemoral views, and full-length bilateral weight-bearing studies that show the hip, knee, and ankle together. Imaging of the spine and hips may also be included. Fluoroscopic images have long been used to evaluate TKAs, and a recent study supported the use of fluoroscopic images in the diagnosis of loosening.[35]

CT and MRI

CT is the preeminent method to quantify rotational positioning of implants in the problem TKA. Although new methods have been proposed to measure rotation

	DIAGNOSIS	Patient:		Implant type:					Note	Y/N
1	Prosthetic Joint Infection	Clinical Suspicion: Y / N Erythema: Swelling: Drainage: SINUS TRACT:*		ESR ( ) CRP ( )	Asp. WBC(<2500) Asp. Diff (<50%)	% PMN	Culture1: Culture2: subcult.	at surgery: pus: Y / N wbc/hpf:	MSIS Criteria Sinus Tract 2 Pos Cultures	
2	Loose	Subside	RadLuc.	BoneScan	Fluoro	Mech axis: o var/val Kennedy Zone:		CT RadLuc / Osteolysis Femur:	Tibia:	
3	Fracture	XR AP fem:	XR AP tib:	XR Lat fem:	XR Lat tib:	XR Lat Patella:	XR Merchant:	CT Fracture: Tib/Fem/Pat		
4	Prosthesis Breakage	Grinding: Y / N		Instab: Y / N		X-Ray: : Y / N		CT Breakage: Tib/Fem/Pat		
5	Extensor Insufficiency	Extensor lag:	PalpDefect:	InsallSalvati:	Avulsed from:	PatFract:	QuadsRupt:	CT Rotation Femur	Tibia	
6	Stiff	ext-flexion	ipsi-hip OK?			tibial slope: femoral size: fem flex/ext: pat thick:		o in/ex TOTAL (fem + tib IR)	o in/ex	
7	Patella & malrotation	Maltrack Y/N	Tilt degrees	Displacement	Pat. Comp					
8	Tibial-femoral instability	VarusValgus Instability arc: Full extension: ° Flexed 30deg: ° End point: Y / N		Flexion Instability Drawer mm Piston @90 mm		Recurvatum var/val Kennedy Zone:				
9	Reoperation- No Revision	Popliteus Impingement: Painful Snap: Y / N	Overhang: Y / N	Low Demand Patient Poly Wear:						
10	No diagnosis-No Surgery	AP pelvis	LS-Spine	BoneScan	RSD	Pre TKA XR: K-L Grade OA:				

FIGURE 3 Worksheet for diagnosis and data collection before revision knee arthroplasty. Modes of failure 1-8 are strong indications for surgery. Number 9 includes conditions that might benefit from surgery but not revision (eg, popliteus tendon impingement). When inadequate data are available to confirm any of 1-9, surgery should be deferred, and additional investigations for sources of referred pain, chronic regional pain syndrome, and inappropriate indications for primary arthroplasty are considered.

on CT scans, the original protocol continues to be reliable and relevant.[36]

CT is also useful to evaluate osteolytic bone defects before revision. Although static mechanical alignment can be reconstructed using CT, these supine studies are less useful in the evaluation of tibiofemoral instability. Single-photon emission computed tomography may be useful in diagnosing loosening and patellofemoral problems.[37] Scintigraphy alone is generally regarded as nonspecific for PJI or loosening.[38]

MRI has not been central to evaluation of the problem TKA because of interference from implants. A 2020 systematic review of 15 studies addressing MRI evaluation of the problem TKA concluded that advanced MRI can be used to diagnose infection, loosening, wear, and malalignment after TKA, but studies on the diagnosis of instability, arthrofibrosis, or patellofemoral complaints using MRI are limited and inconclusive.[39] The role of MRI is likely to increase as the technology improves.

Selection of Patient, Technique, and Implant

An organized evaluation of the problem TKA is necessary to determine whether revision is appropriate for an individual and to identify the causes of failure that require correction. Accordingly, both patient and technique must be selected for surgery. Evaluations that begin with the question "what implant is required?" are generally asking the wrong question. The type of failure and underlying causes are more important. It is important to review revision surgery for specific modes of failure, including the prevalent technical challenges for a particular mode.

SURGICAL TECHNIQUES: SPECIFIC TO DIAGNOSIS

Periprosthetic Joint Infection

Infection is prominently a biologic failure of TKA that increases costs, complexity, and complications. Data from a 2020 study show that the rates for blood transfusion, postoperative complications, and in-hospital mortality (P = 0.0001) were higher after revisions for PJI ($P < 0.0001$). Length of stay was longer for patients undergoing revision for septic failure ($P < 0.0001$).[40] Mortality is increased after revision for infection or fracture in both the short and long term.[41]

Major current issues include the efficacy of surgery without prosthesis removal and whether, if this fails, subsequent treatments are compromised.[42-44] Single-stage revision and two-stage revision protocols are both used for selected cases of PJI. The literature comparing these strategies is difficult to evaluate because of researcher bias and inconsistent criteria for patient selection. The clinical problem is fraught with innumerable variables, to the point where far more sophisticated methods of analysis have been proposed to resolve issues of patient selection, efficacy, and cost.[45-47]

Aseptic Loosening

Osteolysis

Osteolysis is a powerful biologic factor contributing to aseptic loosening, but the technical challenges of an arthroplasty with failed fixation are structural. Loosening typically presents several years after implantation and results from the generation of (mainly) polyethylene wear particles that incite osteolysis and bone loss. Most cases of aseptic loosening result from osteolysis, and the technical problems in revising a loose prosthesis and one affected by osteolysis (usually loose) are similar.[48]

Loosening was originally seen as a mechanical problem and the main impediment to workable knee replacements. The solution to loosening evolved as some unspecified amount of valgus TKA alignment. The relevance of a precisely neutral mechanical axis (a straight line from the hip through the knee to the ankle) has been challenged.[49] This coincides with new ideas about arthroplasty alignment that prioritize soft-tissue tension and the patient's personal knee alignment before arthroplasty over surgical correction. Whether prearthritic alignment is constitutional or pathologic (a contributing factor to arthritic degeneration of cartilage and wear of an arthroplasty) is controversial.[50] Although variations in alignment within limits may not be important for most successful TKAs, malalignment is often important in TKAs that fail.

Numerous factors contribute to aseptic loosening from osteolysis. Varus alignment and medial load patterns are observed in most cases. Wear from the undersurface of modular tibial polyethylene implants (backside wear) is probably the major source of the small and most active particles contributing to osteolysis. This phenomenon is likely more significant in posterior-stabilized arthroplasties and may explain marginally higher failure rates with these designs across all manufacturers.[51] The cam-spine mechanism shunts the tibial insert in the locking mechanism with each flexion cycle, abrading the nonarticular side of the polyethylene, with the greatest wear in the areas of greatest load (medial). Modular implants with older polyethylene production and sterilization methods, nonrigid locking mechanisms, and more abrasive metal surfaces will be at greatest risk. Improved polyethylene and better designs reduce wear particle production in TKA.

Debonding

It is possible that the metal tibial tray might debond from the cement mantle during aseptic loosening, suggesting that pain may result from a lack of adhesion between the two structures. Some very successful hip implants are designed specifically to allow the femoral prosthesis to subside unbonded into the cement mantle.[52]

Most case series have identified early painful failure of specific implant designs without objective diagnostic findings. Revisions performed on speculation were associated with a finding of a tibial tray that could easily be extricated from the cement mantle.[53] It is difficult to know whether debonding might be present in many satisfactorily functioning arthroplasties; cement viscosity may be a factor. The association of one popular high-viscosity cement with slightly higher rates of revision for aseptic failure does not prove the debonding mechanism.[54] An argument has been made that mechanical loosening without increases in inflammatory markers, that is, nonosteolytic loosening, presumably from debonding, is plausible.[55] The current unresolved debate surrounds specific implants and surgical techniques in addition to specific cement products. The danger to a patient with a painful arthroplasty is that debonding might be overdiagnosed without objective evidence, effectively leading to a revision for unexplained pain, which is known to yield poor results.

ASEPTIC LOOSENING—FIRST CHALLENGE: FIXATION

The first challenge in revision for loosening is restoring fixation. Most cases require fixation techniques beyond what was practiced during the primary surgery, illustrating the principle that revision surgery should never simply be a redo procedure. The quality and location of fixation must be considered. Augmented fixation typically

extends to the metaphysis or diaphysis, demonstrating the importance of revision implant systems.[56]

The description of fixation zones in a 2015 study focused attention on the standard anatomic regions of the tibia and femur where fixation is possible, suggesting reasonably that fixation should be achieved in two of the three anatomic zones for revision arthroplasty[57] (**Figure 4**). Given that epiphyseal fixation is often undependable after failed arthroplasty, only the metaphysis and diaphysis are left. It was concluded that a long intramedullary stem must be asymmetric or offset if it is to engage the diaphyseal canal and yet be centered over the tibia or femur at the joint. Epiphyseal fixation, as with primary arthroplasty, requires flat cut bone surfaces and methacrylate cement. Even then, however, quality is often compromised, with little cancellous texture for cement intrusion. Recuts to establish a flat surface may mean sacrificing good bone and attempting fixation distally where the circumference of the tibia is small and there is only cortex. Methacrylate has traditionally been used for fixation in the metaphysis; keeled primary implants depend on it. Porous metals now provide superior metaphyseal fixation for revision TKA. Precisely what constitutes reliable fixation is difficult to define. For example, press-fit diaphyseal engaging stems have been used successfully for decades, but it is not clear to what extent fixation occurs.

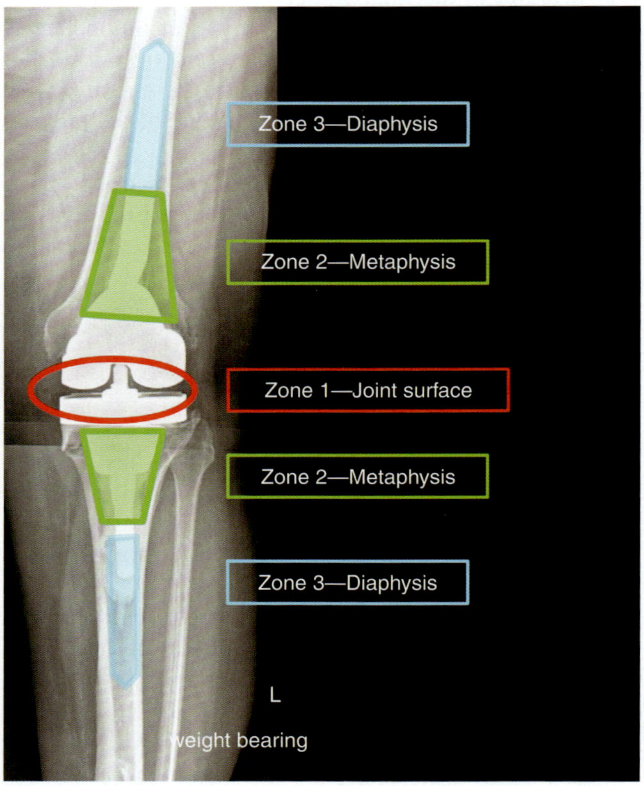

FIGURE 4 Postrevision radiograph showing zonal fixation. These zones correspond to the three anatomic regions of the long bones. In this patient, a long press-fit diaphyseal engaging stem has been used in the femur. Whether this represents solid fixation has not been established. Cement extends around the stem extension in the metaphysis of the femur and has been applied to the residual bone surface as well, but the epiphyseal surface would have been of poor quality in both the femur and tibia. A trabecular metal cone provides secure noncemented fixation to the tibial metaphysis, and a relatively narrow stem extension has been fully cemented into the tibia. A portion of this stem might be construed as diaphyseal fixation. (Reproduced with permission from Morgan-Jones R, Oussedik SI, Graichen H, Haddad FS: Zonal fixation in revision total knee arthroplasty. *Bone Joint J* 2015;97-B[2]:147-149. Copyright © The British Editorial Society of Bone and Joint Surgery.)

Fixation: Stem Extensions

Stem extensions were features of pioneering primary and revision knee prostheses. Most were fully cemented, with techniques borrowed from hip arthroplasty. Fully cemented, long-stem extensions provide solid fixation, but almost insurmountable problems for removal, especially in the presence of infection, when all cement must come out. The alternative, press-fit intramedullary stems were first associated with higher failure rates, but relatively short (metaphyseal length) and narrow stems that did not engage the endosteum were initially used. Superior results have been reported when press-fit stem extensions actually reach the diaphysis, thereby engaging the endosteum. No differences in micromotion were detected using roentgen stereogrammetric analysis when hybrid (press-fit stem) fixation was compared with fully cemented stems.[58] Failure of press-fit stem extensions has been associated with poor fit, in particular narrow diameters.[59] Press-fit stems might need to be combined with metaphyseal fixation in the form of porous metals for more challenging cases.[60] The best use of intramedullary stem extensions has not been determined, but some lessons have been learned. Extremely long, fully cemented stems are not required for durable fixation, but they cause problems during removal. Small-diameter and/or short press-fit stem extensions are associated with loosening.

ASEPTIC LOOSENING—SECOND CHALLENGE: BONE LOSS

Fixation and Bone Loss: Metaphyseal Cones and Sleeves

The problem with bone loss is not devising some structure that can be shaped to fit the defect. This is easily done with methacrylate cement, variously shaped metal blocks, or structural allograft. The problem with bone loss is fixation.[61] Furthermore, many revisions have depended on fully constrained implants in the face of significant bone loss, in cases where restoration of structure would

contribute heavily to restoration of stability. Constraint inevitably stresses fixation. Superior options, such as porous metals, that both restore damaged bone and ensure fixation should also improve surgical techniques to restore stability without resorting to linked, constrained devices.

Residual metaphyseal bone in revision knee arthroplasty is often sclerotic endosteum. Even contained defects are poorly suited for cement fixation. The first porous metal cones were construed mainly as augments to restore deficient bone. These implants were fabricated from tantalum and intended for large contained defects. They have increasingly been used for noncontained defects where part of the device sits above the level of missing bone (**Figure 5**). Most can be used with knee replacements from almost any manufacturer because they are implanted before the knee prosthesis and separate from it. Once in place, the knee prosthesis is cemented inside the cone, as if the cone were an extension of the residual tibia or femur. Anatomically shaped devices are used in the tibia and femur.[62,63] A minimum 10-year follow-up produced encouraging results, with failure due to sepsis in 3 of 32 cases (9.4%) and loosening in 5 of 32 cases (15.6%).[64] Subsequent innovations have included titanium porous devices created by three-dimensional printing.[65] Despite broad appeal, the efficacy of using porous metal cones in all revisions has been questioned, especially in consideration of cost.[66,67]

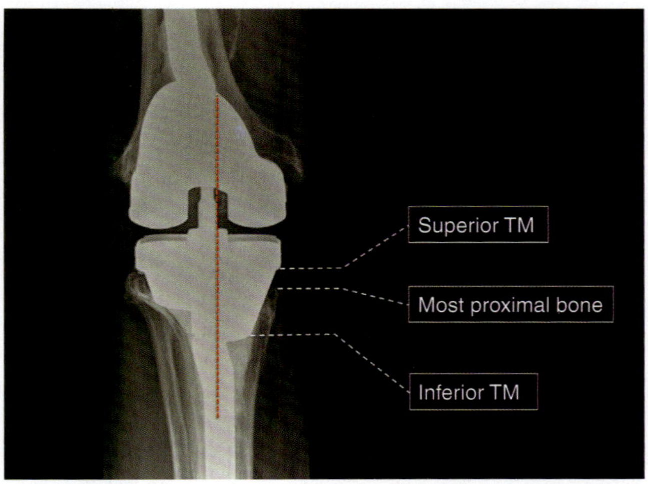

FIGURE 5 An AP radiograph of a postrevision arthroplasty, where extensive noncontained bone defects were present on the tibia. A step-shaped tibial cone has been implanted. As confidence has grown with these devices, they have been used to compensate for severe, noncontained defects as seen here, where the cone projects above the level of the residual bone surface. The dotted red vertical line indicates the tibial axis as part of a study to quantify the extent to which the cone projects above the residual tibia. Porous metal devices are not only augments to substitute for missing bone but they are also probably most useful to ensure fixation. TM = trabecular metal.

Later devices are described as sleeves because they fit directly around the revision prosthesis, functioning as part of it and often attached by Morse tapers.[68] Unlike cones, the location of the sleeve in the bone determines precisely the location of the knee replacement. Sleeves can be used in the presence of minimal bone defects, without removing large amounts of bone, primarily to aid fixation. Similar to cones, sleeves have been used successfully in revisions for septic failure.[69]

Recent attempts to evaluate both devices are fraught with difficulties,[70] mainly from inconsistent indications across clinical reports. The percentage of septic cases varies, and interpretation of bone defects is problematic. One attempt to distinguish between the loosening rates of cones and sleeves was informative but inconclusive, again because of inconsistent patient selection in studies reviewed.[71] It is impossible to compare these results with those of historical control patients because of the vagaries of past reporting on revision TKA.

The commonly used classification system for bone defects is problematic, and attempts are underway to develop more practical treatment-based systems to describe bone defects in failed TKAs.

ASEPTIC LOOSENING—THIRD CHALLENGE: ALIGNMENT

Every device intended to improve fixation and restore bone structure (stems, sleeves, cones, etc) has implications for alignment. Knee alignment has significance for load transfer, fixation, and stability. In turn, all implants that mechanically enhance joint stability have increased requirements for robust fixation.

Frontal plane (varus-valgus) stability affects the load transfer function of alignment because stability limits variations in alignment. The unstable arthroplasty undergoes an arc of alignment angles, always the worst alignment for the loading pattern. An unstable TKA loaded in varus assumes its maximum varus alignment. Published studies of alignment typically do not report data on knee stability. Static alignment is less relevant than alignment under load. If new ideas about TKA alignment technique (kinematic alignment) based on soft-tissue tension and anatomy limit deformity under load, then stability will exert a salutary effect on alignment and fixation.

The classic concern, albeit from data based on short radiographs, has been that preoperative varus deformity is a risk factor for failure due to loosening, especially if undercorrected at arthroplasty, and that valgus deformity is a risk factor for tibiofemoral instability and patellar maltracking.[72] Simple biomechanical calculations confirm that increasing knee varus increases medial

compartment load. Correspondingly, valgus increases tension in the medial collateral ligament. Instrumented TKAs demonstrate that the medial compartment bears more compressive load than the lateral compartment during most activities.[73] Increased varus angulation is associated with increased medial load.[74] If loosening results from osteolysis, osteolysis results from wear, and wear results from load, then alignment should reasonably be considered in revision TKA to reduce medial load. In addition, if fixation is compromised in the revision arthroplasty, simple nonosteolytic mechanical loosening may ensue if medial loads are multiplied by varus deformity.

How much varus alignment is dangerous is yet to be determined. If a prosthesis has failed from aseptic loosening with medial subsidence, whatever the prefailure varus alignment was, it should be reduced.

Target Alignment

If there is no consensus on target alignment among surgeons performing revision knee arthroplasty, the efficacy of new techniques to guide implant position and ensure accurate alignment will be difficult to assess. Several strategies for frontal plane alignment in revision TKA are possible. Repeating the alignment of the failed arthroplasty, especially if it has failed from loosening, seems to ignore a potential cause of failure. Aligning at revision to some version of the patient's native alignment, if it could be calculated from the contralateral limb or prearthroplasty images, seems to pose similar risks of failure, unless the primary arthroplasty was aligned at an angle quite different from the original anatomy (eg, a patient with neutral alignment whose TKA was implanted in varus and failed). The most common strategy is to align every revision to an arbitrary axis, usually a neutral mechanical axis. For many patients with constitutional varus, this would represent slight overcorrection into valgus and might benefit the revision by unloading the medial side. The same strategy might not be as beneficial to the patient whose TKA has failed because of valgus instability. The current techniques of kinematic alignment where implants are oriented to restore desired soft-tissue tension could be precarious in clinical situations where the soft-tissue environment may be compromised, resulting in bizarre alignments.

Means to Achieve Alignment

A study was proposed in 2014 to evaluate computer-assisted revision surgery, in terms of implant position. The proposal did not define target alignment, stating only that results would be compared with those of conventional surgical techniques. No data have been published from this study as of mid 2020. Patient-specific instruments seem to have been limited to revision of failed unicompartmental arthroplasties, where some anatomic landmarks persist.[75]

Periprosthetic Fracture

Supracondylar femur fractures are the most common periprosthetic fractures complicating TKA. Most patients are best treated with open reduction and internal fixation. Revision TKA is preferred for very distal fractures using conventional stemmed implants if possible. A recent study from a center that pioneered the development of large structural allograft reconstruction compared experiences with allograft-implant composites, standard revision implants, and distal femoral arthroplasty prosthesis. These comparisons are hampered by patient selection bias. Nevertheless, these experienced surgeons noted less surgical time with standard revision implants and distal femoral arthroplasty prosthesis and comparable results at 6-month follow-up. Distal femoral replacement is an expensive but time-efficient option in the hands of an experienced surgeon, and it is used more often for difficult supracondylar fractures above TKA.[76] This is a salvage option and may also be used with trepidation for failed implants because of loosening when osteolysis or multiple revisions have destroyed large amounts of distal femoral bone. Many patients with periprosthetic fracture will also have sustained extensive bone weakening because of osteolysis. According to a 2020 study of long-term results of distal femoral arthroplasty prosthesis, the incidence of revision and revision surgery was high.[77]

Prosthesis Breakage

Loosening, periprosthetic fracture, and implant breakage are structural rather than kinematic failures and are related to osteolysis and bone loss. Instances of total knee prosthesis breakage because of poor design, material, or manufacturing are now rare. Even catastrophic polyethylene failure, more common with earlier designs, is seen infrequently. Metal baseplates rarely break, unless polyethylene inserts wear through first, creating abundant debris and eventually a metal-on-metal articulation.[78] The contemporary record is limited to case reports. Most implants that break only do so when the supporting bone has been lost to osteolysis.[79]

Fracture of the tibial spine in posterior-stabilized implants is unusual after normal function; estimates are 0.52% and attributed by some to cross-linked polyethylene, which has superior wear characteristics but may be susceptible to breakage.[80] Most that break are in knees with recurvatum, such that the most distal edge of the femoral trochlear groove impinges on the anterior portion of the base of the polyethylene spine. This can result from poor surgical technique, quadriceps insufficiency requiring a back-kneed gait, or subsidence of a loose femoral implant. Recurvatum may be relative: the knee joint may not hyperextend, but the implants will hyperextend with respect to each other, if the tibial implant is with excess posterior slope and the femoral implant is in a flexed position (**Figure 6**).

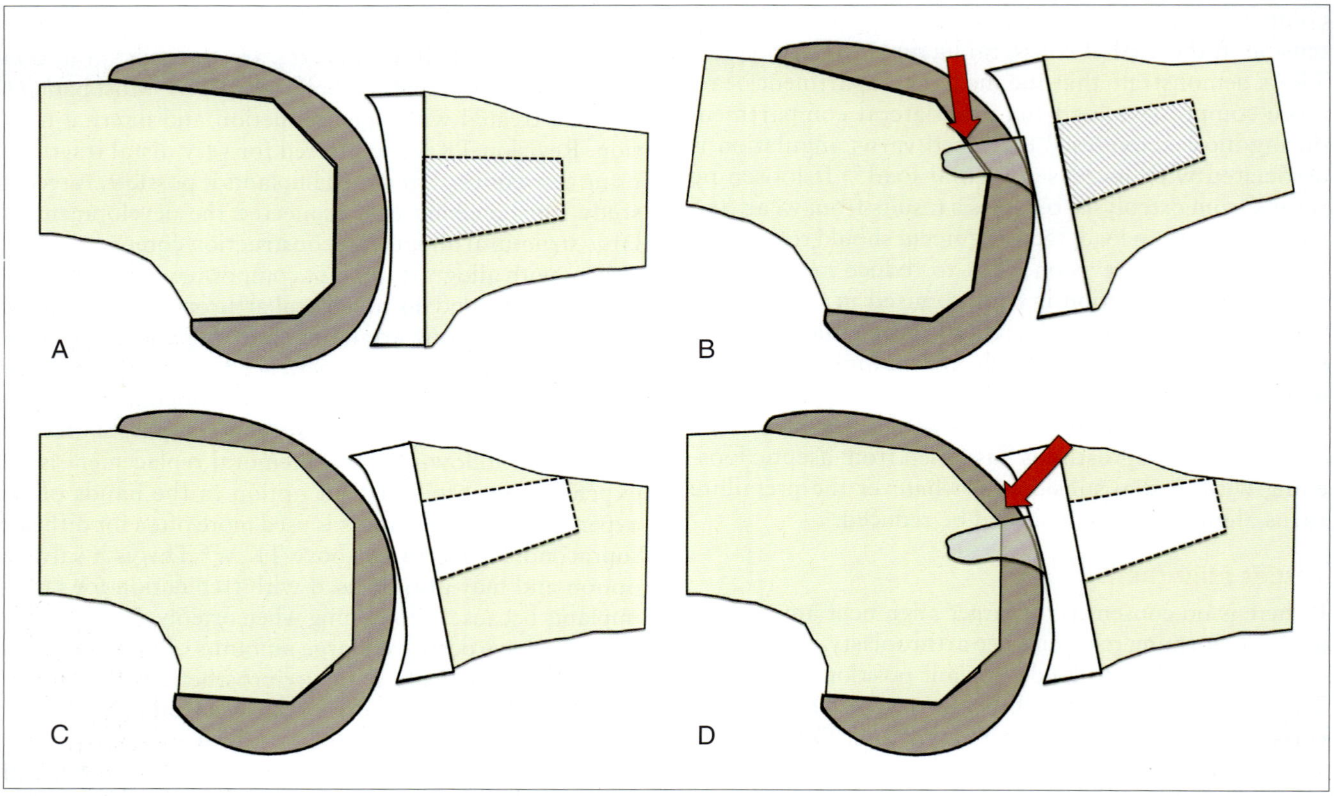

FIGURE 6 Schematic lateral views of a total knee arthroplasty (TKA). **A**, TKA is in full extension, with implants satisfactorily positioned in the sagittal plane. **B**, TKA with suitable femoral implant flexion and tibial slope but in a joint that hyperextends, usually because of ligamentous laxity, specifically the posterior structures. This is a frequent response to extensor mechanism weakness and a back-kneed gait; a tibial spine from a posterior-stabilized implant will be at risk of fracture, where the trochlear edge strikes the anterior post (arrow). **C**, Increased flexed position of the femoral implant relative to the femur and increased posterior slope of the tibial implant. The soft-tissue balance in extension is such that a cruciate-retaining implant is unlikely to be affected. The increased tibial slope may contribute to other problems, such as flexion instability. **D**, Increased flexed position of the femoral implant relative to the femur and increased posterior slope of the tibial implant becomes problematic for posterior-stabilized devices. Although the knee may not hyperextend, the implants are relatively hyperextended with respect to each other, placing the tibial spine in jeopardy as its anterior base will strike the leading edge of the trochlea in full extension (arrow), which may lead to breakage of the spine. In the absence of this effect, tibial spine failure is rare.

When prosthetic posterior condyles break from fatigue failure, it is generally at the transition from distal to posterior curves. The mechanism is inevitably loss of fixation and osseous support of the prosthetic condyle, with a femoral implant that is otherwise well fixed. This mechanism was originally described to explain femoral implant loosening (**Figure 7**).

Mechanical constraint increases load on implants and would be expected to result in more broken implants. Again, this risk increases when implants are not supported by the bone.[81] Revision of an arthroplasty where the implants have been broken requires the same analysis of causation as previously discussed. Given the importance of structural support for implants, elimination of the factors responsible for osteolysis will be key to the successful revision. Recurvatum is similarly destructive. When it occurs as the result of extensor mechanism insufficiency, arthrodesis might logically be considered.

Extensor Insufficiency

Extensor mechanism problems are common in knee arthroplasty but do not always result in revision arthroplasty or repeat surgery. Maltracking is a distinct problem that requires evaluation of the rotational position of implants. Failure of the extensor mechanism to prevent spontaneous flexion or buckling during normal activities risks progressive recurvatum deformity as the patient forces the knees backward to prevent falls. Extensor insufficiency may result from complete mechanical disruption of the extensor mechanism, decreased efficiency due to patellectomy, or even relative weakness in the face of morbid obesity. When the problem is neurologic deficiency, arthrodesis may be considered, although hinged arthroplasty with specific technical considerations has been proposed (**Figure 8**).

Many cases of extensor rupture are managed with repeat surgery, not revision surgery. Close evaluation, including CT, may reveal rotational problems and

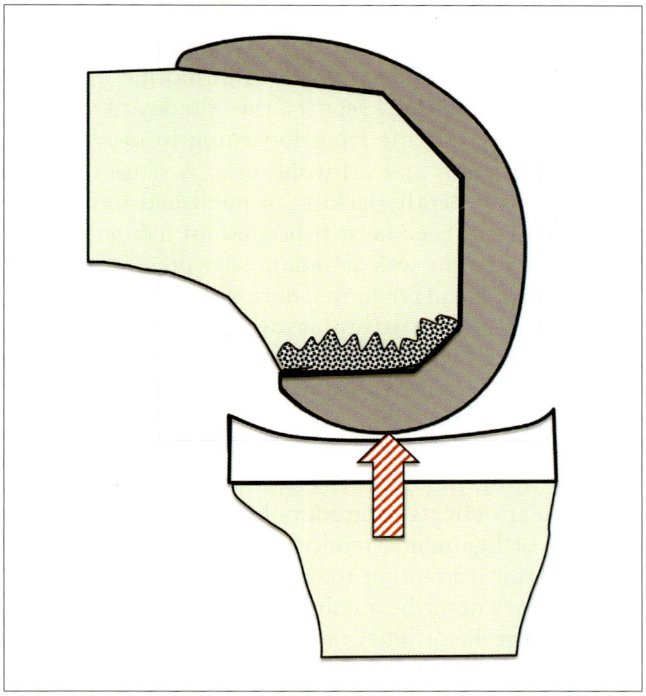

FIGURE 7 Schematic drawing shows that osteolysis forms prominently in the posterior femoral condyle. On rising from a seated position, the femoral implant is driven against the deficient bone (arrow); a common mechanism of femoral implant loosening. Failure to fit the implant or poor cementing technique could lead to the same problem. This is a common reason that posterior augmentation is required in revision total knee arthroplasty. The defects may not be obvious and surgeons may neglect to augment, leading to implantation of a small femoral implant. To balance the flexion and extension gaps with small femoral implant, additional bone will have to be resected from the distal femur, elevating the joint line. (Based upon King TV, Scott RD: Femoral component loosening in total knee arthroplasty. *Clin Orthop Relat Res* 1985;194:285-290.)

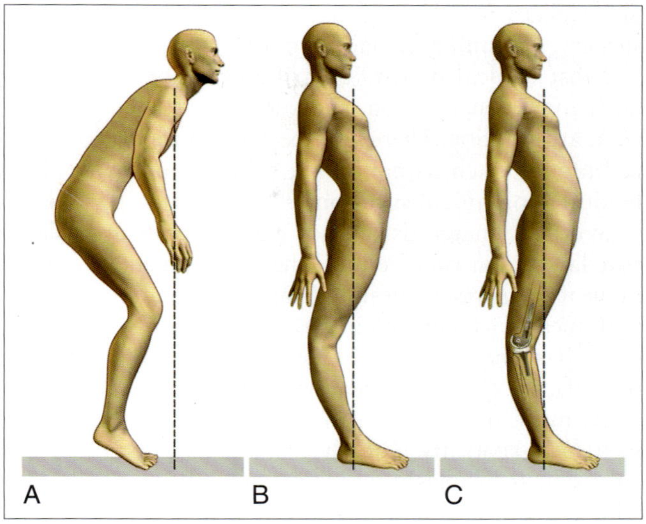

FIGURE 8 Schematic drawing illustrating how patients without functioning quadriceps may benefit for a period from a hinged arthroplasty with a hyperextension stop. **A**, If the knee is loaded when flexed, it will buckle and the patient will fall. **B**, The patient without a functioning quadriceps, as may occur after poliomyelitis, the knee must be locked in hyperextension to prevent spontaneous flexion and falling. **C**, To reproduce this effect, a knee arthroplasty must also permit some hyperextension. A hinge device can provide a "mechanical stop" or limit. Ultimately the forces of hyperextension will break the devices or the fixation. If these patients have surgery that eliminates the recurvatum that enables them to stabilize the knee, they will suffer recurrent buckling and falls. (Reprinted from *The Knee* 16[6]. Tigani D, Fosco M, Amendola L, et al. Total knee arthroplasty in patients with poliomyelitis, 501-506. Copyright © 2009, with permission from Elsevier.)

varying degrees of tibiofemoral instability that should be revised concomitantly. Disruptions may occur anywhere from the tibial tubercle to the quadriceps muscle and usually require surgery to restore function. Tibial tubercle fractures are usually amenable to open reduction and internal fixation, whereas avulsion of the distal patellar tendon, such as rupture of the tendon, generally requires substitution for the tendon. Some quadriceps tendon tears might be amenable to repair.[82]

The original description of extensor mechanism allograft reconstruction for patellar tendon rupture was a significant improvement over simple repair. The indications were expanded to disabling extensor lag in the TKA with patellectomy and previously infected TKA with tendon ruptures. Poor results have been reported, clarifying the importance of creating a disturbingly tight extensor at surgery. Disabling laxity ensues otherwise as the contracted quadriceps muscle recovers length rapidly after the procedure.

Enthusiasm for allograft reconstruction has been tempered by failure rates that predictably increase with time. The largest series, with some cases followed up to 10 years, reported 38% failures.[83] Characteristic of most reports, few cases underwent revision arthroplasty when the allograft was performed. If the cause of extensor failure is inherent in the arthroplasty itself, those flaws will persist after the allograft is placed. Most case series of allograft reconstruction describe the surgical technique and report empirical clinical outcomes, but without critical assessment of the quality of the surgery, for example, by radiographic analysis.

Case reports that describe dislocation of a constrained implant and dissociation of a tibial insert after failure of the extensor mechanism suggest that extensor mechanisms fail for a reason.[84,85] In both cases, the extensor mechanism played an inordinate role in stabilizing the joint; when it ruptured, the joint dislocated. Another report of impingement on a patellar tendon that ruptured identifies a problem in the arthroplasty beyond the vulnerability of the extensor tissue.[86] Any allograft will likely fail under these circumstances. A ruptured extensor may be the symptom of an underlying cause of arthroplasty failure that requires correction with revision surgery, not simply replacement of the ruptured tissue.

Most clinical reports describe extensor mechanism allograft reconstruction, suggesting that it became the standard solution. There have been fewer reports of other techniques, such as hamstring substitution or Achilles tendon allograft substitution.[87,88]

Synthetic materials did not play a significant role in patellar tendon rupture until the development of a technique using surgical mesh.[89] A larger population repaired with mesh was reported in 2018 by surgeons who developed the technique, showing promising results. Of the 77 patients, the quadriceps tendon had ruptured in 27 (35%) (a site more amenable to surgery) and the patellar tendon in 40 (52%) patients. Notably, 59 of 77 patients (77%) had a revision arthroplasty at the time of mesh reconstruction, which may be an important difference over earlier studies. At 2 years, 65 of 77 patients (84.4%) were still in place and functional. Also important to note is that in 10 of 77 patients (13%), the mesh reconstruction was used for patellar fractures.[90] Although disruption of the extensor mechanism through the patella implies that open reduction and internal fixation might be indicated, it has been shown that this complication is best addressed as a ruptured extensor because open reduction and internal fixation is associated with a high rate of serious complications.[91,92]

Mesh reconstructions have been used successfully during two-stage reimplantations for PJI.[93] A multicenter Canadian study reviewed 27 cases comparing synthetic reconstruction with allografts. Superior results were found in the synthetic group, at substantially less cost.[94] Published case series of mesh reconstruction are enthusiastic about the potential of this technique. A 2019 meta-analysis concluded that there were no significant differences in overall failures, infections, functional outcomes, or revision reconstructions between allograft and synthetic material extensor mechanism reconstructions.[95] Another systematic review arrived at similar conclusions, observing that more mesh reconstructions were performed concurrent with a revision arthroplasty. The advantages of synthetic reconstruction included lower cost, better availability, lack of disease transmission, and potential reduction of the (hypothetical) graft stretchout.[96]

Stiffness Challenge: Exposure

Satisfactory results are difficult to achieve with revision of the stiff TKA. When an arthroplasty has not had normal flexion in months, there is no alternative to surgery that is likely to improve motion. No strict definition exists as to what constitutes stiffness: some series have used thresholds in degrees of motion, whereas others have allowed patients to define when they are dissatisfied with motion. Stiff knees generally have poor flexion, but inability to fully extend may be part of the clinical picture, with or without pain.

A recent review searched only for article titles including the word 'stiffness' but not the word 'stiff'.[97] Most studies reported modest increases in motion and pain relief. Across published reports, the etiology of stiffness is speculative, ranging from loosening to overstuffing to scar formation and arthrofibrosis. A sense of cause and effect is generally lacking in published series: Has an arthroplasty become stiff because of formation of a pathologic scar, or was abundant scar present in a stiff TKA because it had not moved normally in many months? If some perfect knee arthroplasties become stiff because of a pathologic formation of collagen scar (arthrofibrosis), they logically should not be revised, as the dominant biology will scar the revision. For the rest, some mechanical impediment to motion exists, which can be improved at revision. By the time the TKA has become stiff, there will be secondary effects from immobility such as profound scarring of ligaments, tendons, and muscles that will require surgical attention and may not recover adequately.

Few series describe a coherent technical strategy for resolution of the primary mechanical causes of stiffness and the secondary biologic results of stiffness. An extensive evaluation and comprehensive surgical procedure will be necessary, as described in a 2018 protocol for management of the stiff TKA, where complete implant revision produced the best results.[98]

Almost any aspect of the primary arthroplasty that induces pain may result in poor motion. This includes malrotation of tibial and/or femoral implants that may not be apparent without CT. A less specific strategy may be effective: release of all scars, to the point of rendering the joint unstable, then revision with mechanically constrained implants to restore stability. This explains the appeal of constrained implants in revisions for stiffness.[99] A 2019 study compared revision of the stiff knee using a nonlinked constrained implant to that achieved with a rotating hinge. A hinged-type prosthetic device was selected in cases with collateral ligament disruption, limited remaining bone stock, and a severe gap imbalance. Better results were observed in the hinge group, and this type of device was recommended to revise the stiff TKA.[100]

Patella Complications Related to Malrotation

Several types of patellar complications can be linked together, as the surgical corrections involve similar techniques for each. The association between implant malrotation, especially internal rotation of the tibial implant, and maltracking has been recognized since the mid 1980s. Because revision surgery was considered difficult in the early days of arthroplasty, early solutions were limited to soft-tissue reconstructions (proximal realignment) or tibial tubercle osteotomies, as might be appropriate in the native knee. Maltracking predisposes to patellar fracture, especially vertical fracture, where the prosthesis is confined to the trochlear groove and yet the patella bone tends to dislocate. The technical problem of patellar maltracking is certainly multifactorial, and successful revision must correct everything that drives the patella out of the femoral groove.

The classic scenario of an internally rotated tibial and/or femoral implant contributing significantly to patellar maltracking and dislocation still stands. Internal rotation of the tibial implant relative to the tibial tubercle is likely with nonasymmetric baseplates when the larger posteromedial tibial plateau is covered or if the implant is aligned with the posterior cortex. Because the extensor attachment is directly in front of the center of the tibia and most surgical exposure is from the medial side, malposition of the tibial implant medial to the extensor can easily occur. Because most contemporary tibial articular surfaces are relatively conforming, the femoral implant sits in a predetermined position in the articular wells of the tibia. If the tibial implant has been internally rotated, the tubercle is accordingly displaced laterally, relative to the tibial implant and the femoral trochlear groove, leading to maltracking, subluxation, and even patellar dislocation.

As with the native knee, if the extensor has been dislocated chronically, the quadriceps muscles will be contracted. Restoring the shortened extensor to the trochlear groove will limit flexion. The short, tight extensor tends to seek the dislocated position: a shorter distance from the tibial tubercle to the origin of the quadriceps. Rotationally nonconstrained implants, such as rotating hinges, may allow the extensor to spin the tibia externally with flexion, re-creating the effect of an internally rotated tibial implant. Rotational constraint, though rarely regarded as beneficial, may be instrumental in keeping the tibial tubercle aligned with the femoral trochlear groove after revision.

Otherwise unexplained anterior knee pain has been associated with internal rotation of the tibial implant as well as stiffness.[101] Revision for pain associated with malrotation can be highly successful if a disciplined prerevision evaluation is combined with CT. Implant malrotation causes the knee to bend during normal function; if the implant has been implanted with laxity, the tibia is likely to rotate and the patella will dislocate. If the implant is implanted with the soft-tissue envelope relatively tight, malrotation is likely to result in pain and stiffness.

Skepticism is appropriate before dismissing the significance of malrotation in TKA.[102] The ultimate effect of rotational position depends on implant design, the general tightness of the knee, and patient expectations. Skepticism is also appropriate when citing minimal amounts of malrotation as a legitimate indication for revision. The precise threshold at which a benefit can be expected from revision is unknown.

Tibiofemoral Instability

True tibiofemoral instability is a distinct mode of failure, resulting from soft tissues disruption or malposition of implants that leaves the soft tissues ineffective. From the perspective of the patient who has undergone TKA, instability is a nebulous symptom; knee joints can give way, buckle, or collapse for many reasons. The symptom of instability (or giving way) is very much like pain; it may accompany any mode of failure. A periprosthetic femur fracture creates instability but would never be diagnosed primarily as a case of instability. Similarly, the grossly loose implant with bone loss will be unstable but is constructively revised as a case of loosening. The dislocating patella renders the knee unstable, but the problem is best solved with correction of rotational positioning and other factors that lead to maltracking. Ultimately any problem, through the mechanism of pain inhibition, may lead the quadriceps to buckle and the patient to experience instability.

Given the equilibrium nature of stability, there are destabilizing as well as stabilizing forces to consider in every unstable TKA. The solution to instability may involve managing the lever arm across the joint as much as restoring ligaments or using mechanical constraint. Valgus malalignment, for example, may be a potent deforming force in cases of valgus instability that needs correction at the time of revision. Ligament reconstruction without revision for TKA instability has long been regarded as misguided because causative factors are not addressed; this strategy should be resisted in most cases.

Given the ease with which ligament function can be substituted by constrained devices and how easily soft-tissue tension can be restored by changing implant size and position, revision for instability should yield the best results of all revisions, if the surgery is properly planned and executed.[103] Instability invariably results from technical errors of malalignment and soft-tissue handling.[104]

Frontal plane instability, most commonly into valgus, is the more common type of instability in published series. The defining issues are usually valgus malalignment and medial collateral ligament incompetence.

CLINICAL SERIES OF REVISION FOR INSTABILITY

A study of revisions for instability in 68 patients reported that all patients had laxity to subjective clinical testing: isolated coronal instability in 31 (45%), isolated flexion instability in 8 (12%), and combined instability in 29 (43%).[105] Cases of secondary instability, such as aseptic loosening, were appropriately excluded. The details of revision prosthesis selection are noted, but little information regarding surgical technique or why the arthroplasty became unstable is provided. Failure, in 22% of cases, was defined as persistent instability or pain and was associated with partial revisions, isolated polyethylene insert exchanges, and overdiagnosis of instability as an explanation for pain.

Flexion Instability

Flexion instability has become an important topic in revision knee arthroplasty, with dramatic increases in the numbers of revision cases and inconsistency in reporting. Instability in flexion was first described for arthroplasties with cruciate-retaining geometry and eventually for posterior-stabilized implants. The posterior-stabilized spine and cam would be expected to provide stability, except that this mechanism does not engage until 70° or more of flexion in most designs. For normal gait and stair or hill descent, the femoral implant moves across the tibial articular surface like a cruciate-retaining knee. The fundamental issue in this mode of instability is a flexion gap that is larger and more lax than the extension gap. If the modular polyethylene insert is selected to achieve full extension, there will be laxity in flexion. These patients initially perform extremely well, achieving above-average flexion, but periarticular tenderness, recurrent effusions, and aversion to stairs and inclines develop. Although the issue is instability in flexion, the functional range when this becomes apparent is the middle range of flexion, during gait (**Figure 9**). The term midflexion instability has been used recently, without distinction from the original description of flexion instability.

A 2014 study described a surgical algorithm for revisions of flexion instability[106] (**Figure 10**). Technical factors contributing to flexion instability were identified and the corrections resulting from revision surgery, as well as clinical outcome, were quantified radiographically. Sixty cases were identified over 10 years from the retrospective review of an institutional database. The diagnosis was made by clinical criteria, and all other cases of instability were excluded (**Table 1**). Radiographs obtained before and after revision were compared. Images obtained during the primary surgery were not included. The focus was on changes resulting from revision, not restoration of normal anatomy. The instability was primarily resolved by decreasing the size of the flexion gap and/or increasing the size of the extension gap, plus reducing posterior slope. Flexion instability is described as a clinical diagnosis that can be subjective and difficult to establish. All patients reportedly had an improved Knee Society Score, and none reported effusions or persistent instability, excluding one with a PJI managed with a two-stage protocol. Three patients required a manipulation under anesthesia for stiffness after revision and presumably achieved a satisfactory result.

Recent Clinical Series on Flexion Instability

A 2015 study reported less salutary results: perceptible improvement in 26 of 37 patients revised for flexion instability.[107]

A 2016 retrospective review compared revision for flexion instability (35 cases) with results after revision for aseptic loosening (32 cases) and PJI (25 cases).[108] Although there were no group differences in Knee Society objective and satisfaction scores at final follow-up and the amount of improvement in function relative to baseline was equivalent in the three groups, the patients with flexion instability were more likely to report that their expectations were not met by revision arthroplasty, attributed in part to the higher function of the patients with flexion instability before revision.

A 2017 study arrived at similar disappointing conclusions: 45 cases revised for isolated flexion instability compared with 53 for aseptic loosening and 43 for PJI.[109] Although all groups improved on average with revision, the improvements were smallest in the flexion instability group. Higher prerevision knee function in the flexion instability group was offered as an explanation.

Patient selection in individual institutional series is difficult to assess. Although flexion instability is a clear mechanical problem, the threshold at which revision would be expected to improve patient satisfaction is unknown. If revisions are performed when flexion instability is slight, or if the diagnosis is applied to patients with unrecognized malrotation, other causes of pain, or simply those who are dissatisfied with what a knee prosthesis affords in terms of normal function, then results will be poor.

A recent comprehensive review of flexion instability considers the problem of poor results for flexion instability, a surgical problem that should be easy to solve.[110] There is a need for reproducible diagnostic criteria, improved biomechanical analysis with motion detection, objective quadriceps strength testing, and computational modeling. Although several series describe poor results, none considers that the cause of flexion instability could be incorrect or incomplete diagnosis or less than perfect revision technique.

Although true cases of flexion instability have unmistakable mechanical origins, researchers have postulated genetic differences associated with collagen and extracellular matrix production in these patients. Why such irregularities should selectively produce instability of the flexed knee is not addressed.[111]

Quantitative diagnostic criteria for flexion instability are missing, although some studies have measured displacement under load radiographically. Most series depend heavily on the clinical experience of tibial excursion anteriorly under the femur with the knee at 90°, as if the problem were identical to an anterior

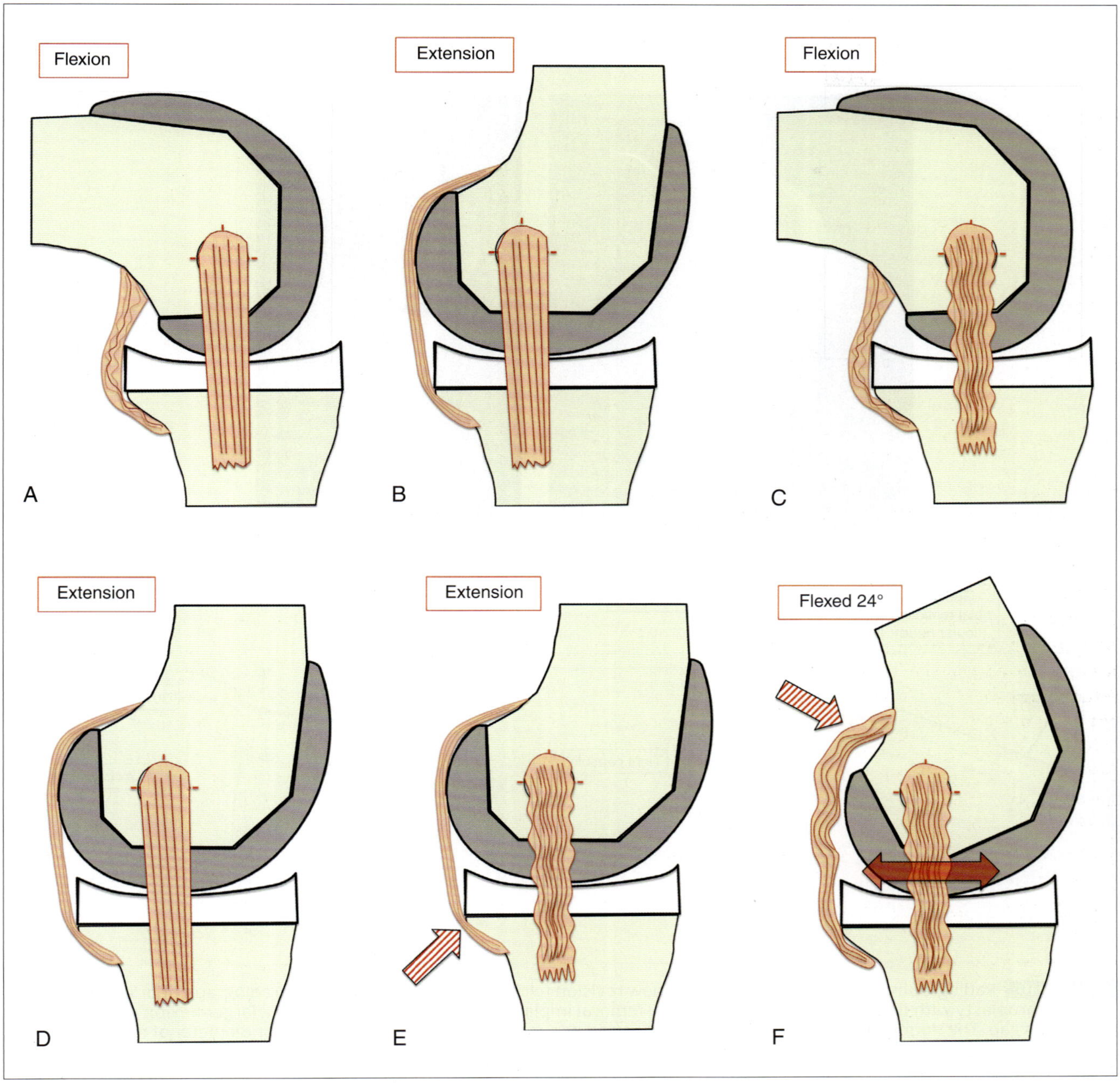

FIGURE 9 Schematic drawings show the preferred status with flexion and extension gaps balanced. **A**, Posterior capsules are relaxed in flexion to 90°, collateral ligament with some tension. **B**, In extension, posterior capsule is tight and collateral ligament under some tension, greater if hyperextension force is applied. **C**, Flexion instability: Flexion gap is more lax. Both posterior capsule and collateral ligaments are lax. The femur is able to slide anterior-posterior on tibial surface. Patient has sense of instability. **D**, Flexion instability, knee extended posterior capsule, and collateral ligaments under physiologic load. **E**, Similar situation to **D** but now collateral tension is decreased and stability in extension, even to varus-valgus loads, is provided by intact posterior capsule under physiologic load (striped arrow). **F**, Even slight flexion eliminates the tension in the posterior structures (striped arrow). Because the collaterals were never under tension, the knee feels unstable in the sagittal plane (double ended arrow), especially on stair or hill descent. The phenomenon is a knee that is unstable in mid-flexion, but it is classic collateral instability with a relatively tight posterior capsule.

cruciate ligament injury (anterior drawer test). This will not be useful, as stated, with posterior-stabilized implants.

There is consensus that the revision technique to correct flexion instability begins with reducing or eliminating excess posterior tibial slope, and increasing the size

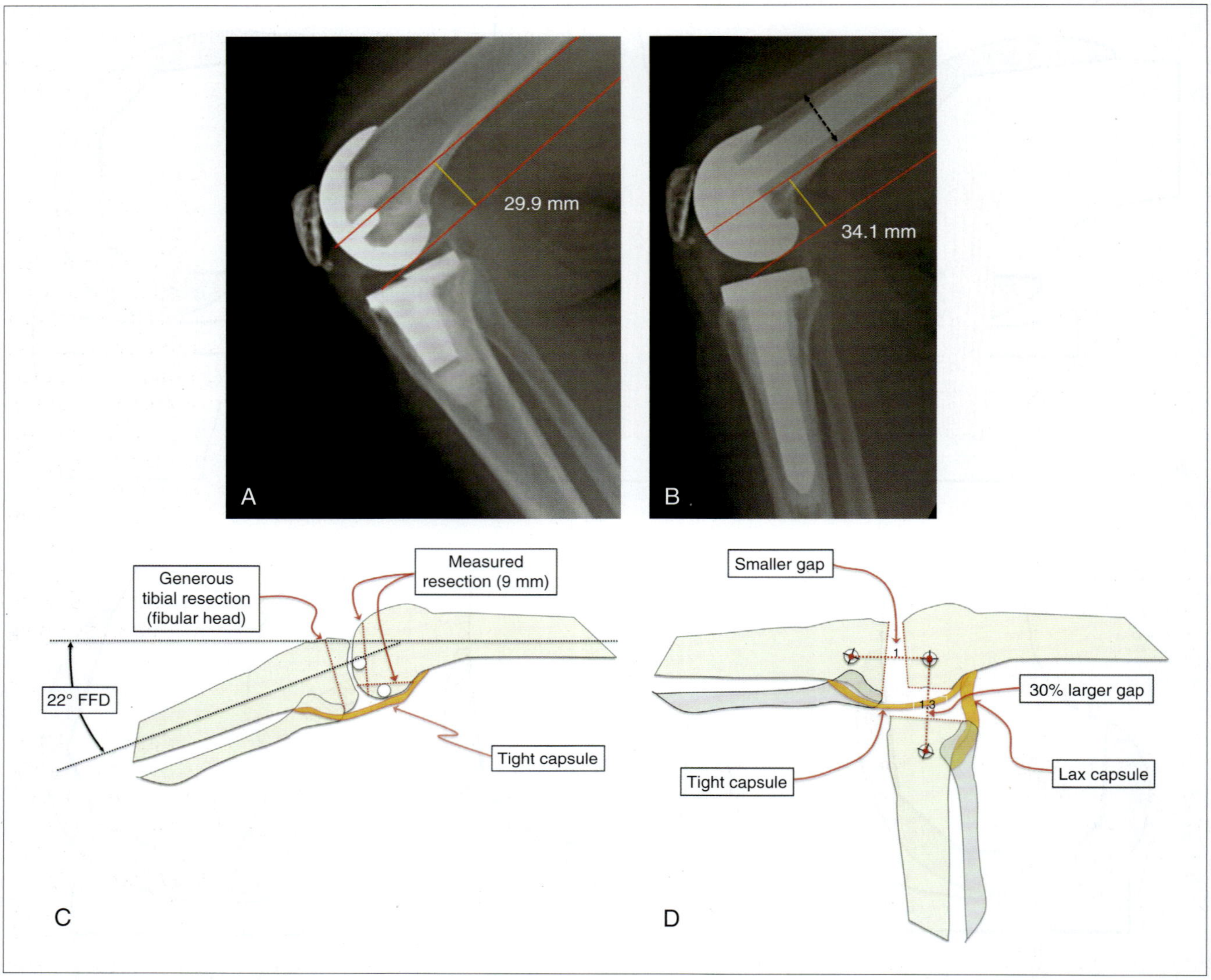

FIGURE 10 Radiographs and schematic drawings show revision for flexion instability. **A**, Lateral radiograph of primary total knee arthroplasty with flexion instability. The primary femoral implant was undersized, leading to a larger flexion gap than extension gap. The double-arrow dotted line has been added as a measure of the anterior-posterior diameter of the femoral shaft to compensate for magnification. This measurement technique later was used to define posterior condylar offset ratio. **B**, The postrevision lateral radiograph where the anterior-posterior dimension of the femoral implant has been increased, to decrease the size of the flexion gap by 4.2 mm. **C**, Schematic diagram of a lateral view of a knee unable to fully extend. The selection of a smaller femoral implant is not the only or perhaps not even the most likely cause of flexion instability. Contracted soft tissues that accompany fixed flexion deformities are frequent. Consider this case with a 22° FFD. If a measured resection or kinematic technique is used to remove a measured amount of bone equal to the thickness of the metal implants, the soft tissues, prominently the posterior capsule, will create an extension gap that is smaller than the flexion gap. It may be possible to fully extend the arthroplasty with a trial implant in place if a generous amount of bone has been removed from the tibia to the level of the fibular head. **D**, When the knee is fully extended, the tight posterior capsule limits the size of the gap in extension. The capsule will not be tight in flexion, so the gap will be defined by collateral ligament. The posterior capsule may be so contracted, which is shorter and tighter than the collateral ligaments in extension. Small amounts of flexion will relax the posterior capsule, and the knee may experience instability in the midrange. FFD = fixed flexion deformity. (A, Technique from Daluga D, Lombardi AV Jr, Mallory TH, Vaughn BK: Knee manipulation following total knee arthroplasty. Analysis of prognostic variables. *J Arthroplasty* 1991;6[2]:119-128 and Johal P, Hassaballa MA, Eldridge JD, Porteous AJ: The posterior condylar offset ratio. *Knee* 2012;19[6]:843-845. Parts A and B adapted with permission from Stambough JB, Edwards PK, Mannen EM, et al.: Flexion Instability After Total Knee Arthroplasty. *J Am Acad Orthop Surg* 2019;27[17]:642-651.)

TABLE 1

Diagnostic Criteria for Flexion Instability

History	
1	Sense of instability without the knee giving way
2	Recurrent swelling
3	Anterior knee pain
Examination	
1	Tibial translation at 90° flexion
2	Effusion
3	Soft-tissue tenderness
Exclude	
1	Varus-valgus instability at limits of extension secondary to collateral incompetence
2	Global instability
3	Infection
4	Genetic
5	Poly wear

Data from Abdel MP, Pulido L, Severson EP, et al.: Stepwise surgical correction of instability in flexion after total knee replacement. *Bone Joint J* 2014;96B[12]:1644-1648.

of the femoral implant to increase the posterior condylar offset and if that fails to restore stability to resect the distal femur to increase the size of the extension gap, which usually elevates the joint line.[106,110]

Partial Revision/Polyethylene Insert Exchange

Isolated polyethylene insert exchange has been identified as a poor solution to stiff and unstable knees. This highlights the multifactorial nature of most TKA problems and the definition of revision TKA: Is a modular exchange a revision? A 2012 study supported isolated polyethylene insert exchange for selected cases, but after limited functional assessment of postoperative outcome where failure was described as revision performed. Wear with osteolysis was considered a poor choice for isolated exchange.[112]

Another report described isolated exchange as successful in more than 90% of highly selected cases of flexion instability. The new insert was either thicker or featured a highly congruent articular geometry.[113] For a thicker insert to succeed, there must be comparable laxity in both flexion and extension, effectively establishing general laxity as the diagnosis. Greater conformity is a logical strategy. Once again, patient selection is a difficult issue in the revision arthroplasty literature.

Partial revision arthroplasty is generally less successful despite the appeal of a smaller procedure. This is generally because the implant that might be easy to revise or loose may not be the one that is responsible for the problem. As the femoral implant controls the balance between flexion and extension, isolated polyethylene insert exchange would not solve problems of flexion instability, with the possible exception of substituting a more deeply conforming polyethylene geometry in these cases.

Instability in the Plane of Motion

Instability in the plane of motion takes the form of recurvatum or spontaneous flexion (buckling). Solutions to these problems come from detailed clinical analysis and understanding of etiology. Recurvatum is usually associated with extensor insufficiency, unless it results from subsidence of a femoral implant, in which case it is the result of loosening. Strictly ligamentous causes are rare, usually associated with global instability or a flexion-extension gap mismatch where there is greater space in extension, but the polyethylene insert was selected to balance the flexion gap preferentially, a rare occurrence. Cases of multidirectional or global instability are best solved by breaking the problem down into the constituent instabilities and correcting each one. Simple recourse to a maximally constrained implant may not only seem like an expedient shortcut but also fail to identify and eliminate the underlying causes, resulting in a disappointing revision.

Revision Surgical Techniques

Many published series of revision TKA lack detailed information on surgical technique, focusing more on how the revision prosthesis was selected; other articles on stiffness and flexion instability identify the causes of failure, describing specific corrective action and analyzing radiographs to confirm whether this was accomplished. Other clinical series identify a surgical diagnosis without criteria, the implant used, a general technique, and then empirical measures of outcome. Revision surgery is not a generic process; the focus on specified corrective technique distinguishes an important development in revision surgery.

Restoration of the Joint Line

Primary implants do not include modular augments. Without posterior augments, the femoral implant must inevitably be undersized to fit the residual AP distal femur. The small femoral implant results in a large flexion gap. The corresponding loss of the bone from the distal femur might result in similar but not necessarily balanced flexion and extension gaps that thick nonmodular, tibial implants might stabilize. The joint line was usually elevated in early revisions.

Two outcomes arise from revision with nonaugmentable primary implants: poor clinical results and an elevated joint line on the AP radiograph. Radiographs demonstrate a more proximal location of the femoral implant and unusually thick polyethylene. The more severe the failure, the greater the bone loss, the higher the joint line, and the worse the result. This will be compounded by soft-tissue derangements. Many studies reported the association between elevated joint line on an AP radiograph and poor results of surgery. It will be increasingly difficult to restore radiographic features when the failure is more severe. This simple relationship evolved into a surgical technique for revision arthroplasty, reestablishing the position of the distal femoral implant on the AP radiograph, the joint line, as the guiding principle of surgery. Numerous methods have been proposed to locate the joint line.[114]

Studies on the joint line in revision knee arthroplasty have focused on distal femoral bone loss without regard for the bone lost from the posterior femur. Distal augments on a small femoral implant may improve the look of the AP radiograph, but the knee will be unstable in flexion. Augments have traditionally been construed as blocks to fill defects in the bone. These defects may not always be obvious; an augment is more accurately used to adjust soft-tissue tension by allowing more choice in implant size and position. There is also confusion in the literature about joint line elevation as opposed to patella baja, a complication resulting from contractures of the patellar tendon.

Distal Augmentation

Early attempts to link postrevision joint line position with clinical outcome were restricted to distal femoral augments. Clinical scores were higher when the postrevision joint line on a lateral radiograph changed less than 8 mm on average. There was no consideration of posterior femoral augmentation. Joint line was measured on the lateral radiograph of the tibia. Using the tibia means there can be no consideration of flexion-extension differences because the tibia is common to both gaps. The tibial articular surface may be at the perfect height, but the locations of the distal and posterior femoral surfaces respectively will determine the motion and stability in extension and flexion. All radiographic measurements are further subject to alterations in tibial slope and the vagaries of radiographic technique and osseous landmarks.

Subsequent reports generally measured joint line on AP radiographs, where aberrations are visually compelling. Measurement techniques are highly susceptible to changes in frontal alignment of the limb and individual implant positions.

Posterior Augmentation

Posterior augments are necessary to ensure fixation of a femoral implant that is sufficiently large to stabilize the flexion gap in the presence of missing bone. Restoration of flexion stability, with incidental consideration of the joint line height, is realistic and functional. If the length or tension in soft tissues has changed, the joint line level will not be relevant. Revision for poor flexion (stiffness) may require a smaller femoral implant and less tight flexion gap, whereas revision for instability requires a larger femoral implant to close and stabilize the gap. Adherence to a specific number of millimeters of posterior condylar offset ratio is less reliable.

Posterior Augments

Postoperative radiographic measurements are often correlated with longevity, but less frequently with clinical function. A 2017 review of 107 revisions for aseptic failures reported an overall rate of satisfaction of 85%, and logistic regression analysis improvement in the Oxford Knee Score ($P = 0.002$) was a significant predictor of patient satisfaction, which is related to posterior condylar offset; however, this was not independently associated with satisfaction.[115] Focusing only on one measurement misses an important point about the many technical objectives that must be satisfied for a revision to be successful, but in this case brings attention to a previously neglected variable.

Wound Care After Revision TKA

A prospectively randomized comparison of standard silver-impregnated dressings with negative pressure wound dressings in patients who have undergone revision surgery with risk factors for wound problems found better wound healing with fewer complications with negative-pressure dressings.[116]

RISK FACTORS FOR COMPLICATIONS AND FAILURE AFTER REVISION TKA

Complication rates are generally low after revision TKA but will be predictably increased by certain risk factors. Non–insulin-dependent diabetes increases the risk of numerous adverse effects, including renal failure and urinary tract infection. Insulin-dependent diabetes increased the risk of septic shock, transfusion, and extended length of stay.[117] Preoperative hyponatremia has been identified as a risk factor for infections, transfusion, pneumonia, extended length of stay, and wound problems. It is also likely to be a marker for poor health status in general. Increasingly severe renal disease predisposes to acute renal failure, return to surgery, extended length of stay, and mortality after revision TKA.[118]

A matched control study of patients with body mass index above and below 40 kg/m^2 identified more revision surgeries and re-revisions in the obese group, as well as decreased survivorship at 10 years. It is difficult to know whether this is due to a physiologic propensity to complications, such as infection, or whether obesity increased the technical difficulty of surgery such that the quality of revision reconstruction was impaired. Most obese patients are not as physically active and do not live as long as their leaner counterparts, so durability of the prosthesis might otherwise be expected to be superior.[119] Smoking predictably and sharply increases the risk of complications after revision TKA.[120]

The younger patient represents a different population of revision patients. The reasons for failure in a 2014 study of surgeries performed between 1999 and 2009 identified aseptic loosening as the more frequent cause of failure in patients aged 50 years or younger compared with PJI in patients between 60 and 70 years. Aseptic failures were more common in the younger patients, identifying that revision reconstructions, at least as performed over a decade ago, may not be sufficiently robust to withstand higher levels of activity.[121] Infection and instability predominate in another population of patients younger than 50 years, with one-third requiring further surgery after revision.[122] In a more recent review of 135 nononcologic aseptic knee revisions for sundry indications, survivorship free of revision at 10 years was 66%. Re-revisions for instability were surprisingly common.[123]

Modes of Failure After Revision TKA

In an audit of 95 failed revision knee arthroplasties, infection was identified as the main cause of failure, followed by aseptic loosening, instability, stiffness, pain, and extensor problems.[9] When stiffness is the mode of failure after revision, the procedure was generally performed because of poor motion.[124] After investigating numerous risk factors for manipulation under anesthesia after revision TKA, young age was identified as the most significant, accounting for a sixfold increase.[125] As with primary arthroplasty, infection and fixation are significant problems; if revision do not fail for these reasons, they are likely to fail for the same reasons that they were originally performed, indicating a fundamental failure to solve the underlying causes of TKA failure.

Salvage

There are cases of intractable infection, extreme bone loss, extensor rupture, and patient fragility where revision may not be feasible. None of the alternatives is particularly appealing, and they have been discussed from an ethical perspective.[126] The literature on scenarios that lead to salvage and options for intervention has been reviewed.[127] There appears to be a decline in the numbers of amputations and fusions after failed TKA, suggesting more aggressive efforts to revise problem joints.[128] Although some reports indicate poor function and higher mortality after amputation,[129] it is the most reliable way to eradicate infection in difficult cases. Arthrodesis may be preferred but is not always possible if infection cannot be eliminated.

SUMMARY

The failed knee arthroplasty places a huge burden on healthcare systems worldwide. The most common indications for revision are PJI and aseptic loosening; these are also the most common reasons that revisions fail. Patient satisfaction may be more difficult to achieve after some types of primary arthroplasty failure. Revision should not be offered on the basis of patient dissatisfaction, however, but only after a recognized cause of failure has been diagnosed with a coherent plan to solve it. Each case requires a systematic and comprehensive evaluation, recognizing that there may be more than one problem: an unstable TKA may also be infected. A disciplined approach to diagnosis of PJI is essential. The underlying cause of failure, whether biologic, structural, or kinematic, must be corrected by the revision procedure; for every case there are causes and solutions, stabilizing and destabilizing forces to be balanced, primary, and secondary effects of failure. The organized approach to the diagnosis of PJI is the most important recent advance to revision TKA. New materials and implants have led to greater success with the procedure but cannot make up for a lack of diagnostic accuracy or surgical technique.

KEY STUDY POINTS

- The literature on revision TKA is abundant and interesting but with notable exceptions of poor quality and being inconclusive, suffering from (1) patient selection bias, (2) ego bias, and (3) bias against publication of poor results.
- Revision knee arthroplasty is a formidable burden on the health care system with numbers expected to rise to unsustainable levels.
- There is neither consistency on what constitutes a revision surgery in the literature nor on the definition of modes of failure.
- The most common indications for revision arthroplasty are prosthetic joint infection and aseptic loosening.
- Accuracy of identification of mode of failure and underlying causes is essential to success of revision TKA. Prerevision diagnosis of infection requires a disciplined approach and strict definition of PJI.

ANNOTATED REFERENCES

1. Delanois RE, Mistry JB, Gwam CU, Mohamed NS, Choksi US, Mont MA: Current epidemiology of revision total knee arthroplasty in the United States. *J Arthroplasty* 2017;32(9):2663-2668.

Data from the Healthcare Cost and Utilization Project National Inpatient Sample database identified infection as the most common etiology for revision TKA (20.4%), followed by mechanical loosening (20.3%). The most common revision TKA procedure performed was all-implant revision (31.3%). The overall mean length of stay was 4.5 days, with arthrotomy for removal of prosthesis without replacement procedures accounting for the longest stays (7.8 days). Without appropriate measures in place, the burden of revision TKAs may become overwhelming and pose a strain on providers and institutions.

2. Koh CK, Zeng I, Ravi S, Zhu M, Vince KG, Young SW: Periprosthetic joint infection is the main cause of failure for modern knee arthroplasty: An analysis of 11,134 knees. *Clin Orthop Relat Res* 2017;475(9):2194-2201.

   New Zealand Joint Registry data identified PJI and aseptic loosening as the two most common forms of TKA failure. The risk of revision or revision surgery for PJI was 2.0% and aseptic loosening was 1.2%. PJI was the dominant reason for failure during the first 15 years after primary TKA. Aseptic loosening became more important with longer follow-up. Level of evidence: III.

3. Schwartz AM, Farley KX, Guild GN, Bradbury TL Jr: Projections and epidemiology of revision hip and knee arthroplasty in the United States to 2030. *J Arthroplasty* 2020;35(6 suppl):S79-S85.

   The incidence of revision TKA is projected to increase, particularly in young patients and for infection. Given the known risk factor profiles and advanced costs, revision-specific protocols will be useful. Level of evidence: IV.

4. Frisch NB, Courtney PM, Darrith B, Della Valle CJ: Do higher-volume hospitals provide better value in revision hip and knee arthroplasty? *Bone Joint J* 2017;99-B(12):1611-1617.

   Although a high-volume hospital is less likely to be a high cost outlier, the higher mean Medicare reimbursements at these facilities may be due to increased case complexity.

5. Halder AM, Gehrke T, Gunster C, et al: Low hospital volume increases re-revision rate following aseptic revision total knee arthroplasty: An analysis of 23,644 cases. *J Arthroplasty* 2020;35(4):1054-1059.

   Five patients received instrumented prostheses that could detect loads in the medial and lateral compartments. The force transferred across the medial compartment was greater than that transferred across the lateral compartment. Varus alignment was associated with greater medial loads.

6. Matar HE, Platt SR, Golish JD, Cameron HU: Overview of randomized controlled trials in total knee arthroplasty (47,675 patients): What have we learnt? *J Arthroplasty* 2020;35(6):1729-1736.

   For most patients, a standard conventional TKA with a surgical approach familiar to the surgeon using standard well-established implants, with or without tourniquet, and without surgical drain leads to satisfactory long-term clinical outcomes.

7. Deehan DJ, Murray JD, Birdsall PD, Pinder IM: Quality of life after knee revision arthroplasty. *Acta Orthop* 2006;77(5):761-766.

8. Klasan A, Magill P, Frampton C, Zhu M, Young SW: Factors predicting repeat revision and outcome after aseptic revision total knee arthroplasty: Results from the New Zealand Joint Registry. *Knee Surg Sports Traumatol Arthrosc* 2020 [Epub ahead of print].

   In this New Zealand National Joint Registry study, 1,720 patients underwent subsequent revision for aseptic indications between 1999 and 2015. Re-revision was recorded in 208 patients (12.1%). Younger patients undergoing a revision and male sex were predictors of re-revision. Level of evidence: III.

9. Agarwal S, Kabariti R, Kakar R, Lopez D, Morgan-Jones R: Why are revision knee replacements failing? *Knee* 2019;26(3):774-778.

   A review of 95 failed revisions showed the most common reasons were infection (32.6%), aseptic loosening (30.5%), instability (12.6%), persistent stiffness (10.5%), ongoing pain (7.3%), extensor mechanism problems (5.2%), and one suspected metal allergy.

10. Khan M, Osman K, Green G, Haddad FS: The epidemiology of failure in total knee arthroplasty: Avoiding your next revision. *Bone Joint J* 2016;98-B(1 suppl A):105-112.

11. Correia J, Kendoff D, Klatte TO, Gehrke T, Citak M: Percutaneous cementation: A case of a failed treatment of a loose revision total knee arthroplasty. *Technol Health Care* 2014;22(4):645-650.

12. Gautreau SJ, Gould ON, Allanach WW, Clark AE, Massoeurs SJ, Forsythe ME: Total knee arthroplasty communication checklist increases patient satisfaction. *J Arthroplasty* 2019;34(3):456-461.

    A TKA communication checklist was developed to help surgeons better understand and manage patients' postoperative expectations to increase satisfaction with TKA. The checklist group reported higher satisfaction on overall TKA satisfaction and expectations met, care and concern shown by the surgeon, surgeons' communication ability, and satisfaction with time spent in follow-ups. Satisfaction with relief from pain and return to function was not significant.

13. Galea VP, Rojanasopondist P, Connelly JW, et al: Changes in patient satisfaction following total joint arthroplasty. *J Arthroplasty* 2020;35(1):32-38.

    For the TKA cohort, anterior (or reverse) tibial implant slope, greater femoral implant valgus angle, less severe osteoarthritis, and lower preoperative health state (odds ratio = −0.02; $P = 0.003$) were associated with lower levels of satisfaction across the study period.

14. Shan L, Shan B, Suzuki A, Nouh F, Saxena A: Intermediate and long-term quality of life after total knee replacement: A systematic review and meta-analysis. *J Bone Joint Surg Am* 2015;97(2):156-168.

15. Kahlenberg CA, Nwachukwu BU, McLawhorn AS, Cross MB, Cornell CN, Padgett DE: Patient satisfaction after total knee replacement: A systematic review. *HSS J* 2018;14(2):192-201.

Section 2: Knee

According to this review, most studies represent lower levels of evidence and use heterogeneous methods for measuring satisfaction. Few studies use validated satisfaction instruments. Most studies report satisfaction rates ranging from 80% to 100%, with postoperative functional outcome and relief of pain being paramount determinants for achieving satisfaction.

16. Ghanem E, Restrepo C, Joshi A, Hozack W, Sharkey P, Parvizi J: Periprosthetic infection does not preclude good outcome for revision arthroplasty. *Clin Orthop Relat Res* 2007;461: 54-59.

17. Meek RM, Dunlop D, Garbuz DS, McGraw R, Greidanus NV, Masri BA: Patient satisfaction and functional status after aseptic versus septic revision total knee arthroplasty using the PROSTALAC articulating spacer. *J Arthroplasty* 2004;19(7):874-879.

18. Barton CB, Wang DL, An Q, et al: Two-stage exchange arthroplasty for periprosthetic joint infection following total hip or knee arthroplasty is associated with high attrition rate and mortality. *J Arthroplasty* 2020;35(5):1384-1389.

This article identified patients who do not make it to the second stage of revision. This documents the unwitting patient selection bias in many series; only patients who survive to undergo reimplantation are reported.

19. Kim YH, Park JW: Long-term (up to 21 years) survival of revision total knee arthroplasty with use of a constrained condylar knee prosthesis: A concise follow-up of a previous report. *J Bone Joint Surg Am* 2020;102(8):674-678.

The purpose of the study was to determine long-term clinical and radiographic results of revision TKA with the Legacy Constrained Condylar Knee prosthesis. At a mean follow-up of 19.2 years (range, 16 to 21 years), re-revision of the prosthesis had been performed in 10 knees (9%). Level of evidence: IV.

20. Kouk S, Rathod PA, Maheshwari AV, Deshmukh AJ: Rotating hinge prosthesis for complex revision total knee arthroplasty: A review of the literature. *J Clin Orthop Trauma* 2018;9(1):29-33.

The authors concluded that rotating hinges have good outcome scores and survivorship but continue to have high complication and revision rates.

21. Pearse AJ, Hooper GJ, Rothwell A, Frampton C: Survival and functional outcome after revision of a unicompartmental to a total knee replacement: The New Zealand National Joint Registry. *J Bone Joint Surg Br* 2010;92(4):508-512.

22. Leta TH, Lygre SH, Skredderstuen A, et al: Outcomes of unicompartmental knee arthroplasty after aseptic revision to total knee arthroplasty: A comparative study of 768 TKAs and 578 UKAs revised to TKAs from the Norwegian Arthroplasty Register (1994 to 2011). *J Bone Joint Surg Am* 2016;98(6):431-440.

23. Woolf CJ: Central sensitization: Implications for the diagnosis and treatment of pain. *Pain* 2011;152(3 suppl):S2-S15.

24. Kim SH, Yoon KB, Yoon DM, Yoo JH, Ahn KR: Influence of centrally mediated symptoms on postoperative pain in osteoarthritis patients undergoing total knee arthroplasty: A prospective observational evaluation. *Pain Pract* 2015;15(6):E46-E53.

25. Koh IJ, Kim MS, Sohn S, Song KY, Choi NY, In Y: Duloxetine reduces pain and improves quality of recovery following total knee arthroplasty in centrally sensitized patients: A prospective, randomized controlled study. *J Bone Joint Surg Am* 2019;101(1):64-73.

A total of 80 patients were identified as being centrally sensitized before primary TKA. Forty patients were randomly assigned to the duloxetine group and 40 to the control group (no duloxetine). The duloxetine group had better performance across pain metrics during the first 2 to 12 weeks postsurgery and a superior quality of recovery 2 weeks after TKA, as indicated by emotional and physical functioning. Level of evidence: I.

26. Kim MS, Koh IJ, Sohn S, Kang BM, Kwak DH, In Y: Central sensitization is a risk factor for persistent postoperative pain and dissatisfaction in patients undergoing revision total knee arthroplasty. *J Arthroplasty* 2019;34(8):1740-1748.

Multivariate logistic regression analysis demonstrated that the odds of dissatisfaction after revision TKAs were increased 39.08 times in patients with Central Sensitization Inventory scores ≥ 40. Level of evidence: III.

27. Baker P, Cowling P, Kurtz S, Jameson S, Gregg P, Deehan D: Reason for revision influences early patient outcomes after aseptic knee revision. *Clin Orthop Relat Res* 2012;470(8):2244-2252.

28. Parvizi J, Tan TL, Goswami K, et al: The 2018 definition of periprosthetic hip and knee infection: An evidence-based and validated criteria. *J Arthroplasty* 2018;33(5):1309-1314.e2.

In this multi-institutional study, the authors provide new criteria for the diagnosis of hip and knee PJI. Two positive cultures or the presence of a sinus tract were considered as major criteria and diagnostic of PJI. The new criteria demonstrated a higher sensitivity of 97.7% compared with the Musculoskeletal Infection Society (79.3%) and International Consensus Meeting definition (86.9%), with a similar specificity of 99.5%.

29. Parvizi J, Della Valle CJ: AAOS clinical practice guideline: Diagnosis and treatment of periprosthetic joint infections of the hip and knee. *J Am Acad Orthop Surg* 2010;18(12):771-772.

30. Yuan J, Yan Y, Zhang J, Wang B, Feng J: Diagnostic accuracy of alpha-defensin in periprosthetic joint infection: A systematic review and meta-analysis. *Int Orthop* 2017;41(12):2447-2455.

This meta-analysis supports alpha defensin as a promising addition to the current methods for diagnosis of PJI.

31. Lonner JH, Fehring TK, Hanssen AD, et al: Revision total knee arthroplasty: The preoperative evaluation. *J Bone Joint Surg Am* 2009;91(suppl 5):64-68.

32. McDowell M, Park A, Gerlinger TL: The painful total knee arthroplasty. *Orthop Clin North Am* 2016;47(2):317-326.

33. Vince KG: The problem total knee replacement: Systematic, comprehensive and efficient evaluation. *Bone Joint J* 2014;96-B(11 suppl A):105-111.

34. Elson DW, Brenkel IJ: A conservative approach is feasible in unexplained pain after knee replacement: A selected cohort study. *J Bone Joint Surg Br* 2007;89(8):1042-1045.

35. Chalmers BP, Sculco PK, Fehring KA, Taunton MJ, Trousdale RT: Fluoroscopically assisted radiographs improve sensitivity of detecting loose tibial implants in revision total knee arthroplasty. *J Arthroplasty* 2017;32(2):570-574.

    The authors reevaluate an old technique that has increased the sensitivity of detecting tibial implant loosening over standard radiographs, but clinical significance is unclear.

36. Yoshino K, Hagiwara S, Nakamura J, Tsukeoka T, Tsuneizumi Y, Ohtori S: Intra- and interobserver reliability and agreement in three-dimensional computed tomography measurements of component positions after total knee arthroplasty. *Knee* 2019;26(5):1102-1110.

    Three-dimensional CT measurements of implant positions after TKA showed good intraobserver and interobserver reliability for the femoral and tibial implants in coronal, sagittal, and rotational positions. The intraobserver and interobserver agreements were favorable for all but the sagittal position of the femur.

37. Murer AM, Hirschmann MT, Amsler F, Rasch H, Huegli RW: Bone SPECT/CT has excellent sensitivity and specificity for diagnosis of loosening and patellofemoral problems after total knee arthroplasty. *Knee Surg Sports Traumatol Arthrosc* 2020;28(4):1029-1035.

    Reasonable sensitivity and specificity for detection of tibial or femoral implant loosening and diagnosis of patellofemoral osteoarthritis with bone single-photon emission computed tomography/CT have been surgically confirmed. Level of evidence: II.

38. Holst DC, Angerame MR, Dennis DA, Jennings JM: What is the value of component loosening assessment of a preoperatively obtained bone scan prior to revision total knee arthroplasty? *J Arthroplasty* 2019;34(7 suppl): S256-S261.

    There is weak agreement regarding implant loosening between a radiologist's opinion of a preoperatively obtained bone scan and the surgeon's preoperative interpretation of clinical and radiographic data. Neither of these reliably predicts what is found at the time of revision.

39. Schroder FF, Post CE, Wagenaar FBM, Verdonschot N, Huis In't Veld RMHA: MRI as diagnostic modality for analyzing the problematic knee arthroplasty: A systematic review. *J Magn Reson Imaging* 2020;51(2):446-458.

    MRI can be used with overall reproducible and accurate results to diagnose infection, loosening, wear, and malalignment after TKA. The diagnosis of instability, arthrofibrosis, or patellofemoral complaints using MRI is limited and inconclusive. Level of evidence: III.

40. Dai WL, Lin Z-M, Shi Z-J, Wang J: Outcomes following revision total knee arthroplasty septic versus aseptic failure: A national propensity-score-matched comparison. *J Knee Surg* 2020 [Epub ahead of print].

    Data from the US Nationwide Inpatient Sample conclude that postoperative complications, blood transfusions, length of stay, in-hospital costs, and in-hospital mortality all are worse for septic versus aseptic revisions.

41. Yao JJ, Hevesi M, O'Byrne MM, Berry DJ, Lewallen DG, Maradit Kremers H: Long-term mortality trends after revision total knee arthroplasty. *J Arthroplasty* 2019;34(3):542-548.

    Mortality is elevated soon after revision TKA for infection and fracture. Mortality is lower than in the general population after revision TKA for loosening and/or bearing wear but gets worse than that of the general population beyond the first postoperative decade.

42. Lizaur-Utrilla A, Asensio-Pascual A, Gonzalez-Parreño S, Miralles-Muñoz FA, Lopez-Prats FA: Negative impact of prior debridement on functional outcome of subsequent two-stage revision for early knee periprosthetic infection. *Knee Surg Sports Traumatol Arthrosc* 2019;27(7):2309-2315.

    The authors studied whether débridement, antibiotics, and implant retention had a negative effect on the functional outcome of a subsequent two-stage revision. Treatment with this procedure for early periprosthetic infection should be used in selected patients, and the first option in patients with *Staphylococcus* organisms should be two-stage revision. Level of evidence: IV.

43. Qasim SN, Swann A, Ashford R: The DAIR (debridement, antibiotics and implant retention) procedure for infected total knee replacement – A literature review. *SICOT J* 2017;3:2.

    Factors contributing to débridement, antibiotics, and implant retention failure are sinus tract, immunocompromised patient, delay between onset of infection and débridement procedure, staphylococcal infection (in particular methicillin-resistant *Staphylococcus aureus*), multiple débridement procedures, retention of exchangeable implants, and short antibiotic duration.

44. Holmberg A, Thórhallsdóttir VG, Robertsson O, W-Dahl A, Stefánsdóttir A: 75% success rate after open debridement, exchange of tibial insert, and antibiotics in knee prosthetic joint infections. *Acta Orthop* 2015;86(4):457-462.

45. Yaghmour KM, Chisari E, Khan WS: Single-stage revision surgery in infected total knee arthroplasty: A PRISMA systematic review. *J Clin Med* 2019;8(2):174.

    Satisfactory outcomes are possible for single-stage revision in the management of infected TKA. The reinfection rates in the studies included in this review varied; however, most reported low reinfection rates and good functional outcomes. Although strict patient selection criteria have yielded successful results, good results were also reported when these criteria were not applied.

46. Pangaud C, Ollivier M, Argenson JN: Outcome of single-stage versus two-stage exchange for revision knee arthroplasty for chronic periprosthetic infection. *EFORT Open Rev* 2019;4(8):495-502.

    This systematic review concluded that single-stage exchange can be a viable alternative to two-stage exchange in patients with chronic knee PJI, as long as no contraindications are present.

47. Srivastava K, Bozic KJ, Silverton C, Nelson AJ, Makhni EC, Davis JJ: Reconsidering strategies for managing chronic periprosthetic joint infection in total knee arthroplasty: Using decision analytics to find the optimal strategy between one-stage and two-stage total knee revision. *J Bone Joint Surg Am* 2019;101(1):14-24.

Despite two-stage revision being considered the current benchmark for infection eradication in patients with PJI following TKA, the optimal decision that produced the highest quality of life was one-stage revision. These results should be considered in shared decision making with patients who experience PJI following TKA. Level of evidence: IV.

48. Gilbert TJ, Anoushiravani AA, Sayeed Z, Chambers MC, El-Othmani MM, Saleh KJ: Osteolysis complicating total knee arthroplasty. *JBJS Rev* 2016;4(7).

49. Parratte S, Pagnano MW, Trousdale RT, Berry DJ: Effect of postoperative mechanical axis alignment on the fifteen-year survival of modern, cemented total knee replacements. *J Bone Joint Surg Am* 2010;92(12):2143-2149.

50. Oussedik S, Abdel MP, Victor J, Pagnano MW, Haddad FS: Alignment in total knee arthroplasty. *Bone Joint J* 2020;102-B(3):276-279.

    The authors present a comprehensive review of current thinking about TKA alignment. This article is used as a means to propose the authors' concept of functional alignment.

51. Vertullo CJ, Lewis PL, Lorimer M, Graves SE: The effect on long-term survivorship of surgeon preference for posterior-stabilized or minimally stabilized total knee replacement: An analysis of 63,416 prostheses from the Australian Orthopaedic Association National Joint Replacement Registry. *J Bone Joint Surg Am* 2017;99(13):1129-1139.

    There was a 45% higher risk of revision for the patients of surgeons who preferred a posterior-stabilized total knee arthroplasty compared with the patients of surgeons who preferred a minimally stabilized total knee arthroplasty. Level of evidence: III.

52. Maggs JL, Smeatham A, Whitehouse SL, Charity J, Timperley AJ, Gie GA: The Exeter Contemporary flanged cemented acetabular component in primary total hip arthroplasty. *Bone Joint J* 2016;98-B(3):307-312.

53. Bonutti PM, Khlopas A, Chughtai M, et al: Unusually high rate of early failure of tibial component in ATTUNE total knee arthroplasty system at implant-cement interface. *J Knee Surg* 2017;30(5):435-439.

    This article represents one of the several recent reports asking whether failure of an adhesive bond between metal implant and cement may result in failure and questioning whether specific designs are at higher risk. The entire phenomenon requires further investigation.

54. Buller LT, Rao V, Chiu Y-F, Nam D, McLawhorn AS: Primary total knee arthroplasty performed using high-viscosity cement is associated with higher odds of revision for aseptic loosening. *J Arthroplasty* 2020;35(6 suppl):S182-S189.

    In this retrospective analysis, whether failure of an adhesive bond between metal implant and cement may result in failure and questioning if specific types of cement are at higher risk was discussed. Some high-viscosity cement types, such as Palacos, are not implicated.

55. Yokhana SS, Bergum C, Ren W, Markel DC: Isolated tibial component failure in total knee arthroplasty: A case series evaluating inflammatory response versus mechanical failure. *J Knee Surg* 2019;32(7):659-666.

    The authors of this article favor debonding of the tibial baseplate from the cement mantle without osteolysis as a completely mechanical mode of loosening because the patients studied had very few elevated inflammatory markers.

56. Meijer MF, Reininga IH, Boerboom AL, Stevens M, Bulstra SK: Poorer survival after a primary implant during revision total knee arthroplasty. *Int Orthop* 2013;37(3):415-419.

57. Morgan-Jones R, Oussedik SI, Graichen H, Haddad FS: Zonal fixation in revision total knee arthroplasty. *Bone Joint J* 2015;97-B(2):147-149.

58. Heesterbeek PJ, Wymenga AB, van Hellemondt GG: No difference in implant micromotion between hybrid fixation and fully cemented revision total knee arthroplasty: A randomized controlled trial with radiostereometric analysis of patients with mild-to-moderate bone loss. *J Bone Joint Surg Am* 2016;98(16):1359-1369.

59. Fleischman AN, Azboy I, Fuery M, Restrepo C, Shao H, Parvizi J: Effect of stem size and fixation method on mechanical failure after revision total knee arthroplasty. *J Arthroplasty* 2017;32(9 suppl):S202-S208.e1.

    Risk for mechanical failure was equivalent for cemented and hybrid stems (relative risk, 0.991; $P = 0.98$). Young age was the single greatest risk factor for mechanical failure ($P = 0.006$). Intramedullary canal fill, not stem length or diameter, was the strongest predictor of failure with hybrid stems, and risk was reduced by 41.2% for each additional 10% canal fill.

60. Bedard M, Cabrejo-Jones K, Angers M, Pelletier-Roy R, Pelet S: The effect of porous tantalum cones on mechanical alignment and canal-fill ratio in revision total knee arthroplasty performed with uncemented stems. *J Arthroplasty* 2015;30(11):1995-1998.

61. Lee SH, Shih H-N, Chang C-H, Lu T-W, Chang Y-H, Lin Y-C: Influence of extension stem length and diameter on clinical and radiographic outcomes of revision total knee arthroplasty. *BMC Musculoskelet Disord* 2020;21(1):15.

    Prosthesis loosening was detected in 17 of 65 patients who had undergone revision TKA. Male sex and severity of the tibial bone defect were associated with loosening. Protective factors included femoral canal fill ratio (CFR) >0.85, CFR >0.7 for >2 cm, and CFR >0.7 for > 4cm, as well as tibial CFR >0.85.

62. Kamath AF, Lewallen DG, Hanssen AD: Porous tantalum metaphyseal cones for severe tibial bone loss in revision knee arthroplasty: A five to nine-year follow-up. *J Bone Joint Surg Am* 2015;97(3):216-223.

63. Potter GD III, Abdel MP, Lewallen DG, Hanssen AD: Midterm results of porous tantalum femoral cones in revision total knee arthroplasty. *J Bone Joint Surg Am* 2016;98(15):1286-1291.

64. Abdelaziz H, Jaramillo R, Gehrke T, Ohlmeier M, Citak M: Clinical survivorship of aseptic revision total knee arthroplasty using hinged knees and tantalum cones at minimum 10-year follow-up. *J Arthroplasty* 2019;34(12):3018-3022.

The authors studied 38 cases of hinged arthroplasty and porous cones. Aseptic loosening complicated (5/32; 15.6%), and peri-PJI (3/32; 9.4%). Four of the five revisions failed because of aseptic loosening; pure hinged knees had been implanted.

65. Denehy KM, Abhari S, Krebs VK, et al: Metaphyseal fixation using highly porous cones in revision total knee arthroplasty: Minimum two year follow up study. *J Arthroplasty* 2019;34(10):2439-2443.

A total of 62 revisions using three-dimensional printed titanium metaphyseal cones showed excellent short-term results with no instances of aseptic loosening.

66. Divano S, Cavagnaro L, Zanirato A, Basso M, Felli L, Formica M: Porous metal cones: Gold standard for massive bone loss in complex revision knee arthroplasty? A systematic review of current literature. *Arch Orthop Trauma Surg* 2018;138(6):851-863.

In this systematic literature review, low rates of aseptic loosening, intraoperative fractures, and infection were noted, along with lower failure rates than the previous treatment methods. Higher quality articles are needed to draw definitive conclusions about porous metal cones.

67. Bohl DD, Brown NM, McDowell MA, et al: Do porous tantalum metaphyseal cones improve outcomes in revision total knee arthroplasty? *J Arthroplasty* 2018;33(1):171-177.

The authors found that metaphyseal cones were not associated with favorable outcomes at short-term follow-up.

68. Angerame MR, Jennings JM, Holst DC, Dennis DA: Management of bone defects in revision total knee arthroplasty with use of a stepped, porous-coated metaphyseal sleeve. *JBJS Essent Surg Tech* 2019;9(2):e14.

The metaphyseal sleeve is an alternative form of porous metal augment that is attached directly to the revision implant. This means that the position of the sleeve in the bone will directly determine the location of the implant.

69. Klim SM, Amerstorfer F, Bernhardt GA, et al: Septic revision total knee arthroplasty: Treatment of metaphyseal bone defects using metaphyseal sleeves. *J Arthroplasty* 2018;33(12):3734-3738.

The authors determined that metaphyseal sleeves are a reliable option for fixation, with promising results regarding osseointegration, clinical scores, and aseptic loosening.

70. Zanirato A, Formica M, Cavagnaro L, Divano S, Burastero G, Felli L: Metaphyseal cones and sleeves in revision total knee arthroplasty: Two sides of the same coin? Complications, clinical and radiological results – A systematic review of the literature. *Musculoskelet Surg* 2020;104(1): 25-35.

Cones and sleeves provided comparable metaphyseal fixation. The aseptic survivorship of the implants was 97.3% in the cone group and 97.8% in the sleeve group. These are viable options in management of type IIb and III Anderson Orthopaedic Research Institute classification of bone defects in aseptic and septic revision TKA with overlapping survival rate.

71. Roach RP, Clair AJ, Behery OA, Thakkar SC, Iorio R, Deshmukh AJ: Aseptic loosening of porous metaphyseal sleeves and tantalum cones in revision total knee arthroplasty: A systematic review. *J Knee Surg* 2020 [Epub ahead of print].

The authors found that rates of aseptic loosening were similar between the sleeve and cone implants, and the rate of revision surgery was nearly double in revision TKAs using tantalum cones. Because of variability in the selected studies and the likely multifactorial nature of failure, no definitive conclusions could be made. Patient selection bias is problematic (regarding which patients were selected for which devices).

72. Ritter MA, Davis KE, Davis P, et al: Preoperative malalignment increases risk of failure after total knee arthroplasty. *J Bone Joint Surg Am* 2013;95(2):126-131.

73. Mundermann A, Dyrby CO, D'Lima DD, Colwell CW Jr, Andriacchi TP: In vivo knee loading characteristics during activities of daily living as measured by an instrumented total knee replacement. *J Orthop Res* 2008;26(9):1167-1172.

74. Halder A, Kutzner I, Graichen F, Heinlein B, Beier A, Bergmann G: Influence of limb alignment on mediolateral loading in total knee replacement: In vivo measurements in five patients. *J Bone Joint Surg Am* 2012;94(11):1023-1029.

75. Schotanus MGM, Thijs E, Boonen B, Kerens B, Jong B, Kort NP: Revision of partial knee to total knee arthroplasty with use of patient-specific instruments results in acceptable femoral rotation. *Knee Surg Sports Traumatol Arthrosc* 2018;26(6):1656-1661.

The hypothesis that patient-specific instruments can reliably restore alignment could not be demonstrated. This technology may be useful for the failed UKA because, in all probability, there are still identifiable osseous landmarks when a UKA has failed, unlike the failure of a TKA. Level of evidence: II.

76. Haidukewych GJ: Role of distal femoral replacement for periprosthetic fractures above a total knee arthroplasty: When and how? *J Orthop Trauma* 2019;33(suppl 6):S33-S35.

Distal femoral replacement may offer a more efficient, facile approach to managing periprosthetic fractures about a loose TKA implant. Failure rates can be high in this technically demanding situation.

77. Wyles CC, Tibbo ME, Yuan BJ, Trousdale RT, Berry DJ, Abdel MP: Long-term results of total knee arthroplasty with contemporary distal femoral replacement. *J Bone Joint Surg Am* 2020;102(1):45-51.

TKAs with contemporary distal femoral replacement had high 10-year cumulative incidences of both revision and revision surgery, underscoring the salvage nature of this procedure as a final reconstructive option.

78. Chatterji U, Ashworth MJ, Smith AL, Brewster N, Lewis PL: Retrieval study of tibial baseplate fracture after total knee arthroplasty. *J Arthroplasty* 2005;20(1):101-107.

79. Cankaya D, Yilmaz S, Deveci A, Ozkurt B: Tibial baseplate fracture associated with polyethylene wear and osteolysis after total knee arthroplasty. *Int J Surg Case Rep* 2014;5(2):49-51.

80. Diamond OJ, Howard L, Basri B: Five cases of tibial post fracture in posterior stabilized total knee arthroplasty using Prolong highly cross-linked polyethylene. *Knee* 2018;25(4):657-662.

Tibial post breakage is extremely rare after normal arthroplasty function. Hyperextension that allows the distal edge of the trochlear flange to strike the base of the post is the usual mechanism.

81. Baral EC, McLawhorn AS, Wright TM, Su EP: Fracture of the femoral adapter bolt and taper adapter in a modern rotating platform knee arthroplasty. *Arthroplasty Today* 2017;3(4):229-233.

The authors present a rare example of implant breakage. Revision scenarios often involve unusual loads on implants. Failure generally is associated with loss of osseous support or in the case of hinges, hyperextension stops and recurvatum.

82. Vajapey SP, Blackwell RE, Maki AJ, Miller TL: Treatment of extensor tendon disruption after total knee arthroplasty: A systematic review. *J Arthroplasty* 2019;34(6):1279-1286.

Reconstruction of patellar tendon rupture has a much lower complication rate than repair. No distinction was made between different types of reconstruction. Surgical repair has long been regarded as an inadequate treatment for extensor tendon disruption by experienced practitioners.

83. Brown NM, Murray T, Sporer SM, Wetters N, Berger RA, Della Valle CJ: Extensor mechanism allograft reconstruction for extensor mechanism failure following total knee arthroplasty. *J Bone Joint Surg Am* 2015;97(4):279-283.

84. Vaishya R, Vijay V, Vaish A: Dislocation of a constrained total knee arthroplasty with patellar tendon rupture after trivial trauma. *Chin J Traumatol* 2015;18(4):241-244.

85. Agarwala S, Vijayvargiya M: Traumatic dissociation of the tibial insert with patellar tendon rupture after high-flex posterior-stabilized Genesis II total knee arthroplasty. *Rev Bras Ortop* 2018;53(5):632-635.

This case report showed that the extensor was the last structure providing stability; when it ruptured, the polyethylene insert dissociated. The study findings demonstrate the frequent need for revision arthroplasty concurrent with extensor reconstruction.

86. Checa A, O'Connor CR: Sonographic evidence of impingement mechanism in a patient with patellar tendon rupture after total knee replacement. *Int J Rheum Dis* 2014;17(2): 221-222.

87. Spoliti M, Giai Via A, Padulo J, Oliva F, Del Buono A, Maffulli N: Surgical repair of chronic patellar tendon rupture in total knee replacement with ipsilateral hamstring tendons. *Knee Surg Sports Traumatol Arthrosc* 2016;24(10):3183-3190.

88. Wise BT, Erens G, Pour AE, Bradbury TL, Roberson JR: Long-term results of extensor mechanism reconstruction using Achilles tendon allograft after total knee arthroplasty. *Int Orthop* 2018;42(10):2367-2373.

Achilles tendon allograft reconstruction is a reliable and durable treatment for patients who sustain not only patellar tendon ruptures but also quadriceps tendon ruptures following TKA. Despite the success of this technique, the injury and procedure have a profound effect on overall function. It should be noted that, when the Achilles tendon graft is used for patellar tendon ruptures, the proximal end of the graft must exit through an opening in the arthrotomy to avoid lying between the articular surface of the patella and the femoral condyles.

89. Browne JA, Hanssen AD: Reconstruction of patellar tendon disruption after total knee arthroplasty: Results of a new technique utilizing synthetic mesh. *J Bone Joint Surg Am* 2011;93(12):1137-1143.

90. Abdel MP, Salib CG, Mara KC, Pagnano MW, Perry KI, Hanssen AD: Extensor mechanism reconstruction with use of Marlex mesh: A series study of 77 total knee arthroplasties. *J Bone Joint Surg Am* 2018;100(15):1309-1318.

A total of 77 mesh reconstructions of extensor mechanisms ruptured at various sites from tubercle to quadriceps. Reconstructions were in place in 84% of cases at follow-up. This method may replace extensor mechanism allograft reconstruction. Level of evidence: IV.

91. Keating EM, Haas G, Meding JB: Patella fracture after post total knee replacements. *Clin Orthop Relat Res* 2003:416:93-97.

92. Berry DJ: Patellar fracture following total knee arthroplasty. *J Knee Surg* 2003;16(4):236-241.

93. Perry KI, Salib CG, Larson DR, Pagnano MW, Abdel MP, Hanssen AD: Two-stage exchange and Marlex-mesh reconstruction for infection with extensor mechanism disruption after total knee arthroplasty. *J Bone Joint Surg Am* 2018;100(17):1482-1489.

Two-stage exchange arthroplasty combined with Marlex mesh reconstruction of the extensor mechanism is a viable alternative to knee arthrodesis or amputation. At 2 years, 75% of mesh reconstructions were in place and without evidence of PJI. Moreover, the functional outcomes were improved, with a negligible extensor lag. Level of evidence: IV.

94. Wood TJ, Leighton J, Backstein DJ, et al: Synthetic graft compared with allograft reconstruction for extensor mechanism disruption in total knee arthroplasty: A multicenter cohort study. *J Am Acad Orthop Surg* 2019;27(12):451-457.

Synthetic reconstruction for extensor mechanism disruption shows benefit in postoperative extensor lag, graft failure, revision surgery, and cost when compared with allograft. Level of evidence: III.

95. Deren ME, Pannu TS, Villa JM, Firtha M, Riesgo AM, Higuera CA: Meta-analysis comparing allograft to synthetic reconstruction for extensor mechanism disruption after total knee arthroplasty. *J Knee Surg* 2019 [Epub ahead of print].

The overall success rate of the synthetic reconstruction was 73.3%. The success rate of allograft (72.8%) was not significantly different from that of synthetic material (78%).

96. Shau D, Patton R, Patel S, Ward L, Guild G III: Synthetic mesh vs. allograft extensor mechanism reconstruction in total knee arthroplasty – A systematic review of the literature and meta-analysis. *Knee* 2018;25(1):2-7.

Results showed equivalent success of allograft and synthetic mesh with approximately 25% failure rate in both groups. PJI remains a common complication and reason for failure in both groups. Mesh showed equivalent success as allograft but with much lower cost, near-universal availability, and lack of disease transmission.

97. Cohen JS, Gu A, Lopez NS, Park MS, Fehring KA, Sculco PK: Efficacy of revision surgery for the treatment of stiffness after total knee arthroplasty: A systematic review. *J Arthroplasty* 2018;33(9):3049-3055.

    Search criteria included stiffness in the title, but not the word stiff. This missed some publications. Reports state that the most common etiologies of stiffness requiring revision TKA were implant malposition, malalignment, overstuffing, aseptic loosening, arthrofibrosis, patella baja, and heterotopic ossification. In cases such as patella baja and stiffness, this fails to discriminate between cause and effect. In general, modest improvements were reported, often in pain reduction, when that is part of pain.

98. Hug KT, Amanatullah D, Huddleston JI III, Maloney WJ, Goodman SB: Protocol-driven revision for stiffness after total knee arthroplasty improves motion and clinical outcomes. *J Arthroplasty* 2018;33(9):2952-2955.

    Isolated polyethylene exchanges, partial revisions, and complete revisions were compared. Complete implant revision may offer the largest improvements in properly selected patients.

99. van Rensch PJH, Heesterbeek PJ, Hannink G, van Hellemondt GG, Wymenga AT: Improved clinical outcomes after revision arthroplasty with a hinged implant for severely stiff total knee arthroplasty. *Knee Surg Sports Traumatol Arthrosc* 2019;27(4):1043-1048.

    Hinged-type revision TKA following a severely stiff TKA renders a significant, although moderate, clinical improvement at 2 years. There was no control group, but the concept of aggressive scar removal, to the point of creating instability, followed by restoration of stability with mechanical constraint is a logical strategy for this challenging technical problem. Level of evidence: IV.

100. Hermans K, Vandenneucker H, Truijen J, Oosterbosch J, Bellemans J: Hinged versus CCK revision arthroplasty for the stiff total knee. *Knee* 2019;26(1):222-227.

    Superior results were reported in the authors' preferred implant. Hinges are generally used for more unstable cases. In cases where extensive releases were performed, hinges would be selected. The releases might be responsible for better results.

101. Barrack RL, Schrader T, Bertot AJ, Wolfe MW, Myers L: Component rotation and anterior knee pain after total knee arthroplasty. *Clin Orthop Relat Res* 2001:392:46-55.

102. Babazadeh S, Dowsey MM, Vasimalla MG, Stoney JD, Choong PFM: Knee arthroplasty component malrotation does not affect function or quality of life in the short to medium term. *J Arthroplasty* 2019;34(7):1382-1386.

    The authors reported that implant malrotation may result in a decreased level of pain improvement in comparison with preoperative levels. Level of evidence: III.

103. Wilson CJ, Theodoulou A, Damarell RA, Krishnan J: Knee instability as the primary cause of failure following Total Knee Arthroplasty (TKA): A systematic review on the patient, surgical and implant characteristics of revised TKA patients. *Knee* 2017;24(6):1271-1281.

    The need for revision due to instability was frequently reported in a younger patient population and most commonly in female TKA patients. Early revision at a younger age highlights the severe implications of an unstable knee.

104. Song SJ, Detch RC, Maloney WJ, Goodman SB, Huddleston JI III: Causes of instability after total knee arthroplasty. *J Arthroplasty* 2014;29(2):360-364.

105. Azzam K, Parvizi J, Kaufman D, Purtill JJ, Sharkey PF, Austin MS: Revision of the unstable total knee arthroplasty: Outcome predictors. *J Arthroplasty* 2011;26(8):1139-1144.

106. Abdel MP, Pulido L, Severson EP, Hanssen AD: Stepwise surgical correction of instability in flexion after total knee replacement. *Bone Joint J* 2014;96-B(12):1644-1648.

107. Kannan A, O'Connell RS, Kalore N, Curtin BM, Hull JR, Jiranek WA: Revision TKA for flexion instability improves patient reported outcomes. *J Arthroplasty* 2015;30(5):818-821.

108. Grayson CW, Warth LC, Ziemba-Davis MM, Michael Meneghini R: Functional improvement and expectations are diminished in total knee arthroplasty patients revised for flexion instability compared to aseptic loosening and infection. *J Arthroplasty* 2016;31(10):2241-2246.

109. Rajgopal A, Panjwani TR, Rao A, Dahiya V: Are the outcomes of revision knee arthroplasty for flexion instability the same as for other major failure mechanisms? *J Arthroplasty* 2017;32(10):3093-3097.

    Patients undergoing revision for isolated flexion instability have less improvement in functional outcome compared with other etiologies. The authors hypothesize this is due to a higher baseline preoperative knee function in the flexion instability group. However, a low threshold for accepting flexion instability as an indication for revision in patients reporting with pain but without other explanation may also be likely.

110. Stambough JB, Edwards PK, Mannen EM, Barnes CL, Mears SC: Flexion instability after total knee arthroplasty. *J Am Acad Orthop Surg* 2019;27(17):642-651.

    The mainstays of surgical management of femoral instability involve increasing the posterior condylar offset, decreasing the tibial slope, raising the joint line in combination with a thicker polyethylene insert, and ensuring appropriate rotation of implants. Advancements in biomechanical analysis with motion detection, isokinetic quadriceps strength testing, and computational modeling are needed to advance the collective understanding of this underappreciated failure mechanism.

111. Lewallen FA, Salib CG, Trousdale WH, et al: Molecular pathology of total knee arthroplasty instability defined by RNA-seq. *Genomics* 2018;110(5):247-256.

    Genes related to collagen production and extracellular matrix degradation were higher in samples from patients with flexion instability.

112. Baker RP, Masri BA, Greidanus NV, Garbuz DS: Outcome after isolated polyethylene tibial insert exchange in revision total knee arthroplasty. *J Arthroplasty* 2012;28(1):1-6.

113. Green CC, Haidukewych GJ: Isolated polyethylene insert exchange for flexion instability after primary total knee arthroplasty demonstrated excellent results in properly selected patients. *J Arthroplasty* 2020;35(5):1328-1332.

Partial revision TKA is generally associated with worse results and isolated polyethylene exchange with the worst result of all. Stringent criteria for selection of patients with flexion instability may lead to satisfactory results after modular polyethylene exchange when an ultracongruent insert is selected.

114. Ozkurt B, Sen T, Cankaya D, Kendir S, Basarır K, Tabak Y: The medial and lateral epicondyle as a reliable landmark for intra-operative joint line determination in revision knee arthroplasty. *Bone Joint Res* 2016;5(7):280-286.

115. Clement ND, MacDonald DJ, Hamilton DF, Burnett R: Posterior condylar offset is an independent predictor of functional outcome after revision total knee arthroplasty. *Bone Joint Res* 2017;6(3):172-178.

This article represents an interesting recognition of the importance of the joint line in flexion. Although failure to restore posterior condylar offset ratio may be a marker of poor revision technique, it could also be a confounding variable for severity of failure.

116. Newman JM, Siqueira MBP, Klika AK, Molloy RM, Barsoum WK, Higuera CA: Use of closed incisional negative pressure wound therapy after revision total hip and knee arthroplasty in patients at high risk for infection: A prospective, randomized clinical trial. *J Arthroplasty* 2019;34(3):554-559.e1.

Closed incisional negative-pressure wound therapy may decrease the rate of postoperative wound complications in patients who are at an increased risk of such wound issues after revision arthroplasty.

117. Gu A, Wei C, Bernstein SA, et al: The impact of gender on postoperative complications after revision total knee arthroplasty. *J Knee Surg* 2020 33(4):387-393.

Multivariate analysis showed male sex as an independent risk factor for four complications and female sex as an independent risk factor for the development of urinary tract infection.

118. Lee D, Lee R, Strum D, Heyer JJH, Swansen T, Pandarinath R: The impact of chronic kidney disease on postoperative complications in patients undergoing revision total knee arthroplasty: A propensity matched analysis. *J Clin Orthop Trauma* 2020;11(1):147-153.

Chronic kidney disease of moderate/severe/failure status was a significant independent risk factor for acute renal failure, blood transfusions, return to the operating room, extended length of stay, and mortality in the 30-day postoperative period.

119. Sisko ZW, Vasarhelyi EM, Somerville LE, Naudie DD, MacDonald SJ, McCalden RW: Morbid obesity in revision total knee arthroplasty: A significant risk factor for Re-operation. *J Arthroplasty* 2019;34(5):932-938.

The authors found that morbidly obese patients had a greater incidence of revision surgery and re-revision, in addition to lower 10-year survivorship for revision surgery.

120. Bedard NA, Dowdle SB, Wilkinson BG, Duchman KR, Gao Y, Callaghan JJ: What is the impact of smoking on revision total knee arthroplasty? *J Arthroplasty* 2018;33(7 suppl):S172-S176.

This study demonstrates that smoking significantly increases the risk of infection, wound complications, and revision surgery after revision TKA. The results are magnified for revision procedures compared with published effects of smoking on primary TKA.

121. Aggarwal VK, Goyal N, Deirmengian G, Rangavajulla A, Parvizi J, Austin MS: Revision total knee arthroplasty in the young patient: Is there trouble on the horizon? *J Bone Joint Surg Am* 2014;96(7):536-542.

122. Stambough JB, Clohisy JC, Barrack RL, Nunley RM, Keeney JA: Increased risk of failure following revision total knee replacement in patients aged 55 years and younger. *Bone Joint J* 2014;96-B(12):1657-1662.

123. Chalmers BP, Pallante GD, Sierra RJ, Lewallen DG, Pagnano MW, Trousdale RT: Contemporary revision total knee arthroplasty in patients younger than 50 years: 1 in 3 risk of re-revision by 10 years. *J Arthroplasty* 2019;34(7 suppl):S266-S270.

Patients aged 50 years or younger undergoing contemporary aseptic revision TKA had a one in three risk of re-revision. Patients specifically revised for instability or with prior TKA revisions had the highest risk of re-revision at 10 years. Level of evidence: IV.

124. Kim GK, Mortazavi SM, Purtill JJ, Sharkey PF, Hozack WJ, Parvizi J: Stiffness after revision total knee arthroplasty. *J Arthroplasty* 2010;25(6):844-850.

125. Dowdle SB, Bedard NA, Owens JM, Gao Y, Callaghan JJ: Identifying risk factors for the development of stiffness after revision total knee arthroplasty. *J Arthroplasty* 2018;33(4):1186-1188.

A total of 1.7% of revision TKAs underwent manipulation under anesthesia after surgery. Young patients (50 years or younger) were six times more likely to have manipulation under anesthesia after revision TKA (6.5, $P < 0.0001$). No difference in odds of manipulation under anesthesia occurred between males and females. A diagnosis of obesity, diabetes, anxiety and/or depression; previous history of narcotic use; or a history of smoking demonstrated no increased risk of manipulation under anesthesia after revision TKA.

126. Capozzi JD, Rhodes R, Chen D: Discussing treatment options. *J Bone Joint Surg Am* 2009;91(3):740-742.

127. Vince KG, Coup R, Morgan-Jones R: The knee arthroplasty endgame: Four options in the face of calamity, in Hirschmann TM, Becker R, eds: *The Unhappy Total Knee Replacement*. Switzerland, Springer, 2015, pp 771-795.

128. Son M-S, Lau E, Parvizi J, Mont MA, Bozic KJ, Kurtz S: What are the frequency, associated factors, and mortality of amputation and arthrodesis after a failed infected TKA? *Clin Orthop Relat Res* 2017;475(12):2905-2913.

The number of arthrodesis and amputation procedures showed a declining trend. Factors associated with arthrodesis include acute renal failure, obesity, and having additional infection-related revisions. Higher Charlson comorbidity score, obesity, deep vein thrombosis, and additional revisions were factors associated with above-knee amputation, which in turn was an independent risk factor for mortality. The risk of death increased with amputation after adjusting for age, comorbidities, and other factors; patients who underwent arthrodesis did not show a change in mortality compared with the patients who did not receive arthrodesis or amputation. A greater number of revisions is associated with a greater risk of subsequent above-knee amputation or arthrodesis. It is not the case, however, that most patients who underwent amputation would have been candidates for arthrodesis. Level of evidence: III.

129. Ryan SP, DiLallo M, Klement MR, Luzzi AJ, Chen AF, Seyler TM: Transfemoral amputation following total knee arthroplasty: Mortality and functional outcomes. *Bone Joint J* 2019;101-B(2):221-226.

The goal of this study was to analyze the factors that lead to transfemoral amputation after TKA, along with mortality rates and functional independence afterward. Patients should be apprised of high mortality rates and poor functional outcomes in those who survive surgery.

SECTION 3

Hip

Section Editor:

Michael Tanzer, MD, FRCSC, FAAOS

CHAPTER 28

Arthroplasty Management of Hip Fractures: Hemiarthroplasty Versus Total Hip Arthroplasty—Results and Complications

MICHAEL TANZER, MD, FRCSC, FAAOS

ABSTRACT

The choice between total hip arthroplasty (THA) and hemiarthroplasty for the management of femoral neck fracture remains a controversial issue in orthopaedic surgery. The recent scientific literature and registry data indicate that THA is associated with improved clinical outcomes, but at the cost of higher dislocation rates. The same data provide conflicting results regarding implant survivorship; therefore, both treatments can be appropriate and management algorithms have been developed to simplify the choice and optimize the results of THA and hemiarthroplasty in the management of femoral neck fractures.

Keywords: femoral neck fracture; hemiarthroplasty; hip fracture; outcomes; total hip arthroplasty

Dr. Tanzer or an immediate family member is a member of a speakers' bureau or has made paid presentations on behalf of Stryker; has received research or institutional support from Stryker; and serves as a board member, owner, officer, or committee member of the American Academy of Orthopaedic Surgeons and the Canadian Arthroplasty Society.

INTRODUCTION

Historically, the management of femoral neck fractures (FNFs) was determined solely by the displacement of the fracture. Fractures with little or no displacement were treated using internal fixation; displaced fractures were treated with hemiarthroplasty. More recently, total hip arthroplasty (THA) has been increasingly used to manage these fractures.[1,2] Because patients who have hip fractures vary from those who are active and healthy to those who are institutionalized and frail, a modern treatment algorithm for FNF needs to account for not only the fracture but also the patient's age and activity level, the presence or absence of coexisting hip arthritis, and medical comorbidities (**Figures 1** and **2**).

In general, internal fixation is performed for minimally displaced FNFs and the management of selected fractures in younger patients. The remaining cases are treated with arthroplasty, either THA or hemiarthroplasty; both are widely accepted for the management of FNF. The optimal treatment option for displaced FNF is currently debated among orthopaedic surgeons.[3-5] Various advantages and disadvantages need to be considered when deciding which type of arthroplasty to use for the management of a displaced FNF in the elderly.

Recent clinical trials and systematic reviews have focused on the survivorship, complications, and clinical outcomes of hemiarthroplasty and THA for the management of FNF. It is important for the

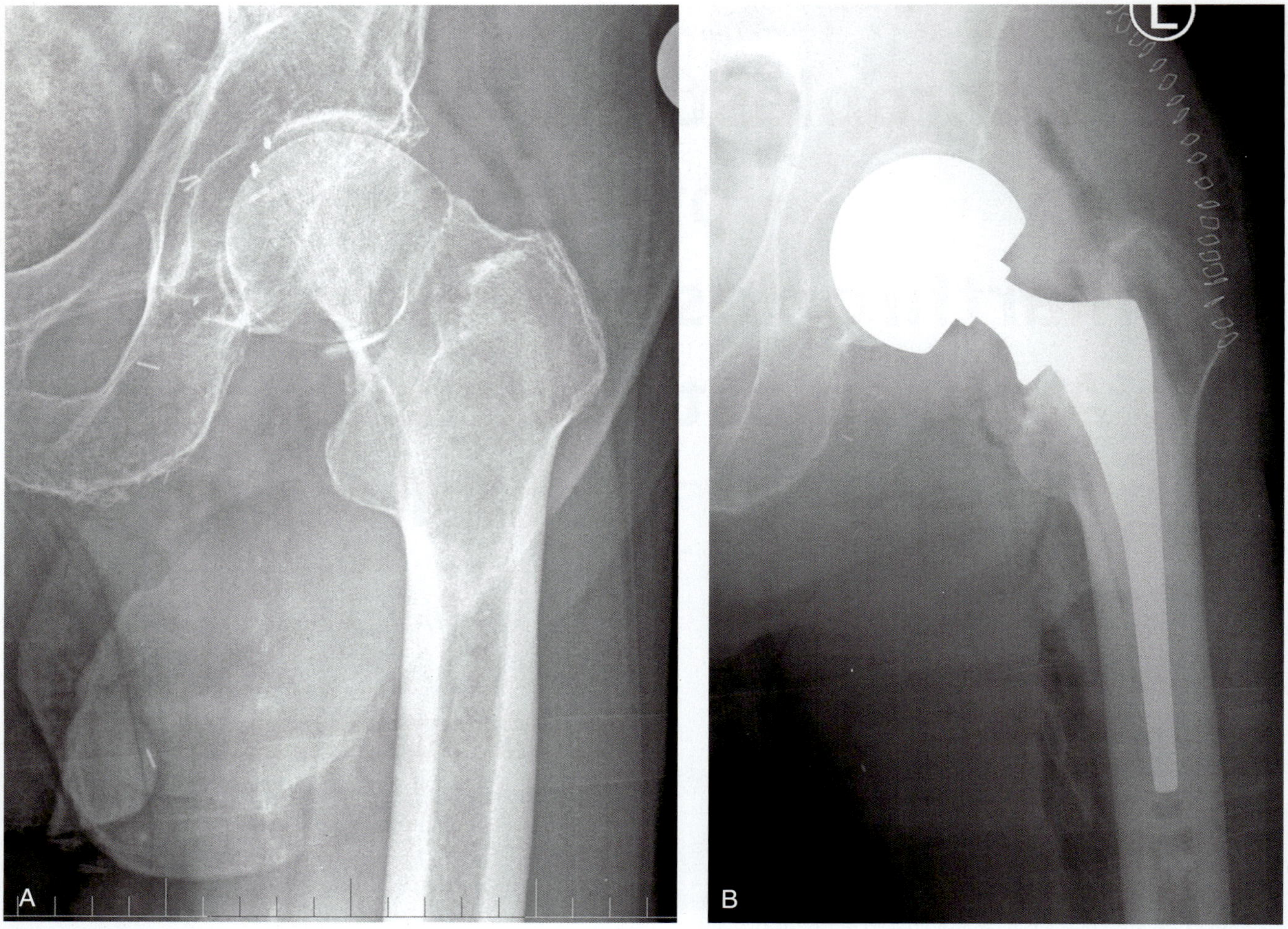

FIGURE 1 **A**, Preoperative AP radiograph of the left hip obtained from an 80-year-old sedentary, frail woman demonstrates a displaced femoral neck fracture. **B**, Immediately postoperative AP radiograph obtained following cemented hemiarthroplasty.

orthopaedic surgeon to have an up-to-date understanding of the indications and results for these two treatment modalities.

REVISION SURGERY AND REVISION RATES

Systematic Reviews and Meta-analyses

Several systematic reviews and meta-analyses have been performed to synthesize the literature and determine the best arthroplasty management of FNFs. Overall, the pooled data demonstrate a trend of fewer reoperations and better functional outcome scores for patients who have FNFs treated with THA compared with hemiarthroplasty.

Recent meta-analyses demonstrated substantially fewer early and late revision surgeries following THA than following hemiarthroplasty. A 2014 meta-analysis reported the risk of revision following hemiarthroplasty was more than twofold higher than following THA for an FNF (relative risk [RR] = 4.14).[4] In part, this resulted from the high prevalence of acetabular erosion, which accounted for 78.1% of revision surgery in patients who underwent hemiarthroplasty. A subsequent study in 2015 analyzed eight randomized controlled trials that included 977 patients.[3] Overall, a 69% reduced risk of revision was reported for patients treated with THA compared with hemiarthroplasty for all follow-up periods up to 13 years (RR = 0.31, P = 0.0003). Similar findings were noted in a 2019 meta-analysis of 17 randomized and quasi-randomized trials comparing hemiarthroplasty with THA in 1,364 patients who have an FNF (Garden III and IV).[6] At a mean follow-up of 5.3 years, the pooled relative risk of revision surgery after hemiarthroplasty compared with THA was 1.54 (P = 0.05). The risk of revision surgery with a hemiarthroplasty was even greater at longer follow-up. A subanalysis of the patients with at least 4 years follow-up (mean follow-up, 8.5 years) showed that hemiarthroplasty had a significantly increased risk of revision surgery compared with THA (RR, 2.49; P = 0.002).

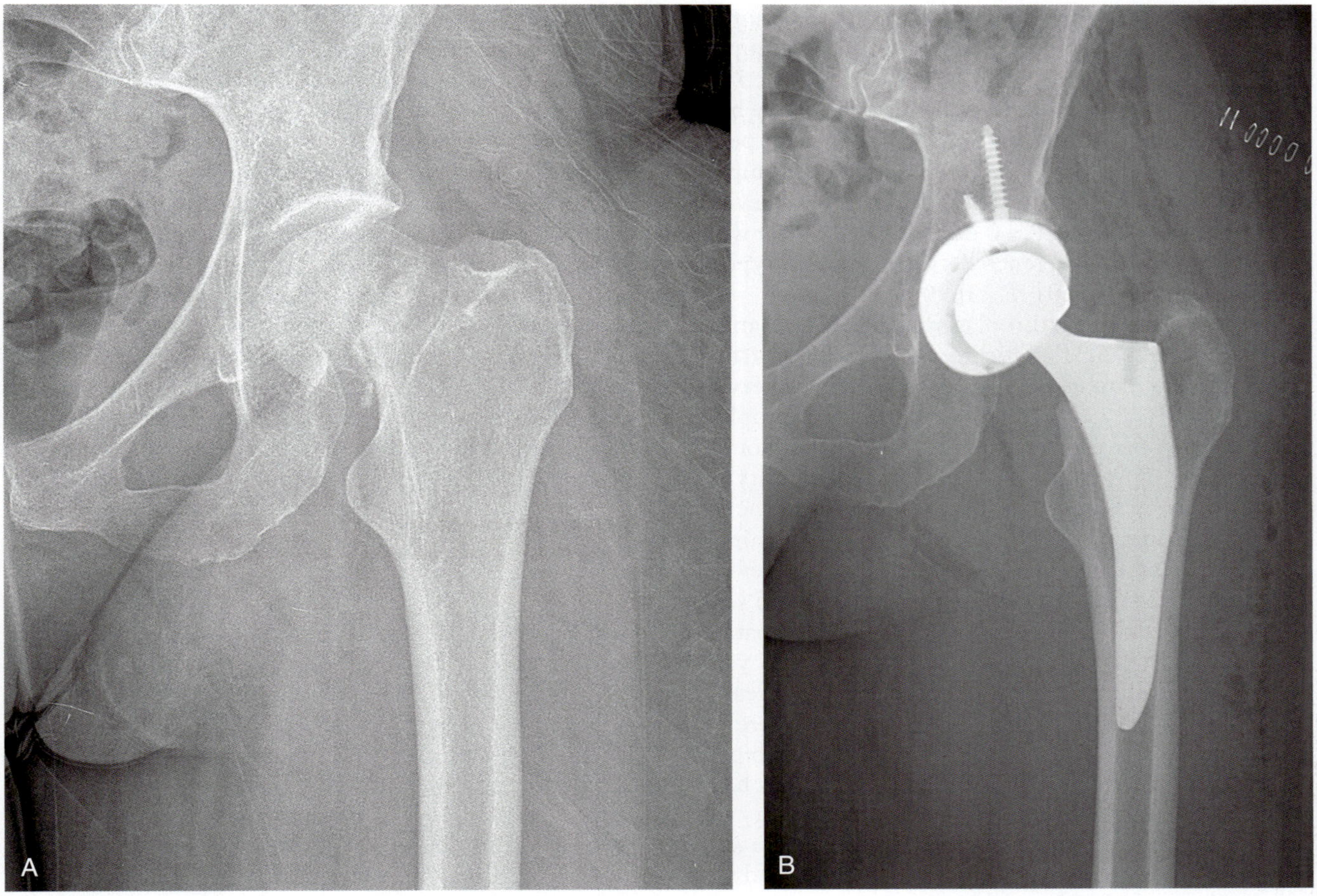

FIGURE 2 **A**, Preoperative AP radiograph of the left hip obtained from a 70-year-old active, healthy man demonstrates a displaced femoral neck fracture. **B**, Postoperative AP radiograph obtained immediately following hybrid total hip arthroplasty.

Conversely, a 2019 meta-analysis of five randomized clinical trials specifically evaluating patients older than 60 years who were independent ambulators, were healthy, and had no cognitive impairment found no difference in the revision rate between THA and hemiarthroplasty for the management of displaced hip fractures.[7]

REGISTRY AND LARGE DATABASES

Data from national registries or from large databases contradict the conclusions from the meta-analyses, generally reporting bipolar hemiarthroplasty revision rates lower than or equal to those of THA when used to manage FNFs.[8] The advantage of using data from these sources is the population-level data from a large number of patients and implants, from surgeons with all levels of experience, and almost no exclusions. Therefore, the data can be considered more representative of community practice.

In 2013, the Australian National Joint Registry first addressed arthroplasties used in the management of FNFs.[2] Overall, the 2019 annual report indicated that in the management of FNF, bipolar hemiarthroplasty had the lowest cumulative revision rate at 10 years (6.2%), followed by unipolar modular hemiarthroplasty (7.4%) and then THA (7.7%).[2] Bipolar hemiarthroplasty had a higher rate of revision compared with THA from 1.5 to 2.5 years postoperatively (hazard ratio [HR] = 1.56; $P < 0.001$). After that time, there was no difference in revision. Unipolar modular hemiarthroplasty had a lower rate of revision than THA for the first 3 months postoperatively (HR = 0.80; $P = 0.001$). From 3 months to 1.5 years there was no difference, but after that time, unipolar modular hemiarthroplasty had a higher rate of revision (HR = 1.61; $P < 0.001$). However, the revision rate of THA and hemiarthroplasty varied depending on the age of the patient. In patients younger than 70 years, no differences were reported in the 10-year cumulative revision when comparing bipolar hemiarthroplasty (10.2%) with THA (9.0%) (HR = 1.10; $P = 0.34$). However, the revision rate was significantly higher with a unipolar modular hemiarthroplasty than with a THA at all times after 3 months postoperatively (HR = 2.68; $P < 0.001$).

In patients aged 70 years and older, the 10-year cumulative revision rate for bipolar hemiarthroplasty, unipolar modular hemiarthroplasty, and THA were 5.4%, 5.9%, and 7.0%, respectively. Bipolar hemiarthroplasty had a lower rate of revision than THA for the entire period (HR = 0.77; $P < 0.001$). Compared with THA, unipolar modular hemiarthroplasty had a lower rate of revision for the first 1.5 years (HR = 0.66; $P < 0.001$), after which time there was no difference between the two types of arthroplasty (HR = 1.01; $P < 0.90$).

The Swedish Hip Arthroplasty Register 2017 annual report evaluated 75,313 patients who underwent arthroplasty for the management of a hip fracture between 2005 and 2017.[9] Unipolar modular hemiarthroplasty and THA had the same risk of a revision throughout the whole follow-up period. Bipolar hemiarthroplasty was found to have a higher risk of revision during the first 2 years postoperatively compared with either unipolar hemiarthroplasty or THA. Overall, the risk of revision varied with age—6.6% in patients younger than 75 years, 5.0% in patients 75 to 85 years old, and 3.9% in patients older than 85 years. In patients younger than 75 years, THA had a lower risk of revision surgery than hemiarthroplasty. In patients aged 75 to 85 years, there was difference in revision rates with a unipolar or bipolar hemiarthroplasty. Patients older than 85 years had a lower revision rate with a unipolar hemiarthroplasty than that with a bipolar hemiarthroplasty. Using the same registry, a study analyzing 38,912 patients who had a hip fracture between 2005 and 2012 and were treated with either a hemiarthroplasty or THA was reported in 2019.[10] The THA group had a reduced risk of revision surgery compared with the hemiarthroplasty group (HR = 0.69).

A study from the Dutch Arthroplasty Register in 2018 evaluated the failure rate and mechanism of hip fractures managed with a hemiarthroplasty and THA.[11] The study included 30,830 acute hip fractures—hemiarthroplasty was performed in 22,675 and a THA was performed in 8,155. The 5-year revision rate of THA was higher (4.3%) compared with the revision rate of hemiarthroplasty (2.5%). Dislocation was the most common reason for revision in both the hemiarthroplasty (29%) and THA (41%) patients.

Using the American College of Surgeons National Surgical Quality Improvement Project database, a 2019 study compared early postoperative outcomes in hip fracture patients older than 65 years treated with a THA or hemiarthroplasty.[12] After propensity score matching, there were 2,795 THAs and 2,795 HAs. At 30-day follow-up, there was no statistically significant relationship for treatment choice between THA and hemiarthroplasty for revision surgery ($P = 0.059$). In a longer term follow-up using propensity score matching of 12,290 independently mobile older adults with hip fractures from the United Kingdom's National Hip Fracture Database, the authors found a 33% lower risk of 12-month revision for THA patients compared with hemiarthroplasty patients.[7] These results are contrary to the findings of a 2017 study of 69,142 hemiarthroplasty and 1,100 THA Medicare patients treated for an FNF.[13] Revision surgery was more common in the THA group than the hemiarthroplasty group (HR = 2.11). At 2 years, 4.5% of the THA group had undergone revision arthroplasty, whereas only 1.6% of the hemiarthroplasty group had undergone revision surgery ($P < 0.0001$).

A 2019 study of Medicare patients who have an FNF compared the revision surgery rate of 275,439 patients treated with a hemiarthroplasty versus 26,017 patients treated with a THA.[14] At 2 years follow-up, patients undergoing hemiarthroplasty had a significantly lower rate of revision (2.48%) compared with those patients treated with a THA (3.85%) (odds ratio = 0.633; $P < 0.0001$).

COMPLICATIONS

Dislocation

The major reported disadvantage of managing an FNF with a THA and not a hemiarthroplasty is the increased risk of dislocation. Recent meta-analyses have shown a substantially greater risk of dislocation following THA for FNF compared with hemiarthroplasty.[3,6,13,14] Two other meta-analyses showed a higher rate of dislocation with a THA; however, the difference between the two types of arthroplasty was not statistically significant.[4,7] Furthermore, two large propensity-matched cohort studies in 2019 have also documented a significantly higher dislocation rate in patients treated with a THA for an FNF, compared with those treated with a hemiarthroplasty.[7,15]

Dislocation after THA is multifactorial in etiology. The meta-analyses comparing THA and hemiarthroplasty for the management of FNF have not addressed femoral head size regarding dislocation. The Australian registry has specifically analyzed the cumulative revision rate for dislocation following THA for the management of FNF and found that a femoral head smaller than 32 mm has a higher rate of revision for dislocation in all age groups (HR = 1.37; $P < 0.001$).[2] Increased femoral head size from 32 to 36 mm or larger does not confer any additional protection against revision for dislocation.[2] There is recent evidence to suggest that compared with conventional THA components, the use of dual mobility cups in FNFs can significantly decrease the risk of dislocation[16-18] (**Figure 3**). This may have an important effect on eliminating the relative risk of dislocation between THA and hemiarthroplasty in the management of FNF. A 2019 study performed a matched-pair analysis of 9,040 cases from the Nordic Arthroplasty Register Association to look at the risk of revision after FNF.[19] After propensity score matching, the authors compared 4,520 THAs with a dual mobility cup and 4,520 THAs

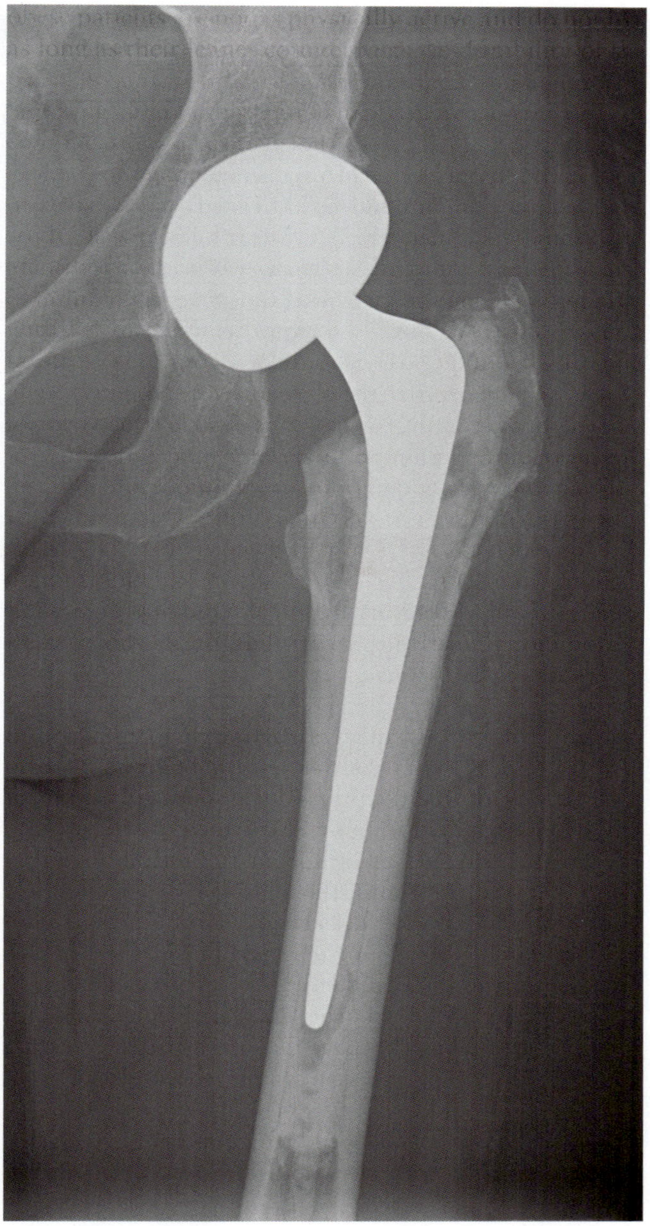

FIGURE 3 Postoperative AP radiograph following hybrid total hip arthroplasty, with a cemented femoral stem and a dual mobility cup, for a displaced femoral neck fracture.

with a conventional cup used to treat an FNF. At 2.4 years follow-up, revision of the cup due to dislocation was lower in the dual mobility group than the conventional group (HR = 0.32; $P < 0.01$).

General Complications

In general, the short-term complication rates appear to be similar following hemiarthroplasty and THA for FNF; however, in-hospital complications may be higher following hemiarthroplasty. A 2014 study using the US National Hospital Discharge Survey database[20] reported on whether in-hospital adverse events, postoperative length of stay, and mortality differed after THA or hemiarthroplasty for isolated FNFs in patients aged 60 years or older. The study included 82,951 patients (74,088 underwent hemiarthroplasty; 8,863 underwent THA) from the United States National Hospital Discharge Survey database who were treated over a 2-year period. Controlling for demographics and comorbidities, patients who underwent hemiarthroplasty had a 40% higher risk of in-hospital adverse events than those who underwent THA ($P < 0.001$). Length of stay and in-hospital mortality did not differ between these groups. It was postulated that these results may reflect the use of hemiarthroplasty in more infirmed patients, and that this was not entirely captured by the analysis of comorbidities.

A 2019 retrospective analysis of the American College of Surgeons National Surgical Quality Improvement Program from 2008 through 2016 was performed to determine the 30-day postoperative outcomes of 2,795 THAs matched with 2,795 hemiarthroplasties used to manage FNFs in patients older than 65 years.[12] Overall, the patients who had undergone THA were at a decreased risk of being in the hospital past 30 days postoperatively and were more likely to be discharged home ($P = 0.017$). When comparing the THA and hemiarthroplasty group, there was no difference in the risk of developing a major complication.

Using the large database of the California Office of Statewide Health Planning and Development, a 2013 study reported that at 90 days postoperatively, patients undergoing THA for FNF had no significant increase in complication rates compared with patients undergoing hemiarthroplasty (14.4% versus 17.4%; $P = 0.06$).[21] Outcomes were influenced by the scores on the Charlson Comorbidity Index, with increased comorbidity increasing the risk of complications. Therefore, with appropriate patient selection, THA was considered to be a safe alternative to hemiarthroplasty following acute FNFs. Also, a meta-analysis of eight trials with 986 patients reported equal rates of major (RR, 1.07) and minor (RR, 0.94) complications in patients undergoing THA or hemiarthroplasty for FNF.[22]

CLINICAL OUTCOMES

Perhaps the greatest impetus to the recent interest in THA for FNF is the reported improvement in functional outcome and quality of life when compared with hemiarthroplasty. This finding is supported by four meta-analyses that analyzed patient clinical outcomes after hemiarthroplasty or THA for the management of FNF.[3,4,6,22] A 2015 study reported that patients who underwent THA had significantly better EQindex-5D (EQ-5D) health outcome scores ($P = 0.01$), higher mobility rates within 5 years of follow-up (RR = 0.76), and significantly lower pain

(RR = 1.44) than patients who underwent hemiarthroplasty.[3] Although no difference was found in Harris Hip Scores (HHS) between the groups, the score tended to be higher after THA. A 2014 study reported that the HHS improved substantially more with THA than with hemiarthroplasty 2 years following treatment for FNF.[4] Another 2012 meta-analysis reported that the mean HHS was 81 points after THA versus 77 points after hemiarthroplasty.[22] The subdomain pain of the weighted mean HHS (42 after THA versus 39 after hemiarthroplasty), the rate of patients reporting mild to no pain (75% versus 56%), and the Western Ontario and McMaster Universities Arthritis Index score (94 versus 78) all favored THA. Quality of life measured using the EQ-5D index (0.69 versus 0.57) also favored THA. A 2019 meta-analysis study of 17 trials comparing hemiarthroplasty with THA in 1,364 patients with an FNF found that the function of patients with a THA, as determined by the HHS and Physical Function component of the SF-36, was significantly better than the function after a hemiarthroplasty.[6] Although the overall HHS in THA patients was significantly greater than the score in hemiarthroplasty patients, subanalysis of those who had a mean age younger than 80 years at the time of surgery conferred an even greater difference. Better still was the benefit in HHS identified in studies with a follow-up of more than 4 years, indicating a prolonged benefit of THA in terms of function over time.

The superiority in functional outcome with THA has recently been corroborated by a large registry study of patient-reported outcomes following surgical management of FNFs.[23] Through collaboration between the Swedish Hip Arthroplasty Register and the Swedish National Hip Fracture Register, 2,204 patients who underwent hemiarthroplasty and 808 who underwent THA for a displaced FNF were surveyed. Overall, patients who underwent THA reported less pain and were more satisfied compared with those who underwent hemiarthroplasty (although the differences between THA and hemiarthroplasty in patients younger than 70 years were not significant). Concerning health-related quality of life, patients in the THA group had the highest mean EQ-5D index (0.70 in patients younger than 70 years; 0.71 in patients older than 70 years). In patients younger than 70 years, the lowest mean EQ-5D index (0.48) was found in the hemiarthroplasty group ($P < 0.001$). Patient-reported pain was significantly higher in the hemiarthroplasty group than the THA group in patients older than 70 years. Moderate to unbearable pain (adjusted for sex and age) for patients older than 70 years was significantly higher in the hemiarthroplasty group (RR, 1.8; $P < 0.001$) than in the THA group. Among patients older than 70 years, those who underwent hemiarthroplasty were not as satisfied as those who underwent THA ($P < 0.001$). For those patients older than 70 years, dissatisfaction with their outcome was higher in the hemiarthroplasty group (RR, 2.3; $P < 0.001$) than in the THA group.

A 2019 prospective, multicenter, randomized clinical trial involving 1,495 patients, who were 50 years of age or older, and had either a THA or hemiarthroplasty for an FNF, specifically addressed health-related quality of life and function following surgery.[24] At 2-year follow-up, the study showed slightly but significantly lower Western Ontario and McMaster Universities Arthritis Index scores (indicating better function) in the THA group, as well as trends that favored THA in EQ-5D, SF-12 scores, and Timed Up and Go test times. However, the differences in Western Ontario and McMaster Universities Arthritis Index scores were deemed clinically unimportant on the basis of the thresholds for the minimal clinically important difference.

TREATMENT ALGORITHM

The goal of hip fracture management is to restore the patient's preoperative function with the lowest possible complication and revision rates. Given the risk/benefit profile of arthroplasty to manage FNFs, an algorithm was proposed to help consider arthroplasty for management of a displaced FNF.[1] THA was recommended in all cases with preexisting osteoarthritis or inflammatory arthritis and in patients older than 65 years who have a displaced FNF. However, because the dislocation rate is higher for THA than for hemiarthroplasty, in the cognitively impaired patient or the patient at high risk of dislocation, unipolar or bipolar hemiarthroplasty or THA with a dual mobility cup is recommended.

In December 2015, the American Academy of Orthopaedic Surgeons (AAOS) Board of Directors adopted the Appropriate Use Criteria for the acute treatment of hip fractures in patients older than 60 years.[25] These criteria were developed to address the most common clinical scenarios to treat hip fractures, to improve patient care, and to obtain the best outcomes while considering the subtleties and distinctions necessary in clinical decision making. Patient scenarios were created based on the fracture type, the patient's preoperative mobility and functional status, and whether there was preexisting hip arthritis. Treatments of 30 various patient scenarios (ie, criteria) were classified as appropriate, may be appropriate, or rarely appropriate. These criteria were developed as guidelines and are not meant to supersede clinician expertise and experience or patient preference.

Overall, strong evidence was presented for the guidelines for displaced FNFs and moderate evidence for the guidelines for stable FNFs, the use of hemiarthroplasty versus THA, and the need to cement the femoral stem. Regarding the use of hemiarthroplasty versus THA, the AAOS Clinical Practice Guideline on the Management

TABLE 1

Indications for the Treatment of Acute Nondisplaced Femoral Neck Fractures

Scenario	Total Hip Arthroplasty	Hemiarthroplasty
Nondisplaced femoral neck, high-functioning/high-demand patient, preexisting and symptomatic arthritis	Appropriate	Rarely appropriate
Nondisplaced femoral neck, moderate-functioning to low-functioning patient, preexisting and symptomatic arthritis	Appropriate	May be appropriate
Nondisplaced femoral neck, nonambulatory/bed-dependent/palliative (low-function/low-demand) patient, preexisting and symptomatic arthritis	May be appropriate	Appropriate
Nondisplaced femoral neck, high-functioning/high-demand patient, no preexisting and symptomatic arthritis	Rarely appropriate	May be appropriate
Nondisplaced femoral neck, moderate-functioning to low-functioning patient, no preexisting and symptomatic arthritis	Rarely appropriate	May be appropriate
Nondisplaced femoral neck, nonambulatory/bed-dependent/palliative (low-function/low-demand) patient, no preexisting and symptomatic arthritis	Rarely appropriate	Rarely appropriate

Adapted from American Academy of Orthopaedic Surgeons. *AAOS Appropriate Use Criteria for the acute treatment of hip fractures in the elderly.* Rosemont, IL: American Academy of Orthopaedic Surgeons; 2015. https://www.aaos.org/globalassets/quality-and-practice-resources/hip-fractures-in-the-elderly/hip-fx-auc_hardcopy-treatment_3.31.161.pdf. Accessed July 14, 2020.

of Hip Fractures in the Elderly indicates that moderate evidence exists to support the benefit to THA in properly selected patients who have unstable (displaced) FNFs.

Regarding specific patient scenarios, the indications for THA or hemiarthroplasty varied for nondisplaced (Garden type 1 or 2) or displaced (Garden type 3 or 4) FNFs (**Tables 1** and **2**). In general, if arthroplasty is chosen to treat a nondisplaced FNF, THA is appropriate if there is concomitant arthritis, except for patients who have low functional demand, in whom hemiarthroplasty is considered appropriate. For displaced FNFs, hemiarthroplasty is appropriate for all cases, and THA is appropriate for those cases of preexisting arthritis and in high-function, high-demand patients who do not have preexisting arthritis.

TABLE 2

Indications for the Management of Acute Displaced Femoral Neck Fractures

Scenario	Total Hip Arthroplasty	Hemiarthroplasty
Displaced femoral neck, high-functioning/high-demand patient, preexisting and symptomatic arthritis	Appropriate	Appropriate
Displaced femoral neck, high-functioning/high-demand patient, no preexisting and symptomatic arthritis	Appropriate	Appropriate
Displaced femoral neck, moderate-functioning to low-functioning patient, preexisting and symptomatic arthritis	Appropriate	Appropriate
Displaced femoral neck, moderate-functioning to low-functioning patient, no preexisting and symptomatic arthritis	May be appropriate	Appropriate
Displaced femoral neck, nonambulatory/bed-dependent/palliative (low-function/low-demand) patient, preexisting and symptomatic arthritis	May be appropriate	Appropriate
Displaced femoral neck, nonambulatory/bed-dependent/palliative (low-function/low-demand) patient, no preexisting and symptomatic arthritis	Rarely appropriate	Appropriate

Adapted from American Academy of Orthopaedic Surgeons. *AAOS Appropriate Use Criteria for the acute treatment of hip fractures in the elderly.* Rosemont, IL: American Academy of Orthopaedic Surgeons; 2015. https://www.aaos.org/globalassets/quality-and-practice-resources/hip-fractures-in-the-elderly/hip-fx-auc_hardcopy-treatment_3.31.161.pdf. Accessed July 14, 2020.

In 2017, National Institute for Health and Care Excellence (NICE) made new recommendations on hip arthroplasties for patients who have a displaced intracapsular fracture.[26] The guidelines recommended offering replacement arthroplasty (THA or hemiarthroplasty) to patients who have a displaced intracapsular hip fracture. It was recommended that a THA, rather than a hemiarthroplasty be used to treat patients who have a displaced intracapsular hip fracture who were able to walk independently out of doors with no more than the use of a stick and are not cognitively impaired and are medically fit for anesthesia and the procedure.

SUMMARY

The choice between THA and hemiarthroplasty for the treatment of FNF remains a controversial issue in orthopaedic surgery. The recent scientific literature and registry data indicate that THA is associated with improved clinical outcomes, but with higher dislocation rates. The same data provide conflicting results regarding implant survivorship. Therefore, both procedures have a role in treatment, and algorithms have been developed to simplify the choice and optimize the results of THA and hemiarthroplasty in the management of FNFs.

KEY STUDY POINTS

- The choice between THA and hemiarthroplasty for the management of FNF remains controversial.
- THA for the management of FNFs results in improved clinical outcomes.
- THA for the management of FNFs can result in a higher risk of dislocation. A femoral head size of at least 32 mm should be used.
- The role of dual mobility cups is still evolving.
- Hemiarthroplasty with a bipolar head continues to have an important role in the management of FNFs. Unipolar heads are best reserved for patients older than 80 years.

ANNOTATED REFERENCES

1. Su EP, Su SL: Femoral neck fractures: A changing paradigm. *Bone Joint J* 2014;96-B(11 suppl A):43-47.

2. Australian Orthopaedic Association National Joint Replacement Registry: Annual Report 2019. Available at: https://aoanjrr.sahmri.com/documents/10180/668596/Hip%2C+Knee+%26+Shoulder+Arthroplasty/c287d2a3-22df-a3bb-37a2-91e6c00bfcf0. Accessed October 26, 2019.

   This 2019 annual report on hip and knee arthroplasty is published by the Australian Joint Registry.

3. Wang F, Zhang H, Zhang Z, Ma C, Feng X: Comparison of bipolar hemiarthroplasty and total hip arthroplasty for displaced femoral neck fractures in the healthy elderly: A meta-analysis. *BMC Musculoskelet Disord* 2015;16:229.

4. Zhao Y, Fu D, Chen K, et al: Outcome of hemiarthroplasty and total hip replacement for active elderly patients with displaced femoral neck fractures: A meta-analysis of 8 randomized clinical trials. *PLoS One* 2014;9(5):e98071.

5. Jonas SC, Shah R, Al-Hadithy N, Norton MR, Sexton SA, Middleton RG: Displaced intracapsular neck of femur fractures in the elderly: Bipolar hemiarthroplasty may be the treatment of choice; a case control study. *Injury* 2015;46(10):1988-1991.

6. Lewis DP, Wæver D, Thorninger R, Donnelly WJ: Hemiarthroplasty vs total hip arthroplasty for the management of displaced neck of femur fractures: A systematic review and meta-analysis. *J Arthroplasty* 2019;34(8):1837-1843.e2.

   This meta-analysis of 17 studies including 1,364 patients (660 THA and 704 hemiarthroplasty) of all randomized and quasi-randomized trials compared hemiarthroplasty with THA in patients with FNF (Garden III and IV).

7. Metcalfe D, Judge A, Perry DC, Gabbe B, Zogg CK, Costa ML: Total hip arthroplasty versus hemiarthroplasty for independently mobile older adults with intracapsular hip fractures. *BMC Musculoskelet Disord* 2019;20(1):226.

   This study is a systematic review and meta-analysis of five randomized clinical trials and an analysis of a propensity score-matched national cohort comparing the outcomes between hemiarthroplasty and THA for independently mobile older adults with hip fractures.

8. Kannan A, Kancherla R, McMahon S, Hawdon G, Soral A, Malhotra R: Arthroplasty options in femoral-neck fracture: Answers from the National Registries. *Int Orthop* 2012;36(1):1-8.

9. Swedish Hip Arthroplasty Register: Annual Report 2017. Available at: https://registercentrum.blob.core.windows.net/shpr/r/Eng_Arsrapport_2017_Hoftprotes_final-Syx2fJPhMN.pdf. Accessed October 26, 2019.

   This 2017 annual report on hip and knee arthroplasty is published by the Swedish Joint Registry.

10. Jawad Z, Nemes S, Bülow E, Rogmark C, Cnudde P: Multistate analysis of hemi- and total hip arthroplasty for hip fractures in the Swedish population – Results from a Swedish National database study of 38,912 patients. *Injury* 2019;50(2):272-277.

    This is a registry study comparing revision rates of hemiarthroplasty and THA for the management of hip fracture.

11. Moerman S, Mathijssen NMC, Tuinebreijer WE, Vochteloo AJH, Nelissen RGHH: Hemiarthroplasty and total hip arthroplasty in 30,830 patients with hip fractures: Data from the Dutch Arthroplasty Register on revision and risk factors for revision. *Acta Orthop* 2018;89(5):509-514.

    This study is an analysis of the rate and failure mechanisms (ie, end-point revision surgery and reasons for revision) of hemiarthroplasties and total hip arthroplasty using data from the national Dutch Arthroplasty Register.

12. Warren JA, Sundaram K, Anis HK, Piuzzi NS, Higuera CA, Kamath AF: Total hip arthroplasty outperforms hemiarthroplasty in patients aged 65 years and older: A propensity-matched study of short-term outcomes. *Geriatr Orthop Surg Rehabil* 2019;10:2151459319876854.

This study is an American College of Surgeons National Surgical Quality Improvement Project database study looking at the 30-day complication rates in patients older than 65 years treated with a THA or hemiarthroplasty for their hip fracture.

13. Wang Z, Bhattacharyya T: Outcomes of hemiarthroplasty and total hip arthroplasty for femoral neck fracture: A Medicare cohort study. *J Orthop Trauma* 2017;31(5):260-263.

This is a Medicare database study comparing hemiarthroplasty and THA for FNF. Level of evidence: III.

14. Eskildsen SM, Kamath GV, Del Gaizo DJ: Age matters when comparing hemiarthroplasty and total hip arthroplasty for femoral neck fractures in Medicare patients. *Hip Int* 2019;29(6):674-679.

In this study, patients who underwent THA for femoral neck fractures had a higher rate of dislocations and infections and increased rates of repeat surgery than those who underwent hemiarthroplasty, but this difference was not significant in patients aged 65 to 69 years.

15. Ravi B, Pincus D, Khan H, Wasserstein D, Jenkinson R, Kreder HJ: Comparing complications and costs of total hip arthroplasty and hemiarthroplasty for femoral neck fractures: A propensity score-matched, population-based study. *J Bone Joint Surg Am* 2019;101(7):572-579.

Among elderly patients with displaced femoral neck fractures, total hip arthroplasty was associated with lower rates of revision surgical procedures and reduced healthcare costs during the index admission and in the year following the surgical procedure, relative to hemiarthroplasty. Level of evidence: III.

16. Ukaj S, Zhuri O, Ukaj F, et al: Dual mobility acetabular cup versus hemiarthroplasty in treatment of displaced femoral neck fractures in elderly patients: Comparative study and results at minimum 3-year follow-up. *Geriatr Orthop Surg Rehabil* 2019;10:2151459319848610.

This is a prospective, comparative interventional single-blinded study looking at the role of dual mobility cups, compared with hemiarthroplasty in the management of femoral neck fractures. Level of evidence: II.

17. Tabori-Jensen S, Hansen TB, Stilling M: Low dislocation rate of Saturne®/Avantage® dual-mobility THA after displaced femoral neck fracture: A cohort study of 966 hips with a minimum 1.6-year follow-up. *Arch Orthop Trauma Surg* 2019;139(5):605-612.

A short-term study assessed the dislocation rate in 966 consecutive patients, with mean age of 80.5 years, with a displaced FNF managed with a dual mobility articulation or a THA.

18. Assi CC, Barakat HB, Caton JH, Najjar EN, Samaha CT, Yammine KF: Mortality rate and mid-term outcomes of total hip arthroplasty using dual mobility cups for the treatment of femoral neck fractures in a Middle Eastern population. *J Arthroplasty* 2019;34(2):333-337.

This study demonstrates a decreased rate of dislocation with dual mobility cups in Middle Eastern patients with an FNF, even in patients having rituals and customs involving extreme hip positions.

19. Jobory A, Kärrholm J, Overgaard S, et al: Reduced revision risk for dual-mobility cup in total hip replacement due to hip fracture: A matched-pair analysis of 9,040 cases from the Nordic Arthroplasty Register Association (NARA). *J Bone Joint Surg Am* 2019;101(14):1278-1285.

This Nordic Registry study demonstrated a significant decrease in the rate of dislocation in THA with a dual mobility cup in the management of femoral neck fractures. Level of evidence: III.

20. Voskuijl T, Neuhaus V, Kinaci A, Vrahas M, Ring D: In-hospital outcomes after hemiarthroplasty versus total hip arthroplasty for isolated femoral neck fractures. *Arch Bone Joint Surg* 2014;2(3):151-156.

21. SooHoo NF, Farng E, Chambers L, Znigmond DS, Lieberman JR: Comparison of complication rates between hemiarthroplasty and total hip arthroplasty for intracapsular hip fractures. *Orthopedics* 2013;36(4):e384-e389.

22. Burgers PT, Van Geene AR, Van den Bekerom MP, et al: Total hip arthroplasty versus hemiarthroplasty for displaced femoral neck fractures in the healthy elderly: A meta-analysis and systematic review of randomized trials. *Int Orthop* 2012;36(8):1549-1560.

23. Leonardsson O, Rolfson O, Hommel A, Garellick G, Åkesson K, Rogmark C: Patient-reported outcome after displaced femoral neck fracture: A National Survey of 4467 patients. *J Bone Joint Surg Am* 2013;95(18):1693-1699.

24. HEALTH Investigators, Bhandari M, Einhorn TA, et al: Total hip arthroplasty or hemiarthroplasty for hip fracture. *N Engl J Med* 2019;381(23):1-10.

This prospective, randomized clinical trial of 1,495 patients shows that the incidence of secondary procedures did not differ significantly between patients who were randomly assigned to undergo THA and those who were assigned to undergo hemiarthroplasty, and THA provided a clinically unimportant improvement over hemiarthroplasty in function and quality of life over 24 months.

25. American Academy of Orthopaedic Surgeons: *Appropriate Use Criteria for the Acute Treatment of Hip Fractures in Patients Over 60 Years of Age.* Rosemont, IL, American Academy of Orthopaedic Surgeons, 2015. Available at: http://www.aaos.org/uploadedFiles/PreProduction/Quality/AUCs_and_Performance_Measures/appropriate_use/Hip%20Fx%20Tx%20AUC.pdf.

26. National Institute for Health and Care Excellence (NICE): *Hip fracture: Management*, in *Clinical Guidelines*. London, National Institute for Health and Care Excellence, 2017. Available at: https://www.nice.org.uk/guidance/cg124/chapter/Recommendations#surgical-procedures. Accessed October 26, 2019.

The National Institute for Health and Care Excellence (NICE) recommends offering replacement arthroplasty (THA or hemiarthroplasty) to patients with a displaced intracapsular hip fracture.

CHAPTER 29

Surgical Approaches for a Primary Total Hip Arthroplasty—Advantages and Disadvantages

MICHAEL TANZER, MD, FRCSC, FAAOS • DYLAN TANZER, MD

ABSTRACT

The choice of surgical approach in primary total hip arthroplasty remains controversial. The recent scientific literature and registry data indicate that although there are advantages and disadvantages of each of the approaches, there is no clear evidence to support the superiority of one approach over all the others. Most surgeons choose a surgical approach based on the experience, comfort, and training, and the surgeons need to balance this against the potential risks and benefits of the preferred approach. Large, randomized clinical trials are required to further clarify this issue.

Keywords: arthroplasty; dislocation; hip; infection; revision; surgical approach

Dr. Michael Tanzer or an immediate family member is a member of a speakers' bureau or has made paid presentations on behalf of Stryker and Zimmer; has received research or institutional support from DePuy, A Johnson & Johnson Company, Stryker, and Zimmer; and serves as a board member, owner, officer, or committee member of the American Academy of Orthopaedic Surgeons and the Canadian Arthroplasty Society. Neither Dr. Dylan Tanzer nor any immediate family member has received anything of value from or has stock or stock options held in a commercial company or institution related directly or indirectly to the subject of this chapter.

INTRODUCTION

Total hip arthroplasty (THA) can be performed through various approaches to the hip. These include the posterior approach and its minimally invasive surgical (MIS) variants, the direct lateral approach, the anterolateral approach, and the direct anterior approach (DAA). Each of the surgical approaches has its own advantages and disadvantages. Presently, there is no consensus in the literature on which is the optimal surgical approach. This is echoed by the American Academy of Orthopaedic Surgery guidelines that state that there are no clinically significant differences in patient-oriented outcomes related to the surgical approach for patients with symptomatic osteoarthritis of the hip undergoing THA.[1] It is important for orthopaedic surgeons to have an up-to-date and evidence-based understanding of the advantages and disadvantages of the various surgical approaches to the hip. The recently published outcomes of the most common surgical approaches to the hip are specifically addressed.

THE INFLUENCE OF SURGICAL APPROACH ON THE RISK OF DISLOCATION

Dislocation after THA is multifactorial, with surgical approach being only one of the factors. Patient factors, implant design, the recent use of larger femoral head size, improved postoperative rehabilitation protocols, and patient education make it difficult to ascertain the direct influence of the surgical approach on the risk of dislocation.

Historically, the posterior approach has been associated with a higher risk of dislocation compared with other approaches. However, the earlier posterior surgical approaches did not include repair or even preservation of the posterior structures, which is now recognized as an important step in reducing the risk of dislocation. Multiple studies now confirm the rate of dislocation with a posterior approach to the hip, and a capsular repair can have a comparable rate of dislocation to those of other surgical approaches. As early as 1990, the surgical technique with repair of the hip capsule and short external rotators was reported in in 259 consecutive cases, resulting in a dislocation rate of less than 1%.[2] The importance of capsular closure was demonstrated in a 2017 multicenter case-control study of 128 unstable and 438 stable hips.[3] An unrepaired joint capsule with a posterior approach was found to be a significant risk factor for instability, with an odds ratio of 6.0.

Although one of the perceived advantages of the DAA is it being superior to other approaches with respect to preventing instability, there is some recent literature that questions this belief. A 2018 systematic review and meta-analysis of prospective studies compared the early, 90-day dislocation rate of THA with those of the posterior approach and the DAA.[4] This review of 13 prospective comparative studies (7 randomized) with THA through a DAA ($n = 524$) or posterior approach ($n = 520$) found no differences between the surgical approaches and the dislocation rates. This finding is supported by a 2016 statewide registry study in which 2,147 patients who underwent DAA THA were propensity score matched with patients undergoing THA with a posterior approach.[5] The 90-day adverse event analysis revealed no differences in dislocation rates between the DAA and posterior approach. A smaller prospective randomized study similarly showed equivalent dislocation rates 12 weeks following DAA and posterior approach for primary THA.[6] Some studies with longer follow-up have shown that the dislocation rate with the posterior approach is higher than the DAA. A 2015 registry review of 22,237 THAs at a median follow-up of 3 years found that the anterolateral approach (adjusted hazard ratio = 0.29) and DAA (adjusted hazard ratio = 0.44) had a lower risk of dislocation relative to the posterior approach.[7] Another cohort registry study of 38,399 primary THA compared the risk of dislocation between posterior approach and the DAA.[8] At 2-year follow-up, after adjusting for covariates, DAA had a lower risk of dislocation compared with posterior approach THA (hazard ratio = 0.39).

The risk of revision THA for dislocation with the posterior approach has been shown to be minimized with the use of larger femoral heads. A 2017 Dutch Arthroplasty Registry analysis of 166,231 THAs (posterior approach: 100,823; direct lateral approach: 35,830; DAA: 14,446; anterolateral approach: 12,744) found that the posterior approach was associated with higher risk of revision for dislocation than the other approaches.[9] At a mean follow-up of 6 years, the risk with a posterior approach was 1.1%, compared with 0.5% to 0.6% for the direct lateral, anterolateral, and direct anterior approaches. However, with 36-mm heads, the risk of revision for dislocation was no different with the posterior approach (0.6%) than with the other approaches.

The lateral approach to the hip has been commonly used, in part, because of its historically low dislocation rate. A 2012 analysis of 78,098 surgeries in the Swedish Hip Arthroplasty Register specifically evaluated the effect of surgical approach on the risk of revision due to dislocation.[10] At a mean follow-up of 2.7 years, the authors found that MIS approaches (relative risk = 4.2) and the posterior approach (relative risk = 1.3) had a higher risk of revision due to dislocation than the direct lateral approach. A 2015 systematic review and meta-analysis of six studies involving 3,377 THAs showed that both DAA and the direct lateral approach were associated with similar risk of dislocation (direct anterior versus lateral approaches, relative risk = 1.15).[11] However, this conclusion has been challenged by a recent population-based retrospective cohort study.[12] The authors compared 2,993 propensity score–matched patients undergoing a DAA with 2,993 matched patients undergoing a direct lateral approach (2,326) or a posterior approach (667) for the THA. At 1 year, patients who had an anterior approach had a significantly greater risk of dislocation, requiring closed or open reduction (0.7% versus 0.3%; hazard ratio = 2.63). Although the lateral approach has historically been associated with a lower risk of dislocation than the posterior approach, this may no longer be the case since the introduction of the modern posterior approach surgical technique that repairs the capsule and posterior structures. This finding was highlighted in a 2019 observational study of 156,979 hips in the Swedish Hip Arthroplasty Register.[13] The authors investigated the risk of revision surgery due to dislocation for the posterior and direct lateral surgical approaches and compared the risk for two periods (1999 to 2006 and 2007 to 2014). At 2 years postoperatively, the posterior approach was found to be associated with a higher risk of revision surgery due to dislocation in the period from 1999 to 2006 (hazard ratio = 2.3), but not in the period from 2007 to 2014 (hazard ratio = 1.2) compared with the lateral approach. This change over time was postulated to be a result of the improved surgical technique for the posterior approach.

The Australian Orthopaedic Association National Joint Replacement Registry (AOANJRR) has been collecting data on revisions for dislocation of primary THA by surgical approach for the past 3 years.[14] Of the 122,345

THAs being followed, the surgical approach was a posterior approach in 65,791, a DAA in 32,086, and a lateral approach in 24,468. Overall, the anterior approach had a lower rate of revision for dislocation compared with the posterior approach (hazard ratio = 1.87) and for the first 6 months compared with the lateral approach (hazard ratio = 1.48). The posterior approach had a higher rate of revision for dislocation compared with the lateral approach (hazard ratio = 1.27). These findings are slightly different than that reported in a 2017 analysis of 21,860 THAs from the Norwegian Arthroplasty Register in which only the posterior approach has a higher risk of revision for dislocation than the direct lateral approach.[15] The cohort consisted of THAs performed through an MIS DAA in 2017: 2,087 through an MIS anterolateral approach; 5,961 through a posterior approach; and 11,795 through a direct lateral approach. The registry data revealed that the relative risk of revision due to dislocation using the posterior approach was more than double (2.1, $P < 0.001$) that of the direct lateral approach. The relative risk was 0.71 ($P = 0.25$) for the MIS DAA and anterolateral approach compared with the direct lateral approach.

Overall, there remains conflicting data regarding the best surgical approach to minimize the risk of dislocation. The historically high dislocation rate with the posterior approach has been markedly decreased with contemporary surgical techniques that include capsular closure and the use of larger femoral heads. Nevertheless, it is not unreasonable to consider that the posterior approach has a slightly higher dislocation rate than the other approaches. The literature regarding the superiority of the DAA versus the direct lateral approach is inconsistent and requires level I studies to clarify.

THE INFLUENCE OF SURGICAL APPROACH ON THE RISK OF INFECTION

Despite some conflicting evidence, it appears that the DAA is associated with a higher risk of wound complications, and possibly infection. This is likely related to the proximity of the incision to the abdominal pannus and inguinal crease. A 2014 cohort study comparing wound complications between the direct anterior (505 hips) and posterior (1,288 hips) approaches found a significantly greater number of DAA THAs that required revision surgery as a result of wound-related complications (1.4% versus 0.2%).[16] The risk of wound complications is even greater with the DAA in obese patients, as shown in a 2015 retrospective cohort study.[17] When comparing the rate of wound infections in 716 DAA THAs with 3,040 posterior THAs, the authors found that obesity (body mass index [BMI] ≥30 kg/m²) was a stronger risk factor for wound complication with patients undergoing DAA (hazard ratio = 4.3) than in patients undergoing posterior approach (hazard ratio = 1.4). This was even more apparent in morbidly obese patients (BMI ≥40 kg/m²) with the hazard ratio being 19.3 in DAA THAs and 3.8 for THAs with a posterior approach. The increased risk of wound complications in obese patients having a DAA has been corroborated in a 2015 study that retrospectively compared the outcomes of 210 obese and nonobese patients undergoing a THA through a DAA.[18] This study demonstrated that obese patients undergoing a DAA have a 3.6 times increase in wound complications compared with patients with a BMI <30 kg/m². Similarly, an earlier study in 2011 of 800 primary THAs performed with a DAA reported a wound complication in 4.6% of the patients.[19] A 2018 study comparing the DAA with the posterior approach found higher rates of superficial wound complications after DAA hip arthroplasty regardless of BMI.[20] This single-center, multisurgeon, retrospective cohort analysis involved 4,651 consecutive primary THAs, in which the surgical approach was the DAA in 2,424 cases and the posterior approach in 2,227 cases. The rate of superficial wound complications for all patients undergoing DAA was 1.07% compared with 0.40% for all patients undergoing posterior approach ($P < 0.01$), with a hazard ratio of 2.7. In contrast to other studies, the rate of wound complications in nonobese (BMI <35 kg/m²) patients was significantly greater in the DAA hips than the posterior approach hips (1.0% and 0.3%, respectively, $P < 0.005$), but there was no difference in the rate of wound complications in the obese patients (BMI ≥35 kg/m²) (1.0% in DAA and 0.3% in posterior approach, $P = 0.10$).

The increased rate of deep infection in obese patients undergoing DAA was first reported in a 2016 study that retrospectively evaluated 1,621 consecutive primary THAs performed with a DAA.[21] The severely obese patients (BMI ≥35 kg/m²) had a deep infection treated with a revision procedure in 2.5% of the THAs, compared with 0.35% of the THAs with a BMI <35 kg/m² ($P = 0.0044$).

Therefore, in this study, obese patients undergoing DAA hip were at 7 times greater risk than the nonobese counterparts to develop a postoperative infection. In a subsequent 2018 follow-up study, the same author found no difference in the infection rate between the DAA THAs (2,424 hips) and the posterior approach THAs (2,227 hips), independent of whether the patients were obese (BMI ≥35 kg/m²) or not (BMI <35 kg/m²).[20] However, the infection rate in the nonobese DAA group was 0.28%, as compared with the obese DAA group (2.35%; $P = 0.0003$). This difference reflects a relative risk of 8.4 for patients undergoing DAA with a BMI ≥35 kg/m². The increased risk of infection in obese patients undergoing a THA with a DAA is supported by a 2018 matched-control, retrospective, clinical study comparing 129 DAA

THAs in obese (BMI ≥35 kg/m^2) patients with 118 DAA THAs in nonobese (BMI <25 kg/m^2) patients.[22] Obese patients were 2.9 times more likely to develop a wound complication than the nonobese patients and 5.8 times more likely to develop an infection. In a 2018 retrospective study comparing 796 posterior approach THAs with 399 DAA THAs, no difference was found in the rates of wound complications or infections leading to revision surgery.[23] However, the rate of prosthetic joint infections (PJIs) following the DAA (1.5%) was double that following the posterior approach (0.75%). The difference was not statistically significant ($P = 0.23$); however, the power analysis done by the authors showed that the study was underpowered.

There is conflicting literature on the effect of the DAA on PJI compared with nonanterior surgical approaches.[12,14,20,24] With this being the case, a 2019 retrospective cohort study specifically evaluated whether PJI rates differed between the DAA and nonanterior approach.[24] The study evaluated 6,086 consecutive patients (1,985 patients in the DAA group, 4,101 patients in the nonanterior group) and found in the multivariate analysis that patients in the DAA group had 2.2 times the odds of experiencing a PJI after THA. Overall, the rate of PJI was significantly higher in the DAA group compared with the nonanterior group (1.2% versus 0.6%; $P = 0.023$). Another 2019 study from the same institution and the author found a higher number of revision surgeries in the anterior group, mainly because of wound drainage and infection.[25] A 2020 population-based retrospective cohort study of 2,993 propensity score–matched patients undergoing a DAA with 2,993 matched patients undergoing a direct lateral or a posterior approach also demonstrated that the DAA had a significantly greater risk of deep infection that required surgery (1.2% versus 0.4%; hazard ratio = 3.27).[12] In contrast to these studies, the 2019 AOANJRR reported a lower rate of revision for infection for the anterior approach compared with the posterior approach (hazard ratio = 1.58) and for the first 3 months compared with the lateral approach (hazard ratio = 1.85).[14]

The 2019 AOANJRR did not find any difference between the posterior and lateral approaches, with respect to revision for infection. This is supported by an earlier 2012 study from the Swedish Hip Arthroplasty Register of 90,662 cemented THAs that found that using a posterior or direct lateral surgical approach had no influence on revision rate due to infection.[26] In contrast, the 2017 analysis of 21,860 THAs from the Norwegian Arthroplasty Register found that revision due to infection was greatest with the direct lateral approach.[15] Compared with the lateral approach, the relative risk of revision for infection was 0.53 ($P = 0.002$) for the DAA and anterolateral approach and 0.57 (0.80, $P = 0.001$) for the posterior approach.

Aside for obese patients, there remains contradictory information regarding the effect of surgical approach on the rate of infection following THA. Future prospective randomized studies with multivariate analysis should be performed to confirm the effect of the approach on infection after THA.

THE INFLUENCE OF SURGICAL APPROACH ON POSTOPERATIVE RECOVERY

Although the postoperative course of a patient undergoing THA is multifactorial, the surgical approach can have an effect on the patient's recovery. Furthermore, the patient's ability to recover quickly after surgery has an important influence on the length of stay in the hospital, and the patient's ability to return to the daily life and work. Several studies have addressed this issue, with particular emphasis on the DAA, which is considered by surgeons using this approach to be one of its advantages.

A 2019 systematic review and meta-analysis of 20 articles comprising 7,377 patients (DAA: 3,728 and posterior approach: 3,649) found the DAA was superior to posterior approach in early functional recovery, activity ability, pain relief, and hospitalization duration.[27] Similarly, the 2018 systematic review and meta-analysis of 13 prospective studies comparing postoperative outcomes of the DAA and posterior approach in the first 90 days found patients treated with the DAA reported less pain, consumed fewer narcotics, and reported better Harris Hip Scores.[4] These results were unchanged when assessing only the seven randomized clinical trials (RCTs) included in this meta-analysis. One of the studies included in this systematic review was a 2018 prospective RCT that specifically addressed the functional recovery of patients undergoing THA through a DAA compared with an MIS posterior approach (MPA).[28] One surgeon performed DAA THAs in 52 hips and three other surgeons performed the 49 THAs in the posterior approach group. All patients were evaluated at 2 weeks, 2 months, and 1 year. At 2 weeks, only activity monitoring and the patient's milestone diary were assessed. The authors found that at 2 weeks, there were small differences in early functional recovery that favored the DAA versus the MPA: time to discontinue walker use (10 days versus 15 days, $P = 0.01$), time to discontinue all gait aids (17 days versus 24 days, $P = 0.04$), time to do stairs with a gait aid (5 days versus 10 days, $P < 0.01$), time to walk six blocks (21 days versus 26 days, $P = 0.05$), and the mean steps per day (3,897 versus 2,235, $P < 0.01$). There were no other differences in the other early functional milestones. Patient-reported outcome scores were first evaluated at 2 months postoperatively, and there was no difference between the groups. Overall, the authors found that patients undergoing the DAA had a slightly faster recovery, as measured by milestones of function and quantified by activity monitor data, but no substantive differences were evident at the second follow-up, 2 months postoperatively.

The difference in the early functional recovery of patients undergoing a DAA or direct lateral approach THA was assessed in a 2016 RCT.[29] When comparing 44 DAA THAs with 40 direct lateral approach THAs, the DAA patients were found to have better function in some early activity outcomes measured, including the measured timed up and go test and the gait speed test ($P = 0.0001$). These differences were no longer apparent at 4 weeks postoperatively. However, the authors did find that the DAA groups had a better Lower Extremity Functional Score, and the difference leveled out at 6 months. Overall, it was concluded that the DAA did provide some benefits in early functional recovery, but not in other measured parameters, compared with the direct lateral approach.

Like the DAA, the anterolateral approach is an intermuscular approach to the hip with the potential benefit of an earlier functional recovery. This was addressed in a 2013 prospective, multicenter RCT that compared the quality of life and patient satisfaction scores of 135 patients undergoing primary THA through either an MIS anterolateral approach (69 hips) or the surgeon's preferred MIS approach (direct lateral approach: 40 hips or posterior approach: 26 hips).[30] The authors found no differences between the anterolateral group and the comparison group at early recovery (Western Ontario and McMaster Universities Osteoarthritis Index, 3 months postoperatively), nor in generic quality of life (SF-36) or patient-reported utility score (PAT5D) and patient-reported satisfaction scores up to 2 years postoperatively.

Overall, the literature supports that the DAA can result in a faster functional recovery of selected activities. However, the accelerated recovery appears to be short lived, and the functional recovery is equivalent to other approaches by 4 to 6 weeks postoperatively.

THE INFLUENCE OF SURGICAL APPROACH ON THE RISK OF REVISION SURGERY

Various studies have looked at the influence of surgical approach on the revision rate following primary THA. Overall, the data suggest that the surgical approach can have an effect on both the early and late risk of revision surgery. Most of the studies indicate that the posterior approach has a higher risk of revision for dislocation, but an overall lower rate of revision than the other surgical approaches.

Surgical approach can have an effect on the early risk of revision following primary THA. This was seen in the 2020 retrospective cohort study that included 5,986 propensity score–matched patients, where the DAA, compared with the posterior approach or direct lateral approach, was significantly associated with a higher risk of revision arthroplasty (1.2% versus 0.7%; hazard ratio = 1.75) within 1 year.[12] This is contrary to the 2018 systematic review and meta-analysis of 13 prospective comparative studies, which found that the 90-day revision surgery rate was no different between the DAA and posterior approach.[4] In addition, the 2018 RCT of 101 hips also found no difference in the complication and revision rate between the DAA and the posterior approach THAs (8% versus 10%) at 1 year postoperatively.[28]

In a 2019 study with slightly a longer mean follow-up of 3.72 years, most of the patients who required revision surgery were in the DAA group (48%).[25] The incidence of revision surgery was 4.7% in the DAA group, 3.3% in the anterolateral approach group, 3.1% in the posterior approach group, and 2.8% in the direct lateral approach group.

Some of the arthroplasty registries have also provided regional data regarding the influence of surgical approach on revision rates following primary THA. The results of these registries were dependent on whether the hazard ratio analysis was adjusted for covariates, with the adjusted studies demonstrating a difference between approaches and the nonadjusted data not showing any correlation. The 2019 AOANJRR analysis of 115,707 THAs found that after adjusting for age, sex, ASA (American Society of Anesthesiologists) score, BMI category, femoral fixation, and head size, the DAA has a significantly higher rate of major revisions when compared with the posterior (hazard ratio = 1.21) and direct lateral approaches (hazard ratio = 1.36).[4] There was a higher rate of revision for aseptic loosening with the DAA compared with both the posterior (hazard ratio = 2.16) and direct lateral approaches (hazard ratio = 1.82). The DAA also had a higher rate of revision for fracture for the first 3 months compared with the posterior (hazard ratio = 2.01) and direct lateral approaches (hazard ratio = 1.94). After 3 months, the DAA had a lower rate of revision for fracture than the posterior approach (hazard ratio = 0.62). There were no differences between the posterior and the direct lateral approaches for these revision etiologies. After adjusting for covariates, a 2020 cohort registry study of 38,399 primary THAs through DAA had a lower risk of revision for instability (hazard ratio = 0.33) and revision for periprosthetic fracture (hazard ratio = 0.57) compared with posterior approach, but a higher risk of revision for aseptic loosening (hazard ratio = 2.26).[8] The 2019 observational study of the Swedish Hip Arthroplasty Register of 96,781 THAs (44,933 direct lateral and 51,848 posterior approach) found that the posterior approach, after adjusting for covariates, was associated with a statistically significantly lower risk of revision surgery due to all causes (hazard ratio = 0.8) compared with the direct lateral approach at 2 years follow-up.[13] Similarly, the 2017

Dutch Arthroplasty Registry analysis of 166,231 THAs found that the posterior approach was associated with a significantly lower risk of revision for all reasons (especially stem loosening) other than dislocation, compared with the anterolateral and anterior approaches (hazard ratio = 1.0 versus 1.2).[9] Without any adjustment for patient and implant factors, the 2018 Norwegian Arthroplasty Register found that in patients who underwent surgery since 2008, there was no difference in prosthetic survival between the direct anterior, anterolateral, posterior, and direct lateral surgical approaches.[31] Some of these registries did find differences in the revision risk between the various surgical approaches with respect to infection and dislocation, as previously discussed.

SUMMARY

There are several surgical approaches that are currently being used successfully in primary THA. The ideal surgical approach continues to be debated and is controversial. The literature demonstrates advantages and disadvantages of each surgical approach, but the literature at times has contradictory findings. Presently, there is no evidence to support the superiority of one approach over all the others. Most surgeons choose a surgical approach based on the experience, comfort, and training. Therefore, adoption of a new surgical approach should be based on definitive evidence in the literature that the approach provides optimal exposure of the hip, minimizes soft-tissue injury, allows ideal implant positioning, and minimizes complications and the need for revision surgery compared with the surgeon's current approach.

KEY STUDY POINTS

- The literature demonstrates advantages and disadvantages of each surgical approach.
- Presently, there is no evidence to support the superiority of one approach over all the others.
- The historically high dislocation rate with the posterior approach has been markedly decreased, but it is not unreasonable to consider that the posterior approach has a slightly higher dislocation rate than the other approaches.
- The DAA has better functional recovery in the first 4 to 6 weeks postoperatively.
- The DAA is associated with a higher risk of wound complications, and possibly infection.
- Overall, the posterior approach has the lowest risk of revision surgery.
- The direct lateral approach is associated with a low dislocation rate and infection rate and a slightly higher revision rate than the posterior approach.

ANNOTATED REFERENCES

1. American Academy of Orthopaedic Surgery. Appropriate Use Criteria for the Management of Osteoarthritis of the Hip. December 8, 2017. Available at: https://aaos.org/globalassets/quality-and-practice-resources/osteoarthritis-of-the-hip/oa-hip-auc.pdf.

   This is the American Academy of Orthopaedic Surgery guidelines for the management of hip arthritis.

2. Hedley AK, Hendren DH, Mead LP: A posterior approach to the hip joint with complete posterior capsular and muscular repair. *J Arthroplasty* 1990;5(suppl):S57-S66.

3. Fessy MH, Putman S, Viste A, et al: What are the risk factors for dislocation in primary total hip arthroplasty? A multicenter case control study of 128 unstable and 438 stable hips. *Orthop Traumatol Surg Res* 2017;103(5):663-668.

   This large comparative study isolated important patient-related factors for dislocation that surgeons must be aware of. Level of evidence: III.

4. Miller LE, Gondusky JS, Bhattacharyya S, Kamath AF, Boettner F, Wright J: Does surgical approach affect outcomes in total hip arthroplasty through 90 days of follow-up? A systematic review with meta-analysis. *J Arthroplasty* 2018;33(4):1296-1302.

   This systematic review included prospective studies comparing postoperative outcomes through 90 days of anterior approach versus posterior approach in primary THA.

5. Maratt JD, Gagnier JJ, Butler PD, Hallstrom BR, Urquhart AG, Roberts KC: No difference in dislocation seen in anterior vs posterior approach total hip arthroplasty. *J Arthroplasty* 2016;31(9 suppl):127-130.

6. Cheng TE, Wallis JA, Taylor NF, et al: A prospective randomized clinical trial in total hip arthroplasty-comparing early results between the direct anterior approach and the posterior approach. *J Arthroplasty* 2017;32(3):883-890.

   This smaller prospective randomized study similarly showed equivalent dislocation rates 12 weeks following DAA and posterior approach for primary THA. Level of evidence: I.

7. Sheth D, Cafri G, Inacio MCS, Paxton EW, Namba RS: Anterior and antero-lateral approaches for THA are associated with lower dislocation risk without higher revision risk. *Clin Orthop Relat Res* 2015;473:3401-3408.

8. Charney M, Paxton EW, Stradiotto R, et al: A comparison of risk of dislocation and cause-specific revision between direct anterior and posterior approach following elective cementless total hip arthroplasty. *J Arthroplasty* 2020;35(6):1651-1657.

   This registry study found that the DAA was associated with a lower risks of dislocation and revision for instability and periprosthetic fracture, but it is associated with a higher revision risk for aseptic loosening.

9. Zijlstra WP, De Hartog B, Van Steenbergen LN, Scheurs BW, Nelissen RGHH: Effect of femoral head size and surgical approach on risk of revision for dislocation after total hip arthroplasty. *Acta Orthop* 2017;88(4):395-401.

Compared with the posterior approach, direct anterior and anterolateral approaches reduce the risk of revision for dislocation, but at the cost of more stem revisions and other revisions. For the posterolateral approach, 36-mm heads can safely further reduce the risk of revision for dislocation.

10. Hailer NP, Weiss RJ, Stark A, Kärrholm J: The risk of revision due to dislocation after total hip arthroplasty depends on surgical approach, femoral head size, sex, and primary diagnosis. An analysis of 78,098 operations in the Swedish Hip Arthroplasty Register. *Acta Orthop* 2012;83(5):442-448.

11. Yue C, Kang P, Pei F: Comparison of direct anterior and lateral approaches in total hip arthroplasty: A systematic review and meta-analysis (PRISMA). *Medicine (Baltimore)* 2015;94(50):e2126-e2136.

12. Pincus D, Jenkinson R, Paterson M, Leroux T, Ravi B: Association between surgical approach and major surgical complications in patients undergoing total hip arthroplasty. *J Am Med Assoc* 2020;323(11):1070-1076.

    This study compared 2,993 propensity score–matched patients undergoing a lateral or posterior approach, with 2,993 matched patients undergoing anterior approach for THA. An anterior approach was associated with a small but statistically significant increased risk of major surgical complications compared with a posterior or lateral surgical approach.

13. Skoogh O, Tsikandylakis G, Mohaddes M, et al: Contemporary posterior surgical approach in total hip replacement: Still more reoperations due to dislocation compared with direct lateral approach? An observational study of the Swedish Hip Arthroplasty Register including 156,979 hips. *Acta Orthop* 2019;90(5):411-416.

    Risk of revision surgery due to dislocation and all-cause for the posterior and direct lateral surgical approaches were compared for two periods (1999 to 2006 and 2007 to 2014) up to 2 years postoperatively. In the period from 1999 to 2006, the posterior approach was associated with increased risk of revision surgery due to dislocation (hazard ratio = 2.3), but there was no difference in the risk of all-cause revision surgery (hazard ratio = 1.1). In the period from 2007 to 2014, there was no statistically significant difference in the risk of revision surgery due to dislocation (hazard ratio = 1.2, confidence interval 0.9 to 1.6), but the risk of all-cause revision surgery was lower for the posterior approach (hazard ratio = 0.8).

14. Australian National Joint Replacement Registry: 2019. Available at: https://aoanjrr.sahmri.com/annual-reports-2019. Accessed April 5, 2020.

    This 2019 annual report on hip and knee arthroplasty is published by the Australian Joint Registry.

15. Mjaaland KE, Svenningsen S, Fenstad AM, Havelin LI, Furnes O, Nordsletten L: Implant survival after minimally invasive anterior or anterolateral vs. conventional posterior or direct lateral approach: An analysis of 21,860 total hip arthroplasties from the Norwegian Arthroplasty Register (2008 to 2013). *J Bone Joint Surg Am* 2017;99(10):840-847.

    The revision rates and risk of revision associated with the MIS anterior and anterolateral approaches were not increased compared with those of the conventional posterior and direct lateral approaches in this study. Level of evidence: III.

16. Christensen CP, Karthikeyan T, Jacobs CA: Greater prevalence of wound complications requiring reoperation with direct anterior approach total hip arthroplasty. *J Arthroplasty* 2014;29(9):1839-1841.

17. Watts CD, Houdek MT, Wagner ER, et al: High risk of wound complications following direct anterior total hip arthroplasty in obese patients. *J Arthroplasty* 2015;30:2296-2298.

18. Russo MW, Macdonell JR, Paulus MC, Keller JM, Zawadsky MW: Increased complications in obese patients undergoing direct anterior total hip arthroplasty. *J Arthroplasty* 2015;30:1384-1387.

19. Jewett BA, Collis DK: High complication rate with anterior total hip arthroplasties on a fracture table. *Clin Orthop Relat Res* 2011;469(2):503-507.

20. Purcell RL, Parks NL, Cody JP, Hamilton WG: Comparison of wound complications and deep infections with direct anterior and posterior approaches in obese hip arthroplasty patients. *J Arthroplasty* 2018;33(1):220-223.

    In the largest available series, there was no difference in deep infection rates between the two approaches. However, anterior hip cases experienced higher rates of superficial wound complications compared with posterior cases across all BMIs.

21. Purcell RL, Parks NL, Gargiulo JM, Hamilton WG: Severely obese patients have a higher risk of infection after direct anterior approach total hip arthroplasty. *J Arthroplasty* 2016;31(9 suppl):162-165.

22. Antoniadis A, Dimitriou D, Flury A, Wiedmer G, Hasler J, Helmy N: Is direct anterior approach a credible option for severely obese patients undergoing total hip arthroplasty? A matched-control, retrospective, clinical study. *J Arthroplasty* 2018;33(8):2535-2540.

    This study showed an increased risk of revision surgery (relative risk = 4.0), mostly due to wound infection and dehiscence, in obese than in nonobese patients.

23. Tissot C, Vautrin M, Luyet A, Borens O: Are there more wound complications or infections with direct anterior approach total hip arthroplasty? *Hip Int* 2018;28(6):591-598.

    In this study of patients undergoing THA, the DAA did not increase the rates of either wound complications leading to revision surgery or early or delayed infection compared with the posterior approach.

24. Aggarwal VK, Weintraub S, Klock J: A comparison of prosthetic joint infection rates between direct anterior and non-anterior approach total hip arthroplasty. *Bone Joint J* 2019;101-B(6 suppl B):2-8.

    This study found a higher rate of PJI in direct anterior versus nonanterior approaches. However, adoption of infection prevention protocols lowered these PJI rates, regardless of approach.

25. Aggarwal VK, Elbuluk A, Dundon J: Surgical approach significantly affects the complication rates associated with total hip arthroplasty. *Bone Joint J* 2019;101-B(6):646-651.

The study indicates that surgical approach plays a role in the incidence of complications. It was found that the posterior approach had a significantly lower overall complication rate compared with the anterior approach, with an equal dislocation rate.

26. Lindgren V1, Garellick G, Kärrholm J, Wretenberg P: The type of surgical approach influences the risk of revision in total hip arthroplasty: A study from the Swedish Hip Arthroplasty Register of 90,662 total hip replacements with 3 different cemented prostheses. *Acta Orthop* 2012;83(6):559-565.

27. Jia F, Guo B, Xu F, Hou Y, Tang X, Huang L: A comparison of clinical, radiographic and surgical outcomes of total hip arthroplasty between direct anterior and posterior approaches: A systematic review and meta-analysis. *Hip Int* 2019;29(6):584-596.

    A systematic review and meta-analysis were used to directly evaluate the DAA and the posterior approach indicating that the DAA presents superior early recovery following THA.

28. Taunton MJ, Trousdale RT, Sierra RJ, Kaufman K, Pagnano MW: John Charnley Award: Randomized clinical trial of direct anterior and miniposterior approach THA. Which provides better functional recovery? *Clin Orthop Relat Res* 2018;476(2):216-229.

    This RCT found that both the DAA and MPA approaches provided excellent early recovery with a low risk of complications. Patients undergoing the DAA had a slightly faster recovery, as measured by milestones of function and quantified by activity monitor data, but no substantive differences were evident at 2 months. Level of evidence: I.

29. Parvizi J, Restrepo C, Maltenfort MG: Total arthroplasty performed through direct anterior approach provides superior early outcome: Results of a randomized, prospective study. *Orthop Clin North Am* 2016;47(3):497-504.

30. Greidanus NV1, Chihab S, Garbuz DS, et al: Outcomes of minimally invasive anterolateral THA are not superior to those of minimally invasive direct lateral and posterolateral THA. *Clin Orthop Relat Res* 2013;471(2):463-471.

31. Norwegian Arthroplasty Register 2018. Available at: http://nrlweb.ihelse.net/eng/Rapporter/Report2018_english.pdf. Accessed April 5, 2020.

CHAPTER 30

Designs, Porous Surfaces, and Bearing Surfaces

MATHIAS PER GUNNAR BOSTROM, MD • EMILE-VICTOR KUYL • BRANDEN R. SOSA

ABSTRACT

Total hip arthroplasty (THA) and total knee arthroplasty (TKA) are highly effective treatment options for patients with debilitating hip and knee arthrosis. The biologic response to implants is constantly under investigative research as physicians and manufacturers strive to design adaptable implant technologies to enhance the rate of successful osseointegration and mitigate the risk of infection following hip or knee replacement surgery. Through an in-depth review of the innovative technologies surrounding implant design, porous surfaces and treatments, and bearing surfaces, comparisons can be made regarding how modifications in implant properties have affected patient outcomes in both the short and long term.

Dr. Bostrom or an immediate family member has received royalties from Smith & Nephew; serves as a paid consultant to or is an employee of Smith & Nephew; has received research or institutional support from Ines Mandl Research Foundation, National Institutes of Health (NIAMS & NICHD), and Smith & Nephew; and serves as a board member, owner, officer, or committee member of the American Austrian Foundation and the Hip Society. Neither of the following authors nor any immediate family member has received anything of value from or has stock or stock options held in a commercial company or institution related directly or indirectly to the subject of this chapter: Mr. Kuyl and Mr. Sosa.

Keywords: bearings; cemented/noncemented; implant design; osseointegration; surface coatings

INTRODUCTION

The clinical success of proper bone ingrowth and adherence to an implant following total joint arthroplasty is dependent on a variety of factors, including implant design, material, and microstructure. Each section of this chapter will provide an overview of the transformation of different components in implant design followed by a detailed update in patient outcomes reported from various studies and registries. The chapter will begin by focusing on the design of the implant itself, specifically highlighting acetabular cups, three-dimensional printing in arthroplasty, and femoral implants. The following section will give an overview of porous metal coatings and treatments, followed by biologic coatings to enhance bone ingrowth and implant coatings to prevent infection. The most recent study results in the growing field of adaptive coatings will be discussed. The last section of this chapter will cover bearings surfaces, along with the effect that bearing design has had on patients undergoing total joint arthroplasty.

DESIGNS

Acetabular Cups

Noncemented acetabular cup design has changed significantly over the past several decades, allowing for better locking mechanisms, compatibility with alternative bearing surfaces, and new enhanced porous ingrowth surfaces.

This chapter is adapted from Hozack W, Duncan C, Herman A, et al: Surgical approaches and bearing surfaces, in Mont MA, Tanzer M, eds: *Orthopaedic Knowledge Update®: Hip and Knee Reconstruction*, ed 5. Rosemont, IL, American Academy of Orthopaedic Surgeons, 2017, pp 345-365 and Gibon E, Goodman SB: The biologic response to bearing materials, in Mont MA, Tanzer M, eds: *Orthopaedic Knowledge Update®: Hip and Knee Reconstruction*, ed 5. Rosemont, IL, American Academy of Orthopaedic Surgeons, 2017, pp 367-365.

First-Generation Acetabular Cups

The first generation of hemispherical cups was designed in the 1980s.[1] The polyethylene bearing surface in these designs extended over the edge of the hemisphere and resulted in significant impingement with the femoral prosthesis. This impingement led to liner damage, causing the already poor locking mechanism to fail and eventually leading the polyethylene liner to dislocate. These cups also suffered from limited congruity between the polyethylene and the metal shell resulting in a gap between the polyethylene liner and the acetabular cup, further stressing the thin peripheral polyethylene and poor locking mechanism.

Second-Generation Acetabular Cups

In the 1990s, second-generation hemispherical acetabular cup designs addressed the impingement caused by the polyethylene from the previous generation.[2] The liners were modified to be much thicker and capable of enduring impingement. These cups also addressed the gap between the acetabular cup and polyethylene liner by improving congruity, which in turn reduced back-side liner wear.

Third-Generation Acetabular Cups

Third-generation hemispherical cups were designed in the 2000s.[3] This generation of acetabular cups addressed impingement by improving the liners and locking mechanisms and further optimizing liner congruity. The introduction of highly cross-linked polyethylene (XLPE) dramatically decreased the incidence of osteolysis and peri-implant bone loss. These are currently the most commonly used designs in total hip arthroplasty (THA). Although the interface between the liner and shell continues to be optimized, major advancements have occurred at the outer porous surface for enhancement of bone ongrowth/ingrowth.

Three-Dimensional Printing in Arthroplasty

Three-dimensional (3D) printing, also known as additive manufacturing, represents an exciting advancement in arthroplasty implant design and manufacturing.[4,5] Three-dimensional printing allows for the design of complex implants that are not limited by the constraints of traditional manufacturing.[6] As the field of orthopaedics strives toward personalized treatment, this technology eliminates the additional cost of complex designs allowing for internal geometries, part assemblies, and part consolidation.[7] Currently, both acetabular cups for total hip replacements and cones and tibial baseplates in total knee replacements use 3D printing. The cost associated with designing larger orthopaedic implants has resulted in a delay in technology adoption. Nonetheless, with the advancement of printer designs and software, this limitation is being addressed and will allow for more widespread use of 3D printing in arthroplasty.[8]

FEMORAL IMPLANTS

Cemented Femoral Stems

Loaded Taper (Exeter)

In this design, the stem is tapered in either two or three planes and is lodged into the cement mantle during axial loading, which reduces stress in the proximal and distal cement mantles.[9] The implant is allowed to subside until radial compressive forces are transferred from the adjacent cement to bone as hoop stress. In loaded taper stems, a polished finish is required to allow for subsidence to a stable position. Over the first 1 to 2 years of implantation, loaded taper stems normally show a mean initial subsidence of 0.7 mm, but tend to gradually subside at a much slower pace over time.[10] This process tends to contribute to a secure fixation in the long term as cement and cement-bone interface are compressed. Long-term studies have shown that despite this initial migration, Exeter and other loaded taper stems are relatively stable over time and have excellent clinical results.[11]

Composite-Beam (Charnley)

In this concept, the stem needs to be rigidly bound to the cement and even limited micromotion can cause damage to the cement and subsequent implant failure.[12] As opposed to loaded taper stems, composite-beam femoral stems achieve better initial stability with a roughened surface to increase cement to stem bonding. However, the roughened surface of the implant increases tensile and shear stresses with the cement that can result in implant failure in suboptimal cementing conditions. Composite-beam stems often have a rectangular surface and can be straight or anatomic.[13]

NONCEMENTED FEMORAL STEMS

Although there are only two basic cemented femoral stem designs, there are numerous noncemented femoral stem designs. These were classified by the authors of a 2011 study into six major types[14] (**Table 1**).

Single-Wedge Stem (Type 1)

Although single-wedge noncemented stems have generally been discouraged in THA for Dorr type C femurs,[15,16] long-term results of type 1 stems show excellent stem survivorship in Dorr type C bone similar to that of other bone types.[17] Other long-term data have shown that the use of type 1 stems in THA demonstrates excellent results but with potentially higher rates of thigh pain and stress-shielding.[18,19]

Double-Wedge Stem (Type 2)

Type 2 stems have been shown to yield the highest risk of periprosthetic femoral fractures (PFF) (3.42%) based

TABLE 1

Classification of Noncemented Femoral Stem Designs

Type	Geometry	Fixation	General Description
1	Straight, single-wedge taper	Proximal fixation at metaphysis	Proximally coated, narrows in medial-lateral plane, flat and thin in AP plane
2	Straight, double-wedge taper	Proximal fixation at metaphysis	Proximally coated, narrows in both medial-lateral and AP planes, fills metaphyseal region because of thicker AP plane
3A	Straight, round taper, conical stem	Proximal fixation at metaphyseal-diaphyseal junction	Coated at proximal two thirds, rounded corners with tapered shape in both planes
3B	Straight, conical stem	Proximal fixation at metaphyseal-diaphyseal junction, distal fixation at proximal diaphysis	Contains raised longitudinal spines along entire length of stem
3C	Straight, rectangular stem	Proximal fixation at metaphyseal-diaphyseal junction, distal fixation at proximal diaphysis	Rectangular cross-section with four-point rotational support, tapered shape in both planes
4	Straight, cylindrical stem	Distal fixation primarily at proximal diaphysis	Extensive coating along full length, proximal bone collar for loading enhancement and axial stability, polished bullet tip
5	Straight, modular stem	Proximal and distal fixation through independent metaphyseal sleeve and diaphyseal stem	Adjustable stem modifications to accommodate for intraoperative adjustment because of femoral abnormalities
6	Curved, anatomic stem	Proximal fixation at metaphyseal fill and distal fixation at diaphysis through anterior bow	Wider in lateral and posterior regions at proximal stem, resulting in right or left femur-specific designs Distal end can be a cylindrical or tapered stem

Classification system based on data from Khanuja HS, Vakil JJ, Goddard MS, Mont MA: Cementless femoral fixation in total hip arthroplasty. *J Bone Joint Surg Am* 2011;93(5):500-509.

on registry data from 22 noncemented stem studies and shown to be significantly higher than type 1 stems and all other types.[20] When examining intraoperative PFF rates in 236 cases from eight different studies, 90.01% occurred with type 2 stems.[20] However, midterm and long-term data have shown that THA success rates with type 2 stems over a mean of 5 and 10+ years after treatment have been high, including in patients who have Dorr type C bone with slight incidences of thigh pain.[21-23]

Tapered Stems (Type 3)

Type 3C stems have shown excellent long-term survival rates and are popular options for THA in patients who have Dorr type C femurs, due to their unique shape. This subtype of tapered stems has been widely used in Europe.[14] Excellent rates of type 3A stem survivorship was observed in both young and elderly patients who have Dorr type C bone with mild thigh pain and stress-shielding.[24,25] Type 3B femoral stems have shown success in complex cases such as hips with dysplasia or prior intertrochanteric osteotomies and are often used in revision cases as opposed to primary surgeries.[26-28]

Cylindrical and Full-Surface Treated Stems (Type 4)

Type 4 stems have been modified (the addition of a full surface coating, medial cutout, and polished bullet tip) from their initial design to limit micromotion, decrease implant stiffness, and prevent pain at the distal portion of the stem with overall high survival rates.[29] With this transition to second-generation designs, incidences of thigh pain have been reduced, but the use for patients with Dorr type C femurs has not currently been addressed.

Modular Stems (Type 5)

One of the main advantages of modular stems is the ability to intraoperatively adjust stem modifications to accommodate for femoral abnormalities, giving the surgeon customizability of femur biomechanics without the worry of implant stability.[30] For example, the use of the S-ROM modular hip system in conjunction with subtrochanteric shortening osteotomy is widely effective for treatment of developmental dysplasia of the hip.[31,32] In addition, modular stems have yielded good to excellent clinical results in THAs for patients undergoing revision surgery and with high hip dislocation secondary to hip pyogenic arthritis.[33,34] The deviation from the classic one-piece stem to multiple combinations of proximal and distal implants is more costly, bringing in economic implications when considering the use of these stems for routine cases.

Anatomic Stems (Type 6)

Type 6 stems, also known as anatomic stems, are curved to match the proximal femur's endosteal geometry.[35,36] The first generation of these stems produced poor results and were associated with higher rates of thigh pain.[14] Since then, modifications have been made to achieve a more reliable fixation.[35] Not many studies have been done with this implant design to address its effect on various bone types.

SHORT FEMORAL STEMS

Most of the implants described earlier achieve fixation through initial bone-implant contact at the metaphyseal region. This has prompted the design of implants with shorter stem length that minimize the loss of femoral bone stock, may result in less postoperative pain, and may minimize stress shielding on the proximal femur. Although these short femoral stems are not a part of the aforementioned Mont classification, the Mont group has divided these short femoral stems into four types based on loading area.[37]

A recent study has found that short stems showed long-term survival rates similar to conventional stems in younger patients who have normal morphologies.[38] The use of this type of stem showed no higher risk of premature aseptic loosening and intraoperative and periprosthetic fractures when compared with conventional stems.

Porous Treatments and Coatings

Highly porous coatings, such as Trabecular Metal and Tritanium, have been used to combine the bone ingrowth properties of a surface coating with the mechanical strength of the underlying implant. Innovative applications of biologic coatings to enhance bone ingrowth and other coatings to mitigate infection have been gaining traction in a field that is constantly seeking to reduce the occurrence of arthroplasty failure (**Table 2**).

Trabecular Metal/Tantalum

Originally referred to as Hedrocel (Implex, Allendale, NJ), Trabecular Metal (Zimmer, Warsaw, IN) is a commercially available highly porous metal coating that offers several advantages for proper bone ingrowth in femoral stems.[39] Materials such as Trabecular Metal with much higher porosity (75%) allow for more bone to form at the interface and therefore higher ultimate fixation strength per unit area. In addition, the microtexture created on the struts is in the range shown to be osteoconductive in in vitro and in vivo studies.[40-43]

Trabecular Metal has the longest clinical history of any of the newer highly porous metals, having been first used in 1995 in a monoblock acetabular cup. Studies have shown that the use of porous tantalum cups, in lieu of titanium fiber-mesh cups or conventional reinforcement rings, has resulted in slightly better initial stability and reduces the risk of aseptic loosening.[44,45] Some reports have indicated that dislocation has been a recurrent issue

TABLE 2

Overview of Physical and Mechanical Characteristics of Various Traditional Porous Metal Implant Treatments[a]

Porous Metal	Porosity	Mean Pore Size (μm)	Compressive Strength (MPa)	Elastic Modulus (GPa)	Porous Coating	Monoblock Implant
Trabecular metal	75%	430	60	3.0	Yes	Yes
Tritanium	72%	546 (major pores), 311 (minor pores)	N/A	2.7	Yes	Yes
Biofoam	69%	530 (major pores), 200 (minor pores)	86	2.7	Yes	Yes
Regenerex	67%	300	157	1.9	Yes	Yes
Gription	64%	220	N/A	N/A	Yes	No
Stiktite	60%	215	N/A	N/A	Yes	No

N/A = not available or not applicable

[a]All materials have received FDA clearance for use in specific implants.

in revision THA with porous tantalum shells.[45,46] One disadvantage of tantalum is the high price of the raw material and the complexity of the manufacturing add to a high total cost of production of these implants.

Tritanium

Tritanium (Stryker, Mahwah, NJ) is material developed to provide similar properties and advantages as described previously for Trabecular Metal, with a simpler manufacturing process that involves mixing sacrificial polymer particles with an appropriate fraction and size of metal particulate. Tritanium has widely been used in acetabular implant designs for its low modulus of elasticity, with greater similarity to bone, which has been shown to reduce stress shielding. However, recent clinical studies have indicated that the use of Tritanium primary acetabular cups in THA has led to early aseptic cup loosening.[47] Short-term to midterm follow-ups of Tritanium primary acetabular implants have also shown that although adequate implant survivorship is common, many Tritanium cups showed multiple zones of radiolucency associated with lower Harris hip scores.[48]

Biofoam

Biofoam (Wright Medical Technology, Arlington, TN) is made of commercially pure titanium and possesses a dodecahedral structure, with the large pores and smaller interconnecting portals with a similar appearance to that of Trabecular Metal.[49] The material possesses a noticeable microtexture on all of the strut surfaces, and the friction coefficient against bone is higher than for titanium plasma spray or sintered beaded surfaces. Transcortical implants placed in metaphyseal and diaphyseal sites have demonstrated substantial bone ingrowth and attachment strength, more than with sintered beaded surfaces. It also has the capacity to be used in a similar manner for bone defect augments in the hip and knee. There are few to no long-term clinical studies performed using Biofoam coating technology.

Regenerex

Regenerex (Biomet, Warsaw, IN) is another form of highly porous metal made of titanium alloy. Because the porosity is somewhat lower than that of either Tritanium or Trabecular Metal, the strength of the bulk material is substantially greater. This material has been incorporated into the design of a fairly wide variety of implants for the hip, knee, and shoulder. It is used both as a porous coating and as a bulk material (for hip and knee augments in revision surgery), the latter once again taking advantage of the low stiffness for better potential load sharing with bone. Animal studies with transcortical implants have confirmed the suitability of Regenerex for bone ingrowth, with comparably high percentage filling with new bone as reported for Tritanium and Trabecular Metal. Regenerex appears to have a somewhat coarser and a more uneven surface structure than the other highly porous metals. This could reduce contact area with bone and create a wider tolerance band of part size that would require careful registry with instrumentation and surgical technique to ensure control over initial implant fixation. Short-term outcomes of THA with a Regenerex acetabular cup proved encouraging, with a 2016 study reporting no loosening or cup failure after an average follow-up of 2.6 years in a registry of 476 hip joints.[50]

Gription

A simple modification in the geometry of the outer layer of sintered titanium particles led to the creation of Gription (DePuy, Johnson & Johnson, Warsaw, IN), a traditional type of porous coating with higher porosity and rougher surface features. Gription cannot be manufactured in bulk form for the fabrication of stand-alone implants, but a similar structure could likely be made in cobalt-based alloy instead of titanium. Currently, Gription is applied only to acetabular cups and short femoral stems. A study has indicated that Gription acetabular cups appear to have very slight micromotion over time when compared with a traditional sintered bead surface in cases of low bone mineral density, both otherwise show no significant difference.[51]

Stiktite

A similar innovation using asymmetric particles to create a sintered porous coating resulted in Stiktite (Smith & Nephew, Memphis, TN). Using a friction and wear testing machine, linear dynamic friction tests against a bone analog material demonstrated the maximum friction coefficient of Stiktite to be equivalent to that of Trabecular Metal and twice that of conventional sintered spherical beads.[52] The benefit of higher interface friction was demonstrated in a radiostereometric analysis of 20 Stiktite acetabular cups that quantified substantially less implant migration in the early postoperative period compared with implants of the same design coated with spherical beads.[53] A preclinical study in an ovine tibial metaphyseal implant model confirmed extensive bone growth into the asymmetric coating and substantial mechanical fixation at 6 and 26 weeks, although not to a significantly greater extent compared with implants having a spherical beaded coating.[54] A 2013 radiostereometric study has indicated that when compared with an older sintered bead porous surface (Roughcoat), Stiktite achieved equally high levels of fixation with a significant reduction in pain reporting. The authors noted, however, that each group exhibited a similar difference in pain scores preoperatively.[55]

BIOLOGIC COATINGS TO ENHANCE BONE INGROWTH

In addition to the relatively traditional porous designs highlighted in the previous section, bioengineers, material scientists, and orthopaedic surgeons have begun, in 2013, to incorporate biologic coatings into orthopaedic implantation in an effort to increase osseointegration and bone ingrowth while simultaneously attempting to mitigate adverse tissue responses to infection.[56]

Hydroxyapatite coatings of orthopaedic implants have been shown to accelerate early bone ingrowth, improve early implant stability and increase long-term implant survival in experimental settings.[57,58] However, a more recent study has indicated that there is seemingly no added value to using hydroxyapatite-coated cups, as opposed to uncoated cups.[59] The study also reported that hydroxyapatite-coated cups seemed to have a higher risk of infection in THA. Recent reports from a large national registry have highlighted that hydroxyapatite coating of femoral stems is associated with a design dependent, but generally lower risk of revision.[60]

Hydrogel coatings draw on the ability to adhere biomolecules of interest, such as growth factors, viruses, or peptides, to an orthopaedic implant surface.[56] A recent study on periprosthetic infection in two-stage hip revision indicated that antibacterial loaded hydrogel coatings provided better infection control and lower hospitalization time with patients receiving this treatment, as opposed to two-stage hip revisions done without the coating.[61]

Layer-by-layer (LBL) coatings offer a solution to the problem that rises when hydrophobic or neutrally charged implant surfaces fail to effectively bind to essential biomolecules. With this method, implants are repeatedly dipped into polyelectrolyte solutions with alternating charges to control the loading efficiency of biomolecules, such as growth factors, or to control the release of drugs. However, because a few hundred layers are often required to prevent a burst release of biomolecules, the LBL technique can be costly and labor intensive.[56] In a 2016 study, LBL coatings of chitosan and diclofenac have been proposed as a controlled method for drug release in a multimechanism manner when applied to hip replacement implants.[62]

Implant Coatings to Prevent Infection

Periprosthetic joint infections continue to be a devastating complication following total joint arthroplasty. In these infections, implants become colonized with bacteria leading to the formation of biofilm and the progression of infection to the surrounding tissue.[63] When bacteria form biofilm on implant surfaces, the bacteria reduce their metabolic activity, making them less susceptible to antibiotic treatments and host immune system defense.[64-68]

Passive surface modification utilizes changes to the topography or chemistry composition of the implants to reduce bacterial adhesion. The physical and chemical properties of the implant surfaces, such as its roughness, hydrophilicity, conductivity, and surface energy, play a significant role in the adhesion of bacteria to these surfaces.[69] Researchers are striving to modify the surfaces of these implants while retaining their essential beneficial properties to prevent periprosthetic joint infection.

Ultraviolet-radiated implants have increased “spontaneous” wettability on titanium dioxide, which can inhibit bacterial surface adhesion.[56,70,71] Crystalline anatase-type titanium oxide layers on implant surfaces can also prevent bacterial growth on implants and prevent the progression of infection.[72] Although some coatings demonstrate antimicrobial activity and reduce bacterial colonization, some can have significant impairment on biologic fixation because of their effect on osteoblasts.[73-75]

Several arthroplasty implants have been coated in silver, an antibacterial metal.[76,77] The authors of a 2015 study found a significant reduction in postoperative infection rate with silver-coated megaendoprostheses.[78] Nonetheless, the use of silver-coated implants is limited by concerns of silver ion toxicity to host cells necessary for osseointegration.[79]

Antibiotic-impregnated polymethyl methacrylate[80] bone cement has also been used as an alternative approach to prevent infection. Gentamicin is a broad-spectrum, thermally stable antibiotic that has been used in these cements, but the widespread use of noncemented THA has minimized its utility as a method to prevent infection.[81,82] Calcium phosphate cements are another form of local antibiotic delivery. These cements have been loaded with a number of antibiotics in porous hydroxyapatite implant coatings,[82,83] but have the limitation of suboptimal kinetic elution properties.[84,85] Biodegradable polymers and sol-gel coatings have also been tested as potential LBL implant surface coatings, as mentioned in the previous section. This LBL formulation improves elution kinetics but has not been easily translated to the clinic.[56]

Future directions in preventing infection will require prolonged local delivery of treatment or improvements to chemical and physical modifications to implant surfaces while ensuring the implants are mechanically stable, durable, and noncytotoxic and allow for osseointegration.

BEARING SURFACES

Metal–on–Cross-Linked Polyethylene

It is clear that the use of metal–on–highly XLPE has resulted in a dramatic decrease in wear and wear-related complications, such as osteolysis and loosening, compared with metal on conventional polyethylene, resulting in a reduction in revision rates.[86]

These wear reductions are associated with improvements in clinical survival. The Swedish Hip Arthroplasty Register reported that 98% of all surgeries using noncemented cups in 2017 were done with XLPE.[87] This follows a report from the 2013 registry that states: "Unlike previous years, when the observation time has increased, a trend toward reduced number of cup/liner revisions concerning the use of XLPE."[88]

Multiple studies have shown that liner thickness does not affect the wear rate of XLPE.[89] Larger femoral heads with XLPE, which originally were associated with more volumetric wear, have since been reported to have low rates of linear and volumetric wear at 5 to 13 years.[90]

No correlation of the magnitude of penetration and head size with evidence of loosening and osteolysis have been found.[91]

The most commonly used metal femoral head is a modular head constructed from a cobalt-chromium (CoCr) alloy. Because most noncemented femoral implants are constructed from a titanium alloy, a situation of mixed metals is created and increases the risk of corrosion at the modular junction. Several reports have been published on corrosion at the trunnion, increased metal wear at the trunnion, and adverse local tissue reactions to products emanating from the trunnion.[92] Although reports of severe reactions have led many to advocate a wholesale change to ceramic femoral heads in all patients, it appears from the national registries that the prevalence of trunnion reactions related to modular CoCr femoral heads resulting in failure is relatively low.[93] The significantly higher cost of ceramic femoral heads has led some investigators to conclude that they are not cost effective for most patients. Certain studies and the 2019 Australian National Joint Replacement Registry have indicated that although ceramicized metal on XLPE has the lowest rate of revision at 10 years, the differences in revision rates for metal/XLPE versus ceramic/XLPE are negligible.[94,95] However, a recent study of the New Zealand Mayo Clinic Joint Replacement Database claims that ceramic-on-highly XLPE remains as the most durable and favorable pairing couple.[96] First-generation highly XLPE formulations are showing excellent long-term survivorship.[86,97]

Most observers have concluded that XLPE acetabular liners are the most tolerant of implant malpositioning, which several studies have suggested occurs in a higher percentage of cases than might be expected (more than 50% in some studies). The improved wear characteristics of XLPE, the comparative low cost of a metal on cross-linked bearing couple, and tolerance of malposition of metal-on-polyethylene bearings suggest that this bearing couple should remain a bearing couple option for THA especially in the elderly despite the potential for trunnion corrosion.[98-103]

Antioxidant Cross-Linked Polyethylene

First-generation XLPE used annealing or melting after irradiation to improve oxidation resistance. Melting effectively eliminated detectable residual free radicals but also decreased crystallinity, resulting in some loss of fatigue strength of the material. Annealing resulted in partial elimination of free radicals and, thus, some oxidation potential, but annealing had better retention of fatigue strength. In 2014, antioxidant stabilization of radiation cross-linked ultra-high–molecular-weight polyethylenes (UHMWPEs) eliminated the need for melting after irradiation for improved oxidation resistance, thereby better retaining the mechanical properties. The addition of antioxidants, such as vitamin E or pentaerythritol tetrakis (3-[3,5-di tertiary butyl-4-hydroxyphenyl] propionate), can substantially improve oxidation resistance of XLPE, while maintaining its strength.[104] The presence of these antioxidants does not alter the wear resistance of the base highly cross-linked material under either adhesive or abrasive conditions. In addition, in vitro and in vivo animal data support lowered functional biologic activity of particulate debris containing antioxidants in terms of their propensity to cause osteolysis.[105,106] Vitamin E-stabilized highly cross-linked UHMWPEs have been in clinical use in hips since 2007 and in knees since 2008. Clinical use of pentaerythritol tetrakis (3-[3,5-di tertiary butyl-4-hydroxyphenyl] propionate) stabilization started in 2011, but only in total knee applications.

In 2015, researchers identified that polyethylene can oxidize in vivo, through not only preexisting residual free radicals from gamma sterilization or radiation cross-linking but also mechanisms accelerated by cyclic loading and/or absorbed lipids. Laboratory evidence shows increased rates of oxidation with different formulations of polyethylene in the presence of cyclic loading.[107] Explanted tibial knee inserts show higher oxidation levels below loaded articular surfaces compared with parts of the implants that are not typically loaded, for example, around the eminence.[108,109] Surgically explanted polyethylene implants typically show a variety of absorbed lipids, namely squalene (a precursor of cholesterol) and esters of cholesterol.[110] Primarily, squalene and other absorbed lipids act as prooxidants. Artificial aging experiments in the presence of such lipids have shown higher rates of oxidation in polyethylene.[111] The incorporation of an antioxidant before or after radiation cross-linking may effectively minimize or even eliminate oxidation caused by preexisting residual free radicals, cyclic loading, and/or absorbed lipids. Antioxidant-stabilized XLPEs are now commonly used in both total knee and THA applications.

Antioxidant stabilization can help continue these excellent outcomes beyond the second decade of use in both THA and total knee arthroplasty, largely by minimizing any potential degradation of properties caused by long-term oxidation and improving the mechanical properties.[93,105]

Ceramic–on–Cross-Linked Polyethylene

The combination of ceramic and UHMWPE provides many advantages as a bearing choice in THA. Surgeons prefer the bearing combination that minimizes the risk of complications, optimizes implant longevity, and achieves cost effectiveness. Previously, ceramic-on-ceramic and metal-on-metal bearings became popular as a means to address the limited implant longevity associated with older-generation polyethylene liners.

When using UHMWPE acetabular bearings, options for the femoral head bearing couple include CoCr, ceramic, and ceramicized metal. Historically, CoCr has been the most commonly used bearing couple with polyethylene, yet the use of ceramic or ceramicized metal for the femoral head has been argued to decrease the rate of polyethylene wear.[112] In 2015, the phenomenon of so-called trunnionosis, most commonly caused by fretting and corrosion between a CoCr femoral head and the femoral implant trunnion, has been recognized as a mode of catastrophic failure in metal-on-polyethylene hips. The process may not be rare, and it is unclear if trunnionosis was previously unrecognized or if it is the result of more recent changes in implant design.[113-115] Although the epidemiology and tribology of the process are becoming better understood with time, the use of a ceramic femoral head may help avoid this mechanism of catastrophic failure.[116]

Certainly, the use of a ceramic femoral head has potential disadvantages. With any ceramic implant, including the ceramic on polyethylene combination, the risk of ceramic fracture exists. To address the risk of ceramic fracture associated with older generations of ceramic, mixed oxide ceramic materials with increased fracture strength were developed. The fracture of such modern ceramic femoral heads is extremely rare.[117] Ceramic femoral heads typically are associated with an increased cost compared with the CoCr alternative. However, the cost-effectiveness of using the former is dependent on the price premium for ceramic and the age of the patient.[118] Randomized controlled trials and national registries show similar short-term to midterm survivorship between ceramic on XLPE and metal on XLPE bearing surfaces. The choice of bearing surface is often viewed as experience-based as opposed to evidence-based.[95,119]

Ceramic-on-Ceramic Bearings

Ceramic-on-ceramic bearings are designed to reduce both wear and osteolysis that are traditionally associated with ceramic-on-polyethylene bearings. The trade-off of the superior tribological properties of ceramic-on-ceramic bearings, such as low wear and low soft-tissue reactions, is their association with noise generation and fracture. Squeaking, wear and the biologic response to the ceramic debris, ceramic fractures, and the results and debate with respect to large-diameter (greater than 36 mm) ceramic-on-ceramic bearings are related issues.

A 2014 meta-analysis that included data acquired from the Australian National Mayo Clinic Joint Replacement Database reported that the rate of squeaking was 4.2%, and the rate of revision for squeaking was 0.2%.[120]

Pathologic squeaking was shown to be associated with anterosuperior edge loading secondary to excessive inclination and anteversion of the acetabular implant; this type of squeaking has a social and psychologic effect on patients, some of whom seek further surgical intervention. Benign squeaking is frequently associated with posterior edge loading and generally can be improved with patient education by avoiding specific positions and reassuring the patient.[121,122]

Although no clear evidence shows that squeaking reduces the overall survival rate of THA, some suggestions associate squeaking with implant wear.[123-125]

Ceramic-on-ceramic bearings have the lowest rate of wear among all the bearings available. The tissue reaction to ceramic debris differs from the reaction to metal or polyethylene debris, especially with respect to the destruction of surrounding soft tissues and bone. This result was derived from an evaluation of synovium and periarticular tissue obtained from revised third-generation ceramic-on-ceramic articulations.[126] The etiology for revision varied among patients, but none had a revision because of osteolysis. The tissue evaluation demonstrated small numbers of macrophages predominantly in the fibrous connective tissue, rare multinucleated giant cells, and minimal necrosis. Overall, the severity of synovial changes did not correlate with either the degree of volumetric wear or the revision diagnosis. Therefore, the inflammatory changes in the pseudocapsule of ceramic-on-ceramic hips may be clinically insignificant.[126] Other authors have suggested that the lack of periprosthetic foreign body reaction, together with the dense fibrous tissue observed during ceramic-on-ceramic revision surgery, has a role in joint stabilization and dislocation prevention.[127]

Ceramic fracture is linked to the internal brittleness of ceramics. With the evolution of ceramic manufacturing and processing, stronger crack resistance materials have been produced, which has further improved the already low rate of ceramic fractures.[128] However, a few reports have now shown that patients undergoing trauma to fourth-generation ceramic heads may be susceptible to delayed fracture, coined "slow crack growth."[129] Contributing factors to head fractures are the cleanliness of the taper, impaction of the head onto the taper, and femoral head size and length. A taper covered with debris and blood and/or insufficient impaction and inadequate bore centralization can result in uneven load distribution on the head, which may facilitate fracture formation. Smaller sizes and shorter heads are observed to have a higher rate of fractures.[130]

The bearing to be used in revision surgery for fractured ceramic implants is still being debated; however, it is generally agreed that a revision to a ceramic-on-ceramic or a ceramic-on-polyethylene bearing is acceptable.[131] A conversion to a metal-on-polyethylene bearing is not recommended because of the scratching effect of the ceramic particles on the metal femoral head, potentially resulting in excessive wear of the head and the polyethylene.

Trunnionosis is a concern when metal heads are used; however, it seems that trunnionosis is not an issue when ceramic heads are used.

Large-diameter monoblock (greater than 36 mm) fourth-generation ceramic-on-ceramic articulations were introduced at the end of 2008. Currently, the literature is limited to short-term clinical follow-up that indicates good clinical functional outcomes.[132] However, the overall rate of squeaking is high, with up to 21.7% seen in a single series.

A recent concern with the use of large femoral head sizes is related to the increased forces acting on the head-Morse taper junction. The evolution of taper design has reduced both the height and the width of the trunnion, resulting in shorter, narrower trunnions. The rationale for these design changes was to reduce impingement by increasing the head-neck ratio. However, the excessive forces generated by the large femoral head on the trunnion, especially in suboptimal lubrication conditions, can amplify the forces acting at the taper junction. The implant-bone interface also will experience high force transmission; however, the clinical implications of these forces are not clearly understood.[133,134]

Ceramicized Metal Heads

The surgeon now has several options for femoral head material, namely, CoCr, alumina ceramic, or ceramicized metal. Ceramicized metal, also known as oxidized zirconium (OxZr), was first used in the nuclear industry before it was adapted THA in approximately 2003.

In essence, the surface is transformed into a ceramic oxide layer and has all the material properties inherent to ceramic, including more scratch resistance, a smoother surface, and increased hardness and wettability compared with CoCr.

The ceramic oxide surface of these OxZr implants has the advantage of improved wear properties against polyethylene because of its resistance to scratching and increased surface hardness, smoothness, and wettability. Fracture of an OxZr femoral head is not possible. In addition, OxZr femoral heads maintain all their modularity (ie, all sizes and lengths), because they are not limited by any mechanical properties. With current concerns about trunnionosis, a further potential advantage of OxZr femoral heads may relate to their relatively high resistance to corrosion and fretting (compared with CoCr), thus potentially decreasing the likelihood of trunnion-related problems.[135] Because OxZr contains no nickel, it is also well suited for use with patients who have a suspected metal allergy.

The main disadvantage of OxZr, as with ceramic heads, relates to its cost compared with CoCr. Also, OxZr is currently manufactured by only one company and therefore should be used only with that manufacturer's femoral stem systems to ensure taper compatibility. Although this material has demonstrated scratch resistance in vitro and in vivo under normal joint conditions, the oxide surface can be damaged if subjected to abnormal contact against other metal surfaces (such as a titanium acetabular shell), especially in the setting of a joint dislocation. Consequently, similar to ceramic femoral heads, care must be taken when reducing the femoral head at the time of the index procedure to avoid damage to the OxZr head or metal transfer to its surface.

Overall, the reported clinical results of OxZr-on-XLPE bearings have been excellent with more than a decade of use. In particular, the Australian Mayo Clinic Joint Replacement Database continues to report the lowest revision rate (3.3% at 11 years) with this bearing couple compared with all other bearing options.[136] However, the registry points out that this result should be interpreted with caution, because this bearing is associated with a single manufacturer and, therefore, has a small number of femoral stem and acetabular implant combinations. Nevertheless, this combination of bearing has performed extremely well and has demonstrated excellent clinical results since its clinical release.

With respect to its measured wear performance in vivo, mixed evidence supports the improved wear performance of OxZr femoral heads compared with CoCr femoral heads against XLPE. Several recent publications have demonstrated no significant difference in femoral head penetration, both in randomized controlled trial study designs, comparing CoCr heads to OxZr heads against XLPE.[137,138] However, other studies have demonstrated either a trend or a statistically significant decrease in wear associated with the use of OxZr against XLPE.[139,140] Perhaps most important, every study has clearly demonstrated that the use of XLPE, rather than conventional polyethylene, has the greatest effect on wear reduction when compared with the femoral head material.

The use of an OxZr femoral head against an XLPE liner is an excellent option for an alternate bearing in a young, active patient who requires THA. This unique material combines the beneficial features of a metal and a ceramic. In addition, it is a good choice for patients in whom a metal allergy is suspected. Furthermore, the corrosion-resistant and fretting-resistant properties of this material, compared with CoCr, may make it beneficial with respect to ameliorating the potential for long-term trunnion-related problems. The outstanding results following a decade of clinical use support its ongoing role as a viable bearing option for THA.[141-143]

Metal-on-Metal Bearings

The use of large metal-on-metal bearings in THA has resulted in reports of soft-tissue reactions that result in implant failure and associated complications. The most compelling evidence indicating that metal-on-metal bearings should be abandoned for THA comes from the National Mayo Clinic Joint Replacement Database for England, Wales.[144] The data included 402,051 THAs and 31,171 stemmed metal-on-metal THAs implanted between 2003 and 2011. Overall, stemmed metal-on-metal articulations had a 5-year revision rate of 6.2% (95% confidence interval = 5.8% to 6.6%).

Patients who are symptomatic and have had a metal-on-metal THA should undergo a thorough clinical history, a detailed physical examination, and radiographic and laboratory tests to rule out causes such as aseptic loosening and infection as a source of pain. These patients should then be considered for revision THA. Patients who are asymptomatic and considered low risk (male, ideal implant placement, and implant design) should be followed up annually. Patients considered to be at moderate risk (whether they are symptomatic or asymptomatic) should undergo serum metal ion assessment and ultrasonography to identify soft-tissue reactions.[145]

It is now clear that metal-on-metal bearings in THA are longer recommended. For an elderly patient, the low cost of a metal on a cross-linked bearing couple and tolerance of malposition of metal-on-polyethylene bearings make a metal-on-XLPE bearing a suitable bearing couple for THA. With the extent of trunnion corrosion still not clear, the use of ceramic or ceramicized metal couple on XLPE is recommended in the younger patient population.

SUMMARY

Innovative implant designs and coatings have led to significant improvements in long-term outcomes for patients. As technology progresses and the cost of manufacturing decreases, implants design will be improved to address limitations of current designs and to serve the needs of each individual patient. Three-dimensional printing will be critical in allowing for the personalized treatment of patients. This manufacturing technology was first used on acetabular cups and have shown excellent results.

Although there are many different femoral implant designs, studies demonstrate good long-term survival across all designs. Younger patients particularly have excellent results following noncemented femoral fixation, but the decision on which implant design to use should be guided by the patient's anatomy, the need for distal fixation, and the surgeon's preference.

In efforts to improve osseointegration and prevent infection, porous surface treatments and coatings have been developed for implants. These surface treatments leverage the unique properties of various metals such as titanium, tantalum, and cobalt to create surfaces conducive to bony ingrowth. Research is currently being performed to develop biologic coatings to further enhance bone ingrowth and to prevent prosthetic joint infection. Choosing an appropriate bearing surface is critical for the success of total joint arthroplasty. There are currently a number of bearing surfaces available, but the choice largely depends on the age and activity of a patient. Each surface has unique reported complications such as trunnionosis, squeaking, and wear that should be assessed when deciding the optimal bearing surface for your patient.

KEY STUDY POINTS

- New porous coatings, many manufactured by 3D printing, are demonstrating good clinical results when used on acetabular implants.
- Many noncemented stem designs are available, which when used in the proper clinical setting will lead to good results.
- Biologic coatings to improve osseointegration and decrease infections are being developed.
- Ceramic on XLPE remains an excellent bearing for most patients.

ANNOTATED REFERENCES

1. Hamilton WG, Calendine CL, Beykirch SE, Hopper RH Jr, Engh CA: Acetabular fixation options: First-generation modular cup curtain calls and caveats. *J Arthroplasty* 2007;22(4 suppl 1):75-81.

2. Min BW, Song KS, Kang CH, Won YY, Koo KH: Polyethylene liner failure in second-generation Harris-Galante acetabular components. *J Arthroplasty* 2005;20(6):717-722.

3. Powers CC, Ho H, Beykirch SE, et al: A comparison of a second- and a third-generation modular cup design: Is new improved? *J Arthroplasty* 2010;25(4):514-521.

4. Jones GG, Clarke S, Jaere M, Cobb J: 3D printing and unicompartmental knee arthroplasty. *EFORT Open Rev* 2018;3(5):248-253.

   This review paper describes the concept of detailed unicompartmental knee arthroplasty planning in 3D and 3D planning technology in patient-specific instrumentation. Level of evidence: V.

5. Bagaria V, Bhansali R, Pawar P: 3D printing-creating a blueprint for the future of orthopedics: Current concept review and the road ahead! *J Clin Orthop Trauma* 2018;9(3): 207-212.

   This paper provides an overview of current developments in the use of 3D printing in orthopaedics such as metal printing and an outlook at the use of 3D bioprinting. Level of evidence: V.

6. Trauner KB: The emerging role of 3D printing in arthroplasty and orthopedics. *J Arthroplasty* 2018;33(8):2352-2354.

   This article provides a review of the emerging role of 3D printing in arthroplasty and orthopaedics and discusses the evolution and value offered by this technology. Level of evidence: V.

7. Lipson H: New world of 3-D printing offers "completely new ways of thinking": Q&A with author, engineer, and 3-D printing expert Hod Lipson. *IEEE Pulse* 2013;4(6):12-14.

8. Toto JM, Chang EI, Agag R, Devarajan K, Patel SA, Topham NS: Improved operative efficiency of free fibula flap mandible reconstruction with patient-specific, computer-guided preoperative planning. *Head Neck* 2015;37(11): 1660-1664.

9. Lim SJ, Park YS, Moon YW, Jung SM, Ha HC, Seo JG: Modular cementless total hip arthroplasty for multiple epiphyseal dysplasia. *J Arthroplasty* 2009;24(1):77-82.

10. Murray DW, Gulati A, Gill HS: Ten-year RSA-measured migration of the Exeter femoral stem. *Bone Joint J* 2013;95-B(5):605-608.

11. Woodbridge AB, Hubble MJ, Whitehouse SL, Wilson MJ, Howell JR, Timperley AJ: The Exeter short revision stem for cement-in-cement femoral revision: A five to twelve year review. *J Arthroplasty* 2019;34(7 suppl):S297-S301.

    This study reviewed 166 cases of cement-in-cement revision using the Exeter short stem to compare its performance with standard length Exeter stems. Level of evidence: III.

12. Scheerlinck T, Casteleyn PP: The design features of cemented femoral hip implants. *J Bone Joint Surg Br* 2006;88(11):1409-1418.

13. Briggs D: The evolution of the femoral stem design in total hip arthroplasty. *UNM Orthop Res J* 2013;2:24-25.

14. Khanuja HS, Vakil JJ, Goddard MS, Mont MA: Cementless femoral fixation in total hip arthroplasty. *J Bone Joint Surg Am* 2011;93(5):500-509.

15. Aro HT, Alm JJ, Moritz N, Mäkinen TJ, Lankinen P: Low BMD affects initial stability and delays stem osseointegration in cementless total hip arthroplasty in women: A 2-year RSA study of 39 patients. *Acta Orthop* 2012;83(2): 107-114.

16. Cooper HJ, Rodriguez JA: Early post-operative periprosthetic femur fracture in the presence of a non-cemented tapered wedge femoral stem. *HSS J* 2010;6(2):150-154.

17. Kim JT, Jeong HJ, Lee SJ, Kim HJ, Yoo JJ: Does proximally coated single-wedge cementless stem work well in Dorr type C femurs? Minimum 10-year followup. *Indian J Orthop* 2019;53(1):94-101.

    This study compares long-term outcomes of proximally coated single-wedge cementless stems according to the type of proximal femoral geometry. Level of evidence: III.

18. Muller LA, Wenger N, Schramm M, Hohmann D, Forst R, Carl HD: Seventeen-year survival of the cementless CLS Spotorno stem. *Arch Orthop Trauma Surg* 2010;130(2):269-275.

19. Hu H, Liu Z, Liu B, et al: Comparison of clinical outcomes, radiological outcomes and bone remodeling outcomes between proximal coated single-wedge new stem and full coated dual-wedge classic stem in 1-stage bilateral total hip arthroplasty. *Med Sci Monit* 2020;26:e921847.

    This retrospective study investigates the clinical outcomes, radiologic outcomes, and bone remodeling patterns associated with a medial/lateral taper stem and link classic uncemented stem in one-stage bilateral THA. Level of evidence: III.

20. Carli AV, Negus JJ, Haddad FS: Periprosthetic femoral fractures and trying to avoid them: What is the contribution of femoral component design to the increased risk of periprosthetic femoral fracture? *Bone Joint J* 2017;99-B(1 suppl A):50-59.

    This paper performs a review of the literature investigating periprosthetic femoral fractures following THA. Level of evidence: III.

21. Epinette JA, Manley MT: Uncemented stems in hip replacement—Hydroxyapatite or plain porous: Does it matter? Based on a prospective study of HA Omnifit stems at 15-years minimum follow-up. *Hip Int* 2008;18(2):69-74.

22. Incavo SJ, Beynnon BD, Coughlin KM: Total hip arthroplasty with the Secur-Fit and Secur-Fit plus femoral stem design a brief follow-up report at 5 to 10 years. *J Arthroplasty* 2008;23(5):670-676.

23. Nebergall AK, Rolfson O, Rubash HE, Malchau H, Troelsen A, Greene ME: Stable fixation of a cementless, proximally coated, double wedged, double tapered femoral stem in total hip arthroplasty: A 5-year radiostereometric analysis. *J Arthroplasty* 2016;31(6):1267-1274.

24. Ellison B, Berend KR, Lombardi AVJ, Mallory TH: Tapered titanium porous plasma-sprayed femoral component in patients aged 40 years and younger. *J Arthroplasty* 2006;21(6 suppl 2):32-37.

25. Reitman RD, Emerson R, Higgins L, Head W: Thirteen year results of total hip arthroplasty using a tapered titanium femoral component inserted without cement in patients with type C bone. *J Arthroplasty* 2003;18(7 suppl 1):116-121.

26. Schuh A, Schraml A, Hohenberger G: Long-term results of the Wagner cone prosthesis. *Int Orthop* 2009;33(1):53-58.

27. Bohm P, Bischel O: Femoral revision with the Wagner SL revision stem: Evaluation of one hundred and twenty-nine revisions followed for a mean of 4.8 years. *J Bone Joint Surg Am* 2001;83(7):1023-1031.

28. Weber M, Hempfing A, Orler R, Ganz R: Femoral revision using the Wagner stem: Results at 2-9 years. *Int Orthop* 2002;26(1):36-39.

29. Hennessy DW, Callaghan JJ, Liu SS: Second-generation extensively porous-coated THA stems at minimum 10-year followup. *Clin Orthop Relat Res* 2009;467(9):2290-2296.

30. Park CW, Lim SJ, Park YS: Modular stems: Advantages and current role in primary total hip arthroplasty. *Hip Pelvis* 2018;30(3):147-155.

This review paper discusses published studies that have investigated the use and advantages of modular femoral stems in THA. Level of evidence: V.

31. Togrul E, Ozkan C, Kalaci A, Gulsen M: A new technique of subtrochanteric shortening in total hip replacement for Crowe type 3 to 4 dysplasia of the hip. *J Arthroplasty* 2010;25(3):465-470.

32. Wang D, Li LL, Wang HY, Pei FX, Zhou ZK: Long-term results of cementless total hip arthroplasty with subtrochanteric shortening osteotomy in Crowe type IV developmental dysplasia. *J Arthroplasty* 2017;32(4):1211-1219.

This study evaluates the 10-year outcomes of transverse subtrochanteric shortening osteotomy in cementless, modular THA in Crowe type IV-Hartofilakidis type III developmental dysplasia of the hip.

33. Rieger B, Ilchmann T, Bolliger L, Stoffel KK, Zwicky L, Clauss M: Mid-term results of revision total hip arthroplasty with an uncemented modular femoral component. *Hip Int* 2018;28(1):84-89.

The aim of this retrospective study is to assess the clinical and radiographic midterm outcome of revision THA using a modular uncemented, tapered, grit-blasted, distal straight stem system. Level of evidence: IV.

34. Yang Y, Yu QP, Wang SL, et al: Outcomes after total hip arthroplasty using a cementless S-ROM modular stem for patients with high hip dislocation secondary to hip pyogenic arthritis. *Orthop Surg* 2019;11(3):460-466.

This retrospective study analyzes the safety and effectiveness of cementless S-ROM modular femoral stems used with subtrochanteric transverse shortening osteotomy for the treatment of high hip dislocation secondary to hip pyogenic arthritis. Level of evidence: IV.

35. Mont MA, Yoon TR, Krackow KA, Hungerford DS: Clinical experience with a proximally porous-coated second-generation cementless total hip prosthesis: Minimum 5-year follow-up. *J Arthroplasty* 1999;14(8):930-939.

36. Noble PC, Alexander JW, Lindahl LJ, Yew DT, Granberry WM, Tullos HS: The anatomic basis of femoral component design. *Clin Orthop Relat Res* 1988;235:148-165.

37. Feyen H, Shimmin AJ: Is the length of the femoral component important in primary total hip replacement? *Bone Joint J* 2014;96-B(4):442-448.

38. Giardina F, Castagnini F, Stea S, Bordini B, Montalti M, Toni A: Short stems versus conventional stems in cementless total hip arthroplasty: A long-term registry study. *J Arthroplasty* 2018;33(6):1794-1799.

This report compares the survival rates and the reasons for revision of short stems versus conventional stems in cementless THAs, in a registry-based population. Level of evidence: III.

39. Cohen R: A porous tantalum trabecular metal: Basic science. *Am J Orthop (Belle Mead NJ)* 2002;31(4):216-217.

40. Kieswetter K, Schwartz Z, Hummert TW, et al: Surface roughness modulates the local production of growth factors and cytokines by osteoblast-like MG-63 cells. *J Biomed Mater Res* 1996;32(1):55-63.

41. Hacking SA, Bobyn JD, Tanzer M, Krygier JJ: The osseous response to corundum blasted implant surfaces in a canine hip model. *Clin Orthop Relat Res* 1999;364:240-253.

42. Kienapfel H, Sprey C, Wilke A, Griss P: Implant fixation by bone ingrowth. *J Arthroplasty* 1999;14(3):355-368.

43. Zhang Y, Ahn PB, Fitzpatrick DC, Heiner AD, Poggie RA, Brown TD: Interfacial frictional behavior: Cancellous bone, cortical bone, and a novel porous tantalum biomaterial. *J Musculoskelet Res* 1999;3(4):245-251.

44. Baad-Hansen T, Kold S, Nielsen PT, Laursen MB, Christensen PH, Soballe K: Comparison of trabecular metal cups and titanium fiber-mesh cups in primary hip arthroplasty. *Acta Orthop* 2011;82(2):155-160.

45. Bruggemann A, Fredlund E, Mallmin H, Hailer NP: Are porous tantalum cups superior to conventional reinforcement rings? *Acta Orthop* 2017;88(1):35-40.

This study investigates the use of porous tantalum metal cups in revision hip surgery with re-revision for aseptic loosening as the primary outcome measure. Level of evidence: III.

46. Laaksonen I, Lorimer M, Gromov K, et al: Trabecular metal acetabular components in primary total hip arthroplasty. *Acta Orthop* 2018;89(3):259-264.

This study compared the survivorship of trabecular metal cups with that of other uncemented cups in primary THA. Level of evidence: III.

47. Long WJ, Nayyar S, Chen KK, Novikov D, Davidovitch RI, Vigdorchik JM: Early aseptic loosening of the Tritanium primary acetabular component with screw fixation. *Arthroplast Today* 2018;4(2):169-174.

This case series reports on the risk of early acetabular cup loosening and its associated clincal presentation, workup, and surgical management in patients with the Tritanium primary cup augmented with screws. Level of evidence: IV.

48. Carli AV, Warth LC, de Mesy Bentley KL, Nestor BJ: Short to midterm follow-up of the Tritanium primary acetabular component: A cause for concern. *J Arthroplasty* 2017;32(2):463-469.

This study compared the clinical and radiographic results of 109 hips in 95 patients using a Tritanium primary cup (Stryker, Mahwah, NJ) to an age-matched, body mass index, and gender-matched cohort of 100 patients that received a contemporary cup (Stryker Trident PSL HA). Level of evidence: III.

49. Scholvin D, Obert R, Moseley J, et al: Highly porous reticulated titanium foam for orthopedic implant applications. *Proc Amer Acad Orthop Surg* 2008:SE40.

50. Sueyoshi T, Keating EM, Ritter MA, Meding JB, Brunsman MJ: Early clinical outcomes with a 3-D porous titanium acetabular cup. *Open J Orthop* 2016;06:121-125.

51. Beckmann NA, Jaeger S, Janoszka MB, Klotz MC, Bruckner T, Bitsch RG: Comparison of the primary stability of a porous coated acetabular revision cup with a standard cup. *J Arthroplasty* 2018;33(2):580-585.

    This study compared the primary stability of two revision cups of the same geometry, yet with different surface properties—porous titanium versus conventional sintered-bead titanium—in an in vitro scenario.

52. Gilmour LJ, Jones R, Dickinson J: Mechanical properties of a sintered asymmetric particle ingrowth coating. *Proc Amer Soc Mater Conference (Materials and Processes for Medical Devices)* 2009:11.2.

53. Bourne RB, McCalden RW, Naudie D, Charron KDJ, Yuan X, Holdsworth DW: The next generation of acetabular shell design and bearing surfaces. *Supplement to Orthopaedics Innovation in Total Hip Arthroplasty*, 2008, pp 92-96.

54. Heuer DA, Williams M, Moss R, et al: A1062. Biologic fixation of an asymmetric titanium particle porous coating in a load-bearing animal model. *Orthop Proc* 2011;93-B(suppl 4):419.

55. Naudie DDR, Somerville L, Korczak A, et al: A randomized trial comparing acetabular component fixation of two porous ingrowth surfaces using RSA. *J Arthroplasty* 2013;28(suppl 8):48-52.

56. Goodman SB, Yao Z, Keeney M, Yang F: The future of biologic coatings for orthopaedic implants. *Biomaterials* 2013;34(13):3174-3183.

57. Thanner J, Kärrholm J, Herberts P, Malchau H: Porous cups with and without hydroxylapatite-tricalcium phosphate coating: 23 matched pairs evaluated with radiostereometry. *J Arthroplasty* 1999;14(3):266-271.

58. Furlong RJ, Osborn JF: Fixation of hip prostheses by hydroxyapatite ceramic coatings. *J Bone Joint Surg Br* 1991;73-B(5):741-745.

59. Lazarinis S, Mäkelä KT, Eskelinen A, et al: Does hydroxyapatite coating of uncemented cups improve long-term survival? An analysis of 28,605 primary total hip arthroplasty procedures from the Nordic Arthroplasty Register Association (NARA). *Osteoarthritis Cartilage* 2017;25(12):1980-1987.

    This study investigates the survival of different uncemented cups that were available with or without hydroxyapatite coatings. Level of evidence: III.

60. Inacio MC, Lorimer M, Davidson DC, De Steiger RN, Lewis PL, Graves SE: What is the risk of revision surgery in hydroxyapatite-coated femoral hip stems? Findings from a large national registry. *Clin Orthop Relat Res* 2018;476(12):2353-2366. Available at: https://journals.lww.com/clinorthop/Fulltext/2018/12000/What_Is_the_Risk_of_Revision_Surgery_in.14.aspx.

    This study evaluates the risk of revision in THAs with hydroxyapatite-coated stems compared with non-hydroxyapatite-coated stems. Level of evidence: II.

61. Zagra L, Gallazzi E, Romano D; Scarponi S; Romano C: Two-stage cementless hip revision for peri-prosthetic infection with an antibacterial hydrogel coating: Results of a comparative series. *Int Orthop* 2019;43(1):111-115.

    This study investigates the hypothesis that a two-stage exchange procedure, performed with an antibiotic-loaded, fast-resorbable hydrogel coating, may provide better infection cure rate than a two-stage procedure without the coating in patients affected by periprosthetic hip infection. Level of evidence: III.

62. Finšgar M, Uzunalić AP, Stergar J, Gradišnik L, Maver U: Novel chitosan/diclofenac coatings on medical grade stainless steel for hip replacement applications. *Sci Rep* 2016;6:26653.

63. Hetrick EM, Schoenfisch MH: Reducing implant-related infections: Active release strategies. *Chem Soc Rev* 2006;35(9):780-789.

64. van de Belt H, Neut D, Schenk W, van Horn JR, van der Mei HC, Busscher HJ: Infection of orthopedic implants and the use of antibiotic-loaded bone cements. A review. *Acta Orthop Scand* 2001;72(6):557-571.

65. Costerton JW, Cheng KJ, Geesey GG, et al: Bacterial biofilms in nature and disease. *Annu Rev Microbiol* 1987;41:435-464.

66. Danon D, Kowatch MA, Roth GS: Promotion of wound repair in old mice by local injection of macrophages. *Proc Natl Acad Sci USA* 1989;86(6):2018-2020.

67. Dunne WMJ: Bacterial adhesion: Seen any good biofilms lately? *Clin Microbiol Rev* 2002;15(2):155-166.

68. Koo H, Allan RN, Howlin RP, Stoodley P, Hall-Stoodley L: Targeting microbial biofilms: Current and prospective therapeutic strategies. *Nat Rev Microbiol* 2017;15(12):740-755.

    This review focuses on current therapeutic strategies and those under development that target vital structural and functional traits of microbial biofilms and drug tolerance mechanisms, including the extracellular matrix and dormant cells. Level of evidence: V.

69. Arciola CR, Campoccia D, Montanaro L: Implant infections: Adhesion, biofilm formation and immune evasion. *Nat Rev Microbiol* 2018;16(7):397-409.

    This review explores the fundamental pathogenic mechanisms underlying implant infections, highlighting orthopaedic implants and *Staphylococcus aureus* as a prime example, and discusses innovative targets for preventative and therapeutic strategies. Level of evidence: V.

70. Yu JC, Ho W, Lin J, Yip H, Wong PK: Photocatalytic activity, antibacterial effect, and photoinduced hydrophilicity of TiO_2 films coated on a stainless steel substrate. *Environ Sci Technol* 2003;37(10):2296-2301.

71. Del Curto B, Brunella MF, Giordano C, et al: Decreased bacterial adhesion to surface-treated titanium. *Int J Artif Organs* 2005;28(7):718-730.

72. Zhang F, Zhang Z, Zhu X, Kang ET, Neoh KG: Silk-functionalized titanium surfaces for enhancing osteoblast functions and reducing bacterial adhesion. *Biomaterials* 2008;29(36):4751-4759.

73. Harris LG, Tosatti S, Wieland M, Textor M, Richards RG: *Staphylococcus aureus* adhesion to titanium oxide surfaces coated with non-functionalized and peptide-functionalized poly(L-lysine)-grafted-poly(ethylene glycol) copolymers. *Biomaterials* 2004;25(18):4135-4148.

74. Kaper HJ, Busscher HJ, Norde W: Characterization of poly(ethylene oxide) brushes on glass surfaces and adhesion of *Staphylococcus epidermidis. J Biomater Sci Polym Ed* 2003;14(4):313-324.

75. Rivardo F, Turner RJ, Allegrone G, Ceri H, Martinotti MG: Anti-adhesion activity of two biosurfactants produced by *Bacillus* spp. prevents biofilm formation of human bacterial pathogens. *Appl Microbiol Biotechnol* 2009;83(3): 541-553.

76. Schmidt-Braekling T, Streitbuerger A, Gosheger G, et al: Silver-coated megaprostheses: Review of the literature. *Eur J Orthop Surg Traumatol* 2017;27(4):483-489.

    This review provides a history and overview of silver-coated megaprotheses and their mechanism of action to prevent periprosthetic joint infections. Level of evidence: V.

77. Hardes J, Henrichs MP, Hauschild G, Nottrott M, Guder W, Streitbuerger A: Silver-coated megaprosthesis of the proximal tibia in patients with sarcoma. *J Arthroplasty* 2017;32(7):2208-2213.

    This study compares the infection rate for patients who received titanium versus silver-coated megaprostheses in patients treated for sarcomas. Level of evidence: III.

78. Wafa H, Grimer RJ, Reddy K, et al: Retrospective evaluation of the incidence of early periprosthetic infection with silver-treated endoprostheses in high-risk patients: Case-control study. *Bone Joint J* 2015;97-B(2):252-257.

79. Mijnendonckx K, Leys N, Mahillon J, Silver S, van Houdt R: Antimicrobial silver: Uses, toxicity and potential for resistance. *Biometals* 2013;26(4):609-621.

80. De Grood MP: Pathology, diagnosis and treatment of subdural empyema. *Arch Chir Neerl* 1951;3(2):128-138.

81. Zhao L, Chu PK, Zhang Y, Wu Z: Antibacterial coatings on titanium implants. *J Biomed Mater Res B Appl Biomater* 2009;91(1):470-480.

82. Stigter M, Bezemer J, de Groot K, Layrolle P: Incorporation of different antibiotics into carbonated hydroxyapatite coatings on titanium implants, release and antibiotic efficacy. *J Control Release* 2004;99(1):127-137.

83. Boyle KK, Sosa B, Osagie L, Turajane K, Bostrom MPG, Yang X: Vancomycin-laden calcium phosphate-calcium sulfate composite allows bone formation in a rat infection model. *PLoS One* 2019;14(9):e0222034.

    This translational animal study compares the efficacy of calcium phosphate–calcium sulphate composite to polymethylmethacrylate for the treatment of osteomyelitis.

84. Gautier H, Daculsi G, Merle C: Association of vancomycin and calcium phosphate by dynamic compaction: In vitro characterization and microbiological activity. *Biomaterials* 2001;22(18):2481-2487.

85. Guillaume O, Garric X, Lavigne JP, Van Den Berghe H, Coudane J: Multilayer, degradable coating as a carrier for the sustained release of antibiotics: Preparation and antimicrobial efficacy in vitro. *J Control Release* 2012;162(3): 492-501.

86. Devane PA, Horne JG, Ashmore A, Mutimer J, Kim W, Stanley J: Highly cross-linked polyethylene reduces wear and revision rates in total hip arthroplasty: A 10-year double-blinded randomized controlled trial. *J Bone Joint Surg Am* 2017;99(20):1703-1714.

    This study compares in vivo wear rates and clinical and radiographic outomes bewteen XLPE and UHMWPE in a prospective double-blinded randomized controlled trial with a minimum of 10 years of follow-up. Level of evidence: I.

87. Garellick G, Kärrholm J, Rogmark C, Herberts P, Rolfson O: *Swedish Hip Arthroplasty Register–Annual Report 2017.* 2018. Available at: https://registercentrum.blob.core.windows.net/shpr/r/Eng_Arsrapport_2017_Hoftprotes_final-Syx-2fJPhMN.pdf. Accessed October 23, 2019.

88. Garellick G, Karrholm J, Lindahl H, Malchau H, Rogmark C, Rolfson O: *Swedish Hip Arthroplasty Register–Annual Report 2013.* 2016. Available at: https://registercentrum.blob.core.windows.net/shpr/r/Annual-report-2013-HJnnK8Tie.pdf. Accessed October 23, 2019.

89. Haw JG, Battenberg AK, Huang D-CT, Schmalzried TP: Wear rates of larger-diameter cross-linked polyethylene at 5 to 13 years: Does liner thickness or component position matter? *J Arthroplasty* 2017;32(4):1381-1386.

    This study investigates the effect of liner thickness, acetabular abduction angle, and acetabular anteversion on large-diameter XLPE wear for THA.

90. Lachiewicz PF, O'Dell JA, Martell JM: Large metal heads and highly cross-linked polyethylene provide low wear and complications at 5-13 years. *J Arthroplasty* 2018;33(7): 2187-2191.

    This study investigated the rates of linear and volumetric wear of acetabular implants and XLPE with large metal heads at mean follow-up of 8 years. Level of evidence: IV.

91. Lachiewicz PF, Soileau ES, Martell JM: Wear and osteolysis of highly crosslinked polyethylene at 10 to 14 years: The effect of femoral head size. *Clin Orthop Relat Res* 2016;474(2):365-371.

92. Wood TJ, Alzahrani M, Langohr D, et al: Catastrophic femoral head trunnion dissociation: A case series with surface wear analysis. *Hip Int* 2019;29(5):NP1-NP5.

    The purpose of this study is to review five cases of catastrophic femoral head trunnion dissociation to better understand clinical and implant-related risk factors for this complication. Level of evidence: IV.

93. de Steiger RN, Muratoglu O, Lorimer M, Cuthbert AR, Graves SE: Lower prosthesis-specific 10-year revision rate with crosslinked than with non-crosslinked polyethylene in primary total knee arthroplasty. *Acta Orthop* 2015;86(6):721-727.

94. Higuchi Y, Seki T, Morita D, Komatsu D, Takegami Y, Ishiguro N: Comparison of wear rate between ceramic-on-ceramic, metal on highly cross-linked polyethylene, and metal-on-metal bearings. *Rev Bras Ortop (Sao Paulo)* 2019;54(3): 295-302.

The aim of this study is to calculate the 5-year to 10-year wear rate and the incidence rate of osteolysis for three types of bearings. Level of evidence: III.

95. Australian Orthopaedic Association National Joint Replacement Registry: *2019 Annual Report*. 2019. Available at: https://aoanjrr.sahmri.com/documents/10180/668596/Hip%2C+Knee+%26+Shoulder+Arthroplasty/c287d2a3-22df-a3bb-37a2-91e6c00bfcf0. Accessed October 23, 2019.

96. Sharplin P, Wyatt MC, Rothwell A, Frampton C, Hooper G: Which is the best bearing surface for primary total hip replacement? A New Zealand Joint Registry study. *Hip Int* 2018;28(4):352-362.

This study investigates the revision rates of all bearing surface combinations for primary total hip replacement registered on the New Zealand Mayo Clinic Joint Replacement Database to determine which coupling has been the most durable and successful over the last 16 years. Level of evidence: III.

97. Hart A, Janz V, Trousdale RT, Sierra RJ, Berry DJ, Abdel MP: Long-term survivorship of total hip arthroplasty with highly cross-linked polyethylene for osteonecrosis. *J Bone Joint Surg Am* 2019;101(17):1563-1568.

The purpose of this study was to compare the long-term implant survivorship, functional outcomes, and radiographic results of contemporary THAs with a highly XLPE liner between patients with osteonecrosis and those with osteoarthritis. Level of evidence: III.

98. Digas G, Karrholm J, Thanner J, Herberts P: 5-year experience of highly cross-linked polyethylene in cemented and uncemented sockets: Two randomized studies using radiostereometric analysis. *Acta Orthop* 2007;78(6): 746-754.

99. Shen FW, Lu Z, McKellop HA: Wear versus thickness and other features of 5-Mrad crosslinked UHMWPE acetabular liners. *Clin Orthop Relat Res* 2011;469(2):395-404.

100. Tower SS, Currier JH, Currier BH, Lyford KA, Van Citters DW, Mayor MB: Rim cracking of the cross-linked longevity polyethylene acetabular liner after total hip arthroplasty. *J Bone Joint Surg Am* 2007;89(10):2212-2217.

101. Bragdon CR, Doerner M, Martell J, Jarrett B, Palm H, Malchau H: The 2012 John Charnley Award: Clinical multicenter studies of the wear performance of highly cross-linked remelted polyethylene in THA. *Clin Orthop Relat Res* 2013;471(2):393-402.

102. Zhang L, Sawae Y, Yamaguchi T, Murakami T, Yang H: Effect of radiation dose on depth-dependent oxidation and wear of shelf-aged gamma-irradiated ultra-high molecular weight polyethylene (UHMWPE). *Tribol Int* 2015;89:78-85.

103. Cooper HJ, Della Valle CJ, Berger RA, et al: Corrosion at the head-neck taper as a cause for adverse local tissue reactions after total hip arthroplasty. *J Bone Joint Surg Am* 2012;94(18):1655-1661.

104. Oral E, Neils AL, Wannomae KK, Muratoglu OK: Novel active stabilization technology in highly crosslinked UHMWPEs for superior stability. *Radiat Phys Chem* 2014;105:6-11.

105. Bichara DA, Malchau E, Sillesen NH, Cakmak S, Nielsen GP, Muratoglu OK: Vitamin E-diffused highly cross-linked UHMWPE particles induce less osteolysis compared to highly cross-linked virgin UHMWPE particles in vivo. *J Arthroplasty* 2014;29(suppl 9):232-237.

106. Bladen CL, Teramura S, Russell SL, et al: Analysis of wear, wear particles, and reduced inflammatory potential of vitamin E ultrahigh-molecular-weight polyethylene for use in total joint replacement. *J Biomed Mater Res B Appl Biomater* 2013;101(3):458-466.

107. Medel F, Kurtz S, MacDonald D, Pascual FJ, Puertolas JA: Does cyclic stress play a role in highly crosslinked polyethylene oxidation? *Clin Orthop Relat Res* 2015;473(3):1022-1029.

108. Reinitz SD, Currier BH, Levine RA, Van Citters DW: Crosslink density, oxidation and chain scission in retrieved, highly cross-linked UHMWPE tibial bearings. *Biomaterials* 2014;35(15):4436-4440.

109. Reinitz SD, Currier BH, Van Citters DW, Levine RA, Collier JP: Oxidation and other property changes of retrieved sequentially annealed UHMWPE acetabular and tibial bearings. *J Biomed Mater Res B Appl Biomater* 2015;103(3):578-586.

110. Costa L, Bracco P, del Prever EB, Luda MP, Trossarelli L: Analysis of products diffused into UHMWPE prosthetic components in vivo. *Biomaterials* 2001;22(4):307-315.

111. Oral E, Ghali BW, Neils A, Muratoglu OK: A new mechanism of oxidation in ultrahigh molecular weight polyethylene caused by squalene absorption. *J Biomed Mater Res B Appl Biomater* 2012;100(3):742-751.

112. Selvarajah E, Hooper G, Grabowski K, Frampton C, Woodfield TBF, Inglis G: The rates of wear of X3 highly cross-linked polyethylene at five years when coupled with a 36 mm diameter ceramic femoral head in young patients. *Bone Joint J* 2015;97-B(11):1470-1474.

113. Tan SC, Teeter MG, Del Balso C, Howard JL, Lanting BA: Effect of taper design on trunnionosis in metal on polyethylene total hip arthroplasty. *J Arthroplasty* 2015;30(7):1269-1272.

114. Plummer DR, Berger RA, Paprosky WG, Sporer SM, Jacobs JJ, Della Valle CJ: Diagnosis and management of adverse local tissue reactions secondary to corrosion at the head-neck junction in patients with metal on polyethylene bearings. *J Arthroplasty* 2016;31(1):264-268.

115. Del Balso C, Teeter MG, Tan SC, Lanting BA, Howard JL: Taperosis: Does head length affect fretting and corrosion in total hip arthroplasty? *Bone Joint J* 2015;97-B(7):911-916.

116. Gaudiani MA, White PB, Ghazi N, Ranawat AS, Ranawat CS: Wear rates with large metal and ceramic heads on a second generation highly cross-linked polyethylene at mean 6-year follow-up. *J Arthroplasty* 2018;33(2):590-594.

This study assessed wear rates with large metal and ceramic heads on a second-generation highly XLPE. Level of evidence: III.

117. Baek SH, Kim WK, Kim JY, Kim SY: Do alumina matrix composite bearings decrease hip noises and bearing fractures at a minimum of 5 years after THA? *Clin Orthop Relat Res* 2015;473(12):3796-3802.

118. Carnes KJ, Odum SM, Troyer JL, Fehring TK: Cost analysis of ceramic heads in primary total hip arthroplasty. *J Bone Joint Surg Am* 2016;98(21):1794-1800.

119. Zagra L, Gallazzi E: Bearing surfaces in primary total hip arthroplasty. *EFORT Open Rev* 2018;3(5):217-224.

The aim of this paper is to evaluate the main advantages and drawbacks of various types of tribology in THA. Level of evidence: V.

120. Owen DH, Russell NC, Smith PN, Walter WL: An estimation of the incidence of squeaking and revision surgery for squeaking in ceramic-on-ceramic total hip replacement: A meta-analysis and report from the Australian Orthopaedic Association National Joint Registry. *Bone Joint J* 2014;96-B(2):181-187.

121. Walter WL, Insley GM, Walter WK, Tuke MA: Edge loading in third generation alumina ceramic-on-ceramic bearings: Stripe wear. *J Arthroplasty* 2004;19(4):402-413.

122. Walter WL, Yeung E, Esposito C: A review of squeaking hips. *J Am Acad Orthop Surg* 2010;18(6):319-326.

123. Walter WL, Kurtz SM, Esposito C, et al: Retrieval analysis of squeaking alumina ceramic-on-ceramic bearings. *J Bone Joint Surg Br* 2011;93(12):1597-1601.

124. Esposito CI, Walter WL, Roques A, et al: Wear in alumina-on-alumina ceramic total hip replacements: A retrieval analysis of edge loading. *J Bone Joint Surg Br* 2012;94(7):901-907.

125. Abdel MP, Heyse TJ, Elpers ME, et al: Ceramic liner fractures presenting as squeaking after primary total hip arthroplasty. *J Bone Joint Surg Am* 2014;96(1):27-31.

126. Esposito C, Maclean F, Campbell P, Walter WL, Walter WK, Bonar SF: Periprosthetic tissues from third generation alumina-on-alumina total hip arthroplasties. *J Arthroplasty* 2013;28(5):860-866.

127. Sedel L, Walter WL, Pitto RP: Clinical faceoff: Ceramic-on-ceramic THA. Do the advantages outweigh the limitations? *Clin Orthop Relat Res* 2014;472(10):2927-2931.

128. Massin P, Lopes R, Masson B, Mainard D: Does Biolox Delta ceramic reduce the rate of component fractures in total hip replacement? *Orthop Traumatol Surg Res* 2014;100(suppl 6):S317-S321.

129. Rankin CS, Robinson PG, Beattie N, Gaston P: Fracture of a BIOLOX delta ceramic femoral head. *JBJS Case Connect* 2019;9(4):e0336.

This case report highlights a patient who had a BIOLOX delta ceramic head fracture following THA. Level of evidence: V.

130. Koo KH, Ha YC, Jung WH, Kim SR, Yoo JJ, Kim HJ: Isolated fracture of the ceramic head after third-generation alumina-on-alumina total hip arthroplasty. *J Bone Joint Surg Am* 2008;90(2):329-336.

131. Traina F, De Fine M, Di Martino A, Faldini C: Fracture of ceramic bearing surfaces following total hip replacement: A systematic review. *Biomed Res Int* 2013;2013:157247.

132. McDonnell SM, Boyce G, Bare J, Young D, Shimmin AJ: The incidence of noise generation arising from the large-diameter Delta Motion ceramic total hip bearing. *Bone Joint J* 2013;95-B(2):160-165.

133. Kraaij G, Zadpoor AA, Tuijthof GJM, Dankelman J, Nelissen RGHH, Valstar ER: Mechanical properties of human bone-implant interface tissue in aseptically loose hip implants. *J Mech Behav Biomed Mater* 2014;38:59-68.

134. Waddell BS, Koch C, Trivellas M, Burket JC, Wright T, Padgett D: Have large femoral heads reduced prosthetic impingement in total hip arthroplasty? *Hip Int* 2019;29(1):83-88.

This study assessed retrieved THA implants for evidence of impingement to determine if large femoral heads reduced the rate of impingement in primary THA. Level of evidence: V.

135. Hampton C, Weitzler L, Baral E, Wright TM, Bostrom MPG: Do oxidized zirconium heads decrease tribocorrosion in total hip arthroplasty? *Bone Joint J* 2019;101-B(4):386-389.

This study aimed to evaluate fretting and corrosion in retreived OxZr and CoCr femoral heads. Level of evidence: III.

136. Duncan CP, Toms A, Masri BA: Minimally invasive or limited incision hip replacement: Clarification and classification. *Instr Course Lect* 2006;55:195-197.

137. Greidanus NV, Chihab S, Garbuz DS, et al: Outcomes of minimally invasive anterolateral THA are not superior to those of minimally invasive direct lateral and posterolateral THA. *Clin Orthop Relat Res* 2013;471(2):463-471.

138. Inaba Y, Kobayashi N, Yukizawa Y, Ishida T, Iwamoto N, Saito T: Little clinical advantage of modified Watson-Jones approach over modified mini-incision direct lateral approach in primary total hip arthroplasty. *J Arthroplasty* 2011;26(7):1117-1122.

139. Martin R, Clayson PE, Troussel S, Fraser BP, Docquier PL: Anterolateral minimally invasive total hip arthroplasty: A prospective randomized controlled study with a follow-up of 1 year. *J Arthroplasty* 2011;26(8):1362-1372.

140. Foucher KC, Wimmer MA, Moisio KC, et al: Time course and extent of functional recovery during the first postoperative year after minimally invasive total hip arthroplasty with two different surgical approaches—A randomized controlled trial. *J Biomech* 2011;44(3):372-378.

141. Morison ZA, Patil S, Khan HA, Bogoch ER, Schemitsch EH, Waddell JP: A randomized controlled trial comparing Oxinium and cobalt-chrome on standard and cross-linked polyethylene. *J Arthroplasty* 2014;29(suppl 9):164-168.

142. Jonsson BA, Kadar T, Havelin LI, et al: Oxinium modular femoral heads do not reduce polyethylene wear in cemented total hip arthroplasty at five years: A randomised trial of 120 hips using radiostereometric analysis. *Bone Joint J* 2015;97-B(11):1463-1469.

143. Jassim SS, Patel S, Wardle N, et al: Five-year comparison of wear using oxidised zirconium and cobalt-chrome femoral heads in total hip arthroplasty: A multicentre randomised controlled trial. *Bone Joint J* 2015;97-B(7):883-889.

144. Smith AJ, Dieppe P, Vernon K, Porter M, Blom AW: Failure rates of stemmed metal-on-metal hip replacements: Analysis of data from the National Joint Registry of England and Wales. *Lancet* 2012;379(9822):1199-1204.

145. Kwon YM, Lombardi AV, Jacobs JJ, Fehring TK, Lewis CG, Cabanela ME: Risk stratification algorithm for management of patients with metal-on-metal hip arthroplasty: Consensus statement of the American Association of Hip and Knee Surgeons, the American Academy of Orthopaedic Surgeons, and the Hip Society. *J Bone Joint Surg Am* 2014;96(1):e4.

CHAPTER 31

Primary Total Hip Arthroplasty—Cemented

MATTHEW J.W. HUBBLE, MBBS, FRCS (TR&ORTH)

ABSTRACT

Although noncemented fixation predominates in North America, there is increasing awareness of the role of cemented implants, particularly cemented stems, in certain patient groups. Multiple national joint registries from around the world, including North America, now report superior results with cemented stems in patients older than 70 years, particularly in terms of reduced periprosthetic fracture and reliability of implant fixation. Growing evidence also supports hybrid fixation, with a noncemented cup and cemented stem, both in terms of results and of cost effectiveness and this combination is increasingly performed. Additional advantages of cemented stems include the intraoperative ease of adjustment of leg length and version and the future option of cement-in-cement revision if necessary. Although cement implantation syndrome is a concern, with the use of an appropriate cementing technique, overall mortality, in fact, is reduced with cemented stems in both hemiarthroplasty and total hip arthroplasty patients. The evidence supports the increasing use of cemented implants in North America and surgeons should familiarize themselves with these principles and undergo training in cementing techniques accordingly.

Dr. Hubble or an immediate family member has received royalties from Stryker; serves as a paid consultant to or is an employee of Stryker; and has received research or institutional support from Stryker.

Keywords: arthroplasty; cement; hip; polymethyl methacrylate

INTRODUCTION

Total hip arthroplasty (THA) continues to be one of the most successful and commonly performed surgical procedures in North America. Although there has been an overall convergence of surgical designs and techniques, controversies still exist. Among these are the indications and pros and cons of cemented versus noncemented fixation. Surgeons are influenced as much by their training as they are by the literature and as a result there are great national and regional variations in the use of cemented and noncemented implants. In addition to the published literature, data from national joint registries is now increasingly relied on as not only do they give an indication of real-world practices and outcomes, but they are also comparatively free from the bias of studies with industry sponsorship, or from designer centers. They also provide insight into these regional and national variations. There is a growing awareness from these data that there is evidence for the increased use of cemented implants, particularly cemented stems, in certain population groups, particularly older patients and those who have osteopenia. Cemented acetabular implants also have a role, although with the improvement in the long-term results of noncemented cups when highly cross-linked polyethylene (XLPE) liners are used, the benefits of cemented fixation are less marked on the acetabular side of the joint. Although cemented cups are indicated in specific situations, there is evidence that for many patients a combination of cemented and noncemented implants, namely a hybrid THA, may be the best of both worlds. In particular there is increasing popularity in many regions

This chapter is adapted from Della Valle CJ, Berry DJ, Bragdon CR, et al: Primary total hip arthroplasty, in Mont MA, Tanzer M, eds: *Orthopaedic Knowledge Update®: Hip and Knee Reconstruction*, ed 5. Rosemont, IL, American Academy of Orthopaedic Surgeons, 2017, pp 377-391.

for the combination of a cemented stem with a noncemented cup, although the converse (a reverse hybrid) may also have its merits in certain circumstances.

FEMORAL IMPLANT SELECTION AND RESULTS

The femoral implant of a THA must effectively restore the biomechanics of the proximal femur and hip joint and achieve and maintain durable fixation to the proximal femur. Both cemented and noncemented femoral implants have demonstrated the capability to achieve reliable and durable fixation with excellent long-term results. However, results vary considerably according to implant design and method of fixation. In North America, noncemented femoral fixation is used in most patients (95%), and it is only in the ninth decade and beyond that cemented stems are used with any regularity (35%)[1] (**Figure 1**). By comparison, cemented femoral fixation is much more common in the United Kingdom, and in the Scandinavian countries. In the United Kingdom in particular, the popularity of hybrid THA (with a cemented stem and noncemented cup) means that most patients (60% in 2019) currently receive a cemented stem (though only 30% a cemented cup).[2] The incidence of cemented stem use is even higher in Sweden (65% in 2017)[3] and in Australia (35%).[4,5]

There is great focus in the literature and at orthopaedic conferences on the younger, high-demand patient. The reality, however, is that most patients undergoing THA are not in this group, and indeed most are 65 years of age or older.[1,2,5] Although data from several sources suggest noncemented THA outperforms cemented in younger patients,[6] most data show that cemented implants have the lowest revision rate in older patients.[7,8] Joint registries provide some of the best high-level information on factors that influence performance of different implant categories in different circumstances.[1-5] As the American Joint Replacement Registry grows and matures, the data from it can be added to that from the more well-established registries around the world, giving an invaluable insight into practices and outcomes in North America.[1] However, as the use of cemented implants is proportionately so small in North America, data from these other countries, where cemented implants are more commonly used, need to be considered if the relative merits of cemented and noncemented implants are to be assessed. Although information from the Australian registry, for example, demonstrates that noncemented THA outperforms cemented and hybrid THA in patients aged 64 years and younger at 10 to 14 years postoperatively, the American, Australian, United Kingdom, and Scandinavian registries all demonstrate that cemented THA has a lower revision rate than noncemented THA in older patients[1-4,7,8] (**Figure 2**). Individual prosthesis design as well as method of fixation will also influence outcome. A recent study therefore looked specifically at the three best noncemented and three best cemented stems in the Australian registry to try to reduce the confounding influence of poorer performing implants on outcome by method of fixation as a class. In patients older than 75

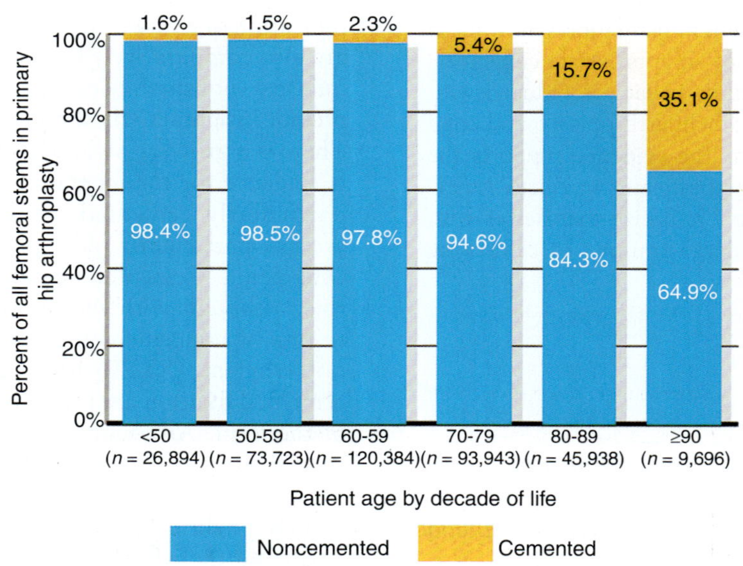

FIGURE 1 A bar graph showing the proportion of noncemented and cemented stems in primary hip arthroplasty by decade in life. (Reprinted with permission from American Joint Replacement Registry (AJRR): *2018 Annual Report*. Rosemont, IL: American Academy of Orthopaedic Surgeons (AAOS), 2018.)

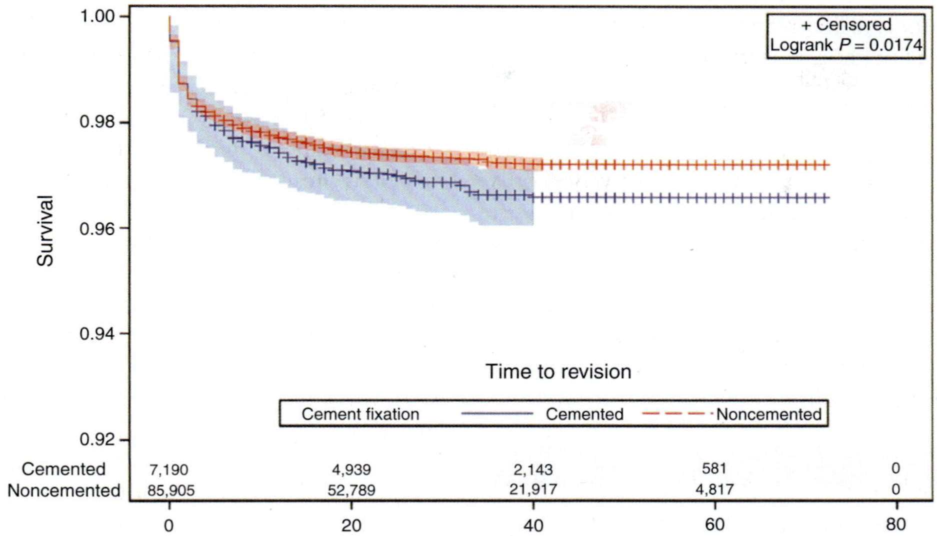

* Total possible patient population: 108,002; after accounting for missing data and exclusions as notes, the number analyzed = 93,095 (85% of total population)

Summary of the number of censored and uncensored values

Stratum	Cement Fixation	% of the Total	Total	Failed	Censored	Percent Censored
1	Cemented	7.7%	7,190	219	6,971	96.0%
2	Noncemented	92.3%	85,905	2,175	83,730	97.5%
Total			93,095	2,394	90,701	97.4%

A

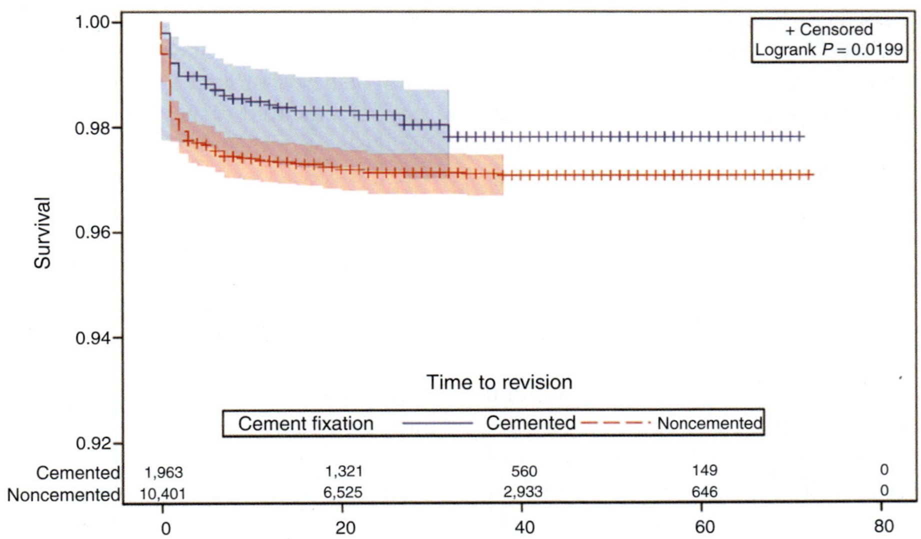

* Total possible patient population: 22,669; after accounting for missing data and exclusions as notes, the number analyzed = 12,364 (54% of total population)

Summary of the number of censored and uncensored values

Stratum	Cement Fixation	% of the Total	Total	Failed	Censored	Percent Censored
1	Cemented	15.9%	1,963	37	1,926	98.1%
2	Noncemeted	84.1%	10,401	290	10,111	97.2%
Total			12,364	327	12,037	97.4%

B

FIGURE 2 Superior results are shown in these graphs for noncemented implants in the cohort as a whole (**A**), but favor cemented implants in older patients, especially females aged 80 years or older (**B**). (Reprinted with permission from American Joint Replacement Registry (AJRR): *2018 Annual Report*. Rosemont, IL: American Academy of Orthopaedic Surgeons (AAOS), 2018.)

years, cemented stems demonstrated superior results in both osteoarthritis and hip fracture patients, due primarily to a lower incidence of periprosthetic fracture and loosening within the first 3 months.[9]

Despite this evidence and the American Joint Replacement Registry showing superior results with cemented stems in patients aged 80 years or older, only 15% of stems in the age group 80 to 89 years were cemented in American Joint Replacement Registry participating hospitals in the 2018 report.[1]

All registries show that 1% to 3% of THAs fail in the first year after surgery, and for noncemented THAs, proportionately more early failures are related to periprosthetic fractures or failure of osseointegration.[9,10]

CEMENTED STEMS

The trend toward noncemented fixation initially began because of concerns of loosening and osteolysis with some early designs of cemented implants, but ultimately became common because noncemented fixation is more efficient and the surgical technique is less demanding.

Four generations of cement technique have been described in the literature. The goal of advancing cement techniques has ultimately been to achieve a 2- to 5-mm symmetrical cement mantle around the implant with interdigitation into the host bone to achieve long-term fixation. As cement techniques have improved, so have survivorship rates, with several studies reporting cemented survivorship rates of 95% at more than 20 years. One such study recently reported similar outcome scores and survivorship rates (98.1% and 99.6%, respectively) for cemented and noncemented fixation using the same femoral implant at 20-year follow-up.[11] Other studies have also reported similar survivorship rates (96% and 95%) at 25-year follow-up in the same patients, all of whom were younger than 50 years.[12] These studies demonstrate that at 20- to 25-year follow-up, both cemented and noncemented fixation can provide excellent survivorship.

In contemporary North American practice, the use of cemented stems has declined substantially. As previously outlined, these stems may have substantial advantages in certain patient demographic groups, including patients older than 70 years and patients whose bone quality is otherwise compromised, in which groups noncemented stems have shown a higher rate of periprosthetic fracture and failure of fixation and cemented stems have shown outstanding durability.

Philosophies of Cemented Femoral Stem Design

It is increasingly apparent that with both noncemented and cemented stems, outcomes are design specific and that arguably more important than the method of fixation (cemented or noncemented) is the particular design or brand of the stem. With cemented stems, there are two broad classes of stem: taper slip (polished collarless tapers) or composite beam designs (rough or matte surfaced, often collared). Each relies on a very different mechanical principle of fixation, with some stems exhibiting greater or fewer of these design features. Within each of these two broad design classes, there are examples of both excellent and poorly performing stems. Long-term outcomes in national joint registries are conflicting, with the United Kingdom and Australian registries tending to favor taper slip designs and the Nordic favoring a composite beam.[13-15] It is critical, therefore, that a surgeon is familiar with the long-term results of the specific stem that they are using, rather than just those of that broad class. In the United Kingdom, the Orthopaedic Data Evaluation Panel (ODEP) was established in 2002 to rate every make of hip prosthesis and each is graded according to the quality of evidence and results supporting their use, with the recent introduction of a 10A* grading, indicating good evidence of a revision rate for all causes of less than 5% at 10 years.[16] Referencing the information available from ODEP gives surgeons and institutions an independent system to help guide their prosthesis selections. Recently, the United Kingdom nationwide Get It Right First Time (GIRFT) program assesses units on the ODEP rating of the prostheses they use in an attempt to reduce variation and raise outcomes at a national level.[17] The GIRFT program also recommends that patients older than 70 years receive cemented rather than noncemented implants on the basis of both results and cost effectiveness.

Periprosthetic Fracture

A number of studies, including large-scale registry reviews of many hundreds of thousands of patients, have found that periprosthetic fracture is significantly more common with noncemented rather than cemented stems. One such study involving over 400,000 cases in the pooled Arthoplasty Register Association database found an increased relative risk of 8.72 for noncemented stems (0.07% versus 0.47%) in the first 2 years after implantation.[11] The risk of periprosthetic fracture also varies by stem design as well as method of fixation, both for cemented and noncemented stems. Of the cemented stems, matt coated composite beam designs appear to have a lower incidence compared with the polished taper stems.[18] The increased incidence seen with noncemented stems is highest in the elderly, in females, and following surgery for hip fracture. This was highlighted in the 2019 supplementary report of the Australian Joint Replacement Registry,[19] which revealed a dramatic difference in the incidence of periprosthetic fracture following bipolar hemiarthroplasty and which increased steadily with time (**Figure 3**).

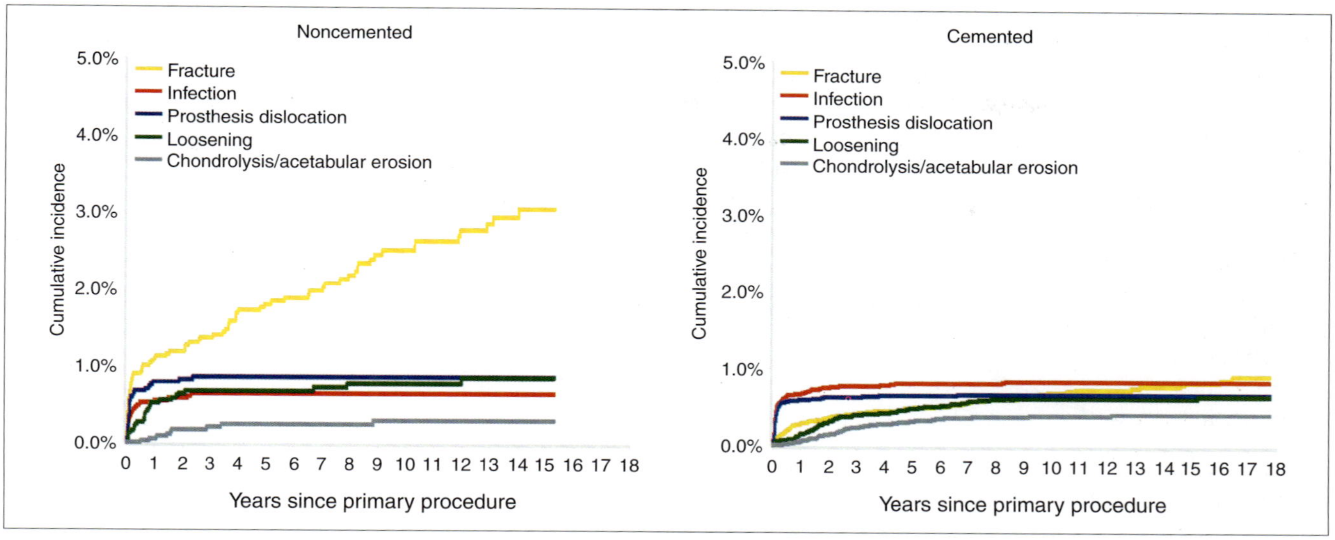

FIGURE 3 Graphs showing a marked increase in the incidence of revision for periprosthetic fracture (yellow line) is seen with the use of noncemented stems (left graph) in patients undergoing bipolar hemiarthroplasty. (Reproduced with permission from Australian Orthopaedic Association National Joint Replacement Registry: *Partial Hip Arthroplasty. Supplementary Report*. Available at: www.aoanjrr.sahmri.com/annual-reports-2019.)

Use of Cement and Data on Mortality

Cement implantation syndrome is a real concern and every effort should be made to minimize this complication. However, with the adoption of appropriate anesthetic and surgical techniques, the incidence of this phenomenon can be dramatically reduced—to the point where even in elderly patients the risk-benefit ratio in terms of overall complications and mortality favors the use of cemented rather that noncemented implants. Previous studies in hemiarthroplasty patients, who by their age and frailty are at the greatest risk of cement implantation syndrome, demonstrated an increased early risk of death in patients undergoing cemented versus noncemented hemiarthoplasty. Perhaps counterintuitively, however, this trend was reversed by day 7 and at all time points thereafter, making cemented fixation the lower risk option in the longer term. This finding has recently been confirmed in THA patients in a large registry study of almost 180,000 patients in Sweden, which showed a 5 in 10,000 (0.05%) increase in mortality in the early postoperative period that was then reversed at 14 days and beyond.[20]

National guidelines have recently been published in Great Britain and Ireland, applicable elsewhere, to highlight the anesthetic and surgical steps that can and should be undertaken to minimize the risk of bone implantation syndrome and protect patients undergoing cemented hip arthroplasty.[21] Clinicians undertaking cemented THA have a responsibility to be familiar with these recommendations. These include early identification of those at risk (older age, significant cardiopulmonary disease, diuretic use, and male sex) and close communication between surgeon and anesthetist, especially just before cementing. Anesthetic steps include adequate preoperative and intraoperative fluid hydration, close blood pressure monitoring and control, aiming for systolioc pressure within 20% of preinduction values, and having vasopressors prepared in case of cardiovascular collapse. Surgeons should thoroughly wash and dry the canal with lavage and suction, use a canal plug and suction catheter, and insert the bone cement with a gun in a retrograde fashion. Undue cement pressurization should be avoided in at-risk groups.

Cement Types

Although there is evidence to show benefit in improved surgical technique and the method and generation of cementing, there is less significant difference in the outcomes with different cement types, or with different levels of viscosity. In terms of long-term fixation and implant survival, the evidence for or against low viscosity or even vacuum mixing of cement in THA is limited. Outside of North America the use of antibiotic-loaded cement is commonplace. The Australian Joint Replacement Registry has recently produced a supplement on the use of different types of bone cement in THA, including a comparison of revision rates with antibiotic loaded and plain cements.[22] This demonstrated approximately a 10% reduction in long-term revision rates with the use of antibiotic-loaded cement at 10 years (6.3% versus 5.7%) (**Figure 4**). Interestingly, the main cause for this difference appeared to be due to aseptic loosening, rather than infection rates. This of course raises the possibility of occult infection as a hidden cause for many cases of apparent aseptic loosening.

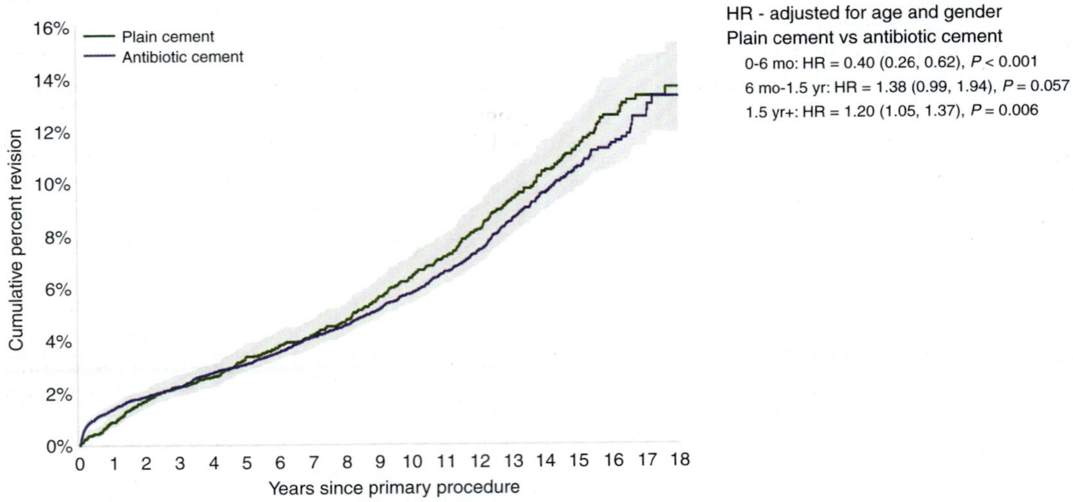

Number at risk	0 yr	1 yr	3 yr	5 yr	10 yr	15 yr	18 yr
Plain cement	5,637	5,420	4,950	4,445	2,796	1,186	157
Antibiotic cement	18,246	17,003	14,629	11,993	5,918	1,463	82

FIGURE 4 Graphs showing revision rates with (blue) and without (green) antibiotic in the bone cement used for total hip arthroplasty. (Reproduced with permission the Australian Orthopaedic Association National Joint Replacement Registry: *Cement in Hip and Knee Arthroplasty. Supplementary Report*. Available at: www.aoanjrr.sahmri.com/annual-reports-2019.)

Restoration of Anatomy and Cemented Stems

One of the advantages of a cemented stem is the flexibility in terms of implant positioning that insertion with cement allows—the depth of insertion can be preplanned and then fine-tuned and adjusted intraoperatively to maximize restoration of leg length or balancing of the soft tissues.[23] Particularly with the collarless polished designs of stem, the absence of a collar adds to the flexibility of positioning and insertion depth into the femur. Likewise, version is much less constrained by the anatomy of the femur than it is with a noncemented stem and can be increased or decreased relative to the native version, within the cement mantle, to maximize stability. Unfortunately, the use of modular necks with noncemented stems, to try to achieve a similar flexibility of anatomic restoration, have been associated with an increased failure rate. Several studies and national registries have highlighted concerns and advised against the use of modular-neck implants accordingly.[24]

Cement-in-Cement Revision

One of the benefits of the use of cemented implants, often underappreciated by surgeons less familiar with cemented THA, is the ability to perform cement-in-cement revision should revision surgery be required in the future. A number of studies have highlighted that all cemented implants, both acetabular and femoral, can be considered to be modular at the cement-prosthesis interface. A well-fixed stem, for example, can be tapped out of a well-fixed cement mantle to facilitate exposure for acetabular revision, and a new stem can then be recemented into the old mantle. This not only improves exposure and facilitates the revision but also allows the position of the new stem to be adjusted to match the newly revised acetabular implant and allow balancing of the joint. A recent report has confirmed that if necessary, this can be successfully repeated on more than one occasion if further revisions are required over the life time of the joint, highlighting the potential for modularity at the cement-prosthesis interface.[25]

Cemented Cups

Although the use of cemented all-polyethylene acetabular implants has reduced dramatically in North America, in many areas of the world, the technique is still common, with excellent reported results. Historically, most North American series showed initial excellent durability through the first decade; however, a higher rate of radiographic loosening and revision was observed beyond 10 years. In the hope of reducing the rate of failure, metal backing was added to cemented polyethylene implants in the early 1980s. Although the metal backing theoretically reduced strains in the cement mantle, the clinical results were worse, and use of these implants was universally abandoned. In North America, the preference then moved increasingly to noncemented acetabular implants, whereas in Sweden, for example, cementing of the acetabulum remains the favored procedure, with 60% of all acetabular implants being cemented in 2017, and over 80% in patients older than 70 years, with results superior to noncemented implants in these age groups.[5] Although reduced cost is also a real benefit, a more demanding surgical technique and the relative lack of modularity are disadvantages to be considered with a cemented all-polyethylene implant.

Current indications for a cemented all-polyethylene implant primarily include patient age older than 70 years or cases in which bone stock is thought to be inadequate to mechanically support a noncemented acetabular implant while ingrowth is occurring. In one study of 2,000 primary Charnley arthroplasties followed for 25 years, age and length of follow-up correlated most strongly with outcomes.[26] Survivorship free of revision for aseptic loosening was poorer for each subsequent decade and varied from 68.2% in patients younger than 40 years to 100% for patients older than 80 years. Males had a twofold higher rate of implant revision for aseptic loosening than females (25-year survivorship was 95% for females and 81% for males; $P < 0.0001$). Similar outcomes have subsequently been observed from the larger European registries and meta-analyses, hence the practice and recommendation that the ideal population for cemented cups is patients older than 70 years. As with noncemented implants, recent evidence shows that longer term results are significantly improved in all age groups with the use of highly XLPE.[27]

The surgical technique includes reaming to subchondral bone; reaming is generally 2 to 4 mm greater than the diameter of the cup to be inserted. The aim is to expose the more porous cancellous bone to maximize interdigitation of cement to host bone. A series of additional pilot holes or footings are then made circumferentially around the rim of the acetabulum, especially in any residual sclerotic areas, to allow better cement intrusion and anchoring of the implant. The acetabulum is cleansed with pulsed lavage to clear the interspaces of blood and fat, followed by the insertion of cement in the earlier stages of hardening. Thumb pressure is used to encourage interdigitation, followed by use of a silicone plunger to further pressurize the cement. The interface is carefully dried, and an implant 2 to 4 mm smaller than the largest reamer used is inserted. To ensure a uniform cement mantle that is 2 to 3 mm thick, cups with polymethyl methacrylate studs/centralizers on the surface can be used.

Cemented cups also have a role in the management of complex primary THA and in the revision setting, in which they have been used successfully in conjunction with impaction bone grafting; or cementation into a well-fixed noncemented cup, a highly porous cup with no locking mechanism, or a reconstruction cage.[28] Cemented dual-mobility acetabular implants are also becoming increasingly popular and positive reports of their use in all of the aforementioned situations have recently been published.[29-31] They are also increasingly used in the setting of hip fractures, such patients being more suited to a cemented implant and at increased dislocation risk.[32] Recent reports have also highlighted the use of a combination of porous metal wedges and cemented cups with or without impaction grafting in both the primary and revision setting[33-35] (**Figure 5**). These include a comparison of the results of using porous metal wedges with both cemented and noncemented cups that concluded that midterm results were similarly good with either.[35]

Cost Effectiveness

Most cemented implants, both femoral and acetabular, are relatively lower cost than noncemented implants. This particularly applies to the acetabular cup, with popular designs with ODEP 10A* ratings being available for a one-fourth the price of most noncemented acetabular implants. The results of recent cost-effectiveness studies are conflicting, but favor a cemented stem.[36] Even allowing for consumables, cement, and theater time costs, a recent study using UK and Swedish Registry data found in favor of fully cemented implants, whereas a previous study of almost 40,000 UK patients found that although fully cemented implants were cheapest, a hybrid THA with a cemented stem and a noncemented cup was the most cost effective.[37]

Hybrid THA

The combination of a cemented stem with a noncemented cup is an increasingly popular combination in

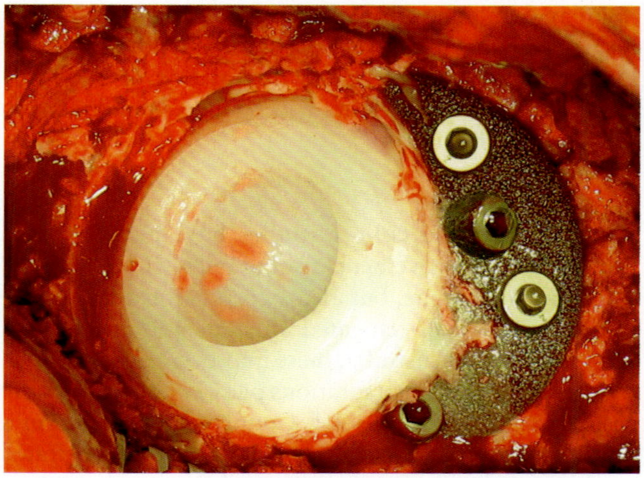

FIGURE 5 Clinical photograph showing a porous metal wedge, fixed with screws, to close a superior uncontained acetabular defect, with a cemented cup inserted below.

Section 3: Hip

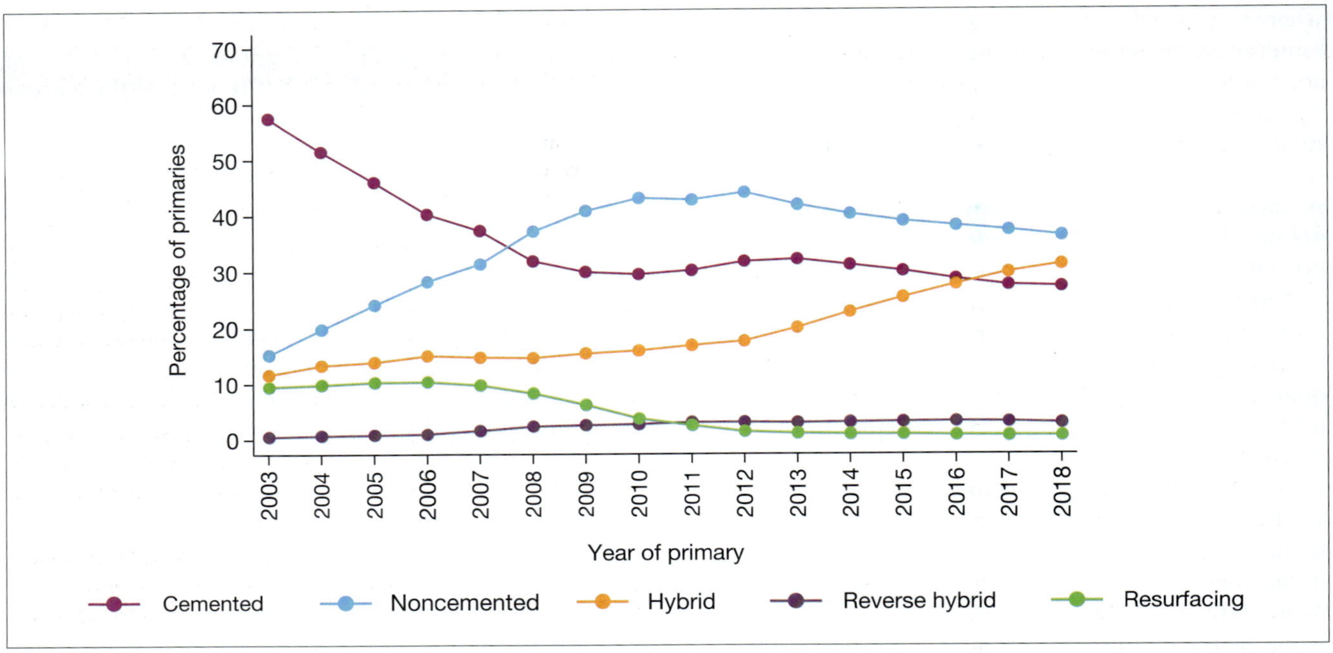

FIGURE 6 Graph shows increasing popularity (yellow line) for hybrid total hip arthroplasty with a combination of a cemented stem with a noncemented cup, with a relative decline in the use of fully cemented (purple) or fully noncemented (blue) implants. (Reproduced with permission from the National Joint Registry for England, Wales, Northern Ireland, the Isle of Man and the States of Guernsey, 2019, p 45, Figure 3.3. Available at: http://www.njrcentre.org.uk.)

many parts of the world. It now represents more than 30% of all arthroplasties, in the UK Joint Replacement Registry, and is also popular in Australia, New Zealand, and other countries (**Figure 6**). As detailed earlier, the use of a cemented stem has been demonstrated to reduce the risks of periprosthetic fractures and failure of fixation and allows flexibility in the intraoperative adjustment of leg length and version. The ease and speed of insertion of a noncemented cup, combined with the low revision rates associated with an XLPE liner has made this a popular combination. As mentioned earlier, long-term results and cost-effectiveness studies support this combination, and it is likely that this pairing of cemented and noncemented implants will be increasingly used in the foreseeable future.

Training and Cementation Skills

Registry data and cohort studies have demonstrated not only an improvement in outcomes with improved cementing technique, but also a correlation between the frequency of use of cemented implants and results. In a 2019 study from Australia, these improvements were seen after as little as 10 implantations per year, although were greater still after 25 cases.[38] Countries that perform a high proportion of cemented implants have demonstrated superior results (the Swedish effect) than countries where cemented prostheses are less frequently used.[5,8] These findings suggest that surgical technique has a significant influence on outcome. This is particularly relevant for North America, where there is an increasing realization that there is a role for cemented implants in certain patient groups, but where many surgeons have little current experience of cementing. These issues support the incorporation of training in cementing techniques into residency programs and continuing education events to minimize the relearning curve of cementing skills in North America.

SUMMARY

Although noncemented fixation predominates in North America, cemented fixation clearly has a role. Superior results, particularly with cemented stems, are reported in patients older than 70 years in multiple national joint registries from around the world including North America. Cemented cups also have a role, particularly in the more elderly. However, hybrid fixation, with a cemented stem and noncemented cup, may for many be the optimum compromise both in terms of results and cost-effectiveness and is increasingly popular. Periprosthetic fractures in particular are less common with cemented stems, notably in the elderly, females, and after hip fracture. Although cement implantation syndrome remains a concern, paradoxically overall mortality with the use of an appropriate cementing technique is in fact lower with cemented stems in both hemiarthroplasty and THA patients. Additional advantages of cemented stems include ease of intraoperative adjustment of leg length and version and the ability to undertake cement-in-cement revision if indicated in the future. The evidence supports the increasing use of cemented implants, particularly cemented stems, in North America and, accordingly, training in cementing techniques.

KEY STUDY POINTS

- Noncemented femoral fixation has proved superior for younger patients; however, overall survivorship for older patients favors cemented femoral fixation.
- Contemporary modular noncemented cups are appropriate for most patients; however, cemented all-polyethylene implants show good results in older patient populations.
- Hybrid THA with a cemented stem and a noncemented cup may be the best combination for many patients in terms of both results and cost effectiveness and is increasingly performed.
- Periprosthetic fracture and failure of osseointegration are less common with cemented implants, particularly in the elderly, females, and after hip fracture.
- With the use of techniques to minimize cement implantation syndrome, cemented stems paradoxically carry a lower risk of overall mortality after both hemiarthroplasty and THA. Surgeons should adopt these techniques.
- Training in cementing technique is encouraged to minimize the relearning curve with cemented implants in North America.

ANNOTATED REFERENCES

1. American Joint Replacement Registry: *Annual Report 2018*. Available at: www.ajrr.net. Accessed October 15, 2019.

   Although only established in 2009, the registry already holds data on 2 million hip and knee arthroplasty procedures.

2. National Joint Registry for England, Wales, Northern Ireland and the Isle of Man: *Annual Report 2019*. Available at: www.njrcentre.org.uk. Accessed October 15, 2019.

   Set up in 2002, and now with more than 3 million procedures recorded, this is the world's largest prosthetic joint registry. It includes data on ankle, shoulder, and elbow arthroplasties as well as hip and knee procedures.

3. Swedish Hip Arthroplasty Register: *Annual Report 2017*. Available at: www.shpr.registercentrum.se/shar-in-english/annual-reports. Accessed October 15, 2019.

   One of the first arthroplasty registries, established in 1979, this now has outcome data to 40 years.

4. Australian Orthopaedic Association National Joint Replacement Registry: *Annual Report 2019*. Available at: www.aoanjrr.sahmri.com/annual-reports-2019. Accessed October 15, 2019.

5. Paxton EW, Cafri G, Nemes S, et al: An international comparison of THA patients, implants, techniques, and survivorship in Sweden, Australia, and the United States. *Acta Orthop* 2019;90(2):148-152.

   Patients, practices, and implant usage in primary THA patients were compared in 159,695 Swedish, 279,693 Australian, and 69,641 United States Registry cases. Cemented fixation predominated in Sweden, noncemented in the United States and Australia. Sweden's 5-year (97.8%) and 10-year survival (95.8%) was higher than those of the United States (97.0% and 95.2%) and Australia (96.3% and 93.5%), with differences in patient characteristics, surgical technique, and implant choice. Level of evidence: III.

6. Pedersen AB, Mehnert F, Havelin LI, et al: Association between fixation technique and revision risk in total hip arthroplasty patients younger than 55 years of age. Results from the Nordic Arthroplasty Register Association. *Osteoarthritis Cartilage* 2014;22(5):659-667.

7. Troelsen A, Malchau E, Sillesen N, Malchau H: A review of current fixation use and registry outcomes in total hip arthroplasty: The uncemented paradox. *Clin Orthop Relat Res* 2013;471(7):2052-2059.

8. Mäkelä KT, Matilainen M, Pulkkinen P, et al: Failure rate of cemented and uncemented total hip arthroplasty: A register study of combined Nordic database of four nations. *Br Med J* 2014;348:f7592.

9. Tanzer M, Graves SE, Peng A, Shimmin AJ: Is cemented or noncemented femoral stem fixation more durable in patients older than 75 years of age? A comparison of the best-performing stems. *Clin Orthop Relat Res* 2018;476(7):1428-1437.

   The outcome of the three most successful cemented and noncemented stems used in patients older than 75 years in the Australian Registry were compared. This included assessing rates of early and late revision for both osteoarthritis and hip fracture patients and by sex. Cemented stems demonstrated superior results in both sexes and for both diagnoses. The difference was most marked in females and after hip fracture. The difference was due to an increased incidence of early failure, predominantly periprosthetic fracture and loosening in the first 3 months, after which time no further increase in difference occurred. Level of evidence: III.

10. Thien TM, Chatziagorou G, Garellick G, et al: Periprosthetic femoral fracture within two years after total hip replacement: Analysis of 437,629 operations in the Nordic Arthroplasty Register Association database. *J Bone Joint Surg Am* 2014;96(19):e167.

11. Meding JB, Ritter MA, Davis KE, Hillery M: Cemented and uncemented total hip arthroplasty using the same femoral component. *Hip Int* 2016;26(1):62-66.

12. Kim YH, Park JW, Kim JS, Kim IW: Twenty-five- to twenty-seven-year results of a cemented vs a cementless stem in the same patients younger than 50 years of age. *J Arthroplasty* 2016;31(3):662-667.

13. Kazi HA, Whitehouse SL, Howell JR, Timperley AJ: Not all cemented hips are the same: A register-based (NJR) comparison of taper slip and composite beam stems. *Acta Orthop* 2019;90(3):214-219.

Section 3: Hip

A total of 292,987 arthroplasties from the National Joint Registry from England and Wales were analyzed. Composite beam stems had a higher rate or revision (1.7% versus 1.3%), and this difference was more pronounced when comparing the most commonly implanted designs of stem. Level of evidence: III.

14. Hoskins W, van Bavel D, Lorimer M, de Steiger RN: Polished cemented femoral stems have a lower rate of revision than matt finished cemented stems in total hip arthroplasty: An analysis of 96,315 cemented femoral stems. *J Arthroplasty* 2018;33(5):1472-1476.

    This study compared the outcomes of matt and polished cemented stems from 96,315 in the Australian Joint Registry. Revision at 14 years was less common with polished (3.6%) than matt (4.9%) stems. Aseptic loosening was the main reason for the difference. Level of evidence: III.

15. Junnila M, Laaksonen I, Eskelinen A, et al: Implant survival of the most common cemented total hip devices from the Nordic Arthroplasty Register Association database. *Acta Orthop* 2016;87(6):546-553.

16. Orthopaedic Data Evaluation Panel (ODEP). Available at: www.odep.org.uk.

17. Getting It Right First Time: *Orthopaedic Surgery*. Available at: www. gettingitrightfirsttime.co.uk/surgical-specialty/orthopaedic-surgery/. Accessed October 15, 2019.

18. Kristensen TB, Dybvik E, Furnes O, Engesæter LB, Gjertsen JE: More reoperations for periprosthetic fracture after cemented hemiarthroplasty with polished taper-slip stems than after anatomical and straight stems in the treatment of hip fractures: A study from the Norwegian Hip Fracture Register 2005 to 2016. *Bone Joint J* 2018;100-B(12):1565-1571.

    The incidence and indication for revision surgery in 20,532 primary cemented bipolar hemiarthroplasties in patients older than 70 years were analyzed. The overall incidence of periprosthetic fractures with these cemented stems was low at 0.2%, with 48 periprosthetic fractures identified over an 11-year period. These were seen more commonly with polished tapered stem designs with the relative risk with the six different stems in the study ranging from 0.09 to 3.19. Level of evidence: III.

19. Australian Orthopaedic Association National Joint Replacement Registry: *Partial Hip Arthroplasty. Supplementary Report*. Available at: www.aoanjrr.sahmri.com/annual-reports-2019. Accessed October 15, 2019.

    This report includes a comparison of revision rates for noncemented and noncemented hemiarthroplasty that identifies periprosthetic fracture as the main cause for the increase in failure seen with noncemented implants.

20. Garland A, Gordon M, Garellick G, et al: Risk of early mortality after cemented compared with cementless total hip arthroplasty: A nationwide matched cohort study. *Bone Joint J* 2017:99-B(1):37-43.

    This is a large registry study of almost 180,000 patients in Sweden, which showed a 5 in 10,000 (0.05%) increase in mortality in the early postoperative period that was then reversed at 14 days and beyond. Level of evidence: III.

21. Association of Anaesthetists of Great Britain and Ireland, British Orthopaedic Association, British Geriatric Society: Safety guideline: Reducing the risk from cemented hemiarthroplasty for hip fracture 2015. *Anaesthesia* 2015;70:623-626.

22. Australian Orthopaedic Association National Joint Replacement Registry: *Cement in Hip and Knee Arthroplasty. Supplementary Report*. Available at: www.aoanjrr.sahmri.com/annual-reports-2019. Accessed October 15, 2019.

    This is a review of the use of bone cement in hip and knee arthroplasty in Australia, including a comparison of THA revision rates with antibiotic loaded and plain cements. This demonstrates approximately 10% reduction in long-term revision rates with the use of antibiotic loaded cement at 10 years (6.3% versus 5.7%).

23. Halai M, Gupta S, Gilmour A, et al: The Exeter technique can lead to a lower incidence of leg-length discrepancy after total hip arthroplasty. *Bone Joint J* 2015;97-B(2):154-159.

24. Graves SE, de Steiger R, Davidson D, et al: The use of femoral stems with exchangeable necks in primary total hip arthroplasty increase the rate of revision. *Bone Joint J* 2017;99-B(6):766-773.

    This paper from the Australian Joint Registry reported on 9,289 femoral stems with exchangeable necks compared with 253,165 fixed-neck prostheses inserted for osteoarthritis between 1999 and 2014. Exchangeable-neck prostheses had a higher revision rate, and this was particularly significant for prostheses with a titanium stem and cobalt-chromium neck (relative risk 1.83 $P < 0.001$). Their continued use is questioned. Level of evidence: III.

25. Sandiford NA, Jameson SS, Wilson MJ, et al: Cement-in-cement femoral component revision in the multiply revised total hip arthroplasty: Results with a minimum follow-up of five years. *Bone Joint J* 2017;99-B(2):199-203.

    This study reports the minimum 5-year results (5 to 20 years) of 24 cases where cement-in-cement femoral revision had been done on at least two occasions in the same hip (in six cases on three occasions, in one, four). Stem survival was 91.7% at 10 years, despite the repeated cement-in-cement procedures—highlighting both the durability of the technique and the modularity at the stem-cement interface. Level of evidence: IV.

26. Berry DJ, Harmsen WS, Cabanela ME, Morrey BF: Twenty-five-year survivorship of two thousand consecutive primary Charnley total hip replacements: Factors affecting survivorship of acetabular and femoral components. *J Bone Joint Surg Am* 2002;84-A(2):171-177.

27. de Steiger R, Lorimer M, Graves SE: Cross linked polyethylene for total hip arthroplasty markedly reduces revision surgery at 16 years. *J Bone Joint Surg Am* 2018;100(15):1281-1288.

    This study from the Australian Joint Registry compared revision rates of 41,171 THAs using conventional polyethylene with 199,131 using XLPE at up to 16 years. XLPE was associated with a lower revision rate by 6 months and this difference increased with time. By 16 years, it was 11.1% for CPE versus 6.2% for XLPE (hazard ratio at 9 years 3.02). This benefit was seen regardless of the method of fixation—noncemented, cemented, or hybrid. Level of evidence: III.

28. Tan TL, LeDuff MJ, Ebramzadeh E, Bhaurla SK, Amstutz HC: Long-term outcomes of liner cementation into a stable retained shell: A concise follow up of a previous report. *J Bone Joint Surg Am* 2015;97(11):920-924.

29. Kavcic G, Mirt P, Bedencic K: Good mid-term clinical results of a cemented dual-mobility cup: A single-centre experience. *Hip Int* 2018;28(1):59-62.

At primary THA, 188 cemented dual mobility cups were inserted. At a mean follow-up of 7.7 years (5 to 10) there were no dislocations, no revisions, and no radiologically loose cups. Level of evidence: IV.

30. Neil Wheelton A, Myatt D, Helm AT: Outcome for cemented dual mobility cups to treat recurrent instability; A UK case series. *J Orthop* 2019;16(3):220-223.

Fifty-four revision THAs using a cemented dual mobility cup, of which 20 were cement-in-cement revisions were reviewed at short-term follow-up (6 months to 5 years, mean 1.9 years). There were no cases of further instability, no cups were radiologically loose, and one case was revised for infection. Level of evidence: IV.

31. Moreta J, Uriate I, Foruria X, Urra I, Aguirre U, Martinez-deLos Mozoz JL: Cementation of a dual-mobility cup into a well fixed cementless shell in patients with high risk of dislocation undergoing revision total hip arthroplasty. *Hip Int* 2019:1120700019873617. [Epub ahead of print].

Ten cases where a dual mobility cup had been cemented into a well fixed cementless shell at the time of revision THA were reviewed at a mean of 3.5 years. There was one case of postoperative dislocation (10%). No intraprosthetic dissociation, loosening of the cementless shell or at the cup-shell interface was seen. Level of evidence: VI.

32. Jobory A, Karrholm J, Overgaard S, et al: Reduced revision risk for dual mobility cup in total hip replacement due to hip fracture: A matched-pair analysis of 9,040 cases from the Nordic Arthroplasty Register Association (NARA). *J Bone Joint Surg Am* 2019;101(14):1278-1285.

In the NARA database, 4,520 hips with a DMC were matched with 4,520 controls. The dual mobility cups had a reduced overall risk of revision with an adjusted hazard ratio of 0.75 and a reduced risk of revision for dislocation (adjusted hazard ratio 0.45) in particular. Level of evidence: III.

33. Gill K, Wilson MJ, Whitehouse SL, Timperley AJ: Results using Trabecular Metal™ augments in combination with acetabular impaction bone grafting in deficient acetabula. *Hip Int* 2013;23(6):522-528.

34. Gehrke T, Bangert Y, Schwantes B, Gebauer M, Kendoff D: Acetabular revision in THA using tantalum augments combined with impaction bone grafting. *Hip Int* 2013;23(4):359-365.

35. Mahmoud AN, Sundberg M, Flivik G: Comparable results with porous metal augments in combination with either cemented or uncemented cups in revision hip arthroplasty: An analysis of one hundred and forty-seven revisions at a mean of five years. *J Arthroplasty* 2017;32(5):1612-1617.

One hundred four cemented and 43 noncemented acetabular revisions with metal augments were reviewed at a mean of 60 months (13 to 112). At latest review three (2.8%) cemented and two (4.6%) noncemented wedges showed features of aseptic loosening with no difference in clinical or radiological outcomes. Level of evidence: IV.

36. Fawcitt CG, Thom HHZ, Hunt LP, et al: Choice of prosthetic implant combinations in total hip replacement: Cost effectiveness analysis using UK and Swedish Hip Joint Registries data. *Value Health* 2019;22(3):303-312.

A Markov model was used to compare the cost effectiveness of a variety of methods of fixation and bearing type against small-headed cemented metal-on-polyethylene implants. Data for over 1 million patients were analysed, including probability of revision and quality adjusted life years. Small-headed metal on polyethylene was found to be the most cost effective overall, with a minor advantage seen with ceramic on polyethylene in patients younger than 65 years. No benefit to noncemented, hybrid, or reverse hybrid fixation was seen. Level of evidence: III.

37. Pennington M, Grieve R, Sekhon JS, Gregg P, Black N, van der Meulen JH: Cemented, cementless and hybrid prostheses for total hip replacement: Cost effectiveness analysis. *Br Med J* 2013;346:f1026.

38. Hanly RJ, Whitehouse SL, Lorimer MF, et al: The outcome of cemented acetabular components in total hip arthroplasty for osteoarthritis defines a proficiency threshold: Results of 22,956 cases from the Australian Orthopaedic Association National Joint Replacement Registry. *J Arthroplasty* 2019;34(8):1711-1717.

The authors looked at the relationship between number of cases performed per annum (10 or less, 11 to 25 or over 25 cases) and revision in a series of 22,956 cemented cups in the Australian Orthopaedic Association National Joint Replacement Registry. Overall survivorship was excellent and improved with volume, over 25 being best and with even a minimum of 10 cases conferring a revision benefit. Level of evidence: III.

CHAPTER 32

Primary Total Hip Arthroplasty—Noncemented

AHMED SIDDIQI, MD, MBA • AMAR S. RANAWAT, MD

ABSTRACT

The results of total hip arthroplasty continue to improve over time, and with careful study of implant performance, more data are available to help guide decision making. Noncemented stem fixation has become more common and proved to have superior results in many patient populations. However, noncemented stem length has recently been debated, and the optimal length for a noncemented stem is unclear given that some short-stemmed designs are associated with excellent results. On the acetabular side, modular noncemented cups are used most frequently with excellent reported results. Although a metal or ceramic femoral head articulating with a highly cross-linked polyethylene liner seems to perform best in most situations, the ideal femoral head size is still unclear and a topic of controversy. Larger femoral head sizes have been associated with a lower risk of dislocation and are used far more commonly in contemporary practice; however, they have their own risks and potential complications.

Keywords: acetabular implant; femoral head size; femoral stems; noncemented THA; primary total hip arthroplasty

Dr. Siddiqi or an immediate family member serves as a paid consultant to or is an employee of Zimmer; serves as an unpaid consultant to AZ Solutions, LLC; and has stock or stock options held in ROM Tech. Dr. Ranawat or an immediate family member has received royalties from DePuy, A Johnson & Johnson Company and Stryker; is a member of a speakers' bureau or has made paid presentations on behalf of ConvaTec, DePuy, A Johnson & Johnson Company, Mako, and Stryker; serves as a paid consultant to or is an employee of Arthrex, Inc., Ceramtec, and DePuy, A Johnson & Johnson Company; has stock or stock options held in ConforMIS and Strathspey Crown; has received research or institutional support from Ceramtec, DePuy, A Johnson & Johnson Company, and Stryker; has received non-income support (such as equipment or services), commercially derived honoraria, or other non–research-related funding (such as paid travel) from DePuy, A Johnson & Johnson Company and Stryker; and serves as a board member, owner, officer, or committee member of the American Association of Hip and Knee Surgeons, the American Academy of Orthopaedic Surgeons, EOA, the Hip Society, and the Knee Society.

INTRODUCTION

Total hip arthroplasty (THA) continues to be one of the most successful and commonly performed surgical procedures in North America. Although there has been an overall convergence of surgical designs and techniques, some controversies still exist. Further advancements, particularly in bearing materials, have improved outcomes and a better understanding of their performance will help surgeons make appropriate choices for their patients.

FEMORAL IMPLANT SELECTION AND RESULTS

The femoral implant of a THA must effectively restore the biomechanics of the proximal femur and hip joint and achieve and maintain durable fixation to the proximal femur. Both cemented and noncemented femoral implants have demonstrated the capability to achieve reliable and durable fixation. However, results vary considerably according to implant design. In North America,

This chapter is adapted from Della Valle CJ, Berry DJ, Bragdon CR, et al: Primary total hip arthroplasty, in Mont MA, Tanzer M, eds: *Orthopaedic Knowledge Update®: Hip and Knee Reconstruction*, ed 5. Rosemont, IL, American Academy of Orthopaedic Surgeons, 2017, pp 377-391.

noncemented femoral fixation is used in most patients, whereas cemented femoral fixation remains common in the United Kingdom and in some Scandinavian countries.

Data from several sources suggest noncemented THA is outperforming cemented and hybrid THA in younger patients, but most data suggest cemented implants have the lowest revision rate in older patients.[1] Joint registries provide some of the best high-level information on factors that influence performance of different implant categories in different circumstances.[2-4] Information from the Australian registry demonstrates that at 10 to 14 years postoperatively, noncemented THA outperforms cemented and hybrid THA in patients aged 64 years and younger. However, information from the Australian, United Kingdom, and Scandinavian registries demonstrate that cemented THA has a lower revision rate than noncemented THA in older patients.

The results of using various femoral implant categories are discussed in the following sections. Although series with level IV evidence are valuable, they are subject to potential selection and publication bias, with perhaps the most successful results being most likely to be reported. Therefore, cross-referencing case series data with large national registry data is important to gain the most comprehensive understanding of the performance of each implant category. It is also important to be aware that each implant category may have unique advantages and disadvantages. For example, some prostheses may be easier to implant with certain surgical approaches, but they may have lower overall long-term fixation rates. Some implants may be associated with higher intraoperative and early postoperative periprosthetic fracture rates, or a different pattern of long-term periprosthetic bone remodeling (stress shielding), or a different degree of thigh pain.

BASIC SCIENCE OF NONCEMENTED FIXATION

Osseointegration is the attachment of bone to metal implants without intervening fibrous tissue.[5] Retrieval analysis studies have shown that osseointegration generally occurs 4 to 12 weeks after implant placement, but may continue up to 3 years postoperatively.[6-8] Biomechanical studies have shown that micromotion of >150 µm leads to fibrous union, between 40 and 150 µm leads to a combination of osseous and fibrous formation, and micromotion <20 µm primarily results in bone formation and ingrowth.[8-10] Excessive micromotion inhibits noncemented implant bony integration, because it is based on new bone ingrowth and ongrowth.[11] Bone growing inside a porous surface is termed ingrowth and bone growing onto a roughened surface is termed ongrowth, which is determined by implant surface characteristics.[11] Therefore, adequate bony contact and firm implant fixation is essential during noncemented THA implantation to minimize micromotion. Initial fixation is generally obtained by press-fitting a slightly oversized implant into the acetabulum and femur.

Standard-Length Noncemented Stems

Standard-length noncemented femoral stems are the most commonly used femoral implants in North America and globally. This preference is attributable to favorable short-term and long-term clinical results with a high rate of implant fixation, ease and consistency of insertion, and broad applicability to most femoral geometries. Standard-length noncemented stems provide early and long-term fixation over a relatively broad surface area, thereby distributing stress and avoiding extreme stress concentration. The stem length also helps the surgeon to attain consistent alignment in the femoral canal, which creates predictable hip biomechanics.

Several different categories of noncemented standard-length femoral implants are in common use. Based on geometry, these include double-tapered stems, single-tapered (blade-shaped) stems, extensively porous-coated stems, and anatomic stems. These stem designs all are engineered to gain initial stability by interference press fit and long-term stability through osseointegration via bone ingrowth or ongrowth to different surface finishes or coatings (including porous coatings, plasma spray, surface roughening with grit blasting, and hydroxyapatite coatings). Early implant stability, which is key to osseointegration and long-term fixation, depends on optimal implant sizing and geometry to achieve stable fixation.

Numerous standard-length noncemented stems from each of the main categories previously listed have shown high rates of fixation and good clinical success in many case series as well as in registry studies. Several combinations of noncemented stems and cups listed in the 2018 Australian registry (which has the most robust data on noncemented implants) report demonstrate cumulative rates of revision at 17 years of less than 10%.[12] Several case series have explored the long-term results of standard-length noncemented implants at 15 to 25 years after surgery.[13,14] These case series demonstrate that the long-term loosening rate of standard-length noncemented stems can be low. Randomized head-to-head comparison of femoral implants from different implant geometry categories is uncommon, and registry data are subject to selection bias, making absolute comparison of results within this general implant category challenging. One study showed tapered wedge femoral stems to have greater axial stability and decreased subsidence in patients who have increasing body mass index compared with traditional fit-and-fill stem design.[15] For implants offered in versions with porous coating or hydroxyapatite coating, clinical series comparing the two surface finishes (including randomized trials) have shown equivalent fixation rates and clinical outcomes.[16]

Standard-length noncemented stems load the femur differently than do short stems or cemented stems, with consequent effects on bone remodeling, which also differs with each stem category.[17] With the exception of extensively porous-coated stems, which exhibit more pronounced bone remodeling changes in some patients, modest bone remodeling changes have not been shown to have notable clinical consequences.

Short Noncemented Stems

Shorter noncemented stems for primary THA has drawn increasing interest, especially with minimally invasive surgery. Optimal femoral stem length for noncemented primary THA has not been determined, and different stem lengths are available. Shorter stem lengths are attractive, because they are less invasive of the femur and require less surgical exposure. Seldom discussed is the ease of revising a shorter stem if it becomes necessary. A shorter stem, in theory, will promote more proximal femoral loading, which may prevent stress shielding from more distal stem fixation. The concern, however, is that the shorter length may be less stable, resulting in a higher rate of failure of osseointegration.

There are two general types of short stems: ultrashort stems, which are placed in the femoral neck and upper metaphysis and are usually less than 90 mm long, and the more common metaphyseal filling short stem, which does not engage the actual diaphysis and varies from 90 to 140 mm in length, which increases proportionally to the size of the stem. Various stem geometries are available, with new and unique designs; other, shorter stem alternatives have been previously available as a longer stem.

As with any other noncemented stem, initial stable fixation must be achieved for osseointegration to occur. This requires sufficient fill of the canal and, ideally, a neutral or valgus stem position, which requires line-to-line fill on the AP radiograph and three-point fixation on the lateral projection. It is important to consider that a shorter stem is less forgiving than a longer stem. Hence, until the surgeon has adequate experience with a shorter stem, an intraoperative radiograph may help ensure that the planned endosteal positioning of the stem has been achieved. For maximal contact of the porous coating on the proximal metaphyseal bone, metaphyseal fill is more important than distal fill. Potting the tip of the stem without proximal fill may result in failure of fixation.

One study reported experience with two different titanium flat-tapered stems, including 849 longer stems (135 to 170 mm) and 902 shorter stems (97.5 to 132.0 mm). At a mean follow-up of 36 months (range, 6 to 88 months), stem survivorship was not significantly different (99% in both groups).[18] Another study compared an ultrashort and a standard stem using dual-energy x-ray absorptiometry at 2 years postoperatively. The results showed reduced bone loss with the short stem in all zones but indicated an especially remarkable difference in zone 1. There was more subsidence of the short stem at 6 weeks, but at 2 years, the clinical outcome was not significantly different.[19] Another study compared a short stem and standard stem in a prospective randomized double-blind study, with 40 hips in each group.[20] Group comparison at 6 weeks showed no difference in clinical scores, Harris hip score, Medical Outcomes Study 36-Item Short Form score, or Western Ontario and McMaster Universities Arthritis Index. Radiographic comparison showed no difference in the restoration of the femoral offset between the two stem groups.

A 2015 bench study with 16 synthetic bones and two sets of matched cadaver femurs assessed the effect of femoral stem length on the torsional resistance to periprosthetic fracture.[21] The specimens were mounted and rapidly rotated to simulate stumbling. Custom three-dimensional cutting guides were created to ensure the accuracy of the placement of the stem. For both models, the shorter stems failed at a significantly higher torque, and the researchers concluded that shorter stems may allow more femoral flexibility and confer a higher resistance to periprosthetic fracture.

Quantifying ease of implant placement is difficult because of varying surgical skill sets. A study compared a series of shorter stems (389 hips) to standard-length wedge-fit stems (269 hips), all placed through an anterolateral approach. A reduced number of intraoperative complications (trochanteric and femoral shaft fractures) was reported with the shorter stem than with the longer stem (0.4% and 3.1%, respectively). No difference was noted in survival or clinical scores at a mean follow-up of 29.2 months.[22]

Reports on shorter femoral stems in the literature have been encouraging; shorter stems compare favorably with standard-length stems for clinical outcomes and anatomic hip restoration. Bone density studies have shown a smaller reduction in bone loss from stress shielding. Importantly, short-stem revision allows for less complex revision surgery. Finally, the stems may be ideal for patients who have certain bony morphologies (such as a narrow diaphysis or an exaggerated bow) that would be hard to fit with a longer stem.

Modular Stems

Restoration of the hip center is crucial for restoring native hip biomechanics following primary THA, which is beneficial for both functional performance and longevity of the implant. In addition to modular femoral heads, several implant systems have incorporated a second modular junction to allow surgeons to independently adjust femoral anteversion, lateral offset, and limb length, along with fit and fill of the proximal or distal femur. These implants provide the surgeon with intraoperative flexibility to accommodate variation among patients' native anatomy and manage complex proximal femoral deformities. Furthermore, these modular features offer the potential advantages of reduced neck-cup impingement, more precise limb length and hip biomechanics restoration, and enhanced fixation in cases of femoral anatomic variances.

All dual-modular stems are not the same, however. Most dual- modular stems used in primary THA have a proximal modular connection, either at the neck-stem junction or within the metaphyseal region of the proximal femur. Modularity at the neck-stem junction is generally proximal to the femoral neck osteotomy and, therefore, unsupported by host bone. This results in different physiologic loads placed on the taper, whereas in other proximal modular stems, the junction lies below the neck osteotomy and within the metaphyseal region of the femur.

Despite theoretical concerns of fretting and junctional failure, long-term clinical results of a metaphyseal modular femoral implant, with a clinical history of more than 30 years of use in the United States, have shown low rates of aseptic loosening or failure at 15 to 20 years.[23] A modular femoral stem has proved particularly useful in complex primary THA in the setting of severe dysplasia in which a concurrent femoral shortening osteotomy is required at the time of THA (**Figure 1**).

In July 2012, an orthopaedic company issued a voluntary recall of its modular neck femoral implants because of higher-than-expected early revision rates for excessive fretting and corrosion at the modular junction resulting in adverse local tissue reactions (ALTRs) and osteolysis. This company's design used a mixed-alloy couple in which the neck was cobalt chromium and the stem was titanium alloy. Some studies have shown that mixed-alloy couples can produce more corrosion and fretting than a single-alloy interface and can be susceptible to galvanic corrosion. A series of 123 of these stems (97 of which were the modular version) reported elevated serum metal levels in 48% of the modular group and a 28% revision rate at a mean follow-up of 2.7 years.[24] Diagnosis of an ALTR associated with a modular stem is generally made by measurement of serum cobalt and chromium levels combined with cross-sectional imaging in the form of ultrasonography or metal artifact reduction sequence MRI. Treatment includes revision surgery with removal of the femoral implant.

Another dual-modular femoral implant with neck-stem modularity has been designed to offer a wide variety of head center options with a variable titanium alloy neck that mates with a titanium stem via a modular taper. Although early reports noted more accurate restoration of the hip center, more recent reports have questioned the clinical significance of these findings. One study reported results from 284 patients who underwent THA with a nonmodular neck and 594 patients in whom a modular

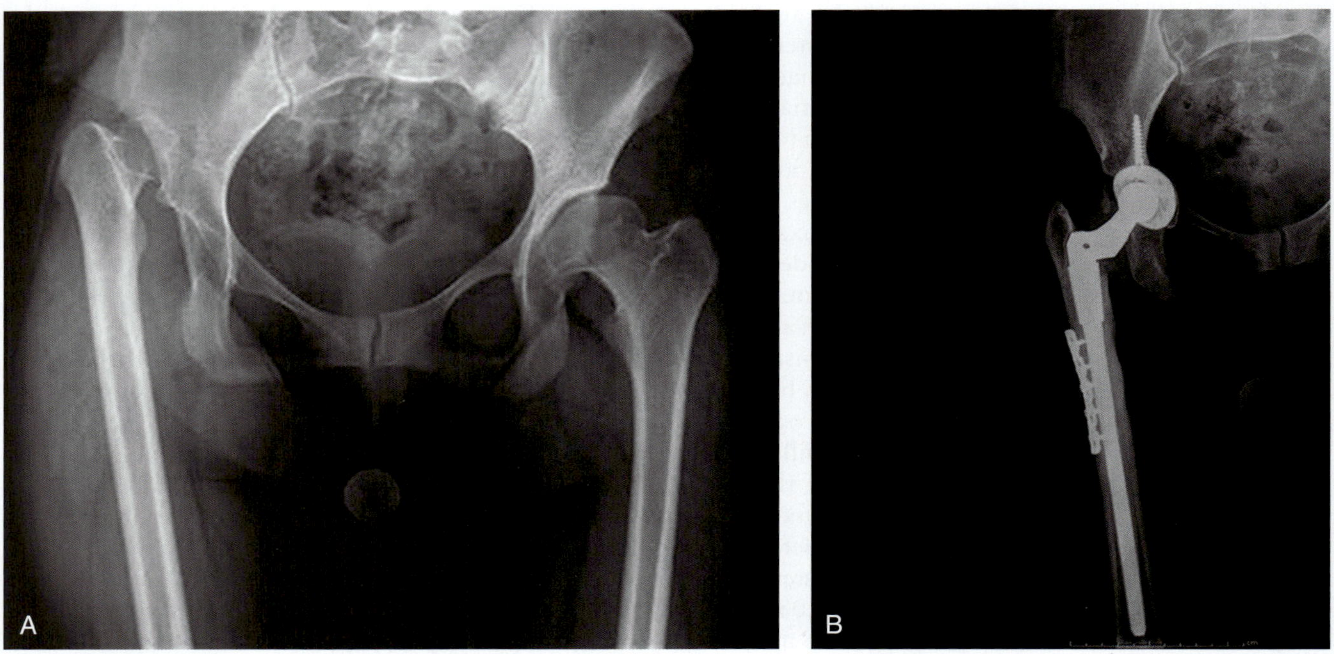

FIGURE 1 AP pelvic radiographs of a patient with developmental dislocation of the hip (Crowe stage 4). **A**, Preoperative view. **B**, View obtained 5 years following total hip arthroplasty with a dual-modular femoral implant.

neck femoral implant was used.[25] Patients in whom the modular femoral implant had been implanted demonstrated a higher percentage of equal radiographic limb lengths and offset restoration, although these results did not translate to differences in clinical outcome scores at 2-year follow-up. No reduction in the incidence of complications or reoperations was observed with modular necks, leading to questioning the use of dual modularity in routine primary THA. However, similar to the 2012 recall, in May 2015 there was a class 1 voluntary recall on this system for increasing reports of corrosion and ALTR.[26,27]

Although corrosive wear appears to be more significant with cobalt-chromium modular necks, resulting in metal ion release and ALTR, titanium modular necks are not without their own unique set of problems. Most reports of fatigue fracture of dual-modular femoral stems have occurred with implants that use a titanium alloy coupling. Titanium alloy implants are also more susceptible to cold welding, which may complicate revision surgery and necessitate complete removal of a well-fixed stem in circumstances in which simple modular head-neck exchange would suffice.

Modular femoral implants offer the surgeon excellent intraoperative flexibility to adjust anteversion, offset, and limb lengths, with the goal of restoring the native hip center in primary THA. Modularity also allows accommodation of complex proximal femoral deformities, especially in the setting of developmental dysplasia of the hip or other proximal femoral deformities. Although some dual-modular devices maintain a strong clinical history of success, recent device recalls secondary to taper corrosion and early breakage have reduced surgeon preferences for dual-modular implants.

ACETABULAR IMPLANT SELECTION AND RESULTS

Whereas THA in North America was initially performed with a cemented, all-polyethylene acetabular implant, most surgeons quickly migrated to use of noncemented acetabular implants in the mid-1980s to late 1980s, given the ease of insertion and the perceived benefits of modularity. Long-term studies have since shown noncemented acetabular cups with survivorship exceeding 90% with aseptic loosening as an end point.[28] However, wear was a problem, and near the year 2000, three options were available to decrease wear-related complications: highly cross-linked polyethylene, ceramic-on-ceramic bearings, and metal-on-metal bearings.

Most large databases support highly cross-linked polyethylene as the preferred option for most patients, given the low wear rates, low risk of complications and subsequent revision, and lower cost when compared with the alternative choices. Although a metal femoral head has traditionally been used as the primary bearing on highly cross-linked polyethylene, ceramic heads have become more common in the past 7 years because of the lower risk of head-neck corrosion, improvements in material strength (which have lowered the risk of head breakage), and a theoretical lower wear rate.[29,30] Demonstrating a lower wear rate, however, has been challenging given the already low wear rates observed with highly cross-linked polyethylene, and demonstrating a clinical benefit in a lower risk of revision has yet to be proved. Ceramic heads remain substantially more costly than their metal counterparts, and in most health models, cost is still an important factor. A recent Markov model study determined that the ability to regain the initial increased expenditure of ceramic heads through a diminished lifetime revision cost burden is dependent on the price differential between ceramic and metal femoral heads and the age of the patient.[30] The cost of ceramic femoral heads continues to decrease among most vendors with its increased widespread use.

Although fixation and wear-related complications appear to have been reduced over time, dislocation continues to be among the most common complications and causes of revisions following THA in North America. In response to the lower wear observed with highly cross-linked polyethylene, many surgeons have started using larger femoral heads. One randomized trial that compared a 36-mm head with a 28-mm femoral head showed a significant reduction in risk.[31] Dual mobility has also become an option that may be appropriate for patients known to be at high risk for instability;[32] however, concerns persist regarding these novel constructs, and more experience is necessary to ensure that the risks of wear and intraprosthetic dislocation have been reduced in comparison with those of earlier designs.

Press-fit Modular Implant With and Without Screws

In contemporary practice, a modular, noncemented acetabular implant is most commonly used (**Figure 2**). Contraindications to use are rare; however, severe osteoporosis that cannot mechanically support a noncemented cup while ingrowth occurs and radiation necrosis of the pelvis are the two most common. Radiation necrosis of the pelvis can be recognized by a chalky appearance of the retroacetabular bone when reamed, indicating avascularity that will not support osseointegration. In these cases, cemented acetabular implants do not perform much better than noncemented ones, and a mechanical construct, such as a reconstruction cage with multiple screws, can be used.

Although several different noncemented designs were produced in the late 1980s and early 1990s, a convergence

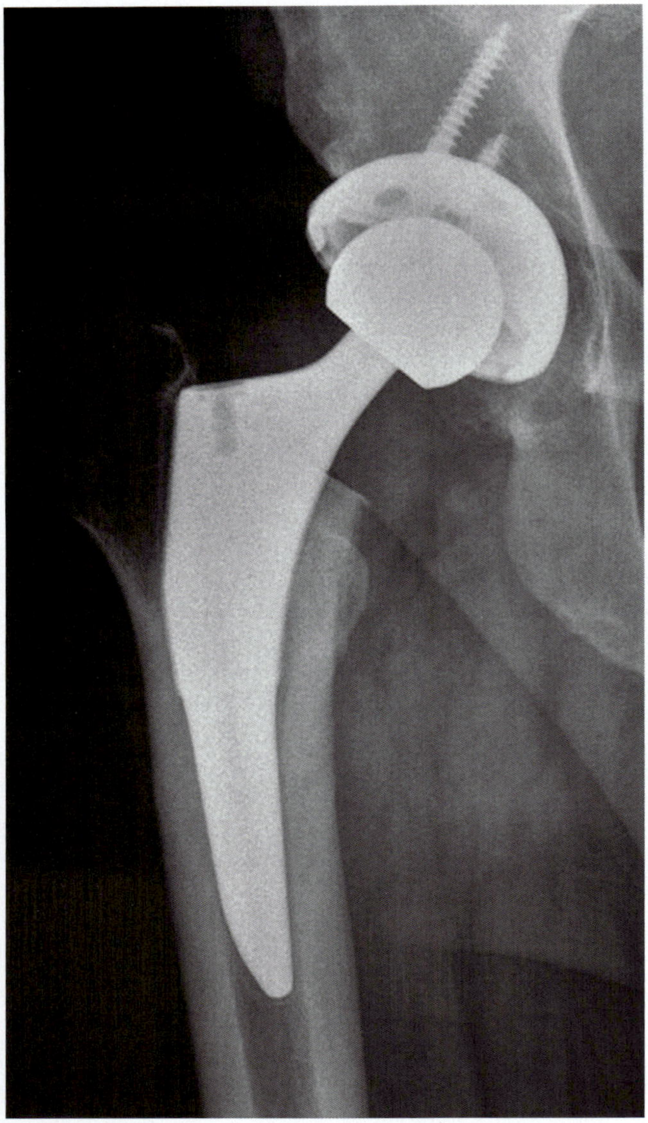

FIGURE 2 AP radiograph obtained following primary total hip arthroplasty performed with a noncemented modular cup with screws and a noncemented stem.

of designs has occurred, and most contemporary implants use a porous titanium surface. Given the high rates of successful osseointegration with these implants, surface coatings such as hydroxyapatite are rarely used because of the cost. Coatings are now primarily reserved for specialized implants, such as monoblock dual-mobility and resurfacing cups; in these cases, the ingrowth surface consists of cobalt-chromium alloy (which has been shown to be inferior to titanium as an ingrowth surface) and the addition of hydroxyapatite may be important to ensure that osseointegration occurs.

Noncemented acetabular cups with varying sizes have all shown to have similar outcomes. One recent study looking at the outcomes of a cohort of patients of short stature (145.0 ± 6.9 cm) compared with a matched cohort of patients of average stature (163.1 ± 8.0 cm) found that the short stature group with smaller cup sizes (50.5 ± 3.50 mm) had outcomes similar to those of individuals of average stature with a greater mean cup size (51.32 ± 2.64 mm) without any risk of higher dislocation.[33] Likewise, studies reporting larger acetabular cups (≥62 mm) also show negligent rates of dislocation with improved functional outcomes.[34-36] However, most of the large-diameter cup studies are based on metal-on-metal bearing surfaces and the results may not be extrapolated to current metal-on-polyethylene or ceramic-on-polyethylene THA.

Although the use of screws has been controversial, with the advent of contemporary bearing surfaces (such as highly cross-linked polyethylene), osteolysis appears to be rare, so concerns about screws and screw holes as access pathways for particulate debris are probably no longer relevant. Screws provide the mechanical stability that is critical for bone ingrowth, and if the surgeon has any doubt regarding the initial mechanical stability of the cup, screws should be used, if not used routinely. The screw holes also allow the surgeon to visualize the floor of the acetabulum, providing confirmation of full implant seating. Similarly, although modularity has been identified to contribute to backside wear of the modular liner among the first iterations of noncemented acetabular implants, lessons learned from these earlier generation implants have resulted in more robust locking mechanisms in contemporary designs. The benefits of modularity are thought by most surgeons to outweigh the potential concerns of the past.

The most important part of the surgical technique for noncemented acetabular reconstruction is adequate exposure; if the femur is not adequately mobilized, and if the field of view is not clear, the accuracy of implantation will be compromised. The amount of underreaming performed is based on surgeon preference; other variables include whether screws will be used, surface roughness and stiffness of the implant, and the differential between the labeled and true size of the implant to be inserted. The true size of the implant is an important variable; the consistent use of one implant is probably beneficial because it results in surgeon comfort with the amount of underreaming that is required to safely insert the cup while obtaining an adequate press fit. With most designs, a 1-mm underream is adequate, although line-to-line reaming may certainly be acceptable (particularly if screws are used for adjunctive fixation), depending on the surface roughness of the implant and the size of the cup inserted. Specifically, in a smaller diameter acetabulum in a female patient, even a 1-mm underream may result in a pelvic fracture during insertion, whereas a large male patient with a much larger diameter acetabulum may easily tolerate 2 mm of underreaming.

Positioning of the acetabular implant is one of the most challenging and difficult problems in contemporary practice. Recent studies have shown a large number of cups placed outside of the safe zone, even by experienced surgeons,[37] whereas other studies have challenged the idea of a safe zone, showing that many hips that subsequently dislocate are within acceptable parameters.[38] Hence, challenges exist both in achieving what is considered an ideal target and in understanding what the ideal target should be (and whether that target is different depending on individual patient anatomic considerations). A 2015 study has also highlighted the complex interplay between the spine and the pelvis, suggesting that these relationships may change over time.[39] Given the importance of cup positioning on the risk of instability and complications related to bearing surface wear, more work is needed in this area.

Monoblock Implants

The predominant failure mode of noncemented acetabular implant fixation has traditionally been osteolysis produced by a biologic reaction to particulate debris. Both metallic and polyethylene wear debris have been implicated as stimuli for an inflammatory response resulting in osteolysis and resorption of bone at the prosthetic interfaces. Although polyethylene debris is generated primarily at the bearing surface, wear can occur secondary to motion at the interface between the liner and the metallic shell. Fretting of screws used for adjunctive fixation can occur, resulting in debris generation. Finally, the locking mechanism itself can potentially produce particulate debris if a ring-type configuration is used.

In the late 1990s, noncemented monoblock acetabular implants were introduced as an alternative to combat these issues. Monoblock cups consist of nonmodular acetabular implants in which the liner is compression-molded directly into the metallic shell framework, eliminating the locking mechanism and dome screw holes and associated concerns with backside wear and access channels for wear debris. The polyethylene thickness also tends to be greater for the same cup diameter and femoral head sizes. Monoblock cups tend to be more difficult to implant because the acetabular floor cannot be visualized through screw holes in the surface of the shell at the time of implantation. Additionally, if revision is necessary for acetabular wear or dislocation, the liner alone cannot be exchanged, and full cup revision is necessary.

The cumulative 10- to 15-year survival rates of several designs of monoblock cups, considering revision for cup loosening as the end point, all are excellent. A 2015 randomized controlled trial reporting the 12-year results of 113 patients receiving either a tantalum monoblock or a porous-coated titanium monoblock cup showed survivorship of 100% in the porous tantalum group, although one cup was revised for aseptic loosening at 12 years after implantation in the porous-coated titanium group; significantly fewer radiolucencies were found in the porous tantalum group.[40]

Highly Porous Cups for Primary and Revision THA

Third-generation highly porous titanium and tantalum surfaces have been developed to further improve osseointegration and longevity (**Figure 3**). These surfaces are rougher, providing greater initial press-fit fixation and stability, and allow greater amounts of bone ingrowth because they are more porous.[41] The generally greater flexibility may reduce the risk of stress shielding while also allowing greater degrees of osseointegration. A 2015 randomized trial suggested improved fixation when highly porous cups were compared with a standard porous-coated titanium cup.[40]

Although highly porous metal acetabular implants have demonstrated excellent durability and clinical results in primary THA, the revision setting represents the greatest opportunity for enhanced fixation surfaces to have a substantial clinical effect because of the frequency with which bone loss and poor bone quality are encountered. In a large clinical database review of 3,448 revision THA procedures with a noncemented acetabular implant, the overall survival rate at 15 years was

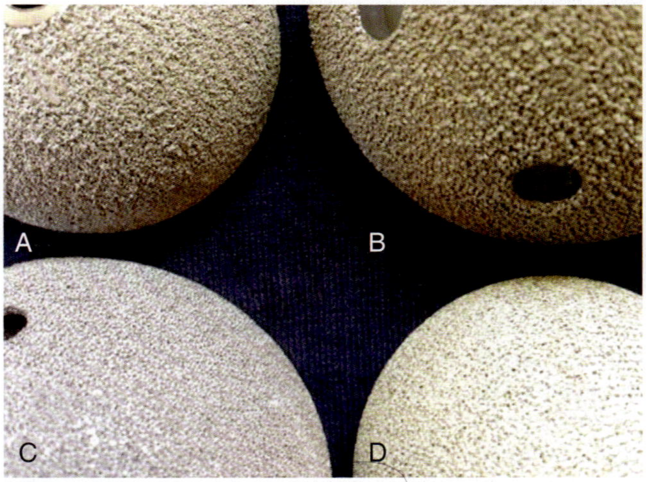

FIGURE 3 Photograph demonstrates four acetabular implants of various highly porous metal fixation surfaces. **A**, P^5 highly porous titanium (DJO Surgical). **B**, Tritanium highly porous revision cup (Stryker). **C**, Tritanium highly porous titanium primary cup (Stryker). **D**, Trabecular Metal highly porous tantalum revision cup (Zimmer Biomet). (Reprinted with permission from Zielinski M, Deckard ER, Meneghini RM. The Fate of Zone 2 Radiolucencies in Contemporary Highly-Porous Acetabular Components: Not All Designs Perform Equally. Presented on Friday, November 3, 2017 at the AAHKS Annual Meeting. https://aahks.scientificposters.com/epsAbstractAAHKS.cfm?id=2)

Section 3: Hip

only 69%.[42] Compared with titanium wire mesh designs, cup revision for aseptic loosening was significantly more common with beaded designs, but less common with highly porous tantalum designs. Similarly, in a 2-year retrospective clinical follow-up of 599 porous tantalum acetabular implants used in the revision setting, no cups were revised for aseptic loosening.[43] These implants can also be combined with highly porous-coated augments, and their use in contemporary practice has superseded the use of structural grafts and reconstruction cages in most centers. There is an exception for the most complex cases, for which the use of combining porous-coated cups and cages has been advocated. Cost, however, is greater with these implants, and further studies will be required to determine in which scenarios the increased costs associated with these highly porous implants are justified.

FEMORAL HEAD SIZE

Early debate concerning the optimal head size in THA focused on those between 22 and 32 mm. This was based on the low frictional torque associated with small femoral heads (ie, frictional torque is related to the radius squared) and the large contact area; hence, low contact stress was associated with large femoral heads (stress = force/area). A classic study showed higher linear wear associated with 22-mm heads and high volumetric wear associated with 32-mm heads.[44] This resulted in 28-mm heads as the most common choice in the 1980 and 1990s. In the 1990s, long-term wear studies demonstrated lower linear and volumetric wear with 22-mm heads. The explanation for the reduction of wear with smaller head sizes was related to the decrease in sliding distance during gait. All of these studies were performed on polyethylene that had been gamma irradiated in air.

In the late 1990s, moderately and highly cross-linked polyethylene became available. With time, cross-linked polyethylene was shown to provide a fivefold to tenfold improvement in wear resistance when compared with polyethylene sterilized by gamma radiation in air. Because dislocation has been recognized as a leading cause of failure, larger femoral heads have been preferred given their association with an increased head-to-neck ratio, an increased primary arc range of motion before implant-to-implant impingement, and an increased jump distance, all of which result in greater THA stability. A randomized trial in patients undergoing primary THA performed via a posterior approach compared 28- and 36-mm femoral heads (on highly cross-linked polyethylene) and showed a significant decrease (five times lower) in incidence of dislocation within the first year after primary THA.[31] A similar benefit has been found with patients undergoing THA with an anterolateral approach and using larger head sizes (36 mm or larger); a lower dislocation rate was reported than for those with heads less than 36 mm in diameter.[45] Finally, in a study of 501 patients undergoing primary THA, all of whom were considered to be at high risk for dislocation, 282 of the patients given 36-mm femoral heads were compared with 219 patients who have anatomic femoral heads larger than 36 mm; a significant difference in dislocation rate was observed between the two groups favoring the anatomic femoral heads (4.6% and 0.5%, respectively).[32]

Larger femoral head size increases range of motion by increasing the primary arc range as well as the jump distance, resulting in greater range of motion before neck-cup impingement occurs. Although an increase in impingement-free range of motion following THA is theoretically advantageous, an improvement in functional outcome through the use of larger heads has limited support in the literature. A prospective study of 726 THAs, investigating functional outcomes at 6 and 12 months postoperatively as measured by the Oxford hip score, Western Ontario and McMaster Universities Arthritis Index, High-Activity Arthroplasty Score, and University of California Los Angeles activity score, compared femoral head size groups: smaller than 36 mm, 36 mm, and larger than 36 mm. Although a significant increase was seen in the High-Activity Arthroplasty Score 3 (overall), University of California Los Angeles, and Western Ontario and McMaster Universities Arthritis Index scores between groups who have the large and smaller heads at 6 months, there was no statistically significant difference seen in any of the functional outcome measures at 12 months. A decrease in dislocation rate was seen in the group with femoral heads 36 mm or larger.[46]

However, concerns exist about larger femoral heads, including the requirement for thinner polyethylene, especially peripherally, at the capturing mechanism of modular acetabular shells. This is especially concerning with highly cross-linked polyethylene, which has decreased strength and decreased fatigue properties related to the cross-linking process. Cups that are positioned vertically, which can increase contact stresses, may be at highest risk for liner fracture. Although rim fractures have been reported with highly cross-linked polyethylene, these reports are rare.

An additional concern is the increased forces at the head-neck junction caused by use of larger heads that may result in a greater risk of corrosion at the modular head-neck junction. One experimental study on biomechanics has demonstrated increased frictional torque with a larger metal head and with a metal head articulating with vitamin E, compared with highly cross-linked polyethylene. This could result in increased stresses at the modular head-neck junction[47] and a concomitant increase in the risk of corrosion that could result in ALTR.[48]

The development and use of highly cross-linked polyethylene liners in THA has resulted in significantly lower long-term wear rates when compared with conventional (ultra-high–molecular-weight) polyethylene. This has allowed for use of larger femoral head sizes, which appear to reduce the risk of dislocation, with wear rates reduced to what is believed to be the threshold for the development of clinically relevant osteolysis. However, a 2016 long-term follow-up study of highly cross-linked polyethylene has demonstrated some osteolysis at 10 to 14 years in 14% of hips and median volumetric wear rates of 3.1, 12.3, 12.9, and 26.1 mm^3/yr with head sizes of 26, 28, 32, and 36 to 40 mm, respectively.[49] A 2018 Nordic Arthroplasty Registry study found no benefits with the use of 36 mm heads over 32 mm, because the transition from 32 to 36 mm was associated with a higher risk of all-cause revision that was not accompanied by a decrease in risk of revision resulting from instability.[50] Given these concerns, a 32-mm head is favored by many surgeons for the patient who is at low risk for dislocation, whereas other surgeons routinely use the largest size femoral head that can be accommodated by the system that they use.

SUMMARY

Improvements in both materials and design continue to improve the durability of noncemented THA. As instability remains among the most common modes of failure for THA, increased interest has been shown in both the routine use of larger femoral head sizes as well as dual-mobility bearings; however, both concepts require further evaluation to ensure durability over the longer term. The continued careful evaluation of implant performance over time will yield even greater clarity on the optimal techniques for optimizing outcomes following THA.

KEY STUDY POINTS

- Contemporary modular noncemented cups and noncemented femoral fixation have proved viable long-term longevity, especially in younger individuals.
- Highly porous metals have the advantages of greater surface roughness, increased porosity, and a modulus of elasticity more similar to that of bone; however, concise advantages over standard titanium ingrowth surfaces have been difficult to demonstrate.
- Highly cross-linked bearings have allowed for the safe use of larger femoral head sizes that have been shown to reduce the risk of dislocation, although concerns remain regarding longer term performance.

ANNOTATED REFERENCES

1. McMinn DJ, Snell KI, Daniel J, Treacy RB, Pynsent PB, Riley RD: Mortality and implant revision rates of hip arthroplasty in patients with osteoarthritis: Registry based cohort study. *Br Med J* 2012;344:e3319.
2. Pedersen AB, Mehnert F, Havelin LI, et al: Association between fixation technique and revision risk in total hip arthroplasty patients younger than 55 years of age. Results from the Nordic Arthroplasty Register Association. *Osteoarthritis Cartilage* 2014;22(5):659-667.
3. Stea S, Comfort T, Sedrakyan A, et al: Multinational comprehensive evaluation of the fixation method used in hip replacement: Interaction with age in context. *J Bone Joint Surg Am* 2014;96(suppl 1):42-51.
4. Wechter J, Comfort TK, Tatman P, Mehle S, Gioe TJ: Improved survival of uncemented versus cemented femoral stems in patients aged <70 years in a community total joint registry. *Clin Orthop Relat Res* 2013;471(11):3588-3595.
5. Albrektsson T, Brånemark PI, Hansson HA, Lindström J: Osseointegrated titanium implants. Requirements for ensuring a long-lasting, direct bone-to-implant anchorage in man. *Acta Orthop Scand* 1981;52(2):155-170.
6. Galante J, Rostoker W, Lueck R, Ray RD: Sintered fiber metal composites as a basis for attachment of implants to bone. *J Bone Joint Surg Am* 1971;53(1):101-114.
7. Zweymüller KA, Lintner FK, Semlitsch MF: Biologic fixation of a press-fit titanium hip joint endoprosthesis. *Clin Orthop Relat Res* 1988;235:195-206.
8. Khanuja HS, Vakil JJ, Goddard MS, Mont MA: Cementless femoral fixation in total hip arthroplasty. *J Bone Joint Surg Am* 2011;93(5):500-509.
9. Engh CA, O'Connor D, Jasty M, Mcgovern TF, Bobyn JD, Harris WH: Quantification of implant micromotion, strain shielding, and bone resorption with porous-coated anatomic medullary locking femoral prostheses. *Clin Orthop Relat Res* 1992;285:13-29.
10. Pilliar RM, Lee JM, Maniatopoulos C: Observations on the effect of movement on bone ingrowth into porous-surfaced implants. *Clin Orthop Relat Res* 1986;208:108-113.
11. Karuppal R: Biological fixation of total hip arthroplasty: Facts and factors. *J Orthop* 2016;13(3):190-192.
12. Australian Orthopaedic Association National Joint Replacement Registry: *Hip, Knee & Shoulder Arthroplasty–Annual Report 2018*. Adelaide, South Australia, Australian Orthopaedic Association, 2018.
13. Capello WN, D'Antonio JA, Jaffe WL, Geesink RG, Manley MT, Feinberg JR: Hydroxyapatite-coated femoral components: 15-year minimum followup. *Clin Orthop Relat Res* 2006;453:75-80.
14. Loughead JM, O'Connor PA, Charron K, Rorabeck CH, Bourne RB: Twenty-three-year outcome of the porous coated anatomic total hip replacement: A concise follow-up of a previous report. *J Bone Joint Surg Am* 2012;94(2):151-155.

15. Grant TW, Lovro LR, Licini DJ, Warth LC, Ziemba-davis M, Meneghini RM: Cementless tapered wedge femoral stems decrease subsidence in obese patients compared to traditional fit-and-fill stems. *J Arthroplasty* 2017;32(3):891-897.

An anatomically designed morphometric tapered wedge femoral stem demonstrated greater axial stability and decreased subsidence with increasing body mass index than a traditional fit-and-fill stem. The resistance to subsidence, irrespective of body mass index, is likely due to the inherent axial stability of a tapered wedge design and may be the optimal stem design for obese patients. Level of evidence: III.

16. Parvizi J, Sharkey PF, Hozack WJ, Orzoco F, Bissett GA, Rothman RH: Prospective matched-pair analysis of hydroxyapatite-coated and uncoated femoral stems in total hip arthroplasty. A concise follow-up of a previous report. *J Bone Joint Surg Am* 2004;86-A(4):783-786.

17. Petis SM, Howard JL, McAuley JP, Somerville L, McCalden RW, MacDonald SJ: Comparing the long-term results of two uncemented femoral stems for total hip arthroplasty. *J Arthroplasty* 2015;30(5):781-785.

18. Barrington JW, Emerson RH Jr: The short and "shorter" of it: >1750 tapered titanium stems at 6- to 88-month follow-up. *J Arthroplasty* 2013;28(8 suppl):38-40.

19. Salemyr M, Muren O, Ahl T, et al: Lower periprosthetic bone loss and good fixation of an ultra-short stem compared to a conventional stem in uncemented total hip arthroplasty. *Acta Orthop* 2015;86(6):659-666.

20. von Roth P, Perka C, Mayr HO, et al: Reproducibility of femoral offset following short stem and straight stem total hip arthroplasty. *Orthopedics* 2014;37(7):e678-e684.

21. Jones C, Aqil A, Clarke S, Cobb JP: Short uncemented stems allow greater femoral flexibility and may reduce periprosthetic fracture risk: A dry bone and cadaveric study. *J Orthop Traumatol* 2015;16(3):229-235.

22. Molli RG, Lombardi AV Jr, Berend KR, Adams JB, Sneller MA: A short tapered stem reduces intraoperative complications in primary total hip arthroplasty. *Clin Orthop Relat Res* 2012;470(2):450-461.

23. Le D, Smith K, Tanzer D, Tanzer M: Modular femoral sleeve and stem implant provides long-term total hip survivorship. *Clin Orthop Relat Res* 2011;469(2):508-513.

24. Meftah M, Haleem AM, Burn MB, Smith KM, Incavo SJ: Early corrosion-related failure of the rejuvenate modular total hip replacement. *J Bone Joint Surg Am* 2014;96(6):481-487.

25. Duwelius PJ, Burkhart B, Carnahan C, et al: Modular versus nonmodular neck femoral implants in primary total hip arthroplasty: Which is better? *Clin Orthop Relat Res* 2014;472(4):1240-1245.

26. Canham CD, Muradov PI, Simpson JB, Incavo SJ: Corrosion and adverse local tissue reaction after total hip arthroplasty with a modular titanium alloy femoral neck. *Arthroplast Today* 2017;3(4):211-214.

ALTR associated with crevice corrosion has involved only modular junctions in which at least one of the two members is fabricated from a cobalt-chromium alloy. Titanium fretting corrosion has been demonstrated in retrieval studies of failed bimodular stems with titanium necks, and elevated serum titanium levels have been found in patients with titanium femoral stems. Level of evidence: V.

27. Shah R, Talmo C, Nandi S: Titanium neck-titanium stem taper corrosion in a modular neck stem. *Arthroplast Today* 2019;5(2):145-147.

Close surveillance for ALTR should be considered in patients with the Zimmer M/L Taper Kinectiv Technology System, particularly in those with a cobalt alloy head. Surgeons should be cautious with regard to the use of modular neck stems due to the risk of mechanically assisted crevice corrosion and ALTR. Level of evidence: V.

28. Long WJ, Nayyar S, Chen KK, Novikov D, Davidovitch RI, Vigdorchik JM: Early aseptic loosening of the Tritanium primary acetabular component with screw fixation. *Arthroplast Today* 2018;4(2):169-174.

Multiple studies and joint registries have reported on outcomes of THA using a wide range of implants. These sources have documented survival rates that exceed 90% at a 10-year follow-up and approach 85% at a 15-year follow-up in patients undergoing THA using a noncemented acetabular implant with supplementary screw fixation. Level of evidence: V.

29. American Joint Replacement Registry: *Fifth AJRR Annual Report on Hip and Knee Arthroplasty Data 2018*. Chicago, IL, American Joint Replacement Registry, 2018.

30. Carnes KJ, Odum SM, Troyer JL, Fehring TK: Cost analysis of ceramic heads in primary total hip arthroplasty. *J Bone Joint Surg Am* 2016;98(21):1794-1800.

31. Howie DW, Holubowycz OT, Middleton R, Large Articulation Study Group: Large femoral heads decrease the incidence of dislocation after total hip arthroplasty: A randomized controlled trial. *J Bone Joint Surg Am* 2012;94(12):1095-1102.

32. Haughom BD, Plummer DR, Moric M, Della Valle CJ: Is there a benefit to head size greater than 36 mm in total hip arthroplasty? *J Arthroplasty* 2016;31(1):152-155.

33. Anis HK, Mcconaghy KM, Charles RJ, et al: Perioperative outcomes and complications after primary total hip arthroplasty in patients with disproportionately short stature: A matched cohort analysis. *J Arthroplasty* 2020;35(3):801-804.

Patients with disproportionately short stature had longer surgical times and slight longer lengths of stay. However, complication and readmission rates were similar. Level of evidence: III.

34. Saragaglia D, Belvisi B, Rubens-Duval B, Pailhé R, Rouchy RC, Mader R: Clinical and radiological outcomes with the Durom™ acetabular cup for large-diameter total hip arthroplasty: 177 implants after a mean of 80 months. *Orthop Traumatol Surg Res* 2015;101(4):437-441.

35. Naal FD, Kain MS, Hersche O, Munzinger U, Leunig M: Does hip resurfacing require larger acetabular cups than conventional THA? *Clin Orthop Relat Res* 2009;467(4):923-928.

36. Schmidutz F, Fottner A, Wanke-Jellinek L, Steinbrück A, Jansson V, Mazzochian F: Hip resurfacing requires larger acetabular cups than conventional hip replacement: A comparative analysis of 100 hips, based on radiographic templating. *Acta Orthop Belg* 2012;78(4):484-491.

37. Callanan MC, Jarrett B, Bragdon CR, et al: The John Charnley Award: Risk factors for cup malpositioning. Quality improvement through a joint registry at a tertiary hospital. *Clin Orthop Relat Res* 2011;469(2):319-329.
38. Abdel MP, von Roth P, Jennings MT, Hanssen AD, Pagnano MW: What safe zone? The vast majority of dislocated THAs are within the Lewinnek safe zone for acetabular component position. *Clin Orthop Relat Res* 2016;474(2):386-391.
39. Buckland AJ, Vigdorchik J, Schwab FJ, et al: Acetabular anteversion changes due to spinal deformity correction: Bridging the gap between hip and spine surgeons. *J Bone Joint Surg Am* 2015;97(23):1913-1320.
40. Wegrzyn J, Kaufman KR, Hanssen AD, Lewallen DG: Performance of porous tantalum vs. titanium cup in total hip arthroplasty: Randomized trial with minimum 10-year follow-up. *J Arthroplasty* 2015;30(6):1008-1013.
41. Meneghini RM, Meyer C, Buckley CA, Hanssen AD, Lewallen DG: Mechanical stability of novel highly porous metal acetabular components in revision total hip arthroplasty. *J Arthroplasty* 2010;25(3):337-341.
42. Kremers HM, Howard JL, Loechler Y, et al: Comparative long-term survivorship of uncemented acetabular components in revision total hip arthroplasty. *J Bone Joint Surg Am* 2012;94(12):e82.
43. Long WJ, Noiseux NO, Mabry TM, Hanssen AD, Lewallen DG: Uncemented porous tantalum acetabular components: Early follow-up and failures in 599 revision rotal hip arthroplasties. *Iowa Orthop J* 2015;35:108-113.
44. Livermore J, Ilstrup D, Morrey B: Effect of femoral head size on wear of the polyethylene acetabular component. *J Bone Joint Surg Am* 1990;72(4):518-528.
45. Stroh DA, Issa K, Johnson AJ, Delanois RE, Mont MA: Reduced dislocation rates and excellent functional outcomes with large-diameter femoral heads. *J Arthroplasty* 2013;28(8):1415-1420.
46. Allen CL, Hooper GJ, Frampton CM: Do larger femoral heads improve the functional outcome in total hip arthroplasty? *J Arthroplasty* 2014;29(2):401-404.
47. Meneghini RM, Lovro LR, Wallace JM, Ziemba-Davis M: Large metal heads and vitamin E polyethylene increase frictional torque in total hip arthroplasty. *J Arthroplasty* 2016;31(3):710-714.
48. Plummer DR, Berger RA, Paprosky WG, Sporer SM, Jacobs JJ, Della Valle CJ: Diagnosis and management of adverse local tissue reactions secondary to corrosion at the head-neck junction in patients with metal on polyethylene bearings. *J Arthroplasty* 2016;31(1):264-268.
49. Lachiewicz PF, Soileau ES, Martell JM: Wear and osteolysis of highly crosslinked polyethylene at 10 to 14 years: The effect of femoral head size. *Clin Orthop Relat Res* 2016;474(2):365-371.
50. Tsikandylakis G, Kärrholm J, Hailer NP, et al: No increase in survival for 36-mm versus 32-mm femoral heads in metal-on-polyethylene THA: A registry study. *Clin Orthop Relat Res* 2018;476(12):2367-2378.

    There were no benefits with the use of 36-mm heads over 32 mm, because the transition from 32 to 36 mm was associated with a higher risk of revision for all reasons, which was not accompanied by a decrease in the risk of revision resulting from dislocation. The use of 32-mm heads appears to offer the best compromise between joint stability and other reasons for revision in metal-on-polyethylene THA. Further studies with longer follow-up, especially of 36-mm heads, as well as better balance of confounders across head sizes and better control of patient-related risk factors for THA revision are needed. Level of evidence: III.

CHAPTER 33

Primary Total Hip Arthroplasty in Challenging Conditions

ELIZABETH B. GAUSDEN, MD, MPH • ROBERT T. TROUSDALE, MD

ABSTRACT

Challenging conditions in the context of total hip arthroplasty are those in which the likelihood of intraoperative technical difficulties, perioperative complications, or premature failure is more likely than usual. Such conditions can be of congenital, genetic, metabolic, endocrine, neurologic, or traumatic origin. Success in managing these conditions requires a thorough understanding of the underlying condition and its implications relevant to total hip arthroplasty. All such conditions require careful preoperative planning, adequate exposure, and familiarity with a variety of adjunctive techniques such as corrective osteotomy, the use of structural allografts, and trochanteric osteotomy. The surgeon must also be familiar with a variety of different femoral and acetabular components including modular stems; bipolar, dual-mobility, and constrained acetabular components; and, occasionally, custom implants. A team approach to assist in the management of the medical comorbidities associated with certain of these conditions may enhance patient care and reduce complications.

Dr. Trousdale or an immediate family member has received royalties from DePuy, A Johnson & Johnson Company; serves as a paid consultant to or is an employee of DePuy, A Johnson & Johnson Company; and serves as a board member, owner, officer, or committee member of the American Association of Hip and Knee Surgeons, the Hip Society, and the Knee Society. Neither Dr. Gausden nor any immediate family member has received anything of value from or has stock or stock options held in a commercial company or institution related directly or indirectly to the subject of this chapter.

Keywords: developmental dysplasia; metabolic bone disease; posttraumatic osteoarthritis; protrusion; spinal fusion

INTRODUCTION

Various difficult, but not necessarily uncommon, conditions result in a challenging primary total hip arthroplasty (THA). The difficulties may involve the femoral and/or the acetabular sides of the hip joint. It is important to be knowledgeable about the general principles and outcomes of these techniques.

DEVELOPMENTAL DYSPLASIA OF THE HIP

Background

Primary THA for management of developmental dysplasia of the hip (DDH) presents unique challenges on both the acetabular and femoral sides. An understanding of the bony and soft-tissue deformities that occur in dysplasia is crucial for the success of the THA and to minimize the risk of complications. The techniques and outcomes of primary THA for dysplasia depend on the severity of DDH. Recent techniques of acetabular and femoral

This chapter is adapted from Glassman AH, Tanzer M, Iorio R, Dundon JM, Sayeed Y, Bostrom M PG, Ries MD, Trousdale RT, Desy NM: *Primary Total Hip Arthroplasty in Challenging Conditions* in Mont MA and Tanzer M, eds. *Orthopaedic Knowledge Update®: Hip and Knee Reconstruction 5*. Rosemont, IL, American Academy of Orthopaedic Surgeons, 2017, pp 393-422.

reconstruction have yielded significant improvements in clinical outcomes with survivorship rates similar to those of THA for osteoarthritis.

Acetabulum

Changes in the acetabular anatomy range from mild dysplasia to subluxation and complete dislocation of the hip. The reconstructive techniques and outcomes are dependent on the severity of these changes.

The acetabulum in DDH has a shallow articular cavity, increased anteversion, insufficient acetabular coverage of the femoral head, and a deficient anterior wall.[1,2] In the case of a low hip dislocation, there is a false acetabulum that partially covers the true acetabulum and the femoral head is typically contained within the false acetabulum. The acetabulum usually has an anterior segmental defect or a posterior wall deficiency, is oval shaped, and has increased anteversion.[1,2] In the case of a high hip dislocation, the femoral head migrates posterosuperiorly and the acetabulum is narrow, shallow, and triangular in shape; the iliac wing is also anteverted and the entire rim of the acetabulum may be deficient.[1-3] Implanting an acetabular implant in patients who have DDH can be challenging because the anatomic landmarks are difficult to identify and the bony anatomy can be severely compromised. As a result, careful preoperative templating is imperative to characterize the patient's individual anatomy and available bone stock. Doing so will minimize the risk of the acetabular implant malposition and unplanned medial wall penetration. Three-dimensional imaging may be helpful to assess version of the acetabulum as well as bony deficiencies in these cases.[3,4] Ideally, the acetabular implant should be placed close to the teardrop, in the true acetabulum, as a platform for the restoration of hip offset and restoration of hip biomechanics. However, depending on the age of the patient and the anatomy, acetabular implant positioning may be modified to provide sufficient acetabular implant coverage.[5]

The typical acetabular reconstructive technique includes several steps.[2,5] The center of rotation should be restored as close as possible to the native hip center. Identifying the native hip center can be challenging, because the cotyloid fossa is commonly covered by soft tissue and contractures can make identifying landmarks difficult.[2] Cementless components should be used, whereby the anterior-posterior dimension of the native acetabulum dictates the size of the cup. In cases of subluxation, slight medialization of the hip center of rotation can be used to avoid the use of a bulk autograft for reconstruction. In cases of low hip dislocation, socket uncoverage (generally >50%) usually requires augmentation with a femoral head autograft (**Figure 1**). In cases of high dislocation, a small cementless acetabular implant (average outside diameter 38 to 44 mm) is placed in the native acetabulum. A femoral head autograft is not required because complete host-bone coverage is usually obtained from the anterior and posterior walls of the true acetabulum. Finally, the acetabular implant should be anteverted based on the combined orientation of both the acetabular and femoral implant to maximize stability and range of motion (ROM).

Acetabular reconstruction with restoration of the hip center is biomechanically advantageous and has yielded good results clinically. The results of 50 Crowe type III and IV hips with mean 6.4-year follow-up (range, 2.2 to 11.5 years) using cementless cups placed in the anatomic position were reported in a 2012 study.[6] No hip had any adjuvant lateral bone graft. At final follow-up, the Harris hip score increased

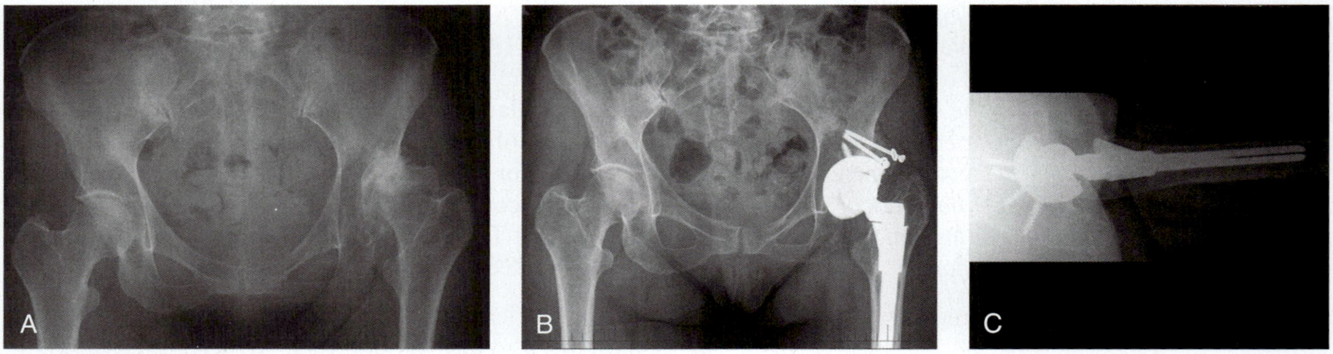

FIGURE 1 **A**, Preoperative AP pelvis radiograph from a 48-year-old woman who has developmental dysplasia of the hip demonstrating severe arthritis of the left hip with superior subluxation of the femoral head. **B**, AP pelvis radiograph 4 year following total hip arthroplasty with a cementless acetabular implant fixed with screws, a bulk femoral head autograft to the pelvis, and a modular femoral stem. **C**, Lateral radiograph of the hip demonstrating that the modular femoral stem is retroverted, relative to the anatomically placed proximal sleeve, to correct the excessive femoral anteversion.

from 40 preoperatively to 86 ($P = 0.03$) and no cups were revised. One study reported the outcome of 52 hips with DDH with 30% to 50% lateral uncoverage of cementless acetabular components at the time of THA.[7] The uncovered portion above the component was reconstructed by filling with particulate bone autograft. At a mean of 4.8 years (range, 3 to 7 years), there were no loose or revised cups. Based on these findings, it was proposed that a cup that has initial stability and up to 17 mm of lateral uncoverage, supplemented with particulate bone grafting, would have an acceptable outcome.

In cases of acetabular deficiency that result in component uncoverage greater than 50%, superolateral bulk autogenous grafting or porous metal augments should be considered. A recent study of 102 THAs in dysplastic hips using bulk bone grafting reported successful bone remodeling without loosening in 101 of 102 cases at 3 year follow-up.[8] However, another study of 115 DDH cases reported a rapid increase in failure rate of this technique at 15 years, bringing into question the long-term results.[9] The overall rate of revision for aseptic loosening was 16%.

It may not always be feasible to re-create the anatomic hip center at the time of THA because of excessive acetabular deficiencies. An alternative technique to obtain acetabular bony coverage is to use a high hip center with superior placement of the cup. The influence of a high hip center on hip abductor strength and the presence of a Trendelenburg sign in patients who have DDH was assessed in a 2015 study.[10] As long as the femoral implant restored the femoral offset and the abductor lever arm, a high center of hip rotation (up to approximately 30 mm from the interteardrop line) resulted in only 10% of the patients who have DDH having a Trendelenburg sign. However, a higher loosening and revision rate of both the femoral and acetabular components has been reported in DDH when a cemented acetabular cup is placed superior and/or lateral to the anatomic position.[9] It would therefore seem prudent to reserve this technique for the elderly patient in whom an anatomic position would leave more than 40% to 50% of the socket surface uncovered or covered by bone graft.[5] If a high hip center is required for reconstruction, it is important to avoid lateral placement of the cup. One study showed no acetabular loosening at 10-year follow-up in their series of 30 cementless cups when the cup is placed at least 20 mm superior, but not lateral to the anatomic hip center.[11]

Femur

In DDH, the femur has a shorter neck, increased anteversion, a smaller canal width, thinner cortices, a straight contour, and the anterior bow of the femur displaced further distally with increasing degrees of dysplasia. The femoral implant and reconstruction technique must take into account these anatomic changes in the femur. Additionally, it must be determined whether femoral shortening will be required if the prosthetic hip center is placed in the anatomic position. Both cemented and cementless stems have been successfully used in DDH. Modular stems, narrow diaphyseal-fixed cone-type tapered stems, and narrow cemented stems are most commonly used to allow correction of the excessive femoral anteversion and to reconcile the metaphyeal-diaphyseal size mismatch seen in DDH (**Figure 1**). Femoral shortening with a subtrochanteric femoral shortening osteotomy and implantation of a cementless stem is most commonly performed in Crowe IV hips to prevent overlengthening of the leg when the hip is brought down to the anatomic hip center. This technique requires that the femur is reamed or broached before the osteotomy. Next, a transverse osteotomy is created in the subtrochanteric region, and a trial component is inserted into the proximal fragment. The hip is reduced, and the amount of femoral shortening necessary is determined intraoperatively by overlapping the two fragments. A second cut is made, removing the overlapping proximal portion of the distal femur. The tip of the trial component is then inserted and reduced into the distal fragment while adjusting for anteversion. The goal of the osteotomy is to avoid overlengthening of the leg and subsequent sciatic nerve injury when the hip is reduced in the anatomic hip center. Two fixation techniques for stabilizing a transverse subtrochanteric osteotomy were compared in 79 hips.[12] Both techniques involved splitting the removed bone segment longitudinally without the removal of any soft tissue, wrapping the bone fragments around the osteotomy site. The fragments were stabilized either with a cable in one group, or with a plate and screws in the second group. Overall, fixation with a cable had an average union time of 113 days and nonunion developed in one hip, whereas the plate technique had an average union time of 152 days and nonunion developed in three hips.[13]

Insufficiency of the hip abductors is classically associated with a limb-length discrepancy in patients who have DDH because of abductor muscle contracture and disuse. Forty-five patients who have unilateral DDH were evaluated before and following their THA.[14] The greatest improvement in abductor strength was seen within the first 6 months after THA. However, in some patients who have a good reconstruction, affected hip abductor muscle strength remained poor because of severely contracted tissues and insufficient abductor strength. Abductor strength was consistently greater in patients who have mild dysplasia (Crowe I and II) than in patients who have severe dysplasia (Crowe III and IV). Overall, in patients who have DDH, the extent of preoperative limb-length discrepancy and the increase in abductor length were related to post-THA abductor strength recovery.

Excellent outcomes have been reported with varying types of femoral implants. In selected patients who have DDH, one study found that an anatomic cementless femoral stem can provide excellent long-term outcomes.[15] The Anatomic Hip (Zimmer) was used in 135 hips with good bone quality, neck-shaft angles less than 160°, femoral anteversion less than 50°, and a canal diameter 10 mm or larger. Intraoperatively, a nondisplaced metaphyseal fracture occurred in 3.7% of the cases. At a mean follow-up of 13.5 years (range, 10 to 18 years), there were no cases of aseptic loosening of the femoral implant.

A 2- to 5-year follow-up of a modular S-ROM stem (DePuy) modified for Asian patients was reported in 220 hips with DDH.[16] In 74% of the hips, the stem required rotational correction so that the version of the stem did not match the version of the femur. Overall, bone ingrowth was achieved in 99.5% of the stems. Another study reported results at a mean follow-up of 18.7 years (range, 15.8 to 21.8 years) in 25 Crowe III and IV hips, in which the S-ROM stem was used in conjunction with a low resection of the femoral neck.[17] Two patients sustained an intraoperative fracture of the calcar, which was stabilized with cerclage wires at the time of surgery. At final follow-up, the mean modified Harris hip score improved from 46 points preoperatively to 90 points ($P < 0.001$), all stems were bone ingrown, and none required revision. The mean postoperative increase in leg length was 21 mm (6 to 56 mm). No patients had a sciatic nerve injury. It was concluded that a low femoral neck osteotomy combined with a cementless, modular femoral implant and anatomic restoration of the hip center is a successful technique of THA for DDH and avoids the need for femoral shortening osteotomy.

THA Following Prior Surgery

It is not uncommon for patients who have DDH to have undergone prior surgical procedures before requiring a THA. Periacetabular osteotomy (PAO) is one of the most effective procedures for reorientation of the acetabulum in patients who have symptomatic dysplasia. When necessary, THA can be performed with reasonable safety and can be expected to result in significant improvement in functional scores in most patients who have undergone previous PAOs.[18] In a 2015 study, 23 hips of patients who underwent a THA after PAO were matched for age, sex, and body mass index with 23 patients who have DDH undergoing THA without a history of PAO.[19] At a mean follow-up of 10 ± 4 years in the osteotomy group and 6 ± 4 years in the nonosteotomy group, there was no difference in the complication or revision rates between the two groups. There was no difference in the mean postoperative Harris hip score at final follow-up between the study groups (93 ± 7 and 95 ± 10, respectively). In this study, 44% of the acetabula with a PAO were found to be retroverted. As a result, trimming of the anterior wall and/or bone grafting of a deficient posterior wall were required to place the acetabular implant in the proper position. Overall, the mean acetabular implant anteversion was decreased by 17° in the PAO group. It was concluded that THA in patients after a PAO offers major improvements in function with acceptable complication and revision rates when compared with THA for DDH in patients without a prior PAO. However, according to a post hoc power analysis, the study was underpowered to detect a difference in the rate of postoperative complications or revision THA.

Similarly, a 2015 study found that 22 patients undergoing a THA for DDH following a successful rotational acetabular osteotomy had results similar to those of 30 matched patients undergoing THA for DDH who had not undergone previous surgery.[10] At an average follow-up of 8.2 years (range, 7 to 11 years), no patient in either group required revision surgery. No significant difference in total Harris hip scores, pain scores, function scores, intraoperative blood loss, and surgical time was found between the two groups. In contrast, a 2018 case-control study compared patients undergoing THA without a prior PAO with patients who have the same Crowe classification who had not undergone prior PAO and found that the osteotomy group demonstrated significantly poorer Harris hip scores for gait and activity.[20]

Results

The results of a 2015 study highlight the potential complications that can occur when performing THA for DDH.[21] Complications developed in 25 of 102 hips (24.5%) and revision surgery was performed in 15 of these patients (14.7%). The possibility of undergoing revision surgery was 5.95 times higher in Crowe IV hips compared with Crowe type I hips. Complications included acetabular implant aseptic loosening (seven hips), dislocation (five hips), delayed union of the subtrochanteric osteotomy (three hips), femoral implant aseptic loosening (two hips), superficial wound infection (two hips), heterotopic ossification (two hips), acetabular and femoral implant loosening (one hip), iliac artery and vein rupture during acetabular cup-screw preparation (one hip), intraoperative femur fracture treated with a cerclage wire (one hip), sciatic nerve palsy that fully recovered (one hip), deep vein thrombosis (one hip), and pulmonary embolism (one hip). In the low dislocations, absence of the superior wall and anterolateral segmental deficiency made acetabular reconstruction challenging and caused the acetabular implant to be partially uncovered. This uncoverage was postulated to have led to the early failures of the acetabular components in this series.[18] In a previous study of the Norwegian Arthroplasty Register, there was no increased risk for revision following THA in patients who have DDH without dislocation (n = 2,425 hips) and patients who have osteoarthritis (n = 5,229 hips) (relative risk = 1.0) following cementless THA.[22] DDH with dislocation (n = 445 hips) had, in fact, less risk for revision than osteoarthritis (relative risk = 0.8).

A 2012 study specifically addressed the long-term results of THA with a shortening subtrochanteric osteotomy in Crowe IV DDH.[23] In all hips, a porous-coated acetabular implant with screws was placed at the true anatomic hip center. Structural femoral head autograft fixed with screws was used in 10 of the acetabular reconstructions to improve superolateral coverage of the cup. Cementless femoral components were used in all cases. A subtrochanteric osteotomy was performed in all hips, with the osteotomy site augmented with cortical autograft struts cut from the resected femoral bone fragment in 20 hips and by cortical allograft struts in 2 hips. At mean follow-up 10 years, there was a significant improvement in the Harris hip score from the preoperative value (43 versus 87). Twenty-nine percent of patients had an early complication, but these did not have long-term deleterious effects on the reconstruction, and there were no revision surgeries for any reason after 7 years. Complications included intraoperative femur fractures (four hips) and dislocations (three hips). There were two femoral nonunions of the osteotomy site (7%). At 10 years, one acetabular implant was revised for aseptic loosening and three stems were revised—two for aseptic loosening and one for fracture. Overall, the survivorship of the components free of revision for aseptic loosening was 89%, with no radiographic evidence of additional loosening. It was concluded that reliable 10-year results could be obtained with cementless THAs and simultaneous shortening subtrochanteric osteotomies in patients who have Crowe IV DDH. Similarly, a 2018 study reported the results of 26 consecutive THAs in Crowe III-IV hips without subtrochanteric osteotomies.[24] They found a mean postoperative leg-length discrepancy of 7 mm, two transient nerve palsies (one sciatic and one femoral), and six hips (23.1%) required revision. At 15 years, there was a 12.5% cumulative incidence of aseptic loosening of the femoral implant. If early complications are managed appropriately, subsequent sequelae or new problems are rare.

Despite the numerous acetabular and femoral complexities inherent to THA in patients who have DDH, a 2013 study demonstrated comparable short-term functional outcomes (Oxford Hip Score) and revision rates in 1,205 hips with DDH compared with 40,589 hips with osteoarthritis at 6 months following THA.[25] Overall, the hips with DDH required bone grafting more frequently (4% versus 0.9%; $P < 0.001$), received cementless implants more often (68.3% versus 28.1%; $P < 0.001$), and required a longer surgical time than the osteoarthritis group (mean time, 94.4 minutes versus 79.7 minutes; $P < 0.001$). Unexpectedly, this analysis of the New Zealand Registry did demonstrate a higher-than-expected 6-month mortality rate in the DDH group. In a subsequent study, registry data were presented on the functional response to THA in patients who have hip dysplasia with a minimum 1-year follow-up.[26] The 33 patients who have DDH undergoing THA reported more severe preoperative impairment of disease-specific functions (Oxford hip score and Western Ontario and McMaster Universities Osteoarthritis Index) and general health measures (Short Form-12 physical health and mental health scores) than the 968 patients who have primary osteoarthritis undergoing THA. Despite their poor preoperative function, and despite the challenges and complexities inherent to THA in hip dysplasia, the DDH patients achieved superior postoperative functional improvements compared with the osteoarthritis patients. It was concluded that patients who have DDH requiring THA could expect comparable function to those patients undergoing THA for primary osteoarthritis (**Figures 2** through **5**).

PROXIMAL FEMUR DEFORMITY AND PROXIMAL FEMUR FRACTURE

Background

Both proximal femur fracture and proximal femur deformity can be challenging in total joint arthroplasty. Proper imaging and preoperative planning help guide surgical treatment and are crucial for success. Moreover,

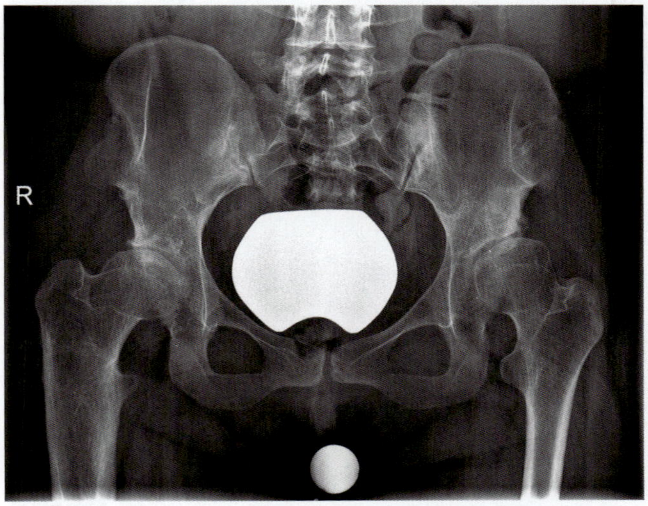

FIGURE 2 AP pelvis radiograph shows developmental dysplasia of the hip bilaterally and right proximal femoral deformity from multiple previous surgeries.

Section 3: Hip

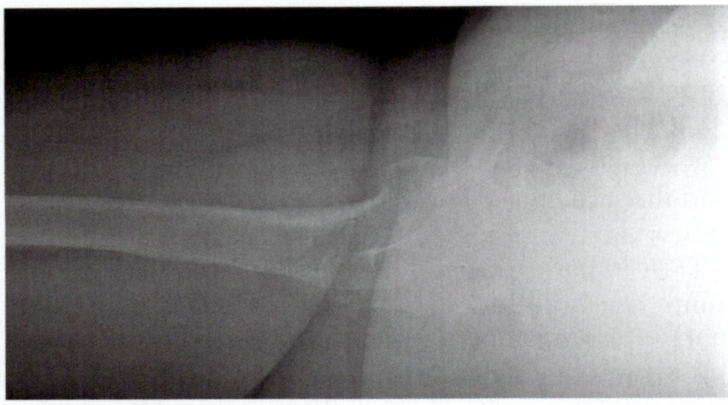

FIGURE 3 Lateral radiograph of the right hip shows developmental dysplasia of the hip bilaterally and right proximal femoral deformity from multiple previous surgeries.

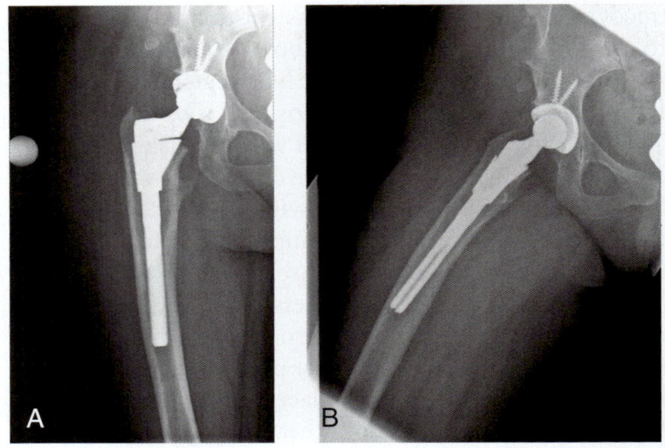

FIGURE 5 **A**, AP radiograph of right hip treated with total hip arthroplasty using a modular stem. **B**, Lateral view of the hip, postarthroplasty.

a physical examination assessing for ROM, abductor strength, and gait is necessary to verify patient status. For failed fixation for femoral neck or intertrochanteric hip fractures, retained hardware must be removed before THA is performed. DDH, Paget disease of bone, hip instability associated with Down syndrome, and achondroplasia all present unique challenges. These cases are individualized, based on the type and degree of femoral deformity. Proximally coated implants may often be used in these patients, but modular and diaphyseal fixation implants should be available for severe deformities. If direct access to the femoral canal is not obtainable, extended trochanteric or diaphyseal osteotomy should be considered to obtain appropriate fixation. As a group, these patients are more technically challenging and have higher complications rates than patients who have uncomplicated osteoarthritis. With thoughtful and carefully planned management, patients who have proximal femur fracture and proximal femur deformity should realize significant pain relief and improved function following THA.

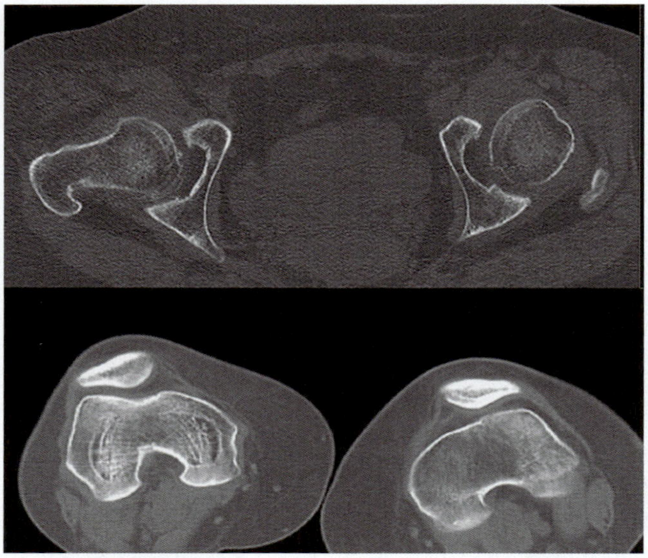

FIGURE 4 CT femoral version study showing retroversion of the right femur.

The aging population is growing, and individuals aged 65 years and older are expected to exceed 77.2 million in the United States by 2040.[27] Concomitantly, the rate of hip fractures is expected to double. An increased number of patients presenting for THA secondary to degenerative arthritis or failure of treatment of hip fractures is therefore expected. Currently, there are 258,000 hip fractures in the United States annually, with a reported rate as high as 957.3 per 100,000 people.[27] THA in patients who have severe proximal femoral deformities and those who have retained proximal femoral hardware will continue to be prevalent and challenging for the orthopaedic surgeon.

Proximal femur deformity is caused by several factors that can be categorized by abnormalities due to development, trauma, metabolic bone disease, or previous surgical intervention (**Table 1**). The Paprosky classification system is commonly used to describe bone stock damage in the revision setting and can be used in these cases. Femoral bone loss is categorized as outlined in **Table 2**.

Another methodology was created for classifying femoral deformity based on the anatomic site[28] (**Table 3**). Subclassifications were determined by geometry. Using an alphabetical system, A represents torsional deformity resulting in excessive anteversion or retroversion, B is angular deformity (varus/valgus or flexion/extension), C is translational deformity, and D represents size alterations (larger or smaller bone than usual) along with the cause of the deformity.

TABLE 1

Etiology of Proximal Femoral Deformity

Previous surgery
Femoral neck nonunion/malunion
Intertrochanteric hip fracture nonunion/malunion
Developmental dysplasia of the hip
Paget disease
Achondroplasia
Multiple epiphyseal dysplasia
Mucopolysaccharidosis
Osteogenesis imperfect
Osteopetrosis
Rickets
Fibrous dysplasia
Down syndrome
Slipped capital femoral epiphysis
Legg-Calvé-Perthes disease
Multiple hereditary exostoses

Contraindications to Arthroplasty

Contraindications to arthroplasty in cases of proximal femur deformity parallel those for primary THA in other conditions. Absolute contraindications would include active infection, a medically unstable condition, and inability to comply with postoperative instructions. Relative contraindications include active Paget disease, uncontrolled diabetes, previous hip infection, uncontrolled rheumatoid arthritis with active use of immunosuppressants, alcoholism, morbid obesity, renal failure, and undiagnosed anemia.

TABLE 2

Paprosky Classification for Femoral Deficiency

Type I	Minimal loss
Type II	Metaphyseal loss with intact diaphysis
Type IIIa	Metadiaphyseal bone loss with at least 4 cm of intact cortical bone in the diaphysis
Type IIIb	Metadiaphyseal bone loss with less than 4 cm of intact cortical bone in the diaphysis
Type IV	Metadiaphyseal bone loss with nonsupportive diaphysis

Adapted with permission from Pak JH, Paprosky WG, Jablonsky WS, Lawrence JM: Femoral strut allografts in cementless revision total hip arthroplasty. *Clin Orthop Relat Res* 1993;295:172-178.

TABLE 3

Berry Classification for Proximal Femoral Deformity

Site of deformity	Greater trochanter Femoral neck Metaphysis Diaphysis
Geometry of deformity	Torsional Angular Translational
Size of abnormality	—
Cause of deformity	Developmental (ie, DDH) Metabolic (ie, Paget disease) Previous osteotomy Previous fracture

DDH = developmental dysplasia of the hip

Adapted with permission from Berry DJ: Total hip arthroplasty in patients with proximal femoral deformity. *Clin Orthop Relat Res* 1999;369:262-272.

Preoperative Planning

As is true for all patients, preoperative workup and planning are essential prerequisites for successful outcomes. A thorough physical examination is required with a focus on hip ROM and leg length inequality. Gait pattern should be observed and assessed. Abductor strength and Trendelenburg status should be recorded. Evaluation of the lower back and lumbar spine of the patient should be documented. Lumbar spine deformities and previous spinal surgery and fusion can alter the pelvic incidence of the patient and functional anteversion of the acetabulum. A fixed pelvic deformity in conjunction with proximal femoral deformity can affect the combined anteversion of the total hip components. Functional status and realistic patient outcomes need to be discussed with patients, many of whom have had surgeries operations on the hip with subsequent poor ROM, and outcomes similar to uncomplicated primary THA may not be realistic.

For patients who have a previous hip operation, the possibility of latent infection is always considered. The erythrocyte sedimentation rate and C-reactive protein level should be obtained. If inflammatory markers are elevated, a hip aspiration and/or biopsy is indicated to rule out infection before hip replacement surgery. Frozen sections and cultures may be indicated if there is any concern at the time of surgery. An antibiotic spacer as a backup plan and preoperative discussion with the patient about a staged procedure is suggested if suspicion of infection is warranted. Medical comorbidities and underlying disease processes must be evaluated. Standard preoperative laboratory studies are performed to screen for anemia, nutritional deficiencies, or uncontrolled diabetes, which may predispose to infection. Disease-specific laboratory studies should also be performed to show adequate control, such as alkaline phosphatase in Paget disease.

Standard AP views of the pelvis, along with AP and lateral views of the hip and proximal femur, should be obtained and are important for a successful outcome. Judet views of the acetabulum can be obtained if there is any concern for an associated anterior or posterior wall deficiency or columnar discontinuity. The proximal femur needs to be assessed for the suspected version alteration or canal disruption and to assess for any varus remodeling of the femur. AP, lateral, and flexion/extension radiographs of the lumbar spine should be obtained if there is a history of previous spinal surgery or lumbar spine deformity. Full-length standing radiographs can also be useful if there is concern for any additional deformity or if there is a limb-length discrepancy that must be addressed during surgery. MRI is typically not useful in these patients.

CT scans are essential if there are concerns regarding abnormal femoral or acetabular anteversion. If there is a limb-length discrepancy, a scanogram or full-length radiographs may be indicated. EOS body imaging (Cambridge, MA) is an evolving, low-radiation dose slot scanning radiograph system allowing the acquisition of radiographic images while the patient is standing, sitting, or squatting. EOS can be used to study spinal deformities simultaneously with pelvic, acetabular, and femoral parameters along with limb-length discrepancy, three-dimensional evaluation, and impingement/dislocation evaluation.[29-32]

Implant choice should be determined preoperatively, and there are multiple options available. Cementless stems have become the mainstay of treatment in the United States and are used in most cases[33] (**Figure 6**). Proximally coated metaphyseal engaging stems can be used in patients who have minimal deformity and good proximal bone stock. Modular implants that allow for metaphyseal fixation and the ability to independently adjust version are useful in proximal femoral deformities. They can also be used to reconcile proximal-distal femoral canal disproportion[34] (**Figure 7**). Extensively porous-coated stems can be used as well, but have higher failure rates when stem sizes are larger than 19 mm in diameter. Monoblock tapered splined stems, such as Wagner type stems, are quite useful in providing initial diaphyseal fixation and rotational control, especially in those patients who have poor metaphyseal bone stock. Monoblock components also avoid the concerns of junctional fretting and fracture associated with modular implants. Modular diaphyseal engaging stems provide good fixation while allowing for independent adjustment of length, offset, and version of the femoral stem, although stem fracture can occur with distally fixed, small-diameter stems.[33-40]

Greater trochanteric deformity may be present in the form of trochanteric overhang or proximal femoral varus malalignment. Either may prevent direct access to the femoral canal or may lead to fracture of the greater trochanter, malalignment of the implant, and/or early failure. To access the femoral diaphysis, an extended trochanteric osteotomy (ETO), trochanteric slide, or a subtrochanteric osteotomy can be used.

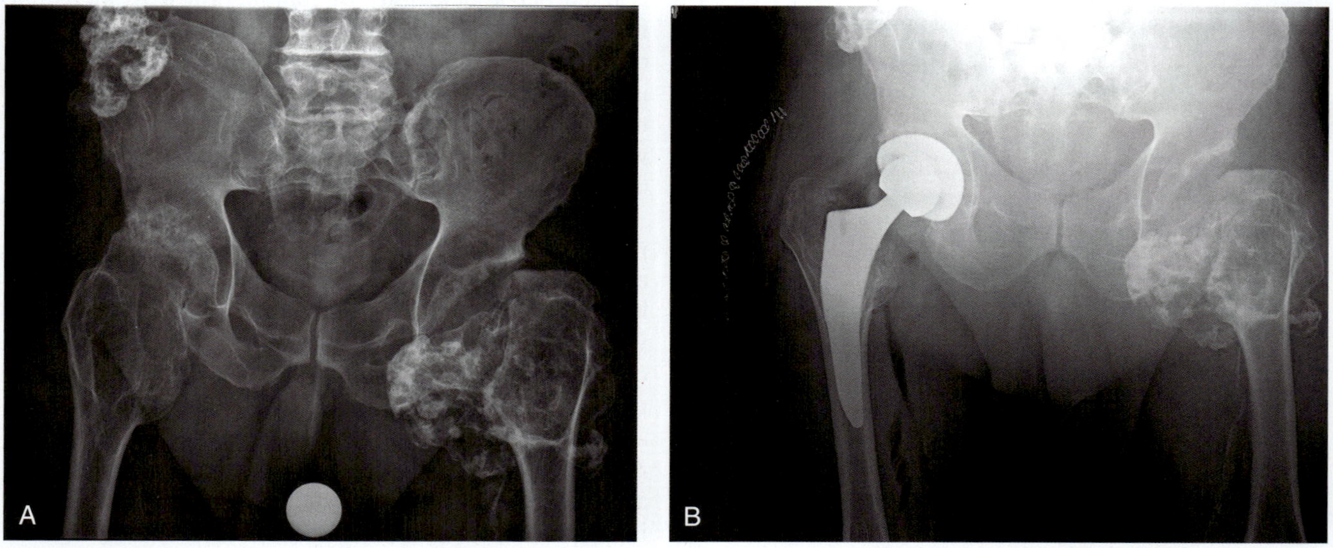

FIGURE 6 **A**, AP pelvis radiograph from a 61-year-old man who has multiple hereditary exostoses and right hip pain. **B**, AP pelvis radiograph after right total hip arthroplasty was performed with a proximally coated femoral stem.

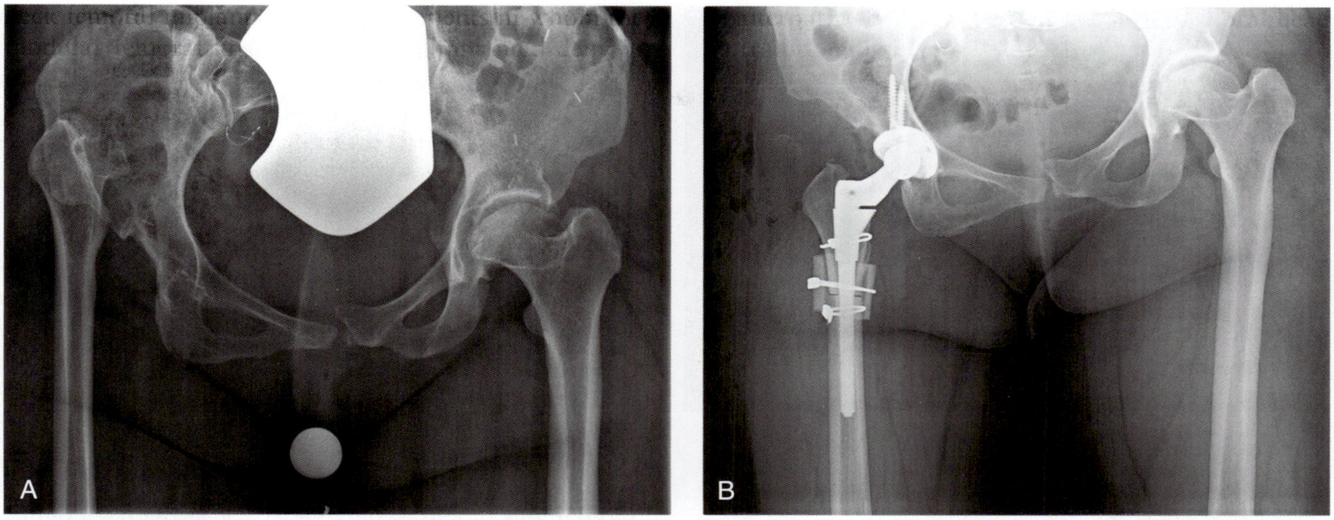

FIGURE 7 **A** and **B**, AP pelvis radiographs from a patient who has Crowe IV developmental dysplasia and a high hip center treated with a modular stem for the proximal femoral deformity.

Technical Considerations

THA after failed fixation for femoral neck or intertrochanteric hip fracture can be technically challenging and has a higher complication rate than primary THA, including an elevated risk of periprosthetic fracture and dislocation.[34] An approach that permits extensile exposure of the femur is recommended. Minimally invasive techniques may need to be avoided because the anatomy and bone are already deformed and the risk of component malposition is high. A posterior or lateral approach provides improved visualization and the ability to expose the femur in the event of fracture or the need for an ETO. Capsulotomy and exposure of the hardware to be removed is accomplished before dislocation of the hip. When exposure is obtained, appropriate gentle dislocation of the hip is then performed before removal of hardware. The hip is then reduced and the implants are removed. The hip can then be dislocated again, and the femoral neck cut can be made (**Figures 8** through **10**).

Failed treatment of femoral neck fracture usually results in a varus deformity and retroversion of the femoral head. Bone quality is often poor.[36] The metaphyseal bone may also be compromised because of the previous surgery. Typically, nonunion or malunion of femoral neck fractures can be managed with a metaphyseal engaging proximally porous-coated stem, or with a cemented stem. If there is severe retroversion or loss of metaphyseal bone stock, a modular or tapered titanium Wagner type stem can be used. These stems can accommodate smaller distal diameters, which may be useful for patients who have small femoral canals and proximal femoral deformity.[33-42]

Failed fixation for intertrochanteric fractures managed with THA is more difficult to manage and is associated with increased surgical time, blood loss, transfusion requirements, and hospital stay than THA for failed femoral neck fractures.[37] Patients who have failed cephalomedullary nail fixation tend to be more difficult to treat than those patients treated with failed sliding hip screws, requiring longer surgical time and greater blood loss.[38] A recent study reported excellent short-term survivorship of conversion hip arthroplasty after surgical management of IT fracture (94% to 95% at 5-years), but those previously treated with an intramedullary nail were at higher risk of intraoperative fracture (12%) compared with those treated with extramedullary fixation devices (1%).[43] Failed fixation of intertrochanteric fractures with

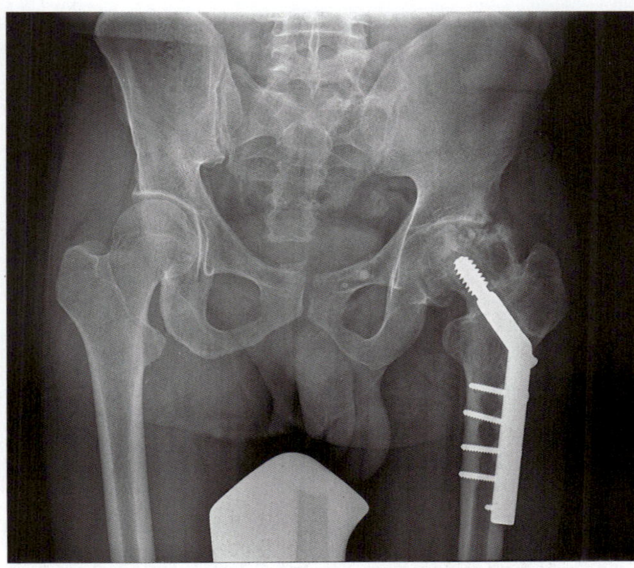

FIGURE 8 AP radiograph shows a previous intertrochanteric hip fracture, in which osteonecrosis developed, treated with a sliding hip screw construct.

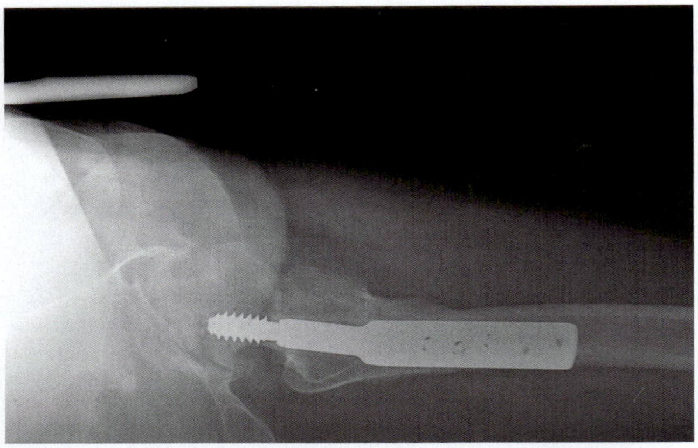

FIGURE 9 Lateral view of previous intertrochanteric hip fracture, in which osteonecrosis developed, treated with a sliding hip screw construct.

a cephalomedullary nail often results in proximal femoral varus and retroversion, and the greater trochanter, along with the abductors, also may be compromised.

Hardware should be removed after dislocation of the hip to prevent fracture propagation through screw or nail tracts. Metaphyseal fixation is not reliable after failed fixation of intertrochanteric fractures. Longer femoral components should be used to bypass the most distal stress riser by at least two cortical diameters. Calcar-replacing stems should be considered in those patients in whom the calcar has been disrupted and is no longer supportive. A diaphyseal engaging, tapered stem can provide good fixation and allow for control of femoral stem

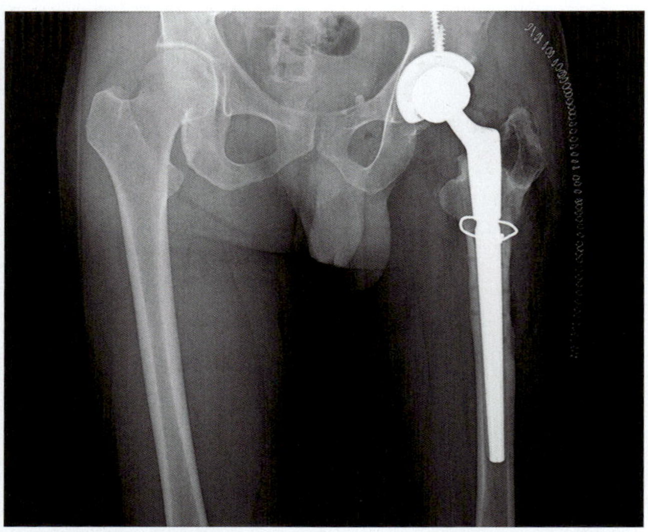

FIGURE 10 AP pelvis radiograph after removal of the sliding hip screw shows left total hip arthroplasty with a modular diaphyseal engaging stem. The most distal screw hole was bypassed by greater than two cortical diameters, and a prophylactic cerclage wire was placed before reaming the femur to prevent fracture.

anteversion. These stems have shown good short-term results.[39,41] Modular stems provide the option to change length and offset in the case of instability and have shown good survivorship at 5-year follow-up.[40] Care should be taken to maintain the continuity of the abductors to the greater trochanter.

Down Syndrome

Patients who have Down syndrome typically have multiple orthopaedic problems. Hip pathology is common in Down syndrome, with hip instability occurring in 2% to 5% of this population. The hip instability typically occurs later than hip dysplasia, occurring in adolescence to adulthood. The typical deformity involves decreased acetabular anteversion, increased femoral anteversion, coxa valga, and a narrow femoral canal. Before surgery, lumbar spine radiographs should be obtained, because there is a significant association with scoliosis and previous spinal fusion, which can alter hip version and stability. EOS imaging may be useful in determining the functional position and acetabular version for these patients. Flexion-extension radiographs of the cervical spine should also be obtained to assess upper cervical spine instability before any surgical procedure. Proximal metaphyseal engaging cementless stems can often be used in these patients as long as care is taken to address the version. Good long-term results have been reported using these stems.[44] Hip instability is a common problem, and constrained liners often are necessary for stability.

Achondroplasia

Achondroplasia is caused by mutations of the gene encoding fibroblast growth factor receptor-3 on chromosome 4, resulting in underdevelopment and shortening of the long bones formed by endochondral ossification. Proximal femoral deformity consisting of a short femur with a very narrow canal can render placement of standard femoral stems difficult or impossible. Significant femoral anteversion may be present, along with significant varus of the tibia with decreased external tibial torsion, altering the perceived normal anatomy of the hip joint. Spine pathology is also common in these patients. Hyperlordosis affects up to 80% of children who have achondroplasia, making lumbar radiographs mandatory before any hip surgery to account for the abnormality in pelvic incidence. Custom femoral implants have been used in this population but failure is common, with 21% requiring revision at an average 36-month follow-up.[45] Some authors have reported good results in the presence of femoral hypoplasia by cementing a small stem instead of using a cementless component. Preoperative assessment is recommended to determine the potential of a metaphyseal engaging wedge-type implant. If the bone is too small or there is too great of a metaphyseal/diaphyseal mismatch,

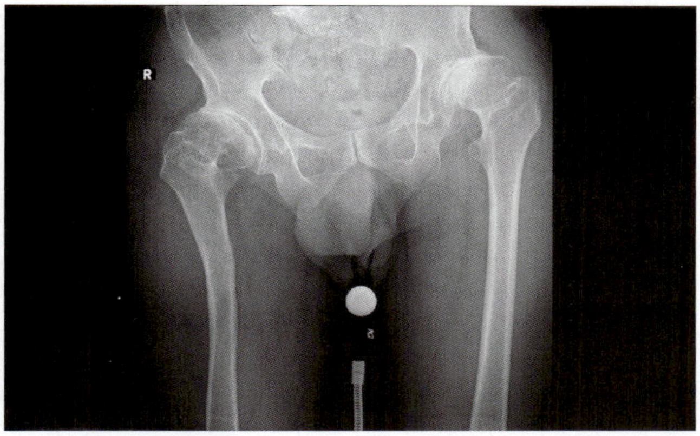

FIGURE 11 AP pelvis radiograph shows achondroplasia in a 59-year-old patient who has bilateral hip pain and a previous right femoral neck fracture that proceeded to malunion.

a modular or tapered titanium Wagner-type cementless stem can be used to achieve fixation and appropriate version (**Figures 11** and **12**).

Fibrous Dysplasia

Fibrous dysplasia is a disease of bone in which the normal lamellar cancellous bone is replaced with immature fibro-osseous tissue, resulting in poorly formed trabeculae of immature woven bone, having a monostotic or polyostotic effect. Deformities of the proximal femur can be severe, with extensive widening and loss of the metaphysis leading to microfracture and pain. This results in the classic shepherd's crook deformity of the proximal femur as it falls into coxa vara. Although coxa vara may be the most common deformity, associated lateral bowing and other deformities of the femur may need to be addressed. Up to 91% of these patients will have proximal femoral pathology.[46] Diphosphonate therapy has been shown to result in major improvements in bone quality, filling of lytic lesions, improved cortical thickness, and improved bone mineral density. Diphosphonate therapy can lead to partial resolution of fibrous dysplasia.[45] The technical difficulty of THA in this population will depend on the severity of the deformity. Implant requirements can range from standard metaphyseal engaging cementless implants to surgery requiring an ETO and diaphyseal engaging implants. The severity of the coxa vara deformity will determine implant choice and requirement for an ETO.

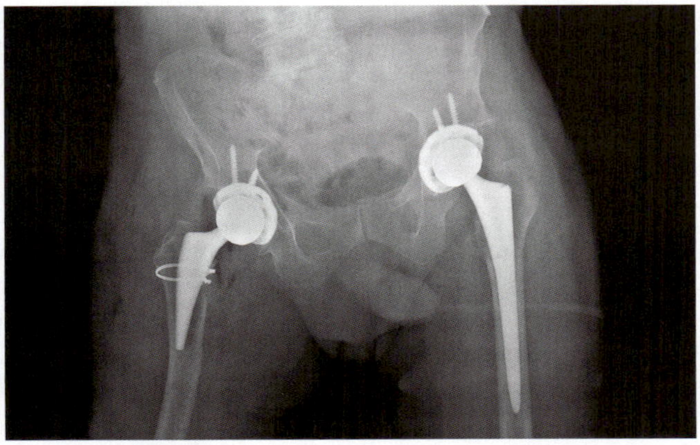

FIGURE 12 AP pelvis radiograph from a 59-year-old patient who has achondroplasia managed with staged bilateral total hip arthroplasty, treated on the left with a metaphyseal engaging stem and on the right treated with a mini stem.

THA IN THE NEUROMUSCULAR HIP

Background

Patients who have neuromuscular hip disorders comprise a rare but challenging population of patients. Because of the different degrees of muscle imbalance or paralysis, the pathology in these hips is quite variable. The severity of spasticity and contractures depends on the underlying neuromuscular disease. These patients are often debilitated and their functional goals may be limited. Treatment goals are to achieve pain relief, optimize physical function, and improve care. Conservative and/or nonarthroplasty treatment options are usually indicated. However, in ambulatory patients who have hip pain and dysfunction, THA with varying degrees of constraint can be an appropriate and successful treatment option with relatively low complication rates.

Neuromuscular diseases resulting in hip pathology in adults include myopathies, muscular dystrophies, upper and lower motor neuron diseases/injuries, neurodegenerative disorders, movement disorders, and diseases of the neuromuscular junction. These patients comprise a heterogeneous group that requires individualized care of their hip disease.

Muscle imbalance about the hip secondary to an underlying neuromuscular disease can result in subluxation and dislocation of the hip in growing children and may predispose adult patients to degenerative joint disease of the hip. Specifically, strong hip flexors and adductors that overpower weaker or absent hip extensors and abductors lead to acquired hip instability and dysfunction. Although the direct cause of the instability is muscle imbalance, the underlying etiology of the hip dysfunction may be either intrinsic or extrinsic factors. Intrinsic muscle imbalance about the hip manifests during childhood and plays a primary role in subsequent hip problems, frequently with osseous abnormalities. Extrinsic causes of neuromuscular imbalance occur in stable hips and play a secondary role in development of osteoarthritis and contractures in later life.

The two basic types of paralysis or paresis are flaccid paralysis, which is caused by injury to the lower motor neurons or peripheral nerves, and spastic paralysis, which is caused by injury to the upper motor neurons or the cortex of the brain. Spastic muscle has increased tone and often functions in both phases of gait (ie, in phase and out of phase). Flaccid muscle has decreased tone, but always functions according to its normal role. Both spastic and flaccid type pareses are found in both intrinsic and extrinsic disorders.

Extrinsic movement disorders, such as dyskinesis, athetosis, Parkinson disease, and multiple sclerosis (which may be more specifically classified as a demyelinating disorder), may have elements of spasticity, but hip subluxation-dislocation is rare in this group of patients because the onset of disease is usually after growth is complete. However, movement disorders are frequently associated with contractures about the hip, and painful degenerative arthritis often develops in these patients.

Children who are born with intrinsic neuromuscular disorders (eg, cerebral palsy, myelomeningocele), or in whom a neuromuscular affliction occurs while the hip is still in early development (eg, poliomyelitis, encephalitis, cerebral vascular accidents, childhood spinal cord injuries, brain trauma), are at increased risk for hip subluxation-dislocation. In these children, frequent examinations and hip radiographs can detect and even predict those hips at risk. Botulinum toxin A injections, early muscle releases or transfers, and appropriate varus rotation femoral osteotomies can improve hip stability. Still, despite treatment, hips can remain subluxated or dislocated and thus can be a source of pain and disability in the adult.

Although sensation in general does not play a role in hip instability, compromised proprioception may play a role in hip instability. Diminished or absent proprioception, whether it existed preoperatively or was compromised as the result of surgery about the hip, may cause instability after THA. Unfortunately, assessing proprioception about the hip is challenging clinically, and accurately assessing its role is therefore difficult.

Intrinsic Disorders

Spasticity

Among the intrinsic neuromuscular hip disorders, the major causes of spasticity are cerebral palsy, cerebral vascular accidents, and spinal cord injuries in the young child. Despite differing etiologies, the hip pathology seen in these patients is quite similar, and thus, their treatment may be approached in a like manner. Early treatment during childhood consists of nonsurgical measures such as physical therapy, bracing treatment, wheelchair modifications, botulinum toxin A injections, and surgical treatment including muscle releases and transfers to obtain muscle balance as well as early varus-rotation femoral osteotomies to better stabilize the hip or hips. When the acetabulum is deficient, acetabuloplasty should also be considered. Although these procedures may be suitable for the growing child, salvage operations are usually necessary in the treatment of adult patients.

The goals of treatment of the adult spastic neuromuscular hip, regardless of the etiology or ambulatory status, include preventing contractures, eliminating pain, and optimizing function. Salvage procedures are often required if contractures result in pain, sitting imbalance, or difficulty with perineal care.

As outlined by the treatment algorithm in **Figure 13**, the three traditional surgical options for managing the painful, dislocated hip in an adult are head-neck resection with or without interposition arthroplasty; hip arthrodesis; and total hip arthroplasty. Although resection arthroplasty or arthrodesis had been advocated in the past, there is currently increasing preference for THA in the ambulatory adult.

Flaccid Paralysis

The intrinsic neuromuscular disorders associated with flaccid paralysis include poliomyelitis, myelomeningocele, and Charcot-Marie-Tooth disease. Fortunately, the incidence of these disorders is decreasing worldwide. In the adult who has a painful arthritic hip, surgical treatment is often necessary. The risk of instability after THA with flaccid paralysis must be addressed. If the muscle weakness is so profound that the arthroplasty is unstable, a constrained device is often necessary to provide stability (**Figure 14**).

Extrinsic Disorders

Extrinsic neuromuscular disorders comprise a diverse group of problems that secondarily involve the hip joint. In these disorders, muscle imbalance with hip subluxation-dislocation plays a secondary role, but contractures about the hip frequently develop. Some of these disorders are associated with spasticity, whereas others have flaccid paralysis as the dominant feature. Each of the disorders will be reviewed individually, although the treatment algorithms are similar.

Charcot Neuropathic Hip Joint

Neuropathic or Charcot joints present a special problem for the orthopaedic surgeon, regardless of the specific joint involved. The critical element in treating a patient who has a neuropathic hip joint is to establish the diagnosis. Charcot joints can be caused by a variety of diseases and disease processes, including tertiary syphilis, diabetes mellitus, and syringomyelia. Any joint presenting with atypical findings such as painless joint dysfunction and radiographic evidence of a relentless destructive process should alert the clinician to the possibility of a neuropathic joint.

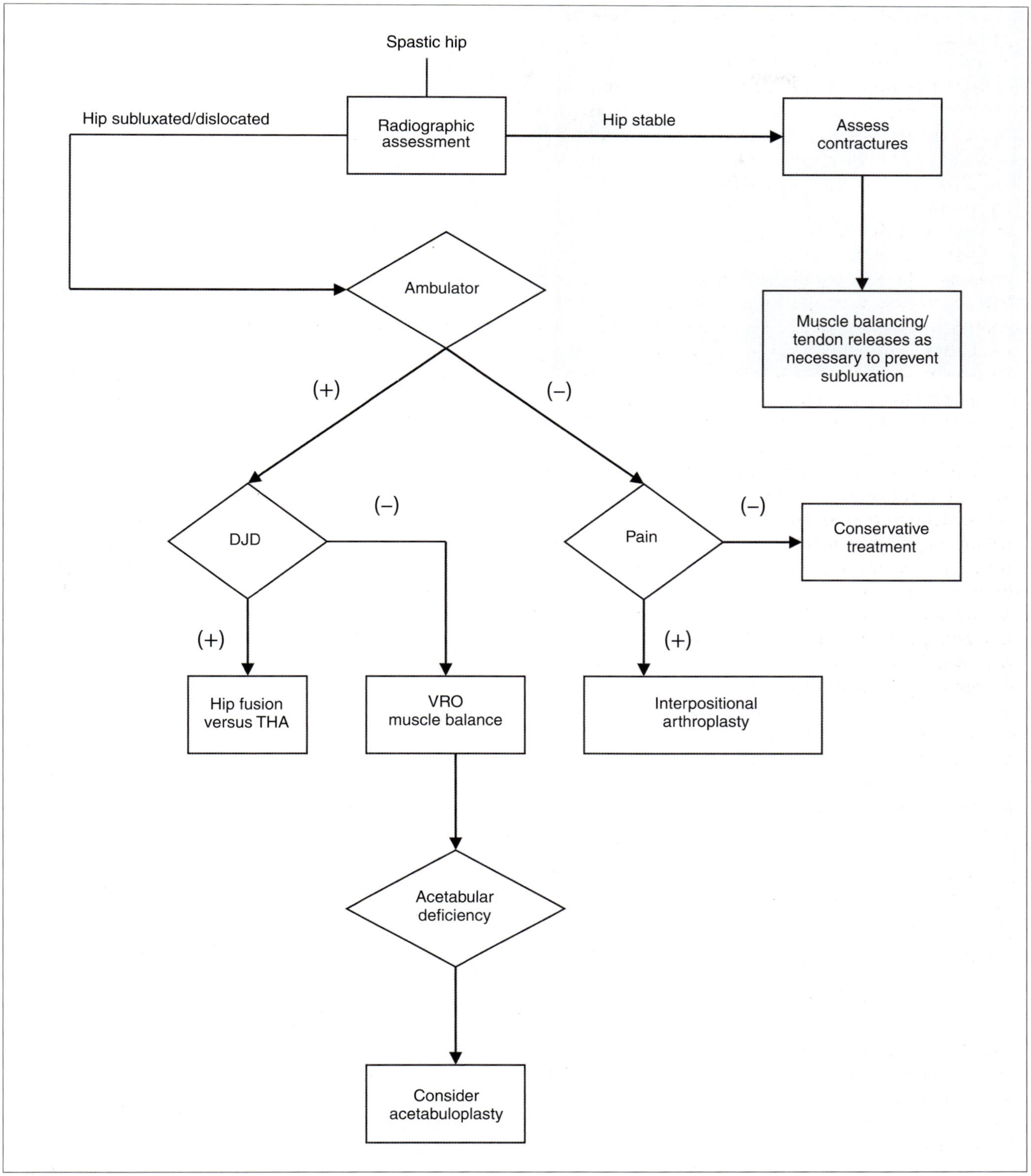

FIGURE 13 Treatment algorithm for the spastic hip. DJD = degenerative joint disease, THA = total hip arthroplasty, VRO = varus rotational osteotomy.

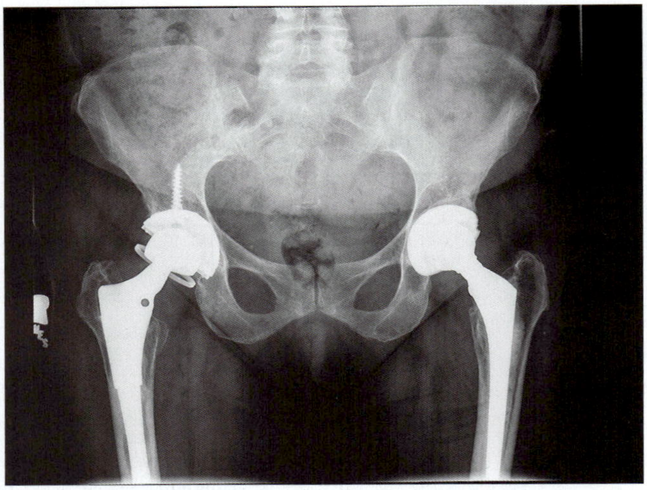

FIGURE 14 AP pelvis radiograph shows flaccid paralysis managed with a constrained acetabular implant.

If the joint remains painless and functional, no treatment is recommended. If pain is present and function is impaired, conservative treatment with protected weight bearing should be extended as long as possible before any type of surgical procedure is considered. If nonsurgical treatment fails, the surgical options available include arthrodesis, THA, and resection arthroplasty. Historically, arthrodesis and THA have demonstrated high failure rates, especially in patients who have significant neurologic findings or ataxia.[47-49] Resorting to a resection arthroplasty may be the only viable solution in the treatment of the painful hip in these patients. One recent study of 12 THAs performed in Charcot hips found that 75% survived free of revision at both 5 years, but the overall complication rate was high at 58%. The complications included three recurrent dislocations, two periprosthetic fractures, one femoral loosening, and one delayed wound healing.[50]

Parkinson Disease

Degenerative arthritis of the hip in patients who have Parkinson disease may occur through natural processes or following hip fractures. The treatment of hip fractures in these patients remains problematic with a high rate of complications, including frequent dislocation of hips treated with hemiarthroplasty. Patients who have Parkinson disease undergoing elective THA are also at increased risk for dislocation.[51] Thus, optimal medical management before elective THA is highly recommended.

Multiple Sclerosis

Painful hip flexion adduction contractures in patients who have advanced multiple sclerosis are very difficult to treat. In the end stages of the disease, treatment is complicated by knee flexion contractures and contracted upper extremities. Early release of contracted hip adductors, flexors, and iliopsoas muscles, as well as hamstrings, is essential to prevent painful fixed joint deformities.

When contractures are fixed and severe, painful decubitus ulcers and/or pelvic obliquity develop, and patients are often unable to sit or even lie down comfortably. Despite the fact that these patients are essentially considered terminally ill, multiple extensive soft-tissue procedures may provide pain relief and some improvement in sitting. Occasionally, a proximal femoral resection or THA is warranted for pain relief. Because of prolonged steroid use and diminished function and strength, fractures about the hip, particularly the femoral neck and trochanter, are also a concern.

Adult-Onset Cerebral Vascular Accident (Stroke), Upper Motor Neuron Spinal Cord Injury, and Head Injury

As noted earlier, hip subluxation-dislocation rarely occurs in adult-onset spasticity due to brain or upper spinal cord injury. Hip joint contractures are frequent, however. Thus, early, intensive physical therapy is important for maintenance of hip ROM. Unless regularly manipulated through a normal ROM, significant contractures will develop in these hips. If the patient survives the initial insult, whether it is due to a traumatic event or a cerebrovascular accident, efforts should be directed toward regaining functional ambulation. Nonetheless, patients who have significant residual neurologic impairment will most likely be rendered wheelchair bound. Simple tenotomies of the involved muscles may be helpful in restoring balance. Balance is critically important in this population to lessen their risk of falls and fragility fractures of the hip or femur. Still, the functional recovery after surgical treatment of hip fractures is similar to that of patients who have not had a prior cerebrovascular accident.

Another problem in these patients, especially those suffering traumatic brain injuries, is the propensity for heterotopic ossification, which can also limit joint motion. This excessive bone must be allowed to fully mature before attempting resection; otherwise, more extensive heterotopic bone formation may occur postresection. After surgical resection of heterotopic ossification, multimodal prophylaxis to prevent recurrence must be instituted, including low-dose radiation, NSAIDs, and early mobilization.

Older patients who have stroke are more prone to degenerative joint disease of the hip and should be treated with the same guidelines as the general population. They may, however, require release of contracted adductor or hip flexor muscles at the time of the THA. Adductor tenotomy can be performed percutaneously just before positioning the patient for the hip arthroplasty, and the iliopsoas can be released from its insertion on the lesser trochanter during the exposure of the joint.

THA is also recommended for younger patients who, in addition to sustaining head injuries, develop painful posttraumatic arthritis or even osteonecrosis.

Spinal Cord Injury

As in juvenile patients, spinal cord injuries in adults can result in significant spasticity of the muscles around the hip. Although subluxation and dislocation are usually not as problematic in the adult patient as they are in children, spasticity can lead to contractures that require appropriate early releases. If degenerative arthritis does develop, THA may be indicated for pain relief. However, if the patient is nonambulatory with severe contractures and skin breakdown, resection arthroplasty may be a more viable option. Although not as prevalent as in traumatic brain injury patients, heterotopic ossification does occur with some frequency and should be approached in a similar fashion.

PRIMARY THA FOLLOWING ACETABULAR FRACTURE

Background

Acetabular fractures may result in considerable damage to the periacetabular bone and soft tissues. Open reduction and internal fixation (ORIF) of acetabular fractures can be associated with extensive soft-tissue dissection. Posttraumatic arthritis requiring THA is a common complication after acetabular fracture, despite improvements in reduction technique and fixation. The technical complexity and results of THA after prior acetabular fracture may be affected by many factors, including bony deformity, prior infection, retained hardware, limb shortening, sciatic nerve palsy, abductor deficiency, and heterotopic bone formation.

Acetabular fractures in young patients are typically high-energy injuries, which can result in damage to the articular cartilage, bony columns, and surrounding soft tissues. Low-energy injuries in elderly patients who have osteoporosis can also result in acetabular fractures, which may have considerable comminution. Nerve and vascular injuries are not uncommon. Treatment with ORIF may require extensive soft-tissue dissection to achieve bony reduction, and the application of multiple plates and screws. Posttraumatic arthritis, osteonecrosis, and heterotopic bone formation are common complications after ORIF of acetabular fractures. THA for posttraumatic arthritis after prior acetabular fracture is effective in improving hip pain and function, but also associated with greater surgical time, blood loss, and complications in comparison with THA for primary osteoarthritis.[52-54]

Preoperative Planning

In addition to an AP pelvis radiograph, Judet views and a CT scan can be helpful to delineate bony deformity, the location of retained hardware, and the presence, extent, and location of any heterotopic bone. Surgical scars and prior medical records are reviewed to determine what surgical approaches have been used and the location of retained hardware. Preoperative templating is performed to determine the implant size and position, and any expected change in leg length and offset.

Pelvic deformity should be considered if nonanatomic reduction or loss of fracture fixation has resulted in malunion. Transverse fractures, both-column fractures, and anterior column with posterior hemitransverse wall fractures that have healed with some displacement typically present with medialization of the inferior pelvis, which creates a protrusio acetabular deformity (**Figure 15**). Restoration of the anatomic hip center, rather than relative medial or lateral cup placement, is associated with a lower risk of aseptic cup loosening after THA for protrusio deformity.[55] Segmental bone defects may require structural augments. A cage may be necessary for large cavitary lesions in osteoporotic bone.

Technical Considerations

Any standard surgical approach can be used, but if posterior hardware requires removal, a posterior approach will provide access to both the acetabulum and the hardware. This approach also permits exposure and identification of the sciatic nerve, which is often surrounded by scar tissue. Mobilization of the nerve may be necessary to remove posterior hardware. Only that hardware protruding into the acetabulum during reaming requires removal (**Figure 16**). However, if there is concern for infection, all hardware should be removed. In aseptic cases, intra-articular screws that are not accessible from the outer surface of the pelvis can be removed with a metal-cutting burr. This avoids unnecessary dissection along the outer pelvic bone or a separate ilioinguinal approach to remove anteriorly placed screws.

Both cementless and cemented acetabular components have been used with successful results.[52] For protrusio defects, a large rim-fit cup provides relative lateralization of the hip to its anatomic center (**Figure 15**). Use of a large-diameter reamer to ream the rim of the acetabular cavity prevents medialization that can occur with a smaller reamer. Morcellized bone obtained from acetabular reamings or the femoral head can be used to fill cavitary defects. Segmental bone loss may require revision THA techniques and implants including augments and cages. Nonunion of acetabular fractures involving both columns may be approached in a similar way to pelvic discontinuity, with the goal of recreating stability

Section 3: Hip

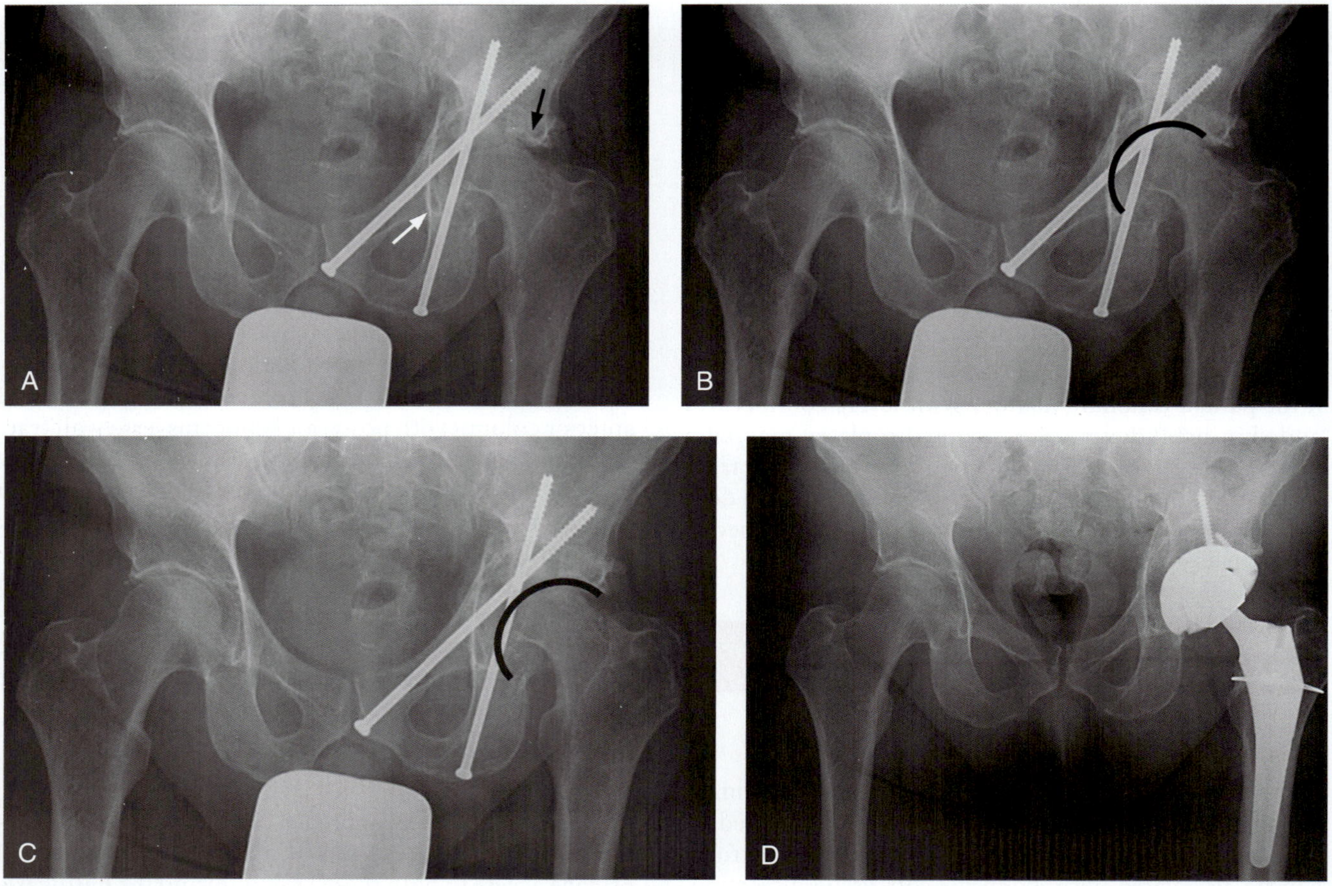

FIGURE 15 AP pelvis radiographs show a transverse acetabular fracture. **A**, After open reduction and internal fixation of a transverse acetabular fracture, the inferior hemipelvis has healed in a medialized position as indicated by the location of the teardrop (white arrow), whereas the superior hemipelvis remains in its normal anatomic relationship to the sacroiliac joint and the lateral acetabulum (black arrow) is not displaced. **B**, If the acetabular implant is templated adjacent to the medial wall, the component will be medialized relative to the upper pelvis. **C**, The acetabular implant should be templated relative to the normally aligned superior acetabular rim and upper pelvis. **D**, A slightly oversized rim fit acetabular implant is used to provide relative lateralization of the component relative to the medial wall and restoration of the anatomic hip center.

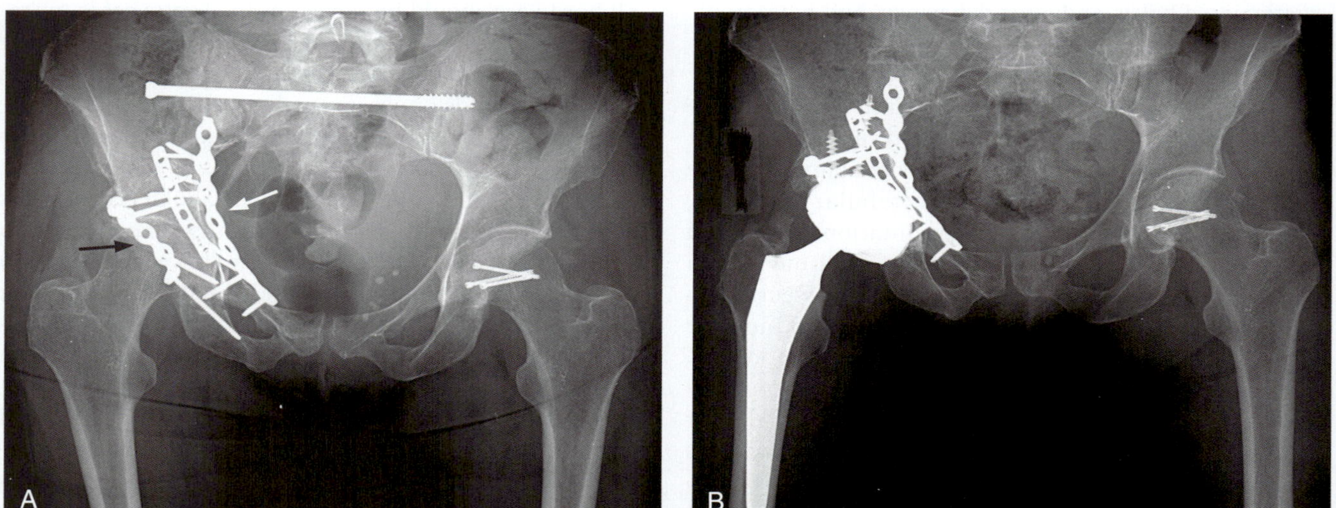

FIGURE 16 **A**, AP pelvis radiograph demonstrates anterior (white arrow) and posterior (black arrow) retained plates. **B**, Postoperative AP radiograph after total hip arthroplasty shows that portions of the posterior hardware were removed while anterior hardware was retained.

and continuity of the hemipelvis. This may be achieved via distraction techniques with jumbo cups, cup-cage constructs, or custom triflanges. If heterotopic bone is removed during THA, perioperative radiation therapy or postoperative treatment with NSAIDs should be considered to minimize the risk of recurrent heterotopic bone formation following THA.

Results

Results of THA after prior acetabular fracture are generally less favorable than for THA for primary osteoarthritis. Surgical time and blood loss are increased. One recent case-control study comparing 74 patients undergoing THA with prior acetabular fracture with patients without prior fracture found a lower 10-year survivorship (70% versus 90%), and a higher likelihood of developing infection (7% versus zero), dislocation (11% versus 3%), and heterotopic ossification (43% versus 16%).[56] In a systematic review of 659 hips (654 patients) with THA after acetabular fracture, the 10-year survivorship with loosening, osteolysis, or revision as the end point was 76% for the acetabular implant and 85% for the femoral implant.[44] Eighty-one percent of the acetabular components and 59% of the femoral components used were cementless. Heterotopic ossification was the most common complication (30%), followed by infection (6%), dislocation (4%), and nerve injuries (2%). These findings demonstrate a more frequent rate of complications than conventional THA for primary osteoarthritis. However, patients who have posttraumatic arthritis are often more debilitated than those who have primary osteoarthritis as a result of leg length inequality, sciatic nerve palsy, limited hip motion, and complications from prior surgery.[53] THA for posttraumatic arthritis is associated with favorable improvements in pain and function. In a retrospective review of 53 patients after THA following prior acetabular fracture, all but 3 were satisfied or very satisfied with the procedure, indicating that despite the technical complexity of the procedure, patient satisfaction with the outcomes is relatively high.[54]

THA IN METABOLIC BONE DISEASE

Background

THA in patients who have metabolic bone disease offers unique challenges to the surgeon to achieve a satisfactory outcome. The bone quality and/or alignment is typically affected to such a degree that it forces the surgeon to adjust surgical technique and implant choice to avoid complications. Such conditions include osteoporosis, osteopetrosis, Paget disease, and renal osteodystrophy. It is important to recognize each disease preoperatively and to specially plan intraoperative precautions and techniques for each scenario (**Table 4**). Preoperative templating is essential to reduce complications and achieve a successful outcome.

THA in Osteoporosis

Osteoporosis is the most common metabolic bone disease, particularly in the elderly population. It is characterized by a decreased bone mineral density that is below 2.5 SD, as measured on a bone dual-energy x-ray absorptiometry scan. Because in many countries people are living longer, osteoporosis is more often seen as a comorbidity in patients undergoing THA. Approximately 26% of patients undergoing THA and total knee arthroplasty for osteoarthritis also have osteoporosis.[57] Furthermore, THA is becoming increasingly used in patients who have low-energy acetabular fractures and femoral neck fractures.[58,59] Osteoporosis is characterized as high turnover or low turnover. High-turnover osteoporosis is seen in postmenopausal women who have declining levels of estrogen, which leads to increased osteoclast-mediated bone resorption. Low-turnover osteoporosis is characterized by diminished osteoblastic activity that can result from medications such as chemotherapy and steroids and some antiosteoporotic medications. Medical management can consist of an adequate intake of calcium and vitamin D as well as antiresorptive medication (eg, diphosphonates) or anabolic agents (eg, teriparatide [parathyroid hormone 1-34]).

Diminished bone quality is of major concern to the orthopaedic surgeon during THA in patients who have osteoporosis. Historically, cemented fixation has been the preferred technique for these patients, especially on the femoral side, to avoid intraoperative iatrogenic femur fractures. Recent evidence has demonstrated efficacy and safety with cementless femoral components.[60-62] In North America, the use of cementless femoral stems is increasing, whereas in Europe cemented femoral components are favored.[63] However, in a large cohort of patients (32,644 primary THAs) intraoperative fractures occur 14 times more often with cementless femoral components, particularly in female patients older than 65 years.[63]

Therefore, in patients who have osteoporosis, it is important to consider cemented femoral components (**Figure 17**) as a strategy to prevent iatrogenic femur fractures. Optimal cement technique is critical to obtaining a proper cement mantle and includes proper preparation of the bony bed of the proximal femur with pulsatile lavage and suction, retrograde filling of the femoral canal using a cement gun and long nozzle, and the maintenance of pressurization during the cementation period and implant insertion.[64] If a cementless femoral implant is chosen, it is important to carefully impact the broaches

TABLE 4

Summary of Surgical Challenges for Total Hip Arthroplasty in Patients Who Have Metabolic Bone Disease With Specific Recommendations for Each Condition

Metabolic Bone Disease	Intraoperative Challenges	Recommendations
Osteoporosis	Weak bone quality	Consideration of a cemented femoral stem Careful proximal femoral preparation and implant insertion with cementless femoral components Screw augmentation of the acetabular implant
Osteopetrosis	Hard, brittle bone quality Obliterated femoral medullary canal	Use of a high-speed burr, drills, and reamers to re-create a medullary canal Use of fluoroscopic guidance during canal preparation Use of smaller femoral stems Screw augmentation of the acetabular implant
Paget disease	Hypervascularity Acetabular protrusio Hard, sclerotic bone Varus deformity of the proximal femur	Appropriate intraoperative fluid and blood management Consideration of a blood salvage system Medial acetabular bone grafting Oversized acetabular hemispherical cup Offset acetabular liners Screw augmentation of the acetabular implant Use of a high-speed burr, drills, and reamers to re-create a medullary canal Use of fluoroscopic guidance during canal preparation Possible need for femoral osteotomy or osteotomies
Renal osteodystrophy	Weak bone quality	Consideration of a cemented femoral stem Use of alternative bearing surfaces in younger patients

during proximal femoral preparation and to cautiously insert the final implant. With proper patient selection, implant choice, and surgical technique, clinical outcomes can be optimized and complications can be avoided.

THA in Osteopetrosis

Osteopetrosis is a rare inherited bone disease that is characterized by decreased function in osteoclasts leading to decreased bone resorption, which results in increased cortical bone and calcified cartilage. Two autosomal recessive types of osteopetrosis are lethal and one autosomal dominant type is nonlethal. Patients who have the nonlethal form typically live a full lifespan; however, they can experience various orthopaedic issues including frequent fractures, coxa vara, osteoarthritis, osteomyelitis, fracture nonunion, and long bone malalignment.

The usual indications for THA in patients who have osteopetrosis are hip osteoarthritis or periarticular hip fracture nonunion. Surgeons need to appreciate the technical difficulties that can be encountered intraoperatively to avoid complications. Bone associated with osteopetrosis is typically brittle, and it often lacks a medullary canal, which can make implantation challenging (**Figure 18**). Techniques to circumvent these obstacles include (1) use of a burr, high-speed drills, and reamers under fluoroscopic guidance to re-create a medullary canal in the proximal femur; (2) use of a smaller femoral implant to obviate the need for the creation of a larger femoral canal; and (3) screw augmentation of the acetabular implant for increased initial stability due to the increased presence of sclerotic bone. Some authors have used computer-assisted navigation for femoral canal preparation[65,66] or customized instrumentation and femoral stems.[65,67] These cases will take more time than primary osteoarthritis THAs, and averaged almost 5 hours in one study.[68] The few reports on the outcomes of THA in patients who have osteopetrosis have consisted of case reports and case series, which have included fully cemented THA, a hybrid construct, or cementless THA. Most patients have experienced significant benefit.

THA for Paget Disease

Paget disease of bone (osteitis deformans) is characterized by a localized osteoclast dysfunction that causes an increase in bone resorption with the subsequent formation of new unorganized woven bone. It is the second most

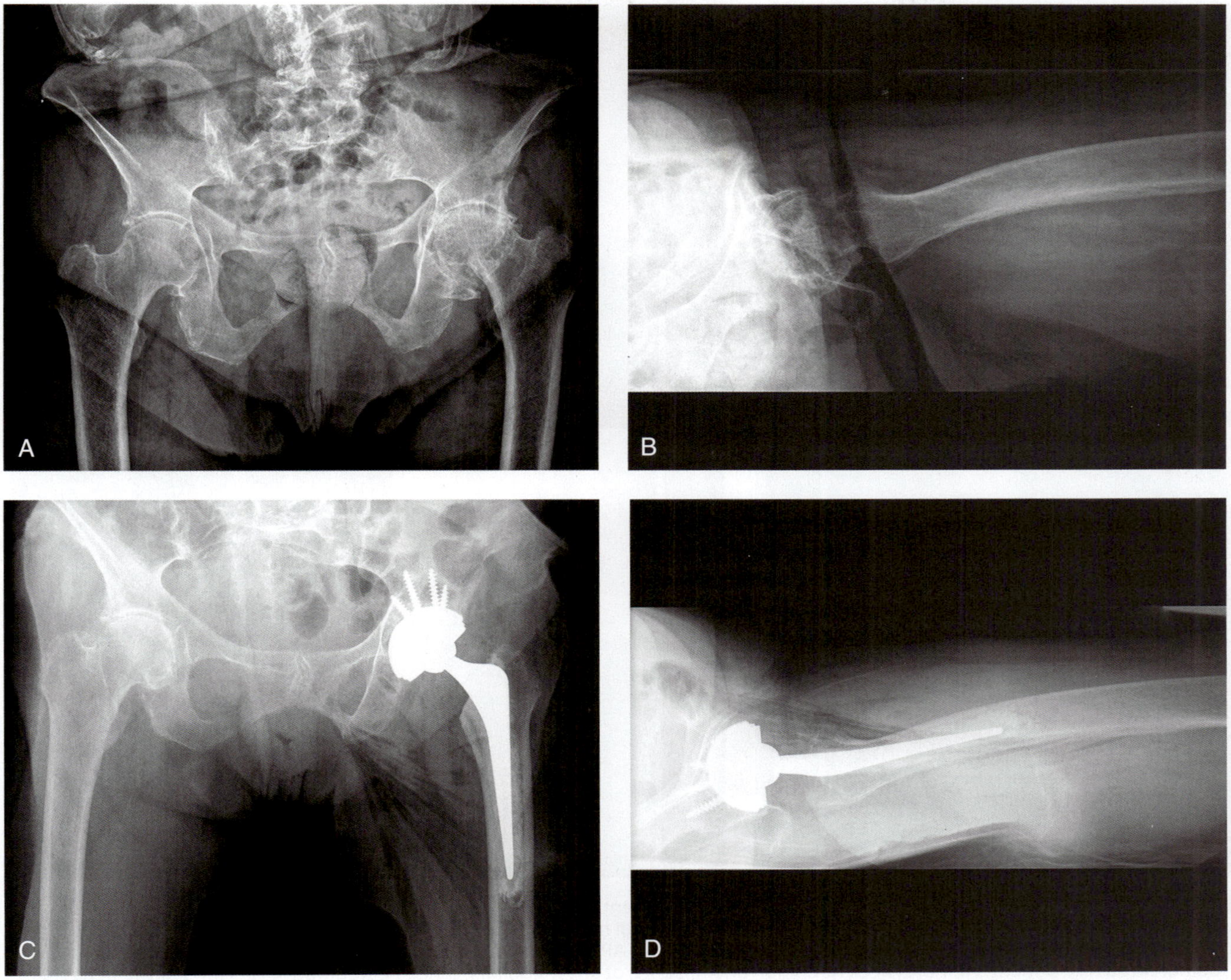

FIGURE 17 Radiographs show total hip arthroplasty (THA) in a patient who has osteoporosis. AP view of the pelvis (**A**) and cross-table lateral radiograph of the left hip (**B**) demonstrate severe osteoarthritis of the left hip. Evidence of osteoporosis can also be seen with loss of the trabeculae in the proximal femur and cortical thinning. Severe lumbar spine osteoarthritis and deformity can also be noted in panel **A**. Postoperative radiograph of the patient's pelvis (**C**) centered over the pubic symphysis and cross-table lateral view of the left hip (**D**) show a left hybrid THA. A cementless acetabular cup was used and reinforced with multiple screws because of the patient's poor bone quality. A dual-mobility articulation was placed to address the patient's risk of instability from the severe spinal deformity. A cemented collarless, polished, double-tapered femoral stem was implanted to minimize the risk of fracture resulting from the weak bone quality.

common metabolic bone disease after osteoporosis and more commonly affects the elderly. Patients can present with monostotic or polyostotic patterns; however, the pelvis and proximal femur are the most common sites involved in 20% to 80% of patients, leading to frequent hip disease. Osseous deformities about the hip joint include coxa vara, femoral bowing, acetabular protrusio, and bone enlargement, which can lead to arthropathy. These patients are also at risk for femoral neck fractures, stress fractures, and nonunions, which can further complicate treatment. Medical management has included the use of nitrogen-containing diphosphonates to inhibit osteoclast-mediated bone resorption and in turn decrease bone turnover in conjunction with analgesics.[69]

Before performing THA in patients who have Paget disease of bone, it is imperative to preoperatively identify the etiology of the hip pain. Although osteoarthritis is a common source of hip pain in these patients, other causes include bone pain, femoral neck stress fracture, spinal radiculopathy, or even Paget sarcoma. If nonsurgical treatment has failed and THA is contemplated (**Figure 19**), it is important to predict potential intraoperative difficulties. Preoperative radiographs should include an AP view of the pelvis as well as AP and cross-table lateral views of

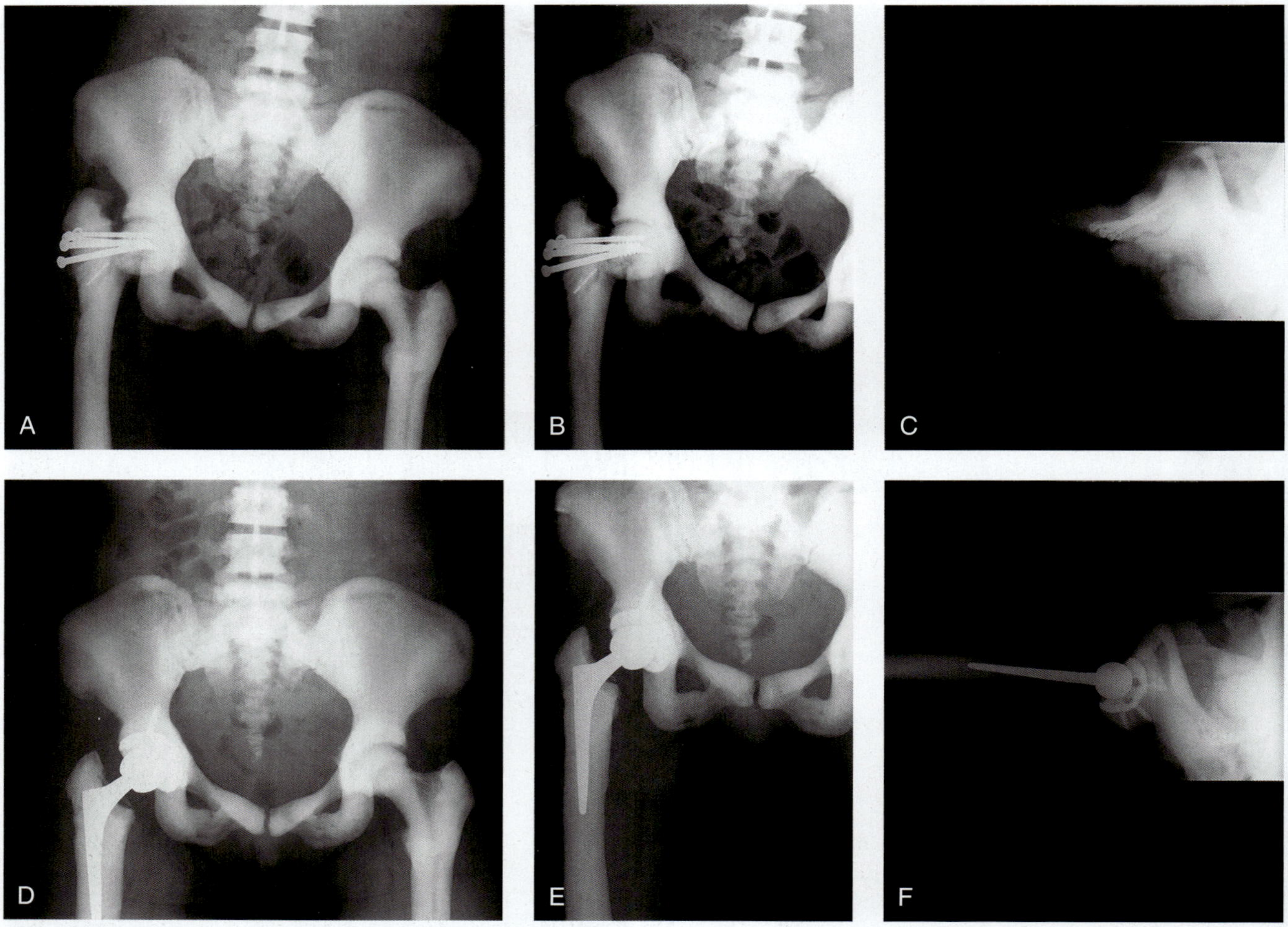

FIGURE 18 Images show total hip arthroplasty (THA) in a patient who has osteopetrosis. AP plain radiograph of the pelvis (**A**) shows osteopetrosis in a patient who also has a right femoral neck fracture nonunion that has progressed to varus. The loss of the medullary canals within both femurs is also evident. AP (**B**) and cross-table lateral (**C**) views of the right hip further demonstrate the patient's femoral neck nonunion and absence of any medullary canal. Postoperative AP views of the pelvis (**D**) and AP (**E**) and cross-table lateral (**F**) views of the right hip demonstrate a right hybrid THA that was performed for the patient's femoral neck nonunion. A cementless acetabular implant was used with augmented screw fixation. The creation of a new femoral intramedullary canal was required with the use of multiple burr sizes and drill bits. Intraoperative fluoroscopy was also used to ensure proper placement of the femoral broach. The smallest cemented collarless, polished, double-tapered femoral implant was ultimately used.

the involved hip. Full-length views of the femur and full-length standing extremity radiographs are important to assess the extent of disease and femoral deformity.

Special intraoperative technical challenges that can be anticipated include hypervascularity, altered bone quality, and bone deformity. It is important to recognize the potential need for increased fluid and blood replacement resulting from the hypervascularity of bone affected by Paget disease. In these cases, an intraoperative blood salvage system can decrease the need for allogeneic blood products.[70] If cemented components are planned, it may be difficult to obtain a dry bony bed for cement interdigitation. Visualization may also be impaired because of the increased hypervascularity and bleeding. Acetabular protrusio can be encountered in these patients, which can in turn lead to medialization of the acetabular implant and hip center. Techniques used to prevent overmedialization include medial acetabular bone grafting or the use of an oversized hemispherical cup. Offset acetabular liners can also be used in situations where the cup has been placed too far medially. Multiple acetabular screws are useful to increase cup stability, especially with compromised bone quality. The choice of cemented versus cementless acetabular components is at the discretion of the treating surgeon. Sclerotic femoral bone and varus deformity are two challenges that must be anticipated. The use of high-speed burrs and reamers in conjunction with intraoperative radiographs can be used to ensure

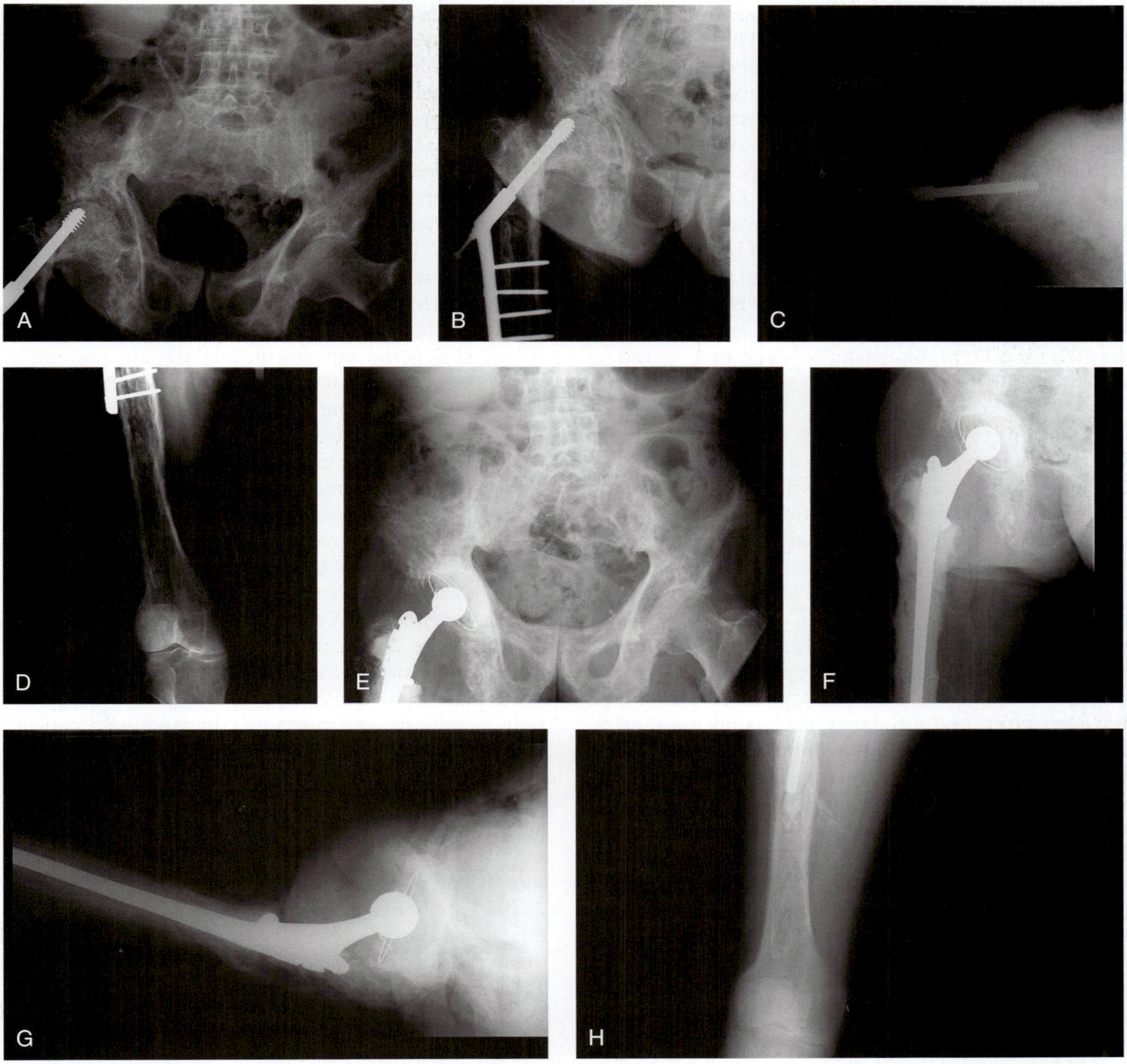

FIGURE 19 Images from a patient with Paget disease who underwent total hip arthroplasty (THA). AP radiograph of the pelvis (**A**) and AP (**B**) and cross-table lateral (**C**) radiographs of the right hip show a femoral neck fracture nonunion that is also in varus in a patient who also has Paget disease, which can be appreciated by the coarsened trabeculae and remodeled cortices. AP view of the distal femur (**D**) demonstrates the distal extent of the disease and a previous united diaphyseal femur fracture. Postoperative AP radiograph of the pelvis (**E**), AP (**F**), and cross-table lateral (**G**) views of the right hip, and an AP view of the distal femur (**H**) demonstrate the cemented THA that was placed for reconstruction. A cemented all-polyethylene acetabular cup and a long cemented femoral implant were placed to address the femoral neck nonunion and underlying bone quality associated with Paget disease. Femoral canal preparation required the use of multiple flexible reamers, a high-speed burr, and conical reamers.

proper preparation of the proximal femur as well as position and fit of the trial components. Simultaneous or staged osteotomy may also be necessary to address any varus deformity that compromises femoral implant placement.

Cemented THA has been traditionally used in patients with Paget disease of bone; however, recently reported midterm to long-term results of cementless components demonstrate satisfactory outcomes.[71] In a 2014 study, results were reported for 14 cementless

THAs in 11 patients who have a mean follow-up of 12.3 years (range, 10 to 17 years).[72] The survival rate at 10-year follow-up for both cup and stem was 86% using revision for any cause as the end point and was 95.5% using aseptic loosening as the end point. However, postoperative heterotopic ossification is also common in these patients, with a reported incidence as high as 56%. Postoperative radiation or chemoprophylaxis should be considered for patients undergoing THA in the setting of Paget disease of bone to prevent heterotopic bone formation. A recent review article that included eight studies and 358 THAs in patients who have Paget disease found that aseptic loosening was the most common reason for revision (5% rate at a mean of 8.6 years).[73]

THA in Renal Osteodystrophy

Chronic kidney disease can lead to an alteration in calcium and phosphate regulation that translates into a deficiency in bone mineralization resulting in renal osteodystrophy. Two forms of renal osteodystrophy have been described: high-turnover renal osteodystrophy and low-turnover renal osteodystrophy. High-turnover renal osteodystrophy is the classic form of this disease and is characterized by an increase in parathyroid hormone secretion, parathyroid gland hyperplasia, increased osteoblast and osteoclast activity, maintenance of high bone turnover, and ultimately osteitis fibrosa cystica. Low-turnover renal osteodystrophy develops following the improved management of renal disease, such as appropriate dialysis. Parathyroid hormone levels are normal with low bone formation and unmineralized bone formation is not increased. Bone density is typically reduced in renal osteodystrophy and adult patients present with bone pain, muscle weakness, skeletal deformity, and heterotopic calcification. Furthermore, with the use of corticosteroids to treat chronic renal disease or for the prevention of renal transplant rejection, osteopenia and osteonecrosis are common in this patient population.

THA for patients who have renal osteodystrophy is usually for management of osteonecrosis or osteoarthritis. In one study, a five to eight times higher incidence of THA was identified in patients following renal transplantation compared with the general population, and osteonecrosis was the most frequent reason for THA (72% of cases).[4,74] Hip replacement surgery in this population requires a multidisciplinary approach, including anesthesia, nephrology, and possibly transplant services (in the setting of renal transplantation) for proper preoperative optimization and postoperative care. Careful preoperative planning and templating are necessary to address any bony malalignment and weakness. Radiographs of the entire femur are helpful to fully appreciate the overall alignment and bone quality. Templating is needed to help choose the appropriate femoral implant that can accommodate the proximal femur. In the face of severely compromised bone density, cemented implants should be considered to avoid intraoperative iatrogenic fractures. Patients who have renal osteodystrophy also present for THA at a younger age, which makes it important to contemplate alternative bearing surfaces for their improved wear rates.

Postoperative care for these patients requires avoidance of perioperative medical complications, such as further kidney injury. Proper postoperative hydration is critical as is the adjustment, cessation, or prevention of the use of any renal toxic agents such as NSAIDs or angiotensin-converting enzyme inhibitors.

Contemporary studies examining the outcomes of THA in patients who have chronic renal disease demonstrate a high postoperative complication rate, including mortality, especially among patients who are dialysis dependent.[75-77] A 2016 study compared the complications and mortality between patients who have chronic renal failure and patients who had a history of renal transplantation who underwent either THA or total knee arthroplasty.[75] These patients were shown to have a statistically significant increase in postoperative complications such as surgical site infections, wound complications, transfusions, deep vein thrombosis, and mortality compared with patients without kidney disease. Furthermore, patients on dialysis had increased rates of surgical site infections, wound complications, transfusions, and mortality compared with patients who had undergone renal transplant. Therefore, some authors have advocated delaying joint arthroplasty surgery until after renal transplantation has taken place.[76] A 2014 study examined the outcomes of hip and knee total joint arthroplasty in patients who have various solid organ transplants.[78] In 97% of patients who underwent THA after a renal transplant, outcomes were good to excellent at a mean follow-up of 35 months. This same cohort had a 28% rate of perioperative medical complications and an 8% revision surgery rate for periprosthetic fractures alone.

THA IN PATIENTS WHO HAVE SPINAL PATHOLOGY

There is a growing body of research demonstrating an increased risk of dislocation in patients who have decreased spinopelvic motion, secondary to either degenerative disease of the lumbar spine or previous spinal fusion[79,80] (**Figure 20**). The increased understanding of the dynamic relationship between hip, pelvis, and spine motion has challenged the classic teaching of positioning the acetabular implant within the safe

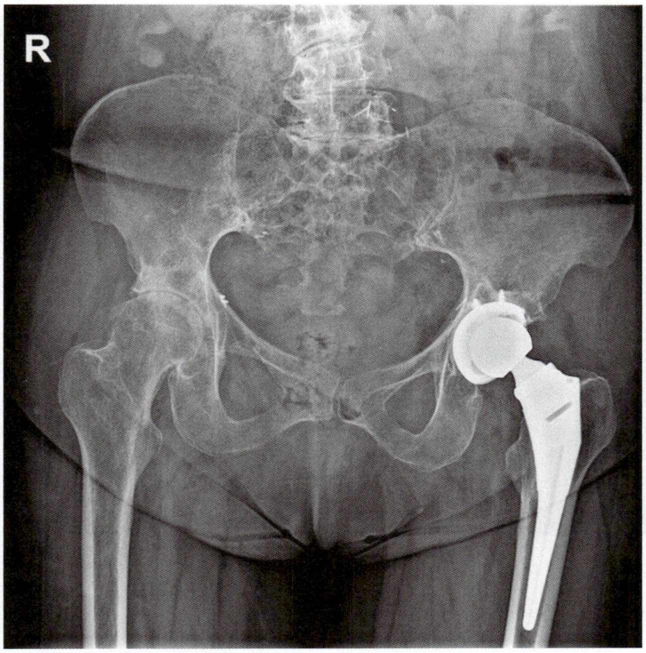

FIGURE 20 Preoperative AP radiograph of a patient who has severe lumbar degenerative disease and deformity. The left total hip arthroplasty was performed elsewhere.

zone of Lewinnek between 15° ± 10° of abduction and 40° ± 10° of inclination.[81,82] In patients who have a known history of spinal fusion, or significant degeneration that can be appreciated on the AP pelvis radiograph, obtaining lateral radiographs of the pelvis in both the seated and the standing position will help to further delineate the spinopelvic pathology present.

A recent study presented a simplified algorithm for treating patients who have spinopelvic pathology.[79] For patients who have normal alignment on the lateral radiograph, as defined by the anterior pelvic plane oriented such that the anterior superior iliac spine is posterior to the pubic symphysis (**Figure 21**), but with a stiff spine, as defined as less than 10° of change in lordosis from sitting to standing, adding additional anteversion to the acetabular implant for a target of 25° to 30° can prevent dislocation. In these patients, the stiff spine prevents the functional posterior pelvic tilting that normally occurs when sitting, putting them at risk for posterior dislocation in this position and making them ideal candidates for slight overanteversion of the acetabular implant at surgery. Patients who stand with excessive posterior pelvic tilt increase their functional anteversion in the standing position, and thus, the functional anteversion

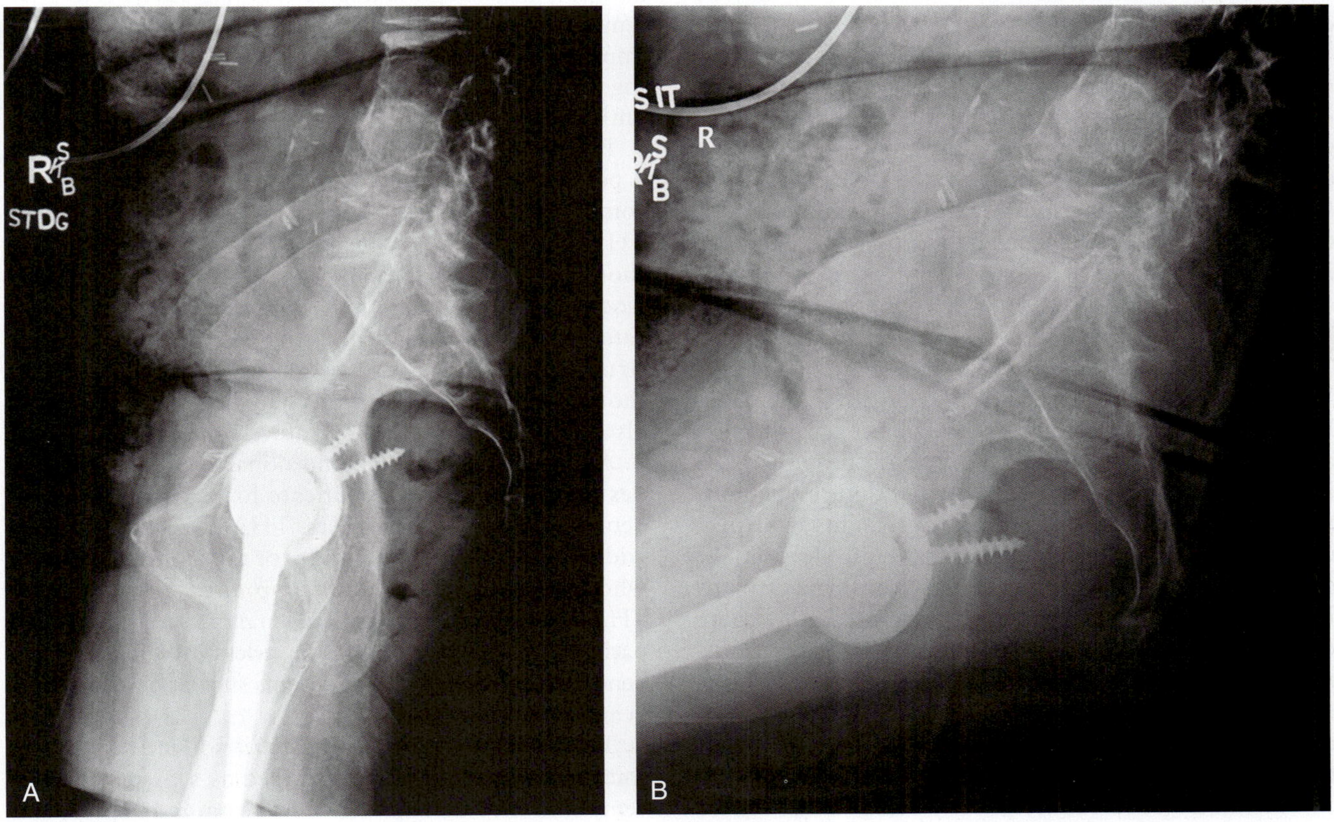

FIGURE 21 Sitting (**A**) and weight-bearing (**B**) lateral radiographs of the pelvis and lumbar spine demonstrating the fixed lumbar deformity.

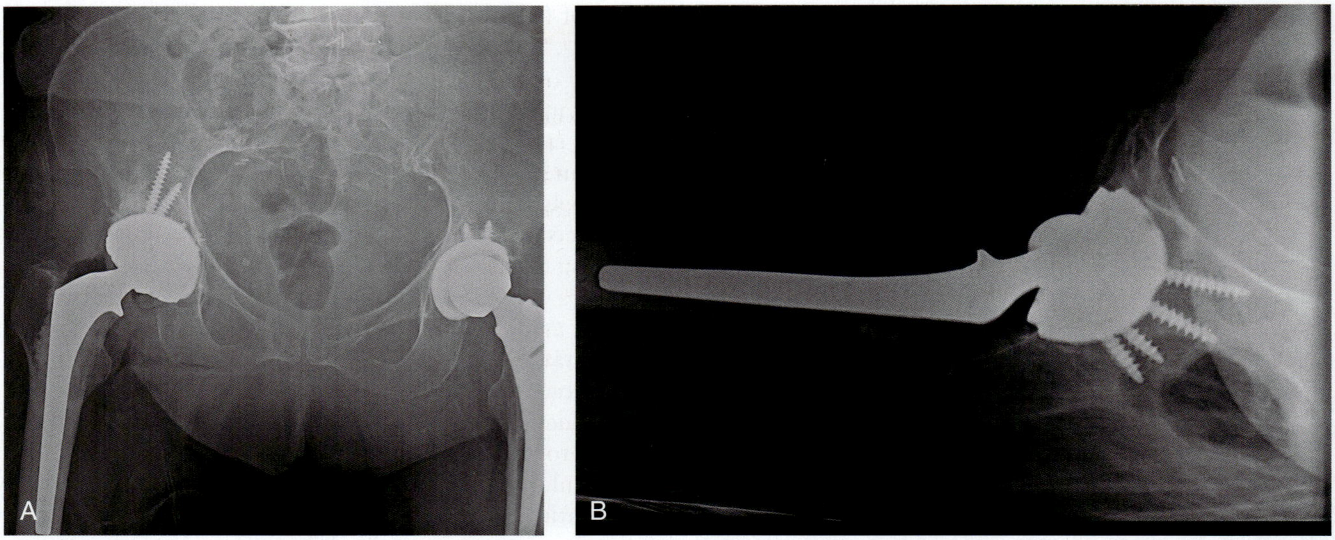

FIGURE 22 Postoperative AP (**A**) and lateral (**B**) radiographs demonstrating the right total hip arthroplasty using a dual-mobility implant.

of the acetabular implant is increased. In such patients, overanteverting the acetabular implant may increase the risk of anterior dislocation, and dual-mobility may be considered (**Figure 22**).

Although this is a developing area of research and concrete recommendations are yet to develop, surgeons should consider obtaining sitting and standing radiographs in patients who have lumbar spine pathology and consider surgical techniques to prevent dislocation in such patients, including adding additional femoral offset, increasing head size, or converting to a dual-mobility implant.

SUMMARY

Various conditions render THA technically challenging. However, favorable outcomes are possible if key principles are followed, including understanding of the pathophysiology and pathoanatomy of the condition, meticulous preoperative planning to ensure the availability of all necessary implants and instruments to execute the primary surgical plan, and having one or more contingency plans if needed. Adequate exposure is imperative. A variety of femoral and acetabular implant designs are available to achieve initial and lasting fixation, navigate deformities, approximate normal leg length and offset, optimize abductor function, and maximize stability against dislocation.

THA in DDH can be technically demanding because of acetabular bone stock deficiency and excessive femoral anteversion. In some cases, high acetabular fixation is possible. In other cases, augmentation with structural allograft or a metallic augment is necessary. Excessive femoral anteversion may require a conical or modular implant. The need for and ability to perform a shortening osteotomy, with or without derotation, should be anticipated.

Prior trauma or corrective osteotomy may result in a proximal femoral deformity, which may be further complicated by retained hardware, which interferes with THA and leaves significant stress risers on removal. There should be a low threshold for performing an extended trochanteric osteotomy to facilitate hardware removal, canal preparation, and corrective osteotomy, and apply structural allograft if necessary. The femoral implant should be of sufficient length to bypass stress risers and also allow for correction of anteversion.

Although conservative and nonarthroplasty modalities remain the mainstays of care for patients who have neuromuscular hip disorders, THA is becoming more widely accepted as appropriate for the ambulatory adult who has painful degenerative hip disease. Constrained THA designs must be considered in more severely affected patients, whereas those who have less involvement may benefit from newer implant designs such as dual-mobility bearings.

THA for posttraumatic arthritis after acetabular fracture is increasingly considered as a primary intervention in the elderly patient who sustains an acetabular fracture and articular impaction injury after low-energy trauma. ORIF is still commonly performed in younger patients after high-energy trauma. Technical challenges of late or secondary THA include bony deformity, prior infection, retained hardware, limb shortening, sciatic nerve palsy, abductor deficiency, and heterotopic bone formation. Favorable results are generally achieved with careful preoperative planning, removal of intra-articular hardware, identification of the sciatic nerve, bone grafting or augmentation of acetabular defects, use of a hemispheric cup or cage, and perioperative radiation therapy or NSAIDs if heterotopic bone excision is required.

Metabolic bone disease comprises a heterogeneous group of conditions. Adherence to the principles of THA is essential; equally important is close collaboration with appropriate medical consultants. The metabolic, endocrine, and renal abnormalities that accompany these conditions are generally outside the expertise of experienced hip surgeons. If possible, THA is deferred until bone quality is optimized and bone turnover minimized. Cement fixation is considered in the face of significant osteopenia.

Regardless of the type of treatment chosen, it is essential to define the goals of treatment: pain relief, optimizing function, and improving care of these challenging and often severely debilitated individuals.

KEY STUDY POINTS

- Meticulous preoperative planning with consideration of physical findings, plain radiographs, and advanced imaging is critical. The need for selective retained hardware is anticipated.
- Adequate exposure is mandatory. Extensile exposure including trochanteric osteotomy/extended trochanteric osteotomy may be required.
- Various femoral implant designs and fixation philosophies are optimum in different situations. One should be experienced in the use of cemented stems, cementless primary components, conical monoblock stems, modular stems including those with distal tapers, and extensively porous coated cylindrical stems.
- When stability against dislocation is of particular concern, jumbo heads, dual-mobility constructs, and constrained components should be considered.
- Close collaboration with medical consultants is important in the management of patients with neuromuscular disease and metabolic bone disease.

ANNOTATED REFERENCES

1. Sakellariou VI, Christodoulou M, Sasalos G, Babis GC: Reconstruction of the acetabulum in developmental dysplasia of the hip in total hip replacement. *Arch Bone Joint Surg* 2014;2(3):130-136.

2. Greber EM, Pelt CE, Gililland JM, Anderson MB, Erickson JA, Peters CL: Challenges in total hip arthroplasty in the setting of developmental dysplasia of the hip. *J Arthroplasty* 2017;32(9):S38-S44.

   This review article outlines the challenges of treating dysplastic hips with THA. Level of evidence: III.

3. Yoshitani J, Kabata T, Kajino Y, et al: Morphometric geometrical analysis to determine the centre of the acetabular component placement in Crowe type IV hips undergoing total hip arthroplasty. *Bone Joint J* 2019;101-B(2): 189-197.

   This was a retrospective study comparing 52 Crowe IV hips with 50 nondysplastic hips undergoing THA that used CT to describe the native acetabulum. They found that Crowe IV hips are triangular and that the ideal position of the acetabular component is superior on the posterior bony wall. Level of evidence: III.

4. Yang Y, Zuo J, Liu T, Xiao J, Liu S, Gao Z: Morphological analysis of true acetabulum in hip dysplasia (Crowe classes I-IV) via 3-D implantation simulation. *J Bone Joint Surg Am* 2017;99(17):e92.

   This study compared dysplastic hips with normal hips with three-dimensional implantation simulation. The mean medial wall was most thick in Crowe II and III hips compared with Crowe I and IV hips, and segmental bone deficiency was most prevalent in Crowe II and III hips. Level of evidence: III.

5. Dapuzzo MR, Sierra RJ: Acetabular considerations during total hip arthroplasty for hip dysplasia. *Orthop Clin North Am* 2012;43(3):369-375.

6. Wu X, Li SH, Lou LM, Cai ZD: The techniques of soft tissue release and true socket reconstruction in total hip arthroplasty for patients with severe developmental dysplasia of the hip. *Int Orthop* 2012;36(9):1795-1801.

7. Li H, Mao Y, Oni JK, Dai K, Zhu Z: Total hip replacement for developmental dysplasia of the hip with more than 30% lateral uncoverage of uncemented acetabular components. *Bone Joint J* 2013;95-B(9):1178-1183.

8. Maruyama M, Wakabayashi S, Ota H, Tensho K: Reconstruction of the shallow acetabulum with a combination of autologous bulk and impaction bone grafting fixed by cement. *Clin Orthop Relat Res* 2017;475(2):387-395.

   This study described a bone grafting method used in 102 THAs in DDH patients with shallow acetabulum. The author used bulk bone grafting from the resected femoral head combined with morselized bone graft with a medial-reduced cemented acetabular component. Level of evidence: IV.

9. Zahar A, Papik K, Lakatos J, Cross MB: Total hip arthroplasty with acetabular reconstruction using a bulk autograft for patients with developmental dysplasia of the hip results in high loosening rates at mid-term follow-up. *Int Orthop* 2014;38(5):947-951.

10. Fukui K, Kaneuji A, Sugimori T, Ichiseki T, Matsumoto T: Does rotational acetabular osteotomy affect subsequent total hip arthroplasty? *Arch Orthop Trauma Surg* 2015;135(3):407-415.

11. Kaneuji A, Sugimori T, Ichiseki T, Yamada K, Fukui K, Matsumoto T: Minimum ten-year results of a porous acetabular component for Crowe I to III hip dysplasia using an elevated hip center. *J Arthroplasty* 2009;24(2):187-194.

12. Stans AA, Pagnano MW, Shaughnessy WJ, Hanssen AD: Results of total hip arthroplasty for Crowe Type III developmental hip dysplasia. *Clin Orthop Relat Res* 1998;348:149-157. Available at: http://www.ncbi.nlm.nih.gov/pubmed/9553547. Accessed February 10, 2020.

13. Çatma MF, Ünlü S, Öztürk A, Aksekili AM, Ersan Ö, Ateş Y: Femoral shortening osteotomy in total hip arthroplasty for severe dysplasia: A comparison of two fixation techniques. *Int Orthop* 2016;40(11):2271-2276.

14. Liu R, Li Y, Bai C, Song Q, Wang K: Effect of preoperative limb-length discrepancy on abductor strength after total hip arthroplasty in patients with developmental dysplasia of the hip. *Arch Orthop Trauma Surg* 2014;134(1):113-119.

15. Kaneuji A, Sugimori T, Ichiseki T, Fukui K, Takahashi E, Matsumoto T: Cementless anatomic total hip femoral component with circumferential porous coating for hips with developmental dysplasia: A minimum ten-year follow-up period. *J Arthroplasty* 2013;28(10):1746-1750.

16. Tamegai H, Otani T, Fujii H, Kawaguchi Y, Hayama T, Marumo K: A modified S-ROM stem in primary total hip arthroplasty for developmental dysplasia of the hip. *J Arthroplasty* 2013;28(10):1741-1745.

17. Imbuldeniya AM, Walter WL, Zicat BA, Walter WK: Cementless total hip replacement without femoral osteotomy in patients with severe developmental dysplasia of the hip: Minimum 15-year clinical and radiological results. *Bone Joint J* 2014;96-B(11):1449-1454.

18. Parvizi J, Burmeister H, Ganz R: Previous Bernese periacetabular osteotomy does not compromise the results of total hip arthroplasty. *Clin Orthop Relat Res* 2004;423:118-122.

19. Amanatullah DF, Stryker L, Schoenecker P, et al: Similar clinical outcomes for THAs with and without prior periacetabular osteotomy. *Clin Orthop Relat Res* 2015;473(2):685-691.

20. Osawa Y, Hasegawa Y, Seki T, Takegami Y, Amano T, Ishiguro N: Patient-reported outcomes in patients who undergo total hip arthroplasty after periacetabular osteotomy. *J Orthop Sci* 2018;23(2):346-349.

This case-control study compared 29 THAs for patients who had previously undergone PAOs with THAs in patients who had not undergone PAOs that were matched by age, sex, and Crowe classification. The previous PAO group reported worse Harris hip scores for gait and activity at the last follow-up. Level of evidence: III.

21. Yildirim T, Guclu B, Karaguven D, Kaya A, Akan B, Cetin I: Cementless total hip arthroplasty in developmental dysplasia of the hip with end stage osteoarthritis: 2-7 years' clinical results. *Hip Int* 2015;25(5):442-446.

22. Ollivier M, Abdel MP, Krych AJ, Trousdale RT, Berry DJ: Long-term results of total hip arthroplasty with shortening subtrochanteric osteotomy in Crowe IV developmental dysplasia. *J Arthroplasty* 2016;31(8):1756-1760.

23. Boyle MJ, Frampton CMA, Crawford HA: Early results of total hip arthroplasty in patients with developmental dysplasia of the hip compared with patients with osteoarthritis. *J Arthroplasty* 2012;27(3):386-390.

24. Hitz OF, Flecher X, Parratte S, Ollivier M, Argenson JN: Minimum 10-year outcome of one-stage total hip arthroplasty without subtrochanteric osteotomy using a cementless custom stem for Crowe III and IV hip dislocation. *J Arthroplasty* 2018;33(7):2197-2202.

This study reported 10-year outcome of THA in Crowe III and IV hips without subtrochanteric osteotomy using a custom cementless stem that matched patients' intramedullary fit as well as offset. They reported 87.5% survival free from aseptic loosening at 15 years. Level of evidence: IV.

25. Boyle MJ, Singleton N, Frampton CMA, Muir D: Functional response to total hip arthroplasty in patients with hip dysplasia. *ANZ J Surg* 2013;83(7-8):554-558.

26. Engesæter LB, Furnes O, Havelin LI: Developmental dysplasia of the hip – Good results of later total hip arthroplasty. 7135 primary total hip arthroplasties after developmental dysplasia of the hip compared with 59774 total hip arthroplasties in idiopathic coxarthrosis followed for 0 to 15 years in the Norwegian Arthroplasty Register. *J Arthroplasty* 2008;23(2):235-240.

27. Roberts KC, Brox WT, Jevsevar DS, Sevarino K: Management of hip fractures in the elderly. *J Am Acad Orthop Surg* 2015;23(2):131-137.

28. Berry DJ: Total hip arthroplasty in patients with proximal femoral deformity. *Clin Orthop Relat Res* 1999;369:262-272.

29. Lazennec JY, Rousseau MA, Rangel A, et al: Pelvis and total hip arthroplasty acetabular component orientations in sitting and standing positions: Measurements reproductibility with EOS imaging system versus conventional radiographies. *Orthop Traumatol Surg Res* 2011;97(4):373-380.

30. Folinais D, Thelen P, Delin C, Radier C, Catonne Y, Lazennec JY: Measuring femoral and rotational alignment: EOS system versus computed tomography. *Orthop Traumatol Surg Res* 2013;99(5):509-516.

31. Buck FM, Guggenberger R, Koch PP, Pfirrmann CWA: Femoral and tibial torsion measurements with 3D models based on low-dose biplanar radiographs in comparison with standard CT measurements. *Am J Roentgenol* 2012;199(5):W607-W612.

32. Journé A, Sadaka J, Bélicourt C, Sautet A: New method for measuring acetabular component positioning with EOS imaging: Feasibility study on dry bone. *Int Orthop* 2012;36(11):2205-2209.

33. Mortazavi SMJ, Restrepo C, Kim PJW, Parvizi J, Hozack WJ: Cementless femoral reconstruction in patients with proximal femoral deformity. *J Arthroplasty* 2011;26(3): 354-359.

34. Kang JS, Moon KH, Kim RS, Park SR, Lee JS, Shin SH: Total hip arthroplasty using S-ROM prosthesis for dysplastic hip. *Yonsei Med J* 2011;52(4):655-660.

35. Archibeck MJ, Carothers JT, Tripuraneni KR, White RE: Total hip arthroplasty after failed internal fixation of proximal femoral fractures. *J Arthroplasty* 2013;28(1): 168-171.

36. Petrie J, Sassoon A, Haidukewych GJ: When femoral fracture fixation fails: Salvage options. *Bone Joint J* 2013;95-B(11): 7-10.

37. DeHaan AM, Groat T, Priddy M, et al: Salvage hip arthroplasty after failed fixation of proximal femur fractures. *J Arthroplasty* 2013;28(5):855-859.

38. Bercik MJ, Miller AG, Muffly M, Parvizi J, Orozco F, Ong A: Conversion total hip arthroplasty. A reason not to use cephalomedullary nails. *J Arthroplasty* 2012;27:117-121.

39. Chu X, Liu F, Huang J, Chen L, Li J, Tong P: Good short-term outcome of arthroplasty with Wagner SL implants for unstable intertrochanteric osteoporotic fractures. *J Arthroplasty* 2014;29(3):605-608.

40. Abouelela AAKH: Salvage of failed trochanteric fracture fixation using the Revitan curved cementless modular hip arthroplasty. *J Arthroplasty* 2012;27(7):1382-1388.

41. Shi X, Zhou Z, Yang J, Shen B, Kang P, Pei F: Total hip arthroplasty using non-modular cementless long-stem distal fixation for salvage of failed internal fixation of intertrochanteric fracture. *J Arthroplasty* 2015;30(11):1999-2003.

42. Reikerås O, Haaland JE, Lereim P: Femoral shortening in total hip arthroplasty for high developmental dysplasia of the hip. *Clin Orthop Relat Res* 2010;468(7):1949-1955.

43. Yuan BJ, Abdel MP, Cross WW, Berry DJ: Hip arthroplasty after surgical treatment of intertrochanteric hip fractures. *J Arthroplasty* 2017;32(11):3438-3444.

    This retrospective review study evaluated 111 patients who converted to THA after a previous intertrochanteric fracture managed with either an extramedullary device or an intramedullary device. They found that risk of intraoperative femoral fracture was higher in patients who had an intramedullary device to manage their fracture. Level of evidence: III.

44. Kosashvili Y, Taylor D, Backstein D, et al: Total hip arthroplasty in patients with Down's syndrome. *Int Orthop* 2011;35(5):661-666. Available at: https://pubmed.ncbi.nlm.nih.gov/?term=Kosashvili+Y%2C+Taylor+D%2C+Backstein+D%2C+et+al%3A+Total+hip+arthroplasty+in+patients+with+Down%27s+syndrome.+. Accessed February 13, 2020.

45. Osagie L, Figgie M, Bostrom M: Custom total hip arthroplasty in skeletal dysplasia. *Int Orthop* 2012;36(3): 527-531.

46. Boyce AM, Kelly MH, Brillante BA, et al: A randomized, double blind, placebo-controlled trial of alendronate treatment for fibrous dysplasia of bone. *J Clin Endocrinol Metab* 2014;99(11):4133-4140.

47. Johnson JT: Neuropathic fractures and joint injuries. Pathogenesis and rationale of prevention and treatment. *J Bone Joint Surg Am* 1967;49(1):1-30. Available at: http://www.ncbi.nlm.nih.gov/pubmed/4163089. Accessed February 13, 2020.

48. Berend ME, Ritter MA, Meding JB, Faris PM, Keating EM, Pierce A: Clinical results of isolated tibial component revisions with femoral component retention. *J Arthroplasty* 2008;23(1):61-64.

49. Robb JE, Rymaszewski LA, Reeves BF, Lacey CJ: Total hip replacement in a Charcot joint: Brief report. *J Bone Joint Surg Br* 1988;70(3):489. Available at: http://www.ncbi.nlm.nih.gov/pubmed/3372580. Accessed February 13, 2020.

50. Chalmers BP, Tibbo ME, Trousdale RT, Lewallen DG, Berry DJ, Abdel MP: Primary total hip arthroplasty for Charcot arthropathy is associated with high complications but improved clinical outcomes. *J Arthroplasty* 2018;33(9): 2912-2918.

    This case series included 12 primary THAs for Charcot arthropathy in 11 patients and found that 75% were free from any revision at 5-year follow-up, but the overall complication rate was high, 58%. The complications included three recurrent dislocations, two periprosthetic fractures, one femoral component loosening, and one delayed wound healing. Level of evidence: IV.

51. Gausden EB, Parhar HS, Popper JE, Sculco PK, Rush BNM: Risk factors for early dislocation following primary elective total hip arthroplasty. *J Arthroplasty* 2018;33(5):1567-1571.e2.

    Researchers used the National Readmissions Database to determine risk factors for patients who dislocated in the first 90 days following THA. Parkinson disease was a strong independent risk factor for dislocation. Level of evidence: IV.

52. Makridis KG, Obakponovwe O, Bobak P, Giannoudis PV: Total hip arthroplasty after acetabular fracture. Incidence of complications, reoperation rates and functional outcomes: Evidence today. *J Arthroplasty* 2014;29(10): 1983-1990.

53. Lai O, Yang J, Shen B, Zhou Z, Kang P, Pei F: Midterm results of uncemented acetabular reconstruction for posttraumatic arthritis secondary to acetabular fracture. *J Arthroplasty* 2011;26(7):1008-1013.

54. Zhang L, Zhou Y, Li Y, Xu H, Guo X, Zhou Y: Total hip arthroplasty for failed treatment of acetabular fractures. A 5-year follow-up study. *J Arthroplasty* 2011;26(8): 1189-1193.

55. Baghdadi YMK, Larson AN, Sierra RJ: Restoration of the hip center during THA performed for protrusio acetabuli is associated with better implant survival. *Clin Orthop Relat Res* 2013;471(10):3251-3259.

56. Morison Z, Moojen DJF, Nauth A, et al: Total hip arthroplasty after acetabular fracture is associated with lower survivorship and more complications. *Clin Orthop Relat Res* 2016;474(2):392-398.

57. Labuda A, Papaioannou A, Pritchard J, Kennedy C, DeBeer J, Adachi JD: Prevalence of osteoporosis in osteoarthritic patients undergoing total hip or total knee arthroplasty. *Arch Phys Med Rehabil* 2008;89(12):2373-2374.

58. Jauregui JJ, Clayton A, Kapadia BH, Cherian JJ, Issa K, Mont MA: Total hip arthroplasty for acute acetabular fractures: A review of the literature. *Expert Rev Med Devices* 2015;12(3):287-295.

59. Miller BJ, Callaghan JJ, Cram P, Karam M, Marsh JL, Noiseux NO: Changing trends in the treatment of femoral neck fractures: A review of the American Board of Orthopaedic Surgery database. *J Bone Joint Surg Am* 2014;96(17):e149.

60. Kim YH, Park JW, Kim JS: Is diaphyseal stem fixation necessary for primary total hip arthroplasty in patients with osteoporotic bone (Class C bone)? *J Arthroplasty* 2013;28(1):139-146.e1.

61. Patel RM, Smith MC, Woodward CC, Stulberg SD: Stable fixation of short-stem femoral implants in patients 70 years and older. *Clin Orthop Relat Res* 2012;470:442-449.

62. Rhyu KH, Lee SM, Chun YS, Kim KI, Cho YJ, Yoo MC: Does osteoporosis increase early subsidence of cementless double-tapered femoral stem in hip arthroplasty? *J Arthroplasty* 2012;27(7):1305-1309.

63. Abdel MP, Watts CD, Houdek MT, Lewallen DG, Berry DJ: Epidemiology of periprosthetic fracture of the femur in 32 644 primary total hip arthroplasties: A 40-year experience. *Bone Joint J* 2016;98B(4):461-467.

64. Sierra RJ, Timperley JA, Gie GA: Contemporary cementing technique and mortality during and after Exeter total hip arthroplasty. *J Arthroplasty* 2009;24(3):325-332.

65. Benum P, Aamodt A, Nordsletten L: Customised femoral stems in osteopetrosis and the development of a guiding system for the preparation of an intramedullary cavity: A report of two cases. *J Bone Joint Surg Br* 2010;92(9): 1303-1305.

66. Egawa H, Nakano S, Hamada D, Sato R, Yasui N: Total hip arthroplasty in osteopetrosis using computer-assisted fluoroscopic navigation. *J Arthroplasty* 2005;20(8):1074-1077.

67. Ramiah RD, Baker RP, Bannister GC: Conversion of failed proximal femoral internal fixation to total hip arthroplasty in osteopetrotic bone. *J Arthroplasty* 2006;21(8): 1200-1202.

68. Strickland JP, Berry DJ: Total joint arthroplasty in patients with osteopetrosis: A report of 5 cases and review of the literature. *J Arthroplasty* 2005;20(6):815-820.

69. Delmas PD, Meunier PJ: The management of Paget's disease of bone. *N Engl J Med* 1997;336(8):558-566.

70. Lewallen DG: Hip arthroplasty in patients with Paget's disease. *Clin Orthop Relat Res* 1999;369:243-250.

71. Tudor F, Ariamanesh A, Potty A, Hashemi-Nejad A: Resurfacing hip arthroplasty in neuromuscular hip disorders – A retrospective case series. *J Orthop* 2013;10(3): 105-110.

72. Imbuldeniya AM, Tai SM, Aboelmagd T, Walter WL, Walter WK, Zicat BA: Cementless hip arthroplasty in Paget's disease at long-term follow-up (average of 12.3 years). *J Arthroplasty* 2014;29(5):1063-1066.

73. Hanna SA, Dawson-Bowling S, Millington S, Bhumbra R, Achan P: Total hip arthroplasty in patients with Paget's disease of bone: A systematic review. *World J Orthop* 2017;8(4):357-363.

The authors review the current trends in THA in patients with Paget disease of bone. Level of evidence: III.

74. Bucci JR, Oglesby RJ, Agodoa LY, Abbott KC: Hospitalizations for total hip arthroplasty after renal transplantation in the United States. *Am J Transplant* 2002;2(10):999-1004.

75. Cavanaugh PK, Chen AF, Rasouli MR, Post ZD, Orozco FR, Ong AC: Complications and mortality in chronic renal failure patients undergoing total joint arthroplasty: A comparison between dialysis and renal transplant patients. *J Arthroplasty* 2016;31(2):465-472.

76. Ponnusamy KE, Jain A, Thakkar SC, Sterling RS, Skolasky RL, Khanuja HS: Inpatient mortality and morbidity for dialysis-dependent patients undergoing primary total hip or knee arthroplasty. *J Bone Joint Surg Am* 2015;97(16): 1326-1332.

77. Warth LC, Pugely AJ, Martin CT, Gao Y, Callaghan JJ: Total joint arthroplasty in patients with chronic renal disease: Is it worth the risk? *J Arthroplasty* 2015;30(9):51-54.

78. Ledford CK, Watters TS, Wellman SS, Attarian DE, Bolognesi MP: Risk versus reward: Total joint arthroplasty outcomes after various solid organ transplantations. *J Arthroplasty* 2014;29(8):1548-1552.

79. Luthringer TA, Vigdorchik JM: A preoperative workup of a "hip-spine" total hip arthroplasty patient: A simplified approach to a complex problem. *J Arthroplasty* 2019;34(7S):S57-S70.

The authors review the body of evidence on performing THA in patients with spinal deformity, lumbar fusion, and abnormal spinopelvic mobility and provide simplified recommendations for component positioning based on spinopelvic parameters. Level of evidence: V.

80. Esposito CI, Carroll KM, Sculco PK, Padgett DE, Jerabek SA, Mayman DJ: Total hip arthroplasty patients with fixed spinopelvic alignment are at higher risk of hip dislocation. *J Arthroplasty* 2018;33(5):1449-1454.

This was a consecutive series of 1,000 patients who underwent lateral sitting and standing radiographs 1 year following THA and found that patients who dislocated had less spine flexion, less change in pelvic tilt, and more hip flexion from standing to sitting positions compared with patients with normal spines. Level of evidence: IV.

81. Lewinnek GE, Lewis JL, Tarr R, et al: Dislocations after total arthroplasties. *J Bone Joint Surg Am* 1978;60(2): 217-220.

82. Abdel MP, von Roth P, Jennings MT, Hanssen AD, Pagnano MW: What safe zone? The vast majority of dislocated THAs are within the Lewinnek safe zone for acetabular component position. *Clin Orthop Relat Res* 2016;474(2): 386-391.

Section 3: Hip

Dual-Mobility Bearings and Large-Diameter Heads for Primary and Revision Total Hip Arthroplasty

DANIEL PINCUS, MD, PhD, FRCSC • CHRISTOPHER PEDNEAULT, MDCM, FRCSC
DONALD S. GARBUZ, MDCM, FRCSC

ABSTRACT

Dual-mobility bearings and large femoral heads (36 and 40 mm) were increasingly used during the last decade in primary and revision total hip arthroplasty to reduce the risk of dislocation. Highly cross-linked polyethylene is key for the safe use of both large heads (which require thinner liners) and dual-mobility bearings (which wear at multiple surfaces). Current literature suggests a small femoral head can either be upsized to a large one or converted to a dual-mobility construct at the time of revision with similar short-term outcomes. Future well-designed observational and randomized studies will be required to compare large heads and dual-mobility bearings in terms of reducing dislocation in both primary and revision settings. Wear with modern dual-mobility bearings and corrosion with modular dual-mobility cups are unexamined areas of concern that need close clinical monitoring and further study. There are also several unique technical considerations of dual-mobility bearings surgeons should be familiar with before using them in the primary or revision setting.

Dr. Garbuz or an immediate family member serves as a paid consultant to or is an employee of Canntab Therapeutics and Stryker and serves as a board member, owner, officer, or committee member of the Hip Society and the Mueller Foundation of North America. Neither of the following authors nor any immediate family member has received anything of value from or has stock or stock options held in a commercial company or institution related directly or indirectly to the subject of this chapter: Dr. Pincus and Dr. Pedneault.

Keywords: dual mobility; head size; large femoral heads; primary; revision; total hip arthroplasty

INTRODUCTION

Despite improvements in surgical technique and implant design, there are still patients who have an increased risk of instability following primary total hip arthroplasty (THA). These patients include those who have cognitive dysfunction, neuromuscular disorders, hip fractures, and spinopelvic fusion, among others.[1] The rate of dislocation following primary THA in these high-risk groups remains elevated at approximately 4.8% to 13%.[1] The etiology of dislocation in the revision scenario is multifactorial, but it is usually related to the extensile exposure required to perform revision surgery and bone/soft-tissue defects.[2] For these reasons, instability also continues to be a common complication following revision THA with an incidence of approximately 10%.[3-6]

For patients at high risk for instability in either the primary or revision setting, it is important to identify this increased risk and attempt to mitigate it. Constrained liners are ideally reserved for ingrown acetabular implants and/or cases of abductor dysfunction. Other implant options that may maximize stability include large femoral heads (considered those ≥36 mm) and dual-mobility bearings. Both constructs have been shown to reduce dislocation risk with a larger head-neck ratio and jump distance that increases stability. Both constructs were also made safer with the introduction of highly cross-linked polyethylene (HXPE). Although these techniques were increasingly used during the last decade, concerns persist about the long-term outcomes.

HISTORY

The first dual-mobility implant, the Novae©-1 (SERF, Décines, France), was developed by Gilles Bousquet in 1979.[7,8] The design was inspired by combining the concepts of Charnley's low-friction arthroplasty[9,10] with the McKee-Farrar[11] large-diameter heads. Although common in France since that time, given worries about wear at multiple surfaces, North American surgeons were reluctant to use dual-mobility bearings until HXPE was incorporated in the design. The latest (third-generation) dual-mobility implants incorporate HXPE and were approved for use in the United States by the FDA in 2009.[12-14]

These third-generation designs include a small-diameter femoral head captured by a HXPE liner that forms both a hard-on-soft bearing with the femoral head and a soft-on-hard bearing with the acetabular implant. The acetabular implant comprises a polished metal liner that is either incorporated into a monoblock cup or impacted inside a tapered porous-coated titanium shell that contains holes for screw fixation. The dual-mobility design improves stability, allowing for a greater arc of impingement-free range of motion. Motion of the HXPE liner occurs at the extremes of motion of the first bearing, which then causes the liner to mobilize, and the maximum range of motion is finally reached when the femoral stem contacts the acetabular implant (**Figure 1**). Dual-mobility implants also benefit from an increased effective head-neck ratio and jump distance where the large head (composed of the femoral ball and HXPE liner) requires a greater distance to travel before dislocation. This distance is equal to the combined radius of both implants (**Figure 2**).

Similarly, HXPE facilitated safer use of fixed-bearing large head sizes (considered those ≥36 mm) in both primary and revision arthroplasty through corresponding decreases in the acceptable thickness of acetabular liners. There have been increases in the average femoral head sizes with associated decreases in dislocation rates.[15] This practice is in contrast to the 28-mm heads that were most commonly implanted by North American surgeons before the 2000s and was based on classic studies of polyethylene gamma irradiated in air having higher linear wear at 22 mm and higher volumetric wear at 32 mm.[16] Because dislocation remains one of the most common complications following THA, particularly in the high-risk scenarios noted previously, larger femoral heads have been increasingly used for the same reasons as

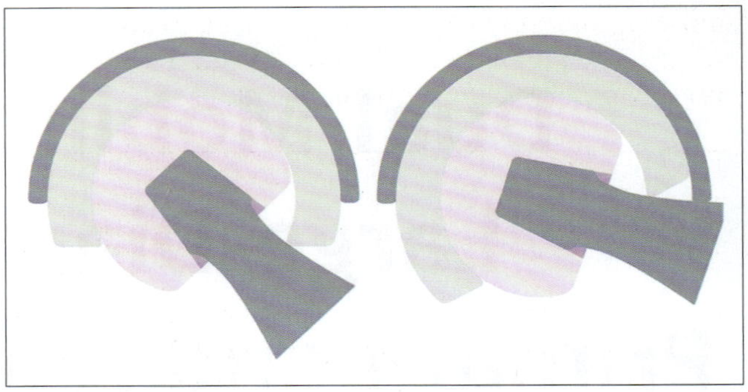

FIGURE 1 Illustration showing the greater arc of impingement-free range of motion with the dual-mobility design. The femoral stem only recruits the polyethylene liner at the extremes of motion of the first bearing, which then causes the liner to mobilize, and the maximum range of motion is finally reached when the femoral stem contacts the acetabular implant. (Republished with permission of British Editorial Society of Bone & Joint Surgery, from Darrith B, Courtney PM, Della Valle CJ: Outcomes of dual mobility components in total hip arthroplasty: A systematic review of the literature. *Bone Joint J* 2018;100B(1):11-19.)

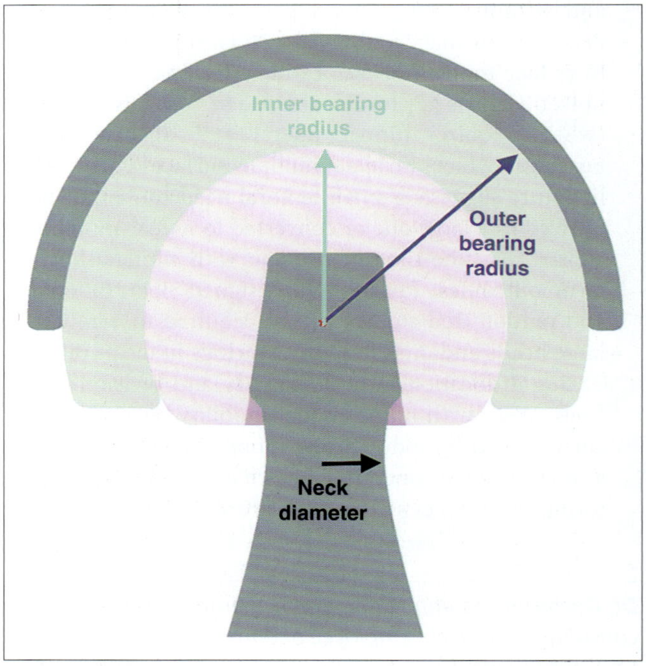

FIGURE 2 Illustration showing the increased head-neck ratio and jump distance where the large head that is composed of the femoral ball and polyethylene liner requires a greater distance to travel before dislocation—the combined radius of both implants. (Republished with permission of British Editorial Society of Bone & Joint Surgery, from Darrith B, Courtney PM, Della Valle CJ: Outcomes of dual mobility components in total hip arthroplasty: A systematic review of the literature. *Bone Joint J* 2018;100B(1):11-19.)

dual-mobility constructs: an increased head-to-neck ratio, an increased jump distance, and an increased range of motion before impingement.

REDUCING DISLOCATION IN PRIMARY THA: EVIDENCE FOR LARGE HEADS AND DUAL-MOBILITY BEARINGS

There is level I evidence that large heads reduce dislocation risk in the short term following primary THA. Well-designed observational studies also show similar findings over the medium-term and long-term irrespective of approach type.

A randomized trial of primary THA cases via a posterior approach found a five times lower rate of dislocation at 1 year for patients who have 36-mm femoral heads compared with 28-mm heads.[17] An observational study with a mean follow-up of 5 years also found improved stability for heads >32 mm versus 32 mm or smaller in THAs performed through a lateral approach.[18] Longer term population-based registry data from the Nordic Arthroplasty Register Association database including 186,231 metal-on-polyethylene primary THAs found the lowest adjusted dislocation risk with 36-mm heads compared with smaller heads.[19] For patients specifically considered at high risk for dislocation, there was an observational study of 501 primary THAs where a significant difference in dislocation rate (4.6% versus 0.5%) was found between patients who have 36- and >36-mm heads.[20]

There are no prospective or randomized studies to our knowledge that examine dual-mobility bearings in the primary setting. Available literature is mostly from case series but supports the use of dual-mobility implants to reduce the risk of dislocation in high-risk primary patients, while being cautious about the potential for higher wear. A total of 59 articles were included in a recent systematic review examining dual-mobility bearings in the primary setting.[21] The risk of dislocation was 0.9% out of 12,844 hips at a mean follow-up of 6.8 years. The risk of intraprosthetic dislocation (IPD) was 0.7%. The average age at time of surgery was 68.8 years. Of the series included in the systematic review, one including 2,480 THAs reported a 0.88% dislocation rate at an average of 7 years.[22] Another recent systematic review of dual-mobility constructs included studies with midterm follow-up (approximately 7 years) and supports the role of reducing the incidence of dislocation in the primary setting.[12]

Although dual-mobility may protect against dislocation, concerns persist about wear, IPD, and other complications unique to dual-mobility that would lead to revision surgery for reasons other than dislocation in the longer term. There is preliminary evidence for this in the available literature. For example, the overall 5-year revision rate in the 2015 Australian Orthopaedic Association National Joint Replacement Registry[23] of primary dual-mobility implants (which included 1,702 dual-mobility THAs) was 4.4% (compared with the 3.3% baseline). Similarly, a recent study from the Nordic Arthroplasty Register Association database of 2,277 propensity score–matched patients found that patients who have dual-mobility bearings had a lower risk of revision due to dislocation, but twice the risk of revision due to infection.[24] Because patients selected for dual-mobility implants in current practice are generally at higher risk for dislocation and potentially other complications, revision rates in these nonrandomized studies may be overestimated. Nevertheless, these observational data suggest concerns about using dual-mobility bearings liberally in the primary setting are not unfounded, particularly when used in young patients and/or outside of those considered at high risk for dislocation.

REDUCING DISLOCATION IN REVISION THA: EVIDENCE FOR LARGE HEADS AND DUAL-MOBILITY BEARINGS

Instability continues to be a common surgical complication (10% incidence) following revision THA.[3-6] Current available implant options to manage this risk include inserting a constrained liner in a well-fixed acetabular shell, large femoral heads, and dual-mobility prostheses.[25] Constrained liners can limit range of motion and experience mechanical failure, as well as develop aseptic loosening as a result of the higher forces being seen through the cup from the constraint, particularly if it is not yet ingrown. Consequently, large femoral heads and dual-mobility constructs recently gained in popularity in revision THA with a greater impingement-free range of motion and a larger head-neck ratio that equates to a greater jump distance before dislocation.

The etiology of dislocation in the revision scenario is multifactorial, but it is usually related to the extensile exposure, soft-tissue damage, and acetabular-femoral head size mismatch.[2] There is level I evidence that large heads reduce this risk in the revision setting. A randomized controlled trial from 2012 found a significantly lower rate of dislocation for patients who have 36- and 40-mm femoral heads (1%; 1 of 92 hips) compared with those with 32-mm heads (9%; 8 of 92 hips) at 5-year follow-up.[26] Another randomized controlled trial from 2012 found a 5% dislocation rate following revision THA with a 36-mm implant and 12% with a 28-mm implant, but the difference was not significant with the sample size available.[17] Longer term follow-up will be required to determine whether large femoral heads cause clinically meaningful accelerated wear and adverse local tissue reactions (ALTRs) (when a large cobalt-chromium [CoCr] head on a titanium stem is used).

Dual-mobility bearings are also increasingly being used in the revision setting to improve stability, particularly in cases where prior dislocation is the indication for revision. In a recent systematic review of nine retrospective studies, including six case series and three cohort studies, all-cause and aseptic survivorship rates, dislocation rates, complications, and clinical outcomes of dual-mobility bearings in revision THA were evaluated.[1] The all-cause survivorship and aseptic survivorship was 94.5% and 97.7%, respectively, at a mean follow-up of 31 months. IPD remains a unique risk for dual-mobility prostheses, where small femoral ball becomes dislodged from the polyethylene liner and requires mandatory revision. However, this risk was only 0.2%, occurring in 2 out of the 693 hips included in this study. The overall risk of dislocation was 2.2%, and when the authors analyzed three studies that directly compared dual-mobility prostheses with fixed-bearing prosthesis, there was a lower odds ratio of dislocation in the dual-mobility cohort (odds ratio = 0.24, 95% confidence interval = 0.10 to 0.59, $P = 0.002$). In addition, the risk of aseptic loosening is 0.7%, which can in part be explained by improvements in the design of the newest generation of dual-mobility prostheses. Modular technology allows the surgeons to directly visualize the dome contact of the shell to determine the possibility of proper seating and screw fixation. Cementless biologic fixation is also improved as many of the dual-mobility implants are coated with plasma-sprayed titanium with hydroxyapatite overlay, which may further reduce the chances of aseptic loosening. Overall, this systematic review demonstrated positive short-term results for the dual-mobility implants in the revision setting, especially in regard to the risk of dislocation. The limitations of this study are the short follow-up, small numbers, and retrospective nature. Another recent systematic review of dual mobility in the revision setting found the risk of dislocation was 3.0% out of 5,064 hips at a mean follow-up of 4.4 years and had the same limitations. The rate of IPD was 1.3%.[21] Individual studies in these reviews included one with 88 cemented dual-mobility liners during revision, which resulted in only one revision for recurrent dislocation at 5 years.[27] Another longer term study assessed 163 dual-mobility bearings with a dislocation rate of 4% at 12 years.[28]

Several studies have examined the role of dual mobility in revision cases where prior dislocation was the indication for revision. There were 228 THA revisions for instability from the Swedish Hip Replacement Registry that used dual mobility. Re-revision for dislocation was only 2% at 2 years.[29] A smaller study of 24 revision THAs using dual-mobility bearings for instability found no recurrent dislocations at 2 years.[30] In terms of longer term follow-up, a series of 51 patients who have cemented dual-mobility bearings for instability found 86% did not re-dislocate by 10 years.[31,32]

COMPARING LARGE HEADS AND DUAL-MOBILITY BEARINGS IN REDUCING DISLOCATION FOLLOWING THA

There are no prospective or randomized studies that directly compare large heads and dual-mobility bearings in either primary or revision THA (**Table 1; Figure 3**). Two recent observational studies from the same patient

TABLE 1

Comparing and Contrasting Dual-mobility Bearings and Large-diameter (36- and 40-mm) Heads for Primary and Revision Total Hip Arthroplasty

	Dual-mobility Bearings	Large-diameter (36 and 40 mm) Heads
Stability	• Evidence from observational studies demonstrate improved stability compared with smaller heads in primary and revision hip arthroplasty	• Level I evidence more stable than smaller heads in primary and revision hip arthroplasty irrespective of approach used
Cost	• Implants more expensive • May be cost saving over longer term if revision rate is reduced	• Implants less expensive
Unique considerations	• Intraprosthetic dislocation • Polyethylene wear at two surfaces (or three if neck and polyethylene included) • Corrosion between metal liner and cup in modular cup designs • Minimum cup size required if using modular cup designs and 28-mm head (52- or 54-mm depending on implant manufacturer) • Potential for long-term wear, osteolysis, fracture, and dislocation largely unexamined	• Polyethylene fracture • Increased volumetric polyethylene wear compared with smaller head sizes • Minimum cup size required (52- or 54-mm cup for a 40-mm head depending on implant manufacturer) • Potential for long-term wear, osteolysis, fracture, and dislocation largely unexamined

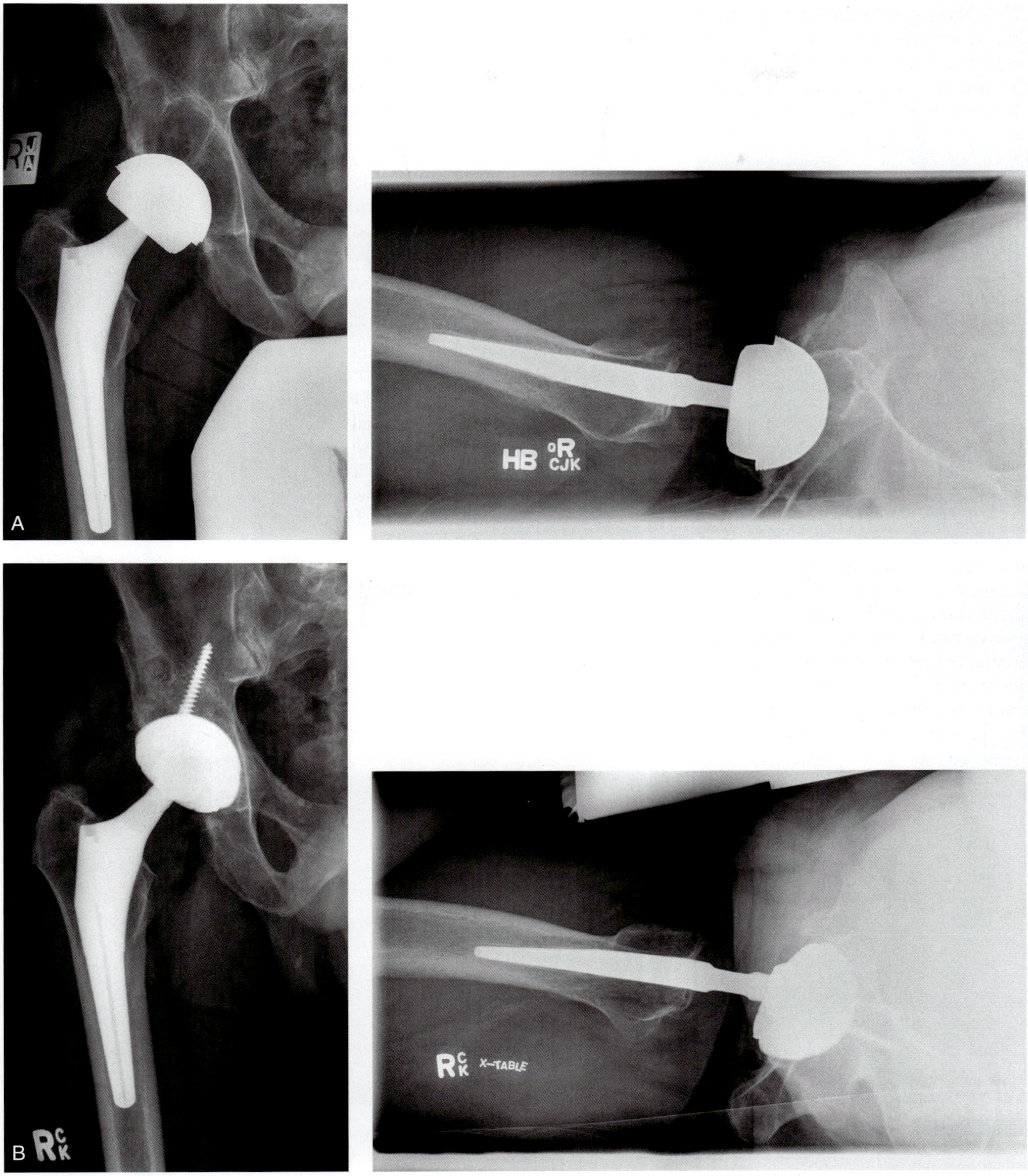

FIGURE 3 AP and lateral radiographs of two different middle-aged patients who have contained acetabular osteolysis following metal-on-metal total hip arthroplasty. **A** and **C**, Preoperative views. **B** and **D**, Views obtained 2 months following acetabular bone grafting and revision to a highly porous cementless cup with screws (Stryker Trident II Tritanium). The dual-mobility bearing (Stryker MDM) in (**B**) and a large 40-mm ceramic head in (**D**) were chosen to improve stability in these revision cases.

Section 3: Hip

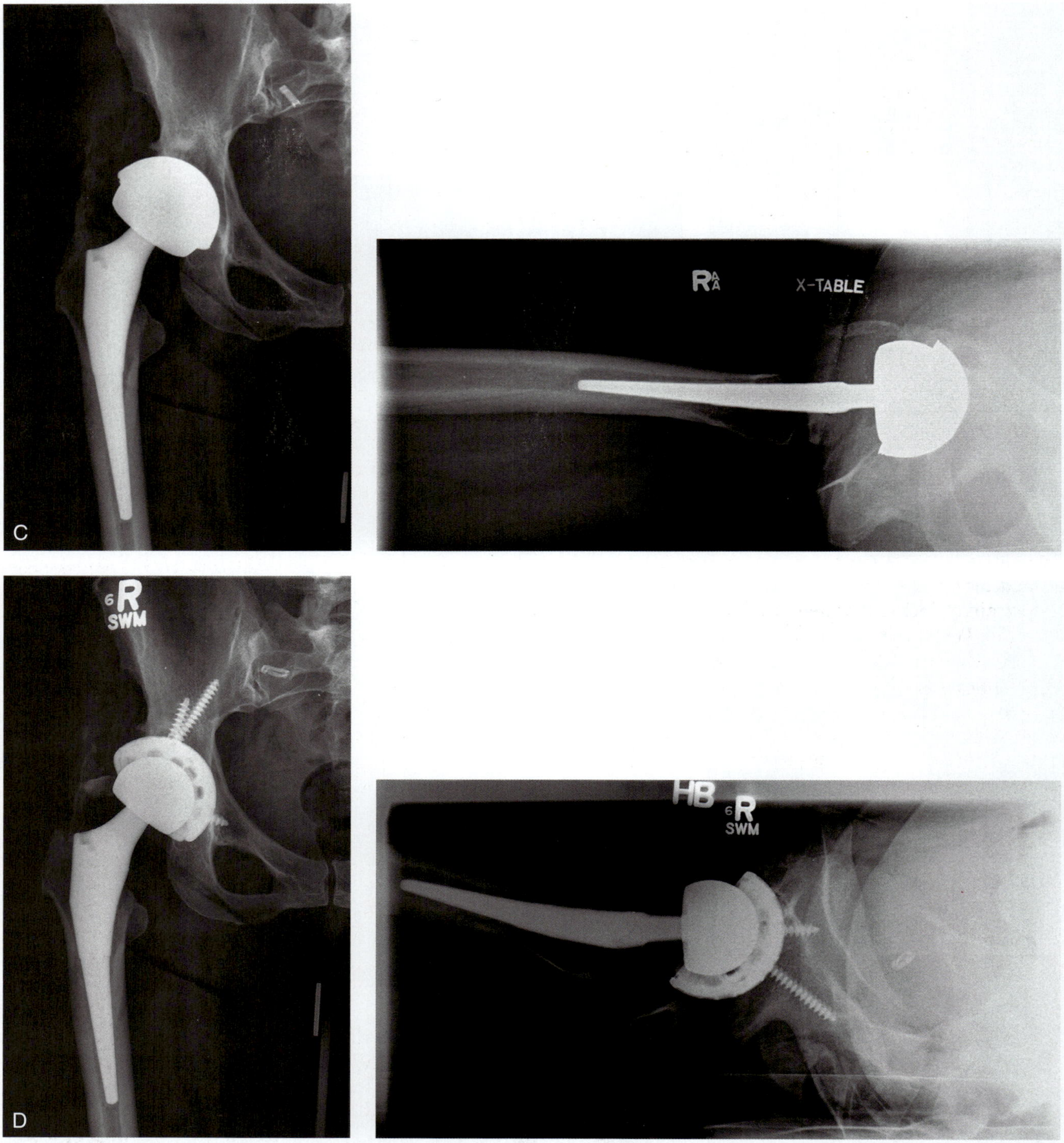

FIGURE 3 Cont'd

cohort have compared large heads and dual-mobility bearings for revision THA in terms of preventing dislocation[33] and reducing medical costs.[34] Subsequent dislocations in the dual-mobility group were lower (3% [4 of 126]) compared with the 40-mm group (10% [17 of 176]) with a hazard ratio = 3.2 [1.1 to 9.4]; P = 0.03).[33] All-cause re-revisions were also lower for dual-mobility bearings leading to lower overall medical costs despite the high initial costs for dual-mobility implants.[34] Based on these findings the authors suggest the role of dual-mobility should be judiciously expanded in contemporary revision THA.[33]

On the one hand, dual-mobility bearings in the study were associated with an impressive threefold lower dislocation rate despite selection bias to use dual mobility in patients at the highest risk for dislocation. On the other hand, follow-up was only 3 years and revisions due to increased wear with dual-mobility bearings would not be captured in this time frame. The 10% dislocation rate in the large head (40 mm) group at 3 years also differs markedly from the 1% dislocation rate at 5 years from prior level I evidence from 2012 on this topic.[26] This 2012 randomized controlled trial also excluded revision cases with abductor dysfunction because prior studies have shown that an increase in head size cannot compensate for abductor deficiency.[35] The same principle has been applied to dual-mobility implants in that abductor dysfunction is regarded as a contraindication. Unfortunately, information on abductor function could not be included in the recent comparative studies discussed in the previous paragraph.[33,34] The 10% dislocation rate among the large head (40 mm) group, and 3% rate in the dual-mobility group, may thus indicate these constructs were being used in cases of abductor dysfunction where many surgeons would argue a constrained liner is indicated. Whether these data can be generalized to cases with intact abductors is up for debate.

To summarize the literature and clinical experience, a small femoral head can either be upsized to a large one or converted to a dual-mobility construct at the time of revision with similar short-term outcomes (**Table 1**; **Figure 3**). Future well-designed observational and randomized studies will be required to compare large heads and dual-mobility bearings in terms of reducing dislocation in primary and revision settings, as well as to compare other reasons for revision, patient-reported outcomes, and costs. Most surgeons still agree that abductor dysfunction necessitates the use of a constrained liner.

UNIQUE CONSIDERATIONS

There are several unique considerations for large heads and dual-mobility bearings that surgeons should be familiar with before using them in the primary or revision setting. Long-term studies of modern large head and dual-mobility bearings are not available, and although these studies offer surgeons an option to improve stability without the downside of constraint, unexpected complications may occur in the future and should be considered. Prospective and randomized research is required to better examine the clinical relevance of each of these unique considerations. Most importantly, large heads and dual-mobility bearings should be used as an adjunct and not replace proper implant positioning, restoration of length and offset, and meticulous soft-tissue repair irrespective of approach.

Intraprosthetic Dislocation

IPD is a complication that is unique to the dual-mobility design. With its aperture being 1 to 2 mm smaller than the femoral ball, the polyethylene liner is designed to capture the smaller femoral head.[36] Consequently, the two implants are assembled together with a mechanical press stand on a back table before impaction on the femoral stem (**Figure 4**). Despite this constraint, the femoral ball can be dislodged from the polyethylene liner in two reported circumstances. Firstly, IPD can occur as a late complication when the retentive rim of the polyethylene liner is damaged secondary to wear and the femoral head becomes dislodged.[37] Secondly, IPD can also occur as an early complication following dislocation of the large head including the polyethylene liner. When forceful closed reduction is attempted, the liner can get caught on the rim of the acetabular cup or bony prominences and the liner gets dislodged from the femoral ball in what is known as the bottle-opener effect.[38] Postreduction radiographs must be carefully inspected and an eccentrically located femoral head should alert the surgeon to the possibility of an IPD (**Figure 5**). When the polyethylene liner remains in the soft tissues following IPD, it can be seen on plain radiographs or CT scan. This radiolucent arc is pathognomonic for IPD and is called the bubble sign.[39] In a recent systematic review of 14 case reports and 2 retrospective case series, there were 19 cases of IPD, where 15 patients sustained early IPDs at a mean follow-up of 3.2 months, whereas 4 patients sustained late IPDs at a mean follow-up of 15.1 months. The authors recommended adequate conscious sedation and the use of fluoroscopic imaging to reduce the chance of IPD and cautioned that a missed diagnosis of IPD can lead to severe damage to both the femoral and acetabular implants. In one instance, the patient also required revision of the acetabular implant because of severe wear.[40]

Corrosion

Corrosion may be an issue for both dual-mobility bearings and large heads, but for different reasons. A complication specific to modular dual-mobility cups, where a CoCr articular surface liner locks into an outer titanium shell, is the potential for corrosion at this interface and resultant ALTRs. One study of 100 patients who have modular dual-mobility cups found elevated cobalt or chromium levels in 25% of patients. Two patients had MRI evidence of a pseudotumor, but none had undergone revision.[41] No other studies have documented ALTRs secondary to modular dual-mobility cups to our knowledge. However, there are unpublished reports of improper seating of CoCr liners into modular titanium shells that may predispose to corrosion. Corrosion with modular dual-mobility cups remains an ongoing and largely unexamined area of concern that requires close clinical monitoring and further study.

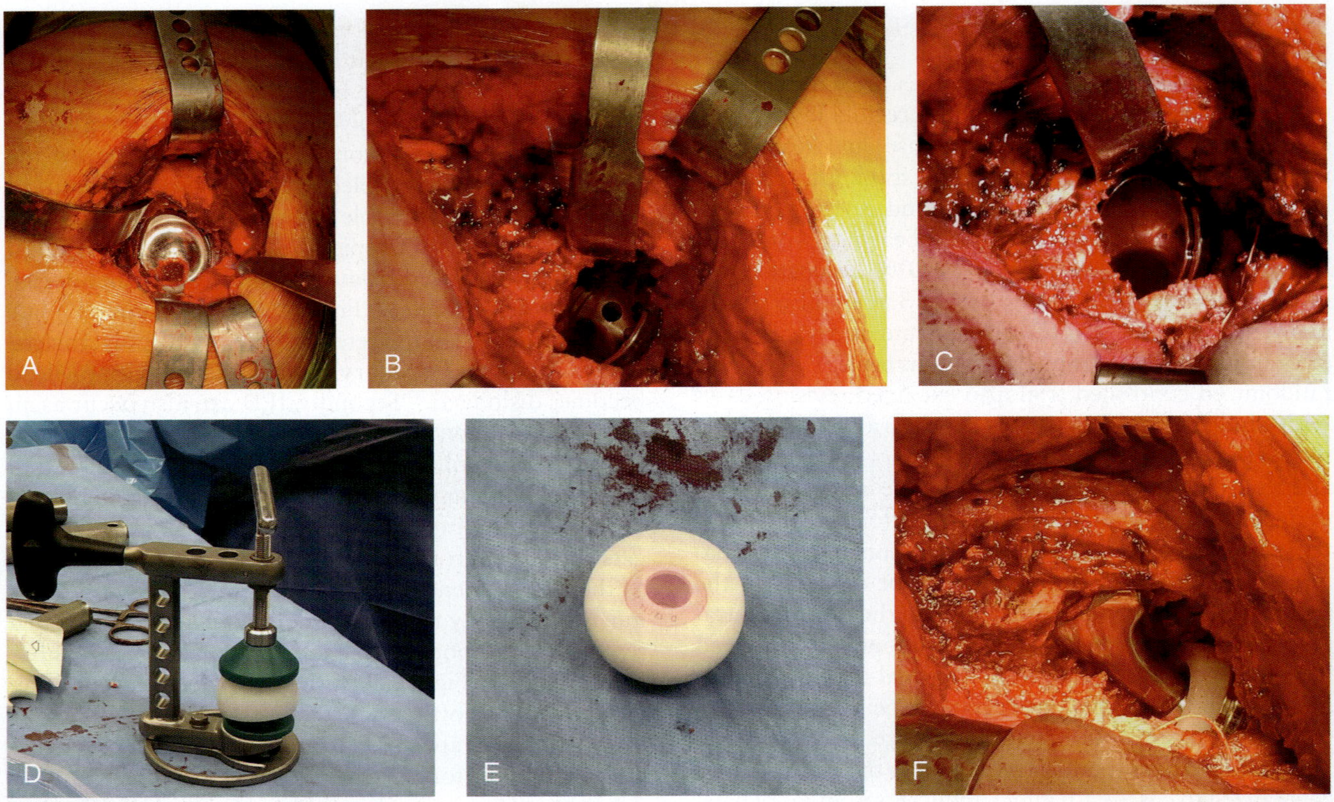

FIGURE 4 Intraoperative photographs of total hip arthroplasty with different dual-mobility bearings. **A**, Example of a nonmodular, cementless cup designed for coupling with a dual-mobility bearing (Stryker ADM). **B**, Example of a modular cementless cup designed for coupling with dual-mobility bearing after insertion of an inner metal (CoCr) liner (Stryker MDM) in (**C**). **D**, Intraoperative device for coupling head/liner. **E**, Assembled dual-mobility bearing. **F**, In situ—cup, metal liner, dual-mobility bearing (ceramic head and polyethylene liner) on an cementless stem.

Trunnion corrosion (or trunnionosis) is a rare, but well-documented, complication of metal (CoCr) femoral heads used with titanium stems. However, there is concern that increased forces at the head-neck junction caused by the use of larger heads may increase baseline corrosion risk. Because trunnionosis is rare, evidence is based mainly on extrapolations from basic science. Biomechanical studies have shown increased frictional torque and stresses at the modular head-neck junction of larger compared with smaller heads[42] with a corresponding increase in the risk of corrosion.[43] However, there is also evidence that ALTR may be an idiosyncratic reaction, regardless of the extent of corrosion or ion levels generated.[44]

Trunnionosis may be avoided altogether by using large ceramic heads instead of metal ones. Large ceramic heads have been shown to be less fracture prone compared with smaller ceramic heads, although the overall risk of modern ceramic head fracture is extremely low in either case at 0.003%.[45] In the revision scenario where a stem is retained, it is important to use a revision ceramic head that contains a titanium sleeve to prevent ceramic head fracture.

Wear

HXPE has facilitated the safer use of larger head sizes through corresponding decreases in the thickness of acetabular liners. The classic studies of polyethylene gamma irradiated in air that showed higher linear wear associated with 22-mm heads and higher volumetric wear associated with 32-mm heads[16] nonetheless continue to give surgeons worries about long-term volumetric wear and osteolysis with larger heads. Clinical studies do not support these concerns extrapolated from basic science, however, and clinically significant wear with large femoral head sizes has not been observed when used with HXPE.

One study with follow-up of 6 years found no association between 28-mm versus 32-mm heads in terms of femoral head penetration or osteolysis.[46] Another study of 768 primary hips patients who underwent primary THA found higher linear and volumetric wear with 36-mm heads compared with 28- and 32-mm heads. However, the wear rate for 36-mm heads in the study was still below the accepted threshold pertaining to the generation of osteolysis and much lower than conventional polyethylene.[47] A more recent study with longer

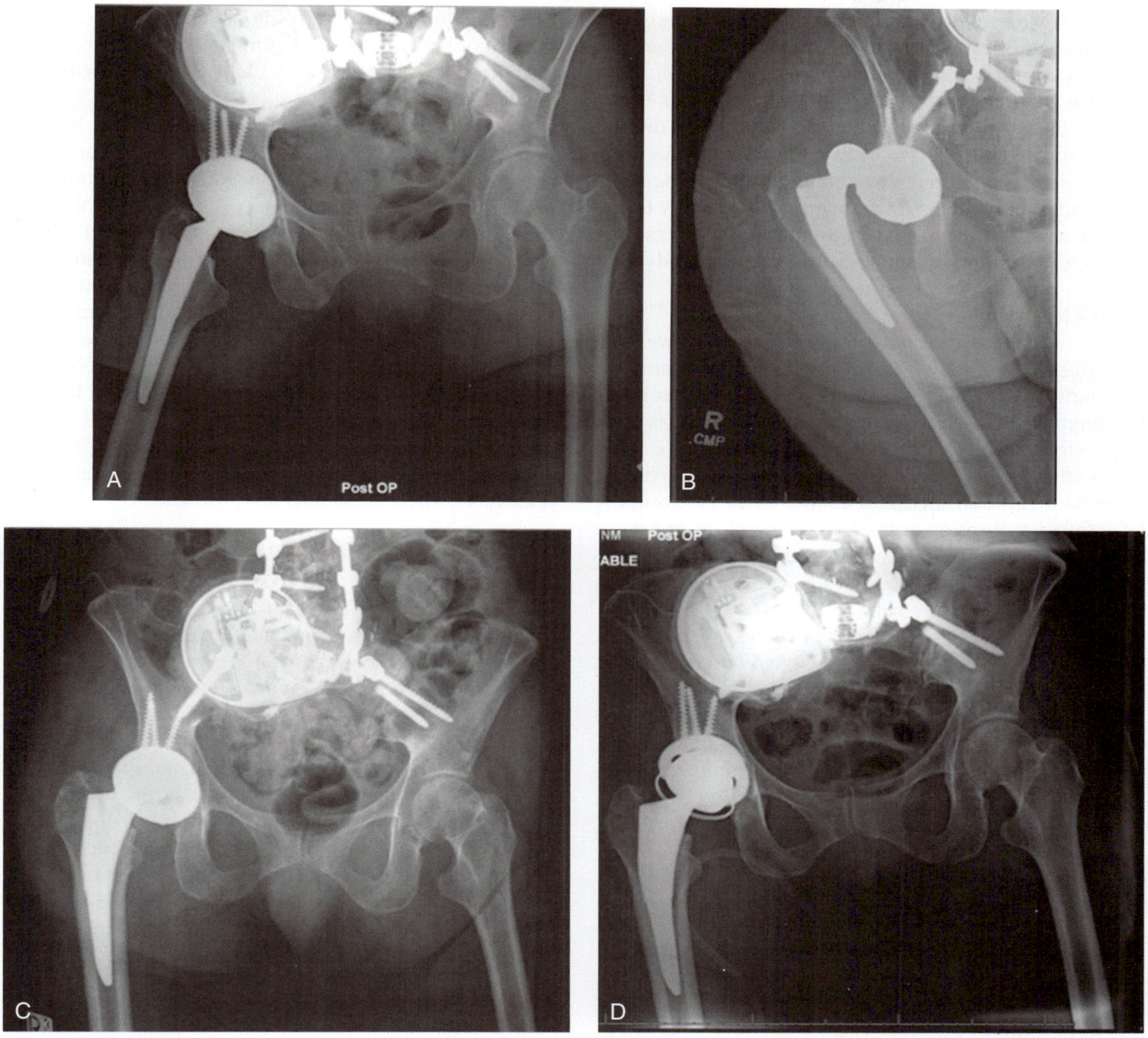

FIGURE 5 Radiographs show revision to a constrained liner following intraprosthetic dislocation of a dual-mobility bearing. **A**, View obtained immediately following initial total hip arthroplasty with a modular cup and dual-mobility bearing (Stryker MDM). The dual-mobility bearing was chosen to improve stability in this patient who previously underwent T5 to pelvis spinal fusion. **B**, View obtained in the emergency department showing the posterior dislocation. Radiolucency around the head shows the liner remains on the femoral ball. **C**, Postreduction view showing the femoral head eccentrically in the cup and the radiolucent liner posterior and lateral to the vastus ridge of the femur. **D**, View obtained immediately following revision to a constrained liner.

follow-up (up to 14 years) of HXPE in 84 hips also found higher volumetric wear in 36- and 40-mm heads compared with smaller ones, but there was no association between head size and the small osteolytic lesions that were noted in 12 cases (14%).[48] Future research should continue to monitor wear rates of large heads on HXPE over the longer term.

Less is known about the longer term performance of modern dual-mobility bearings that were only approved for use in the United States in 2009. However, there are several theoretical reasons to be concerned about the wear properties of these new bearings. Concerns for increased polyethylene wear in dual-mobility implants mainly arise from the added modularity of the implant design. In addition to the traditional hard-on-soft bearing, the convex surface of the polyethylene liner also articulates with the concave surface of the polished metal surface of the acetabular implant, which may lead to increased wear. Another source of polyethylene wear is from the neck of the femoral stem impinging on the liner at extremes of motion. Short-term studies of wear rates for third-generation dual-mobility bearings (with HXPE) have found head penetration and wear double those reported for HXPE in fixed bearings.[49] As with corrosion with modular dual-mobility cups, long-term wear and osteolysis remain an ongoing and largely unexamined area of concern for dual-mobility bearings that require close clinical monitoring and further study.

Liner Fracture

Related to wear is the concern for catastrophic wear or *liner fracture*. This is especially concerning with smaller acetabuli when large heads and very thin HXPE is used. Although the cross-linking process decreases the fatigue properties of HXPE, very few liner fractures have actually been reported. One known risk factor is a vertically positioned cup that increases contact stresses. To minimize this complication as discussed previously, one must be particularly careful to avoid excessive cup abduction angles when combining large heads with small-diameter cups, particularly those between 50- and 54-mm outer diameter. In these cases, the polyethylene is very thin at 45° and is at risk of fracture.[26] Although 6 mm is generally considered the minimum thickness threshold for HXPE, future research should help determine empirically what constitutes an acceptable minimum thickness of an HXPE acetabular liner with regard to both long-term wear and liner fracture.

Technical Considerations

As mentioned, dual-mobility bearings and large heads should be used as an adjunct to proper implant positioning, restoration of length and offset, and meticulous soft-tissue repair. Implanting a large femoral head does not require any special techniques other than those already mentioned, except for understanding a minimum cup size is required and the caveat to avoid a vertical cup position. Surgeons unfamiliar with dual-mobility bearings, however, should be aware of a number of technical nuances with third-generation dual-mobility designs.

The acetabular implant of a dual-mobility construct comprises a polished metal liner that is either incorporated into a monoblock cup or impacted inside a tapered porous-coated titanium shell that contains holes for screw fixation (**Figure 4**). Advantages of the modular technology is that it allows surgeons to directly visualize the dome contact of the shell to determine proper seating and use screws if desired. Disadvantages of the modular design are the potential for corrosion between the CoCr liner and titanium shell, and a minimum cup size depending on the implant manufacturer. It is also important to check circumferentially for adequate liner seating following impaction into the modular cups because there are unpublished reports of improper seating of CoCr liners into modular titanium shells that may predispose to corrosion.

The monoblock acetabular implants do not have an option for screw fixation, but avoid potential corrosion, and may be used in smaller acetabuli. Surgeons may seat a trial cup intraoperatively to get a sense of where the final monoblock cup (without screw holes) will sit in relation to the native acetabulum. Some monoblock acetabular implants (Stryker ADM) have a sidedness that surgeons should be aware of and can be marked with a sterile pen intraoperatively to ensure the anterior recess is aligned to avoid psoas tendon impingement. The polyethylene liner is designed to capture the smaller femoral head and so the two implants are assembled together intraoperatively with a custom mechanical press stand on a back table before impaction on the femoral stem[36] (**Figure 4**).

Patient-reported Outcomes

Although the literature has focused on the role of dual-mobility bearings and large heads in reducing dislocation, if these constructs enable an increase in impingement-free range of motion (**Figure 2**), then improvements in patient-reported outcomes may also be expected. One prospective observational study of 726 THAs found no differences in any functional outcome measurements assessed between different head sizes despite a lower dislocation rate in the larger head group (36 mm or greater).[50] One explanation for this finding is that improvements in patient-reported outcomes following THA are driven by improvements in pain control rather than range of motion. Another explanation is that further study in this area is required, including studies of patients who have dual-mobility designs.

SUMMARY

Despite improvements in surgical technique and implant design, there remains a subset of patients who have an increased risk of instability following THA including those who have cognitive dysfunction, neuromuscular disorders, hip fractures, and spinopelvic fusion, among others.[1] The etiology of dislocation in the revision scenario is multifactorial, but it is usually related to the extensile exposure required to perform revision surgery, soft-tissue damage, and acetabular-femoral head size mismatch.[2] For patients at high risk for instability in either the primary or revision setting, dual-mobility bearings and large femoral heads (36 and 40 mm) were increasingly used during the last decade to reduce the risk of dislocation. Clinical vignettes in which implanting these novel constructs was felt to be advantageous are provided (**Figures 5 through 8**).

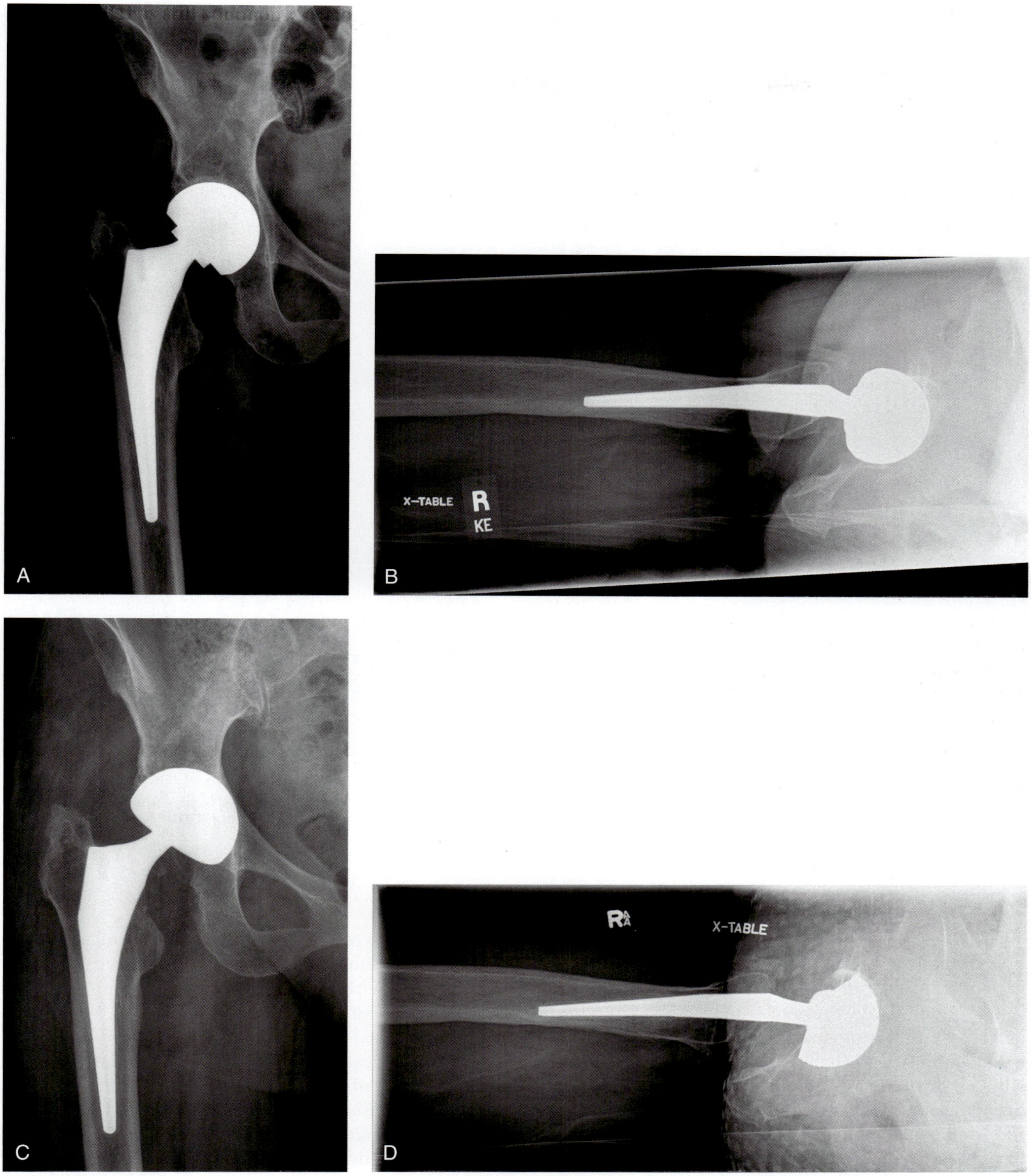

FIGURE 6 AP and lateral radiographs of an elderly patient who developed acetabular erosion and pain after being treated with a hemiarthroplasty for a hip fracture. **A**, Preoperative view. **B**, View obtained 2 months following revision to a total hip arthroplasty. A dual-mobility bearing (Stryker ADM) was chosen because the patient's cementless stem was found to be well ingrown in 5° of retroversion at the time of revision surgery and retained.

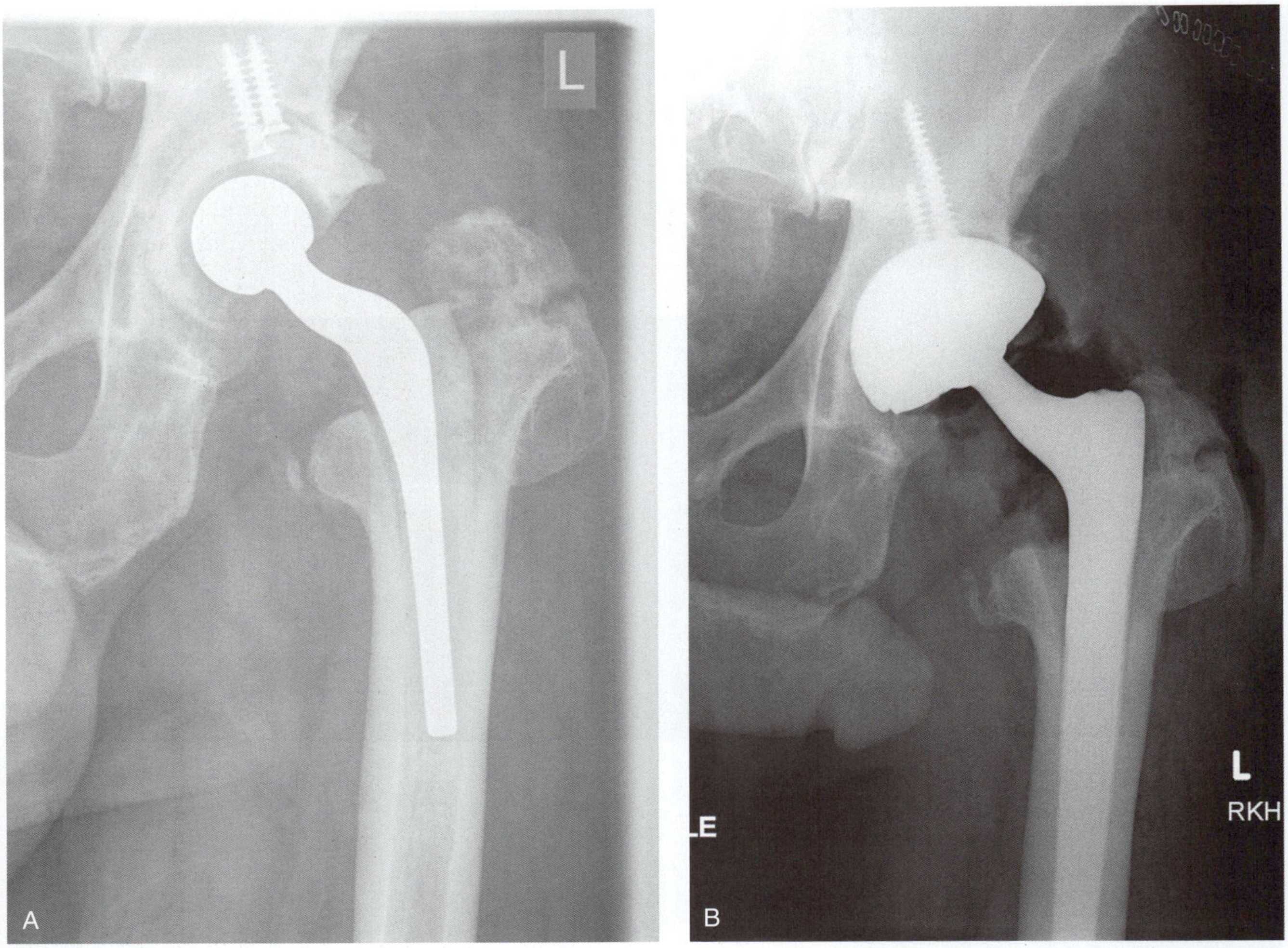

FIGURE 7 AP and lateral radiographs of a patient undergoing a two-stage revision for an infected total hip arthroplasty. **A**, Following stage-one. **B**, View obtained immediately following stage two with re-implantation of a highly porous cementless cup with screws and a dual-mobility bearing. The dual-mobility bearing was chosen to improve stability in this infected revision case.

HXPE is key for the safe use of both large heads (which require thinner liners) and dual-mobility bearings (which wear at multiple surfaces). Current literature and clinical experience suggest a small femoral head can either be upsized to large one or converted to a dual-mobility construct at the time of revision, with similar short-term outcomes. Future well-designed observational and randomized studies will be required to compare large heads and dual-mobility bearings in terms of reducing dislocation in both primary and revision settings. Wear with modern dual-mobility bearings and corrosion with modular dual-mobility cups remain ongoing and largely unexamined areas of concern that need close clinical monitoring and further study. There are also several unique technical considerations of dual-mobility bearings surgeons should be familiar with before using them in the primary or revision setting.

Overall, dual-mobility bearings and large heads may decrease dislocation risk in the primary and revision setting but are not a panacea. These constructs should be used as an adjunct to proper implant positioning, restoration of length and offset, and meticulous soft-tissue repair irrespective of approach. These should also be used for the correct indication—primary cases at high risk for dislocation and revision cases with intact abductors. Most surgeons still agree that abductor dysfunction necessitates the use of a constrained liner.

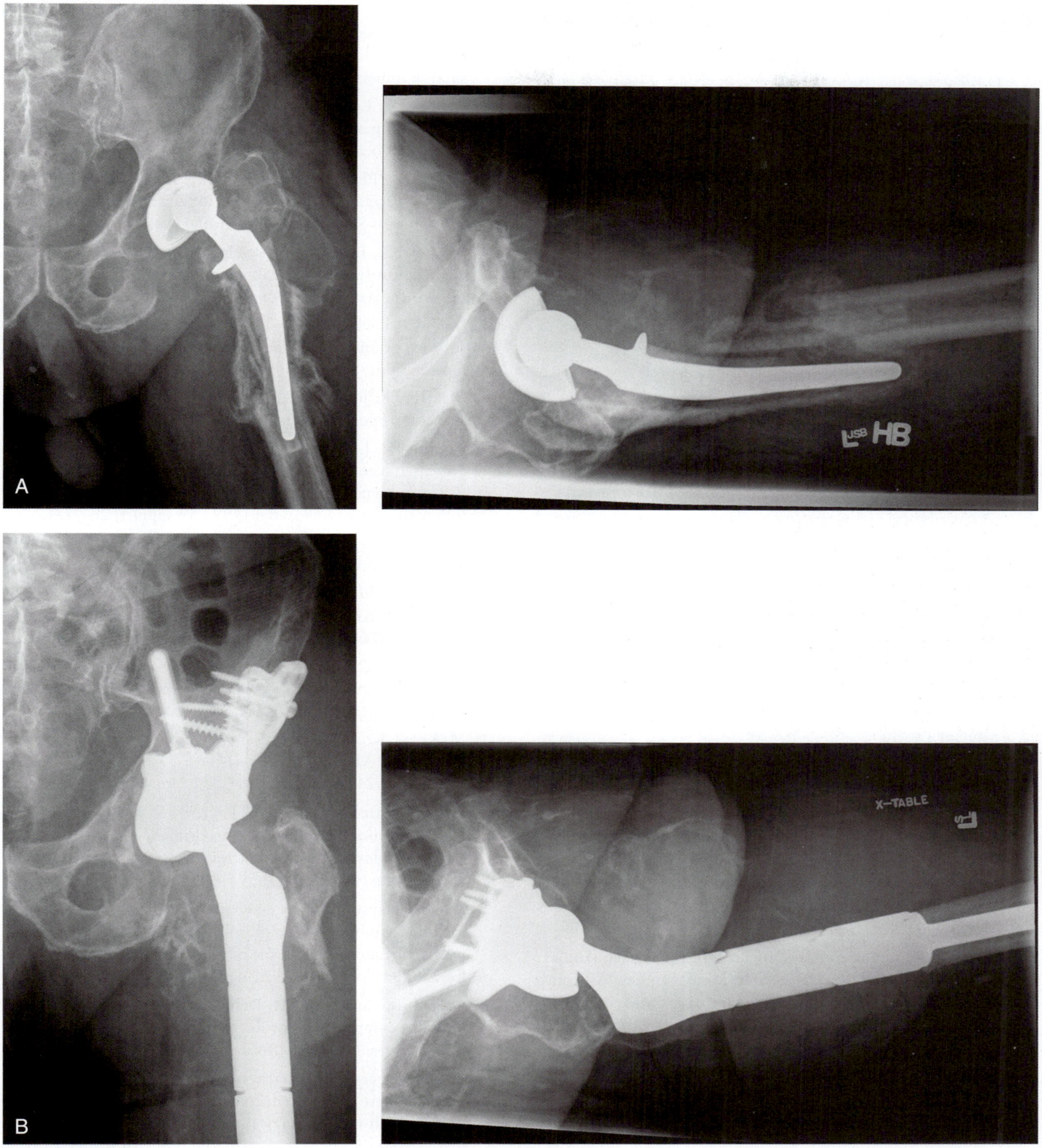

FIGURE 8 AP and lateral radiographs of an elderly patient undergoing revision hip arthroplasty for aseptic cup loosening and periprosthetic femur fracture (Vancouver B3) in the context of acetabular and femoral osteolysis from polyethylene wear. **A**, Preoperative view. **B**, View obtained 2 months postoperatively. Acetabular reconstruction performed using a custom triflange cup into which was cemented a cementless cup with dual-mobility bearing (Stryker ADM). The dual-mobility bearing was chosen to improve stability in this patient with abductor dysfunction in the context of femoral reconstruction with a proximal femoral replacement. A constrained liner was avoided to allow for ingrowth of the custom triflange cup.

KEY STUDY POINTS

- HXPE is key in enabling the safe use of large heads (which require thinner liners) and dual-mobility bearings (which wear at multiple surfaces).
- Dual-mobility bearings and large heads may decrease dislocation risk in the primary and revision setting but are not a panacea. These constructs should be used as an adjunct to proper implant positioning, restoration of length and offset, and meticulous soft-tissue repair irrespective of approach, as well as for the correct indication: primary cases at high risk for dislocation and revision cases with intact abductors.
- A small femoral head can either be upsized to large one or converted to a dual-mobility construct at the time of revision, with similar short-term outcomes. Future well-designed observational and randomized studies will be required to compare dislocation rates of large heads and dual-mobility bearings in the high-risk primary and revision settings, as well as in terms of other reasons for revision, patient-reported outcomes, and costs.
- There are unique technical considerations of dual-mobility bearings surgeons should be familiar with before using them in the primary or revision setting. Wear with modern (HXPE) dual-mobility bearings and corrosion with modular dual-mobility cups remain ongoing and largely unexamined areas of concern that need close clinical monitoring and further study.

ANNOTATED REFERENCES

1. Levin JM, Sultan AA, O'Donnell JA, et al: Modern dual-mobility cups in revision total hip arthroplasty: A systematic review and meta-analysis. *J Arthroplasty* 2018;33(12):3793-3800.

   This is a systematic review of nine retrospective studies, including six case series and three cohort studies. All-cause and aseptic survivorship rates, dislocation rates, complications, and clinical outcomes of dual-mobility bearings in revision THA were evaluated. The all-cause survivorship and aseptic survivorship were 94.5% and 97.7%, respectively, at a mean follow-up of 31 months. IPD was only 0.2%, occurring in 2 out of the 693 hips included in this study. The overall risk of dislocation was 2.2%, and when the authors analyzed three studies that directly compared dual-mobility prostheses with fixed-bearing prosthesis, there was a lower odds ratio of dislocation in the dual-mobility cohort (odds ratio = 0.24, 95% confidence interval = 0.10 to 0.59, $P = 0.002$). In addition, the risk of aseptic loosening is 0.7%, which can in part be explained by improvements in the design of the newest generation of dual-mobility prostheses. Overall, there are positive short-term results for the dual-mobility implants in the revision setting, especially in regard to the risk of dislocation, but the limitations of this study are the short follow-up, small numbers, and retrospective nature.

2. Kelley SS, Lachiewicz PF, Hickman JM, Paterno SM: Relationship of femoral head and acetabular size to the prevalence of dislocation. *Clin Orthop Relat Res* 1998;355:163-170.
3. Lachiewicz PF, Soileau ES: Fixation, survival, and dislocation of jumbo acetabular components in revision hip arthroplasty. *J Bone Joint Surg Am* 2013;95(6):543-548.
4. Whaley AL, Berry DJ, Scott Harmsen W: Extra-large uncemented hemispherical acetabular components for revision total hip arthroplasty. *J Bone Joint Surg Am* 2001;83(9):1352-1357.
5. Jones CP, Lachiewicz PF: Factors influencing the longer-term survival of uncemented acetabular components used in total hip revisions. *J Bone Joint Surg Am* 2004;86(2):342-347.
6. Meldrum R, Johansen RL: Safe screw placement in acetabular revision surgery. *J Arthroplasty* 2001;16(8):953-960.
7. Aubriot JH, Lesimple P, Leclercq S: Study of Bousquet's non-cemented acetabular implant in 100 hybrid total hip prostheses (Charnley type cemented femoral component). Average 5-year follow-up. *Acta Orthop Belg* 1993;59(suppl 1):267-271.
8. Farizon F, de Lavison R, Azoulai JJ, Bousquet G: Results with a cementless alumina-coated cup with dual mobility. A twelve-year follow-up study. *Int Orthopaedics* 1998;22(4):219-224.
9. Charnley J: Arthroplasty of the hip. A new operation. *Lancet* 1961;1(7187):1129-1132.
10. Charnley J: The long-term results of low-friction arthroplasty of the hip performed as a primary intervention. *J Bone Joint Surg Br* 1972;54(1):61-76.
11. McKee GK, Watson-Farrar J: Replacement of arthritic hips by the McKee-Farrar prosthesis. *J Bone Joint Surg Br* 1966;48(2):245-259.
12. Reina N, Pareek A, Krych AJ, Pagnano MW, Berry DJ, Abdel MP: Dual-mobility constructs in primary and revision total hip arthroplasty: A systematic review of comparative studies. *J Arthroplasty* 2019;34(3):594-603.

    A recent systematic review of dual-mobility constructs included studies with midterm follow-up (approximately 7 years) and supports the role of reducing the incidence of dislocation in the primary setting. Level of evidence: III.

13. Darrith B, Courtney PM, Della Valle CJ: Outcomes of dual mobility components in total hip arthroplasty: A systematic review of the literature. *Bone Joint J* 2018;100-B(1):11-19.

    Another recent systematic review of DM constructs supporting their role of reducing the incidence of dislocation in both high-risk primary and revision settings. The review included studies with mid-term follow-up for primary (mean 8.5 years) and revision cases (mean 5.4 years) and short-term follow-up for DM bearings used in femoral neck fractures (1.3 years).

14. De Martino I, Triantafyllopoulos GK, Sculco PK, Sculco TP: Dual mobility cups in total hip arthroplasty. *World J Orthop* 2014;5(3):180-187.

15. Malkani AL, Ong KL, Lau E, Kurtz SM, Justice BJ, Manley MT: Early- and late-term dislocation risk after primary hip arthroplasty in the Medicare population. *J Arthroplasty* 2010;25(6 suppl):21-25.

16. Livermore J, Ilstrup D, Morrey B: Effect of femoral head size on wear of the polyethylene acetabular component. *J Bone Joint Surg Am* 1990;72(4):518-528.

17. Howie DW, Holubowycz OT, Middleton R, Large Articulation Study Group: Large femoral heads decrease the incidence of dislocation after total hip arthroplasty: A randomized controlled trial. *J Bone Joint Surg Am* 2012;94(12):1095-1102.

18. Stroh DA, Issa K, Johnson AJ, Delanois RE, Mont MA: Reduced dislocation rates and excellent functional outcomes with large-diameter femoral heads. *J Arthroplasty* 2013;28(8):1415-1420.

19. Tsikandylakis G, Kärrholm J, Hailer NP, et al: No increase in survival for 36-mm versus 32-mm femoral heads in metal-on-polyethylene THA: A registry study. *Clin Orthop Relat Res* 2018;476(12):2367-2378.

    Longer term population-based registry data from the Nordic Arthroplasty Register Association database including 186,231 metal-on-polyethylene primary THAs found the lowest adjusted dislocation risk with 36-mm heads compared with smaller heads. Level of evidence: III.

20. Haughom BD, Plummer DR, Moric M, Della Valle CJ: Is there a benefit to head size greater than 36 mm in total hip arthroplasty? *J Arthroplasty* 2016;31(1):152-155.

21. De Martino I, D'Apolito R, Soranoglou VG, Poultsides LA, Sculco PK, Sculco TP: Hip technologies dislocation following total hip arthroplasty using dual mobility acetabular components a systematic review. *Bone Joint J* 2017;99-B(1): 18-24.

    A total of 59 articles were included in this recent systematic review examining dual-mobility bearings in the primary setting. The risk of dislocation was 0.9% out of 12,844 hips at a mean follow-up of 6.8 years. The risk of IPD was 0.7%.

22. Combes A, Migaud H, Girard J, Duhamel A, Fessy MH: Low rate of dislocation of dual-mobility cups in primary total hip arthroplasty. *Clin Orthop Relat Res* 2013;471(12):3891-3900.

23. Australian Orthopaedic Association National Joint Replacement Registry (AOANJRR): Australian Orthopaedic Association National Joint Replacement Registry.

24. Kreipke R, Rogmark C, Pedersen AB, et al: Dual mobility cups: Effect on risk of revision of primary total hip arthroplasty due to osteoarthritis. A matched population-based study using the Nordic Arthroplasty Register Association database. *J Bone Joint Surg Am* 2019;101(2):169-176.

    A recent study from the Nordic Arthroplasty Register Association database of 2,277 propensity score–matched patients found that patients with dual-mobility bearings had a lower risk of revision due to dislocation, but twice the risk of revision due to infection. Level of evidence: III.

25. Plummer DR, Christy JM, Sporer SM, Paprosky WG, Della Valle CJ: Dual-mobility articulations for patients at high risk for dislocation. *J Arthroplasty* 2016;31(9):131-135.

26. Garbuz DS, Masri BA, Duncan CP, et al: The Frank Stinchfield Award: Dislocation in revision THA. Do large heads (36 and 40 mm) result in reduced dislocation rates in a randomized clinical trial? *Clin Orthop Relat Res* 2012;470(2):351-356.

27. Langlais FL, Ropars M, Gaucher F, Musset T, Chaix O: Dual mobility cemented cups have low dislocation rates in THA revisions. *Clin Orthop Relat Res* 2008;466(2):389-395.

28. Philippot R, Adam P, Reckhaus M, et al: Prevention of dislocation in total hip revision surgery using a dual mobility design. *Orthop Traumatol Surg Res* 2009;95(6):407-413.

29. Hailer NP, Weiss RJ, Stark A, Kärrholm J: Dual-mobility cups for revision due to instability are associated with a low rate of re-revisions due to dislocation: 228 patients from the Swedish Hip Arthroplasty Register. *Acta Orthopaedica* 2012;83(6):566-571.

30. Mohammed R, Hayward K, Mulay S, Bindi F, Wallace M: Outcomes of dual-mobility acetabular cup for instability in primary and revision total hip arthroplasty. *J Orthop Traumatol* 2015;16(1):9-13.

31. Hamadouche M, Ropars M, Rodaix C, et al: Five to thirteen year results of a cemented dual mobility socket to treat recurrent dislocation. *Int Orthop* 2017;41(3):513-519.

    This is another case series examining the role of dual mobility in revision cases where prior dislocation was the indication for revision. This study has longer term follow-up; a series of 51 patients with cemented dual-mobility bearings for instability found 86% did not re-dislocate by 10 years.

32. Hamadouche M, Biau DJ, Huten D, Musset T, Gaucher F: The use of a cemented dual mobility socket to treat recurrent dislocation. *Clin Orthop Relat Res* 2010;468(12):3248-3254.

33. Hartzler MA, Abdel MP, Sculco PK, Taunton MJ, Pagnano MW, Hanssen AD: Otto Aufranc Award: Dual-mobility constructs in revision THA reduced dislocation, rerevision, and reoperation compared with large femoral heads. *Clin Orthop Relat Res* 2018;476(2):293-301.

    Two recent observational studies from the same patient cohort have compared large heads and dual-mobility bearings for revision THA in terms of preventing dislocation and reducing medical costs. Subsequent dislocations in the dual-mobility group were lower (3% [4 of 126]) compared with the 40-mm group (10% [17 of 176]) with a hazard ratio = 3.2 [1.1 to 9.4]; $P = 0.03$). All-cause re-revisions were also lower for dual-mobility bearings leading to lower overall medical costs despite the high initial costs for dual-mobility implants. Based on these findings, the authors suggest the role of dual mobility should be judiciously expanded in contemporary revision THA. Because these studies included patients with abductor deficiency, whether these data can be generalized to cases with intact abductors is up for debate. Level of evidence: III.

34. Abdel MP, Miller LE, Hanssen AD, Pagnano MW: Cost analysis of dual-mobility versus large femoral head constructs in revision total hip arthroplasty. *J Arthroplasty* 2019;34(2):260-264.

    Two recent observational studies from the same patient cohort have compared large heads and dual-mobility bearings for revision THA in terms of preventing dislocation and reducing medical costs. Subsequent dislocations in the dual-mobility group were lower (3% [4 of 126]) compared with the 40-mm group (10% [17 of 176]) with a hazard ratio = 3.2 [1.1 to 9.4]; *P* = 0.03). All-cause re-revisions were also lower for dual-mobility bearings, leading to lower overall medical costs despite the high initial costs for dual-mobility implants. Based on these findings, the authors suggest the role of dual mobility should be judiciously expanded in contemporary revision THA. Because these studies included patients with abductor deficiency, whether these data can be generalized to cases with intact abductors is up for debate.

35. Kung PL, Ries MD: Effect of femoral head size and abductors on dislocation after revision THA. *Clin Orthop Relat Res* 2007;465:170-174.

36. Farizon F, Caton J: *La cupule à double mobilité de Gilles Bousquet. Un concept révolutionnaire dans la prothèse totale de hanche. Un siècle d'innovations françaises en chirurgie orthopédique et traumatologique*. 2019.

    French-language summary of the history of dual mobility bearings in total hip arthroplasty.

37. De Martino I, D'Apolito R, Waddell BS, McLawhorn AS, Sculco PK, Sculco TP: Early intraprosthetic dislocation in dual-mobility implants: A systematic review. *Arthroplasty Today* 2017;3(3):197-202.

    IPD is a complication that is unique to the dual-mobility design. With its aperture being 1 to 2 mm smaller than the femoral ball, the polyethylene liner is designed to capture the smaller femoral head. Despite this constraint, the femoral ball can be dislodged from the polyethylene liner in two reported circumstances. First, IPD can occur as a late complication when the retentive rim of the polyethylene liner is damaged secondary to wear and the femoral head becomes dislodged. Second, IPD can also occur as an early complication following dislocation of the large head including the polyethylene liner. In this recent systematic review of 14 case reports and 2 retrospective case series, there were 19 cases of IPD where 15 patients sustained early IPDs at a mean follow-up of 3.2 months, whereas 4 patients sustained late IPDs at a mean follow-up of 15.1 months. The authors recommended adequate conscious sedation and the use of fluoroscopic imaging to reduce the chance of IPD and cautioned that a missed diagnosis of IPD can lead to severe damage to both the femoral and acetabular implants.

38. Loubignac F, Boissier F: Cup dissociation after close reduction of a dislocated bipolar hemiarthroplasty. *Rev Chir Orthop Reparatrice Appar Mot* 1997;83(5):469-472.

39. Waddell BS, De Martino I, Sculco T, Sculco P: Total hip arthroplasty dislocations are more complex than they appear: A case report of intraprosthetic dislocation of an anatomic dual-mobility implant after closed reduction. *Ochsner J* 2016;16(2):185-190.

40. Schirmers J, Horazdovsky R, Marston S: Early intraprosthetic dislocation of dual-mobility total hip arthroplasty implant following attempted closed reduction: A case report. *Reconstructive Rev* 2014;5(2).

41. Matsen Ko LJ, Pollag KE, Yoo JY, Sharkey PF: Serum metal ion levels following total hip arthroplasty with modular dual mobility components. *J Arthroplasty* 2016;31(1):186-189.

42. Meneghini RM, Lovro LR, Wallace JM, Ziemba-Davis M: Large metal heads and vitamin E polyethylene increase frictional torque in total hip arthroplasty. *J Arthroplasty* 2016;31(3):710-714.

43. Plummer DR, Berger RA, Paprosky WG, Sporer SM, Jacobs JJ, Della Valle CJ: Diagnosis and management of adverse local tissue reactions secondary to corrosion at the head-neck junction in patients with metal on polyethylene bearings. *J Arthroplasty* 2016;31(1):264-268.

44. Kilb BKJ, Kurmis AP, Parry M, et al: Frank Stinchfield Award: Identification of the at-risk genotype for development of pseudotumors around metal-on-metal THAs. *Clin Orthop Relat Res* 2018;476(2):230-241.

    This genotyping study suggests trunnion corrosion and ALTR in large head metal-on-metal prostheses may be due to genetic differences in the immune system.

45. Massin P, Lopes R, Masson B, Mainard D: Does Biolox Delta ceramic reduce the rate of component fractures in total hip replacement? *Orthop Traumatol Surg Res* 2014;100(6):S31 7-S321.

46. Bragdon CR, Kwon YM, Geller JA, et al: Minimum 6-year followup of highly cross-linked polyethylene in THA. *Clin Orthop Relat Res* 2007;465:122-127.

47. Bragdon CR, Doerner M, Martell J, et al: The 2012 John Charnley Award: Clinical multicenter studies of the wear performance of highly crosslinked remelted polyethylene in THA. *Clin Orthop Relat Res* 2013;471(2):393-402.

48. Lachiewicz PF, Soileau ES, Martell JM: Wear and osteolysis of highly crosslinked polyethylene at 10 to 14 years: The effect of femoral head size. *Clin Orthop Relat Res* 2016;474(2):365-371.

49. Deckard ER, Azzam KA, Meneghini RM: Contemporary dual mobility head penetration at five years: Concern for the additional convex bearing surface? *J Arthroplasty* 2018;33(7):S28 0-S284.

    This study found wear rates and head penetration for third-generation dual-mobility bearings (with HXPE) to be double compared with those reported for HXPE in fixed bearings.

50. Allen CL, Hooper GJ, Frampton CMA: Do larger femoral heads improve the functional outcome in total hip arthroplasty? *J Arthroplasty* 2014;29(2):401-404.

CHAPTER 35

Computer Navigation and Robotics in Total Hip Arthroplasty

JUSTIN S. CHANG, MBBS, MRCS, FRCSC • BABAR KAYANI, MBBS, BSc, MRCS
BRADFORD S. WADDELL, MD • DOUGLAS E. PADGETT, MD
FARES S. HADDAD, BSc, MD (Res), FRCS

ABSTRACT

Computer navigation and robotics play substantial roles in total hip arthroplasty. It is important for orthopaedic surgeons to have an understanding of the types of navigation currently used, as well as newer technologies, such as robotic assistance and precision-manufactured aligning guides. A review of the recently published data confirms the precision advantages of these enabling technologies compared with freehand techniques. Evolving technologies have the potential to improve surgical accuracy and reproducibility in a time-efficient and cost-efficient manner.

Dr. Waddell or an immediate family member serves as a paid consultant to or is an employee of OrthAlign and Smith & Nephew. Dr. Padgett or an immediate family member has received royalties from DJ Orthopaedics; is a member of a speakers' bureau or has made paid presentations on behalf of DJ Orthopaedics; serves as a paid consultant to or is an employee of DJ Orthopaedics; has stock or stock options held in Evolve Orthopaedics, Orthophor, Parvizi Surgical Innovations, and Tangen; and serves as a board member, owner, officer, or committee member of the Hospital for Special Surgery and the Hip Society. Dr. Haddad or an immediate family member has received royalties from Corin, Matortho, Smith & Nephew, and Stryker; serves as a paid consultant to or is an employee of Smith & Nephew and Stryker; has received research or institutional support from Smith & Nephew and Stryker; and serves as a board member, owner, officer, or committee member of BOSTAA. Neither of the following authors nor any immediate family member has received anything of value from or has stock or stock options held in a commercial company or institution related directly or indirectly to the subject of this chapter: Dr. Chang and Dr. Kayani.

Keywords: computer-assisted; haptics; hip arthroplasty; navigation; robotics

INTRODUCTION

Optimization of implant orientation in total hip arthroplasty (THA) has been known for some time to maximize long-term success. Suboptimal position has been associated with instability, accelerated bearing wear, and the potential for impingement at nonintended interfaces, all of which result in early failure. Although some latitude exists in the placement of femoral implants in THA performed with or without cement, femoral geometry often determines the ultimate position of the stem. Despite the use of anatomic landmarks or external guides, the acetabular implant position is the factor most susceptible to suboptimal position.[1,2] Variation in the acetabular position has been attributed to numerous factors, ranging from patient position on the operating table (supine versus lateral), pelvic movement during the procedure (affecting spatial orientation), and the effect of the lumbosacral spine. In addition to implant orientation, changes in the longitudinal direction (hip or limb length) as well as the lateral direction (offset) are known to affect performance and satisfaction after THA. These observations have inspired studies exploring the potential of supporting technologies, such as computer-assisted (CAS) navigation and robotics, to overcome the limitations of freehand techniques. It is important to review some basic concepts of navigation and robotics relevant to THA, recent results of these technologies, and future directions.

NAVIGATION

Computer navigation is a useful means to accurately determine the location in the space of the pelvis and/or femur during THA. Recognizing that hip kinematics rely on proper spatial orientation of the implants to each other and to the body is key to proper implant preparation and insertion. Several methods of navigation have evolved to address the requirements for both tracking and imaging for rigid bodies, such as bone, instruments, or implants.

TYPES OF NAVIGATION

Tracking is essential for all aspects of CAS surgery. The computer must be able to recognize where in space the patient and instruments are located relative to one another. The most common type of tracking is optical tracking (**Figure 1**), which uses infrared stereoscopic technology in which a light source emits a signal that is reflected back and captured. Although simple and reliable, optical tracking is limited by line-of-sight issues (eg, drapes or personnel) that block the signal and disrupt the workflow. Alternatively, some systems use electromagnetic tracking systems, which have the distinct advantage of avoiding line-of-sight issues. However, these systems have fallen out of favor because of numerous issues with noise created by instruments and power tools that distort the electromagnetic signal.

CAS surgery can be split into two major categories: image-based and imageless. Image-based systems can use CT (preoperative CT is required), fluoroscopy, or more recently, ultrasonography.[3] Imageless systems do not require preoperative or intraoperative radiologic studies and rely on the identification of the anterior pelvic plane, which is typically done with the patient supine. After a reference tracking device is attached to the pelvis (typically at the iliac crest), anatomic landmarks are digitized (ie, points obtained from the anterior superior iliac spine [ASIS] and pubic symphysis) to allow the computer to determine the plane of the pelvis (**Figure 2**), which is used to reference instrument and implant positions.

One advantage of an imageless system is that the cost of preoperative imaging is negated. In addition, intraoperative procedures involving fluoroscopy or ultrasonography are not needed. Imageless systems are relatively simple to use, and surgeons can quickly adapt to them. However, imageless systems have several distinct disadvantages. First, initial reference points are typically acquired in the supine position. Subsequently, the patient must be reprepped and redraped if the procedure is performed in the lateral position. However, methods of registration have been described without the need to register the anterior pelvic plane, allowing surgeons to accurately register points in the lateral position and avoid reprepping and redraping.[4] Second, errors in point acquisition can occur during digitization.

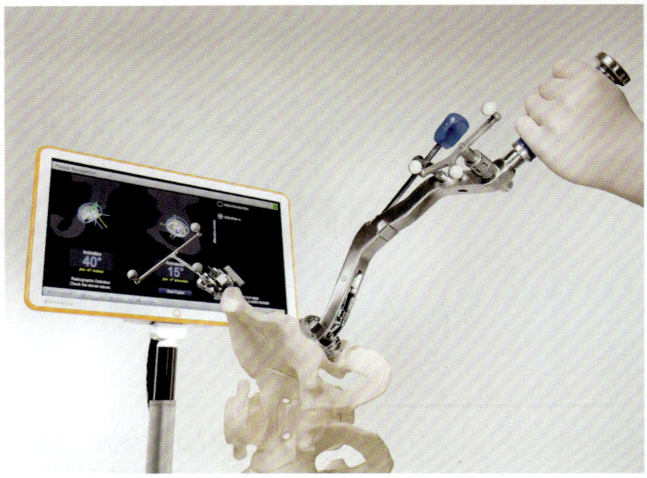

FIGURE 1 Illustration shows a standard infrared sensor and reflectors based on the intraoperative instruments. (Reproduced with permission from Smith+Nephew.)

Landmarks are difficult to confirm in patients who have obesity, which can result in errors in establishing the coordinate plane and incorrect version and abduction values. Because no reference images exist, these errors can go undetected.

Image-based techniques have been promoted to improve the precision and accuracy of computer navigation. Fluoroscopically based navigation (**Figure 3**) uses real-time images of anatomic landmarks coupled with tracking of the pelvis or femur to facilitate accurate determination of spatial orientation. In addition, fluoroscopically based navigation can help confirm position, and reacquisition can be performed at any time during surgery to ensure optimal positioning. Although preoperative imaging is not needed with fluoroscopically based navigation, access to fluoroscopic equipment and disruption of workflow while obtaining images are distinct disadvantages of this method.

Ultrasonography-based navigation has gained popularity in some centers as an alternative to fluoroscopy-based and imageless systems. Although no preoperative planning is necessary, the main advantage of ultrasonography-based navigation is the more precise determination of anatomic landmarks, such as the anterior pelvic spines and pubic symphysis. Patients are placed in a supine position and a pelvic tracking device is placed, and ultrasonographic capture of the pelvic points is performed. Care should be taken to ensure that the ultrasonography probe is vertical to the bony landmark being captured. Compared with manual palpation of bony landmarks, ultrasonographic digitization is not affected by overlying adipose tissue, resulting in more precise measurements of acetabular position, especially version.[5] The limitations of

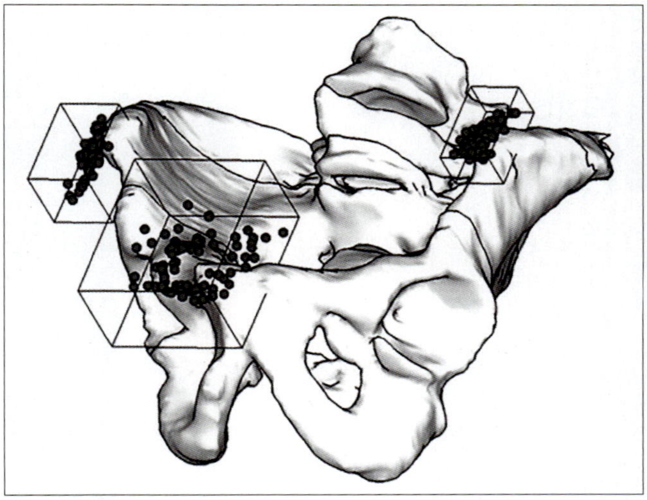

FIGURE 2 Illustration shows registration points on the pelvis. (Reproduced with permission from British Editorial Society of Bone & Joint Surgery. Spencer JMF, Day RE, Sloan KE, Beaver RJ: Computer navigation for the acetabular component: A cadaver reliability study. *J Bone Joint Surg Br* 2006;88[7]:972-975.)

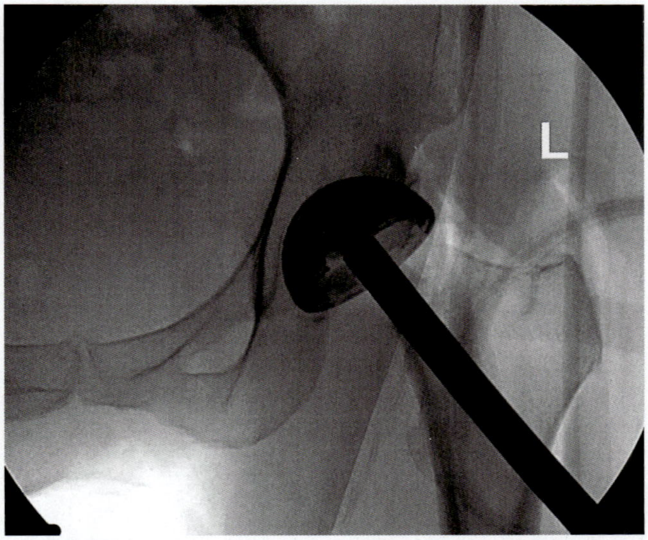

FIGURE 3 Intraoperative fluoroscopic view demonstrates an implanted acetabular cup.

ultrasonography-based navigation include user experience; the need for intraoperative ultrasonographic equipment; and the need to adhere to sterile techniques during prepping, draping, and registration. In addition, registration in the lateral decubitus position can be challenging and can also be a barrier to acceptance of this technique by some surgeons.

CT-based navigation is considered by many to be the benchmark for both navigation and robotics. Precise computer models are generated from the preoperative CT scan, providing in-depth assessment of morphology and orientation. CT-based systems have the greatest capacity in preoperative planning for implant sizing and positioning, which ultimately affect limb length, offset, and virtual range of motion (ROM). The key element in CT-based navigation is to couple the virtual bone model with the patient's actual anatomy at the time of surgery. This linkage is accomplished via the process of registration. Using an instrumented pointer for discrete locations or an instrumented probe to identify a larger area for surface registration, this process maps the registered points on the computer model (**Figure 4**). The degree of accuracy of this matching process can be quantified by placing a probe on the bone surface and determining the distance between the model position and actual position. If the registration error is too large, the registration process can be repeated to reduce error. CT-based navigation is the most accurate method of computer navigation and does not require intraoperative equipment or intraoperative imaging. CT-based navigation can be performed in both supine and lateral positions without affecting precision. However, the time and cost of any CT-based technology will always be a concern.

RESULTS OF NAVIGATION

A large body of literature supports the theory that both the precision and accuracy of acetabular implant positioning are improved when using navigation. Most of the recent literature focuses on the use of imageless techniques, which have been favored over CT-based systems because of the cost associated with preoperative imaging.

Several early clinical experiences with imageless techniques have been reported. A 2009 study reported that 192 THAs using conventional imaging guidance and 450 THAs using computer navigation (125 CT-based and 325 imageless procedures) exhibited similar abduction and anteversion measurements.[6] However, when the transverse acetabular ligament was registered for version alignment, a substantial improvement was reported in acetabular version alignment with navigation. This observation resulted in discussion of the learning curve associated with novel technologies, such as navigation.

The learning curve for navigation was similarly reported in a 2009 study.[7] This study reviewed the surgeon's ability to implant the cup in 45° abduction and 20° to 30° of anteversion based on patient-specific anatomy. Implant position was compared in three groups: 55 cases using conventional guides, the initial experience of 50 cases using an imageless navigation system, and the next 50 cases using the same system. Cup abduction and version were measured using postoperative cross-table lateral radiographs. For the initial

Section 3: Hip

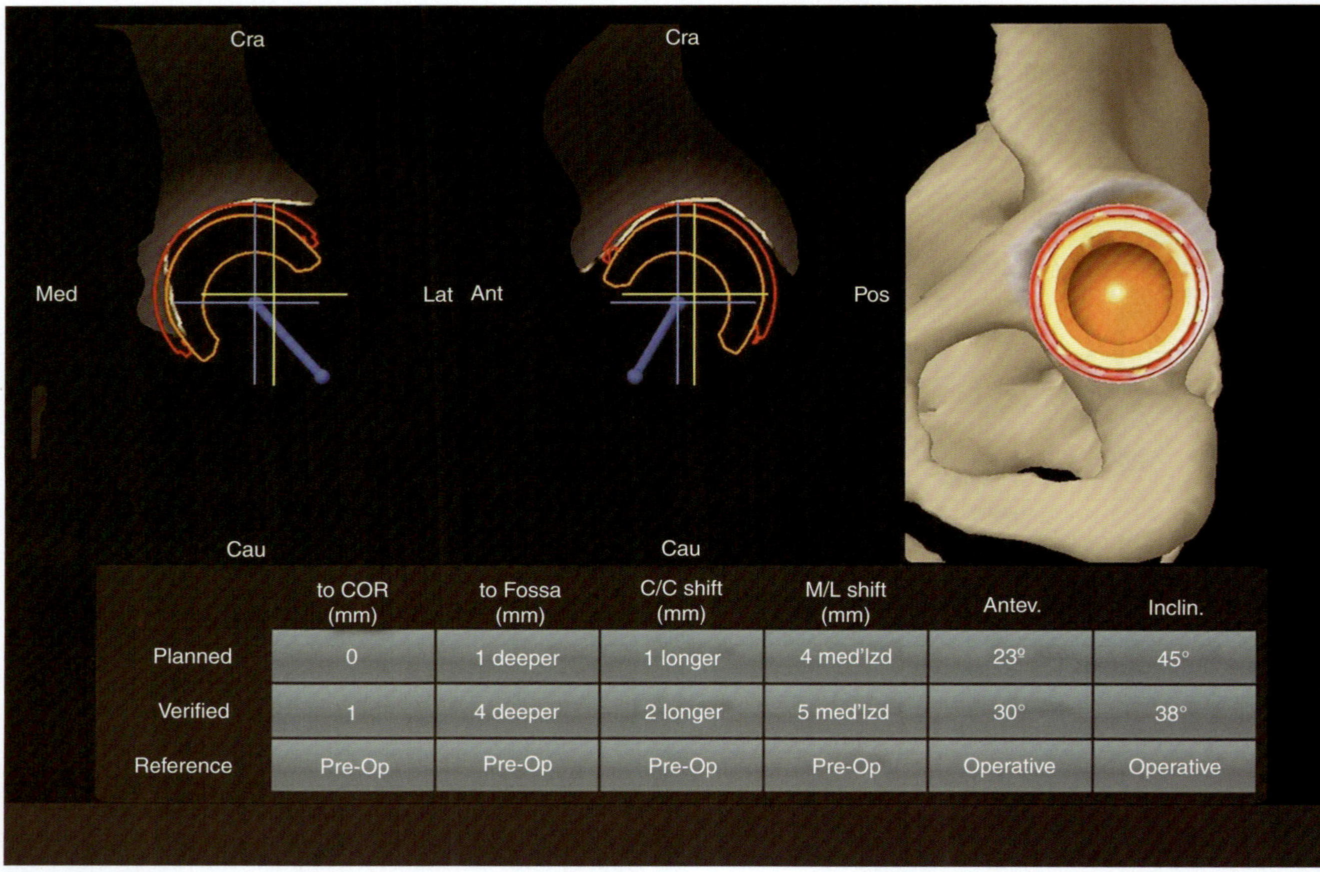

FIGURE 4 Illustration demonstrates CT-based hip navigation. (Reproduced with permission from Kelly TC, Swank ML: Role of navigation in total hip arthroplasty. *J Bone Joint Surg Am* 2009;91(suppl 1):53-58.)

50 cases with imageless navigation, variation was significantly reduced in both abduction and anteversion compared with conventional mechanical guides. A further decrease in variation was demonstrated in the second group of 50 cases with imageless navigation compared with the initial 50 cases ($P < 0.01$). A 2019 study analyzed the accuracy of cup orientation and learning curve of a accelerometer-based portable navigation system (HipAlign) for THA in the supine position.[8] Seventy-five patients were categorized into sequential surgical time periods: initial cases (1 to 25), intermediate (26 to 50), and recent group (51 to 75). The accuracy of acetabular inclination and anteversion was compared. In addition, the time required for navigation and total surgical time were recorded. No significant differences were identified for cup inclination and anteversion, with an average absolute error of 2.6° ± 2.7° and 2.8° ± 2.7°, respectively. The required time for navigation and total surgical time were constant except for the initial five patients.

Although cohort studies provide insight into the applicability of new technologies, the ultimate challenge is to test the results in the context of a randomized clinical trial.[9] A prospective randomized clinical trial compared imageless navigation with a freehand conventional technique for cementless THA: 65 patients were enrolled in each group, with target goals of 40° of cup inclination and 15° of anteversion. Postoperative assessment of cup position was performed using a multislice CT scan. Outcome measures included a modified hip score, Western Ontario and McMaster Universities Osteoarthritis Index score, and surgical time. No differences were reported between the groups. The mean surgical time was 18.1 minutes longer in the navigation group, which can be attributed to tracker placement and registration. Regarding cup position, no significant difference was reported in mean cup abduction between the navigated and freehand group (38.6° versus 37.7°), but a significant difference was reported in anteversion (19.5° versus 17.3°, $P = 0.007$). In addition, there was a significant reduction in deviation from target position between the navigated and freehand group. This study is one of the first to confirm the use of navigation, especially in the reduction of outliers, and it also demonstrated that improvement in cup position may not be manifested by early clinical improvement.

A 2007 randomized controlled study of 60 patients undergoing THA compared the accuracy of acetabular implant position in an anterolateral approach with and without the use of CAS navigation.[10] The anteversion and abduction angles were not substantially different between the CAS and freehand-placed acetabular cups. However, the standard deviations in the CAS group were smaller, indicating a more homogenous group of angles compared with the freehand-placed group. In addition, only 6 of 30 (20%) were outliers in the CAS group compared with 17 of 30 (57%) in the freehand-placed group, according to the safe zone described by Lewinnek.[8] In 2016, 10-year results were subsequently published for this randomized controlled trial.[11] No differences were identified between the groups regarding Harris hip score (HHS) at last follow-up (95.3 ± 5.9 [CAS] versus 96.2 ± 4.5, $P = 0.6$). There was also no difference in mean acetabular linear wear at 10 years (0.71 ± 0.52 mm [CAS] versus 0.77 ± 0.52 mm, $P = 0.54$). There was no identified difference in rates of aseptic loosening in either group, with equivalent survivorship.

A 2012 study evaluated the postoperative cup position of 39 hips in 38 patients following computer-navigated THA.[12] The average intraoperative navigated versus postoperative abduction angles were 41.5° and 40.8°, respectively. Similarly, intraoperative navigated and postoperative anteversion angles were 23.7° and 21.4°, respectively. Overall, the navigation system demonstrated 90% accuracy for abduction and 87% accuracy for anteversion.

A 2011 study compared acetabular position in 25 computer-navigated THAs with 25 conventionally placed THAs.[13] The computer navigation was abandoned intraoperatively in three patients because of excessive pelvic tilt and unreliable registration. In the other 22 patients who underwent computer-guided THA, the mean (±SD) abduction and anteversion angles were 40.0° ± 2.9° and 17.7° ± 3.5°, respectively; for the 25 patients who underwent conventional placement, the angles were 42.5° ± 6.3° and 20.3° ± 7.6°, respectively. The mean (±SD) placement error for abduction and anteversion in the computer-navigated group was 2.3° ± 1.5° and 3.4° ± 2.7°, respectively; for the conventional placement group, the error was 5.5° ± 3.8° and 7.3° ± 5.7°, respectively. The placement error was significantly less for the computer-navigated group than that for the conventionally placed group for both the abduction and anteversion angles. The study authors concluded that navigation results in less variance in the placement of the acetabular implant of THA but cautioned that pelvic morphology may necessitate abandoning the use of navigation under certain circumstances.

In a study that used an imageless CAS surgery system, the postoperative abduction and anteversion angles of acetabular implants placed with computer guidance were measured in 25 patients.[14] The mean (±SD) angles measured intraoperatively for abduction and anteversion using the navigation system were 39.4° ± 4.0° and 32.6° ± 7.0°, respectively, whereas postoperative CT measurements were 38.8° ± 3.5° and 32.2° ± 6.8°, respectively. The accuracy of the guidance system (the absolute difference between the angles measured by the navigation and the angles measured on postoperative CT) was 1.8° ± 1.2° for abduction and 2.0° ± 2.0° for anteversion. Furthermore, precision was 3.4° for abduction and 5.5° for anteversion.

Another study of computer-navigated assistance in THA investigated the accuracy of acetabular implant positioning.[15] The study included 30 patients with 30 hips undergoing CAS THA compared with 101 hips in 99 patients undergoing THA with surgeon-guided acetabular placement. CAS navigation was accurate within 5° for all cases, with a precision of 4.4° for abduction and 4.1° for anteversion. For all angles, the intraoperative navigation angle estimates were within 1° of the angles measured on postoperative CT. When the computer-navigated and surgeon-guided acetabular angles were compared, the computer and the experienced surgeon had similar abduction estimates, but the computer estimate of anteversion was more accurate.

There has been concern that navigation is not as reliable in obese patients. A 2018 study compared the accuracy and precision of imageless navigation in obese (body mass index [BMI] ≥30) and nonobese patients using superficial landmark registration. A retrospective review of 459 THAs from a single surgeon's database was conducted. Inclination precision was better for nonobese patients. However, there was no difference in inclination accuracy, anteversion precision, or anteversion accuracy. Eighty-three percent of implants were placed within the acceptable target zone. There was no relationship between obesity and implant position outside Lewinnek safe zones for inclination or anteversion. The authors concluded that utilization of superficial landmark registration in obese patients is achievable, and imageless navigation improves acetabular implant position in both obese and nonobese patients.

There is promise that navigation can be helpful in cases of severe pelvic deformities. A retrospective review compared the accuracy of cup size and position in patients who have Crowe type I dysplasia and Crowe type IV dysplasia. CT-based navigation was used for 34 THAs in each group. There was no statistically significant difference in accuracy of cup size for Crowe type I (79.4%) and type IV (94.1%, $P = 0.075$). The mean deviations of the cup angle and three-dimensional position were comparable in both groups. It was concluded that a CT-based navigation system is accurate with severe pelvic deformities.

A retrospective cohort study analyzing the Medicare database of 803,732 THAs, including 14,540 navigated THAs, suggested CAS navigation was associated with decreased rates of dislocation and acetabular implant revision.[16] A multivariate regression was used to control for potential confounders. Navigation was associated with a decreased rate of dislocation (1.0% versus 1.7%, $P < 0.001$) and aseptic revision of the acetabular implant (1.03% versus 1.55%, $P < 0.001$). It was not associated with aseptic revision of the femoral implant (1.54% versus 1.87%, $P = 0.064$) or prosthetic joint infection at 30 days (0.34% versus 0.45%, $P = 0.121$) and 90 days (0.50% versus 0.66%, $P = 0.458$). The study authors advised caution when interpreting the results because of the potential of unmeasured confounders.

A retrospective review comparing clinical outcomes and polyethylene wear after 5 to 7 years follow-up suggested no difference between conventional THA and navigated CAS THA with an imageless system.[17] The Hip Osteoarthritis Outcome Score and HHS were obtained in 25 patients who underwent CAS THA and 25 patients who underwent conventional THA. No statistically significant difference was found for the Hip Osteoarthritis Outcome Score, HHS, and polyethylene wear. Cup inclination was more precise in the navigated group. It was concluded that cup-first navigation with an imageless system did not lead to improved midterm functional outcomes or polyethylene wear.

A 2015 randomized controlled trial compared impingement-free ROM and acetabular implant cover between patients who were treated with femur-first navigated THA (66 patients) and conventional THA (69 patients).[18] The Hip Osteoarthritis Outcome Score, HHS, EuroQol-5D, and Mancuso THA expectation scores were also assessed. Desired ROM boundaries without prosthetic impingement was present in 84% of the navigated THA group and 65% in the conventional THA group ($P = 0.016$). Acetabular implant cover was >87% in both groups. There were no differences in clinical outcomes at 6 months and 1 year postoperation. The authors concluded that the navigated femur-first technique improves the potential ROM for activities of daily living but did not lead to observed improved clinical outcomes.

A retrospective review of 152 consecutive THAs analyzed how accurately leg length and hip offset were restored in navigated THA. Compared with the contralateral hip, 95.39% of patients had hip offset restored within 6 mm and 96.04% had leg length restored within 6 mm. The authors concluded that navigation can accurately restore native hip offset and leg length.

A 2017 study compared the incidence of noise after ceramic-on-ceramic THA using navigation (68 THAs) and conventional methods (118 THAs).[19] Patients younger than 65 years and those who have 32-mm heads were included. The risk of noise was significantly increased in the conventional group (28% versus 10%, $P = 0.005$) and the relative risk was 2.7 ($P = 0.1$). Squeaking THAs had decreased anteversion compared with silent THAs (13.4° ± 5.2° versus 17.6° ± 6.9°, $P = 0.01$).

ROBOTICS IN THA

Although interest remains steady in the use of CAS navigation in joint arthroplasty, the application of robotic technology in joint arthroplasty has entered an exciting period. The features that differentiate robotics from navigation are bone preparation and implant insertion. All robotic-guided surgery requires preoperative CT scanning. As with CT-based navigation, tracking of the pelvis and/or femur is required, along with exact bone registration. Robotic-assisted surgery then combines three-dimensional preoperative planning with a precisely guided bone resection and implant placement. Robotic guidance falls into two main categories: active or passive. Active robotic systems used in surgical practice are best thought of as automated. Cutting tools and instruments are controlled by the robotic arm, with no need for surgeon control. Registration accuracy is of paramount importance for active robotic systems. Passive, or haptic, systems require surgical guidance: if deviation beyond the boundaries created by the surgical plan occurs, tactile, auditory, or visual feedback alerts the surgeon to the possibility of error. Haptic systems allow the surgeons to drive the robot, thereby allowing surgeons to retain some element of control.

The first robot that aided in hip surgery was the ROBODOC® (THINK Surgical®)[20,21] (**Figure 5**). This active robotic system was designed to be used with the ORTHODOC software (IBM) and was used on the basis of a preoperative CT scan. The five-axis robot used sensors and a high-speed cutting tool to prepare the bone for the femoral prosthesis. One disadvantage of this robot was the use of pins placed preoperatively (before the CT scan) in the greater trochanter and distal femur. Although early results were encouraging, the system gained little popularity in the United States.

Another active robotic system available for hip arthroplasty is the CASPAR (Computer Assisted Surgical Planning and Robotics system; URS Ortho).[22] This system also uses a preoperative CT scan and sensors attached to the patient to help prepare the bone for the femoral prosthesis. Although this system was once commonly used in Germany, it failed to gain traction in the United States.

The introduction of haptic-guided robotic technology has had global success. This technology has been used in both partial knee arthroplasty and THA. The surgical protocol starts with three-dimensional preoperative planning (**Figure 6**) based on the preoperative CT scan. Preoperative limb-length discrepancy and native femoral

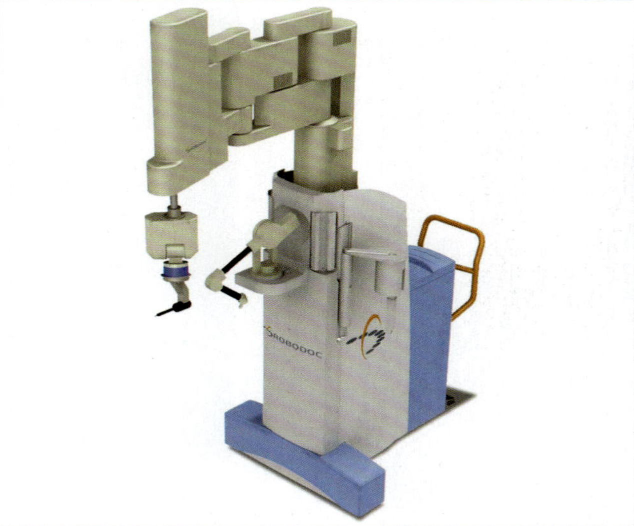

FIGURE 5 Illustration of the ROBODOC® surgical system. (Courtesy of THINK Surgical®.)

version are noted. Planning of the implant position begins with virtual placement of the acetabular socket in the model with preferred abduction and version angles. The virtual center of rotation (COR) can be compared with the native COR, and any effect, such as medialization or cephalization, is noted. A virtual femoral stem is placed, and the resultant effect of length and offset is noted (**Figure 7**). The level of neck osteotomy and/or type or size of the femoral stem can be adjusted to achieve the intended length and offset target.

Following placement of a femoral tracking array, femoral registration and navigated resection level of the femoral neck is performed. The femur is prepared, tracking array is placed on the trial femoral implant, and the femoral version is calculated. Based on the femoral version, the planned acetabular version can be adjusted accordingly to obtain an adequate combined version. Acetabular preparation begins with the application of a pelvic tracking array, followed by acetabular registration of multiple points around the bony socket (**Figure 8**). The robot is registered, and the end effector (working end of the robotic arm) is verified. Acetabular reaming in the preferred degree of abduction and version is performed with visual feedback showing real-time bone removal. Reaming is permitted within the confines of a virtual haptic cone, allowing the robotic arm small degrees of freedom to work outside of the preferred target. After the planned acetabular reaming diameter is reached, the acetabular implant is inserted. Unlike reaming, which allows some latitude during bone resection, robotic cup insertion is performed with the haptics fully engaged, corresponding to the final planned cup position, including depth of insertion (**Figure 9**). Final cup position is confirmed using a tracking probe, accessing multiple points around the periphery of the acetabular implant (**Figure 10**).

ROBOTIC RESULTS

In a 2015 study, 54 patients undergoing THA were randomly assigned to either THA with manual rasping (27 patients) or THA augmented with the ROBODOC® system (27 patients):[23] Twenty-four patients completed follow-up in the robotic group, as did 25 in the manual group. Mean surgical time was longer in the robotic group than in the manual group (103 minutes versus 78 minutes; $P < 0.012$). At follow-up, no significant difference between the robot-assisted and manual groups was found in HHSs (mean, 93; range, 85 to 100 versus mean, 95; range, 89 to 100; $P = 0.0512$) or Western Ontario and McMaster Universities Osteoarthritis Index scores (mean, 11; range, 6 to 17 versus mean, 12; range, 5 to 15; $P = 0.30$). No dislocations were reported in either group at 24 months. The robot-assisted group had better mean varus-valgus alignment (0.3° versus 2.2° for the manual group) and less limb-length discrepancy (1.9 versus 4.9 mm for the manual group).

A 2017 study followed up patients from two separate clinical trials undergoing conventional manual THA versus robotic THA augmented with the ROBODOC® system.[24] The study included 22 patients undergoing conventional manual THA and 45 patients receiving robotic THA augmented with the ROBODOC® system, comparing pain scores, radiographic outcomes, and patient-reported outcome measures between the two groups at 14 years follow-up. Patients undergoing THA with ROBODOC® augmentation had better Health Status Questionnaire pain (62.65 ± 16.21 versus 83.75 ± 20.40, respectively, $P = 0.19$), Harris pain scores (39.09 ± 7.37 versus 41.81 ± 5.05, respectively, $P = 0.25$), and improved Western Ontario and McMaster Universities Osteoarthritis Index scores (11.32 ± 11.92 versus 8.44 ± 11.48, respectively, $P = 0.34$) compared with conventional manual THA. Despite the previously reported improvements in femoral stem fit and alignment in the robotic group, there was no statistically significant difference in probability of a revision for wear between the groups and no revisions for loosening in either group at 14 years follow-up.

HAPTIC RESULTS

The role of haptically guided hip arthroplasty requires preclinical validation to demonstrate the precision and accuracy of the implant placement. A 2013 experiment used a robot (Stryker) for placement of an acetabular prosthesis

Section 3: Hip

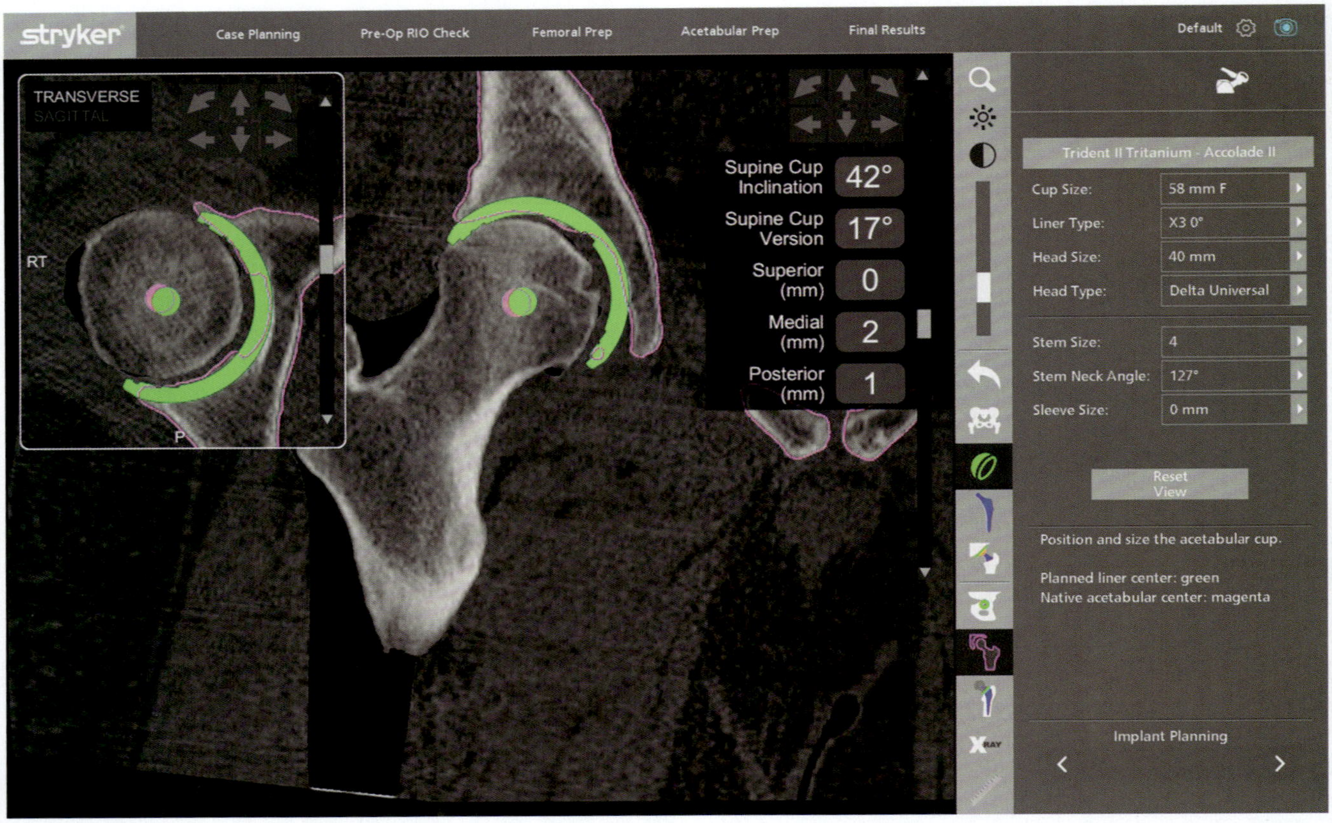

FIGURE 6 Illustration demonstrates preoperative CT-based acetabular planning with Mako SmartRobotics™. (Courtesy of Stryker.)

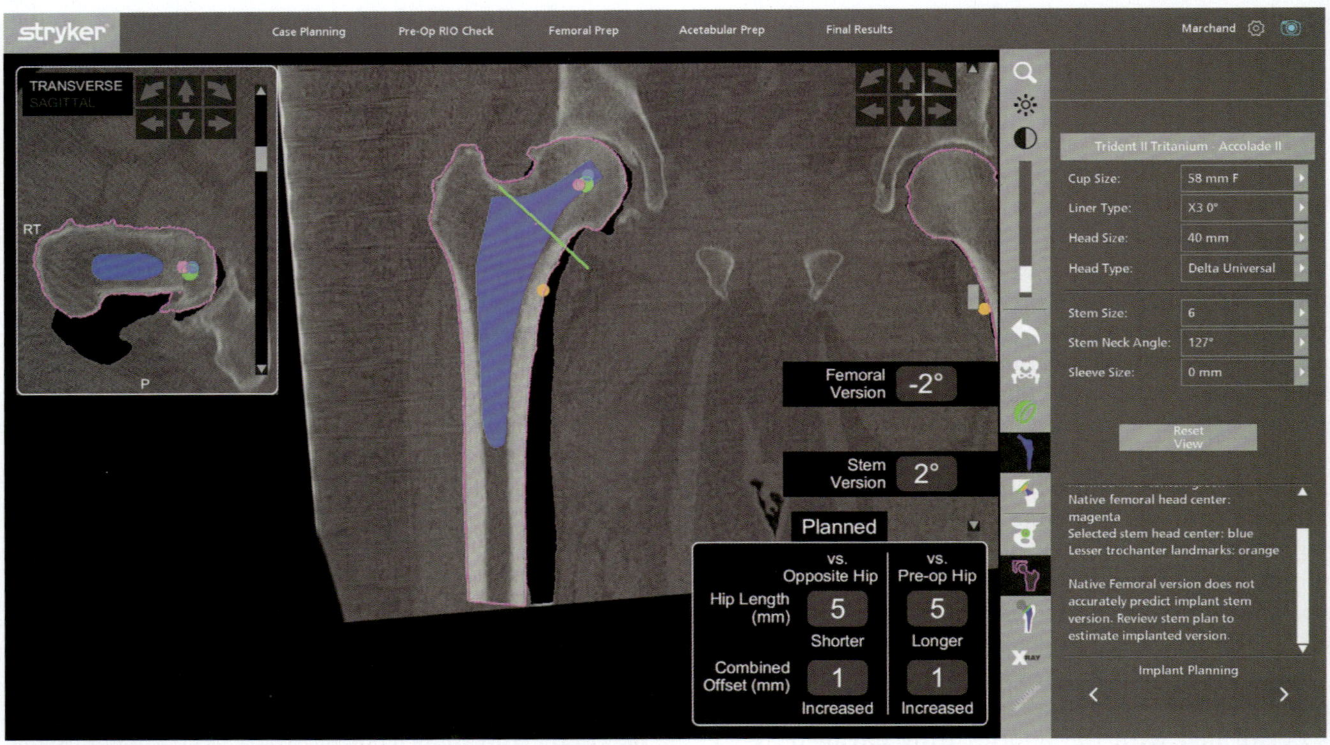

FIGURE 7 Illustration demonstrates preoperative CT-based femoral planning with Mako SmartRobotics™. (Courtesy of Stryker.)

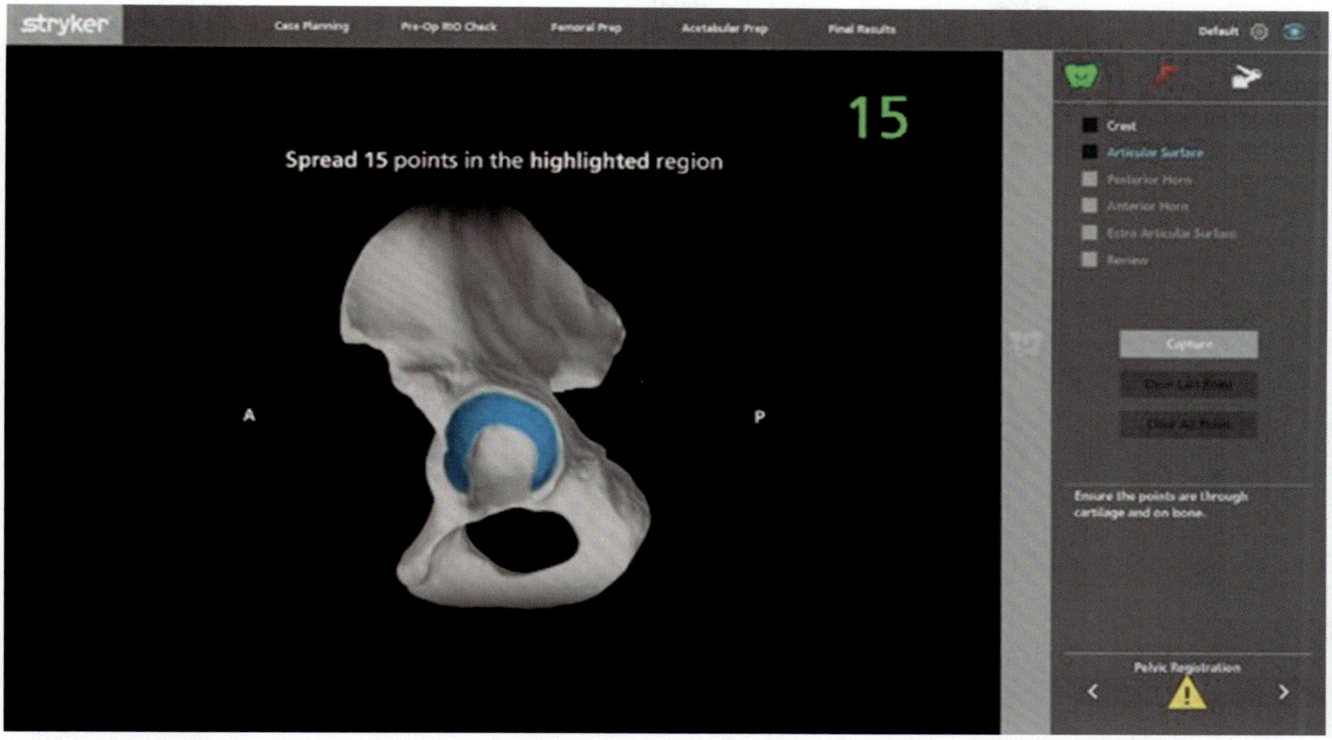

FIGURE 8 Illustration demonstrates acetabular registration points with Mako SmartRobotics™. (Courtesy of Stryker.)

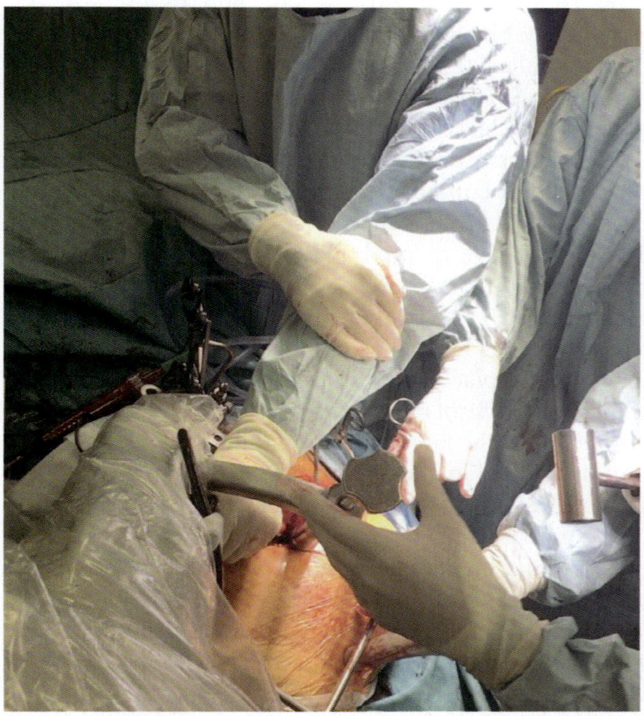

FIGURE 9 Illustration demonstrates the acetabular component insertion using Mako SmartRobotics™. (Courtesy of Stryker.)

in 12 cadaver pelvises: the acetabular implant was placed with the robot on one side and manually on the other side.[25] In all cases, surgery was performed using a posterior approach by an experienced surgeon. Measures included mediolateral, anterior-posterior, and superoinferior COR compared with the native socket. In addition, the abduction and anteversion angles were compared with respect to the Lewinnek safe zones. The robot was more accurate than the experienced surgeon for all COR measurements: for cup abduction, the mean error between the planned and actual cup abduction was 2.31° and 11.6°, respectively ($P < 0.01$); the mean anteversion error between the planned and actual cup position was 2.63° and 8.94°, respectively ($P < 0.01$).

A 2015 study evaluated acetabular placement with Mako SmartRobotics™ using postoperative CT scans to assess cup position and compared it with the position measured in the operating room using the Mako sensors.[26] Although the use of the Mako robotic arm was abandoned in five hips in three patients because of soft-tissue constraints, the Mako sensors were used to evaluate cup position on insertion in these patients. Excluding these patients, 43 hips in 40 patients were evaluated using postoperative CT scans. The planned mean inclination (±SD) for the hips was 39.9° ± 0.8° (range, 35° to 40°); the intraoperative robotic measurement was

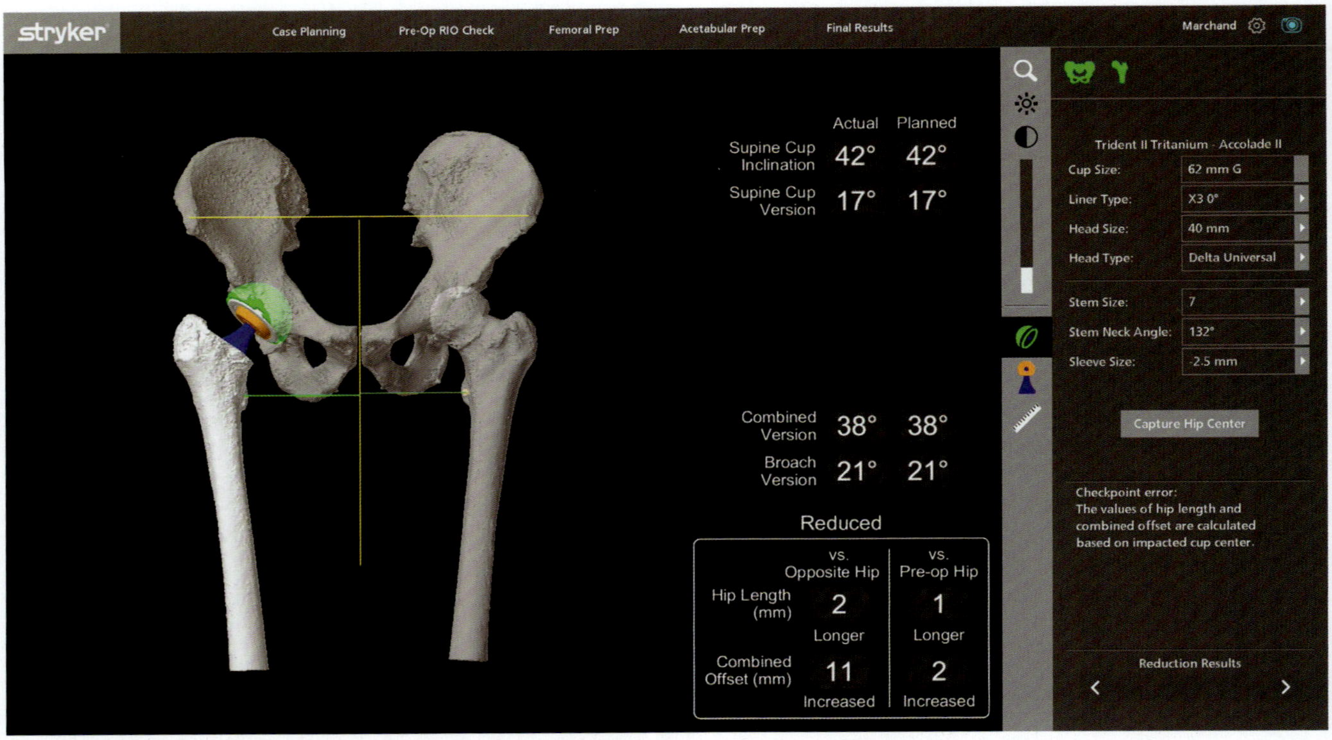

FIGURE 10 Illustration demonstrates the postreduction results with Mako SmartRobotics™. (Courtesy of Stryker.)

38.8° ± 1.6° (range, 25° to 43°). The mean abduction (±SD) on postoperative CT scans was 39.1° ± 3.8° (range, 33° to 48°). Five outliers (12%) were noted between 5° and 10°; none that exceeded 10° were reported. For anteversion, the planned mean angle (±SD) for the hips was 21.2° ± 2.4° (range, 15° to 25°); the intraoperative robotic measurement was 20.7° ± 2.4° (range, 16° to 26°). The mean abduction (±SD) on postoperative CT scans was 18.9° ± 4.1° (range, 7° to 26°). Seven outliers (16%) were reported between 5° and 10°; none that exceeded 10° were reported. COR measurements compared with preoperative measurements were within a mean of 3 mm vertical (superior) and 5 mm horizontally (medial).

Another 2015 study used the Mako SmartRobotics™ system to augment THA in obese patients to address problems with acetabular cup placement.[27] Acetabular positioning can be difficult in obese patients because soft-tissue interposition can affect the tools used to align the cup. A total of 105 patients were prospectively followed in three groups: those who have a BMI less than 30 kg/m^2, those who have a BMI of 30 to 35 kg/m^2, and those who have a BMI greater than 35 kg/m^2. No difference was noted in the number of cases outside the safe zones of Lewinnek or Callanan across the three groups ($P > 0.63$). The mean inclination angles (±SD) for the patients in the groups who have BMI less than 30 kg/m^2, BMI from 30 to 35 kg/m^2, and BMI greater than 35 kg/m^2 were 39.9° ± 3.0°, 39.72° ± 3.29°, and 41.02° ± 2.27°, respectively. The mean (±SD) version angles were 16.8° ± 4.0°, 17.02° ± 3.6°, and 16.73° ± 2.74°, respectively. No significant differences were reported in any of these values ($P > 0.75$). The study authors concluded that Mako SmartRobotics™ can be used reliably in obese patients to achieve accurate acetabular cup position.

A 2017 retrospective cohort study compared accuracy of acetabular cup positioning in 300 consecutive THAs performed by a single surgeon.[28] This included an initial 100 consecutive manual THAs, the last 100 consecutive manual THAs before the introduction of robotic arm–assisted THA, and the first 100 consecutive robotic arm–assisted THAs. The authors reported that acetabular implant placement within Lewinnek safe zone was achieved in 77% of robotic arm–assisted group compared with 45% in the late conventional manual THA group, and only 20% in the early conventional manual THA group ($P < 0.001$). Robotic arm–assisted THA was associated with an additional 71% improvement in accuracy of acetabular implant positioning compared with conventional manual THA in the first year of use ($P < 0.001$). At a minimum of 2 years of follow-up, dislocation rate was zero in the robotic arm–assisted THA group compared with 5% in the early conventional manual THA group, and only 3% in the late conventional manual THA group.

A 2016 retrospective cohort study compared accuracy of achieving the planned acetabular cup positioning and femoral COR in 12 robotic arm–assisted THAs versus 14 conventional manual THAs.[29] All patients underwent CT scans to create virtual three-dimensional models to help assess and quantify anteversion, inclination, and hip joint center in the native hip and implanted THA. Robotic arm–assisted THA was associated with increased combined anteversion (19.1° ± 11.7° versus 23.5° ± 23.6°, respectively, $P < 0.001$) and decreased cup inclination (16.5° ± 6.0° versus 10.2° ± 6.8°, $P < 0.001$) compared with conventional manual THA. Overall, variation in the difference of the implant orientations was 11.1° in the robotic arm–assisted THA group compared with 18.3° in the conventional manual THA group ($P = 0.005$). Variation in the femoral head center was 4.5 mm in the robotic arm–assisted group versus 6.3 mm in the conventional manual THA ($P = 0.204$). The authors concluded that both techniques failed to restore native hip geometry, but robotic arm–assisted surgery was associated with reduced outliers in restoring the planned hip biomechanics.

A 2019 prospective cohort study compared accuracy of achieving the planned hip biomechanics and acetabular cup positioning in conventional manual THA versus robotic arm–assisted THA.[30] In both treatment groups, preoperative planning was undertaken using CT scans and three-dimensional virtual reconstructions of the hip joint. All surgical procedures were undertaken by a single surgeon, and study outcomes were recorded using plain radiography. The study found that robotic arm–assisted THA was associated with improved accuracy in restoring the native horizontal and vertical CORs ($P < 0.001$) and achieving the planned combined offset compared with conventional manual THA ($P < 0.001$). Robotic THA also improved accuracy of acetabular cup positioning within Lewinnek (96% versus 68%, respectively, $P = 0.02$) and Callanan (92% versus 64%, respectively, $P = 0.01$) safe zones compared with conventional manual THA. Furthermore, robotic arm–assisted THA helped to reduce horizontal outliers of greater than 5 mm (4% versus 28%, respectively, $P < 0.001$) and vertical outliers of greater than 3 mm (4% versus 20%, respectively, $P < 0.001$) compared with conventional manual THA. There was no difference between the two treatment groups with respect to correction of leg-length discrepancy.

Patient-specific safe zones based on preoperative assessments of pelvic kinematics have recently gathered momentum as an avenue for improving stability and reducing complications following THA.[31] Pelvic tilt was assessed in 1,517 patients undergoing THA in the supine, standing, and flexed-seated positions. Mean pelvic tilt was 4.2° (range, −20.5° to 24.5°), −1.3° (range, −30.2° to 27.9°), and 0.6° (range, −42.0° to 41.3°) in the three positions, respectively. Mean sagittal pelvic rotation from supine to standing was −5.5° (range, −21.8° to 8.4°), from supine to flexed seated was −3.7° (range, −48.3° to 38.6°), and from standing to flexed seated was 1.8° (range, −51.8° to 39.5°). Preoperative spinopelvic radiographs or CT scans to assess individualized pelvic kinematics during functional activities could help to determine patient-specific safe zones for implant positioning. Robotic technology offers an avenue for executing implant positioning into these patient-specific safe zones with a high-level of accuracy.

EMERGING TECHNIQUES AND TECHNOLOGIES

Many technologies investigating alternatives to traditional navigation and robotics have been recently introduced. The HipXpert (Surgical Planning Associates) is a navigation system that combines CT-based preoperative planning with an intraoperative mechanical alignment tool (**Figure 11**). The alignment guide is tuned in accordance with the preoperative plan's pelvic tilt–adjusted, patient-specific targets for anteversion and inclination. For anterior approaches, place the HipXpert by docking the basepoint leg on the central portion of the ischium just below the inferior acetabular rim and the two footed cannulas on the ASIS. For posterior and lateral approaches, use the drill guide to place a 2.8-mm guidewire posterior to the rim of the acetabulum and superior to the infracotyloid notch. Then slide the HipXpert and basepoint cannula until it docks to the bone. Next, palpate the ASIS and dock the trocar to the bone percutaneously. Repeat the percutaneous docking for the third leg. Assistants should hold both the anterior and lateral tools firmly in place. Once docked, the surgeon should align the cup parallel to the direction indicator and begin impaction. The surgeon may then finalize the impaction with the parallel guide to achieve preferred anteversion and inclination (**Figure 11**).

In a study of 54 THAs performed with this device, the HipXpert eliminated all outliers exceeding 10° from the preoperative plan's patient-specific goals for anteversion and inclination.[32] However, 12.8% of cups were outside 5° of the individual plan targets for inclination,[6] and 23.4% of cups were outside 5° of the individual plan targets for anteversion.[11] This technology, which was designed as a simple tool to use in the navigation of the acetabular cup, now provides leg length and offset navigation. In addition, the company has morphed into a cloud-based THA system that augments the intraoperative navigation tool. Although this technology offers a promising alternative to expensive robotic systems, the use of a preoperative CT scan is required, which exposes the patient to radiation.

Another new technology is the Intellijoint (Intellijoint Surgical). This device uses a camera attached to a standard pin near the ASIS, which then obtains measurements based on a small platform attached to the greater trochanter.

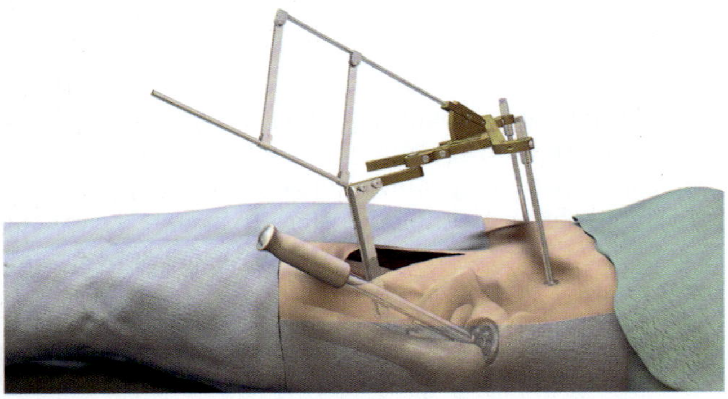

FIGURE 11 Illustration shows an adjustable, patient-specific intraoperative alignment tool for anterior surgery. (Courtesy of HipXpert.)

Measurements are obtained before cutting the femoral neck. After implant insertion, measurements are obtained again to ensure that appropriate leg length and offset have been restored. This second measurement also can allow the surgeon to add or subtract offset or leg length based on preoperative planning. Furthermore, the technology can be added to the acetabular implant insertion handle to precisely measure anteversion and inclination angles.

OrthAlign (OrthAlign) is a new device that uses a gyroscope-based system that was initially used for total knee arthroplasty (**Figure 12**). Since the device received FDA approval for hip arthroplasty in 2014, studies have been underway to test its capability and accuracy in acetabular cup placement, leg length restoration, and offset restoration. This system uses a disposable gyrometer fixed to the patient via a standard pelvic pin. The system uses arms and sensors that attach to the gyrometer and the patient's femur to measure offset, leg length, and cup position. Although this device is in the early stages of its development, this product should be available in the near future.

Another technology on the horizon is a patient-specific guide that assists in the correct placement of the acetabular implant for THA. This guide is prefabricated based on a preoperative CT scan and sterilized for use in surgery. The guide is made using Visualization Toolkit libraries (Kitware) and is initially placed inside the native acetabular position before cup insertion, and a Kirschner wire is placed into the pelvis inside the surgical wound. Based on the preoperative planning and guide construction, this wire will have the planned anteversion and inclination so that during insertion, the handle can be aligned with this wire for proper cup orientation. The guide was tested in 2010 in a prospective series of 31 patients in which the guide was used, compared with 38 patients who underwent standard THA without the guide.[33] The guide reduced outliers (greater than 10° from the safe zones as described by Lewinnek) from 23% in the standard group to zero in the CT-based model-guided group.

Computer-navigated and robotic THAs have several limitations that must be acknowledged when interpreting the findings of any studies comparing outcomes with these technologies and conventional manual THA. Computer-navigated and robotic THAs are associated with substantive costs for installation of the navigation or robotic device, updating and servicing computer software, and training the surgical team to become familiar

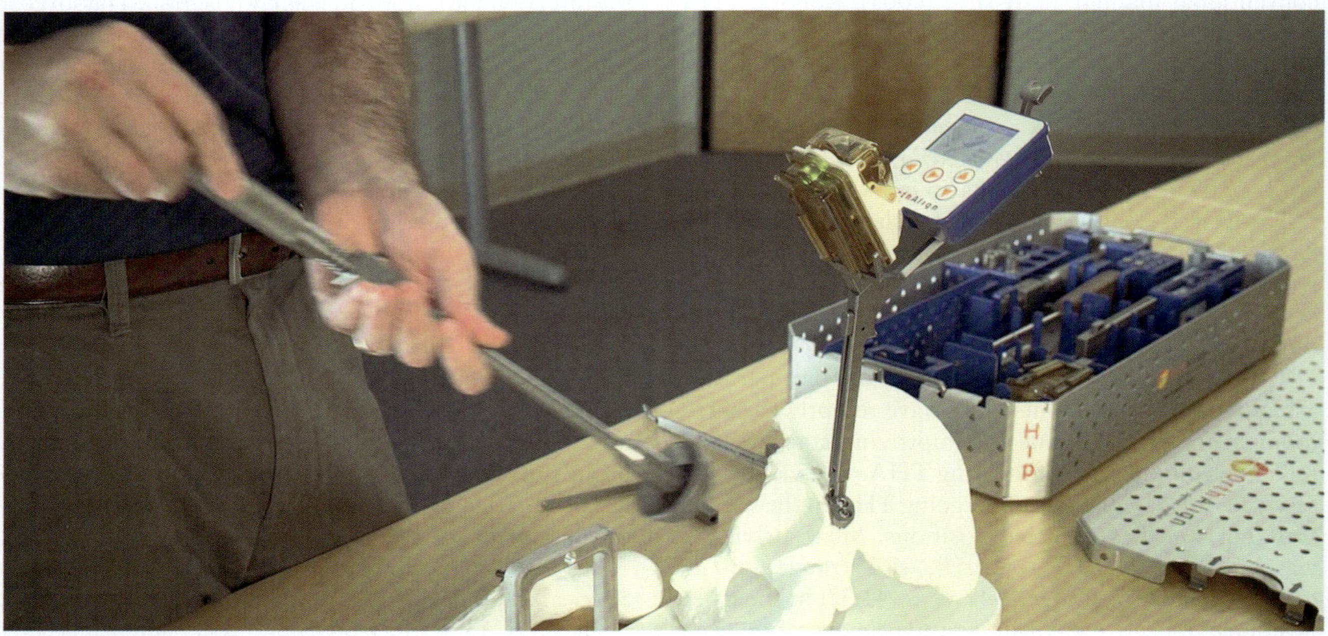

FIGURE 12 Clinical photograph shows the OrthAlign Plus system (OrthAlign). (Reproduced with permission from OrthAlign.)

with the new instruments and workflow. The technology may only be compatible with a selected number of implant designs from the manufacturer. There is a steep learning curve for the operating surgeon, with additional surgical times and surgical delays until surgical proficiency is achieved. Image-based computer navigation and robotic THA are associated with additional costs for preoperative scanning and lead to additional radiation exposure. Malfunctioning of the computer navigation system or robotic device may require intraoperative conversion to conventional manual THA. There are also limited data on the cost effectiveness of computer-navigated and robotic THA compared with conventional manual THA. Further trials assessing the effects of computer-navigated and robotic THAs on patient satisfaction, functional outcomes, implant survivorship, and cost effectiveness compared with conventional manual THA are required before these technologies are adopted into mainstream arthroplasty practice.

SUMMARY

Implant position in THA has been shown to affect dislocation rates and the longevity of the prosthesis. Several studies have shown that standard methods for cup placement are less accurate when positioning the acetabular implant. Over the past decade, many technologies have emerged to aid in the orientation of the acetabular implant. Several computer-based navigation systems have been shown to reduce errors in the placement of the acetabular implant, leg length, and offset. Furthermore, robotic-assisted surgery has been introduced to aid in the preparation and placement of the implants. This technology offers an avenue for improving the accuracy of achieving patient-specific safe zones for implant positioning based on preoperative dynamic assessments of spinopelvic alignment. Although these systems continue to evolve, surgeon reliance on these devices will increase as these devices become more affordable, as well as faster and easier to use in the operating room. In addition, although some technologies have emerged for preparation and insertion of the femoral implant, these technologies are not commonly used in the United States.

KEY STUDY POINTS

- Despite the use of anatomic landmarks or external guides, acetabular implant position is most susceptible to errors.
- Computer navigation systems currently available for clinical use help reduce errors in implant placement.

ANNOTATED REFERENCES

1. Padgett DE, Hendrix SL, Mologne TS, Peterson DA, Holley KA: Effectiveness of an acetabular positioning device in primary total hip arthroplasty. *HSS J* 2005;1(1):64-67.
2. Digioia AM, Jaramaz B, Plakseychuk AY, et al: Comparison of a mechanical acetabular alignment guide with computer placement of the socket. *J Arthroplasty* 2002;17(3):359-364.
3. Parratte S, Kilian P, Pauly V, Champsaur P, Argenson JN: The use of ultrasound in acquisition of the anterior pelvic plane in computer-assisted total hip replacement: A cadaver study. *J Bone Joint Surg Br* 2008;90(2):258-263.
4. Davis ET, Schubert M, Wegner M, Haimerl M: A new method of registration in navigated hip arthroplasty without the need to register the anterior pelvic plane. *J Arthroplasty* 2015;30(1):55-60.
5. Hasart O, Perka C, Tohtz S: Comparison between pointer-based and ultrasound-based navigation technique in THA using a minimally invasive approach. *Orthopedics* 2008;31(10 suppl 1):orthosupersite.com/view.asp?rID=35540.
6. Kelley TC, Swank ML: Role of navigation in total hip arthroplasty. *J Bone Joint Surg Am* 2009;91(suppl 1):153-158.
7. Najarian BC, Kilgore JE, Markel DC: Evaluation of component positioning in primary total hip arthroplasty using an imageless navigation device compared with traditional methods. *J Arthroplasty* 2009;24(1):15-21.
8. Kamenaga T, Hayashi S, Hashimoto S, et al: Accuracy of cup orientation and learning curve of the accelerometer-based portable navigation system for total hip arthroplasty in the supine position. *J Orthop Surg (Hong Kong)* 2019;27(2):2309499019848871.

   This study assessed the accuracy of acetabular implant positioning and learning curve with the disposable accelerometer-based portable navigation system (HipAlign). Seventy-five patients who underwent THA through the anterolateral approach were analyzed retrospectively. The average absolute error was 2.6° ± 2.7° for inclination and 2.8° ± 2.7° for anteversion. The time required for HipAlign navigation and surgical time was constant apart from the initial five patients. Level of evidence: III.
9. Lass R, Kubista B, Olischar B, Frantal S, Windhager R, Giurea A: Total hip arthroplasty using imageless computer-assisted hip navigation: A prospective randomized study. *J Arthroplasty* 2014;29(4):786-791.
10. Parratte S, Argenson JN: Validation and usefulness of a computer-assisted cup-positioning system in total hip arthroplasty. A prospective, randomized, controlled study. *J Bone Joint Surg Am* 2007;89(3):494-499.
11. Parratte S, Ollivier M, Lunebourg A, Flecher X, Argenson JN: No benefit after THA performed with computer-assisted cup placement: 10-year results of a randomized controlled study. *Clin Orthop Relat Res* 2016;474(10):2085-2093.
12. Snyder GM, Lozano Calderón SA, Lucas PA, Russinoff S: Accuracy of computer-navigated total hip arthroplasty. *J Arthroplasty* 2012;27(3):415-420.

13. Lin F, Lim D, Wixson RL, Milos S, Hendrix RW, Makhsous M: Limitations of imageless computer-assisted navigation for total hip arthroplasty. *J Arthroplasty* 2011;26(4):596-605.

14. Ryan JA, Jamali AA, Bargar WL: Accuracy of computer navigation for acetabular component placement in THA. *Clin Orthop Relat Res* 2010;468(1):169-177.

15. Dorr LD, Malik A, Wan Z, Long WT, Harris M: Precision and bias of imageless computer navigation and surgeon estimates for acetabular component position. *Clin Orthop Relat Res* 2007;465:92-99.

16. Bohl DD, Nolte MT, Ong K, Lau E, Calkins TE, Della Valle CJ: Computer-assisted navigation is associated with reductions in the rates of dislocation and acetabular component revision following primary total hip arthroplasty. *J Bone Joint Surg Am* 2019;101(3):250-256.

This is a retrospective study comparing computer navigation and conventional THA using a Medicare database. A total of 803,732 THAs were identified, including 14,540 (1.81%) using navigation. Navigation was associated with a lower dislocation rate (1% versus 1.7%) and aseptic revision of the acetabular implant (1.03% versus 1.55%). No other differences were identified. Level of evidence: III.

17. Keshmiri A, Schröter C, Weber M, Craiovan B, Grifka J, Renkawitz T: No difference in clinical outcome, bone density and polyethylene wear 5-7 years after standard navigated vs. conventional cementfree total hip arthroplasty. *Arch Orthop Trauma Surg* 2015;135(5):723-730.

18. Renkawitz T, Weber M, Springorum HR, et al: Impingement-free range of movement, acetabular component cover and early clinical results comparing “femur-first” navigation and “conventional” minimally invasive total hip arthroplasty: A randomised controlled trial. *Bone Joint J* 2015;97-B(7):890-898.

19. Shah SM, Deep K, Siramanakul C, Mahajan V, Picard F, Allen DJ: Computer navigation helps reduce the incidence of noise after ceramic-on-ceramic total hip arthroplasty. *J Arthroplasty* 2017;32(9):2783-2787.

This is a retrospective study analyzing 375 patients who underwent ceramic-on-ceramic THAs. About 202 patients underwent navigated THA and 173 underwent conventional THA. Navigated THAs were 2.7 times less likely to have noise compared with conventional THAs. Patients with decreased anteversion and those older than 65 years also had an increased incidence of squeaking. Level of evidence: III.

20. Bargar WL, Bauer A, Börner M: Primary and revision total hip replacement using the Robodoc system. *Clin Orthop Relat Res* 1998;354:82-91.

21. Paul HA, Bargar WL, Mittlestadt B, et al: Development of a surgical robot for cementless total hip arthroplasty. *Clin Orthop Relat Res* 1992;285:57-66.

22. Thomsen MN, Breusch SJ, Aldinger PR, et al: Robotically-milled bone cavities: A comparison with hand-broaching in different types of cementless hip stems. *Acta Orthop Scand* 2002;73(4):379-385.

23. Lim SJ, Ko KR, Park CW, Moon YW, Park YS: Robot-assisted primary cementless total hip arthroplasty with a short femoral stem: A prospective randomized short-term outcome study. *Comput Aided Surg* 2015;20(1):41-46.

24. Bargar WL, Parise CA, Hankins A, Marlen NA, Campanelli V, Netravali NA: Fourteen year follow-up of randomized clinical trials of active robotic-assisted total hip arthroplasty. *J Arthroplasty* 2018;33(3):810-814.

This study reports 14-year follow-up of randomized clinical trials comparing robotic-assisted THA using the ROBODOC® and conventional manual THA. Patients in the robotic-assisted group had higher Health Status Questionnaire pain and Harris pain scores as well as lower Western Ontario and McMaster Universities Osteoarthritis Index scores. There was no difference in probability of a revision for wear and no revisions for loosening in either group. The authors concluded that there are small but potentially important improvements in clinical outcomes in the robotic-assisted group. Level of evidence: I.

25. Nawabi DH, Conditt MA, Ranawat AS, et al: Haptically guided robotic technology in total hip arthroplasty: A cadaveric investigation. *Proc Inst Mech Eng H* 2013;227(3):302-309.

26. Kanawade V, Dorr LD, Banks SA, Zhang Z, Wan Z: Precision of robotic guided instrumentation for acetabular component positioning. *J Arthroplasty* 2015;30(3):392-397.

27. Gupta A, Redmond JM, Hammarstedt JE, Petrakos AE, Vemula SP, Domb BG: Does robotic-assisted computer navigation affect acetabular cup positioning in total hip arthroplasty in the obese patient? A comparison study. *J Arthroplasty* 2015;30(12):2204-2207.

28. Illgen RL, Bukowski BR, Abiola R, et al: Robotic-assisted total hip arthroplasty: Outcomes at minimum two-year follow-up. *Surg Technol Int* 2017;30:365-372.

This is a retrospective study comparing acetabular implant position and postoperative complications following manual THA and robotic THA. Three groups were compared: the initial 100 consecutive manual THAs in one surgeon's practice, the last 100 consecutive manual THAs before robotic introduction, and the first 100 consecutive robotic THAs. The rate of acetabular implant placement within the Lewinnek safe zone was 30% in the early manual THA group, 45% in the late manual THA group, and 77% in the robotic THA group. At 2-year follow-up, the dislocation rate was 5% in the early manual THA group, 3% in the late manual THA group, and zero in the robotic THA group. Level of evidence: III.

29. Tsai TY, Dimitriou D, Li JS, Kwon YM: Does haptic robot-assisted total hip arthroplasty better restore native acetabular and femoral anatomy? *Int J Med Robot* 2016;12(2):288-295.

30. Kayani B, Konan S, Thakrar RR, Huq SS, Haddad FS: Assuring the long-term total joint arthroplasty: A triad of variables. *Bone Joint J* 2019;101-B(1 suppl A):11-18.

This prospective cohort study compared accuracy in restoring the native hip center in patients undergoing manual THA and robotic-assisted THA. Fifty patients undergoing manual THA were compared with 25 patients undergoing robotic-assisted THA. Robotic-assisted THA was associated with improved accuracy in restoring the native hip center, preservation of natural offset, and planned leg length correction. Level of evidence: II.

31. Pierrepont J, Hawdon G, Miles BP, et al: Variation in functional pelvic tilt in patients undergoing total hip arthroplasty. *Bone Joint J* 2017;99-B(2):184-191.

    In this study, pelvic tilt was measured in 1,517 patients undergoing THA in three functional positions: supine, standing, and flexed seated (the moment patients initiate rising from a seated position). The mean pelvic tilt was 4.2° supine, −1.3° standing, and 0.6° flexed seated. The mean sagittal pelvic rotation was −5.5° from supine to standing, −3.7° from supine to flexed seated, and 1.8° from standing to flexed seated. Sagittal pelvic rotation could lead to functional malorientation of the acetabular implant in 17% of patients. The authors concluded that optimal acetabular implant positioning is patient specific and requires an evaluation of functional pelvic tilt preoperatively. Level of evidence: IV.

32. Jennings JM, Randell TR, Green CL, Zheng G, Wellman SS: Independent evaluation of a mechanical hip socket navigation system in total hip arthroplasty. *J Arthroplasty* 2016;31(3):658-661.

33. Hananouchi T, Saito M, Koyama T, Sugano N, Yoshikawa H: Tailor-made surgical guide reduces incidence of outliers of cup placement. *Clin Orthop Relat Res* 2010;468(4):1088-1095.

CHAPTER 36

Complications of Total Hip Arthroplasty

MICK P. KELLY, MD • NATHANAEL HECKMANN, MD • JOSHUA J. JACOBS, MD

ABSTRACT

Total hip arthroplasty (THA) is one of the most successful surgical procedures developed in the past century. The number of revision THAs has risen along with the increased demand for THAs, and this has occurred at a time of greater national attention to readmission and complication rates to demonstrate accountability in health care and to reduce costs. Because complications seriously affect patient outcomes, and public reporting of complication rates is often used as a proxy for quality of care, it is vital to examine complications to prevent their occurrence.

Keywords: complications after THA; heterotopic ossification; instability; leg-length discrepancy; trunionosis

Dr. Heckmann or an immediate family member serves as a paid consultant to or is an employee of Intellijoint Surgical and MicroPort Orthopedics and serves as a board member, owner, officer, or committee member of the American Academy of Orthopaedic Surgeons. Dr. Jacobs or an immediate family member serves as a paid consultant to or is an employee of Zimmer; has stock or stock options held in Hyalex; has received research or institutional support from Medtronic Sofamor Danek, Nuvasive, and Zimmer; and serves as a board member, owner, officer, or committee member of the American Board of Orthopaedic Surgery, Inc., the Hip Society, and the Orthopaedic Research and Education Foundation. Neither Dr. Kelly nor any immediate family member has received anything of value from or has stock or stock options held in a commercial company or institution related directly or indirectly to the subject of this chapter.

INTRODUCTION

Although an uncommon occurrence, serious complications after total hip arthroplasty (THA) can delay or hinder complete functional recovery. Even though major medical complications, such as myocardial infarction or pulmonary embolism, can occur and should be on the surgeon's radar, they are less frequent and are often related to the patient's comorbidities, medications, allergies, and so on. It is important to be knowledgeable about potential surgical complications, including instability, trunionosis, limb-length discrepancy, heterotopic ossification, and neurovascular injuries. Please note that periprosthetic joint infection and periprosthetic fractures are covered in separate chapters.

INSTABILITY AFTER THA

Dislocation is the number one indication for revision hip arthroplasty.[1] Despite the overwhelming success of THA, instability remains a challenging problem. Reports on the incidence of dislocation vary widely, from 0.3% to 10.0% after primary THA and up to 28% after revision THA. There are patient-specific and surgery-specific risk factors for dislocation, and managing this problem requires a clear diagnosis and an understanding of the etiology of instability. Although many dislocations can be managed with closed reduction alone, revision for recurrent instability may be necessary. Success requires an algorithmic approach as well as appropriate expectations from both the surgeon and patient.

Hip instability after THA is a particularly challenging problem for the adult reconstruction surgeon. Patient-specific risk factors for dislocation include prior hip surgery, neuromuscular or cognitive disorders,

This chapter is adapted from Kheir MM, Parvizi J, Fleischman AN, et al: Complications of total hip arthroplasty, in Mont MA, Tanzer M, eds: *Orthopaedic Knowledge Update®: Hip and Knee Reconstruction*, ed 5. Rosemont, IL, American Academy of Orthopaedic Surgeons, 2017, pp 473-505.

noncompliance, alcoholism, and THA for femoral neck fracture. Surgery-specific risk factors include the surgical approach, inadequate soft-tissue balancing, implant malpositioning, impingement (bony and/or implant), smaller head size, and surgeon experience. Appropriate management of dislocation after THA requires a clear understanding of the cause of dislocation, which begins with a detailed history, physical examination, and radiographic evaluation. Although most early dislocations can be managed with closed reduction, revision surgery may be necessary; however, it should be undertaken when the cause of the dislocation is apparent and a clear surgical plan has been developed. Occasionally, the management of recurrent dislocation is required even though investigations do not demonstrate an apparent etiology.

Epidemiology and Financial Effect

Although hip revision for instability has decreased significantly, instability remains a major cause for revision. A query of the National Inpatient Sample database from 2009 to 2013 found that hip instability accounted for approximately 17% of all revision hip surgery and remains the most common indication for revision surgery.[2] Additionally, revision for instability continues to have higher failure rates. One study found the cumulative risk of redislocation in 539 patients who had revision for instability to be 34.5% at 15 years.[3] This problem has substantial financial effect. The cost of a closed reduction was found to be 19% of the cost of primary THA in one study,[4] and the overall cost of a single dislocation was shown to increase the cost of THA by 342% in another study.[5] Recurrent dislocation is exceedingly expensive, costing 300% more than a single dislocation according to a study by another group of authors.[6] Notably, the authors found that surgical intervention for current dislocation was significantly less expensive (40%) than continued closed treatment.

Pathophysiology of Instability

It is important to recognize that the cause of instability is often multifactorial. Two classifications of instability may prove useful: temporal and anatomic. The classification related to timing is grouped as early, intermediate, and late. An early dislocation occurs within the first 6 months, an intermediate dislocation occurs between 6 months and 5 years, and a late dislocation occurs after 5 years. Early and intermediate dislocations have distinct pathologic features and are more likely related to preexisting neuromuscular disorders, patient noncompliance, implant malposition, or impingement. Late dislocation is more likely related to wear and osteolysis, implant loosening, trochanteric osteolysis or stress shielding, a new-onset neuromuscular disorder, or muscle atrophy. Early and intermediate dislocations are more likely to be successfully managed with closed reduction, whereas late dislocation more often requires surgery.[7] One anatomic classification system categorized instability into six types[8] (**Table 1**). Regardless of classification system, the primary focus for successful treatment is identifying the specific source of the dislocation and careful planning, should revision surgery be undertaken.

TABLE 1

Classification System for Instability

Type	Etiology
I	Isolated acetabular malposition
II	Isolated femoral malposition
III	Abductor deficiency
IV	Impingement
V	Polyethylene wear
VI	Unknown

Patient Risk Factors

Patient-related risk factors, although not always modifiable, are important to identify because they may contribute to instability. Gender is a risk factor for dislocation after primary THA, with a higher incidence in women. However, gender does not predict success for revision and is therefore unlikely to contribute to a treatment plan.[9] A history of prior hip surgery has been found to significantly increase the risk for dislocation.[10] Alcoholism and cognitive disorders that increase the risk of falls and noncompliance with restrictions can also increase the risk. Age may be a risk factor for dislocation, although studies show varying risk, and it is possible that the increased risk is related to the increased incidence of neuromuscular and cognitive deficits, as well as increased prevalence of arthroplasty related to femoral neck fractures in the elderly.

It is important to identify anatomic and neuromuscular patient-related risk factors because they directly affect treatment decisions. The primary soft-tissue restraints to dislocation are the abductor mechanism of the gluteus medius and minimus, and the hip capsule (iliofemoral, pubofemoral, and ischiofemoral ligaments). A history of hip dysplasia and femoral or acetabular osteotomies can contribute to muscle imbalance and changes in anatomy that increase the risk of instability. Spinopelvic relationship is critical to hip biomechanics and may contribute to hip instability (see next section). Conditions that result in soft-tissue laxity, including rheumatoid arthritis, hypermobility, and ligamentous laxity, have been shown to increase the risk of dislocation. Significant weight loss can also change soft-tissue tension, leading to dislocation. Additionally, conditions that require THA in which the normal soft-tissue contractures associated with hip osteoarthritis are absent (eg, femoral neck fracture, osteonecrosis) are also associated with a higher rate of dislocation.[11] Neuromuscular disorders, including cerebral palsy, muscular dystrophy, myasthenia gravis, Parkinson disease, multiple sclerosis, and severe spinal stenosis, also increase the risk of dislocation, presumably because of abductor weakness. Higher preoperative range of motion has been shown to be an independent risk factor for instability after primary THA.

Surgical Risk Factors

Surgical Approach

Although not modifiable, the surgical approach for primary THA may have an effect on the cause of dislocation. Surgical approaches that disrupt the posterior soft-tissue envelope (capsule and external rotators) have a higher risk of dislocation, although meticulous attention to posterior capsular repair has greatly reduced this risk. A published meta-analysis that included more than 13,000 patients found a dislocation rate of 3.20% for the posterior approach, 2.18% for the anterolateral approach, 1.27% for the transtrochanteric approach, and 0.55% for the direct lateral approach.[12] Other studies evaluating posterior and direct lateral approaches indicate that dislocation rates are not statistically different when the posterior approach includes a posterior soft-tissue repair.[13] The direct anterior approach may be associated with few dislocations because the posterior soft-tissue structures are often not disrupted. An analysis of a large arthroplasty registry between 2001 and 2011 including 22,237 patients who have minimum 3 years' follow-up demonstrated a lower dislocation rate in the direct anterior group compared with the posterior approach cohort (adjusted HR, 0.44; 95% CI, 0.22 to 0.87, $P = 0.017$).[14] However, another study at a single institution with 3,574 consecutive patients between 2011 and 2016 found a dislocation rate of 0.84% (14/1,657) with the posterior approach compared with 1.28% (17/1,329) with the anterior approach ($P = 0.32$). A 2017 meta-analysis stated there is inconclusive evidence to demonstrate a lower dislocation rate with the direct anterior approach.[15]

Impingement

Impingement is a broad diagnosis that takes multiple issues into account. It is often related to implant position, inadequate offset, head size, and liner choice. Impingement is a result of the contact of two nonarticular prosthetic surfaces during extremes of motion (most commonly the trunnion and the liner), from unresected osteophytes (most commonly anteriorly), from heterotopic ossification, contact of the ischium with the posterior femur, or capsular scar tissue. Greater femoral head-neck ratio and larger femoral heads increase range of motion before the occurrence of this type of impingement and increase the jump-distance to dislocation once impingement occurs. Skirted necks, larger trunnions, and smaller femoral heads decrease the range of motion.

Implant Positioning

Implant malposition (acetabular, femoral, or both) is one of the most common causes of dislocation. Malposition leads to a lack of restraint and/or impingement from the implant, soft-tissue, or bone. The prior surgical approach may give clues to acetabular positioning. Excessive anteversion of the acetabulum may result in anterior instability, perhaps more commonly in an anterior-based or anterolateral approach. In contrast, underanteverted or retroverted acetabular implants may risk posterior dislocation, perhaps more commonly in posterior approaches. Excessive abduction may result in late dislocation secondary to increased edge loading and subsequent accelerated wear at the superior edge of the liner.

Evaluation of acetabular implant position should be done carefully. However, it should also be noted that many dislocations occur with implants positioned within the established safe zones (abduction 40° ± 10°, and anteversion 20° ± 5°). One study of 206 THA dislocations found that most (58%) had a socket within the safe zone for both abduction and anteversion, 84% were within the safe zone for abduction, and 69% were within the safe zone for anteversion.[16] A safe zone based solely on these measurements gives a false sense of security because the true safe zone is different for each patient and likely depends on anatomic relationships that have yet to be fully quantified (such as spinopelvic parameters).

Dislocation is also related to femoral position, and combined anteversion helps determine stability. Combined anteversion is determined with the cup and stem in place. The lower limb is positioned in neutral (or slight hip flexion) and is internally rotated until the femoral head is symmetrically seated (coplanar) in the cup. The amount of internal rotation in degrees needed to produce a coplanar head and cup is the combined anteversion. One study recommended combined anteversion of 45° in women and 20° to 30° in men.[17] Femoral implants can be malrotated, particularly in hip replacements that use modular implants; this is difficult to determine on plain radiographs but can be ascertained from either a lateral view of the femur or a CT scan.

Head Size

Femoral head size has a significant effect on dislocation risk secondary to both range of motion before impingement (related to the head-neck ratio) and increased jump distance (**Figure 1**). The acceptable thickness of acetabular

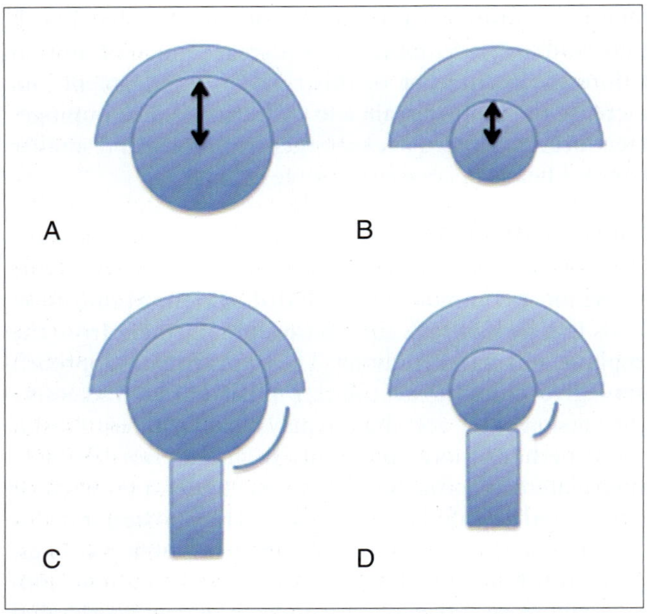

FIGURE 1 Schematic drawings of femoral head in the acetabular cup. An increase in head size affects both jump distance (**A** and **B**) and range of motion before impingement (**C** and **D**).

liners has decreased with the introduction of highly cross-linked polyethylene. Although the appropriateness of this trend is debatable, average head sizes have increased recently, and a corresponding decrease in dislocations has been observed.[18]

Liners

Acetabular liners can help make minor changes to acetabular position (with elevated rims or increased offset through lateralized liners) and their use has become commonplace in primary THA. When an elevated rim liner is present in a patient prone to dislocation, it is important to remember that elevated rims decrease range of motion to impingement, as the trunnion contacts the elevated rim. This may increase the risk of instability. Face-changing or oblique-type liners may decrease the risk of impingement by providing coverage without decreasing range of motion. Different types of liners are shown in **Figure 2**.

Diagnosis

Defining the cause of a dislocation event is critical for management. A thorough history should be obtained that includes the patient position and action at the time of dislocation. This can give clues regarding the direction of dislocation, possible impingement, or implant malposition. Physical examination should include abductor strength testing, assessment of limb length and gait, and neurologic status, as well as evaluation for soft-tissue laxity or hypermobility disorders. Infection should always be ruled out with appropriate laboratory testing, including aspiration.

Adequate radiographs are also critical, both prereduction and postreduction. Additionally, radiographs from the index procedure should be obtained, if possible, to determine signs of wear or changes in implant position. Cross-sectional imaging with CT scans can also be useful. Imaging should start with an AP view of the pelvis and an AP view of the hip. The orientation of the face of the acetabulum in these two radiographs can help determine if the cup is retroverted. It is important to note that an AP view of the pelvis can give a false appearance of cup anteversion compared with an AP of the hip, as shown in **Figure 3**. Lateral radiographs are also helpful in determining version of the cup, and several measurement techniques have been described. One study described the anteversion on a lateral radiograph as an angle formed between the line parallel to the plane of the radiograph and a line tangential to the face of the acetabulum; however, wide standard deviations exist with this method because it depends on the radiograph being perfectly positioned.[10] Another study attempted to improve on this method and described the ischiolateral method as an angle formed between a line parallel to the long axis of the ischium and a line tangential to the face of the acetabulum.[19] The mean SD between this technique and the technique described earlier[10] was found to be 3.7° ($P < 0.001$).

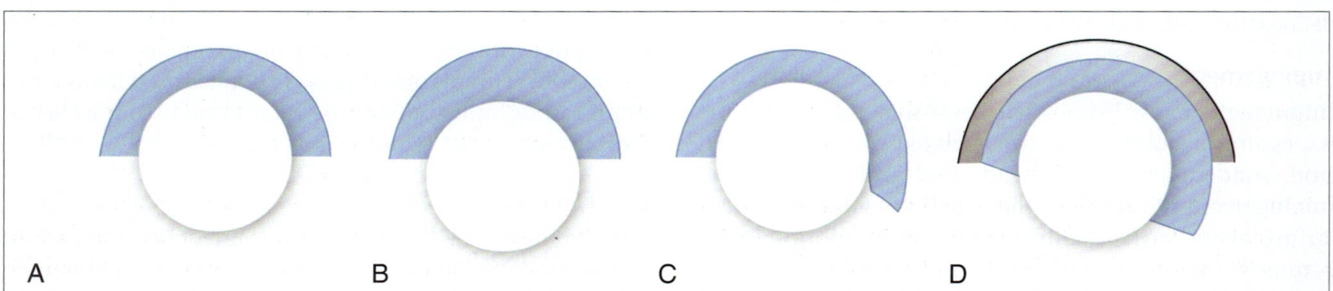

FIGURE 2 Schematic drawings of liner options: neutral (**A**), lateralized (**B**), elevated rim (**C**), and face-changing (**D**).

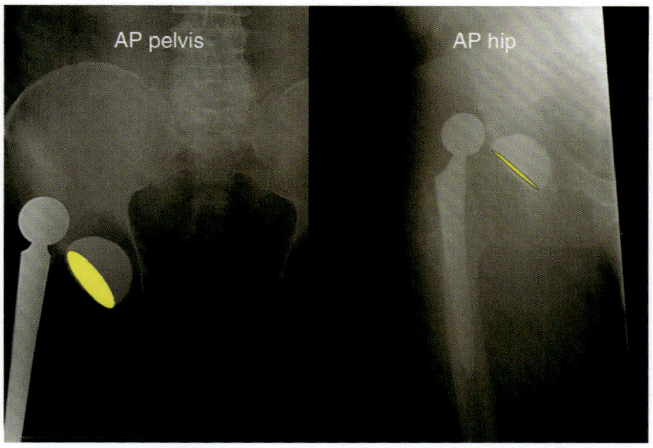

FIGURE 3 AP radiographs of the pelvis and right hip of the same patient after dislocation, demonstrating an underanteverted acetabular implant. This is much more clearly appreciated on the hip radiograph.

Lateral radiographs can give clues to relative version but cannot be used in isolation for diagnosis, and cross-sectional imaging can be very useful.

Management

Early dislocations can often be managed successfully with closed reduction. Dislocations that occur within the first 6 weeks and that are successfully relocated have a more than 80% likelihood of maintaining reduction.[7] Conversely, for dislocations that occur three or more times, or occur at a late stage, the failure rate is high (33% to 55%) with closed reduction, and revision should be strongly considered.[11] If closed reduction is successful, patients should be counseled extensively on positions to avoid and the use of bracing treatment (although evidence supporting the use of bracing treatment is limited). In noncompliant patients or those who have cognitive or neuromuscular disorders, a spica cast can be applied (however, this option should be performed with caution, because of hygiene issues).

Surgical management should be undertaken when appropriate—after the surgeon has gained a clear understanding of the possible cause of dislocation and has created a management plan. Attempts should be made to obtain the prior surgical report or to contact the prior surgeon to determine the implants used. Multiple surgical options should be available, and the surgeon should be prepared to revise the implants if necessary.

Surgical management should focus on the cause of dislocation. Type I dislocations should be treated with revision of the acetabular implant. If the implant is close to optimum position, then an elevated or face-changing liner can be considered; however, this should be used to correct only minor degrees of malposition. Isolated liner exchange was an independent predictor ($P = 0.004$) for recurrent dislocation after revision for instability in a study of 156 revisions.[9] Type II dislocations usually necessitate revision of the femoral implant unless the primary implant is a modular implant that allows for changes in version. Combined malposition should address the most malpositioned implant first. Type III dislocations are the most challenging to treat, and multiple strategies may be used (discussed later in this section), including implant revision if malposition is noted, dual-mobility and constrained liners, and soft-tissue procedures in some cases. It is important to note that studies have shown that an increase in head size cannot make up for abductor deficiency.[20] Revision of type IV dislocations should address any impingement found intraoperatively, and revision of the implants may be necessary. A lateralized liner and increased neck length can be used to improve offset. Elevated and face-changing liners can also be used in combination with other options or to make minor corrections. General strategies to decrease impingement via the implants include increasing the head-neck ratio (usually through increased head size) and increasing offset. Type V dislocations should be treated as one would treat wear and osteolysis, with possible revision of the implants. Isolated liner exchange can be considered, but this may not make the hip stable and, as mentioned earlier, is predictive of recurrent failure. Type VI dislocations should be carefully examined intraoperatively and any pathologic conditions treated. If no pathology is identified, dual-mobility constrained liners or salvage procedures can be considered. Close attention to hip biomechanics should be observed in all cases. A systematic intraoperative approach is warranted, and the algorithm in **Figure 4** should be followed.

Dual Mobility

Please note that this topic is more extensively covered in a separate chapter. An important option in the management of THA instability has been the widespread introduction of dual mobility liners. Adding an articulation increases the range of motion to impingement and several series have examined the results of dual mobility. One study, using the Swedish hip replacement registry, examined 228 hip revisions for instability using a dual-mobility liner. Rerevision for dislocation at a median follow-up of 2 years was 2% (four hips). The study did not examine closed reductions for dislocations.[21] A study of 88 THA revisions using dual-mobility liners resulted in one revision for recurrent dislocation and two for aseptic loosening at 2-year follow-up.[22] Another study examined acetabular revision surgery in 163 hips with a dual-mobility cup, which showed a dislocation rate of 4% at a mean follow-up of 12 years.[23] A 2015 study examined 24 revision THAs using dual-mobility liners for dislocation (18 revisions) or instability (6 revisions with a diagnosis

Section 3: Hip

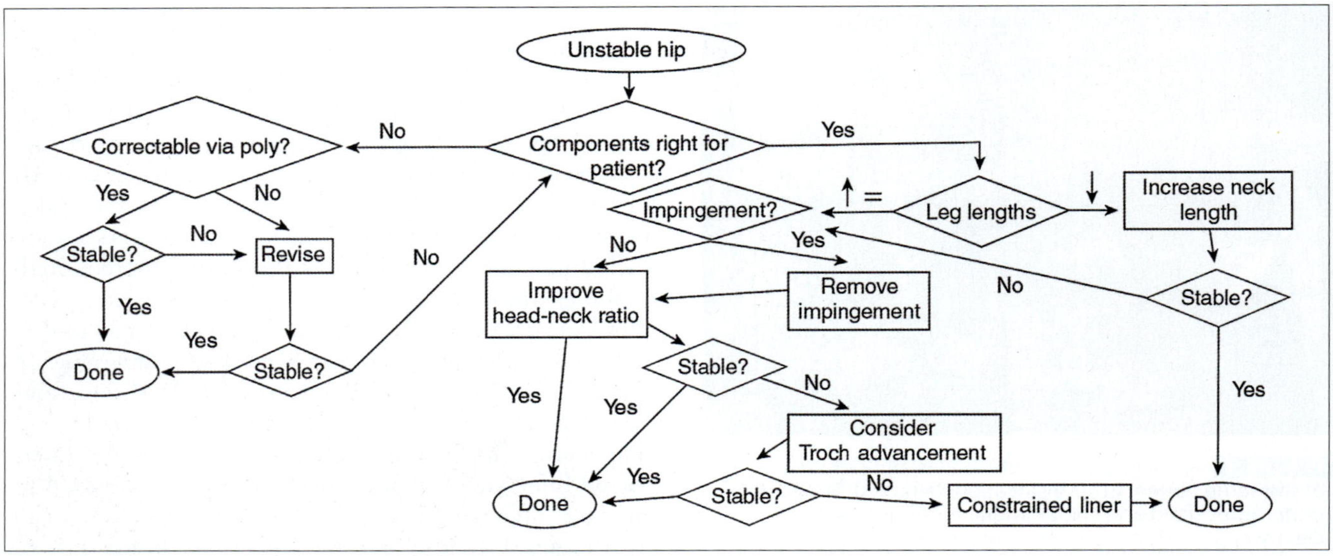

FIGURE 4 Algorithm for intraoperative assessment and management of the unstable total hip arthroplasty. Troch = trochanteric

requiring revision THA combined with abductor deficiency). At a mean follow-up of 22 months, no recurrent dislocations were seen.[24]

Although dual mobility offers the surgeon an option without the downside of constraint, no long-term studies are available, and unforeseen problems may appear in the future. A study of 100 patients who have dual mobility articulations found elevated cobalt levels in 21 patients (21%) and elevated chromium levels in four patients (4%). Two patients who have a painful THA and elevated cobalt levels had MRI results consistent with adverse soft-tissue reactions; however, at the time of the study, none of the patients had undergone revision.[25]

Bipolar and Tripolar Treatment

Bipolar hemiarthroplasty with removal of the acetabular implant has been reported in small series and is a salvage option for treatment of dislocation, but its use is limited because of groin pain and acetabular erosion.[26,27] A study reported on eight patients treated with tripolar articulars (a large acetabular implant with a bipolar hemiarthroplasty) with no recurrent dislocations at an average of 4.2 years' follow-up.[28] As with dual mobility, this treatment strategy has a high failure rate in the presence of abductor deficiency.

Trochanteric Advancement and Soft-tissue Augmentation

Trochanteric advancement is an option for patients who have well-positioned implants but poor abductor tension or abductor insufficiency with an intact tendon. Some small series have reported reasonable outcomes. One study reported 81% success in 21 hips with chronic dislocation and well-positioned implants, but no large series appear in the literature.[29] Given the risk of trochanteric nonunion and escape, this technique is rarely used. Several different soft-tissue augmentation techniques have been described, including using Achilles tendon allograft, advancement of the gluteus medius, and rerouting of the tensor fasciae latae.[30] Small case series have shown moderate success; however, no large studies or long-term outcomes have been reported. In general, these techniques are reserved for the challenging scenario of abductor insufficiency.

Constrained Liners

Constrained liners are an important option and can either be implanted into a previously placed acetabular implant de novo or cemented in place; however, they have limitations and should be used selectively. Several series have reported on the use of constrained liners with a moderately high success rate (84% to 98%) at midterm follow-up, but failure due to loosening (3.6% to 14%) or redislocation (up to 17.5%) poses substantial concerns. Long-term studies show lower success rates in preventing redislocation (70%) with failure rates higher than 40%. This failure rate does not reflect poor surgical choices, but rather the complex nature of the problem. In general, constrained liners are placed in patients at very high risk for dislocation, in cases of abductor insufficiency, or for idiopathic dislocation. These cases exhibit both a predilection for recurrent dislocation and extremely high bone-implant stress. One group reported on the placement of 755 consecutive constrained implants in 720 patients who have minimum 10-year follow-up. Of these, 138 were cases of recurrent instability. Overall Kaplan-Meier survivorship for revision for the entire cohort was 68.5% at 5 years and 51.7% at 10 years. Of the 138 cases treated for recurrent instability, 28.9% failed with recurrent dislocation.[31] Short-term and midterm results are somewhat more encouraging, but they also suggest caution. A 2016 study reported on an average of 3.5 years' follow-up in 58 hips revised with a constrained liner. Eleven hips (19%) redislocated, and 14 hips (24%) required revision for any reason.[32] Another study reported a redislocation rate of 16% (9 hips) at 2 years in 55 patients treated with constrained liners during THA revision. Of the nine dislocations, eight occurred in patients who did not have acetabular implant revision, suggesting that position may not have been optimized.[33]

In general, it is ideal to place a constrained liner in an already well-fixed acetabular implant. When approaching the cup, all screws should be removed and thorough testing performed for osseous ingrowth. If the acetabular implant has to be revised and constraint used, two options exist: (1) placing the cup and allowing ingrowth, and then placing the constrained liner in a staged fashion, or (2) using multiple screws for augmentation, after which the patient's weight bearing and activities are limited for a prolonged period postoperatively. The first option may be preferable because it theoretically has better long-term outcomes because of lower loosening rates; however, this has yet to be shown in the literature. Failure of a constrained liner can be catastrophic, and the patient should be counseled on the risks of constraint and the likelihood of a need for further revision surgery (**Figure 5**).

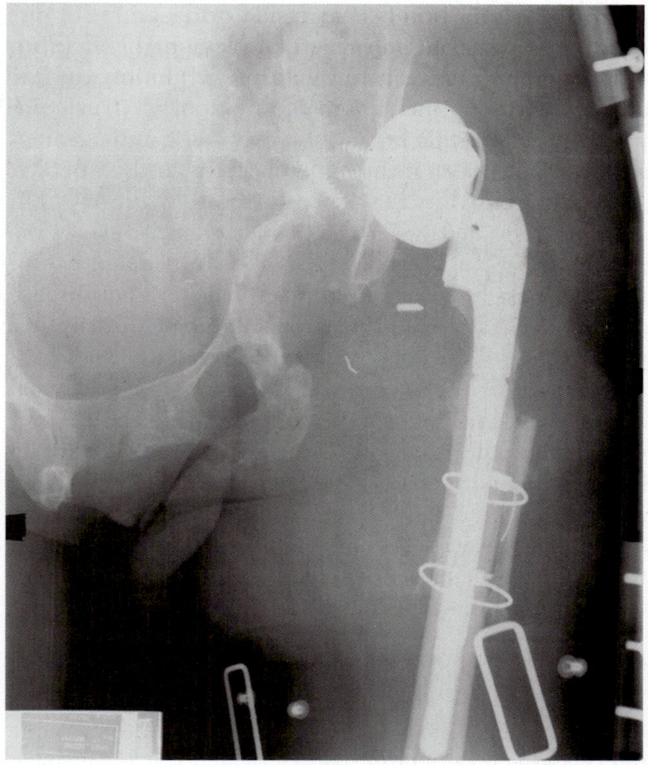

FIGURE 5 AP radiograph of the left hip of a patient who had multiple revisions demonstrating catastrophic failure of a constrained acetabular implant.

Resection Arthroplasty

When dislocation continues to recur after all of the already-discussed strategies have failed, then resection arthroplasty (Girdlestone procedure) is the final salvage surgery. This has poor functional results and should be avoided if possible, but patients should be counseled that it may be a necessary option in the long term.

SPINOPELVIC RELATIONSHIP

In recent years, abnormal spinopelvic motion has been identified as a risk factor for hip instability following primary THA. Several studies have documented the increased rates of dislocation in patients who have a prior spinal fusion following THA.[34-37] Recently, a study assessing approximately 200,000 THAs performed in the United States identified a prior spinal fusion as the strongest predictor of subsequent hip instability necessitating a revision surgery.[38] In this study, a history of spinal fusion was a stronger independent risk factor for instability than Parkinson disease and dementia, underscoring the importance of identifying this high-risk patient population. Furthermore, recent epidemiologic data suggest that the proportion of Medicare patients undergoing primary THA with a prior fusion is increasing. A recent study found that the proportion of Medicare beneficiaries with a prior fusion increased by approximately 300% between 2002 and 2014, from approximately 1.5% of THAs performed in 2002 to almost 4.5% of THAs performed in 2014.[39] Last, other pathologies that affect spinopelvic mechanics may also place patients at increased risk of dislocation including ankylosing spondylitis, lumbar herniation, spondylolisthesis, and degenerative disk disease.[40,41]

Pathoanatomy

Several independent yet related mechanisms are responsible for the increased risk of dislocation observed in THA patients who have abnormal spinopelvic mechanics. In patients without spine disease, changes in posture, such as moving between standing and sitting positions, require the coordinated motion between the hip joint and lumbosacral junction. Normally, when a patient moves from a standing to seated position, lumbar lordosis decreases as the pelvis tilts posteriorly approximately 20° to 30°. While this occurs, the hip flexes approximately 55° to 70°, allowing the upper trunk and the femur to assume approximately 90° of total flexion. However, when the lumbosacral

Section 3: Hip

junction loses motion from a fusion or degenerative disease, there is compensatory increased femoral flexion such that for every 1° decrease in spinopelvic motion, there is approximately 1° increase in hip motion.[42,43] This compensatory increase in hip motion may cause impingement and instability even if the implants are placed optimally.

In addition to increased compensatory hip motion, a spinopelvic deformity may cause a previously well-positioned implant to become malpositioned. For example, if a patient develops lumbar degenerative disease after a THA, the resulting loss of lumbar lordosis and posterior tilt of the pelvis may cause excessive functional anteversion of the acetabular implant when standing, increasing the risk of posterior impingement and anterior instability. Conversely, if a patient is fused surgically in lordosis, the patient's sacrum may lose the ability to tilt posteriorly when sitting, thereby decreasing the patient's functional anteversion and inclination in the seated position, placing the patient at risk of anterior impingement and posterior instability.

Diagnosis

The diagnosis of abnormal spinopelvic motion starts with a thorough history and physical examination. While interviewing a patient, a history of sciatica, lower back pain, lower extremity radiculopathy, or a prior spine surgery should prompt the orthopaedic surgeon to consider further imaging. On physical examination, a hunched posture may be a sign of positive sagittal balance and may be indicative of spinal pathology. Common physical examination findings such as a positive straight leg raise may be a sign of more severe lumbar pathology. When the orthopaedic surgeon has an index of suspicion for spinopelvic pathology, standing and sitting lateral lumbar-pelvis-hip radiographs may allow the surgeon to quantify spinopelvic motion, hip motion, and characterize pelvic and acetabular position in both the sitting and standing positions.[43,44]

Management of Hip Instability With Concomitant Spinal Disease

The management of hips instability in high-risk patients who have spinopelvic disease is a subject of ongoing study.[45-47] Regardless of the patient's spinal deformity, the surgeon should aim to optimize offset, maximize head size, and judiciously assess for soft-tissue and bony impingement when trialing at the time of surgery. Dual-mobility articulations may be considered in this high-risk group to optimize functional head size and minimize the risk of instability. When patients have a fixed anterior tilt of the pelvis, increasing anteversion of the acetabular implant may avoid anterior impingement during sitting because posterior tilt of the pelvis may be limited in this patient population. Conversely, patients who have a flat-back deformity from degenerative lumbar changes that cause loss of lumbar kyphosis may be at risk of posterior impingement and anterior instability while standing. As such, these patients may benefit from decreased anteversion or avoidance of excessive anteversion. However, when considering altering acetabular implant position based on a spinal deformity, knowledge of a patient's preoperative standing and sitting pelvic position is paramount. To achieve a specific acetabular target, robotic-assistance or computer navigation may allow for more precise implant positioning. However, the utilization of these technologies to address this cohort is currently being investigated.

TRIBOCORROSION

Mechanically assisted crevice corrosion (MACC) causing an adverse local tissue reaction has recently been recognized as a mode of failure in patients who have metal on polyethylene bearing surfaces. MACC was first described in the 1990s along with introduction of modularity in the femoral head. However, this process decreased significantly after design improvements from the implant manufacturers. Then with the popularity of metal-on-metal bearing surfaces, there was another increase in metal-induced adverse local tissue reactions (ALTR). Despite almost complete abandonment of metal-on-metal bearings in THA, similar ALTR occur in patients undergoing THA with metal-on-polyethylene bearings because of corrosion at the head-neck junction.

Diagnosis

The diagnosis of MACC-associated ALTR can be challenging. Patients typically present with a painful hip after many years of a well-functioning implant. Standard radiographs should be obtained and are often normal without evidence of loosening, wear, or osteolysis. Workup should include serum laboratory values of erythrocyte sedimentation rate and C-reactive protein to screen for periprosthetic joint infection. Hip aspiration of synovial fluid aids in the diagnosis, and a manual cell count is often required for accurate values. Surgeons should have a low threshold to obtain serum metal ion markers if the diagnosis is uncertain following imaging, screening laboratory markers, and aspiration. A 2017 study investigated cut-off values for interpretation of serum metal ions and concluded that serum cobalt level greater than 1.0 ng/mL had a sensitivity of 100%, specificity of 90%, positive predictive value of 96%, and negative predictive value of 100%. Serum chromium levels and ratio of cobalt to chromium were less diagnostic.[48] If cobalt level is greater than 1.0 ng/mL, a metal artifact reduction sequence MRI should be performed for evaluation of adverse local tissue reaction. Revision surgery is typically recommended, but each decision should be made in context of magnitude of disease, clinical symptoms, and health of the patient. At the time of surgery, the diagnosis of MACC can be confirmed by visible corrosion at the head-neck junction. A histopathologic analysis demonstrating dense infiltrates of perivascular lymphocytes as well as areas of tissue necrosis is consistent with adverse local tissue reaction.

Treatment

Revision surgery for MACC-associated ALTR require extensive workup and thoughtful planning. First, the surgeon must determine the extent of damage caused by adverse local tissue reaction. A complete synovectomy and débridement of necrotic tissue should be performed. The femoral head is inspected for obvious corrosion, and multiple fluid and tissue samples should be obtained for histopathology and cultures. The authors recommend insertion of a titanium sleeve over the taper followed by placement of a ceramic femoral head to decrease likelihood of ongoing taper corrosion. Last, concomitant pathology such as instability secondary to abductor destruction should be addressed at the surgeon's discretion.

LIMB-LENGTH DISCREPANCY AFTER THA

Limb-length discrepancy is one of the most common complications, is a major source of patient dissatisfaction, and is the most common cause for litigation after THA.[49,50] In addition to patient dissatisfaction, a significant limb-length discrepancy can result in functional disabilities, including limp, scoliosis, trochanteric bursitis, and low back pain.[51] Although the definition of what constitutes a substantial limb-length discrepancy is debated, lengthening or shortening the surgical limb as little as possible should be the goal. Limb lengthening that occurs at the time of surgery can be either intentional or inadvertent. Intentional lengthening may be used to correct a preoperative discrepancy or for increased soft-tissue tension to achieve dynamic hip stability at the time of surgery. Because soft-tissue tension is directly related to both length and offset, it is important to consider both when evaluating intraoperative soft-tissue tension. Inadvertent lengthening may occur when the acetabular or femoral implants do not restore the native center of rotation, leading to either lengthening or shortening. The multiple radiographic and intraoperative measurement methods, surgical techniques, and devices that have been developed speak to the difficulty of accurately assessing limb-length intraoperatively.

During the preoperative consultation, the challenges associated with obtaining equal length should be discussed with the patient. Additionally, any preoperative limb-length discrepancy must be identified and documented. Hip abduction and adduction motion should be assessed for the presence of contractures. The Thomas test, in which both hips are flexed to 90° and the surgical leg is extended, helps to identify hip flexion contractures. If a pelvic obliquity is present, it is important to determine whether it is flexible or fixed. A flexible pelvic obliquity will correct in the seated position.[52] Block testing, in which wedges of known widths are placed under the affected extremity until the patient perceives equal leg lengths, best quantifies the functional limb-length discrepancy.

The assessment of limb-length discrepancy can be done radiographically or by measuring from the anterior superior iliac spine to the medial malleolus. However, the most accurate method is the use of blocks, because the patient's perception of limb length is much more important than any measured value.[53] Sources of limb-length discrepancy include cartilage and bone loss from disease processes, previous surgery, or pediatric hip conditions (eg, slipped capital femoral epiphysis, congenital hip dysplasia, or Legg-Calvé-Perthes disease). Limb-length discrepancy can also be extra-articular. A previous femoral or tibial fracture, infection, congenital deformity, or epiphyseal plate arrest can all result in extra-articular limb length inequalities.

In addition to structural abnormalities, limb-length discrepancies can also arise from a functional difference in limb length from a pelvic tilt, scoliosis, or periarticular soft-tissue contractures around the hip or knee.[54] As the hemipelvis elevates, the ipsilateral limb shortens, and the contralateral hemipelvis tilts inferiorly, creating functional shortening and contralateral lengthening. The actual limb-length difference can represent a combination of both the structural difference in limb length and the apparent functional difference due to pelvic position or soft-tissue contracture.

In routine cases with minimal limb-length discrepancies, the center of rotation of the acetabular implant should match that of the normal contralateral side, and the location of the femoral implant should match the center of rotation of the native femoral head. If this is achieved, the prosthetic implants will have reproduced the prearthritic limb length postoperatively. Patients who have functional limb-length discrepancy secondary to soft-tissue contracture may see it resolve over a few months. Compensatory lumbar scoliosis or pelvic tilt secondary to a structural limb-length discrepancy should also correct once limb-length inequality is surgically corrected. However, a fixed pelvic obliquity (from degenerative scoliosis or lumbar fusion) will not correct unless specifically addressed with a separate procedure.

Preoperatively, both patient and surgeon should agree and understand that the ultimate goal of THA is to accurately restore the intra-articular biomechanics of the joint. However, correct soft-tissue tension may occasionally have to take precedence over equal leg lengths to optimize abductor function and maintain dynamic hip stability. Patients should also be counseled preoperatively as to the types of limb-length discrepancies that can be reliably addressed at the time of surgery, those that will likely correct over time, and those that will persist and require treatment with a shoe lift or alternative treatment methods.

Standing AP pelvic radiographs should be obtained for all patients to assess standing pelvic tilt and to identify any pelvic obliquity that would affect limb length. Ideally, the femur should be internally rotated 15° when taking the radiograph to allow for an accurate assessment of femoral offset. However, disease progression may limit internal rotation and underestimate offset. If the opposite hip has normal motion, femoral offset can be estimated from the normal side.

Radiographic limb-length differences can be calculated on a standing AP pelvis radiograph by drawing a horizontal line between two symmetrical pelvic landmarks. The three most common anatomic pelvic landmarks include the base of the acetabular teardrop, the superior aspect of the inferior obturator foramen, and the bottom of the ischial tuberosities.[55] The vertical distance between these lines and a reproducible landmark on the femur, usually the apex or most medial aspect of the lesser trochanter, can then be calculated and the two limbs are compared to determine intra-articular limb-length discrepancy.[56] Note that this radiographic calculation may be influenced by a hip flexion contracture. In a patient who has a clinically significant hip flexion contracture, the lesser trochanter moves cephalad on the radiographs and will appear as a shortened extremity. When the flexion contracture is corrected during surgery, inadvertent leg lengthening will ensue if this is not taken into account. Therefore, it is important to link the clinical and radiographic findings. If a clinically significant flexion contracture is present, it is best to create a template from the normal side to prevent inadvertent limb lengthening. Extra-articular sources of limb-length discrepancy will not be identified on the AP pelvis radiograph; these will be identified on block measurements. A hip-knee-ankle radiograph, CT scanogram, or weight-bearing AP thoracolumbar radiograph should be obtained to clarify the source of the length discrepancy.

Preoperative templating is critical to prevention of postoperative limb-length discrepancy. Preoperative templating should also include a measurement of limb-length discrepancy. Templating provides not only a better understanding of acetabular and femoral implant sizes but also the need for a standard or high offset femoral stem and determines the level of the femoral neck resection.[55] The sequence of templating should begin with the acetabular implant. The inferior aspect of the acetabular implant is positioned slightly below the base of the acetabular teardrop, with the medial aspect of the implant adjacent to the medial wall. Superiorly, the acetabular implant should have superolateral bony coverage, with the dome of the cup resting just above the subchondral bone of the acetabular sourcil.

After the acetabular center of rotation has been established, the center of rotation of the native femoral head is marked on the preoperative AP radiograph. The difference between these two centers of rotation is measured and compared with the preoperative limb-length discrepancy calculated, as occasionally one can either shorten or lengthen the limb through the acetabulum. The femoral template is then dropped down to the appropriate level to accurately restore both length and offset. If it is desired to lengthen the limb by 1 cm, and the limb is lengthened 0.5 cm with the location of the template acetabular implant, the femoral implant would be templated 0.5 cm above the acetabular center of rotation for a cumulative lengthening of 1 cm. A standard or high-offset template is then selected to match the offset, and either the distance from the femoral head center to the proposed neck resection or the distance above the top of the lesser trochanter to the proposed neck resection is noted.[57] If appropriate femoral offset is not restored, the leg is at risk of excessive lengthening to achieve the appropriate soft-tissue tension that should have been addressed with increased offset. Conversely, if too much offset is placed into the system, the patient may experience lateral hip pain secondary to trochanteric bursitis. Another sequela of increasing offset is a perceived limb-length discrepancy whereby the increased offset leads to abductor tightness and tilting of the pelvis to the ipsilateral side. The patient will feel that the leg is long in this situation, even if the radiographic measurement is similar to the other side. In cases with a significant external rotational contracture or deformity, the contralateral hip can be used to assist with native hip geometry and preoperative templating. Electronic templating systems are now available to help with the process and provide accurate measurements of length and offset.

Several methods, surgical techniques, and caliper devices have been developed to help produce accurate limb-length restoration intraoperatively. Several caliper devices have been developed that measure the distance between a fixed point on the ilium and the greater trochanter.[58,59] This measurement is performed before and after placement of trial implants to detect any intraoperative changes in leg length. The difficulty with this technique is that the pelvic fixation point is usually away from the center of rotation of the femur. Small deviations in leg position may result in significant errors in the calculated length between the pelvic and greater trochanteric fixation points.[60] To determine intraoperative leg length in the lateral position, a pin is placed near the infracotyloid fossa before neck resection and compared during implant trial. The pin is temporarily placed outside the bone next to the ischium, at the junction with the posterior aspect of the transverse acetabular ligament. A corresponding mark is made on the greater trochanter, with the patient's knees and heels together. After a trial, these steps are repeated and compared with the previous mark on the trochanter to determine changes in leg length. The advantage of this technique is that it incorporates length changes that occur with both acetabular and femoral implants. This technique may reduce the error associated with changes in leg position because it is closer to the center of rotation of the hip.

A soft-tissue trial is another way to grossly assess soft-tissue tension that reflects a combination of leg length and offset.[61] Commonly used soft-tissue tests include the shuck test, the drop-kick test, the Ober test, and direct heel-to-heel comparison. The shuck test involves direct axial traction on the surgical leg with the hip at 30° flexion and detects axial laxity; the lateral shuck test detects offset laxity. Less than 50% of the reduced femoral head should clear the acetabular rim with manual traction. The drop-kick test is performed with the hip extended just past neutral and the knee flexed to 90°. The amount of leg recoil is used to determine soft-tissue tension, as a leg with excessive kick-back may have been inadvertently lengthened.[61] The Ober test assesses for lateral iliotibial band tightness. A positive test occurs when the femur abducts with knee flexion and slight adduction. With any of these soft-tissue maneuvers, the patient's intrinsic ligamentous laxity and the type of anesthesia must be taken into consideration to avoid significant lengthening because the use of paralytic agents will cause overestimation of ligamentous laxity. The patella of the surgical and nonsurgical extremity can be compared side-by-side, both preoperatively and after placement of the trial implants, allowing for gross assessment of any change in leg position. For the anterolateral or direct anterior approaches performed in the supine position, the medial malleoli can be directly compared. In addition, intraoperative fluoroscopy can be used to assess leg length, offset, and implant position. Computer navigation and robotic THA have both been shown to accurately restore leg length, but the literature has yet to demonstrate a significant difference in the accuracy of this technique when compared with manual methods.[62]

With accurate preoperative planning and a systematic approach to intraoperative execution, significant limb-length discrepancies can be avoided. Patient education is essential to avoid postoperative dissatisfaction from residual limb-length discrepancies that cannot be addressed with THA. Patients should be aware that small increases in leg length and/or offset may be necessary to optimize overall hip stability. Additionally, they should be reassured that functional limb-length discrepancies secondary to soft-tissue contractures and flexible pelvic obliquity should correct gradually over time. Shoe lifts should be discouraged if contracture resolution is anticipated. A careful preoperative plan is essential and will enhance the accuracy of surgical execution.

HETEROTOPIC OSSIFICATION

Heterotopic ossification, or bone formation in abnormal locations, can occur following soft-tissue trauma, fracture, head injury, burns, elective surgery (eg, hip or knee replacement), or as a result of genetic abnormalities (eg, fibrodysplasia ossificans progressiva, progressive osseous heteroplasia).[63-67] The incidence of heterotopic ossification following THA is between 5.2% and 87.0%, with 0.5% to 12.3% of cases exhibiting some level of clinical significance.[68,69]

Basic Science

One study has suggested that the following three conditions must be present for de novo formation of ectopic bone: (1) an inducing agent, (2) an osteogenic precursor cell, and (3) an environment permissive to osteogenesis.[70] Bone morphogenetic proteins (BMPs) have been shown to govern chemotaxis, mitosis, and differentiation in bone formation and can be used to induce heterotopic ossification in vivo.[71] An upregulation in the normal BMP pathway is now thought to be responsible for conversion of progenitor cells to osteogenic precursor cells. Mesenchymal stem cells are believed to play a major role in the formation of heterotopic ossification.[65] Local oxygen tension, pH, micronutrients, and mechanical stimuli also may be substantial determinants in ectopic bone formation.[65] In the genetic condition fibrodysplasia ossificans progressiva, a mutation of the gene *ACVR1/ALK2* has been found.[63,65,67] The *ACVR1/ALK2* gene is a receptor for BMPs, which may lead to osteogenic differentiation and widespread heterotopic bone formation.[67]

Incidence and Risk Factors

A meta-analysis of studies regarding heterotopic ossification found the incidence after THA to be between 5% and 90%, with an accumulated incidence of about 30%.[69] Occurrence of heterotopic ossification is much more frequent after THA than after knee arthroplasty, with rates between 5% and 40% after total knee arthroplasty.[72]

Male sex, cemented prostheses, bilateral THA, ankylosing spondylitis, history of heterotopic ossification, and an ankylosed hip have been identified as risk factors after THA, whereas rheumatoid arthritis is negatively correlated with the development of heterotopic ossification.[65,69]

Physical and Radiographic Evaluation

Occurrence of heterotopic ossification following THA is usually asymptomatic and is often found incidentally on postoperative radiographs. Pain is rarely the chief report, although it can be present. More often, decreased range of motion at the surgical hip is noted, which may create limitations in postoperative rehabilitation or functional deficits. Edema, erythema, and warmth have also been reported in association with heterotopic ossification.[73]

Standard AP and lateral radiographs are usually adequate to determine the existence and degree of heterotopic ossification.[65] Both CT and MRI studies may be obtained if it is necessary to more clearly define the extent and location of heterotopic ossification.[74] Radiographs and CT may only define more mature heterotopic bone. Investigations into radiologic techniques that identify heterotopic ossification at an earlier point in the postoperative period, including three-phase bone scintigraphy with or without single-photon emission CT, near-infrared optical imaging, and transcutaneous Raman spectroscopy, have been studied.[64,65,74]

Classification

The Brooker classification of heterotopic ossification is graded on a supine AP radiograph of the hip, with grades as follows: grade 1, islands of bone within the soft tissues about the hip; grade 2, bone spurs from the pelvis or proximal end of the femur, leaving at least 1 cm between opposing bone surfaces; grade 3, bone spurs from the pelvis or proximal end of the femur, with less than 1 cm between opposing bone surfaces; grade 4, bony ankylosis of the hip.[75] One study found that intraobserver reliability using the Brooker classification was poor, and a modified classification using three grades was proposed: grade A, absence of heterotopic ossification or islands of bone less than 1 cm in length; grade B, 1 cm or more of islands of bone spurs with at least 1 cm between opposing surfaces; grade C, bone spurs with less than 1 cm between opposing surfaces or bony ankylosis.[76]

Prophylaxis

Prophylaxis is the preferred method of management for patients at high risk of development of heterotopic ossification following THA, with NSAIDs and radiation the primary modalities used; the use of diphosphonates has been explored. Prostaglandins are known to be strong costimulating molecules with BMPs in the development of heterotopic ossification.[77] NSAIDs decrease prostaglandin production and may reduce heterotopic ossification. Many studies have successfully demonstrated the efficacy of NSAIDs in decreasing rates of heterotopic ossification, although a single agent, dosage, and duration of treatment have not been agreed on.[65,78,79]

Perioperative radiation has also been shown to effectively decrease rates of heterotopic ossification following THA. Radiation stops the differentiation of osteogenic precursor cells that mature into osteoblasts.[73] A single 7- to 8-Gy fraction, which may be given during a period of 4 hours preoperatively to 72 hours postoperatively, is recommended for prophylaxis.[65]

No studies have shown a significant difference in the effectiveness of NSAIDs versus radiation.[65] For this reason, prophylaxis decisions should be made on an individual basis with consideration given to cost, access, and adverse effects. NSAIDs can lead to increased bleeding and gastrointestinal issues, whereas radiation has a theoretical malignancy risk and can be accompanied by soft-tissue contracture and delayed wound healing.[65]

Treatment

After heterotopic ossification has developed following THA, treatment options are limited; no current pharmacologic intervention is available to treat heterotopic ossification, but late radiation therapy may prevent heterotopic ossification from progressing.[80] Because heterotopic ossification frequently presents as decreased range of motion, a trial period of physical therapy is reasonable to attempt to increase range of motion to acceptable limits. For heterotopic ossification that is painful, limits daily activities, or for which a trial of physical therapy has failed, surgical excision may be considered. Waiting for heterotopic bone to fully mature before excision has been recommended; however, early excision, while preserving tissue planes, has also been suggested.[65] Studies have shown improvements in range of motion following resection; however, pain relief is less predictable.[81,82] Resection is usually combined with radiation or NSAIDs to prevent recurrence of heterotopic ossification following the procedure.

NEUROVASCULAR INJURIES

The incidence of neurovascular injuries in primary hip replacement has been reported to be 0.04% to 0.2% for vascular injuries and 0.09% to 3.7% for nerve injuries.[83-86] In revision arthroplasty, however, these injuries are more frequent and have been reported to be up to 5% for vascular injuries and 7.6% for nerve injuries.[84,86,87] Vascular injuries are less common than nerve injuries, but they result in worse outcomes.[83-85,88] These injuries are more common in the left hip, with the external iliac, femoral, and obturator vessels the most frequently injured.[83-85] Nerve injuries are more common in women and in those with a preoperative diagnosis of posttraumatic arthritis or developmental dysplasia of the hip (DDH).[84] The sciatic, femoral, and superior gluteal nerves (SGNs) are most frequently at risk.[84] Injury to the lateral femoral cutaneous nerve has also been reported, particularly with the recent increase in the use of the anterior surgical approach. In revision cases, a vascular ultrasonography, magnetic resonance angiogram, or CT angiogram may be required preoperatively or recommended postoperatively. These studies may have to be ordered emergently after surgery if internal bleeding is suspected.[86,88] Knowledge of neurovascular anatomy, preoperative planning, appropriate intraoperative techniques, and management of postoperative complications is critical.

Vascular Injury

The incidence of vascular injury (requiring surgery, bypass grafting, or stenting) is 0.04% to 0.2% after primary THA and increases to 5% in revision cases.[84-86,89] Although vascular injuries have a low prevalence in hip surgery, when they occur they are associated with a 7.3% overall reported rate of death, a 1.6% rate of amputation, and permanent disability.[83-86] The external iliac, femoral, and obturator vessels are most frequently injured.[84] In revision cases, the external iliac artery and the femoral artery and vein have been reported to be at an increased risk for injury.[86]

Direct, immediate vascular injury can be caused by intraoperative laceration with a surgical instrument or a sharp piece of bone. A sudden intraoperative drop in blood pressure during reaming or after insertion of acetabular screws should lead to suspicion of an intrapelvic vascular injury.[86] Late damage can occur with chronic erosion of a vessel by protruding screws, extruded cement, or the migration of a loose implant, leading to the formation of a false aneurysm or thrombus.[85] Indirect injuries can result from joint manipulation that stretches atherosclerotic arteries causing tears and detachment of plaques, as well as thrombus formation. Injuries can also occur from thermal damage as a result of the polymerization of cement.[85] Approximately 25% of all intraoperative vascular lesions are identified during the procedure and 50% within 24 hours of surgery; the remaining 25% present days or months later, and possibly up to 1 year or more postoperatively.[85,86] If the patient begins to experience restriction of movement, pain, swelling of the ipsilateral limb, or a decrease in hemoglobin level, diagnostic imaging should be considered to rule out bleeding.[86] Duplex sonography, CT, CT angiogram, or magnetic resonance angiogram can be used; according to one author group, CT is the imaging modality of choice.[86]

The quadrant acetabular system is an established approach to guiding safe transacetabular screw placement. A study reported use of three-dimensional CT angiogram to visualize pelvic vessels in relation to the acetabulum.[90] The external iliac vein was closer to the pelvis on the left side both in the elderly and in females. In 26% of the 200 hips studied, the external iliac veins were directly on the osseous surface of the pelvis. Three anatomic variations of the iliac arteries were described (straight, curved, and tortuous). The mean distance from the pelvis to the external iliac and femoral vessels in the curved and tortuous groups was shorter than in the straight group. The curved and tortuous types were more commonly identified in elderly patients (mean age, 67.9 years), whereas the straight type was more commonly identified in younger patients (mean age, 45.5 years). Because curved and tortuous vessels tend to be closer to the pelvis, elderly patients who have curved or tortuous types had the greatest potential risk of injury. Obturator vessels were located just behind the acetabulum near the obturator foramen, allowing the possibility of damage or avulsion during preparation of the acetabulum.

A case report was presented of an uncommon vascular complication following a failed revision THA that led to injury of the superficial femoral artery, that in turn eventually led to a thromboembolism and transmetatarsal amputation.[88] While the patient in the case report awaited a custom triflange prosthesis, intractable foot pain with diminished pulses developed. A CT angiographic study demonstrated a left superficial femoral artery thrombus adjacent to a migrated screw. If there is the slightest suspicion of vascular injury preoperatively in patients presenting with a failed revision arthroplasty, a vascular surgery consultation and a vascular ultrasonography or CT angiogram should be routine during preoperative planning to avoid catastrophic complications.

A study compared the distance of five common THA acetabular retractor positions (three anterior, one posterior, and one superior) with the closest neurovascular structures measured on hip CT.[84] The inferior retractor position to the obturator neurovascular bundle was not measured because it was not reliably identified on CT. The anterior retractor at the level of the anterior inferior iliac spine had the farthest mean distance (2.65 cm) from the femoral artery, but as the anterior retractor moved inferiorly along the anterior wall, the mean distance to the femoral artery decreased to 0.95 cm. All five retractor positions had shorter distances to the structures in females.

Traditionally, vascular repair has been conducted with open exploration, but more recently there has been a trend toward percutaneous endovascular repair with angioplasty, stenting, or grafting, when possible.[85] Endovascular repair is a quicker procedure that allows faster recovery, lower rates of complication, and higher probability of success, and it may provide superior patient satisfaction.[83,85] For active arterial hemorrhage, open repair is still favored over endovascular treatment.[83]

Neurologic Injury

Nerve injury is defined as a postoperative sensory or motor neural deficit related to the index THA.[89] The incidence is 0.09% to 3.7% after primary THA and up to 7.6% after revision.[84,87] Known causes of nerve injury are intraoperative direct nerve injury, limb lengthening, improper retractor placement, cement-related thermal damage, patient positioning, manipulation, and hematoma. Risk factors include being female, having DDH, having posttraumatic arthritis, and undergoing revision.[91]

The sciatic nerve is the most commonly injured nerve during THA, but the femoral and SGNs are also frequently injured.[84,86] With the aid of CT scans, the proximity of five commonly placed acetabular retractors to neurovascular structures in THA was identified.[84] The anterior inferior iliac spine retractor had the farthest mean distance from the femoral nerve (2.65 cm), and the anterior-inferior retractor distance was the closest (mean distance, 0.95 cm). The superior retractor had a 2.03-cm mean distance from the SGN. The posterior retractor had a 1.75-cm mean distance from the sciatic nerve. All five retractor positions had shorter distances to the structures in females.

A cadaver and a CT angiographic study were performed to analyze the relationships between the superior gluteal neurovascular pedicle and the greater trochanter to identify the site of incision with the lowest risk of injury during THA with the Hardinge direct lateral approach.[92] Results showed that during direct lateral access, a very small safe zone exists, which is even smaller if the SGN presents in a branching pattern. The safe zone was identified as 4.7 cm from the greater trochanter to the SGN and 3.5 cm to its lower ramus. Proximal extension of the incision should be restricted to 3.5 cm from the trochanteric apex with an anterior cranial direction.

Lateral femoral cutaneous nerve injury during THA may occur with use of the anterior surgical approach.[93] In a study to quantify the incidence and functional effect of lateral femoral cutaneous nerve neurapraxia in 132 patients who underwent an anterior approach for THA and hip resurfacing,[94] an incidence of 67% was reported for the THA group, which is higher than the 2.0% and 31.9% incidences reported in other studies. It is suspected that lateral femoral cutaneous nerve neurapraxia is underreported.[95,96] Although a low rate of complete resolution was noted, a decrease in symptoms occurred over time, with no functional limitations reported.[94]

A fivefold increased rate of nerve palsy is reported when lengthening a limb in a patient who had DDH as compared with the general population.[91] A shortening subtrochanteric osteotomy or iliofemoral distraction of the hip joint is often used to supplement THA to prevent nerve palsy after limb lengthening.[91] These techniques have good results but high complication rates.[91] Another technique was presented in a case report of three patients who have Crowe type IV DDH with an average 43 months' follow-up.[91] The technique involved inserting noncemented total hip implants through an anterior approach, leaving the implants unreduced and applying traction until desired alignment of the implants was reached, after which delayed closed reduction was performed. The average hospital stay was 9 days. All three patients reported excellent pain relief and significant improvement of daily living without signs of neurologic deficit. At the last follow-up examinations, radiographs demonstrated all implants to be well fixed in satisfactory position. This technique is not indicated when significant limb-length discrepancy is present.

Intraoperative continuous multimodal monitoring (electromyography, motor-evoked potentials, and somatosensory evoked potentials) have been used during revision and complex THA to minimize the risk of nerve injury.[87] A retrospective review of the 69 procedures of complex hip surgery with adjunctive multimodal intraoperative monitoring showed that in 24 procedures (35%), the surgeon was alerted by a neurophysiologist of a possible nerve lesion, which allowed the surgeon to modify the intraoperative approach. Only one true positive nerve injury was reported postoperatively.

Complete remission of nerve injury by 2 years occurs in 50% of cases.[97] According to another study, 91% of light lesions reach full recovery, and 43% of severe lesions reach full recovery at 2 years; an improvement beyond 2 years is unlikely and independent of the nerve affected.[97] Obesity has been identified as a negative prognostic factor.[98]

Neurovascular injuries are rare complications of THA. Vascular injury is less common than nerve injury, but it has higher morbidity and increased mortality.[83-85] Knowledge of neurovascular anatomy, preoperative planning, appropriate intraoperative techniques, and management of postoperative complications is critical for every surgeon.

SUMMARY

Although it is a very reliable surgical procedure, THA may be burdened by perioperative complications. The surgeon and patient should be cognizant of the risks of the most common complications after THA. It is crucial that the surgeon be familiar with the available evidence on prevention, diagnosis, treatment, and prognosis of variable complications after THA. Instability after THA is problematic; however, advances in management such as the use of dual-mobility implants and constrained constructs may yield positive results. Understanding spinopelvic relationship is crucial for implant placement in THA and should be considered in all cases of instability. MACC at the head-neck junction may cause ALTR in patients who have metal-on-polyethylene bearing surfaces. A serum cobalt level of greater than 1 ng/mL is consistent with adverse local tissue reaction. Limb-length discrepancy can be avoided with accurate preoperative planning and a systematic approach to intraoperative execution. Although prophylactic methods for heterotopic ossification exist, there are limited treatment options available after THA, including resection, which may lead to functional improvement but variable pain relief. Knowledge of neurovascular anatomy, preoperative planning, appropriate intraoperative techniques, and management of postoperative complications is critical for avoiding nerve and vascular injuries that are associated with significant morbidity and mortality.

KEY STUDY POINTS

- There are both patient-specific and surgery-specific risk factors for dislocation; although many dislocations can be managed with closed reduction alone, revision for recurrent instability may be necessary in some cases, and its success requires an algorithmic approach.
- Tribocorrosion can occur at the modular head-neck junction in metal on polyethylene THA. Treatment includes thorough débridement of adverse local tissue reaction and insertion of a titanium sleeve on the taper followed by ceramic head.
- Limb-length discrepancy is a major source of patient dissatisfaction and litigation after THA; with accurate preoperative planning and a systematic approach to intraoperative execution, significant limb-length discrepancies can be avoided.
- Although prophylaxis with NSAIDs and radiation may prevent occurrence of heterotopic ossification, limited treatment options are available after THA. Resection leads to improvements in range of motion; however, pain relief is less predictable.
- Vascular injury is less common than nerve injury but carries a higher risk of morbidity and mortality.

ANNOTATED REFERENCES

1. Kurtz SM, Lau E, Watson H, Schmier JK, Parvizi J: Economic burden of periprosthetic joint infection in the United States. *J Arthroplasty* 2012;27(8 suppl):61-65.e1.
2. Gwam CU, Mistry JB, Mohamed NS, et al: Current epidemiology of revision total hip arthroplasty in the United States: National Inpatient Sample 2009 to 2013. *J Arthroplasty* 2017;32(7):2088-2092.

   This is a retrospective analysis of 539 hips demonstrating a high rate of 35% dislocation at 15 years for hips revised for instability.
3. Jo S, Jimenez Almonte JH, Sierra RJ: The cumulative risk of re-dislocation after revision THA performed for instability increases close to 35% at 15 years. *J Arthroplasty* 2015;30(7):1177-1182.
4. Sanchez-Sotelo J, Haidukewych GJ, Boberg CJ: Hospital cost of dislocation after primary total hip arthroplasty. *J Bone Joint Surg Am* 2006;88(2):290-294.
5. de Palma L, Procaccini R, Soccetti A, Marinelli M: Hospital cost of treating early dislocation following hip arthroplasty. *Hip Int* 2012;22(1):62-67.
6. Abdel MP, Cross MB, Yasen AT, Haddad FS: The functional and financial impact of isolated and recurrent dislocation after total hip arthroplasty. *Bone Joint J* 2015;97-B(8):1046-1049.
7. Joshi A, Lee CM, Markovic L, Vlatis G, Murphy JC: Prognosis of dislocation after total hip arthroplasty. *J Arthroplasty* 1998;13(1):17-21.
8. Wera GD, Ting NT, Moric M, Paprosky WG, Sporer SM, Della Valle CJ: Classification and management of the unstable total hip arthroplasty. *J Arthroplasty* 2012;27(5):710-715.
9. Carter AH, Sheehan EC, Mortazavi SM, Purtill JJ, Sharkey PF, Parvizi J: Revision for recurrent instability: What are the predictors of failure? *J Arthroplasty* 2011;26(6 suppl):46-52.
10. Woo RY, Morrey BF: Dislocations after total hip arthroplasty. *J Bone Joint Surg Am* 1982;64(9):1295-1306.
11. Sanchez-Sotelo J, Berry DJ: Epidemiology of instability after total hip replacement. *Orthop Clin North Am* 2001;32(4):543-552.
12. Masonis JL, Bourne RB: Surgical approach, abductor function, and total hip arthroplasty dislocation. *Clin Orthop Relat Res* 2002;405:46-53.
13. Hummel MT, Malkani AL, Yakkanti MR, Baker DL: Decreased dislocation after revision total hip arthroplasty using larger femoral head size and posterior capsular repair. *J Arthroplasty* 2009;24(6 suppl):73-76.
14. Sheth D, Cafri G, Inacio MC, Paxton EW, Namba RS: Anterior and anterolateral approaches for THA are associated with lower dislocation risk without higher revision risk. *Clin Orthop Relat Res* 2015;473(11):3401-3408.
15. Meermans G, Konan S, Das R, Volpin A, Haddad FS: The direct anterior approach in total hip arthroplasty: A systematic review of the literature. *Bone Joint J* 2017;99-B(6):732-740.

    This is a systematic review of literature evaluating the potential long-term benefit of direct anterior approach in THA but did not find significant benefit.
16. Abdel MP, von Roth P, Jennings MT, Hanssen AD, Pagnano MW: What safe zone? The vast majority of dislocated THAs are within the Lewinnek safe zone for acetabular component position. *Clin Orthop Relat Res* 2016;474(2):386-391.
17. Ranawac C, Maynard M: Modern technique of cemented total hip arthroplasty. *Tech Orthop* 1991;6(3):17-25.
18. Malkani AL, Ong KL, Lau E, Kurtz SM, Justice BJ, Manley MT: Early- and late-term dislocation risk after primary hip arthroplasty in the Medicare population. *J Arthroplasty* 2010;25(6 suppl):21-25.
19. Pulos N, Tiberi Iii JV III, Schmalzried TP: Measuring acetabular component position on lateral radiographs-ischio-lateral method. *Bull NYU Hosp Jt Dis* 2011;69(suppl 1):S84-S89.
20. Kung PL, Ries MD: Effect of femoral head size and abductors on dislocation after revision THA. *Clin Orthop Relat Res* 2007;465:170-174.

21. Hailer NP, Weiss RJ, Stark A, Kärrholm J: Dual-mobility cups for revision due to instability are associated with a low rate of re-revisions due to dislocation: 228 patients from the Swedish Hip Arthroplasty Register. *Acta Orthop* 2012;83(6): 566-571.

22. Langlais FL, Ropars M, Gaucher F, Musset T, Chaix O: Dual mobility cemented cups have low dislocation rates in THA revisions. *Clin Orthop Relat Res* 2008;466(2):389-395.

23. Philippot R, Adam P, Reckhaus M, et al: Prevention of dislocation in total hip revision surgery using a dual mobility design. *Orthop Traumatol Surg Res* 2009;95(6):407-413.

24. Mohammed R, Hayward K, Mulay S, Bindi F, Wallace M: Outcomes of dual-mobility acetabular cup for instability in primary and revision total hip arthroplasty. *J Orthop Traumatol* 2015;16(1):9-13.

25. Matsen Ko LJ, Pollag KE, Yoo JY, Sharkey PF: Serum metal ion levels following total hip arthroplasty with modular dual mobility components. *J Arthroplasty* 2016;31(1):186-189.

26. Parvizi J, Morrey BF: Bipolar hip arthroplasty as a salvage treatment for instability of the hip. *J Bone Joint Surg Am* 2000;82-A(8):1132-1139.

27. Ries MD, Wiedel JD: Bipolar hip arthroplasty for recurrent dislocation after total hip arthroplasty. A report of three cases. *Clin Orthop Relat Res* 1992;278:121-127.

28. Grigoris P, Grecula MJ, Amstutz HC: Tripolar hip replacement for recurrent prosthetic dislocation. *Clin Orthop Relat Res* 1994;304:148-155.

29. Kaplan SJ, Thomas WH, Poss R: Trochanteric advancement for recurrent dislocation after total hip arthroplasty. *J Arthroplasty* 1987;2(2):119-124.

30. Whiteside LA: Surgical technique: Transfer of the anterior portion of the gluteus maximus muscle for abductor deficiency of the hip. *Clin Orthop Relat Res* 2012;470(2): 503-510.

31. Berend KR, Lombardi AV Jr, Mallory TH, Adams JB, Russell JH, Groseth KL: The long-term outcome of 755 consecutive constrained acetabular components in total hip arthroplasty: Examining the successes and failures. *J Arthroplasty* 2005;20(7 suppl 3):93-102.

32. Chalmers BP, Arsoy D, Sierra RJ, Lewallen DG, Trousdale RT: High failure rate of modular exchange with a specific design of a constrained liner in high-risk patients undergoing revision total hip arthroplasty. *J Arthroplasty* 2016;31(9):1963-1969.

33. Della Valle CJ, Chang D, Sporer S, Berger RA, Rosenberg AG, Paprosky WG: High failure rate of a constrained acetabular liner in revision total hip arthroplasty. *J Arthroplasty* 2005;20(7 suppl 3):103-107.

34. Bedard NA, Martin CT, Slaven SE, Pugely AJ, Mendoza-Lattes SA, Callaghan JJ: Abnormally high dislocation rates of total hip arthroplasty after spinal deformity surgery. *J Arthroplasty* 2016;31(12):2884-2885. PubMed PMID: 27612605.

35. Salib CG, Reina N, Perry KI, Taunton MJ, Berry DJ, Abdel MP: Lumbar fusion involving the sacrum increases dislocation risk in primary total hip arthroplasty. *Bone Joint J* 2019;101-B(2):198-206. PubMed PMID: 30700125.

    This is a retrospective review evaluating if lumbar fusion increases risk of hip dislocation with conclusion that prior fusion does raise short-term risk of dislocation within the first 6 months.

36. Buckland AJ, Puvanesarajah V, Vigdorchik J, et al: Dislocation of a primary total hip arthroplasty is more common in patients with a lumbar spinal fusion. *Bone Joint J* 2017;99-B(5):585-591. PubMed PMID: 28455466.

    This study reviewed Medicare database of over 14,000 patients and concluded that dislocation of a primary THA is more common in patients with a prior fusion.

37. Sing DC, Barry JJ, Aguilar TU, et al: Prior lumbar spinal Arthrodesis increases risk of prosthetic-related complication in total hip arthroplasty. *J Arthroplasty* 2016;31(9 suppl):227-232.e1.

38. Gausden EB, Parhar HS, Popper JE, Sculco PK, Rush BNM: Risk factors for early dislocation following primary elective total hip arthroplasty. *J Arthroplasty* 2018;33(5):1567-1571.e2. PubMed PMID: 29395718.

    This is a nationwide database study that demonstrated spinal fusion as most significant independent risk factor for dislocation within the first 6 months after THA.

39. Malkani AL, Garber AT, Ong KL, et al: Total hip arthroplasty in patients with previous lumbar fusion surgery: Are there more dislocations and revisions? *J Arthroplasty* 2018;33(4):1189-1193. PubMed PMID: 29174406.

    This is a Medicare database study that demonstrated increased risk of dislocation, fracture, infection, and revision THA among patients with preoperative lumbar spine diagnosis code.

40. Blizzard DJ, Sheets CZ, Seyler TM, et al: The impact of lumbar spine disease and deformity on total hip arthroplasty outcomes. *Orthopedics* 2017;40(3):e520-e525. PubMed PMID: 28358974.

    This is a Medicare database review that demonstrated increased rate of hip dislocation in patients with a variety of spinal procedures.

41. Blizzard DJ, Penrose CT, Sheets CZ, Seyler TM, Bolognesi MP, Brown CR: Ankylosing spondylitis increases perioperative and postoperative complications after total hip arthroplasty. *J Arthroplasty* 2017;32(8):2474-2479. PubMed PMID: 28438449.

    This is a Medicare database review of patients with ankylosing spondylitis that demonstrated an increased risk of dislocation at 90 days and 2 years postoperatively.

42. Esposito CI, Miller TT, Kim HJ, et al: Does degenerative lumbar spine disease influence femoroacetabular flexion in patients undergoing total hip arthroplasty? *Clin Orthop Relat Res* 2016;474(8): 1788-1797. PubMed PMID: 27020429; PubMed Central PMCID: PMC4925410.

43. Heckmann N, McKnight B, Stefl M, Trasolini NA, Ike H, Dorr LD: Late dislocation following total hip arthroplasty: Spinopelvic imbalance as a causative factor. *J Bone Joint Surg Am* 2018;100(21):1845-1853. PubMed PMID: 30399079.

This is a retrospective review of late dislocations in THA that evaluated spinopelvic motion parameters that may place patients at risk for instability. Level of evidence: IV.

44. Stefl M, Lundergan W, Heckmann N, et al: Spinopelvic mobility and acetabular component position for total hip arthroplasty. *Bone Joint J* 2017;99-B(1 suppl A):37-45. PubMed PMID: 28042117.

    This is a radiographic study of 160 hips in 151 patients who prospectively had evaluation of cup placement in patients with complex spine disease.

45. Luthringer TA, Vigdorchik JM: A preoperative workup of a "hip-spine" total hip arthroplasty patient: A simplified approach to a complex problem. *J Arthroplasty* 2019;34(7S):S57-S70. PubMed PMID: 30755374.

    This study offers a basic workup of hip-spine patients with three radiographic views and provides case examples to illustrate how those radiographs guide your surgical plan.

46. Feng JE, Anoushiravani AA, Eftekhary N, Wiznia D, Schwarzkopf R, Vigdorchik JM: Techniques for optimizing acetabular component positioning in total hip arthroplasty: Defining a patient-specific functional safe zone. *JBJS Rev* 2019;7(2):e5. PubMed PMID: 30817692.

    This paper provides multiple intraoperative tools to increase the likelihood of acetabular placement within the patients' unique safe zone.

47. Ike H, Dorr LD, Trasolini N, Stefl M, McKnight B, Heckmann N: Spine-pelvis-hip relationship in the functioning of a total hip replacement. *J Bone Joint Surg Am* 2018;100(18): 1606-1615. PubMed PMID: 30234627.

    This paper describes basic hip-spine biomechanics and specific implications to hip surgery.

48. Fillingham YA, Della Valle CJ, Bohl DD, et al: Serum metal levels for diagnosis of adverse local tissue reactions secondary to corrosion in metal-on-polyethylene total hip arthroplasty. *J Arthroplasty* 2017;32(9S):S272-s277.

    This is a retrospective review of patients who underwent metal-on-polyethylene THA with concern for adverse local tissue reaction and found a cobalt level of 1.0 to be concerning for adverse local tissue reaction.

49. Xue E, Su Z, Chen C, Wong PK, Wen H, Zhang Y: An intraoperative device to restore femoral offset in total hip arthroplasty. *J Orthop Surg Res* 2014;9:58.
50. Woolson ST, Hartford JM, Sawyer A: Results of a method of leg-length equalization for patients undergoing primary total hip replacement. *J Arthroplasty* 1999;14(2):159-164.
51. Whitehouse MR, Stefanovich-Lawbuary NS, Brunton LR, Blom AW: The impact of leg length discrepancy on patient satisfaction and functional outcome following total hip arthroplasty. *J Arthroplasty* 2013;28(8):1408-1414.
52. Sarin VK, Pratt WR, Bradley GW: Accurate femur repositioning is critical during intraoperative total hip arthroplasty length and offset assessment. *J Arthroplasty* 2005;20(7):887-891.
53. Röder C, Vogel R, Burri L, Dietrich D, Staub LP: Total hip arthroplasty: Leg length inequality impairs functional outcomes and patient satisfaction. *BMC Musculoskelet Disord* 2012;13:95.
54. Ranawat CS, Rodriguez JA: Functional leg-length inequality following total hip arthroplasty. *J Arthroplasty* 1997;12(4):359-364.
55. Ranawat CS: The pants too short, the leg too long! *Orthopedics* 1999;22(9):845-846.
56. Parvizi J, Sharkey PF, Bissett GA, Rothman RH, Hozack WJ: Surgical treatment of limb-length discrepancy following total hip arthroplasty. *J Bone Joint Surg Am* 2003;85(12):2310-2317.
57. Ogawa K, Kabata T, Maeda T, Kajino Y, Tsuchiya H: Accurate leg length measurement in total hip arthroplasty: A comparison of computer navigation and a simple manual measurement device. *Clin Orthop Surg* 2014;6(2):153-158.
58. Nam D, Sculco PK, Abdel MP, Alexiades MM, Figgie MP, Mayman DJ: Leg-length inequalities following THA based on surgical technique. *Orthopedics* 2013;36(4):e395-e400.
59. Meermans G, Malik A, Witt J, Haddad F: Preoperative radiographic assessment of limb-length discrepancy in total hip arthroplasty. *Clin Orthop Relat Res* 2011;469(6):1677-1682.
60. Della Valle AG, Padgett DE, Salvati EA: Preoperative planning for primary total hip arthroplasty. *J Am Acad Orthop Surg* 2005;13(7):455-462.
61. Lambers A, Jennings R, Bucknill A: Does computer navigation help the surgeon to achieve pre-operative leg length and offset targets in total hip arthroplasty? *Bone Joint J* 2013;95-B(suppl 15):110.
62. Maloney WJ, Keeney JA: Leg length discrepancy after total hip arthroplasty. *J Arthroplasty* 2004;19(4 suppl 1): 108-110.
63. Kaplan FS, Chakkalakal SA, Shore EM: Fibrodysplasia ossificans progressiva: Mechanisms and models of skeletal metamorphosis. *Dis Model Mech* 2012;5(6):756-762.
64. Peterson JR, Okagbare PI, De La Rosa S, et al: Early detection of burn induced heterotopic ossification using transcutaneous Raman spectroscopy. *Bone* 2013;54(1):28-34.
65. Ranganathan K, Loder S, Agarwal S, et al: Heterotopic ossification: Basic-science principles and clinical correlates. *J Bone Joint Surg Am* 2015;97(13):1101-1111.
66. Sakellariou VI, Grigoriou E, Mavrogenis AF, Soucacos PN, Papagelopoulos PJ: Heterotopic ossification following traumatic brain injury and spinal cord injury: Insight into the etiology and pathophysiology. *J Musculoskelet Neuronal Interact* 2012;12(4):230-240.
67. Shore EM, Kaplan FS: Role of altered signal transduction in heterotopic ossification and fibrodysplasia ossificans progressiva. *Curr Osteoporos Rep* 2011;9(2):83-88.
68. Aubut J-A, Mehta S, Cullen N, Teasell RW, ERABI Group, Scire Research Team: A comparison of heterotopic ossification treatment within the traumatic brain and spinal cord injured population: An evidence based systematic review. *NeuroRehabilitation* 2011;28(2):151-160.
69. Zhu Y, Zhang F, Chen W, Zhang Q, Liu S, Zhang Y: Incidence and risk factors for heterotopic ossification after total hip arthroplasty: A meta-analysis. *Arch Orthop Trauma Surg* 2015;135(9):1307-1314.

70. Chalmers J, Gray DH, Rush J: Observations on the induction of bone in soft tissues. *J Bone Joint Surg Br* 1975;57(1):36-45.

71. Balboni TA, Gobezie R, Mamon HJ: Heterotopic ossification: Pathophysiology, clinical features, and the role of radiotherapy for prophylaxis. *Int J Radiat Oncol Biol Phys* 2006;65(5):1289-1299.

72. Dalury DF, Jiranek WA: The incidence of heterotopic ossification after total knee arthroplasty. *J Arthroplasty* 2004;19(4):447-452.

73. Board TN, Karva A, Board RE, Gambhir AK, Porter ML: The prophylaxis and treatment of heterotopic ossification following lower limb arthroplasty. *J Bone Joint Surg Br* 2007;89(4):434-440.

74. Perosky JE, Peterson JR, Eboda ON, et al: Early detection of heterotopic ossification using near-infrared optical imaging reveals dynamic turnover and progression of mineralization following Achilles tenotomy and burn injury. *J Orthop Res* 2014;32(11):1416-1423.

75. Brooker AF, Bowerman JW, Robinson RA, Riley LH Jr: Ectopic ossification following total hip replacement. Incidence and a method of classification. *J Bone Joint Surg Am* 1973;55(8):1629-1632.

76. Della Valle AG, Ruzo PS, Pavone V, Tolo E, Mintz DN, Salvati EA: Heterotopic ossification after total hip arthroplasty: A critical analysis of the Brooker classification and proposal of a simplified rating system. *J Arthroplasty* 2002;17(7):870-875.

77. Kaplan FS, Glaser DL, Hebela N, Shore EM: Heterotopic ossification. *J Am Acad Orthop Surg* 2004;12(2):116-125.

78. Kan S-L, Yang B, Ning G-Z, et al: Nonsteroidal anti-inflammatory drugs as prophylaxis for heterotopic ossification after total hip arthroplasty: A systematic review and meta-analysis. *Medicine (Baltimore)* 2015;94(18):e828.

79. Vasileiadis GI, Sakellariou VI, Kelekis A, et al: Prevention of heterotopic ossification in cases of hypertrophic osteoarthritis submitted to total hip arthroplasty. Etidronate or indomethacin? *J Musculoskelet Neuronal Interact* 2010;10(2):159-165.

80. Morcos M, Smith K, Tanzer M: The effect of late radiotherapy on the progression of heterotopic ossification following total hip arthroplasty. *Eur J Orthop Surg Traumatol* 2018;28(6):1125-1131.

    This is a small case series that demonstrates late low-dose radiation may be useful in preventing progression of heterotopic ossification in patients who develop heterotopic ossification after THA.

81. Cobb TK, Berry DJ, Wallrichs SL, Ilstrup DM, Morrey BF: Functional outcome of excision of heterotopic ossification after total hip arthroplasty. *Clin Orthop Relat Res* 1999;361:131-139.

82. Wick M, Müller EJ, Hahn MP, Muhr G: Surgical excision of heterotopic bone after hip surgery followed by oral indomethacin application: Is there a clinical benefit for the patient? *Arch Orthop Trauma Surg* 1999;119(3-4):151-155.

83. Troutman DA, Dougherty MJ, Spivack AI, Calligaro KD: Updated strategies to treat acute arterial complications associated with total knee and hip arthroplasty. *J Vasc Surg* 2013;58(4):1037-1042.

84. Shubert D, Madoff S, Milillo R, Nandi S: Neurovascular structure proximity to acetabular retractors in total hip arthroplasty. *J Arthroplasty* 2015;30(1):145-148.

85. Alshameeri Z, Bajekal R, Varty K, Khanduja V: Iatrogenic vascular injuries during arthroplasty of the hip. *Bone Joint J* 2015;97-B(11):1447-1455.

86. Dietze S, Perka C, Baecker H: Blood vessel and nerve damage in total hip arthroplasty [German]. *Orthopade* 2014;43(1):64-69.

87. Sutter M, Hersche O, Leunig M, Guggi T, Dvorak J, Eggspuehler A: Use of multimodal intra-operative monitoring in averting nerve injury during complex hip surgery. *J Bone Joint Surg Br* 2012;94(2):179-184.

88. Hussain WM, Hussain HM, Hussain MS, Manning DW: A late vascular complication due to component migration after revision total hip arthroplasty. *J Arthroplasty* 2011;26(6):976.e7-976.e10.

89. Healy WL, Iorio R, Clair AJ, Pellegrini VD, Della Valle CJ, Berend KR: Complications of total hip arthroplasty: Standardized list, definitions, and stratification developed by the Hip Society. *Clin Orthop Relat Res* 2016;474(2):357-364.

90. Kawasaki Y, Egawa H, Hamada D, Takao S, Nakano S, Yasui N: Location of intrapelvic vessels around the acetabulum assessed by three-dimensional computed tomographic angiography: Prevention of vascular-related complications in total hip arthroplasty. *J Orthop Sci* 2012;17(4):397-406.

91. Flanagin BA, Dushey CH, Rubin LE, Keggi KJ: Total hip arthroplasty followed by traction and delayed reduction for Crowe IV developmental dysplasia of the hip. *J Arthroplasty* 2013;28(6):1052-1054.

92. Stecco C, Macchi V, Baggio L, et al: Anatomical and CT angiographic study of superior gluteal neurovascular pedicle: Implications for hip surgery. *Surg Radiol Anat* 2013;35(2):107-113.

93. Bhargava T, Goytia RN, Jones LC, Hungerford MW: Lateral femoral cutaneous nerve impairment after direct anterior approach for total hip arthroplasty. *Orthopedics* 2010;33(7):472.

94. Goulding K, Beaulé PE, Kim PR, Fazekas A: Incidence of lateral femoral cutaneous nerve neuropraxia after anterior approach hip arthroplasty. *Clin Orthop Relat Res* 2010;468(9):2397-2404.

95. Restrepo C, Parvizi J, Pour AE, Hozack WJ: Prospective randomized study of two surgical approaches for total hip arthroplasty. *J Arthroplasty* 2010;25(5):671-679.e1.

96. Homma Y, Baba T, Sano K, et al: Lateral femoral cutaneous nerve injury with the direct anterior approach for total hip arthroplasty. *Int Orthop* 2016;40(8):1587-1593.

97. Zappe B, Glauser PM, Majewski M, Stöckli HR, Ochsner PE: Long-term prognosis of nerve palsy after total hip arthroplasty: Results of two-year-follow-ups and long-term results after a mean time of 8 years. *Arch Orthop Trauma Surg* 2014;134(10):1477-1482.

98. Park JH, Hozack B, Kim P, et al: Common peroneal nerve palsy following total hip arthroplasty: Prognostic factors for recovery. *J Bone Joint Surg Am* 2013;95(9):e55.

CHAPTER 37

Revision Total Hip Arthroplasty

DAVID G. LEWALLEN, MD

ABSTRACT

The goals of revision total hip arthroplasty are to achieve both a stable mechanical construct and joint and durable fixation and function to improve quality of life for patients. Many reconstruction options are available for both acetabular and femoral reconstruction. Various options are available to achieve these goals, each with distinct advantages and potential limitations.

Keywords: acetabular reconstruction; femoral reconstruction; revision total hip arthroplasty

INTRODUCTION

Current revision hip arthroplasty tends to reflect the failure and limitations of earlier techniques and technology. Future revisions or repeat re-revisions of any present-day hip arthroplasties will be affected by the hopefully improved methods and technologies used at the time of revision surgery. Thus, revision total hip arthroplasty (THA) treatment goals are an ever-evolving target. In a 2019 review of more than 2,500 revision cases from a single center operated between 2005 and 2015, indications for the index revision were aseptic loosening (socket 21%, femur 15%, both 5%), polyethylene wear 18%, instability 13%, and fracture 11%. With the use of highly cross-linked inserts and improved acetabular designs at the time of index revision, subsequent re-revisions were required for instability in over half (52%), followed by fracture (11%), femoral loosening (11%), and acetabular aseptic loosening (9%). Repeat revisions for wear were reduced to 3%, all of which where an original conventional polyethylene liner had been left in place.[1] These results not only provide an index for current treatment but also help provide guidance for prioritization of efforts aimed at further improvement in the results of revision THA moving forward.

Dr. Lewallen or an immediate family member has received royalties from Zimmer Biomet; serves as a paid consultant to or is an employee of Zimmer Biomet; has stock or stock options held in Acuitive Technologies and Ketai Medical Devices; has received research or institutional support from Corin USA; and serves as a board member, owner, officer, or committee member of the American Joint Replacement Registry and the Orthopaedic Research and Education Foundation.

ACETABULUM

Acetabular revision has continued to evolve over the past 10 to 15 years, with the introduction of techniques designed to help treat large bone defects, improve fixation, and reduce the risk of dislocation. A variety of currently available multihole hemispherical cups can be used successfully in most acetabular revision cases. More recent techniques introduced with the goal of reducing the more common causes of failure of revision surgery include the use of highly porous materials to try to improve fixation; dual mobility articulations to reduce instability; and acetabular augments, cup-cage constructs, and even custom triflange cups for management of massive bone loss.

NONCEMENTED HEMISPHERICAL IMPLANTS

The noncemented hemispherical acetabular cup with adjunctive screws is the most widely used, reproducible, and reliable technique for acetabular revisions. Many

This chapter is adapted from Albers A, Carli A, Daivajna S, Griffin WL, Russell R, Gross AE, Lachiewicz PF, Ledford CK, Padgett DE, Rambani R, Garbuz D, Lewallen DG: *Revision Total Hip Arthroplasty* in Mont MA and Tanzer M, eds. *Orthopaedic Knowledge Update®: Hip and Knee Reconstruction 5*. Rosemont, IL, American Academy of Orthopaedic Surgeons, 2017, pp 453-471.

acetabular revisions require an extra large or jumbo size noncemented hemispherical implant. The accepted parameters for this implant, defined by surgeons at the Mayo Clinic, are as follows: 62 mm or greater in women and 66 mm or greater in men.[2] This definition was based on a size that is 10 mm greater than the mean size of acetabular implants used in primary THA. Use of the jumbo cup has numerous advantages over other techniques.[2,3] Weight bearing occurs over a large area of the pelvis, and surface contact is maximized. Because the acetabulum remains somewhat spherical, even with a loose or migrated implant, the techniques for preparation and insertion are relatively simple. With the large implant, the need for bone graft material, especially bulk allograft, is minimized. This technique is more likely to normalize the center of rotation of the hip joint compared with a high hip center placement or other techniques.

This technique also has specific disadvantages when used for revision. It does not restore acetabular bone structure, as is described with other techniques (such as impaction grafting). The center of rotation of the hip may be elevated 10 mm or more.[4] Preparation of the acetabular bone for a jumbo cup will require some reaming of the anterior and posterior walls or columns, and without careful technique, excess bone from the posterior column could be removed inadvertently. Some surgeons may consider the need for modular acetabular implants and screws, for secure fixation, to be a disadvantage of the jumbo cup. However, modular implants and screws are generally used in all revision THAs.[3,5] The amount of bone that will grow into the porous coating from the damaged acetabular surface is unknown, and less is expected than in primary hip arthroplasty. It is unclear whether a relatively small amount of bone ingrowth will provide durable fixation or will predispose to late loosening.

Technique

Because the implantation of the noncemented hemispherical acetabular cup requires preparation and insertion of an implant much larger than a primary implant, good exposure is recommended, with a longer skin and fascial incision. The posterolateral approach involves release of the femoral insertion of the gluteus maximus tendon to facilitate and improve the retraction of the femur or retained femoral implant anterosuperior to the acetabulum. Occasionally (such as in a stiff or protruded hip), some types of greater trochanteric osteotomy (either a slide or extended osteotomy) may be necessary to provide adequate exposure of the entire rim of the acetabulum. Other exposures, such as the direct lateral approach or even the direct anterior approach, have been used for revision surgeries as well, but extensile versions of each, including companion femoral osteotomies, may be needed in cases of more difficult exposure. After removal of the failed acetabular implant and any residual membrane or bone cement, the acetabulum should be evaluated carefully for pelvic discontinuity by inspection and performing manual tests. If there is no discontinuity, the surgeon may proceed with preparation for using a jumbo cup. If pelvic discontinuity is present, then techniques described later will likely need to be used.

Repetitive reaming of the acetabulum for a noncemented hemisphere is unnecessary, as the surgeon should be conservative in bone preparation. Often, minimal reaming or localized use of a high-speed burr at the periphery of the acetabulum is all that is needed to remove a sclerotic bony edge, and maximize contact of the hemispherical reamer or trial shells on host bone. This serves as a guide for proper sizing of the jumbo cup. Forceful reaming could destroy the damaged or deficient remaining bone. The goal of the technique is to fill the acetabulum from the ilium to the acetabular teardrop (from top to bottom) with the new porous metal shell, for which some bone from the anterior and posterior acetabulum may need to be removed to create a hemispherical acetabular cavity. A trial acetabular implant or reamer shell is then inserted to determine if rim stability can be obtained. Depending on the design of the implant (hemispherical or elliptical), the type of porous coating, and the bone quality, a multihole implant that is 0 to 2 mm larger than the final reamer shell is selected. Before inserting the new implant, all fibrous membrane should be curetted, and any cavitary defects should be packed with allograft bone or bone substitute to improve bone stock. Screw fixation is important for both initial and long-term fixation of the noncemented revision cup.[3,5,6] The intrapelvic neural and vascular structures may be more at risk when a jumbo cup is used.[6] The so-called safe zones for insertion of multiple acetabular screws in the superior and posterior quadrants are used routinely. In addition, screw fixation in an array into the ischium, posterior column, and base of the ilium (superior, posterior, and inferior) should be performed routinely in nearly all revisions; this is recommended to prevent late cup breakout or pulling away from the inferior acetabulum. After placement of a minimum of three to four screws, the empty screw holes can also be filled with allograft before modular liner trial placement or real acetabular insert placement.

There are a few specific contraindications to the isolated use of a noncemented hemispherical cup. This technique usually cannot be used alone in the presence of pelvic discontinuity, when the surgeon is unable to obtain stability on host bone with a large reamer shell or trial implant because of severe bone loss, or rarely if adequate screw fixation cannot be achieved. Additional implants and techniques are required in these scenarios.[7] Historically, it has been reported that host bone–acetabular cup contact of less than 50% may be a contraindication to the use of a jumbo noncemented cup alone.[8,9] However, with the availability of enhanced (or second-generation) highly porous surfaces, this may no longer be the case. In an early 2012 study of 53 hips in which an enhanced surface jumbo acetabular implant was implanted, and there was less than 50% host bone–cup contact, the rate of failure was only 7.5% at a mean follow-up of 72 months (range, 60 to 102 months).[8] Two other earlier studies have also reported successful fixation using cups with this enhanced porous surface in difficult acetabular revisions.[10,11]

Recent Results

Overall results of reported revision series using standard ingrowth surfaces have historically yielded a low overall rate of aseptic loosening. Three earlier studies have reported results of noncemented jumbo acetabular implants being implanted without highly porous materials or augments or cages in revision hip arthroplasty. A 2014 study reported on a group of 196 jumbo implant revisions, with a minimum follow-up of 2 years and mean follow-up of 10 years.[12] Only three patients had revision for acetabular loosening at 7 months, 9 years, and 11 years, respectively. In a 2013 study of 129 acetabular revisions with jumbo implants with failure defined as acetabular revision for loosening or definite radiographic evidence of loosening, 10-year survival was 97.3% (95% confidence interval, 89.6 to 99.3) and 15-year survival was 82.8% (95% confidence interval, 59.0 to 97.6). In 2015, an updated review of the Mayo Clinic jumbo acetabular revision study was published, with a mean follow-up time of 20 years.[13] Cup survival, with failure defined as need for acetabular revision or definite radiographic evidence of loosening, was 85% at 20 years.

The question of whether these historical results can be improved on by more modern highly porous coated acetabular designs and reconstructive techniques is difficult to determine from available evidence. Level I evidence comparing large numbers of cases with different porous materials is lacking. Direct comparisons of data from different single implant studies are problematic because of the wide variation possible in revision cases especially with regard to the severity of bone loss encountered. There can often also be potential selection bias introduced by individual surgeons who frequently choose to use different implants or methods for different revision challenges.

Reports from large national registries are a valuable alternative source of data in that they give a real-world picture of results in the broad community. There are two such reports that provide some insight into the question of the general effect of highly porous materials in acetabular revisions. In a 2017 collaborative study reporting on data drawn from the Swedish Hip Registry and the Australian Orthopaedic Association National Registry, no difference in aseptic or septic revision rates were seen between more than 2,400 first-time revisions using porous tantalum cups and more than 4,400 first-time revisions using other cup designs.[14] In another 2018 study reporting on data from the National Mayo Clinic Joint Replacement Database for England and Wales, the authors used propensity scoring based on multiple potential patient and surgical confounding variables to match 1,931 porous tantalum cup cases with 1,931 nonporous tantalum cups.[15,16] This study was restricted to two porous tantalum designs and two standard noncemented cup designs all from the same manufacturer. Acetabular implant survivorship analysis out to 6 years showed no statistical difference between the porous tantalum designs and the standard noncemented designs in all-cause re-revision rates (2.5% versus 2.6%) or in re-revision for aseptic loosening (0.92% versus 0.97%). No difference was observed in re-revision for infection between the porous tantalum and standard cup designs (1.1% versus 1.4%). On balance, the aforementioned data suggest that there may be limited if any benefit for these highly porous materials when used for large numbers of routine cases with good remaining bony support. But these studies still fail to resolve the question of any benefits that may exist in cases where more severe bone loss is present. This is something that is very difficult to assess in registry studies of revision arthroplasty, which lack information on bone defect severity or radiographic assessment of the outcomes of the reconstructions, and it will likely require other types of studies for resolution of this issue. Even more difficult to answer is the question of whether differences exist between the various highly porous materials now available from multiple manufacturers. Studies directly comparing alternative highly porous ingrowth surfaces are lacking and many newer materials by definition lack long-term follow-up. A 2020 systematic review of 16 studies of highly porous titanium acetabular implants used for revision surgery generated data on 11,366 cases followed up from 2 to 7 years. Overall acetabular implant survivorship was 93% with an aseptic loosening rate of 2.1%.[17] These data certainly do not suggest any improvement in outcome when compared with the aforementioned larger registry-based results on alternative earlier highly porous and standard porous materials. Longer term follow-up and improved comparisons between alternative ingrowth surfaces will be needed to resolve the question of whether long-term benefit is provided by any of these specific highly porous materials across the wide range of revision hip arthroplasty problems encountered clinically.

Careful comparative studies with stratification of results by the severity of bone defects treated will be essential in resolving these questions.

Complications

Dislocation is the most frequent complication after revision hip arthroplasty in which a noncemented hemispherical cup, usually of jumbo size, is implanted. The frequency has been generally reported to be 10% to 15% in several studies.[2,3,5,6] In a recent large series of over 2,500 revision cases published in 2019, more than 50% of subsequent re-revisions were performed for instability.[1] The etiology of dislocation with the jumbo cup is multifactorial and may be related to the usually extensile exposure required for implantation as well as the acetabular implant–femoral head size mismatch.[18] It has been confirmed that acetabular revisions using a larger femoral head may have a lower risk of dislocation.[3,19] These data have influenced subsequent surgical technique with information from the most recent American Joint Replacement Registry annual report documenting a steady increase in head size for both primary and revision hip procedures between 2012 and 2018, with 36-mm heads currently the most frequent head diameter used. In revision cases reported to the American Joint Replacement Registry in 2018, a 36-mm head was used in 45.7% of revision cases and fixed heads larger than 32 mm accounted for over 75% of the total.[20] Recently, dual mobility articulations have also been increasingly used as an alternative to large fixed head bearings not only in the management of dislocation but also for the prevention of instability in high-risk primary and revision hip arthroplasty procedures. In a 2018 single institutional series, 146 revision cases where a dual mobility articulation was used were compared with 209 cases where the treating surgeon instead chose a 40-mm fixed head.[21] Subsequent dislocation was lower in the dual mobility group (3% versus 10%), and revision for dislocation was only 1% in the dual mobility group versus 6% in the 40-mm head group. Multiple other studies have confirmed these same results with a systematic review of dual mobility versus fixed head articulations in 2019 showing a composite dislocation rate of 2.2% versus 7.1%.[22] Nationwide US data from the American Joint Replacement Registry show a rise in the usage of dual mobility articulations for revision THA since 2012 with 16.3% usage of dual mobility sockets for revision cases overall in 2018, and 21% usage for revision procedures performed for instability.[20]

ACETABULAR AUGMENTS

The number of revision hip arthroplasty procedures is increasing steadily, as are complex cases needing more specialized reconstruction.[23] One of the challenges in revision of acetabular implants is bone loss. Bone loss defects are frequently classified with the Paprosky classification, which categorizes the acetabulum into three types, depending on the degree of osteolysis affecting the acetabular teardrop and ischium and the amount and direction of implant migration.[24] Different techniques, mainly cemented or noncemented, have been described to manage these defects. Common cemented techniques involve either impaction bone grafting or bulk allograft with a cemented implant or reconstruction reinforcement rings with allograft and a cemented cup. These techniques produce acceptable results but can be difficult to execute, and reports of early failure have been published, especially in type III defects.[25,26] Noncemented acetabular sockets have good results in primary THA, and similar technology has been used in revision scenarios. They can be used in the form of a jumbo cup, bilobed cup, cup-in-cup stacking, or reconstruction cages.[2,27-32] Challenges related to these techniques include development of adequate healthy host bone to achieve bone ingrowth; replacement of segmental bone loss (Paprosky type IIIA and IIIB defects); and reproduction of a normal or close-to-normal hip center of rotation.

To optimize the likelihood for biologic fixation of the interface, techniques in surface technology, such as hydroxyapatite and porous coatings, have been used. One material used is porous metal with characteristics that are similar to those of bone (strength, flexibility, three-dimensional infrastructure). Porous metal has a high coefficient of surface friction, which assists the surgeon in achieving initial interface stability. It also has impressive bone ingrowth and incorporation characteristics, best demonstrated in the canine model.[33] In addition to using a highly porous coated shell, porous metal augments can replace bone loss, resulting in less reliance on structural allografts to reduce the risk of graft resorption and potential disease transmission. The first example of this technology available for general use was highly porous tantalum or Trabecular Metal (Zimmer). Subsequently, other manufacturers have developed highly porous acetabular implants with augments.

Indications and Technique of Using Trabecular Metal Cup and Augment

Trabecular Metal is available in the form of a variety of acetabular shells and augments. The three types of cups are the jumbo cup as a modular titanium/Trabecular Metal shell for ring lock liner fixation; the revision Trabecular Metal shell for cemented liner fixation; and the continuum titanium/Trabecular Metal shell for internal taper lock liner fixation. The types of Trabecular Metal augments available are the roof and rim pure Trabecular

Metal semilunar augments and the column buttress pure Trabecular Metal semilunar and keel augments for severe defects.

Any of the three cups can be used alone in the jumbo cup configuration, although the revision Trabecular Metal shell has the advantage of allowing independent alignment of the cemented liner if optimal alignment of the shell itself is difficult to achieve because of the location and severity of bone loss. In addition, in the presence of pelvic discontinuity, the revision Trabecular Metal shell can be used with a reconstruction cage (cup-cage technique).[34]

The most commonly used augment is the semilunar, almost always in combination with a revision Trabecular Metal shell. Rarely, the column buttress augment or a combination of stacked augments may be considered in difficult cases.

The main indications for using an augment with a cup are Paprosky acetabular defects types IIB, C, and IIIA and IIIB. The most common locations of the defects are in the superolateral and posterosuperolateral parts of the acetabulum. They affect the superomedial segment less commonly, in which setting it is imperative to rule out pelvic discontinuity before surgery. This will profoundly influence management and outcome and will often necessitate a cup-cage reconstruction. The need for an augment is anticipated on the basis of preoperative templating on an AP pelvis radiograph; however, a definitive decision to use an augment intraoperatively can be made if an oblong bone defect that cannot be supported by the hemispherical implant without augmentation by acetabular bone stock is recognized. When dealing with segmental bone loss, Judet views are useful preoperatively to help characterize the location and extent of bone loss. In cases of greater complexity, CT may be required.

To effectively insert an augment, the normal acetabulum is prepared in its normal location, and the shell size is determined based on the AP dimension, not the oblong superior inferior dimension. The trial cup is positioned, and the location and extent of the segmental defect is characterized. The defect is then prepared to accept an augment of suitable size, such that it has good contact with the remaining host bone and provides the required support for the hemispherical trial cup. This often requires secondary but gentle reaming with a hemispherical reamer to maximize the augment-bone interface contact and stability. This reaming is done with a reamer that matches the diameter of the augment chosen. The metal augment is then secured with a minimum of two 4.5-mm titanium cortical screws. If the location of the screw hole within the augment is inconvenient, a new screw hole can be created in the augment using a 4-mm high-speed burr. Particulate allograft, or bone from reamings, if available, is then packed within the augment. Any additional small contained bone defects can be packed by impaction grafting using cancellous allograft while maintaining adequate contact with host bone.[35] After the augment is secured, the revision Trabecular Metal shell is inserted and fixed with screws. The Trabecular Metal augment and shell can be unitized with cement either when the shell is inserted or later, when the definitive polyethylene liner is cemented in place. Care should be taken to achieve appropriate alignment of the cemented liner independent of the shell if some malalignment of the shell has to be accepted, so as to maximize host bone contact and secure screw fixation.

Results of Using a Cup-Augment Construct

Studies have been published on the use of porous metal cups with augments since 2004. A longer term study presented 53 patients (mean follow-up, 110 months; range, 88 to 128 months) with survival of 92% at 10 years.[36] The survivorship for this construct was 94% to 100% at 2 years, 92% to 100% at 5 years, and 92% at 10 years. Revision for implant loosening or radiolucencies have been associated with concurrent pelvic discontinuity. In a 2017 study of 57 cases involving a high proportion of Paprosky 3A (48%) or 3B (38%) defects, there were also 11 cases of pelvic discontinuity (19%). In this series at a minimum of 5 years follow-up, aseptic loosening occurred in two cases (3%) and partial zone 3 radiolucencies were seen in six cases (10%). But associated pelvic dissociation was present in one of the loosening cases and five of six cases with zone 3 radiolucencies.[37] This suggests the potential for additional fixation methods or alternative implant designs to improve outcomes in cases of pelvic discontinuity.

Discussion

Acetabular bone defects have been managed in many different ways over the past few decades. Cemented acetabular implants have been used with allograft techniques, reconstruction meshes, or reinforcement rings. However, results of these constructs have not been quite successful because of resorption of allograft and failure of the reconstruction rings, in some cases up to 12% at 5 years and 21% to 37% at 10 to 15 years.[38,39] A systematic review comparing the results of Trabecular Metal implants with those of reinforcement rings has shown that Trabecular Metal results are significantly better.[25] A Trabecular Metal cup with an augment has several advantages, including that it can be conformed to the type of defect and custom built to suit a patient's anatomy. There is less reliance on bulk allografts, and expensive computer-generated implants are not required. One article has reported two cases with loosening of the shell, which has created metal debris, suggesting that cup-augment junction failure may occur if there is no ingrowth of host bone into the acetabular shell.[32] Rigid initial fixation is needed to allow initial bone ingrowth over the weeks following surgery to prevent gradual later mechanical failure. Based on the available information, acetabular augments appear to continue to have a valuable role in selected cases of segmental acetabular bone deficiency where stable mechanical support on host bone is difficult to achieve with a hemispherical cup alone.

Cup-Cage Construct

Major acetabular deficiency and pelvic discontinuity in revision THA procedures mandate acetabular reconstruction that can provide initial stability and the potential for durable fixation.[40] Antiprotrusio cage and ring techniques have historically been used in revision settings with significantly deficient bone stock to protect the healing of bulk or cancellous allograft. Midterm survivorship free from revision has been reported at between 72% and 80% with the use of a variety of rings and cages.[41-43] However, the use of such methods independently has decreased with the advent of alternative specially fabricated porous metal ingrowth hemispherical acetabular implants, porous metal acetabular augments, and even custom triflange noncemented implants. Cup-cage reconstruction is another option when major bone deficiency or pelvic dissociation is encountered. This technique was first reported in 2004 as an alternative to traditional cages.[44] The development of the cup-cage technique evolved from previous acetabular reconstructive techniques, by combining a highly porous metal acetabular implant with an antiprotrusio cage. Initially, off-the-shelf antiprotrusio cages were used to provide fixation advantages of the cage in combination with the longer term bone ingrowth and more durable fixation of the ingrowth cup. Subsequently, made-for-purpose cages have become available for use with porous tantalum acetabular implants in a range of cage sizes that match those of the available acetabular implants.

The main indication for the use of an ilioischial cage in combination with a porous ingrowth cup is inadequate initial acetabular implant support or fixation. This can be due to poor bone quality, the size and location of bone defects, or the presence of associated pelvic dissociation. In many cases, a combination of these factors prompts selection of a cup-cage construct during the course of the reconstruction. Cup-cage constructs are most commonly used in select cases of marked superolateral (Paprosky type IIIA) or superomedial (Paprosky type IIIB) acetabular bone loss, with or without pelvic discontinuity. Other indications include the presence of pelvic discontinuity with less severe bone loss or markedly impaired bone quality, as is sometimes seen following therapeutic pelvic radiation.

After adequate, usually extensile, surgical exposure and removal of implants, a decision must be made about sufficiency of the available bone stock for use of a hemispherical cup with multiple screws, with or without an augment. If the pattern of bone deficiency and quality of the bone requires additional support, a cup-cage construct can be added. Reconstruction usually begins with cancellous bone grafting of residual cavitary deficiencies, and even some segmental defects, followed by placement of a highly porous acetabular implant. This implant must allow for multiple screws in an array across the dome, down the posterior column, and into the base of the ischium. It is especially important in all reconstructions with significant bone loss, with or without a cage, to achieve inferior fixation in zone 3 to prevent early separation of the cup from the inferior aspect of the acetabulum, as well as subsequent migration and frank loosening (**Figure 1**). Acetabular augments may be used for segmental defects or elliptical acetabular cavities to improve host bone contact before placement of the cage. A slot must be created in the ischium for the ischial flange of the cage; this is best done early in the case to allow positional adjustment of the acetabular implant and access by the ischial flange into the ischial slot. Occasionally, the cup requires repositioning in a slightly more horizontal and neutral position to uncover the ischium. In other cases, modest superior migration of the hip center of 1 cm or so may allow for lack of coverage of the ischium, despite standard cup version and inclination. After the acetabular implant has been fixed into position with multiple screws, trials for the cage system of choice are used to determine the proper bend of the ischial and iliac flanges to achieve slotting into the ischium and contact against the outer table of the ilium, while also providing for seating of the cage into the cup. The use of cage trials is especially helpful as a template to minimize contouring of the flanges of the real cage. The real cage is impacted into position beginning with the ischial flange, seating the cage into the cup, and then impacting the iliac flange down into position on the outer table of the ilium. A screw is then placed through the cage and through the dome of the cup into the host bone. When an existing screw hole lines up with that of the cage, this screw hole can be used if a screw is not already present within the cup. If a screw is present, the cage may be removed, the screw backed out, the cage replaced, and the screw repositioned into the original hole. The presence of the dome screw unites the reconstruction and brings the cage into good contact against the cup for subsequent iliac flange fixation. The screw holes in the iliac flange are then filled with screws (generally at least three or four screws used in a transverse manner to provide rigid fixation) in combination with the dome screws in the cup, which run relatively perpendicular to the transverse iliac flange screws. It is sometimes possible to place a screw through the shoulder region of the cage and into the base of the

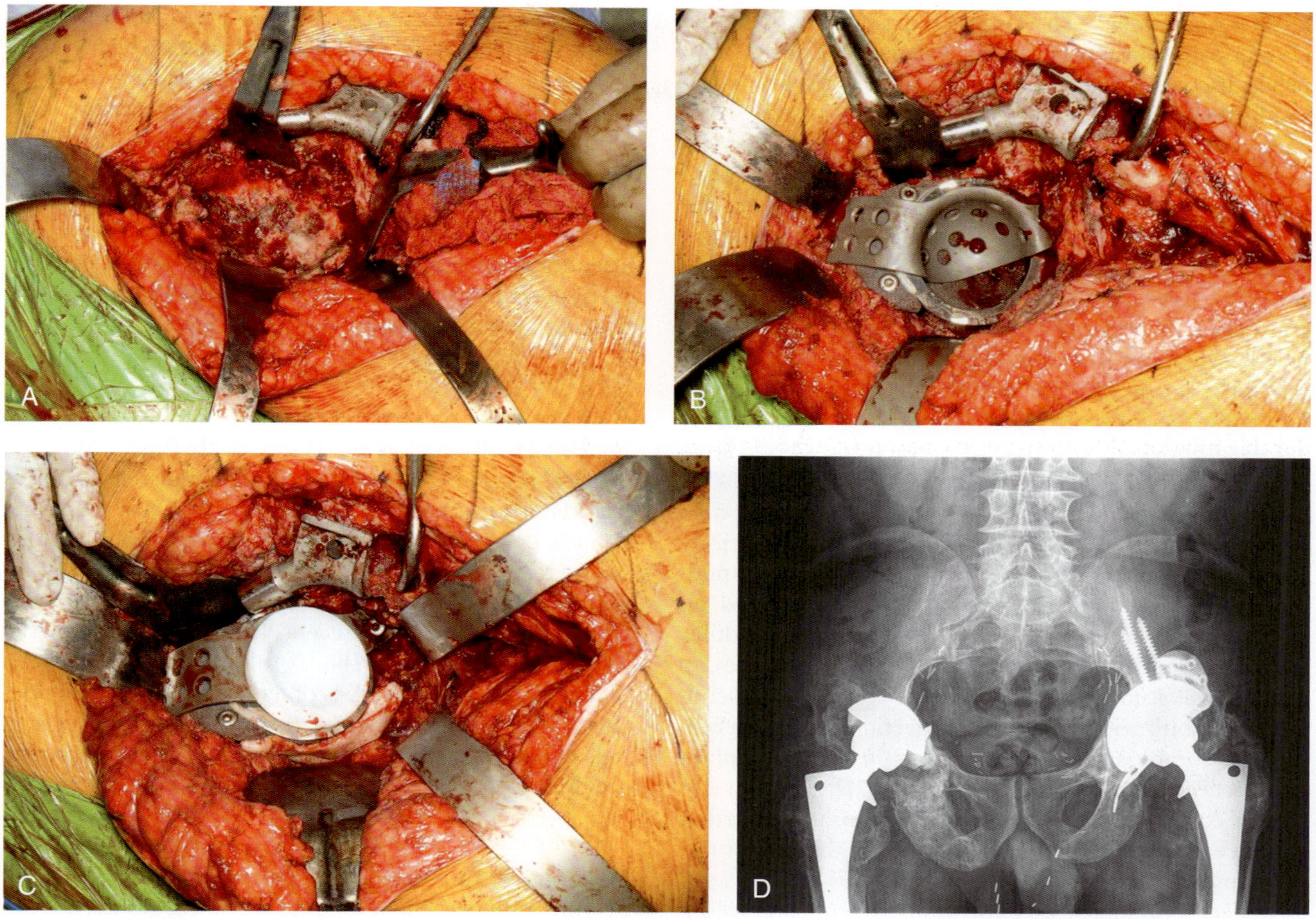

FIGURE 1 Images of a revision total hip arthroplasty. Intraoperative photograph (**A**) demonstrates a Paprosky type IIIA acetabular defect treated by using Trabecular Metal revision shell and superior buttress augment with multiple pelvic screws (**B**), followed by ilioischial cage placement on top of the construct. **C**, The polyethylene liner is cemented within, unitizing the construct. **D**, Postoperative AP left hip radiograph shows cup-cage construct.

ischium through the quadrilateral surface. This inferior screw can add additional important inferior ischial fixation, especially in the presence of pelvic dissociation. A more recent variation of the cup-cage technique involves the use of a half cup-cage construct to ease insertion; one of the flanges of the cage (usually the ischial flange) is removed with a carbide burr to allow added screws to be used into the base of the ischium in the area that would have been filled by the flange. In this case, the iliac portion of the cage is contoured to fit the outer table, and the half cage is rotated into position and fixed with screws through the iliac flange of the dome in a manner similar to that used for the full cage construct. The half cup-cage technique is most useful when large cavitary ischial defects preclude fixation of the iliac flange alone. It may also be useful with an intact acetabulum that has a major defect and a tenuous residual bony bridge, in which case impaction of the cage may cause pelvic dissociation. Hence, the insertion of the half cage can be accomplished in a much more atraumatic manner, with less surgical exposure. This evolution of the cup-cage technique has been documented in a 2017 review of 57 cases performed over a 10-year period from 2002 to 2012, with 30 full cup cages and 27 half cup cages used with ischial screw fixation instead of the inferior flange.[45]

Outcomes of cup-cage constructs have been reported in clinical series of small to moderate numbers with good clinical results and durable fixation in most patients despite major acetabular defects at intermediate-term follow-up. One study reported on 26 consecutive acetabular revision cases with a cage and Trabecular Metal implant used for pelvic discontinuity.[34] No clinical or radiographic evidence of loosening was seen in 89% of hips at 4 years, with only three implants migrating farther than 5 mm and requiring revision surgery. Midterm follow-up comparison studies of the same cohort confirmed that cup-cage reconstruction performed significantly better than conventional cages, with septic or aseptic loosening failure rates of 15% versus

68%, respectively.[46] The largest retrospective review of 67 cup-cage constructs for large acetabular defects and pelvic discontinuity has demonstrated the most promising results thus far.[47] Only four revisions (9%) for aseptic loosening were performed in the 45 pelvic discontinuity cases at 6-year average follow-up. Additionally, postoperative patient outcome scores improved significantly, and the 10-year survival rate was 85%. The rate of complications, most commonly infection and instability, was 12%. In the 2017 series of both full cup-cage and half cup-cage constructs, 57 cases were followed up a mean of 4.6 years with survivorship free of all-cause revision of 89% overall, and 83% versus 96% for the 30 full cup-cage versus 27 half cup-cage constructs. However, fixation was reliably achieved with only one case of revision for aseptic loosening observed in a full cup-cage case.[45]

Further acetabular stabilization techniques may also be applied to the cup-cage reconstruction, especially when additional initial stability is preferred. A small cohort of cup-cage reconstructions demonstrated no short-term failure from aseptic loosening when modular buttress augments were used in conjunction with the cup cage.[48] One study described a successful pelvic discontinuity stabilization technique of acetabular distraction used in combination with a porous ingrowth implant and, if needed, acetabular augments.[49] Distraction can also be combined with the cup-cage technique to further enhance stability and initial fixation, with good survivorship in chronic pelvic discontinuity cases.

Longer term follow-up of the results of cup-cage reconstruction, as well as study of the various adjunctive measures used, including augment, distraction, and half cup cage, would be of interest. However, available data suggest that the cup-cage technique provides a useful tool for selective application in revision hip arthroplasty; it also appears to offer reliable alternatives for major acetabular defects with pelvic discontinuity, where stable fixation cannot be obtained using standard porous hemispherical acetabular implants with multiple screws.

Custom Triflange Acetabular Implants

Another alternative for pelvic discontinuity and selected cases of massive acetabular bone loss is the use of a custom triflange device modeled off CT images of the acetabulum and pelvis.[50] Advantages include the availability of a preoperative bone model for inspection and orientation of the surgeon, and both the accurate fit of the implant and the planned and guided screw placement that results from the three-dimensional CT modeling. Disadvantages include the several weeks delay in surgery required for fabrication of the implant, the time and cost required for imaging, planning and custom manufacturing, and the wide exposure required for placement of a large one-piece implant. However, in the hands of experienced surgeon, excellent fixation has been reported in the face of the most severe bone defects. In a 2018 report from two high-volume centers in 73 patients at 5 to 12 years follow-up, there was a 20.5% acetabular revision rate for instability (8%) and infection (11%) but only a single case of recognized implant loosening.[51] These results suggest that the use of advanced imaging and rapidly advancing custom manufacturing methods deserve continued development and attention as efforts are made to further evolve acetabular revision techniques, especially for patients who have pelvic discontinuity and massive acetabular bone loss.

The Femur

With the aging cohort and the increasing number of hip implants, revision rates are on the rise. In North America, femoral revision with fully porous coated stem implants has historically been the benchmark. In cases of larger femoral bone defects (such as Paprosky type IV), cylindrical stems cannot achieve fixation and proximal femoral replacement with metal and bone has been the historical treatment of choice. In recent years, modular tapered stems have emerged as the workhorse for treatment in North America for all types of femoral deficiency in revision THA. These techniques, as well as impaction grafting (which is much more common in parts of Europe), are described in the following paragraphs.

Fully Porous Coated Stems in Revision THA

Historically, fully porous coated cylindrical stems have demonstrated excellent long-term clinical results in revision THA. Mechanical failure rates of less than 5% have been reported at a mean follow-up of 14 years.[52,53] Long-term fixation is dependent on rigid initial stability of the femoral implant. Fully porous coated stems bypass the deficient proximal bone and gain fixation in the relatively intact isthmus. Initial stability of these stems requires a scratch fit over a minimum of 5 cm of intact isthmus. Therefore, fully porous coated stems are indicated in revision THAs with mild or moderate femoral defects, such as Paprosky type II or IIIA defects[54-56] (**Figure 1**). Clinical scenarios in which fully porous coated stems have higher failure rates include femoral bone defects with less than 4 cm of intact diaphysis and canal diameters greater than 19 mm.[52,53,55,57] Clinical failure rates of 18% have been reported for fully porous coated stems in type IIIB defects and canal diameters greater than 19 mm; this rate increases to 37.5% for type IV defects.[53]

Despite the long-term success of fully porous coated stems, there are concerns. The surgical technique relies on a 0.5-mm underream of the femur to achieve a tight fit in the isthmus. In cases of damaged bone, the margin for error between a tight fit and an intraoperative femoral fracture is small. In addition, longer straight stems are at risk for anterior femoral perforation. An extended trochanteric osteotomy may be required for accurate access down the canal for femoral preparation. Two studies have reported intraoperative fracture rates of 13% and 15% and occurrence of anterior perforations of 4% and 10%.[58,59]

There are long-term concerns regarding stress shielding and implant fracture. With diaphyseal fixation, a well-fixed stem transfers load through the distal portion of the stem directly to the distal femur, resulting in proximal bone resorption, or stress shielding. This process typically occurs within the first 2 years after surgery, then stabilizes.[60] In a series of 208 fully porous coated implants reviewed at a mean of 13.9 years, the rate of stress shielding was 23%.[60] Risk factors for radiographically evident stress shielding included female sex, type C bone, and large stem diameter.[60] Moreover, because the stems are fixed distally, they are subject to cantilever bending, and the potential exists for implant fracture. Stem fractures are rare and tend to occur in smaller implant sizes (less than 13.5-mm diameter).

The inability of fully porous coated cylindrical stems to gain reliable fixation in the more severe Paprosky type IIIB and IV femoral defects, along with the other concerns outlined, has resulted in greater use of modular (or monoblock) tapered fluted titanium stems in the revision setting.

Current indications for potential use of a fully porous coated cylindrical stem include patients who have type II or IIIA bone loss (**Figure 2**).

Tapered Fluted Titanium Stems

Tapered fluted titanium stems of both modular and monoblock designs are increasingly used in all revision settings, even when the proximal femoral bone stock is deficient, of poor quality, or both. Their tapered geometry is designed to provide axial stability, and the flutes/splines allow for rotational stability. Tapered fluted titanium stems are typically used in Paprosky type II, IIIA, and IIIB femoral defects. Although they are also used to reconstruct Paprosky type IV defects, achieving adequate femoral fixation can be difficult. In cases in which adequate axial and rotational stability cannot be achieved with tapered stems, reconstruction may require a proximal femoral replacement or use of more demanding techniques, such as impaction grafting or an allograft-prosthetic composite. Although many different tapered fluted stems are now available for use, no prospective studies comparing different designs are present in the literature to recommend the use of one over another.

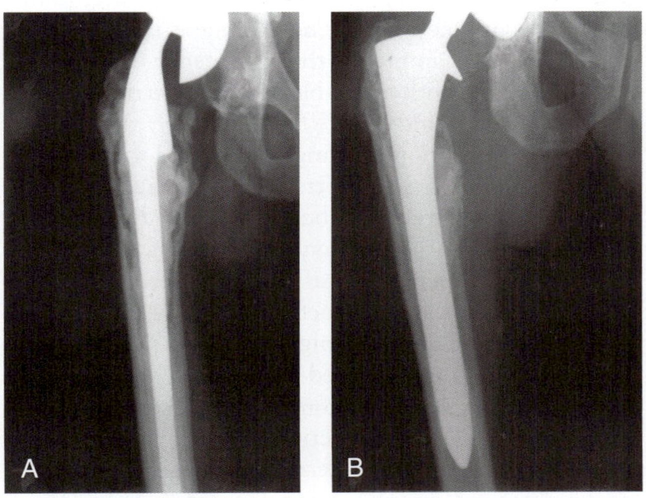

FIGURE 2 AP radiographs of the right femur with loose cemented femoral implant and type IIIA bone deficiency. **A**, Preoperative view. **B**, Postoperative view shows an extensively porous coated stem for type IIIA bone loss.

Compared with extensively porous coated cylindrical monoblock stems, tapered fluted titanium stems are more versatile and more reliable in patients with advanced femoral defects.[53] Tapered fluted stems, especially the modular type, allow the surgeon to readily re-create anatomic leg length, femoral offset, and version, which can result in better functional outcomes. A 2010 study comparing a tapered fluted modular stem with a fully porous coated monolithic cylindrical stem showed improved functional outcomes and increased patient satisfaction in the former, despite more significant preoperative femoral defects.[61] When severe femoral bone loss leaves the proximal stem unsupported, tapered fluted titanium designs have the advantage of minimizing stress shielding and decreasing the risk of implant fatigue failure seen with extensively porous coated cylindrical stems.[52]

Several studies have demonstrated successful diaphyseal osseointegration and good long-term survivorship using monoblock tapered fluted titanium stems for revision THA. A 2014 literature review of medium-term to long-term results of the Wagner self-locking stem (Zimmer), a nonmodular tapered fluted titanium stem, showed excellent survivorship (at least 92% to 15.8 years), high rates of implant stability (83.5% to 97.0% osseointegration and 8% to 15% fibrous stability), good clinical and functional results, and even regeneration of proximal femoral bone stock in cases without major proximal femoral deficits.[62] Although long-term survival and osseointegration have not been a problem with these stems, leg length inequality, periprosthetic fracture, and subsidence have been quite common, resulting from the difficulty of seating the tapered cone in the correct station without fracturing the femur. A 2011 study examining 10- to 15-year follow-up of the Wagner self-locking stem showed subsidence greater than 10 mm in 20% of cases. This is thought to be due to achieving three-point fixation as the mode of initial fixation. In most of these cases, however, subsidence was limited to the first 12 months postoperatively, and although subsidence was quite common, few stems required revision.[63]

Modularity between the distal diaphyseal fitting portion and the proximal stem body facilitates stem insertion and increases the implant's versatility in the revision setting. Specifically, the advantage of modularity is the ability to achieve optimal diaphyseal fixation and then to independently size the metaphyseal segment for optimal leg length, femoral offset, version, and soft-tissue tension. This intraoperative customization has resulted in decreased rates of stem subsidence and is thought to contribute to the reconstitution of proximal femoral bone stock by allowing better contact between the proximal femoral bone and stem body. Several authors have reported favorable clinical and radiologic outcomes at midterm follow-up for various pathologies requiring complex revision THA.[64-66] As widespread experience with modular tapered stems has increased, excellent results in a full range of femoral defects have been documented. In a 2017 review of a large single-center experience, 519 aseptic femoral revision cases were followed up for a mean of 4.5 years (range 2 to 14 years), and the 10-year survivorship was 96% free of all-cause revision.[67] Only 6 of the 16 observed femoral revisions in this series were performed for aseptic loosening. Radiographically, 12 stems showed initial subsidence, but all except one had stabilized at the time of final follow-up. Modular tapered fluted designs have also shown superior results in the face of severe femoral bone loss when directly compared with modular cylindrical femoral stems. A 2013 study comparing these two designs in Paprosky type IIIB/IV femoral defects showed clinically significant superiority of the tapered fluted modular stem in recurrent femoral implant loosening, re-revision surgery, and stem-related failures, despite more severe femoral defects in the tapered fluted group.[68] This portends the tapered designs gaining better stability within a shorter segment of bone (less than 4 cm), which likely favors osseointegration in compromised diaphyseal bone. Similar findings have also been confirmed in cadaver and biomechanical studies in which identical axial and torsional loads resulted in significantly less axial and rotational displacement with tapered fluted stems.[69] Few biomechanical studies have looked at the effect of different tapered fluted designs on implant stability. A 2015 biomechanical study showed that increasing the taper angle and broadening spline geometry exhibited significantly greater axial stability, but had little effect on initial torsional stability.[70]

Despite the cited benefits of implant modularity, earlier concerns that existed regarding long-term implant survivorship of modular stems because of reports of fracture at the modular stem/body junction have driven renewed interest in nonmodular fluted tapered stems. Furthermore, although there are no published data, the theoretical risk of corrosion and adverse local tissue reaction arising from the taper junction is concerning. Early failures at the modular junction seemed to be related to smaller dimension stems (less than 19 mm), which are unsupported in patients who have deficient proximal bone stock, after an extended trochanteric osteotomy, in patients who have higher body mass index, and in those with first-generation taper designs.[71,72] Despite much stronger newer generation modular stem junctions, sporadic implant failures have still been described. For this reason, certain high-volume centers migrated back to the nonmodular tapered fluted design in hopes of avoiding modular stem fractures.[73] In a 2019 study of 146 femoral revision cases where 103 were modular fluted tapered titanium stems and 43 were nonmodular fluted tapered implants, there was no difference in re-revision rate, revision surgery rate, dislocation, fracture, or length of stay between the two groups. The modular stems were significantly more expensive (120%) while the surgical time was longer for the nonmodular implant cases (193 minutes versus 163 minutes).[74] Although this report documents the excellent results achievable with monoblock stems, detailed preoperative planning, careful intraoperative trials, and experience with nonmodular stems are requirements for avoiding the aforementioned complications of monoblock implants. Gaining this experience requires a higher volume of revision cases; thus, for the surgeon with a lower volume of cases, modular stems may still be the best and most forgiving option.

Impaction Grafting

Impaction grafting involves using milled allograft bone to reconstitute a deficient medullary canal. Cement is then inserted within the reconstituted canal followed by a collarless double-tapered polished stem. This technique permits femoral bone stock restoration resulting from incorporation and remodeling of the impacted graft by the host skeleton. Although technically demanding, refinement in technique and the development of specialized instruments have improved the consistency of impaction grafting results, with favorable outcomes in independent clinical centers worldwide.[75,76]

Femoral impaction grafting is indicated for Paprosky type IIIC and IV femoral defects in which the replenishment of bone stock is preferred, but insufficient intact diaphysis is available for noncemented interference (**Figure 3**). Furthermore, impaction grafting should be considered when medullary canal diameters exceed 18 mm, a limit that is associated with a higher risk of postoperative thigh pain with noncemented fixation.[77] The need for an extended trochanteric osteotomy for implant removal does not preclude the use of impaction grafting, with one study finding no difference in midterm results when an extended trochanteric osteotomy was performed.[78] Although no absolute contraindications exist, femoral impaction grafting is not ideal in elderly or medically unfit patients, cases in which recovery of bone stock is either not required or

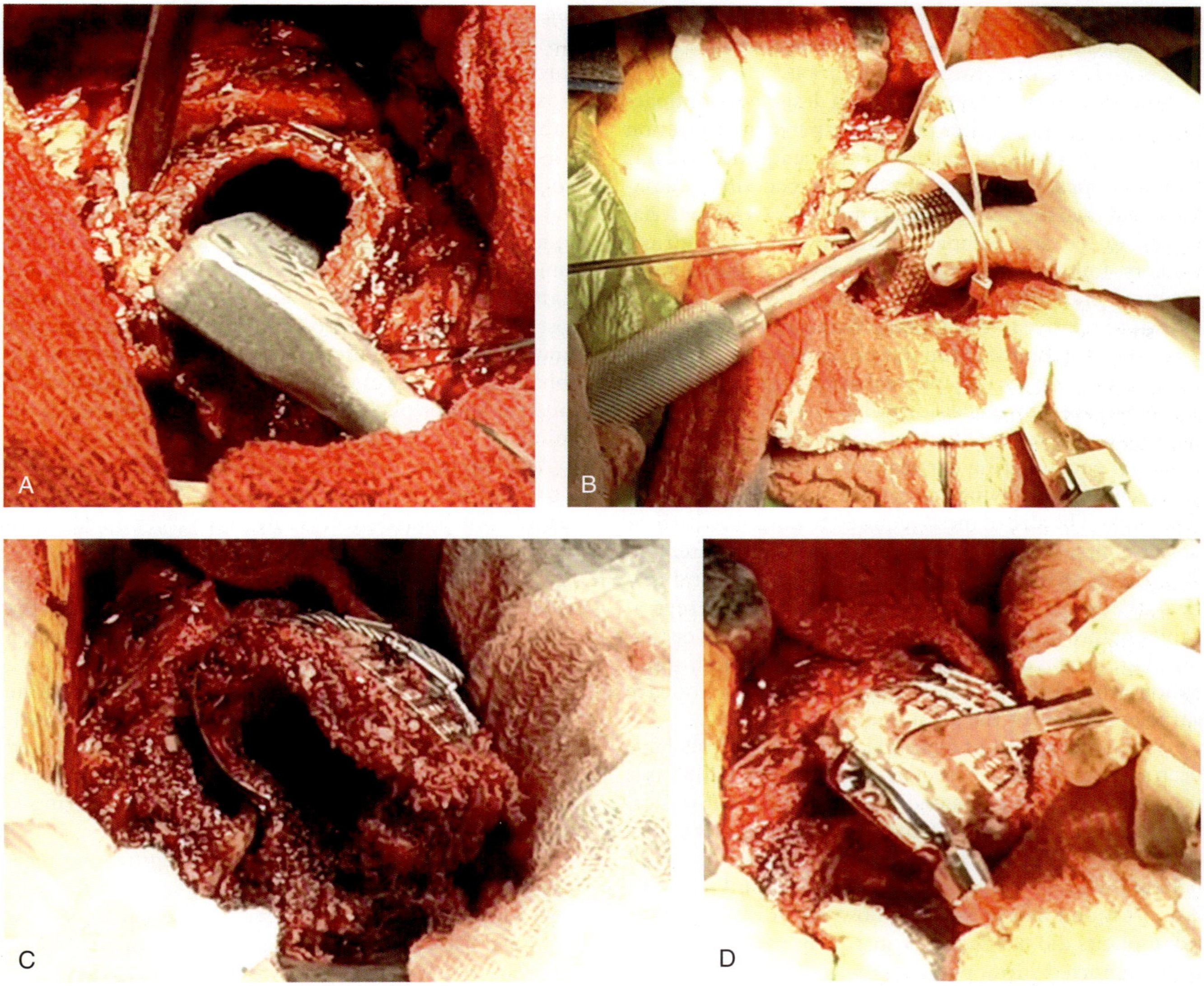

FIGURE 3 Intraoperative photographs of a revision total hip arthroplasty. **A**, A capacious femoral canal with 5 cm proximal posterior tenuous cortical defect. **B**, Following distal bone grafting, steel mesh is applied and secured with cables. A Cobb elevator is used to preserve space for the graft and cement mantle. **C**, Proximal bone grafting is performed, reconstituting the femoral canal. **D**, Cement and the double-tapered, polished femoral stem are inserted.

biologically infeasible. Furthermore, small cortical defects can be managed through careful placement of steel mesh, whereas cortical defects larger than 10 cm may preclude the use of impaction grafting.

Detailed preoperative planning is necessary, including high-quality radiographs from which stem length, size, and offset can be templated. Cortical defects involving more than 50% of femoral circumference on two radiographic views must be bypassed by the prosthesis by at least two cortical diameters. The threaded femoral plug should also be templated, and it usually lies at least 2 cm distal to the tip of the stem to permit adequate distal graft filling. Multiple fresh-frozen femoral head allografts should be ordered from a bone bank; other necessary equipment includes a bone mill and additional reconstruction implants, including metallic mesh, cerclage cables, and femoral plates.

Following adequate exposure of the proximal femur, removal of the previous femoral implant, and removal of intramedullary cement or membrane, the threaded femoral plug can be placed, and the bone graft can be inserted. Appropriate graft preparation has been shown to be critical to the success of femoral impaction grafting. Although optimal size remains contentious, the presence of allograft bone chips greater than 4.5 mm in diameter has been found to provide improved stability within in vitro models,[79,80] and having some heterogeneity in chip size provides higher shear resistance across the entire graft structure.[81] Bone chips should be washed to remove fat particles, reduce lubrication, increase frictional resistance, and improve graft interdigitation.[82]

Several instrument sets have been designed for impaction grafting. A collarless polished taper stem impaction system, which uses cannulated instruments and modular femoral tamps, permits easy, reliable impaction of diaphyseal and then metaphyseal graft material. Graft material is introduced and compacted distally with cylindrical packers, followed by additional diaphyseal and metadiaphyseal graft impaction using femoral tamps that are oversized relative to the actual prosthesis; this permits a 2-mm cement mantle. Modular proximal tamps are then used to re-create the metaphyseal canal without affecting what has been produced distally. The final result is a reconstructed, tapered femoral canal (**Figure 3**).

When encountering cortical bone loss, a reconstruction technique involving use of metallic mesh can be used (**Figure 3**). The size of mesh required to cover the cortical defect is first determined using a flexible template, and then the mesh itself is cut with scissors. For a distal cortical defect, the mesh is applied and secured with several cables before impaction grafting. For a proximal defect, distal grafting is completed first, followed by mesh application around the proximal tamp, taking care to leave sufficient space for the graft and cement mantle.

Long-term results of femoral impaction grafting have been satisfactory. A prospective cohort study of 208 cases implanted with a cemented polished Exeter (Stryker) stem reported a 10-year femoral implant survival rate of 94.9%.[83] An additional retrospective study of 37 patients who have a preoperative Endo-Klinik score of 3 or 4[84] found that at 9-year follow-up, 96.3% of femoral implants did not require subsequent revision.[85] Both series reported intraoperative fracture rates of 15.9% and 5.7%, respectively, a complication that has been reported in 5% to 12% of patients in most studies. This finding reinforces the importance of regularly assessing cortical integrity during the grafting procedure. Another series of 41 patients followed up for 19 years reported a femoral implant survival rate for any reason of 93%, and the rate of aseptic loosening was 98%.[76] Given these findings, femoral impaction bone grafting has a high survival rate in long-term follow-up and continues to be an attractive option in select patients presenting with challenging femoral revisions in which there is severe bone loss.

Allograft-Prosthetic Composite and Proximal Femoral Replacement

Femoral reconstruction with an allograft-prosthetic composite has been in use since the 1980s.[86] The technique of allograft-prosthetic composite reconstruction uses a long-stem prosthesis that spans the host-allograft bone junction. A femoral prosthesis is placed distally within the medullary canal of the host femur, whereas the proximal portion of the stem is positioned and cemented within a proximal femur allograft. The allograft provides initial stability by acting as a strut graft and enhances future bone stock. The potential for enhanced future bone stock may simplify future additional revision surgery and provides an attachment surface for soft tissue and bone. Current understanding of the allograft-prosthetic composite is that the allograft femur provides an organic scaffold for the prosthesis. Bone ingrowth occurs at the host-allograft bone junction and at the greater trochanter junction. Initial stability is achieved with a step-cut or oblique osteotomy and can be augmented with a cortical strut and/or plate. This initial stability is crucial for union.

A 2014 meta-analysis identified 16 studies with a total of 498 patients and a mean follow-up of 8.1 years.[87] The pooled success rate was 81%; pooled structural failure rate, 15%; and pooled infection rate, 8%. The ability to revise an allograft-prosthetic composite adds strength to the decision to initially choose the allograft-prosthetic composite as the surgical solution in a situation in which bone loss is significant. In young and active patients who have proximal femoral bone loss, allograft-prosthetic composite should be considered a preferred option, whereas it is contraindicated in elderly patients who have multiple comorbidities for whom immediate mobilization and weight bearing is necessary and infection is present.[88]

Several studies have outlined encouraging long-term results following the use of an allograft-prosthetic composite for femoral reconstruction. The evidence supports the use of allograft-prosthetic composites when the technique is performed by trained and experienced surgeons in institutions with the facilities to support such complex surgery. With the advent of modular femoral implants, the use of allograft-prosthetic composites has decreased, but it is a viable option for the young patient or when bone loss extends well into the diaphysis.

The use of a proximal femoral replacement for non-neoplastic indications, such as periprosthetic femoral fractures, massive proximal femoral bone loss, and aseptic loosening, was extended after the success of megaprostheses in neoplastic surgery.[89] A proximal femoral replacement has the advantages of no host bone interface allograft healing; no problems of graft fracture, resorption, or disease transmission; relative ease of reconstruction; and no adverse effects from chemotherapy or irradiation to the implant. The ideal patient for proximal femoral replacement is an elderly person who has a sedentary lifestyle. A sufficient amount of bone must be present distally to allow for secure noncemented or cemented fixation of the megaprosthesis. This form of reconstruction is much easier and faster and allows for reduced surgical time and blood loss.[89]

The failure modes of proximal femoral replacement include instability (because of poor soft-tissue and trochanteric attachment), aseptic loosening, severe stress shielding with adaptive bone remodeling, infection, difficulty with revision due to destruction of soft tissues and limited remaining host bone, and mechanical failure. The incidence of mechanical failure decreased significantly in polyaxial endoprostheses compared with uniaxial endoprostheses.[90]

A retrospective review of 403 proximal femoral arthroplasties (endoprosthetic reconstructions) from five institutions after tumor resection reported a 10- and 15-year survival rate of 75%, with mechanical causes being the most common mode of failure.[90]

Proximal femoral bone loss continues to be a challenging condition for the arthroplasty surgeon, which is compounded by the fact that most patients have already had multiple hip surgeries, have severe abductor muscle loss and possible acetabular bone stock deficiency, and are commonly elderly persons who have preexisting comorbidities. Allograft-prosthetic composites and proximal femoral replacements are useful options in severe proximal femoral deficiencies. Postoperative instability remains a concern and can be treated by using a dual mobility cup or a constrained liner.

SUMMARY

Revision THA can be categorized into a series of steps. Adequate exposure and safe implant removal are critical to success. Once these are accomplished, several techniques are available for reconstruction of both the acetabulum and femur. On the acetabular side, hemispherical cups with screws can be used to treat at least 90% of cases. In patients who have larger segmental defects, midterm results of augments used to enhance cup stability have been excellent. Results into the second decade will be viewed with great interest to determine whether augments are as durable as or better than allografts, which were previously used, but for the most part have been replaced by augments. Pelvic dissociation continues to be a challenge, but short-term to midterm results of use of the cup-cage technique and custom triflange implants are both encouraging for this indication. The leading complication of revision hip arthroplasty is dislocation, but the use of dual mobility articulations at the time of revision especially in those with prior instability or otherwise at higher risk for dislocation is increasing and may help reduce dislocation rates in the future.

Tapered fluted modular stems have become the accepted technique for femoral reconstruction. Other techniques, such as fully porous coated stems and impaction grafting, can still be used with high rates of success. In bigger defects (Paprosky types IIIB and IV), tapered stems have become invaluable. Over the next decade, the role of nonmodular tapered titanium stems will become clearer. Although these stems can be used in most cases in which a modular stem had been used, for the low-volume surgeon, modular stems will be technically easier. However, for surgeons who are comfortable performing femoral revisions, nonmodular tapered titanium stems will likely become more common in the next decade. As midterm to long-term results of the newer techniques become available, the benchmark in acetabular and femoral revision will continue to evolve.

KEY STUDY POINTS

- Hemispherical cups with screws can be used to treat at least 90% of cases.
- Dislocation is the leading complication of revision hip arthroplasty, but dual mobility articulations have been adopted widely as a means of combating this in high risk patients.
- In cases with larger segmental defects, midterm results of augments used to enhance cup stability have been excellent.
- The cup-cage reconstruction involves placement of a spanning ilioischial cage on top of a highly porous metal revision acetabular implant. The construct provides acute stabilization of major acetabular defects or pelvic discontinuity to potentially allow for long-term healing and biologic fixation.
- Early to midterm clinical results of cup-cage constructs are encouraging, with low rates of aseptic loosening and excellent long-term implant survivorship.
- Custom triflange acetabular implants, while technically demanding, both preoperatively and intraoperatively have documented excellent fixation results at intermediate-term follow-up of massive acetabular bone defect and pelvic discontinuity cases.
- Tapered fluted modular stems have become the accepted technique for femoral reconstruction.
- Other techniques, such as fully porous coated stems and impaction grafting, can still be used with high rates of success.
- Allograft-prosthetic composites and proximal femoral replacements are useful options in cases of severe proximal femoral deficiencies.

ANNOTATED REFERENCES

1. Goldman AH, Sierra RJ, Trousdale RT, Lewallen DG, Berry DJ, Abdel MP: The Lawrence D. Dorr surgical techniques & technologies award: Why are contemporary revision total hip arthroplasties failing? An analysis of 2500 cases. *J Arthroplasty* 2019;34(7):S11-S16.

   This is a retrospective review of 2,589 cases of revision THA performed between 2000 and 2015. Reasons for index revision were aseptic loosening (21% acetabular, 15% femoral, and 5% both), polyethylene wear or lysis 18%, instability 13%, and fracture 11%. At a mean of 6 years follow-up, subsequent failure requiring re-revision was due to instability in 52%, fracture in 11%, femoral loosening in 11%, and acetabular loosening in 9%. Infection occurred in 6%, and survivorship at 2, 5, and 10 years was 94%, 92%, and 88%.

2. Whaley AL, Berry DJ, Harmsen WS: Extra-large uncemented hemispherical acetabular components for revision total hip arthroplasty. *J Bone Joint Surg Am* 2001;83-A(9):1352-1357.

3. Lachiewicz PF, Soileau ES: Fixation, survival, and dislocation of jumbo acetabular components in revision hip arthroplasty. *J Bone Joint Surg Am* 2013;95(6):543-548.

4. Nwankwo CD, Ries MD: Do jumbo cups cause hip center elevation in revision THA? A radiographic evaluation. *Clin Orthop Relat Res* 2014;472(9):2793-2798.

5. Jones CP, Lachiewicz PF: Factors influencing the longer-term survival of uncemented acetabular components used in total hip revisions. *J Bone Joint Surg Am* 2004;86-A(2):342-347.

6. Meldrum R, Johansen RL: Safe screw placement in acetabular revision surgery. *J Arthroplasty* 2001;16(8):953-960.

7. Sheth NP, Nelson CL, Springer BD, Fehring TK, Paprosky WG: Acetabular bone loss in revision total hip arthroplasty: Evaluation and management. *J Am Acad Orthop Surg* 2013;21(3):128-139.

8. Sternheim A, Backstein D, Kuzyk PR, et al: Porous metal revision shells for management of contained acetabular bone defects at a mean follow-up of six years: A comparison between up to 50% bleeding host bone contact and more than 50% contact. *J Bone Joint Surg Br* 2012;94(2):158-162.

9. Lakstein D, Backstein D, Safir O, Kosashvili Y, Gross AE: Trabecular metal cups for acetabular defects with 50% or less host bone contact. *Clin Orthop Relat Res* 2009;467(9):2318-2324.

10. Jafari SM, Bender B, Coyle C, Parvizi J, Sharkey PF, Hozack WJ: Do tantalum and titanium cups show similar results in revision hip arthroplasty? *Clin Orthop Relat Res* 2010;468(2):459-465.

11. Lachiewicz PF, Soileau ES: Tantalum components in difficult acetabular revisions. *Clin Orthop Relat Res* 2010;468(2):454-458.

12. Gustke KA, Levering MF, Miranda MA: Use of jumbo cups for revision of acetabulae with large bony defects. *J Arthroplasty* 2014;29(1):199-203.

13. von Roth P, Abdel MP, Harmsen WS, Berry DJ: Uncemented jumbo cups for revision total hip arthroplasty: A concise follow-up, at a mean of twenty years, of a previous report. *J Bone Joint Surg Am* 2015;97(4):284-287.

14. Laaksonen I, Lorimer M, Gromov K, et al: Does the risk of rerevision vary between porous tantalum cups and other cementless designs after revision hip arthroplasty?. *Clin Orthop Relat Res* 2017;475(12):3015-3022.

    This study reports the combined registry data from the Swedish Hip Arthroplasty Register and the Australian Orthopaedic Association National Joint Replacement Registry from January 1, 2006 to December 2014. First-time acetabular revision procedures were studied comparing porous tantalum designs with the five most common standard noncemented designs used in revision from each registry, yielding six control cup designs. About 2,442 porous tantalum revision cups (1,456 from Swedish Hip Arthroplasty Register, 981 from Australian Orthopaedic Association National Joint Replacement Registry) were compared with 4,401 standard noncemented cups (1,793 Swedish Hip Arthroplasty Register Joint Replacement Registry, 2,608 Australian Orthopaedic Association National). Overall survivorship up to 7 years was similar between groups: 86% for porous tantalum cup and 87% for the standard designs. However, re-revision for aseptic cup loosening was slightly lower for the porous tantalum designs (1.5% versus 2.4%), whereas dislocation was slightly higher (3.6% versus 2.5%). No difference was seen in septic revision between groups. Level of evidence: III.

15. Matharu GS, Judge A, Murray DW, Pandit HG: Trabecular metal versus non-trabecular metal acetabular components and the risk of re-revision following revision total hip arthroplasty: A propensity score-matched study from the National Joint Registry for England and Wales. *J Bone Joint Surg Am* 2018;100(13):1132-1140.

    This is a National Joint Registry study of acetabular revision using propensity score matching of patients between groups comparing two porous tantalum designs and two standard noncemented cup designs all from the same manufacturer. Acetabular implant survivorship analysis out to 6 years showed no statistical difference between the porous tantalum designs and the standard noncemented designs in all-cause re-revision rates (2.5% versus 2.6%) or in re-revision for aseptic loosening (0.92% versus 0.97%). No difference was observed in re-revision for infection between the porous tantalum and standard cup designs (1.1% versus 1.4%). Level of evidence: III.

16. Matharu GS, Judge A, Murray DW, Pandit HG: Trabecular metal acetabular components reduce the risk of revision following primary total hip arthroplasty: A propensity score matched study from the National Joint Registry for England and Wales. *J Arthroplasty* 2018;33(2):447-452.

    This is a National Joint Registry study of 18,200 primary acetabular implants using propensity score matching of patients between groups comparing two porous tantalum designs and two standard noncemented cup designs all from the same manufacturer. Porous tantalum designs had lower all-cause revision (1.0% versus 1.8%), aseptic revision (0.1% versus 0.2%), and revision for infection (0.5% versus 0.9%). The authors note these statistical differences are small but may be clinically significant, especially if the porous tantalum cups were used in more complex cases not accounted for in the propensity matching process.

17. Malahias MA, Kostretzis L, Greenberg A, Nikolaou VS, Atrey A, Sculco PK: Highly porous titanium acetabular components in primary and revision total hip arthroplasty: A systematic review. *J Arthroplasty* 2020;35(6):1737-1749.

    PubMed/MEDLINE and Cochrane Database of Systematic reviews were queried for highly porous titanium acetabular implants. Of 16 studies with 11,366 total cases and 2 to 7 years follow-up, 8 studies included data on 480 acetabular revision procedures. Overall survival in revision arthroplasties for highly porous titanium cups was 93.5% with an aseptic loosening rate of 2.1%.

18. Kelley SS, Lachiewicz PF, Hickman JM, Paterno SM: Relationship of femoral head and acetabular size to the prevalence of dislocation. *Clin Orthop Relat Res* 1998;355:163-170.

19. Garbuz DS, Masri BA, Duncan CP, et al: The Frank Stinchfield Award: Dislocation in revision THA. Do large heads (36 and 40 mm) result in reduced dislocation rates in a randomized clinical trial? *Clin Orthop Relat Res* 2012;470(2):351-356.

20. American Academy of Orthopaedic Surgeons: American Joint Replacement Registry 2019 Annual Report. http://connect.ajrr.net/2019-ajrr-annual-report. Accessed October 14, 2020.

21. Hartzler MA, Abdel MP, Sculco PK, Taunton MJ, Pagnano MW, Hanssen AD: Otto Aufranc Award: Dual-mobility constructs in revision THA reduced dislocation, rerevision, and reoperation compared with large femoral heads. *Clin Orthop Relat Res* 2018;476(2):293-301.

    This is a retrospective review of 355 revision hip arthroplasty cases performed between 2011 and 2014, where the treating surgeon chose to use either a 40-mm head (209 cases) or a dual mobility articulation (146) to attempt to reduce the risk of dislocation following revision. Subsequent dislocation rates were significantly lower for the dual mobility articulation patients (3%) than for the 40-mm head group (10%), as was the re-revision for dislocation (1% versus 6%) with a hazard ratio of 7.1. Level of evidence: III.

22. Reina N, Pareek A, Krych AJ, Pagnano MW, Berry DJ, Abdel MP: Dual-mobility constructs in primary and revision total hip arthroplasty: A systematic review of comparative studies. *J Arthroplasty* 2019;34(3):594-603.

    This is a systematic review including six studies of revision THA where the overall dislocation rate at a mean of 4.1 years was 7.1% for the control group versus 2.2% for the dual mobility group. The odds ratio (control versus dual mobility) for dislocation was 3.59 and for repeat revision for dislocation, it was 4.88. Level of evidence: III.

23. Kurtz S, Ong K, Lau E, Mowat F, Halpern M: Projections of primary and revision hip and knee arthroplasty in the United States from 2005 to 2030. *J Bone Joint Surg Am* 2007;89(4):780-785.

24. Paprosky WG, Perona PG, Lawrence JM: Acetabular defect classification and surgical reconstruction in revision arthroplasty. A 6-year follow-up evaluation. *J Arthroplasty* 1994;9(1):33-44.

25. Beckmann NA, Weiss S, Klotz MC, Gondan M, Jaeger S, Bitsch RG: Loosening after acetabular revision: Comparison of trabecular metal and reinforcement rings. A systematic review. *J Arthroplasty* 2014;29(1):229-235.

26. Garcia-Cimbrelo E, Cruz-Pardos A, Garcia-Rey E, Ortega-Chamarro J: The survival and fate of acetabular reconstruction with impaction grafting for large defects. *Clin Orthop Relat Res* 2010;468(12):3304-3313.

27. Perka C, Ludwig R: Reconstruction of segmental defects during revision procedures of the acetabulum with the Burch-Schneider anti-protrusio cage. *J Arthroplasty* 2001;16(5):568-574.

28. Ng TP, Chiu KY: Acetabular revision without cement. *J Arthroplasty* 2003;18(4):435-441.

29. Park DK, Della Valle CJ, Quigley L, Moric M, Rosenberg AG, Galante JO: Revision of the acetabular component without cement. A concise follow-up, at twenty to twenty-four years, of a previous report. *J Bone Joint Surg Am* 2009;91(2):350-355.

30. Dearborn JT, Harris WH: Acetabular revision arthroplasty using so-called jumbo cementless components: An average 7-year follow-up study. *J Arthroplasty* 2000;15(1):8-15.

31. Chen WM, Engh CA Jr, Hopper RH Jr, McAuley JP, Engh CA: Acetabular revision with use of a bilobed component inserted without cement in patients who have acetabular bone-stock deficiency. *J Bone Joint Surg Am* 2000;82(2):197-206.

32. Blumenfeld TJ, Bargar WL: Surgical technique: A cup-in-cup technique to restore offset in severe protrusio acetabular defects. *Clin Orthop Relat Res* 2012;470:435-441.

33. Bobyn JD, Stackpool GJ, Hacking SA, Tanzer M, Krygier JJ: Characteristics of bone ingrowth and interface mechanics of a new porous tantalum biomaterial. *J Bone Joint Surg Br* 1999;81(5):907-914.

34. Kosashvili Y, Backstein D, Safir O, Lakstein D, Gross AE: Acetabular revision using an anti-protrusion (ilio-ischial) cage and trabecular metal acetabular component for severe acetabular bone loss associated with pelvic discontinuity. *J Bone Joint Surg Br* 2009;91(7):870-876.

35. Grappiolo G, Loppini M, Longo UG, Traverso F, Mazziotta G, Denaro V: Trabecular metal augments for the management of Paprosky type III defects without pelvic discontinuity. *J Arthroplasty* 2015;30(6):1024-1029.

36. Whitehouse MR, Masri BA, Duncan CP, Garbuz DS: Continued good results with modular trabecular metal augments for acetabular defects in hip arthroplasty at 7 to 11 years. *Clin Orthop Relat Res* 2015;473(2):521-527.

37. Jenkins DR, Odland AN, Sierra RJ, Hanssen AD, Lewallen DG: Minimum five-year outcomes with porous tantalum acetabular cup and augment construct in complex revision total hip arthroplasty. *J Bone Joint Surg Am* 2017;99(10):e49.

This is a study of 57 cases involving a high proportion of Paprosky 3A (48%) or 3B (38%) defects. Eleven cases (19%) had an associated pelvic discontinuity. In this series at a minimum of 5 years follow-up, aseptic loosening occurred in two cases (3%) and partial zone 3 radiolucencies were seen in six cases (10%). But associated pelvic dissociation was present in one of the loosening cases and five of six cases with zone 3 radiolucencies. Level of evidence: IV.

38. Trumm BN, Callaghan JJ, Liu SS, Goetz DD, Johnston RC: Revision with cementless acetabular components: A concise follow-up, at a minimum of twenty years, of previous reports. *J Bone Joint Surg Am* 2012;94(21):2001-2004.
39. Abolghasemian M, Tangsataporn S, Sternheim A, Backstein D, Safir O, Gross AE: Combined trabecular metal acetabular shell and augment for acetabular revision with substantial bone loss: A mid-term review. *Bone Joint J* 2013;95-B(2):166-172.
40. Berry DJ, Lewallen DG, Hanssen AD, Cabanela ME: Pelvic discontinuity in revision total hip arthroplasty. *J Bone Joint Surg Am* 1999;81(12):1692-1702.
41. Zehntner MK, Ganz R: Midterm results (5.5-10 years) of acetabular allograft reconstruction with the acetabular reinforcement ring during total hip revision. *J Arthroplasty* 1994;9(5):469-479.
42. Goodman S, Saastamoinen H, Shasha N, Gross A: Complications of ilioischial reconstruction rings in revision total hip arthroplasty. *J Arthroplasty* 2004;19(4):436-446.
43. Regis D, Sandri A, Bonetti I, Bortolami O, Bartolozzi P: A minimum of 10-year follow-up of the Burch-Schneider cage and bulk allografts for the revision of pelvic discontinuity. *J Arthroplasty* 2012;27(6):1057-1063.e1.
44. Hanssen AD, Lewallen DG: Acetabular cages: A ladder across a melting pond. *Orthopedics* 2004;27(8):830-832, 832.
45. Sculco PK, Ledford CK, Hanssen AD, Abdel MP, Lewallen DG: The evolution of the cup-cage technique for major acetabular defects: Full and half cup-cage reconstruction. *J Bone Joint Surg Am* 2017;99(13):1104-1110.

    Fifty-seven cup-cage cases (30 full cup-cage and 27 half cup-cage constructs) were performed for major bone loss (2B to 3B and 60% associated pelvic discontinuity). Documentation of the technique for both variations is provided. Patients were followed up a mean of 4.6 years with survivorship free of all-cause revision 89% overall (83% full versus 96% half). Partial zone 3 lucency was noted in eight cases (two full cage, six half cage). There was one case of revision for aseptic loosening in a full cup-cage case. Seven of the eight cases with lucencies and the revision for loosening were in patients with pelvic discontinuity. Level of evidence: III.

46. Abolghasemian M, Tangsaraporn S, Drexler M, et al: The challenge of pelvic discontinuity: Cup-cage reconstruction does better than conventional cages in mid-term. *Bone Joint J* 2014;96-B(2):195-200.
47. Amenabar T, Rahman WA, Hetaimish BM, Kuzyk PR, Safir OA, Gross AE: Promising mid-term results with a cup-cage construct for large acetabular defects and pelvic discontinuity. *Clin Orthop Relat Res* 2016;474(2):408-414.
48. Ballester Alfaro JJ, Sueiro Fernández J: Trabecular metal buttress augment and the trabecular metal cup-cage construct in revision hip arthroplasty for severe acetabular bone loss and pelvic discontinuity. *Hip Int* 2010;20(suppl 7):S119-S127.
49. Sporer SM, Bottros JJ, Hulst JB, Kancherla VK, Moric M, Paprosky WG: Acetabular distraction: An alternative for severe defects with chronic pelvic discontinuity? *Clin Orthop Relat Res* 2012;470(11):3156-3163.
50. Christie MJ, Barrington SA, Brinson MF, Ruhling ME, DeBoer DK: Bridging massive acetabular defects with the triflange cup: 2- to 9-year results. *Clin Orthop Relat Res* 2001;393:216-227.
51. Gladnick BP, Fehring KA, Odum SM, Christie MJ, DeBoer DK, Fehring TK: Midterm survivorship after revision total hip arthroplasty with a custom triflange acetabular component. *J Arthroplasty* 2018;33(2):500-504.

    This is a retrospective report from two high-volume centers in 73 patients at 5 to 12 years follow-up. There was a 20.5% acetabular revision rate for instability (8%) and infection (11%), but only a single case of recognized implant loosening.

52. Weeden SH, Paprosky WG: Minimal 11-year follow-up of extensively porous-coated stems in femoral revision total hip arthroplasty. *J Arthroplasty* 2002;17(4 suppl 1):134-137.
53. Sporer SM, Paprosky WG: Revision total hip arthroplasty: The limits of fully coated stems. *Clin Orthop Relat Res* 2003;417:203-209.
54. Nadaud MC, Griffin WL, Fehring TK, et al: Cementless revision total hip arthroplasty without allograft in severe proximal femoral defects. *J Arthroplasty* 2005;20(6):738-744.
55. McAuley JP, Engh CA Jr: Femoral fixation in the face of considerable bone loss: Cylindrical and extensively coated femoral components. *Clin Orthop Relat Res* 2004;429:215-221.
56. Aribindi R, Barba M, Solomon MI, Arp P, Paprosky W: Bypass fixation. *Orthop Clin North Am* 1998;29(2):319-329.
57. Egan KJ, Di Cesare PE: Intraoperative complications of revision hip arthroplasty using a fully porous-coated straight cobalt-chrome femoral stem. *J Arthroplasty* 1995;10(suppl 1):S45-S51.
58. Lachiewicz PF, Soileau ES: What is the survivorship of fully coated femoral components in revision hip arthroplasty? *Clin Orthop Relat Res* 2015;473(2):549-554.
59. Russell RD, Pierce W, Huo MH: Tapered vs cylindrical stem fixation in a model of femoral bone deficiency in revision total hip arthroplasty. *J Arthroplasty* 2016;31(6):1352-1355.
60. Sporer SM, Paprosky WG: Extensively coated cementless femoral components in revision total hip arthoplasty: An update. *Surg Technol Int* 2005;14:265-274.
61. Richards CJ, Duncan CP, Masri BA, Garbuz DS: Femoral revision hip arthroplasty: A comparison of two stem designs. *Clin Orthop Relat Res* 2010;468(2):491-496.
62. Konan S, Garbuz DS, Masri BA, Duncan CP: Non-modular tapered fluted titanium stems in hip revision surgery: Gaining attention. *Bone Joint J* 2014;96-B(11 suppl A):56-59.

63. Regis D, Sandri A, Bonetti I, Braggion M, Bartolozzi P: Femoral revision with the Wagner tapered stem: A ten- to 15-year follow-up study. *J Bone Joint Surg Br* 2011;93(10): 1320-1326.

64. Munro JT, Garbuz DS, Masri BA, Duncan CP: Tapered fluted titanium stems in the management of Vancouver B2 and B3 periprosthetic femoral fractures. *Clin Orthop Relat Res* 2014;472(2):590-598.

65. Rodriguez JA, Deshmukh AJ, Robinson J, et al: Reproducible fixation with a tapered, fluted, modular, titanium stem in revision hip arthroplasty at 8-15 years follow-up. *J Arthroplasty* 2014;29(9 suppl):214-218.

66. Houdek MT, Perry KI, Wyles CC, Berry DJ, Sierra RJ, Trousdale RT: Use of a modular tapered fluted femoral component in revision total hip arthroplasty following resection of a previously infected total hip: Minimum 5-year follow-up. *J Arthroplasty* 2015;30(3):435-438.

67. Abdel MP, Cottino U, Larson DR, Hanssen AD, Lewallen DG, Berry DJ: Modular fluted tapered stems in aseptic revision total hip arthroplasty. *J Bone Joint Surg Am* 2017;99(10):873-881.

This is a large single center report of 519 aseptic femoral revision cases treated with modular tapered femoral implants and followed up for a mean of 4.5 years (range 2 to 14 years). The 10-year survivorship was 96% free of all-cause revision. Level of evidence: IV.

68. Revision Total Hip Arthroplasty Study Group: A comparison of modular tapered versus modular cylindrical stems for complex femoral revisions. *J Arthroplasty* 2013;28(8 suppl): 71-73.

69. Kirk KL, Potter BK, Lehman RA Jr, Xenos JS: Effect of distal stem geometry on interface motion in uncemented revision total hip prostheses. *Am J Orthop (Belle Mead NJ)* 2007;36(10):545-549.

70. Pierson JL, Small SR, Rodriguez JA, Kang MN, Glassman AH: The effect of taper angle and spline geometry on the initial stability of tapered, splined modular titanium stems. *J Arthroplasty* 2015;30(7):1254-1259.

71. Lakstein D, Eliaz N, Levi O, et al: Fracture of cementless femoral stems at the mid-stem junction in modular revision hip arthroplasty systems. *J Bone Joint Surg Am* 2011;93(1):57-65.

72. Van Houwelingen AP, Duncan CP, Masri BA, Greidanus NV, Garbuz DS: High survival of modular tapered stems for proximal femoral bone defects at 5 to 10 years followup. *Clin Orthop Relat Res* 2013;471(2):454-462.

73. Sandiford NA, Duncan CP, Garbuz DS, Masri BA: Tapered, fluted titanium stems in revision total hip arthroplasty: Role and results in contemporary practice. *Instr Course Lect* 2015;64:359-366.

74. Clair AJ, Cizmic Z, Vigdorchik JM, et al: Nonmodular stems are a viable alternative to modular stems in revision total hip arthroplasty. *J Arthroplasty* 2019;34(7):S292-S296.

This is a retrospective review of 146 femoral revision cases where 103 were modular fluted tapered titanium stems and 43 were nonmodular fluted tapered implants. There was no difference in re-revision rate, revision surgery rate, dislocation, fracture, or length of stay between the two groups. Modular stems were significantly 120% more expensive than nonmodular implants; however, surgical time was longer for the nonmodular implant cases by 30 minutes.

75. Gehrke T, Gebauer M, Kendoff D: Femoral stem impaction grafting: Extending the role of cement. *Bone Joint J* 2013;95-B(11 suppl A):92-94.

76. Garvin KL, Konigsberg BS, Ommen ND, Lyden ER: What is the long-term survival of impaction allografting of the femur? *Clin Orthop Relat Res* 2013;471(12):3901-3911.

77. Blake SM, Gie GA, Howell JR: Impaction grafting of the femur, in Cui B, Mihalko S, eds: *Arthritis and Arthroplasty: The Hip*. Philadelphia, PA, Saunders, 2009.

78. García-Rey E, Cruz-Pardos A, Madero R: The evolution of the technique of impaction bone grafting in femoral revision surgery has improved clinical outcome: A prospective mid-term study. *J Arthroplasty* 2015;30(1):95-100.

79. Eldridge JD, Smith EJ, Hubble MJ, Whitehouse SL, Learmonth ID: Massive early subsidence following femoral impaction grafting. *J Arthroplasty* 1997;12(5):535-540.

80. Wallace I, Ammon P, Day R, et al: Does size matter? An investigation into the effects of particle size on impaction grafting in vitro. *J Bone Joint Surg Br* 1997;79-B(suppl 3):366.

81. Brewster NT, Gillespie WJ, Howie CR, Madabhushi SP, Usmani AS, Fairbairn DR: Mechanical considerations in impaction bone grafting. *J Bone Joint Surg Br* 1999;81(1):118-124.

82. Höstner J, Hultmark P, Kärrholm J, Malchau H, Tveit M: Impaction technique and graft treatment in revisions of the femoral component: Laboratory studies and clinical validation. *J Arthroplasty* 2001;16(1):76-82.

83. te Stroet MA, Rijnen WH, Gardeniers JW, van Kampen A, Schreurs BW: The outcome of femoral component revision arthroplasty with impaction allograft bone grafting and a cemented polished Exeter stem: A prospective cohort study of 208 revision arthroplasties with a mean follow-up of ten years. *Bone Joint J* 2015;97-B(6):771-779.

84. Gie GA, Linder L, Ling RS, Simon JP, Slooff TJ, Timperley AJ: Impacted cancellous allografts and cement for revision total hip arthroplasty. *J Bone Joint Surg Br* 1993;75(1):14-21.

85. Te Stroet MA, Bronsema E, Rijnen WH, Gardeniers JW, Schreurs BW: The use of a long stem cemented femoral component in revision total hip replacement: A follow-up study of five to 16 years. *Bone Joint J* 2014;96-B(9):1207-1213.

86. Head WC, Berklacich FM, Malinin TI, Emerson RH Jr: Proximal femoral allografts in revision total hip arthroplasty. *Clin Orthop Relat Res* 1987;225:22-36.

87. Sternheim A, Drexler M, Kuzyk PR, Safir OA, Backstein DJ, Gross AE: Treatment of failed allograft prosthesis composites used for hip arthroplasty in the setting of severe proximal femoral bone defects. *J Arthroplasty* 2014;29(5):1058-1062.

88. Maury AC, Pressman A, Cayen B, Zalzal P, Backstein D, Gross A: Proximal femoral allograft treatment of Vancouver type-B3 periprosthetic femoral fractures after total hip arthroplasty. *J Bone Joint Surg Am* 2006;88(5):953-958.

89. Al-Taki MM, Masri BA, Duncan CP, Garbuz DS: Quality of life following proximal femoral replacement using a modular system in revision THA. *Clin Orthop Relat Res* 2011;469(2):470-475.

90. Henderson ER, Groundland JS, Pala E, et al: Failure mode classification for tumor endoprostheses: Retrospective review of five institutions and a literature review. *J Bone Joint Surg Am* 2011;93(5):418-429.

Index

Note: Page numbers followed by "*f*" indicate figures and "*t*" indicate tables.

A

B

G

H

I

J

K

L

M

P

Q

R

U

V

W

X